Clinico-Investigative Ophthalmology

Modern System of Ophthalmology (MSO) Series

Clinico-Investigative Ophthalmology

Editor-in-Chief

AK Khurana MS, FAICO, CTO (London)
Fellow, Moorfields Eye Hospital, London
Senior Professor and Head
Squint and Oculoplasty Services
Regional Institute of Ophthalmology
Postgraduate Institute of Medical Sciences
Rohtak, Haryana

Editors

Aruj K Khurana DNB, FICO
Fellow, Vitreo-Retina
Narayana Nethralaya, Bengaluru
Consultant, Vitreo-Retina Services
Nirmal Ashram Eye Institute
Rishikesh (Dehradun)

Bhawna P Khurana MS, DNB, FICO
Fellow, Orbit, Oculoplasty and Ocular Oncology
Narayana Nethralaya, Bengaluru
Consultant, Oculoplasty and Orbit Services, and
Deputy Medical Superintendent
Nirmal Ashram Eye Institute
Rishikesh (Dehradun)

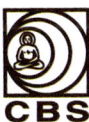

CBS

CBS Publishers & Distributors Pvt Ltd

New Delhi • Bengaluru • Chennai • Kochi • Kolkata • Mumbai
Bhubaneswar • Hyderabad • Jharkhand • Nagpur • Patna • Pune • Uttarakhand

Modern System of Ophthalmology (MSO) Series

Clinico-Investigative Ophthalmology

ISBN: 978-93-87964-18-1

First Edition 2018

Published by Satish Kumar Jain and Produced by Varun Jain for
CBS Publishers & Distributors Pvt Ltd
4819/XI Prahlad Street, 24 Ansari Road, Daryaganj, New Delhi 110 002, India.
Ph: 23289259, 23266861, 23266867   Fax: 011-23243014   Website: www.cbspd.com
e-mail: delhi@cbspd.com; cbspubs@airtelmail.in.
Corporate Office: 204 FIE, Industrial Area, Patparganj, Delhi 110 092, India
Ph: 4934 4934   Fax: 4934 4935   e-mail: publishing@cbspd.com; publicity@cbspd.com

Branches

- **Bengaluru:** Seema House 2975, 17th Cross, K.R. Road, Banasankari 2nd Stage, Bengaluru 560 070, Karnataka
  Ph: +91-80-26771678/79   Fax: +91-80-26771680   e-mail: bangalore@cbspd.com
- **Chennai:** 7, Subbaraya Street, Shenoy Nagar, Chennai 600 030, Tamil Nadu
  Ph: +91-44-26680620/26681266   Fax: +91-44-42032115   e-mail: chennai@cbspd.com
- **Kochi:** Ashana House, No. 39/1904, AM Thomas Road, Valanjambalam, Ernakulam 682 016, Kochi, Kerala
  Ph: +91-484-4059061-65   Fax: +91-484-4059065   e-mail: kochi@cbspd.com
- **Kolkata:** 6/B, Ground Floor, Rameswar Shaw Road, Kolkata-700 014, West Bengal
  Ph: +91-33-22891126, 22891127, 22891128   e-mail: kolkata@cbspd.com
- **Mumbai:** 83-C, Dr E Moses Road, Worli, Mumbai-400018, Maharashtra
  Ph: +91-22-24902340/41   Fax: +91-22-24902342   e-mail: mumbai@cbspd.com

Representatives

- **Bhubaneswar** 0-9911037372   • **Hyderabad** 0-9885175004   • **Jharkhand** 0-9811541605   • **Nagpur** 0-9021734563
- **Patna** 0-9334159340   • **Pune** 0-9623451994   • **Uttarakhand** 0-9716462459

Printed at: Nutech Print Services - India

to
the teachers and residents in ophthalmology for
their endeavour to dissipate and acquire knowledge
to our parents and teachers for their blessings
to our families for their understanding and encouragement
to our patients for letting us learn

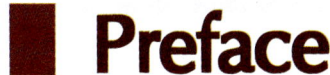

Preface

Modern System of Ophthalmology (MSO) series comprises separate volumes on different subspecialties of ophthalmology. Each volume is planned with a very specific aim to cater to the needs of postgraduate students in ophthalmology.

Salient Features of MSO Series

- Each volume is edited by different editors, yet the layout and organization has been kept identical.
- Editors of different volumes are masters in their subspecialty with an uncanny knack of picking up the right perspectives.
- Text matter is designed to meet the needs of residents in ophthalmology with a comprehensive coverage in a concise manner. Text is complete and up-to-date with recent advances incorporated.
- Text is organized in such a way that the students can easily understand, retain and reproduce it. Various levels of headings, subheadings, bold face and italics given in the text will be helpful for a quick revision of the subject.
- A brief list of chapter contents given in the beginning of each chapter provides a clear layout of the text.
- Text has been profusely illustrated with high quality coloured photographs and computer drawn colour diagrams which provide vivid details.
- Exposition of the text is such that an average postgraduate student will find it easy to glean through and assimilate the facts for longer retention.

Clinico-Investigative Ophthalmology. The present day medical practice in general and ophthalmic practice in particular is impossible without the help of sophisticated investigative tools. However, inspite of the availability of high tech gadgets and speedily changing investigative equipment; the art of painstaking meticulous history taking and accurate illicitation of clinical signs by the skilled physicians and surgeons cannot be overemphasized. Therefore, in this volume on 'Clinico-Investigative Ophthalmology'the fundamental clinical evaluation techniques and the sophisticated investigative techniques have been skillfully intermingled to the advantage of present day ophthalmic residents, optometry students, optometry and ophthalmic teachers and the practicing ophthalmologists and optometrists.

Text matter of the book has been organized in ten sections:

Section I: Clinical Methods in Ophthalmology: General Considerations describes in six chapters, the skill of history taking and basic examination techniques which are central to the practice of ophthalmology and optometry.

Section II: Clinical Evaluation and Investigative Techniques in Cornea is devoted to the Evaluation of Corneal Diseases. It describes the essential investigations for corneal disorders such as Specular Microscopy, Confocal Microscopy, Corneal Pachymetry, Hysteresis, Keratometry, Corneal Topography and Aberrometry.

Section III: Clinical Evaluation and Investigative Techniques in Glaucoma includes Tonometry, Gonioscopy, Optic Nerve Head evaluation techniques, Imaging techniques and Visual Field Examination.

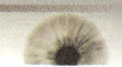

Section IV: Clinical Evaluation and Investigations in Uveitis includes three chapters one each on Clinical Approach, Investigations and Pathological Diagnostic Tests in Uveitis.

Section V: Clinical Evaluation and Investigations for Disorders of Ocular Motility includes methods of clinical work up for concomitant and incomitant strabismus as well as nystagmus.

Section VI: Clinical Evaluation and Investigations for Disorders of Ocular Adnexa includes methods for work up of a case of Ptosis, Watering Eye, Proptosis and Enophthalmos.

Section VII: Clinical Evaluation and Investigations for Cataract Surgery includes a chapter each on Preoperative Evaluation and Biometry: Calculation of IOL Power.

Section VIII: Special Investigations for Retina, Vitreous and Optic Nerve includes three chapters, one each on 'Fundus Angiography and Autofluorescence, Macular Optical Coherence Tomography, and Electrophysiological Tests for Retina.

Section IX: Imaging Techniques in Ophthalmology comprises five chapters one each on X-rays, Ultrasonography, Ultrasound Biomicroscopy, CT Scan and MRI in Ophthalmology.

Section X: Determination of Refractive Errors is devoted to ''Clinical Refraction'' which includes both objective and subjective methods of refraction.

Editorial team of this volume comprises ophthalmologists dedicated to academics in ophthalmology. The Editor of this volume Dr Aruj K Khurana, trained at Sankara Nethralaya, Chennai and Narayana Nethralaya, Bengaluru is consultant, Vitreo-Retina specialist at Nirmal Ashram Eye Institute, Rishikesh. Because of his interest in writing, he is deeply associated with each volume of MSO series. Another Editor, Dr Bhawna P Khurana, an enthusiastic oculoplastic surgeon, is trained at Guru Nanak Eye Centre (GNEC), New Delhi and Fellow of Orbit, Oculoplastic Surgery and Ocular Oncology, at Narayana Nethralaya, Bengaluru. Presently, she is consultant Oculoplasty and Orbit Services at Nirmal Ashram Eye Institute, Rishikesh.

Acknowledgement needs to be made to all those who have been instrumental in making this volume a reality. The generous help received from the faculty and residents of Regional Institute of Ophthalmology, PGIMS, Rohtak is duly acknowledged. The co-operation received from Dr Kamal Garg and Dr Garima Gupta is worth appreciating. My special thanks are due to the editorial team and the selfless contributors of various chapters. I want to express my gratitude to Prof OP Kalra, Vice-Chancellor, UHS, Rohtak; Prof MC Gupta, Dean, PGIMS; and Prof CS Dhull, Head, RIO, PGIMS, Rohtak; for providing an atmosphere conducive to such academic activities.

I want to put on record the remarkable assistance rendered by Dr Aruj Kumar Khurana and Dr Bhawna P Khurana in compiling the whole MSO series. The affection and moral support received from my daughter Dr Arushi and son-in-law Dr Gurukripa, Fellows, Virginia Commonwealth University (VCU), USA and my wife Prof Indu Khurana, Dean-cum-Principal, World College of Medical Sciences and Research, Gurawar, Jhajjar made my task untiring.

The enthusiastic co-operation received from Mr SK Jain, Managing Director; Mr YN Arjuna, Senior Vice President—Publishing, Editorial and Publicity, and Mrs Ritu Chawla, AGM, Production; CBS Publishers & Distributors, New Delhi, needs special acknowledgement. Mr Sanju and Mr Neeraj, Graphic artists, Mrs Sunita Rautela, DTP operator and Mr Mukund Kumar, Proofreader need special mention because of their efforts to provide considerable beauty to this volume.

In spite of the best efforts, a venture like this is unlikely to be error-free. Constructive criticism and suggestions from the readers are invited for further improvement in this volume.

AK Khurana
Editor-in-Chief

Editorial Board

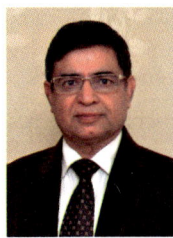
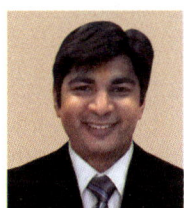
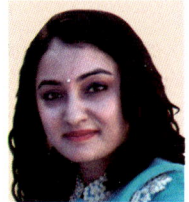

List of Contributors

AK Khurana MS, FAICO, CTO (London)
Senior Professor and Head
Squint and Oculoplasty Services
Regional Institute of Ophthalmology
PGIMS, Rohtak, Haryana, India

Aruj K Khurana DNB, FICO
Consultant, Vitreo-Retina Services
Nirmal Ashram Eye Institute
Rishikesh (Dehradun)

Bhawna P Khurana MS, DNB, FICO
Consultant, Oculoplasty and Orbit Services, and Deputy
Medical Superintendent
Nirmal Ashram Eye Institute
Rishikesh (Dehradun)

Jyotirmay Biswas
Director of Uveitis and Ocular Pathology Department
Sankara Nethralaya
Chennai

Rashmin A Gandhi DNB, FRCS
Managing Director, Beyond Eye Care and
Visiting Consultant, Center for Sight
Hyderabad

Hansa Harshad Thakkar
Professor of Ophthalmology
MJM Institute of Ophthalmology
BJ Medical College, Ahmedabad

Shreya Shah DOMS
Administrative Director
Drashti Netralaya
Dahod, Gujarat

Tanuj Dada MD
Professor, Glaucoma Services
Dr RP Centre for Ophthalmic Sciences
AIIMS, New Delhi

Sushmita Kaushik MS
Associate Professor, Glaucoma Services
Advanced Eye Centre
PGIMER, Chandigarh

Prateep Vyas MS
Medical Director and Head
Glaucoma Services
Centre for Sight, Indore

Shaloo Bageja DNB, MBBS
Senior Consultant
Department of Ophthalmology
Sir Ganga Ram Hospital, New Delhi

Amod Gupta
Former Professor and Head
Advanced Eye Center, and
Dean, PGIMER, Chandigarh

Ashok K Grover MD, MNAMS, FRCS, FIMSA, FICO
Chairman, Department of Ophthalmology
Sir Ganga Ram Hospital and Vision Eye Centres
New Delhi

Indu Khurana MD
Dean-cum-Principal, and
Professor of Physiology
World College of Medical Sciences and Research
Gurawar, Jhajjar

Sunandan Sood MS
Former Professor and Head
Department of Ophthalmology
GMCH, Chandigarh

MR Dogra MS
Professor
Advanced Eye Centre
PGIMER, Chandigarh

Mehul Shah MS, FMRF
Medical Director
Drashti Netralaya
Dahod, Gujarat

SS Pandav MS
Professor and Head, Glaucoma Services
Advanced Eye Center
PGIMER, Chandigarh

Subina Narang MS
Associate Professor, Vitreo-Retina and Uvea
Department of Ophthalmology
Government Medical College and Hospital
Chandigarh

Parthopratim Dutta Majumder
Consultant, Department of Uveitis
and Intraocular Inflammation
Sankara Nethralaya
Chennai

Parul Ichpujani MS
Associate Professor
Govt. Medical College and Hospital
Chandigarh

Reena Gupta MS
Associate Professor
RIO, PGIMS, Rohtak

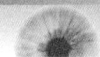

Chekitan Singh DNB
Consultant, Ishwar Eye Center
Rohtak

Pradeep Venktesh MS
Associate Professor, Vitreo-Retina, RPCOS
AIIMS, New Delhi

Radha Annamalai
Associate Professor of Ophthalmology and
Senior Consultant
Sri Ramachandra University
Chennai

Neha Adlakha
Assistant Professor of Ophthalmology
SHKM, GMC
Nalhar, Nuh, Haryana

Shweta Goel MS
Fellow, Glaucoma Services
Venu Eye Institute
New Delhi

Garvit Bhutani
Fellow, Corneal Diseases
LVPI, Vizaik

Ankur Singh MS
Senior Resident
Advanced Eye Centre
PGIMER, Chandigarh

Shibal Bhartiya MS
Consultant, Department of Ophthalmology
Fortis Hospital
Gurgaon

Sukanya MS
Sankara Nethralaya
Chennai

Mohit Dogra MS
Assistant Professor
Advanced Eye Centre
PGIMER, Chandigarh

Avirupa Ghosh MS
Senior Resident
Department of Uveitis
Aditya Birla Sankara Nethralaya
Kolkata

Contents

Preface   vii

List of Contributors   xi

Section I: Clinical Methods in Ophthalmology: General Considerations

1. History Taking and Scheme of Examination and Investigation of an   3
   Ophthalmic Case
   AK Khurana, Aruj K Khurana, Bhawna P Khurana

2. Evaluation of Visual Acuity, Contrast Sensitivity, and Colour Vision   30
   AK Khurana, Aruj K Khurana, Bhawna P Khurana

3. Slit-lamp Biomicroscopy   53
   AK Khurana, Aruj K Khurana, Bhawna P Khurana

4. Examination of Posterior Segment   65
   AK Khurana, Aruj K Khurana, Bhawna P Khurana

5. Evaluation and Assessment of Traumatized Eye   103
   AK Khurana, Mehul Shah, Shreya Shah, S Sood, Aruj K Khurana

6. Examination of a Neuro-ophthalmic Case   111
   Rashmin A Gandhi, AK Khurana, Reena Gupta, Chekitan Singh

Section II: Clinical Evaluation and Investigative Techniques in Cornea

7. Clinical Evaluation and Investigations for Corneal Diseases   135
   Neha Adlakha, AK Khurana, Bhawna P Khurana

8. Specular Microscopy and Confocal Microscopy of Cornea   162
   AK Khurana, Aruj K Khurana, Bhawna P Khurana

9. Corneal Pachymetry, Hysteresis and Keratometry   171
   AK Khurana, Aruj K Khurana, Bhawna P Khurana

10. Corneal Topography and Aberrometry   189
    AK Khurana, Aruj K Khurana, Bhawna P Khurana

Section III: Clinical Evaluation and Investigative Techniques in Glaucoma

11. Clinical Evaluation of Glaucoma: An Overview   225
    AK Khurana, Prateep Vyas, Aruj K Khurana, Shweta Goel

12. Tonometry   233
    AK Khurana, Aruj K Khurana, Bhawna P Khurana

13. Gonioscopy   246
    Tanuj Dada , Aruj K Khurana, Bhawna P Khurana

14. Evaluation of Optic Nerve Head   263
Sushmita Kaushik, Ankur Singh, SS Pandav

15. Imaging in Glaucoma   272
Sushmita Kaushik, Ankur Singh, SS Pandav

16. Perimetry and Other Psychophysical Tests in Glaucoma   306
Parul Ichpujani, Aruj K Khurana, AK Khurana

Section IV: Clinical Evaluation and Investigations in Uveitis

17. Clinical Approach to Uveitis   329
Parthopratim Dutta Majumder, J Biswas, Radha Annamalai

18. Investigations in Uveitis   339
J Biswas, Parthopratim Dutta Majumder, Sukanya, Aruj K Khurana

19. Pathological Diagnostic Tests in Uveitis   365
Avirupa Ghosh, J Biswas

Section V: Clinical Evaluation and Investigations for Disorders of Ocular Motility

20. Evaluation of a Case of Strabismus and Orthoptic Instruments   377
AK Khurana, Bhawna P Khurana

21. Evaluation and Investigations in Paralytic Squint   435
AK Khurana, Bhawna P Khurana

22. Evaluation and Investigations of a Case of Nystagmus   456
AK Khurana, Bhawna P Khurana

Section VI: Clinical Evaluation and Investigations for Disorders of Ocular Adnexa

23. Evaluation of a Case of Ptosis   467
AK Khurana, AK Grover, Bhawna P Khurana, Shaloo Bageja

24. Evaluation of a Case of Watering Eye   481
Bhawna P Khurana, AK Khurana, Aruj K Khurana

25. Evaluation of a Case of Proptosis and Enophthalmos   489
AK Khurana, Bhawna P Khurana, Aruj K Khurana

Section VII: Clinical Evaluation and Investigations for Cataract Surgery

26. Preoperative Evaluation for Cataract Surgery   521
AK Khurana, Aruj K Khurana, Bhawna P Khurana

27. Biometry: Calculation of IOL Power   529
AK Khurana, Aruj K Khurana, Bhawna P Khurana

Section VIII: Special Investigations for Retina, Vitreous and Optic Nerve

28. Fundus Angiography and Autofluorescence   553
Amod Gupta, Subina Narang, Pradeep Venktesh, Mohit Dogra, MR Dogra

29. Macular Optical Coherence Tomography   577
    Subina Narang, Pradeep Venktesh, Mohit Dogra, MR Dogra

30. Electrophysiological Tests in Ophthalmology   590
    Parul Ichpujani, Shibal Bhartiya, Indu Khurana

Section IX: Imaging Techniques in Ophthalmology

31. Plain X-rays in Ophthalmology   601
    AK Khurana, Bhawna P Khurana, Garvit Bhutani

32. Ultrasonography in Ophthalmology   608
    AK Khurana, Neha Adlakha, Aruj K Khurana, Bhawna P Khurana

33. Ultrasound Biomicroscopy (UBM) in Ophthalmology   640
    Hansa Harshad Thakkar

34. Computed Tomography Scanning in Ophthalmology   656
    AK Khurana, Neha Adlakha, Aruj K Khurana, Bhawna P Khurana

35. Magnetic Resonance Imaging in Ophthalmology   678
    Neha Adlakha, AK Khurana, Aruj K Khurana, Bhawna P Khurana

Section X: Determination of Refractive Errors

36. Clinical Refraction: Determination of the Errors of Refraction   701
    AK Khurana, Aruj K Khurana, Bhawna P Khurana

    Index   737

Section

I

Clinical Methods in Ophthalmology: General Considerations

1. History Taking and Scheme of Examination and Investigation of an Ophthalmic Case
2. Evaluation of Visual Acuity, Contrast Sensitivity, and Colour Vision
3. Slit-lamp Biomicroscopy
4. Examination of Posterior Segment
5. Evaluation and Assessment of Traumatized Eye
6. Examination of a Neuro-ophthalmic Case

1

History Taking and Scheme of Examination and Investigation of an Ophthalmic Case

Chapter Outline

HISTORY AND EXAMINATION

History

General physical and systemic examination

Ocular examination

- Testing of visual acuity
- External ocular examination
- Fundus examination
- Visual field examination
- Colour vision testing

Record of ophthalmic case

- Ophthalmic clinical case sheet

TECHNIQUES OF OCULAR EXAMINATION AND DIAGNOSTIC TESTS

- Oblique illumination
- Gonioscopy
- Tonometry
- Techniques of fundus examination
- Perimetry
- Fundus fluorescein angiography
- Electroretinography and electro-oculography
- Ocular ultrasonography
- Optical coherence tomography

HISTORY AND EXAMINATION

HISTORY

The importance of painstaking meticulous history cannot be overemphasized. The patient's history is the first and many times the most important aspect of an ophthalmological examination. It assists in restracting the various stages of the disease. The information gathered from history guides about the specific examination and diagnostic tests to be performed. The information gained also helps in planning the management. Last but not the least, history-taking provides an opportunity to develop appropriate docter–patient relationship.

During history-taking, one should be precise and pertinent. Questions should be asked in an organized manner and a fixed routine followed,

so that the complete required information is obtained. The complete history-taking should be structured as:

- Demographic data
- Chief presenting complaints
- History of present illness
- History of past illness
- Family history.

Demographic data

Demographic data should include patient's name, age, sex, occupation and religion.

Name and address. Name and address are primarily required for patient's identification. It also proves useful for demographic research.

Age and sex. In addition to the utility in patient's identification, knowledge of age and sex of the patient is also useful for noting down and ruling

out the particular diseases pertaining to different age groups and a particular sex.

Occupation. An information about patient's occupation is helpful since ophthalmic manifestations due to occupational hazards are well known, e.g.:

- *Ocular injuries and trauma due to foreign bodies* have typical pattern in factory workers, lathe workers, farmers and sport persons.
- *Computer vision syndrome* is emerging as a significant ocular health problem in computer professionals.
- *Heat cataract* is known in glass factory workers.
- *Photophthalmitis* is known in welders not taking adequate protective measures.

In addition, information about the patient's occupation is useful in providing ocular health education and patient's visual rehabilitation.

Religion. Recording the religion of the patient may be helpful in ascertaining the diseases which are more common in a particular community. It also helps in knowing the aptitude and practices prevalent in different communities for various common eye problems.

Chief presenting complaints

The patient should be encouraged to narrate his complaints in detail and the examiner should be a patient listner. The relevent and important enquiries should be made by the examiner depending upon the patient's compliants. An enquiry should be made about mode of onset, duration, severity and accompaniment of each symptoms.

Some relevant features of the common ocular symptoms and their causes are described:

- Defective vision
- Watering and/or discharge from the eyes
- Redness
- Asthenopic symptoms
- Photophobia
- Burning/itching/foreign body sensation
- Pain (eyeache and/or headache)
- Deviation of the eye
- Diplopia
- Black spots in front of eyes
- Coloured halos
- Distorted vision.

History of present illness

The patients should be encouraged to narrate their complaints in detail and the examiner should be a patient listener. While taking history, the examiner should try to make a note of the following points about each complaint:

- Mode of onset with duration
- Severity
- Progression
- Accompaniment of each symptom.

Treatment history

A detail information about the treatment taken for the present symptoms including its effect on the symptoms is very important.

Leading questions to explore etiology

Leading questions to ascertain the probable cause of the disease should be part to the patient. For example, if a patient gets up at night with history of marked discomfort, pain and watering from the eyes; an enquiry should be made to know where the patient looked at welding are with marked eye in the evening. Similarly, if a patient present with subconjunctival haemorrhage without any history of trauma; an enquiry should be made about atleast of sneezing, coughing or any other cause of straining.

Medical history

A detailed history should be taken to explore the other associated medical diseases which may affect the management plan or final outcome of the treatments. For example, if a patient into operated for cataract the associated diabetes mellitus, hypertension, chronic bronchitis, any source of systemic infection should be explored and treated before the cataract operation is contempulated.

It is also important to know whether the patient is on any medication for some systemic disease or is known to be allergic to some drug.

History of past illness

A probe into history of past illness should be made to know:

- *History of similar ocular complaint in the past.* It is specially important in recurrent conditions

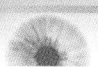

such as *herpes simplex keratitis, uveitis* and *recurrent corneal erosions.*

- *History of similar complaints in other eye* is important in bilateral conditions such as *uveitis, senile cataract* and *retinal detachment.*
- *History of trauma to eye in the past* may explain occurrence of lesions such as delayed rosette cataract and retinal detachment.
- It is important to know about *history of any ocular surgery in the past.*
- *History of any systemic disease in the past* such as tuberculosis, syphilis, leprosy may sometimes explain the occurrence of present ocular disease.
- *History of drug intake and allergies* is also important.

Family history

Efforts should be made to establish familial predisposition of inheritable ocular disorders like congenital cataract, ptosis, squint, corneal dystrophies, glaucoma and refractive error.

Common ocular symptoms and their causes

1. *Defective vision.* It is the commonest ocular symptom. Enquiry should reveal its onset (sudden or gradual), duration, whether it is painless or painful, whether it is more during the day, night or constant, and so on. Important causes of defective vision can be grouped as under:

Sudden painless loss of vision
- Central retinal artery occlusion
- Massive vitreous haemorrhage
- Retinal detachment involving macular area
- Ischaemic central retinal vein occlusion.

Sudden painless onset of defective vision
- Central serous retinopathy
- Optic neuritis
- Methyl alcohol amblyopia
- Nonischaemic central retinal vein occlusion.

Sudden painful loss of vision
- Acute congestive glaucomas (primary or secondary)
- Acute iridocyclitis
- Chemical injuries to the eyeball
- Mechanical injuries to the eyeball.

Gradual painless defective vision
- Progressive pterygium involving papillary area
- Corneal degenerations
- Corneal dystrophies
- Developmental cataract
- Senile cataract
- Optic atrophy
- Chorioretinal degenerations
- Age-related macular degeneration
- Diabetic retinopathy
- Refractive errors.

Gradual painful defective vision
- Chronic iridocyclitis
- Corneal ulceration
- Chronic simple glaucoma.

Transient loss of vision (amaurosis fugax)
- Carotid artery disease
- Papilloedema
- Giant cell arteritis
- Migraine
- Raynaud's disease
- Severe hypertension
- Prodromal symptom of CRAO.

Night blindness (nyctalopia)
- Vitamin A deficiency
- Retinitis pigmentosa and other tapetoretinal degenerations
- Congenital night blindness
- Pathological myopia
- Peripheral cortical cataract.

Day blindness (hamaropia)
- Central nuclear or polar cataracts
- Central corneal opacity
- Central vitreous opacity
- Congenital deficiency of cones (rarely).

Diminution of vision for near only
- Presbyopia
- Cycloplegia
- Internal or total ophthalmoplegia
- Insufficiency of accommodation.

2. *Other visual symptoms.* Visual symptoms other than the defective vision are as follows:

- *Black spots or floaters in front of the eyes may* appear singly or in clusters. They move with the

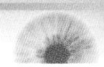

movement of the eyes and become more apparent when viewed against a clear surface, e.g. the sky. Common causes of black floaters are:

- Vitreous haemorrhage
- Vitreous degeneration, e.g.
  - Senile vitreous degeneration
  - Vitreous degeneration in pathological myopia
- Exudates in vitreous
- Lenticular opacity.

Flashes of light in front of the eyes (photopsia). Occur due to traction on retina in following conditions:

- Posterior vitreous detachment
- Prodromal symptom of retinal detachment
- Vitreous traction bands
- Sudden appearance of flashes with floaters is a sign of a retinal tear
- Retinitis
- Migraine.

Distortion of vision

- Central chorioretinitis
- Central serous chorioretinopathy
- ARMD
- CNVM
- Keratoconus
- Corneal irregularity.

Glare

- Early cataract
- Corneal oedema
- Status postrefractive surgery.

Photophobia

- Corneal abrasion
- Acute conjunctivitis
- Keratitis
- Anterior uveitis
- Dilated pupil.

Coloured halos. Patient may perceive coloured halos around the light. It is a feature of:

- Acute congestive glaucoma
- Corneal oedema, e.g. bullous keratopathy
- Early stages of cataract
- Mucopurulent conjunctivitis.

Diplopia, i.e. perceiving double images of an object is a very annoying symptom. It should

be ascertained whether it occurs even when the normal eye is closed (uniocular diplopia) or only when both eyes are open (binocular diplopia). Common causes of diplopia are:

Uniocular diplopia

- Subluxated lens
- Double pupil
- Incipient cataract
- Keratoconus
- Eccentric IOL.

Binocular diplopia

- Paralytic squint
- Myasthenia gravis
- Diabetes mellitus
- Thyroid disorders
- Blow-out fracture of floor of the orbit
- Anisometropic glasses (e.g. uniocular aphakic glasses)
- After squint correction in the presence of abnormal retinal correspondence (paradoxical diplopia).

3. **Watering from the eyes.** Watering from the eyes is another common ocular symptom. Its causes can be grouped as follows:

Excessive lacrimation, i.e. excessive formation of tears occurs in multiple conditions. *Epiphora,* i.e. watering from the eyes due to blockage in the flow of normally formed tears somewhere in the lacrimal drainage system.

4. **Discharge from the eyes.** When a patient complains of a discharge from the eyes, it should be ascertained whether it is mucoid, mucopurulent, purulent, serosanguinous or ropy. Discharge from the eyes is a feature of conjunctivitis, corneal ulcer, stye, burst orbital abscess, and dacryocystitis.

5. **Itching, burning and foreign body sensation in the eyes.** These are very common ocular symptoms. Their causes are:

- Conjunctivitis (e.g. allergic, chronic simple, and GPC)
- Blepharitis
- Dry eye
- Trachoma and other conjunctival inflammations
- Trichiasis and entropion.

6. *Redness of the eyes.* It is a common presenting symptom in many conditions, such as conjunctivitis, keratitis, iridocyclitis, acute glaucomas, conjunctival or corneal foreign body, trichiasis, episcleritis, scleritis, sub-conjunctival haemorrhage, endophthalmitis.

7. *Ocular pain.* Pain in and around the eyes should be probed for its onset, severity, and associated symptoms. It is a feature of ocular inflammations and acute glaucoma. Ocular pain may also occur as referred pain from the inflammation of surrounding structures, such as sinusitis, dental caries and abscess.

8. *Asthenopic symptoms.* Asthenopia refers to mild eyeache, headache and tiredness of the eyes which are aggravated by near work. Asthenopia is a feature of extraocular muscle imbalance and uncorrected mild refractive errors especially astigmatism.

9. *Other ocular symptoms* include:
- Deviation of the eyeball (squint)
- Protrusion of the eyeball (proptosis)
- Drooping of the upper lid (ptosis)
- Retraction of the upper lid
- Sagging down of the lower lids (ectropion)
- Swelling on the lids (e.g. chalazion and tumours).

GENERAL PHYSICAL AND SYSTEMIC EXAMINATION

General physical and systemic examination should be carried out in each case. Sometimes it may help in establishing the etiological diagnosis, e.g. ankylosing spondylitis may be associated with uveitis. Further, it is essential to treat associated diseases like bronchial asthma, hypertension, diabetes and urinary tract problems before taking up the patient for cataract surgery.

OCULAR EXAMINATION

- Testing of visual acuity
- External ocular examination
- Fundus examination
- Visual field examination
- Test for colour vision.

I. TESTING OF VISUAL ACUITY

Visual acuity should be tested in all cases, as it may be affected in numerous ocular disorders.

In real sense, acuity of vision is a retinal function (to be more precise of the macular area) concerned with the appreciation of form sense.

Distant and near visual acuity should be tested separately.

Distant visual acuity

Snellen's test types. The distant central visual acuity is usually tested by Snellen's test types. The fact that two distant points can be visible as separate only when they subtend an angle of 1 minute at the nodal point of the eye, forms the basis of Snellen's test-types. It consists of a series of black capital letters on a white board, arranged in lines, each progressively diminishing in size. The lines comprising the letters have such a breadth that they will subtend an angle of 1 min at the nodal point. Each letter of the chart is so designed that it fits in a square, the sides of which are five times the breadth of the constituent lines. Thus, at the given distance, each letter subtends an angle of 5 min at the nodal point of the eye (Fig. 1.1). The letters of the top line of Snellen's chart (Fig. 1.2) should be read clearly at a distance of 60 m. Similarly, the letters in the subsequent lines should be read from a distance of 36, 24, 18, 12, 9, 6 and 5 m, respectively.

Procedure of testing. For testing distant visual-acuity, the patient is seated at a distance of 6 m from the Snellen's chart, so that the rays of light are practically parallel and the patient exerts minimal accommodation. The chart should be properly illuminated (not less than 20 ft candles). The patient is asked to read the chart with each eye separately and the visual acuity is recorded as a fraction, the numerator being the distance

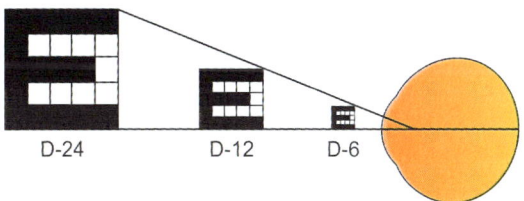

D-24   D-12   D-6

Fig. 1.1: *Principle of Snellen's test types.*

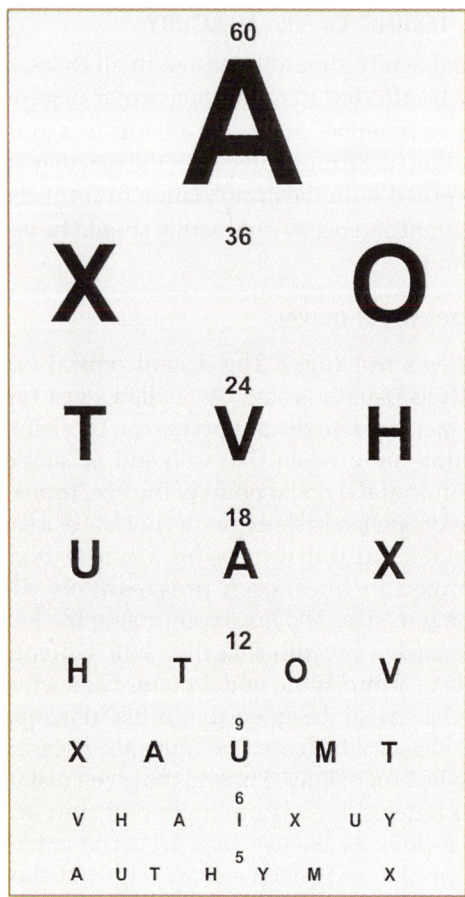

Fig. 1.2: *Snellen's test types.*

the distance at which the patient is able to count fingers. When the patient fails to count fingers, the examiner moves his hand close to the patient's face. If he can appreciate the hand movements (HM), visual acuity is recorded as HM +ve. When the patient cannot distinguish the hand movements, the examiner notes whether the patient can perceive light (PL) or not. If yes, vision is recorded as PL +ve and if not it is recorded as PL –ve.

Other tests which are based on the same principle as Snellen's test types are as follows:
a. Simple picture chart: Used for children >2 years
b. Landolt's C-chart: Used for illiterate patients
c. E-chart: Used for illiterate patients

Visual acuity equivalents in some common notations are depicted in Table 1.1.

Visual acuity for near

Near vision is tested by asking the patient to read the near vision chart (Fig. 1.3), kept at a distance of 35 cm in good illumination, with each eye separately. In near vision chart, a series of different sizes of printer type are arranged in increasing order and marked accordingly. Commonly used near vision charts are as follows:

1. *Jaeger's chart.* In this chart, prints are marked from 1 to 7 and accordingly patient's acuity is labelled as J1 to J7 depending upon the print he can read.

of the patient from the letters, and the denominator being the smallest letters accurately read.

When the patient is able to read up to 6 m line, the visual acuity is recorded as 6/6, which is normal.

Similarly, depending upon the smallest line which the patient can read from the distance of 6 m, his vision is recorded as 6/9, 6/12, 6/18, 6/24, 6/36 and 6/60, respectively. If he cannot see the top line from 6 m, he is asked to slowly walk towards the chart till he can read the top line. Depending upon the distance at which he can read the top line, his vision is recorded as 5/60, 4/60, 3/60, 2/60 and 1/60, respectively.

If the patient is unable to read the top line even from 1 m, he is asked to count fingers (CF) of the examiner. His vision is recorded as CF-3', CF-2', CF-1' or CF close to face, depending upon

Table 1.1 *Visual acuity equivalents in some common notations*

Decimal-reso- lution system	Snellen 6-m table	Snellen 20- foot table	Angle table
1.0	6/6	20/20	1.0
0.8	5/6	20/25	1.3
0.7	6/9	20/30	1.4
0.6	5/9	15/25	1.6
0.5	6/12	20/40	2.0
0.4	5/12	20/50	2.5
0.3	6/18	20/70	3.3
0.1	6/60	20/200	10.0

J. 1(Sn. 0.5) N5.

As she shoke Moses came slowy), on foot, and sweathing under the deal box which he had strapt round his shoulders like a pediar "Welcome, welcome, Mosesi well, myboy, what have you brought us from the fair" MI have brought

J. 2 (Sn, 0.6) N6

Five shillings and twopence is no bad day's work. come, let us have itthen."—"I have brought back no money," cried Moses again. "1 have laidit all out in a bargain and here it is, "pulling out a bundle from his

J. 4 (Sn. 0.8) N9

mother," cried the boy. "why won 't you listen to reason. I had them a dead bargain, or I should not have brought them. The silver rims alone will sell for double the money"—"A fig for

J.6 (Sn. I) N12

The rims, for they are not worth sixpence; for I perceivethey are only copper varnished over. "-"What! Criedmy wife," not silver! the rims not silver?"—"No,"

J.8 (Sn. 1.25) N18

with copper rims and shagreen cases? A murrain take such trumpery! The blockhead has been imposed upon, and should have know his

J.10 (Sn. 1.5) N24

The idiot!" returned she, "to bring me such stuff: if I had them I would throw them in the fire. "-"There again you are wrong, my

J. 12 (SN. 1.75) N36

By this time the unfortunate Moses was undeceived. He now saw that

J.14 (Sn. 2.25) N48

asked the circumstances of his deception. He sold the

Fig. 1.3: *Near vision chart.*

2. *Roman test types.* According to this chart, the near vision is recorded as N5, N8, N10, N12 and N18 (Printer's point system) (Fig. 1.3).

3. *Snellen's near vision test types.*

Note: For details see chapter 2.

II. EXTERNAL OCULAR EXAMINATION

External ocular examination should be carried out as follows:

A. *Inspection in diffuse light* should be performed first of all for a preliminary examination of the eyeballs and related structures, viz. lids, eyebrows, face and head.

B. *Focal (oblique) illumination examination* should be carried out for a detailed examination under magnification. It can be accomplished using a magnifying loupe (uniocular or binocular) and a focussing torch light or preferably a slit-lamp.

C. *Special examination* is required for measuring intraocular pressure (tonometry) and for examining angle of the anterior chamber (gonioscopy).

Scheme of External Ocular Examination

Scheme of external ocular examination is described here. Scheme of examination includes the structures to be examined and the signs to be looked for. Further, the important causes of the common signs are also listed to fulfill the prerequisite that *'the eyes see what the mind knows'*. Both eyes should be examined in each case.

The external ocular examination should proceed in the following order:

1. Examination for the head posture. Position of the head and chin should be noted first of all. Head posture may be abnormal in a patient with paralytic squint (head is turned in the direction of the action of paralysed muscle to avoid diplopia) and incomplete ptosis (chin is elevated to uncover the pupillary area in a bid to see clearly).

2. Examination of forehead and facial symmetry:

- *Forehead may show increased wrinkling* (due to overaction of frontalis muscle) in patient with ptosis.
- *Complete loss of wrinkling* in one-half of the forehead is observed in patients with lower motor neuron facial palsy.
- *Facial asymmetry* may be noted in patient with Bell's palsy and facial hemiatrophy.

3. Examination of eyebrows

- *Level* of the two eyebrows may be changed in a patient with ptosis (due to overaction of frontalis).
- *Cilia* of lateral one-third of the eyebrows may be absent (madarosis) in patients with leprosy or myxoedema.

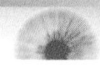

4. Examination of the eyelids. All the four eyelids should be examined for their position, movements, condition of skin and lid margins.

i. *Position.* Normally the lower lid just touches the limbus while the upper lid covers about/1/6th (2 mm) of cornea.

- *In ptosis*, upper lid covers more than 1/6th of cornea.
- Upper limbus is visible due to lid retraction as in thyrotoxicosis and sympathetic over-activity.

ii. *Movements of lids.* Normally the upper lid follows the eyeball in downward movement but it lags behind in cases of thyroid ophthalmopathy.

■■ *Blinking* is involuntary movement of eyelids. Normal rate is 12–16 blinks per minute. It is increased in local irritation. Blinks are decreased in trigeminal anaesthesia and absent in those with 7th nerve palsy.

■■ *Lagophthalmos* is a condition in which the patient is not able to close his eyelids. Causes of lagophthalmos are:

- Facial nerve palsy
- Extreme degree of proptosis
- Symblepharon.

iii. *Lid margin.* Note presence of any of the following:

■■ *Entropion* (inward turning of lid margin).

■■ *Ectropion* (outward turning of lid margin).

■■ *Eyelash abnormalities* such as:

- *Trichiasis*, i.e. misdirected cilia rubbing the eyeball. Common causes are trachoma, blepharitis, stye and lid trauma.
- *Distichiasis*, i.e. an abnormal extra row of cilia taking place of meibomian glands.
- *Madarosis*, i.e. absence of cilia may be seen in patients with chronic blepharitis, leprosy and myxoedema.
- *Poliosis*, i.e. greying of cilia is seen in old age and also in patients with Vogt-Koyanagi-Harada disease.

■■ *Scales* at lid margins are seen in blepharitis.

■■ *Swelling* at lid margin may be stye, papilloma or marginal chalazion.

iv. *Abnormalities of skin.* Common lesions are herpetic blisters, molluscum contagiosum lesions, warts, epidermoid cysts, ulcers, traumatic scar, etc.

v. *Palpebral aperture.* The exposed space between the two lid margins is called *palpebral fissure* which measures 28–30 mm horizontally and 8–10 mm vertically (in the centre). Following abnormalities may be observed:

■■ *Ankyloblepharon* is usually seen following adhesions of the two lids at angles, e.g. after ulcerative blepharitis and burns. It results in horizontally narrow palpebral fissure.

■■ *Blepharophimosis* (all around narrow palpebral fissure) is usually a congenital anomaly.

■■ *Vertically narrow palpebral fissure* is seen in:

- Inflammatory conditions of conjunctiva, cornea and uvea due to blepharospasm
- Ptosis (drooping) of upper eyelid
- Enophthalmos (sunken eyeball)
- Anophthalmos (absent eyeball)
- Microphthalmos (congenital small eyeball)
- Phthisis bulbi
- Atrophic bulbi.

■■ *Vertically wide palpebral fissure* may be noted inpatients with:

- Proptosis
- Large-sized eyeball (e.g. buphthalmos)
- Retraction of upper lid
- Facial nerve palsy.

5. Examination of lacrimal apparatus. A thorough examination of lacrimal apparatus is indicated in patients with epiphora, corneal ulcer and in all patients before intraocular surgery. The examination should include:

- *Inspection of lacrimal sac area* for redness, swelling or fistula.
- *Inspection of the lacrimal puncta,* for any defect such as eversion, stenosis, absence or discharge.
- *Regurgitation test.* It is performed by pressing over the lacrimal sac area just medial to the medial canthus and observing regurgitation of any discharge from the puncta. Normally it is negative. A *positive regurgitation test* indicates dacryocystitis. A *false negative regurgitation test* may be observed in internal fistula, wrong method of performing regurgitation test, patient might have emptied the sac just before coming to the examiner's chamber, encysted mucocele.

- *Lacrimal syringing.* It is done to locate the probable site of blockage in patients with epiphora (*see* page 483).
- *Other tests* such as *Jone's dye test I and II,* dacryocystography, etc. can be performed when indicated (*see* page 484).

6. Examination of eyeball as a whole observe the following points:

i. *Position of eyeballs.* Normally, the two eyeballs are symmetrically placed in the orbits in such a way that a line joining the central points of superior and inferior orbital margins just touches the cornea.

Abnormalities of the position of eyeball can be:

a. *Proptosis/exophthalmos,* i.e. bulging of eyeballs; note whether proptosis is:

- Axial or eccentric
- Reducible or nonreducible
- Pulsatile or nonpulsatile.

b. *Enophthalmos* (sunken eyeball)

ii. *Visual axes of eyeballs.* Normally the visual axes of the two eyes are simultaneously directed at the same object which is maintained in all the directions of gaze. Deviation in the visual axis of one eye is called *squint* (complete evaluation of a case of squint is as pecialised examination).

iii. *Size of eyeball.* Obvious abnormalities in the size of eyeball can be detected clinically. However, precise measurement of size can only be made by ultrasonography (A-scan). The size of eyeball is increased in conditions like buphthalmos and unilateral high myopia. *The causes of small-sized eyeball are:* congenital microphthalmos, phthisis bulbi, and atrophic bulbi.

iv. *Movements of eyeball* should be tested uniocularly (ductions) as well as binocularly (versions) in all the six cardinal directions of gaze.

7. Examination of conjunctiva

i. *Bulbar conjunctiva* can be examined by simply retracting the upper lid with index finger and lower lid with thumb of the left hand.

ii. *Lower palpebral conjunctiva and lower fornix* can be examined by just pulling down the lower lid and instructing the patient to look up (Fig. 1.4).

iii. *Upper palpebral conjunctiva* can be examined only after everting the upper eyelid. Eversion of upper lid can be carried out by one-hand or two-hand technique.

- *One-hand* technique. In it patient looks down and the examiner grasps the lid margin along with lashes with left index finger and thumb. Then swiftly everts the upper lid by making index finger a fulcrum. This, however, requires some practice.
- *Two-hand technique.* It is comparatively easier. Procedure is same as above, except that here the lid is rotated around a fixed probe which is held above the level of tarsal plate with right hand (Fig. 1.5). In slight modification of

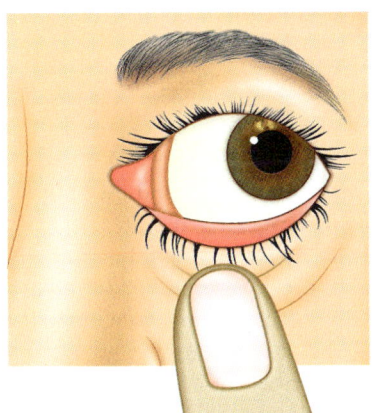

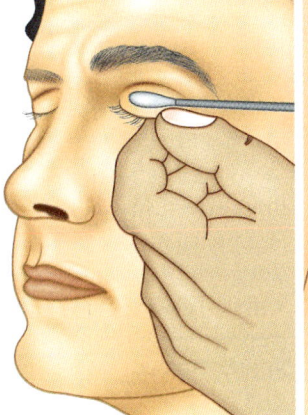

Fig. 1.4: *Examination of the lower fornix and lower palpebral conjunctiva.*

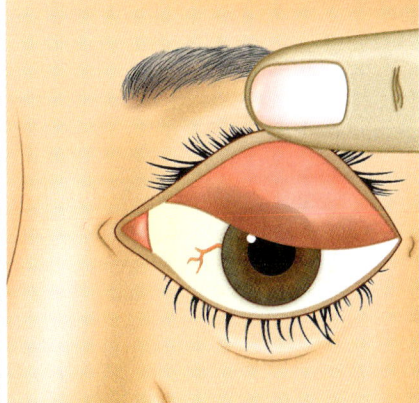

Fig. 1.5: *Two-hand technique of upper lid eversion.*

two-hand technique, index finger of right hand can be used instead of probe.

iv. *Examination of superior fornix* requires double eversion of upper lid using Desmarre's lid retractor.

Conjunctival signs: Normal conjunctiva is a thin semitransparent structure. A fine network of vessels is distinctly seen in it. Following signs may be observed:

■■ *Discolouration* of conjunctiva may be brownish in melanosis and argyrosis (silver nitrate deposits), greyish due to *surma* deposits, pale in anaemia, bluish in cyanosis and bright red due to subconjunctival haemorrhage.

■■ *Congestion of vessels.* Congestion may be superficial (in conjunctivitis) or ciliary/circumcorneal/deep (in iridocyclitis, and keratitis) or mixed (in acute congestive glaucoma). Differences between conjunctival and ciliary congestion are depicted in Table 1.2.

■■ *Conjunctival chemosis* (oedema) may be observed in allergic and infective inflammatory conditions.

■■ *Follicles.* These are seen as greyish white raised areas (mimicking boiled sago-grains) on fornices and palpebral conjunctiva. Follicles represent areas of aggregation of lymphocytes. Follicles may be seen in following conditions:

• Trachoma
• Acute follicular conjunctivitis
• Chronic follicular conjunctivitis
• Benign (school) folliculosis.

■■ *Papillae* are seen as reddish raised areas with flattops and velvety appearance. These represent areas of vascular and epithelial hyperplasia. Papillae are seen in the following conditions:

• Trachoma
• Spring catarrh
• Allergic conjunctivitis
• Giant papillary conjunctivitis.

■■ *Concretions* are seen as yellowish-white hard-looking raised areas, varying in size from pin-point to pin-head. They represent inspissated mucous and dead epithelial cells in glands of Henle. Common causes of concretions are trachoma, conjunctival degeneration and idiopathic.

■■ *Foreign bodies* are commonly lodged in fornices and sulcus subtarsalis on palpebral conjunctiva.

■■ *Scarring on the conjunctiva* may be in the form of a single line in the area of sulcus subtarsalis (*Arlt's line*), irregular, or star-shaped. Common causes of scarring are:

• Trachoma
• Healed membranous or pseudomembranous conjunctivitis
• Healed traumatic wounds
• Surgical scars.

■■ *Pinguecula* is a degenerative condition of conjunctiva observed in many adult patients. It is seen on the bulbar conjunctiva, near the limbus, in the form of a yellowish triangular nodule resembling a fat drop.

■■ *Pterygium* is a degenerative conjunctival fold which encroaches on the cornea in the palpebral area. It must be differentiated from

S. no.	Feature	Conjunctival congestion	Ciliary congestion
Table 1.2 *Differences between conjunctival and ciliary congestion*			
1.	Site	More marked in the fornices	More marked around the limbus
2.	Colour	Bright red	Purple or dull red
3.	Arrangement of vessels	Superficial and branching	Deep and radiating from limbus
4.	On moving conjunctiva	Congested vessels also move	Congested vessels do not move
5.	On mechanically squeezing out the blood vessels	Vessels fill slowly from fornix towards limbus	Vessels fill rapidly from limbus towards fornices
6.	Blanching, i.e. putting one drop of 1 in 10000 adrenaline	Vessels immediately blanch	Do not blanch
7.	Common causes	Acute conjunctivitis	Acute iridocyclitis, keratitis (corneal ulcer)

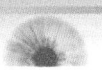

pseudopterygium (an inflammatory fold of conjunctiva encroaching the cornea).

▪▪ *Conjunctival cysts* which may be observed are:
- Retention cyst
- Implantation cyst
- Lymphatic cyst
- Cysticercosis.

▪▪ *Conjunctival tumours.* A few common tumours are dermoids, papillomas and squamous cell carcinoma.

8. Examination of sclera. Normally anterior part of sclera covered by bulbar conjunctiva can be examined under diffuse illumination. Following abnormalities may be seen:

i. *Discolouration.* Normally sclera is white in colour. It becomes yellow in jaundice. Bluish discolouration may be seen as an isolated anomaly or in association with osteitis deformans, Marfan's syndrome, pseudoxanthoma elasticum. Pigmentation of sclera is also seen in naevus of Ota and melanosis bulbi.

ii. *Inflammation.* A superficial localised pink or purple circumscribed flat nodule is seen in *episcleritis.* While a deep, dusky patch associated with marked inflammation and ciliary congestion is suggestive of *scleritis.*

iii. *Staphyloma* is a thinned out bulging area of sclera which is lined by the uveal tissue. Depending upon its location, scleral staphylomas may be intercalary, ciliary, equatorial and posterior.

iv. *Traumatic perforations* in blunt trauma are usually seen in the region of limbus or at the equator.

9. Examination of cornea. Loupe and lens examination or preferably slit-lamp biomicroscopy is a must to delineate corneal lesions. While examining the cornea, a note of following points should be made:

i. *Size.* The anterior surface of normal cornea is elliptical with an average horizontal diameter of 11.7 mm and vertical diameter of 11 mm. Abnormalities of corneal size can be:
- *Microcornea,* when the anterior horizontal diameter is less than 10 mm. It may occur isolated or as a part of microphthalmos.

- Corneal size also decreases in patients with phthisis bulbi.
- *Megalocornea* is labelled when the horizontal diameter is more than 13 mm. Common causes are congenital megalocornea and buphthalmos.

ii. *Shape (curvature).* Normal cornea is like a watchglass with a uniform posterior curve in its central area. In addition to biomicroscopy, keratometry and corneal topography is required to confirm changes in corneal curvature. Abnormalities of corneal shape (curvature) are:
- *Keratoglobus.* It is an ectatic condition in which cornea becomes thin and bulges out like a globe.
- *Keratoconus.* It is an ectatic condition in which cornea becomes cone shaped.
- *Cornea plana,* i.e. flat curvature of cornea which may occur in patients with severe hypotony and phthisis bulbi and rarely as a congenital anomaly.

iii. *Surface.* Smoothness of corneal surface is disturbed due to abrasions, ulceration, ectatic scars and facets. Changes in smoothness of surface can be detected by slit-lamp biomicroscopy, window reflex test and Placido's disc examination.

Placido's keratoscopic disc. It is a disc painted with alternating black and white circles (Fig. 1.6). It may be used to assess the smoothness and curvature of corneal surface. Normally, on looking through the hole in the centre of disc a uniform sharp image of the circles is seen on the cornea (Fig. 1.7). Irregularities in the corneal surface cause distortion of the circles (Fig. 1.8).

iv. *Sheen.* Normal cornea is a bright shining structure. Sheen of corneal surface is lost in 'dry eye' conditions. A loss of the normal polish of the corneal surface causes loss in the sharpness of the outline of the image of circles on *Placido's disc test.*

v. *Transparency* of cornea is lost in corneal oedema, opacity, ulceration, dystrophies, degenerations, vascularization and due to deposits in the cornea.

Examination for corneal ulcer. Once corneal ulcer is suspected, a thorough biomicroscopic

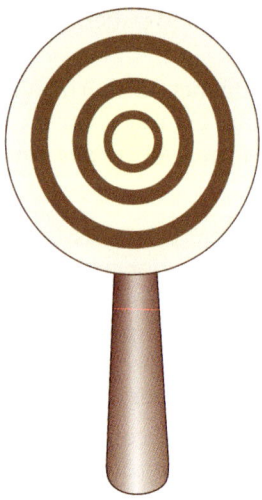

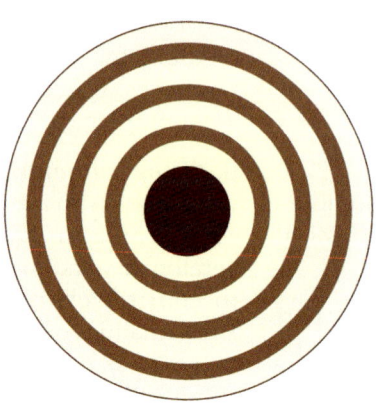

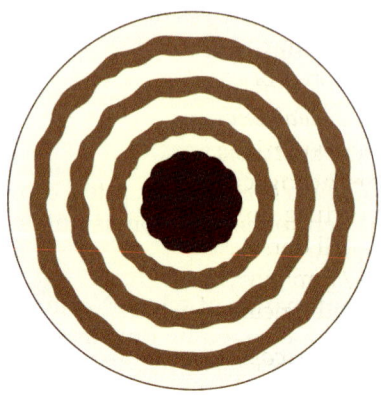

Fig. 1.6: *Placido's disc.*

Fig. 1.7: *Placido's disc reflex from normal cornea.*

Fig. 1.8: *Placido's disc reflex from irregular corneal surface.*

examination before and after fluorescein staining should be performed to note the site, size, shape, depth, floor and edges of the corneal ulcer.

Examination for corneal opacity is best done with the help of a slit-lamp. Note the number, site, size, shape, density (nebular, macular or leucomatous) and surface of the opacity.

vi. Corneal vascularization. The cornea is an avascular structure but its vascularization may occur in many diseases. When vessels are present, an exact note of their position, whether superficial or deep and their distribution whether localised, general, or peripheral should be made.

Differences between superificial and deep vascularization of cornea are shown in Table 1.3.

vii. Corneal sensations. Cornea is a very sensitive structure, being richly supplied by the nerves. The sensitivity of cornea is diminished in many affections of the cornea, viz. herpetic keratitis, neuroparalytic keratitis, leprosy, diabetes mellitus, trigeminal block for postherpetic neuralgia and absolute glaucoma.

■■ *Testing corneal sensations.* Patient is asked to look ahead; the examiner touches the corneal surface with a fine twisted cotton wick (which is brought from the side to avoid menace reflex) and observes the blinking response. Normally, there is a brisk reflex closure of lids. Always compare the effect with that on the opposite side. The exact qualitative measurement of corneal sensations is made with the help of an aesthesiometer.

Table 1.3 *Differences between superficial and deep corneal vascularization*	
Superficial corneal vascularization	*Deep corneal vascularization*
1. Corneal vessels can be traced over the limbus into the conjunctiva.	Corneal vessels abruptly end at the limbus.
2. Vessels are bright red and well-defined.	Vessels are ill-defined and cause only a diffuse reddish blush.
3. Superficial vessels branch in an arborescent manner.	Deep vessels run parallel to each other in a radial fashion.
4. Superficial vessels raise the epithelium and make the corneal surface irregular	Deep vessels do not disturb the corneal surface.

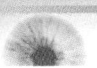

viii. *Back of cornea* should be examined for keratic precipitates (KPs) which are cellular deposits and a sign of anterior uveitis.

KPs can be of different types such as fine, pigmented or mutton fat.

ix. **Corneal endothelium**. It is examined with specular microscope which allows a clear morphological study of endothelial cells including photographic documentation. The cell density of endothelium is around 3000 cells/mm^2 in young adults, which decreases with advancing age.

Biomicroscopic examination after staining of cornea with vital stains is as below:

i. **Fluorescein staining** of cornea is carried out either using one drop of 2 percent freshly prepared aqueous solution of the dye or a disposable autoclaved filter paper strip impregnated with the dye. The area denuded of epithelium due to abrasions or corneal ulcer when stained with fluorescein appear brilliant green. When examined using cobalt blue light, the stained area appears opaque green.

ii. **Bengal rose** (1%) stains the diseased and devitalized cells red, e.g. as in superficial punctate keratitis and filamentary keratitis. Bengal rose dye is very irritating. Therefore, a drop of 2% xylocaine should be instilled before using this dye.

iii. **Alcian blue** dye stains the excess mucus selectively, e.g. as in keratoconjunctivitis sicca.

10. Examination of anterior chamber. It is best done with the help of a slit-lamp.

i. Depth of anterior chamber. Normal depth of anterior chamber is about 2.5 mm in the centre (slightly shallow in childhood and in old age). On slit-lamp biomicroscopy, an estimate of depth is made from the position of iris. Anterior chamber may be normal, shallow, deep or irregular in-depth.

Causes of shallow anterior chamber
- Primary narrow angle glaucoma
- Hypermetropia
- Postoperative shallow anterior chamber (after intraocular surgery due to wound leak or ciliochoroidal detachment)
- Malignant glaucoma

- Anterior perforations (perforating injuries or perforation of corneal ulcer)
- Anterior subluxation of lens
- Intumescent (swollen) lens.

Causes of deep anterior chamber
- Aphakia/pseudophakia
- Total posterior synechiae
- Myopia
- Keratoglobus
- Buphthalmos
- Keratoconus
- Anterior dislocation of lens into the anterior chamber
- Posterior perforation of the globe.

Causes of irregular anterior chamber
- Adherent leucoma
- Iris bombe formation due to annular synechiae
- Tilting of lens in subluxation.

ii. Contents of anterior chamber: Anterior chamber contains transparent watery fluid—the aqueous humour. Any of the following abnormal contents may be detected on examination:

- *Aqueouts flare* in anterior chamber occurs due to collection of inflammatory cells and protein particles in patients with iridocyclitis. Aqueous flare is demonstrated in fine beam of slit-lamp light as fine moving (Brownian movements) suspended particles. It is based on the Tyndall phenomenon (*see* page 155).
- *Hypopyon,* i.e. *Pus* in the anterior chamber may be seen in cases of infectious corneal ulcer, iridocyclitis, toxic anterior segment syndrome (TASS), endophthalmitis and panophthalmitis.
- *Pseudohypopyon* due to collection of tumour cells in anterior chamber and seen in patients with retinoblastoma.
- *Foreign bodies*—wooden, iron, glass particles, stone particles, cilia, etc. may enter the anterior chamber after perforating trauma.
- *Crystalline lens* may be observed in anterior chamber after anterior dislocation of lens.
- *Lens particles* in anterior chamber after trauma, planned extracapsular cataract extraction (ECCE) is a frequent observation.

- *Blood* in the anterior chamber is called *hyphaema* and may be seen after ocular trauma, surgery, herpes zoster and gonococcal iridocyclitis, blood dyscrasias, clotting disorder and intraocular tumours (e.g. retinoblastoma, angioma).
- *Parasitic cyst,* e.g. cysticercus cellulosae has been demonstrated in anterior chamber.
- *Artificial lens.* Anterior chamber intraocular lens may be observed in patients with pseudophakia.

iii. *Examination of angle of anterior chamber* is performed with the help of a gonioscope and slit-lamp. Gonioscopy is a specialized examination required in patients with glaucoma (*see* Chapter 13).

11. Examination of the iris. It should be performed with reference to following points:

i. *Colour of the iris.* It varies in different races; it is light blue or green in caucasians and dark brown in orientals. Heterochromia iridum (different colour of two iris) and heterochromia iridis (different colour of sectors of the same iris) may be present in some individuals. Heterochromia may be either due to involved iris being lighter or darker than the normal.

- *Causes of iris lighter than normal* are: congenital heterochromia, congenital Horner's syndrome, Fuch's heterochromic iridocyclitis, atrophic patches in chronic uveitis, juvenile xanthogranuloma, metastatic carcinoma and Wardenburg syndrome.
- *Causes of darker iris* include, iris naevi, ocular melanocytosis or oculodermal melanocytosis, haemosiderosis, siderosis bulbi, retained iris foreign body, malignant melanoma of iris and lymphoma.
- *Darkly pigmented spots (naevi)* are common freckles on the iris.

ii. *Pattern of normal iris* is peculiar due to presence of collarette, crypts and radial striations on its anterior surface. This pattern is disturbed due to 'muddy iris' in acute iridocyclitis and due to atrophy of iris in healed iridocyclitis.

iii. *Persistent pupillary membrane* (PPM) is seen sometimes as abnormal congenital tags of iris tissue adherent to the collarette area.

iv. *Synechiae,* i.e. adhesions of iris to other intraocular structures may be seen. Synechiae may be anterior (in adherent leucoma) or posterior (in iridocyclitis). Posterior synechiae may be total, annular (ring), or segmental.

v. *Iridodonesis* (tremulousness of the iris). It is observed when its posterior support is lost as in aphakia and subluxation of lens.

vi. *Nodules on the iris surface.* These are observed in granulomatous uveitis (Koeppe's and Busacca's nodules), melanoma, tuberculoma and gumma of the iris.

vii. *Rubeosis iridis* (new vessel formation on the iris). It may occur in patients with diabetic retinopathy, central retinal vein occlusion (CRVO), branch retinal vein occlusion (BRVO), ocular ischaemic syndrome, chronic uveitis, chronic retinal detachment, intraocular tumours, e.g. retinobalstoma.

viii. *A gap or hole in the iris.* It may be congenital coloboma or due to iridectomy (surgical coloboma). Separation of iris from ciliary body is called *iridodialysis.*

ix. *Aniridia or irideremia* (complete absence of iris). It is a rare congenital condition.

x. *Iris cyst.* It may be seen near the pupillary margin in patients using strong miotic drops.

12. Examination of pupil. Note the following points:

i. *Number.* Normally there is only one pupil. Rarely, there may be more than one pupil. This congenital anomaly is called *polycoria.*

ii. *Location.* Normally pupil is placed almost in the centre (slightly nasal) of the iris. Rarely, it may be congenitally eccentric (corectopia).

iii. *Size.* Normal pupil size varies from 3 to 4 mm depending upon the illumination. But it may be abnormally small (*miosis)* or large (*mydriasis).*

Causes of miosis
- Effect of local miotic drugs (parasympathomimetic drugs)
- Effect of systemic morphine
- Iridocyclitis (narrow, irregular, nonreacting pupil)
- Horner's syndrome
- Head injury (pontine haemorrhage)
- Senile rigid miotic pupil

- Due to effect of strong light
- During sleep pupil is pinpoint.

Causes of mydriasis
- Effect of topical sympathomimetic drugs (e.g. adrenaline and phenylephrine)
- Effect of topical parasympatholytic drugs (e.g. atropine, homatropine, tropicamide and cyclopentolate)
- Acute congestive glaucoma (vertically oval large immobile pupil)
- Absolute glaucoma
- Optic atrophy
- Retinal detachment
- Internal ophthalmoplegia
- 3rd nerve paralysis
- Belladonna poisoning.

■■ *Evaluation of anisocoria* (*see* Chapter 6).

iv. Shape. Normal pupil is circular in shape.
- *Irregular narrow, pupil* is seen in iridocyclitis
- *Festooned pupil* is the name given to irregular pupil obtained after patchy dilatation (effect of mydriatics in the presence of segmental posterior synechiae)
- *Vertically oval pupil* (pear-shaped pupil or updrawn pupil) may occur postoperatively due to incarceration of iris or vitreous in the wound at 12 o'clock position.

v. Colour. Of course, pupil is a hole in the iris, but the pupillary area does exhibit colour depending upon the condition of the structures located behind it. Pupil looks:
- *Greyish black* normally
- *Jet black* in aphakia
- *Greyish white* in immature senile cortical cataract
- *Pearly white* in mature cortical cataract
- *Milky white* in hypermature cataract
- *Brown* in cataracta brunescens
- *Brownish black* in cataracta nigra.
- *Leucocoria* (white reflex in pupil) in children is seen in congenital cataract, retinoblastoma, retrolental fibroplasia (retinopathy of prematurity), persistent primary hyperplastic vitreous and toxocara endophthalmitis. The yellowish white, semidilated, non-reacting

pupil seen in retinoblastoma and pseudoglio-mas is also called *amaurotic cat's eye reflex.*
- *Greenish hue* is observed in pupillary area in some patients with glaucoma.
- *Dirty white exudates* may occlude the pupil (*occlusio pupillae*) in patients with iridocyclitis.

vi. Pupillary reactions. Note as follows:

■■ *Direct light reflex.* To elicit this reflex the patient is seated in a dimly-lighted room. With the help of a palm one eye is closed and a narrow beam of light is shown to other pupil and its response is noted. The procedure is repeated for the second eye. A normal pupil reacts briskly and its constriction to light is well-maintained.

■■ *Consensual light reflex.* To determine consensual reaction to light, patient is seated in a dimly-lighted room and the two eyes are separated from each other by an opaque curtain kept at the level of nose (either hand of examiner or a piece of cardboard). Then one eye is exposed to a beam of light and pupillary response is observed in the other eye. The same procedure is repeated for the second eye. Normally, the contralateral pupil should also constrict when light is thrown on to one pupil.

■■ *Swinging flash light test.* It is performed when relative afferent pathway defect is suspected in one eye (unilateral optic nerve lesion with good vision). To perform this test, a bright flash light is shone on to one pupil and constriction is noted. Then the flash light is quickly moved to the contralateral pupil and response is noted. This swinging to and fro of flash light is repeated several times while observing the pupillary response. Normally, both pupils constrict equally and the pupil to which light is transferred remains tightly constricted. In the presence of relative afferent pathway defect in one eye, the affected pupil will dilate when the flash light is moved from the normal eye to the abnormal eye. This response is called 'Marcus Gunn pupil' or a relative afferent pupillary defect (RAPD). It is the earliest indication of optic nerve disease even in the presence of normal visual acuity.

■■ *Near reflex.* In it pupil constricts while looking at a near object. This reflex is largely determined by the reaction to convergence but accommodation also plays a part.

To determine the near reflex, patient is asked to focus on a far object and then instructed suddenly to focus at an object (pencil or tip of index finger) held about 15 cm from patient's eye. While the patient's eye converges and focuses the near object, observe the constriction of pupil.

■■ *Abnormal pupillary reactions include:* (i) amaurotic pupil, (ii) efferent pathway defect, (iii) Wernicke's hemianopic pupil, (iv) Marcus Gunn pupil, (v) Argyll Robertson pupil, and (vi) the tonic pupil.

13. Examination of the lens. A thorough examination of the lens can be accomplished with the help of oblique illumination, slit-lamp biomicroscopy and distant direct ophthalmoscopy with fully-dilated pupils. Following points should be noted:

i. *Position.* A normal lens is positioned in the patellar fossa (space between the vitreous and back of iris) by the zonules. Abnormalities of position may be:

• *Dislocation of lens,* i.e. lens is not present in its normal position (i.e. patellar fossa) and all its supporting zonules are broken. In *anterior dislocation* the intact lens (clear or cataractous) is present in the anterior chamber. While in *posterior dislocation* the lens is present in vitreous cavity where it might be floating *(lensa nutans)* or fixed to the retina *(lensa fixata).*

• *Subluxation of lens,* i.e. lens is partially displaced from its position. Here zonules are intact in some quadrant and lens is shifted on that side. With dilated pupil, edge of the subluxated lens is seen as shining golden crescent on focal illumination and as a dark line (due to total internal reflection) on distant direct ophthalmoscopy. In the presence of substantial degree of subluxation, half pupil may be phakic and half aphakic (and patient may experience unilateral diplopia). Common causes of subluxation of lens are trauma. Marfan's syndrome, homocystinuria, Weill-Marchesani syndrome.

• *Aphakia* (absence of lens) is diagnosed by jet black pupil, deep anterior chamber, empty patellar fossa on slit-lamp biomicroscopy, hypermetropic eye on ophthalmoscopy, retinoscopy and absence of 3rd and 4th Purkinje images.

• *Pseudophakia.* When posterior chamber IOL is present it is diagnosed by a black pupil, deep anterior chamber, shining reflexes from the anterior surface of IOL and presence of all the four Purkinje's images. Examination after dilatation of pupil confirms pseudophakia.

ii. *Shape of lens.* Normal lens is a biconvex structure, which is nicely demonstrated in an optical section of the lens on slit-lamp examination (Fig. 1.9). The optical section of the lens shows from within outward embryonic, foetal, infantile and adult nuclei, cortex and capsule. An anterior Y-shaped and posterior inverted Y-shaped sutures may also be seen.

Abnormalities of the lens shape include:

• Spherophakia, i.e. spherical lens.

• Lenticonus anterior, i.e. an anterior cone-shaped bulge in the lens as seen in Alport syndrome.

• Lenticonus posterior, i.e. a cone-shaped bulge in the posterior aspect of lens.

• Coloboma of lens, i.e. a notch in the lens.

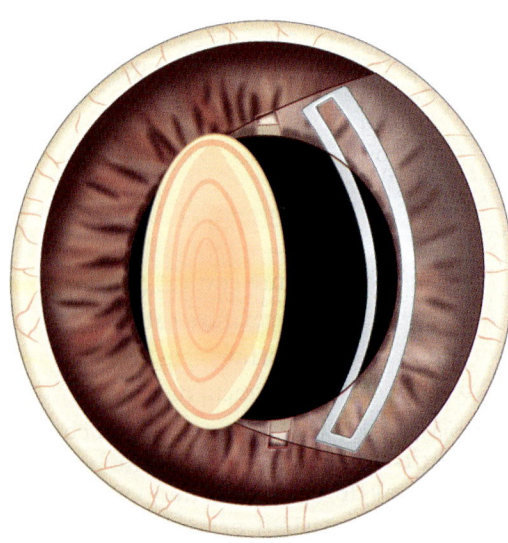

Fig. 1.9: *Optical section of the cornea and adult lens as seen on slit-lamp examination.*

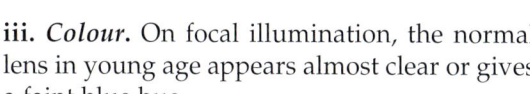

iii. *Colour.* On focal illumination, the normal lens in young age appears almost clear or gives a faint blue hue.

- *In old age,* even the clear lens gives greyish white, hue due to marked scattering of light as a result of increased refractive index of the lens with advancing age. It is usually mistaken for cataract.
- *In cortical cataract,* lens may be greyish white, pearly white or milky white in colour in immature, mature and hypermature cataracts, respectively.
- *In nuclear cataract,* lens may look amber, brown or black in colour.
- *A rusty (orange) discolouration* is seen in cataractous lens with siderosis bulbi (due to retained intraocular iron foreign body).

iv. *Transparency.* Normal lens is a transparent structure. Any opacity in the lens is called *cataract,* which looks greyish or yellowish white on focal illumination. On *distant direct ophthalmoscopy,* the lenticular opacities appear black against a red fundal reflex. On slit lamp biomicroscopy, the morphology of cataract can be studied in detail:

- *Complicated cataract* in the early stages exhibits polychromatic lustre and gives breadcrumbs appearance
- *True diabetic cataract* presents *'snow flake'* opacities
- *Sunflower cataract* is typically seen in disorder of copper metabolism (Wilson's disease)
- *Rosette-shaped cataract,* early as well as late, is typical of concussion injury of lens.

v. *Deposits on the anterior surface of lens* may be:

- *Vossius ring.* It is a small ring-shaped pigment dispersal seen on the anterior surface of lens after blunt trauma. It corresponds in shape and size to the miosed pupil, i.e. smaller than the pupil.
- *Pigmented clumps* may be deposited on the anterior surface of lens in patients with iridocyclitis.
- *Dirty white exudates* may be present on the anterior surface of lens in patients with uveitis and endophthalmitis.

- *Rusty deposits,* i.e. deposition of ferrous ions just below the anterior capsule is seen in siderosis bulbi.
- *Greenish deposits,* i.e. deposition of copper ions is seen in chalcosis.

vi. *Purkinje images test.* This test does not have much significance and thus is not frequently employed in clinical practice. However, it is described as a tribute to the original worker who used this test to diagnose mature cataract and aphakia. Normally, when a strong beam of light is shown to the eye, four images (Purkinje images) are formed from the four different reflecting surfaces, viz. anterior and posterior surfaces of cornea and anterior and posterior surfaces of lens (Fig. 1.10). In patients with mature cataract, fourth image (formed by posterior surface of the lens) is absent, i.e. three Purkinje images are formed. In aphakia, third and fourth Purkinje images (formed by anterior and posterior surface of lens) are absent, i.e. only two images are formed.

14. The intraocular pressure (IOP). The measurement of IOP (ocular tension) should be

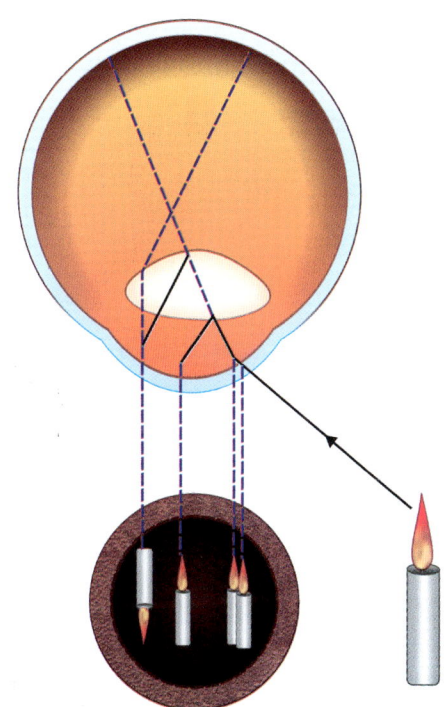

Fig. 1.10: *Purkinje images.*

made in all suspected cases of glaucoma and in routine after the age of 40 years. A rough estimate of IOP can be made by *digital tonometry*. For this procedure patient is asked to look down and the eyeball is palpated by index fingers of both the hands, through the upper lid, beyond the tarsal plate. One finger is kept stationary which feels the fluctuation produced by indentation of globe by the other finger (Fig. 1.11). It is a subjective method and needs experience. When IOP is raised, fluctuation produced is feeble or absent and the eyeball feels firm to hard. When IOP is very low eye feels soft like a partially filled water bag.

The exact measurement of IOP is done by an instrument called tonometer. Indentation (Schiotz tonometer) and applanation (e.g. Goldmann's tonometer) tonometers are frequently used.

- Normal IOP *range* is 10–21 mmHg with an average tension of 16 ± 5.0 mmHg.
- *Hypotony* is labelled when IOP is less than 10 mmHg. Causes of hypotony include ruptured globe, phthisis bulbi, retinal/choroidal detachment, iridocyclitis, ocular ischaemia, postoperative wound leak and traumatic ciliary body shutdown.

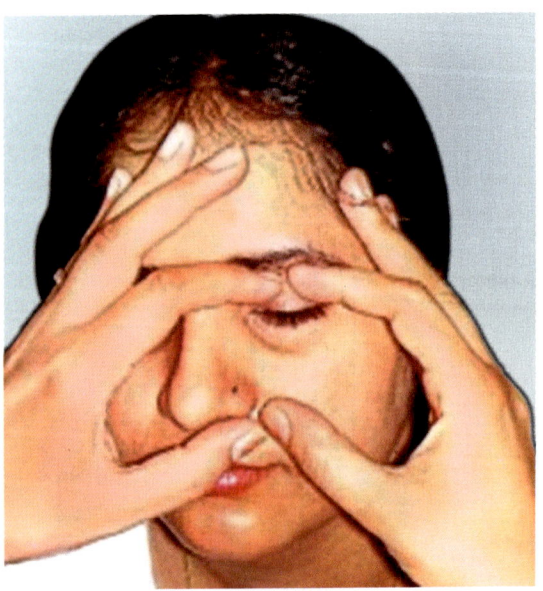

Fig. 1.11: *Technique of digital tonometry.*

- Glaucoma should be suspected when IOP is more than 21 mmHg and such patients should be thoroughly investigated.

III. FUNDUS EXAMINATION

This is essential to diagnose the diseases of the vitreous, optic nerve head, retina and choroid. For thorough examination of the fundus pupils should be dilated with 5% phenylephrine and/or 1% tropicamide eye drops. The fundus examination can be accomplished by ophthalmoscopy and slit-lamp biomicroscopic examination.

Observations during fundus examination

During fundus examination following observations should be made:

1. *Media.* Normally the ocular media is transparent. Opacities in the media are best diagnosed by distant direct ophthalmoscopy, where the opacities look black against the red glow.

Causes of opacities in media are corneal opacity, lenticular opacity, vitreous opacities (may be exudates, haemorrhage, degeneration, foreign bodies and vitreous membranes).

2. *Optic disc*

- *Size (diameter)* of the optic disc is 1.5 mm which looks roughly 15 times magnified during direct ophthalmoscopy. Disc is slightly smaller in hypermetropes and larger in myopes.
- *Shape* of the normal disc is circular. In very high astigmatism, disc looks oblong.
- *Margins* of the disc are well-defined in normal cases. Blurring of the margins may be seen in papilloedema, papillitis, postneuritic optic atrophy and in the presence of opaque nerve fibres.
- *Colour.* Normal disc is pinkish with central pallor area. (i) Hyperaemia of disc is seen in papilloedema and papillitis, (ii) Paler disc is a sign of partial optic atrophy, (iii) Chalky-white disc is seen in primary optic atrophy, (iv) Yellow-waxy disc is typical of consecutive optic atrophy.
- *Cup-disc ratio.* Normal cup disc ratio is 0.3. (i) Large cup may be physiological or

glaucomatous, (ii) cup becomes full in papilloedema and papillitis.

- *Splinter haemorrhages* on the disc may be seen in primary open angle glaucoma, normal tension glaucoma and papilloedema.
- *Neovascularization* of the disc may occur in diabetic retinopathy, CRVO and sickle cell retinopathy.
- *Opticociliary shunt* is a sign of orbital meningioma.
- *Peripapillary* crescent is seen in myopia.
- *Kesten-Baum index* refers to ratio of large blood vessels versus small blood vessels on the disc. Normal ratio is 4:16. This ratio is decreased in patients with optic atrophy.

3. Macula. The macula is situated at the posterior pole with its centre (foveola) being about 2 disc diameters lateral to temporal margin of disc. Normal macula is slightly darker than the surrounding retina. Its centre imparts a bright reflex (foveal reflex). Following abnormalities may be seen on the macula:

- *Macular hole.* It looks red in colour with punched-out margins.
- *Macular haemorrhage* is red and round.
- *Cherry red spot* is seen in central retinal artery occlusion, Tay-Sach's disease, Niemann-Pick's disease, Gaucher's disease and Berlin's oedema.
- *Macular oedema* may occur due to trauma, intraocular operations, uveitis and diabetic maculopathy.
- *Pigmentary disturbances* may be seen after trauma, solar burn, age-related macular degeneration (ARMD), central chorioretinitis and chloroquine toxicity.
- *Bull's eye macular lesions* are seen in ARMD, Stargardt disease, chloroquine retinopathy and cone dystrophy.
- *Hard exudates.* These may be seen in hypertensive retinopathy, exudative diabetic maculopathy, Coat's disease, CNVM.
- *Macular scarring.* It may occur following trauma and disciform macular degeneration.

4. Retinal blood vessels. Normal arterioles are bright-red in colour and veins are purplish with a caliber ratio of 2:3. Following abnormalities may be detected:

- *Narrowing of arterioles* is seen in hypertensive retinopathy, arteriosclerosis, and central retinal artery occlusion.
- *Tortuosity of veins* occurs in diabetes mellitus, central retinal vein occlusion and blood dyscrasias.
- *Sheathing* of vessels may be seen in periphlebitis retinae (Eale's disease, sarcoidosis, syphilis, tuberculosis, Behcet's disease, AIDS) and hypertensive retinopathy.
- *Vascular pulsations. Venous pulsations* may be seen at or near the optic disc in 10–20% of normal people and can be made manifest by increasing the intraocular pressure by slight pressure with the finger on the eyeball. Venous pulsations are conspicuously absent in papilloedema. *Arterial pulsations* are never seen normally and are always pathological. The true arterial pulsations may be noticed in patients with aortic regurgitation, aortic aneurysm and exophthalmic goitre. True arterial pulsations are not limited to disc. While a pressure arterial pulse which is seen in patients with very high IOP or very low blood pressure is limited to the optic disc.

5. General background. Normally the general background of fundus is pinkish red in colour.

▪▪ Physiological variations include dark red background in black races and tessellated or tigroid fundus due to excessive pigment in the choroid.

▪▪ Following abnormal findings may be seen in various pathological states:
- *Superficial retinal haemorrhage* may be found in hypertension, diabetes, trauma, venous occlusions, and blood dyscrasias.
- *Deep retinal haemorrhages* are typically seen in diabetic retinopathy.
- *Cotton wool spots (old name soft exudates)* appeares whitish fluffy spots with indistinct margins. These may occur in hypertensive retinopathy, toxaemic retinopathy

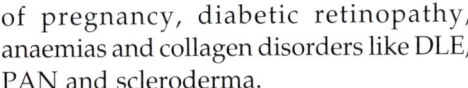

of pregnancy, diabetic retinopathy, anaemias and collagen disorders like DLE, PAN and scleroderma.

- *Hard exudates* are small, discrete yellowish, waxy areas with crenated margins. Common causes are diabetic retinopathy, hypertensive retinopathy, Coats' disease and circinate retinopathy.
- *Colloid bodies* also called *drusens* occur as numerous minute, whitish, retractile spots, mainly involving the posterior pole. They are seen in senile macular degeneration and Doyne's honeycomb dystrophy.
- *Pigmentary disturbances* may be seen in tape to retinal dystrophies, e.g. retinitis pigmentosa and healed chorioretinitis.
- *Microaneurysms* are seen as multiple tiny dot-like dilatations along the venous end of capillaries.

  They are commonly found in diabetic retinopathy. Other causes include hypertensive retinopathy, retinal vein occlusions, Eales' disease and sickle cell disease.
- *Neovascularization of retina* occurs in hypoxic states like diabetic retinopathy, Eales' disease, sickle-cell retinopathy, and following central retinal vein occlusion.
- *Tumours of fundus* include retinoblastoma, astrocytoma and melanomas.
- *Peripheral retinal degenerations* include lattice degeneration, paving stone degeneration, white areas with and without pressure.
- *Retinal holes* are seen as punched out red areas with or without operculum. These may be round or horseshoe in shape or giant tears.
- *Proliferative retinopathy* is seen as disorganized mass of fibrovascular tissue in patients with proliferative diabetic retinopathy, sickle cell retinopathy, following trauma, in Eales' disease and retinopathy of prematurity.
- *Retinal detachment:* Retina looks grey, raised and folded.

IV. VISUAL FIELD EXAMINATION

Examination of visual fields is important in many eye diseases. Technique of visual field examination is described on Chapter 16. Common types of field defects and their causes are mentioned below:

- *Altitudinal field defects:* Ischaemic optic neuropathy, optic disc disease, high myopia and optic neuritis.
- *Enlargement of blind spot:* Glaucoma, papilloedema, optic disc drusen, coloboma of optic disc, medullated nerve fibers, and myopic disc with a crescent.
- *Central scotoma:* Macular disease, optic neuritis, toxic amblyopia, tumours compressing the nerve.
- *Constriction of peripheral fields:* Glaucoma, retinitis pigmentosa, after panretinal photocoagulation, central retinal artery occlusion with cilioretinal artery sparing, and chronic papilloedema.
- *Homonymous hemianopia:* Lesion of the optic-tract, lateral geniculate body, optic radiations in temporal, parietal or occipital lobe lesions of the brain such as stroke, tumours, aneurysm and trauma.
- *Bitemporal hemianopia:* Lesions involving optic chiasma, such as pituitary adenoma, meningioma, craniopharyngioma and glioma.
- *Binasal field defects:* Tumours or aneurysm-compressing both optic nerves, or chiasma, chiasmatic arachnoiditis, bilateral occipital disease, bitemporal retinal disease (e.g. retinitis pigmentosa) and glaucoma.
- *Arcuate scotoma:* Glaucoma, optic disc drusen, high myopia, ischaemic optic neuropathy and optic neuritis.

V. COLOUR VISION TESTING

Colour sense in the ability of the eye to discriminate between colours excited by light of different wavelengths. An individual with normal colour vision is known as 'trichromate'. In colour blindness, faculty to appreciate one or more primary colours in either defective (anomalous) or about (anopia). It may be congenital or acquired.

Tests for colour vision are designed for:

1. Screening defective colour vision from normals;
2. Qualitative classification of colour blindness, i.e. proton, deutron and triton
3. Quantitative analysis of degree of deficiency, i.e. mild, moderate or marked.

Details about the colour vision and its testing are described in Chapter 2.

SPECIALISED OCULAR DIAGNOSTIC TESTS

The specialiged ocular diagnostic tests have their specific indication and are not infrequently performed. A few ommon such tests, listed below are described in separate chapters given in the parenthesis.

- Ocular fluorescein angiograhy (Chapter 28)
- Electrophysiologicats tests (Chapter.30)
  - Electro-retinography (ERG)
  - Electro-oculography (EOG)
  - Visually evoked response (VER)

IMAGING TECHNIQUES IN OPHTHALMOLOGY

Roentgen examination techniques have occupied an important place in the mark-up of an ophthalmic case. These are indespensable both for intraocular and intraoptical lesions. These described in Chapters 31 to 35, include the following:

- Plain X-ray
- Conventional tomography
- Ultrasonography
- CT scanning
- Magnetic Resonance Imaging (MRI)
- Protone.

HISTOPATHOLOGICAL STUDIES IN OPHTHALMOLOGY

In spite of the exaussive clinical mark-up and advanced ocular diagnostic tests, the exact diagnosis in many ocular lesions (especially orbital and adnexal lesions) cannot be made without the help of histopathological studies which can be accomplished by gine needle aspiration biopath incisional biopsy and excisional biopsy.

RECORD OF OPHTHALMIC CASE

Both right and left eye should be examined and findings should be recorded in ophthalmic clinical case sheet (depicted below).

OPHTHALMIC CLINICAL CASE SHEET

Name and Address

Age and Sex

Occupation

Religion

Chief Presenting Complaints

History of Present Illness

Past History

Contd...

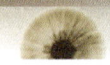

OPHTHALMIC CLINICAL CASE SHEET (Contd...)

Personal History

Family History

General Physical and Systemic Examination

Facial Symmetry

Head Posture

Forehead

Ocular Examination

	Right Eye	**Left Eye**

Visual Acuity

- Distance (with and without glasses)
- Near

Eyebrows

- Level
- Cilia

Orbit

- Inspection
- Palpation

Eyeballs

- Position
- Size
- Alignment
- Movements

Uniocular

Biocular

Eyelids

- Position
- Movements
- Lid Margin
- Eyelashes
- Skin of Lids

Contd...

OPHTHALMIC CLINICAL CASE SHEET (*Contd...*)

Palpebral Aperture

- Width

- Height

- Shape

LACRIMAL Apparatus

- Puncta

- Lacrimal Sac Area

- Regurgitation Test

- Lacrimal Syringing

Conjunctiva

- Bulbar Conjunctiva

- Palpebral Conjunctiva

- Fornices

Limbus

Sclera

- Discoloration

- Nodule

- Ectasia

- Any Other Abnormality

Cornea

- Size

- Shape

TECHNIQUES OF OCULAR EXAMINATION AND DIAGNOSTIC TESTS

OBLIQUE ILLUMINATION

Oblique illumination also known as focal illumination, is a method for examination of the structures of the anterior segment of the eye. Karl Himly (1806) was the first to employ the technique of oblique illumination examination. In it, a zone of light is made to fall upon the structure to be examined so that it is brilliantly illuminated and stands out with special clarity as compared to the surroundings which remain in shadow.

There are two main methods of focal illumination:

- Loupe and lens examination
- Slit-lamp examination.

Loupe and lens examination

Optical principle. It is based on the principle that when an object is placed between a convex lens and its focal point, its image formed is virtual, erect, magnified and on the same side as the object.

Prerequisites. (1) Darkroom, (2) source of light, (3) condensing lens of +13 D, (4) corneal loupe of +41 D, made with two planoconvex lenses each of 20.5 D (×10 magnification) (Fig. 1.12).

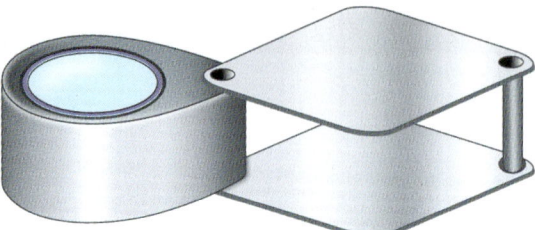

Fig. 1.12: *Corneal loupe.*

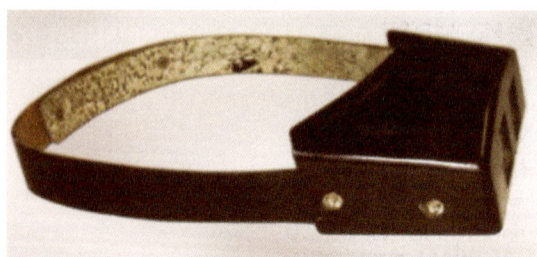

Fig. 1.14: *Binocular loupe.*

Procedure. (1) Light source is placed about 2 feet away, laterally and slightly in front of the patient's eye; (2) Light is focused on the structure to be examined with the help of +13 D condensing lens, held in one hand; (3) The examination is carried out with the help of corneal loupe. The loupe is held between thumb and forefinger of the second hand, the fourth and fifth fingers are supported on the patient's forehead, while the middle finger is used for elevating the upper lid (Fig. 1.13). The loupe is brought close to the patient's eye till the illuminated area is focused. The observer should also move his or her eyes as close to the loupe as possible to have a better view (4) By changing the position of the condensing lens and loupe, various structures of the anterior segment can be examined one by one.

Use of binocular loupe. The corneal loupe may be replaced by a binocular loupe (Fig. 1.14), which gives the added advantage of stereoscopic view and easy manoeuvering, as normally it is fixed to the examiner's head by a band. However, the magnification achieved with binocular loupe is much less than that of uniocular corneal loupe.

SLIT-LAMP EXAMINATION

Note: *For details see Chapter 3.*

■ GONIOSCOPY

Owing to lack of transparency of corneoscleral junction and total internal reflection of light (emitted from angle structures) at anterior surface of cornea it is not possible to visualize the angle of anterior chamber directly. Therefore, a device (goniolens) is used to divert the beam of light and this technique of biomicroscopic examination of the angle of anterior chamber is called *gonioscopy.*

Note: *For details see Chapter 13.*

■ TONOMETRY

The intraocular pressure (IOP) is measured with the help of an instrument called *tonometer.* Two basic types of tonometers available are: indentation and applanation.

Note: *For details see Chapter 12.*

■ TECHNIQUES OF FUNDUS EXAMINATION

A. Ophthalmoscopy
B. Slit-lamp biomicroscopic examination of the fundus by:
- Indirect slit-lamp biomicroscopy
- Hruby lens biomicroscopy
- Contact lens biomicroscopy.

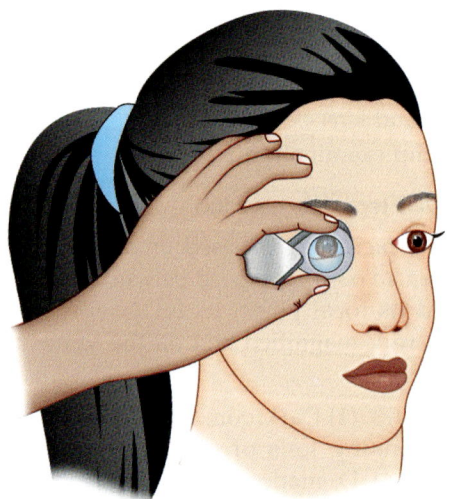

Fig. 1.13: *Technique of loupe and lens examination.*

Note: *For details see Chapter 4.*

PERIMETRY

Visual field is a three-dimensional area of a subject's surroundings that can be seen at any one time around an object of fixation. Traquair described it as an "island of vision surrounded by a sea of darkness". The extent of normal visual field with a 5 mm white colour object is superiorly 50°, nasally 60°, inferiorly 70° and temporally 90° (Fig. 1.15). The field for blue and yellow is roughly 10° less and that for red and green colour is about 20° less than that for white. Perimetry with a red colour object is particularly useful in the diagnosis of bitemporal hemianopia due to chiasmal compression and in the central scotoma of retrobulbar neuritis.

The visual field can be divided into central and peripheral field (Fig. 1.15):

Central field includes an area from the fixation point to a circle 30° away. The central zone contains physiologic blind spot on the temporal side.

Peripheral field of vision refers to the rest of the area beyond 30° to outer extent of the field of vision.

Isopter. Visual field, i.e. the three-dimensional hill of vision can be divided into many isopters depending upon the perception sensitivity. Thus each isopter can be defined as a threshold line forming points of equal sensitivity on a visual field chart.

Scotoma refers to an area of loss of vision totally *(absolute scotoma)* or partially *(relative scotoma)* in the visual field.

Methods of estimating the visual fields

Perimetry. It is the procedure for estimating extent of the visual fields. It can be classified as below:

Kinetic versus static perimetry

Kinetic perimetry. In this, the stimulus of known luminance is moved from a peripheral non-

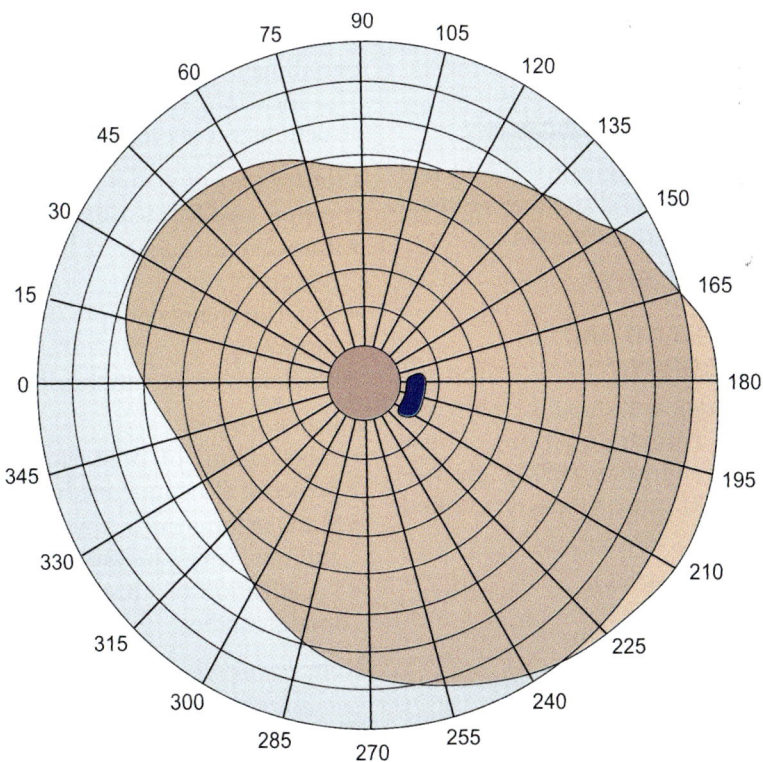

Fig. 1.15: *Extent of normal visual field.*

seeing point towards the centre till it is perceived to establish the isopters. Various methods of kinetic perimetry are: Confrontation method, Lister's perimetry, tangent screen scotometry and Goldmann's perimetry.

Static perimetry. This involves presenting a stimulus at a predetermined position for a preset duration with varying luminance in the field of vision. Various methods of static perimetry adopted are Goldmann perimetry, Friedmann perimetry, automated perimetry.

Peripheral versus central field charting

Peripheral field charting
- Confrontation method
- Perimetry: Lister's, Goldmann's and automated *central field charting*
- Campimetry or scotometry
- Goldmann's perimetry
- Automated field analysis.

Manual versus automated perimetry

- Manual perimetry
- Automated perimetry.

Note: *For details see Chapter 16.*

FUNDUS FLUORESCEIN ANGIOGRAPHY

Fundus fluorescein angiography (FFA) is a valuable tool in the diagnosis and management of a large number of fundus disorders.

Note: *For details see Chapter 28.*

ELECTRORETINOGRAPHY AND ELECTRO-OCULOGRAPHY

The electrophysiological tests allow objective evaluation of the retinal functions. These include: electroretinography (ERG), electro-oculography (EOG), and visually evoked response (VER).

Note: *For details see Chapter 30.*

OCULAR ULTRASONOGRAPHY

Ultrasonography has become a very useful diagnostic tool in ophthalmology. The diagnostic ophthalmic ultrasound is based upon 'pulse-echo' technique. Ultrasonic frequencies in the range of 10 MHz are used for ophthalmic

diagnosis. Rapidly repeating short bursts of ultrasonic energy are beamed into the ocular and orbital structures. A portion of this signal is returned back to the examining probe (transducer) from areas of reflectivity. The echoes detected by the transducer are amplified and converted into display form. The processed signal is displayed on cathode ray tubes in one of the two modes: A-scan or B-scan .

A-scan (time amplitude). The A-scan produces a unidimensional image and echoes are plotted as spikes.

Interpretation of A-scan.
  i. *Distance between the two echo spikes* provides an indirect measurement of tissue such as eyeball length or anterior chamber depth and lens thickness.
  ii. *The height of the spike* indicates the strength of the tissue sending back the echo. The cornea, lens and sclera produce very high amplitude spikes, while the vitreous membrane and vitreous haemorrhage produce lower spikes.

B-scan (intensity modulation). B-scan produces two-dimensional dotted section of the eyeball. The location, size and configuration of the structures is easy to interpret.

Clinical uses of ocular ultrasound

A-scan is used for measurement of:
- Axial length, mainly for IOL power calculation (biometry)
- Anterior chamber depth and other intraocular distances
- Thickness of the intraocular mass.

B-scan is used for:
- Assessment of posterior segment in the presence of opaque media
- Study of intraocular tumours, orbital tumours, and other mass lesions
- Localization of intraocular and intraorbital foreign bodies.

Note: *For details see Chapter 32.*

OPTICAL COHERENCE TOMOGRAPHY

Optical coherence tomography (OCT) is a diagnostic tool that can perform cross-sectional or tomographic images of biological tissues within less than 10 mm axial resolution using light waves. The operation of OCT is analogous to USG B-mode imaging or radar except that light is used rather than acoustic or radiowaves. OCT is specially suited for diagnostic applications in ophthalmology because of the ease of optical access to the anterior and posterior segment of the eye. The information provided by OCT is akin to *in vivo* histopathology of the structure.

Principle. *OCT* utilizes the interferometry and low coherence light in near infrared range.

OCT machine comprises: Fundus viewing unit, interferometric unit, computer display, control panel and colour inkjet printer.

OCT machine is available as:
• Anterior segment OCT machine
• Posterior segment OCT machine
• Combined anterior segment and posterior segment OCT machine.

Types of OCT machines are:
• Time domain OCT (TD-OCT)
• Frequency domain OCT (FD-OCT)

• Specially encoded frequency domain OCT (SEFD-OCT)
• Time encoded frequenc y domain OCT (TEFD-OCT).

Note: *For details see Chapters* 14 *and* 29.

BIBLIOGRAPHY

1. Keeney AH. Ocular examination: basis and techniques. 2nd ed. St. Louis: CV Mosby, 1976.
2. Newell FW. Ophthalmology: principles and concepts. 6th ed. St. Louis: CV Mosby, 1986.
3. Paton D, Goldberg MF. Injuries of the eye, the lids, and the orbit. Philadelphia: WB Saunders, 1968.
4. Robinett DA, Kahn JH. The physical examination of the eye. Emerg Med ClinNorth Am. 2008 Feb;26(1):1–16.
5. Scheie HG, Albert DM. Textbook of ophthalmology. 9th ed. Philadelphia: WB Saunders, 1977:169–98.
6. Stein HA, Slatt BJ. Ophthalmic assistant. 4th ed. St. Louis: CV Mosby. 1982.
7. Vaughan D, Asbury T. General ophthalmology. 11th ed. Los Altos: Appleton and Lange, 1986.

Evaluation of Visual Acuity, Contrast Sensitivity, and Colour Vision

Chapter Outline

VISUAL ACUITY
General Considerations
• Visual angle
Components of Visual Acuity
• Minimum visible
• Resolution
• Recognition
• Hyperacuity
Measurement of Visual Acuity
• Milestones in development of vision
• Tests for visual acuity assessment
• Measurement of visual acuity in infants
• Assessment of visual acuity from 1 to 3 years

• Measurement of visual acuity in preschool children (3–5 years)
• Measurement of visual acuity in school children (above 5 years) and adults
• Measurement of visual acuity for near
CONTRAST SENSITIVITY
• Introduction
• Types of contrast sensitivity
• Measurement of contrast sensitivity
TESTS FOR COLOUR VISION
• Plate tests
• Arrangement tests
• Anomaloscopes

VISUAL ACUITY

GENERAL CONSIDERATIONS

The vision or visual perception is a complex integration of light sense, form sense, contrast sense and colour sense. *Visual acuity* is considered a measure of form sense, so it refers to the spatial limit of visual discrimination. Technically speaking, visual acuity measurement involves the determination of a threshold. In terms of visual angle, the visual acuity is defined as the reciprocal of the minimum resolvable visual angle measured in minutes of arc for a standard test pattern. Therefore, to understand visual acuity, the knowledge about visual angle is essential.

VISUAL ANGLE

Visual angle is the angle subtended at the nodal point of the eye by the physical dimensions of an object in the visual field (Fig. 2.1). Visual angle is a useful and convenient mode of specifying the spatial extent of objects or elements in the visual field.

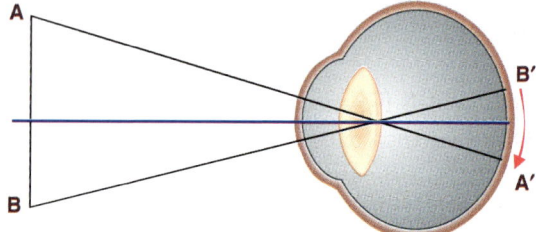

Fig. 2.1: *Visual angle (ANB) subtended at the nodal point by the physical dimensions (AB) of the object.*

It has been observed that the two adjacent points can be seen clearly and discretely only when these two points (say A and B in Fig. 2.1) produce a visual angle not less than 1 minute. The dimensions of the visual angle depend upon the size of the object as well as its distance from the eye. Therefore, to be seen clearly either the object should be large enough or it should be placed near the eye (at an appropriate distance). In terms of the length of the retinal image, it has been seen that the two points (A and B) will be seen clearly when their image size (A'B') is more than 4.5 μ. This is so, because the diameter of individual cone stimulated by the image points A' and B' is 1.5 μ each and at least one cone in between (of 1.5 μ diameter) must be unstimulated. The retinal image size for a given visual angle may vary slightly with changes in viewing distance and associated changes in accommodation of the lens, but this effect is relatively small.

COMPONENTS OF VISUAL ACUITY

In clinical practice, measurement of the threshold of discrimination of two spatially separated targets (a function of the fovea centralis) is termed visual acuity. However, in theory, visual acuity is a highly complex function that consists of the following components:

- Minimum visible,
- Resolution,
- Recognition, and
- Minimum discriminable.

MINIMUM VISIBLE

The ability to determine whether or not an object is present in an otherwise empty visual field is termed *visibility* or *detection*. This kind of task is referred to as the *minimum visible* or *minimum detectable*.

RESOLUTION (ORDINARY VISUAL ACUITY)

Discrimination of two spatially separated targets is termed resolution. The minimum separation between the two points, which can be discriminated, is known as *minimum resolvable*. Measurement of the threshold of discrimination is essentially an assessment of the function of the fovea centralis and is termed *ordinary visual acuity*. The distance between the two targets is specified by the angle subtended at the nodal point of the eye. The normal angular threshold of discrimination for resolution measures approximately 30–60 seconds of an arc; it is usually called the minimum angle of resolution (MAR). The clinical tests determining visual acuity measure the form sense or reading ability of the eye. Thus, broadly, resolution refers to the ability to identify the spatial characteristics of a test figure. The test targets in these tests may either consist of letters (Snellen's chart) or broken circles (Landolt's ring). More complex targets include gratings and checkerboard patterns.

RECOGNITION

It is that faculty by virtue of which an individual not only discriminates the spatial characteristics of the test pattern but also identifies the patterns with which one has had some experience. Recognition is thus a task involving cognitive components in addition to spatial resolution. For recognition, the individual should be familiar with the set of test figures employed in addition to being able to resolve them. The most common example of recognition phenomenon is identification of faces. An average adult can recognize thousands of faces.

MINIMUM DISCRIMINABLE OR HYPERACUITY

Minimum discriminable refers to spatial distinction by an observer when the threshold is much lower than the ordinary acuity. The best example of minimum discriminable is *vernier acuity*, which refers to the ability to determine whether or not two parallel and straight lines are aligned in the frontal plane. The threshold values of vernier acuity (Fig. 2.2) are in the range of only a few seconds (2–10) of arc. Hyperacuity should not be confused with the threshold for the minimum visible, where merely the presence or absence of a target is being judged. The mechanism subserving hyperacuity is not clearly known, but so much is clear; no contradiction is involved with the optical and receptor mosaic factors that limit ordinary visual acuity.

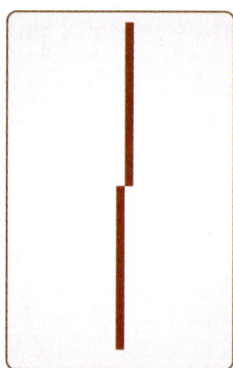

Fig. 2.2: *Typical target configuration for detecting vernier acuity.*

MEASUREMENT OF VISUAL ACUITY

As discussed earlier, the visual acuity is a highly complex function that consists of:

- *Minimum visible,* i.e. detection of presence or absence of stimulus,

- *Minimum separable,* i.e. judgement of location of a visual target relative to another element of the same target, and

- *Minimum resolvable* (ordinary visual acuity), i.e. the ability to distinguish between more than one identifying feature in a visible target.

In clinical practice, the measurement of visual acuity is considered synonymous with the measurement of 'minimum resolvable'. (However, in theory, it is not so, as is clear from the above.) The threshold of the minimum resolvable is between 30 seconds and 1 minute of arc. Therefore, all the clinical tests employed to measure the visual acuity are designed taking into consideration the threshold of the one minimum resolvable. Based on this basic principle, many visual acuity charts have been developed.

MILESTONES IN DEVELOPMENT OF VISION

Before discussing the various methods of visual assessment in infants, children, and adults, it will be worthwhile to have a quick look on the visual development. Important milestones in development of vision are summarized in Table 2.1.

TESTS FOR VISUAL ACUITY ASSESSMENT

Various visual acuity tests available can be grouped as follows:

I. *Detection acuity tests.* These assess the ability to *detect* the smallest stimulus without recognizing correctly. Common detection acuity tests are:

1. Dot visual acuity test
2. Catford drum test
3. Boek candy bead test
4. STYCAR graded ball's test
5. Schwarting metronome test

II. *Recognition acuity tests.* These are designed to assess the ability to recognize the stimulus or to distinguish it from other competing stimuli. These include:

A. *Direction identification tests*
1. Snellen's E-chart test
2. Landolt's C-chart test
3. Sjögren's hand test
4. Arrows test

B. *Letter-identification tests*
1. Snellen's letter chart test
2. Sheridan's letter test
3. Flook's symbol test
4. Lipman's HOTV test

C. *Picture identification charts (miniature toy test)*
1. Allen's picture cards test
2. Beale Collins picture charts test
3. Domino cards test
4. Lighthouse test
5. Miniature toy test of Sheridan

D. *Tests based on picture identification on behavioural pattern*
1. Cardiff acuity cards test
2. Bailey Hall cereal test

III. *Resolution acuity tests*
1. Optokinetic nystagmus (OKN) test
2. Preferential looking test (PLT)
   i. Two-alternative forced choice test
   ii. Operant variation looking test
   iii. Teller acuity cards test
3. Visually evoked response (VER)

Table 2.1 *Milestones in the development of vision*

Age	Visual milestone	Visual acuity
Newborn	• Pupillary reaction to light • Blinking to light stimulus • Conjugate horizontal gaze developed	6/360 to 6/120 (by OKN)
1 week	• Vestibulo-ocular reflex	
2 weeks	• Small saccades develop • Follows horizontal moving objects	
1 month	• Fixation developing • Can watch mother's face for prolonged time	6/480–6/120 (by PL tests)
2 months	• Bifoveal fixation • Large saccades • Pursuits and convergence movements • Conjugate vertical gaze developed	6/120–6/60
3 months	• Watches movements of own hands and reaches out towards interesting objects • Prefers photographs to patterns	
4 months	• Foveal differentiation complete • Sensory fusion and accommodation begins to develops	6/120–6/30
5 months	• Blink response to visible threat (menace response) • Grasps and explores objects • Stereopsis begins to develop	6/90–6/24 6/12–6/6 (by VER)
6 months	• Accommodation well-developed • Fusionalvergence well-developed	6/90–6/24 6/12–6/6 (by VER)
9 months	• Visual differentiation of objects • Picks up small objects	6/48–6/12 6/6 (by VER) 18
18 months	• Visual acuity at adult levels on paediatric acuity card • Myelination of optic nerve completed	6/18–6/7.5
2–3 years	• Best visual acuity approaches near adult levels, but may not be 6/6 • Can play picture or letter recognition games • Can respond to some binocular vision tests • Contrast sensitivity well-developed	6/12–6/6 (36 months)
5 years	• Stereopsis fully developed	6/6–6/5
8–10 years	• Critical period of monocular deprivation ends	6/6–6/5

Tests employed for visual acuity assessment at various age groups are summarized in Table 2.2.

◼ MEASUREMENT OF VISUAL ACUITY IN INFANTS

ASSESSMENT OF VISUAL ACUITY FROM BIRTH TO 3 MONTHS

At birth, visual acuity is 1/60 which improves very fast to 2/60 at 1 month and 6/60 at 4 months. With 1/60 vision, the child is able to fix a face moving within one metre. The fixation reflex and following reflexes take about 6–8 weeks to develop before which an infant may fix for a few seconds and give up. There are a few bizarre movements which appear till the development of definite fixation reflex. Neonates have sporadic jerky movements made up of saccadic eye movements without smooth pursuit. So, visual acuity in a newborn and infant up to 3 months of age can be determined by the tests given below:

1. Blink reflex test. Blink reflex is present since birth (after 30 weeks of gestational age). It is

	Table 2.2 *Commonly used visual assessment tests at various age groups*	
Age	*Tests for assessment of vision*	*Type of visual acuity*
Birth–3 months	• Blink reflex • Pupillary light reflex • Vestibulo-ocular reflex test • Eye popping test • OKN • VER	Resolution acuity
3–6 months	• Fixation and following of objects or small toys • CSM (central, steady and maintained) fixation • Response to occlusion • OKN • VER	Resolution acuity
6–12 months	• Preferential looking tests (Teller acuity tests) • Catford drum test	Resolution acuity Detection acuity
1–3 years	• Cardiff acuity tests • Marble game test • TYCAR ball test • E game test • Boeck candy test	Resolution + Recognition acuity Detection acuity
3–5 years	• Broken wheel test • Landolt C test • Isolated hand figure test • Pictorial vision chart tests • Tumbling E test • HOTV test • Snellen's numbers • Snellen's letters	Recognition acuity
Above 5 years	• Snellen's numbers • Snellen's letters chart • LogMAR chart	Recognition acuity

occasionally present in decorticate infants as well. When bright light is shown, a normal infant should respond by blinking.

2. Pupillary light reflex test. Presence of pupillary light reflex indicates intact afferent visual neurologic pathways to the level of the brachium of the superior colliculus and efferent pathways to the iris sphincter. This reflex is present in premature babies over 29–31 weeks of gestational age. *This is most reliable test to determine presence of vision except in cortical blindness.* The test is best performed in a semi-darkened room because the infant's pupils are smaller than that of a normal adult and constrict in the presence of bright light in the room. In the semi-dark room, the pupil comes to a state of semi-dilatation that reacts briskly. The light used should be small, well-focused and bright. Visualization in very young children sometimes requires a magnifying glass, as their pupils are smaller than those of the older children (because of decreased sympathetic tone) and the light responses are of small amplitude.

3. Vestibulo-ocular reflex. The vestibulo-ocular reflex (VOR) is generally tested by turning the newborn's head on his/her long axis and observing for the doll's eyes response (the eyes deviate opposite to the direction of head rotation).

4. Eye popping test. Another behaviour that is unique to babies is *eye popping*. Sometimes, for a variety of reasons, very young infants do not show any distinguishable visual behaviour at all. In this case, the eye popping reflex indicates at least the baby's ability to detect changes in the room illumination. When the room lights are suddenly dimmed, the baby's upper eyelids should pop open wide for a moment. The baby will often close its eyes when the lights are brought up back, but will again pop its eyes open when the lights are dimmed. This behaviour is documented as 'positive eye popping'.

5. Optokinetic nystagmus (OKN) test. It is an objective method of visual assessment in infants and uncooperative children as well as adults. In this test, nystagmus is elicited by passing a succession of black and white stripes by means of OKN drum of the size 10 × 8 inches diameter, which is rotated at 8–10 rpm through the patient's field of vision (Fig. 2.3). Eyes respond with a slow movement in the direction of drum lasting about 0.2 sec and fast phase in the reverse direction of 0.1 sec. The visual angle subtended by the smallest strip width that still elicits an eye movement (minimum separable) is a measure of visual acuity. The only cooperation required in this test is that the infant be awake and should hold both eyes open. It is reported that OKN acuity is at least 6/120 in the newborns and improves fairly rapidly during the first few months of life, reaching to a level of 6/60 at 2 months, 6/30 at 6 months and 6/6 by 20–30 months. OKN is asymmetric in newborns and becomes symmetric by 4–6 months of age.

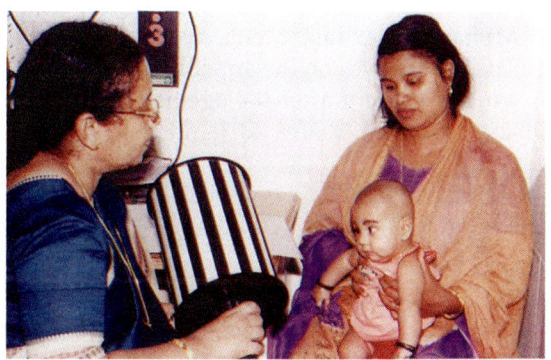

Fig. 2.3: *Optokinetic nystagmus test for visual acuity* (Courtesy: Dr Elizabeth Joseph).

6. Visual evoked response (VER). It refers to electroencephalographic (EEG) recording made from the occipital lobe in response to visual stimuli. VER is the only clinically objective technique available to assess the functional state of the visual system beyond the retinal ganglion cells. It is quite useful in assessing visual function in infants. It reflects acquity from the central retina and thus forms a good macular function test.

Flash VER is usually preformed in very young children or those incapable of fixing on a target. It just tells about the integrity of the macular and visual pathway.

Pattern reversal VER is recorded using some patterned stimulus, as in the checkerboard (Fig. 2.4). In it, the pattern of stimulus is changed (e.g. black squares go white and white become black), but the overall illumination remains the same. The pattern reversal VER depends on form sense and thus gives a rough estimate of the visual acuity. VER studies have shown visual acuity in infants to be 6/120 at the age of 1 month, which reaches to 6/60 at 2 months and 6/6–6/12 at the age of 6 months to 1 year.

Drawbacks of VER include:
- Expensive
- Time consuming
- Limited availability
- Not standardized
- Little clinical relevance

Note: The discrepancy between estimated visual acuity values with optokinetic nystagmus, preferential looking test and visually evoked response at 6 months of age must be kept in mind while performing these tests (Table 2.3).

ASSESSMENT OF VISUAL ACUITY FROM 3 TO 6 MONTHS

Since the fixation develops to moving objects by 3–4 months of age, the visual acuity in this age group can be assessed, in addition to the above mentioned tests, the help of following tests based on fixation behaviour of the infant.

1. Fixation behaviour test. Ability of the child to fix and follow the face of the examiner, toys or interesting object. The test is done first with both eyes open followed by monocular testing by

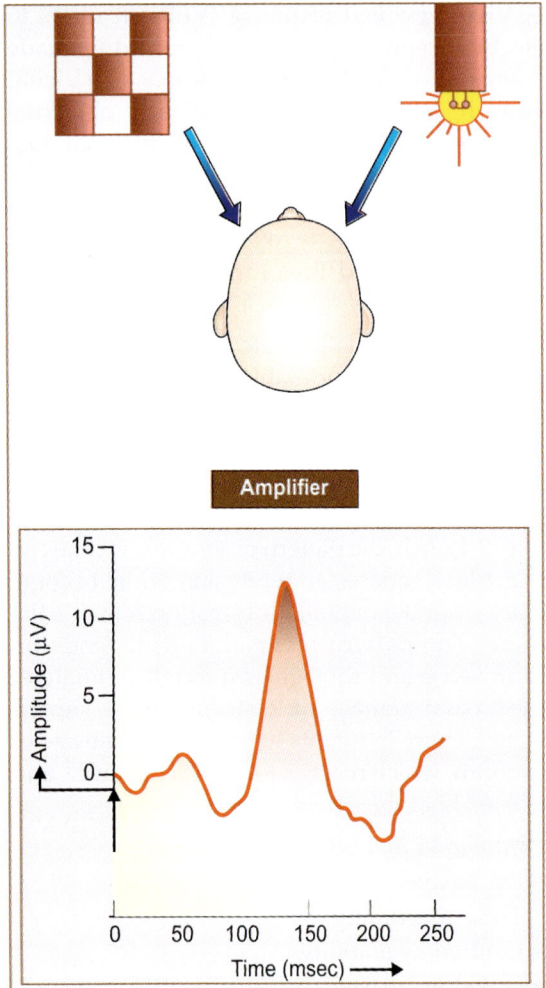

Fig. 2.4: *Technique of recording visually evoked response (VER) and record of normal VER pattern.*

occluding the other eye by hand. If the child habitually fixates with one eye, it indicates poor vision in the non-fixating eye and hence he or she will violently resist occlusion of the better eye.

2. Central, steady, maintained (CSM) method. CSM method is a useful test in this age groups. It implies:

- *Central.* The infant is asked to fixate on penlight and then the examiner looks at the corneal light reflex from a fixation light which is falling at the centre of the pupil. The reflex is considered central, if it falls in the same location in both the eyes in monocular condition.
- *Steady.* This is tested with a small target (thumb-sized toy) which is coupled with light held in front of the child and moved slowly. Nystagmus or oscillation results in unsteady fixation.
- *Maintained.* The ability to keep the eye fixed when either eye is covered.

Results of this test can be interpreted as below:
- CSM: 6/9 to 6/6
- CSNM: 6/36 to 6/60
- Unsteady central fixation: <6/60

3. Brückner's red reflex test. Brückner's reflex is helpful in children uncooperative to the cover test when an assessment is being carried out for small angle strabismus. In this test, fixation and binocular comparison of the red reflex is done. The examiner should stay far enough to illuminate both pupils by the same direct ophthalmoscope beam. The examination should be carried out in dim illumination and the child's attention to be fixed at a distance. Assess the red reflex both before and after dilatation to see how much of the pupillary space is obscured. An overall whitening of the red reflex across the entire pupil of one eye indicates strabismus or anisometropic amblyopia. While the absence of a Brückner reflex is not a good indication of alignment, the presence of a Brückner reflex is considered a positive result, and is a good indication of strabismus, even of small amounts.

4. Menace reflex test. Menace reflex, i.e. reflex closure of the eyes on the approach of an object, is usually present after the age of 5 months, if vision is normal.

Table 2.3 *Estimated visual acuity at different ages*			
Age (months)	*Optokinetic nystagmus*	*Preferential looking test*	*Visually evoked response*
1	6/120	6/120	6/120
2	6/60	6/60	6/60
6	6/30	6/30	6/6–6/12
Age (months) at which 6/6 is achieved	20–30	24–36	6–12

5. Cover test. By 3–6 months, infants have adequate refixation reflex to permit cover test. This test is needed, if there is a concern about strabismus. In patients with normal vision, both eyes look at an object at the same time. Therefore, if one eye is occluded, the opposite eye should not move. In patients with strabismus, one eye is deviated. If the straight eye is covered, the other eye will make a movement to line up the visual target. If a patient is exotropic, the eye will make an inward movement. If an eye is esotropic, it will make an outward movement.

ASSESSMENT OF VISUAL ACUITY FROM 6 TO 12 MONTHS

In addition to the above mentioned tests, the tests described below are more useful in 6–12 months age group.

1. Preferential looking test (PLT). This test is based on the observation that when presented with two adjacent stimulus fields, one of which is striped and the other is homogeneous, the infant will tend to look at the striped pattern for a greater portion of the time. Test procedures have been developed in which an examiner is hidden behind a screen on which one projects a homogeneous surface on one side and black and white stripes on the other side. These two stimuli are alternated randomly. The observer is able to look at the eyes of the infant through a hole in the screen but is unaware of which target, stripes or homogeneous field is presented on which side of the screen.

Teller acuity cards (TAC) test. This is the most commonly used preferential looking test in clinical practice. TAC is recommended to test visual acuity in infants from 1 month to 1 year of age. This test is modification of preferential looking test. This is simple to perform and very reliable and efficient test. The testing distance varies with age of the child, like the test being performed at 36 cm in infants and toddlers, at 54 cm in children up to 3 years and at 84 cm in adults. Estimates of visual acuity, using the TAC grating targets, show a rapid increase in acuity during the first six months of life from 1.0 cycle per degree at one month of age to five cycles per degree by six months of age, then a gradual increase to 40 cycles per degree. Adult like levels are reached at 5 years of age. The results are obtained in *cycles* which can be converted to *Snellen's equivalent*. There are 17 cards, on one half of each card is a set of vertical black-and-white bars of varying size which form the pattern stimulus and on the other half, a uniform gray background which is the blank target (Fig. 2.5). In the centre of each card, there is a small hole through which the examiner observes the infant's fixation. In this by varying the spatial frequency of the bars shown, the finest bar which can no longer be resolved by the infant is used to determine the vision as the infant no longer shows the preference for patterned stimulus. This test can be used effectively on neurologically impaired children.

Visual acuity determined with this method has been reported to range from approximately 6/240 in the newborns to 6/60 at 3 months and 6/6 at 36 months of age. It must be well understood that grating acuity testing cannot automatically be equated with acuity testing based on recognition task, such as naming pictures or Snellen's letters. In normal children, grating acuity is better than recognition acuity. Further, it has been suggested that different neural processing mechanisms in the brain are involved with spatial discrimination and recognition tasks. Hence, it is not advisable to equate grating acuity with recognition acuity (Snellen's).

Limitations. TAC are relatively expensive and less cost effective. Therefore budget versions of FPL acuity testing have emerged in the form of spatial frequency paddles.

2. Catford drum test. It is a *detection acuity test*, useful in infants and children less than 2 years

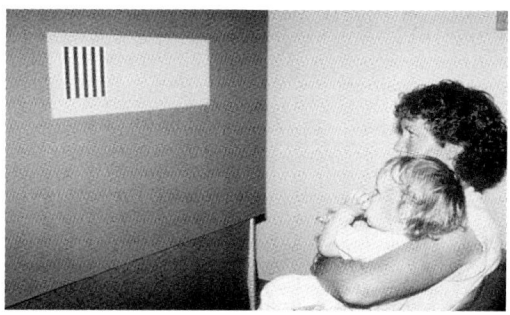

Fig. 2.5: *Teller acuity cards test (a type of preferential looking test).*

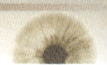

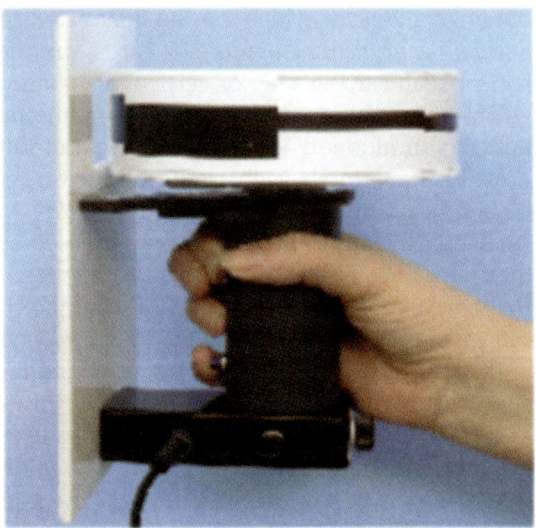

Fig. 2.6: *Catford drum for visual acuity.*

of age. In this test, the child is made to observe an oscillating drum with black dots of varying sizes ranging from 0.5 to 15 mm in diameter representing vision between 6/6 and 2/60 (Fig. 2.6). Rotation of disc at a distance of 60 cm evokes pendular movements. The smallest dot that evokes pendular eye movements (not an OKN) denotes the level of visual acuity. This test is unreliable since it overestimates the vision.

ASSESSMENT OF VISUAL ACUITY FROM 1 TO 3 YEARS

Above 1 year of age, the child is able to visually differentiate the small objects and is able to reach out for toys. So, in addition to the above-mentioned tests, the following detection acuity tests are more useful in this age group.

1. *Cardiff acuity cards test.* Cardiff acuity cards test or vanishing optotypes test (Fig. 2.7) is used to measure visual acuity in this age group. The

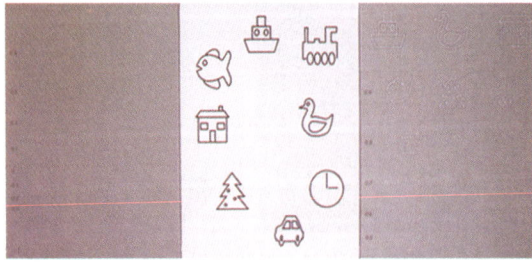

Fig. 2.7: *Cardiff acuity cards test.*

principle is that as long as the child can see the optotype (line drawings of pictures of fish, car, etc.), the child will show a preference for the picture as compared with the plain grey background. The black and white lines forming the pictures become finer with each set of three cards, until the picture cannot be seen (vanishing optotype) and the preference for fixation to the picture is lost. The pictures are presented on cards with the optotype appearing either on the top or the bottom of the card. The rest of the card is a homogeneous grey that matches with the mean luminance of the picture. A total of 11 sets of cards are available, with acuity values ranging from 20/400 to 20/20, which have been calibrated for two presentation distances—0.5 m and 1 m. The patient is presented with one sets of cards at a particular acuity equivalence, one card at a time. By observing the child's eye movements and fixations, the examiner must decide if the optotype is on the top or bottom of the card.

The acuity is determined by the narrowest white band for which the target is visible to the child and correct response is obtained at least 75% of the time when the particular finest line drawing is shown to the child.

Advantages include:
- It is an excellent way to determine minimum separable acuity in a child 1–3 years of age, unless the child can respond to recognition acuity chart.
- The fixations of the child to the pictures on the Cardiff cards are relatively easy to assess.
- CAC is a child friendly test.

Limitations include:
- May miss some cases of visually significant refractive errors.
- TAC is more dependable test to assess amblyogenic conditions despite the use of gratings.

1. *Marble game test.* In children of 6–12 months of age, reaching or placing games can be used to estimate visual function. One such game is the 'marble game'. In it, the child is asked to place marbles in the holes of a card or in a box. This test is not intended to measure visual acuity

of each eye, but rather to compare the functioning of the child's eye when one or the other is closed. The vision of an eye is then noted as being 'useful' or 'less useful'.

2. Sheridan's ball test. Mary Sheridan (1960) used a series of styrofoam balls of progressively smaller sizes. One records the smallest ball that the infant can fixate and follow at a distance of 10 feet. Rolling the ball on a white or grey background and asking the child to pick it up, and noting the smallest size to which the child gives a good response is a rough way of estimating visual acuity.

3. Worth's ivory ball test. Ivory balls ranging in size from 0.5 to 2.5 inches in diameter are rolled on the floor in front of the child who is asked to retrieve each ball. Acuity is estimated on the basis of smallest size of the ball for the test distance.

4. Dot visual acuity test. Child is shown an illuminated box with black dots of different sizes printed on it. The smallest dot identified denotes the visual acuity of the child.

5. Coin test. In this test, the child is asked to identify the two faces of coins of different sizes held at different distances.

6. Miniature toy test. In this test, the child is shown a miniature toy from a distance of 10 ft and is asked to name or pick the pair from the assortment.

▰ MEASUREMENT OF VISUAL ACUITY IN PRESCHOOL CHILDREN (3–5 YEARS)

At this age, the child is able to verbalize and recognize well, so in addition to the above mentioned test, the following tests (based mainly on recognition acuity) are more useful for visual assessment.

1. Landolt C test. This test attempts to test minimum separable acuity in young children who can understand the concept of break in the circle. Landolt Cs are presented with the opening of the optotype at 3, 6, 9 or 12 o'clock. The child has to tell where the opening is. The separation at the break in the C represents 1 minute of arc and the entire C subtends 5 minutes of arc at the eye for 20/20. (For further details *see* page 42).

2. Broken wheel test. This test is another subjective assessment of visual acuity in toddlers and preschoolers who are not able to perform matching tasks. A pair of cars in progressively smaller sizes, one of which has a wheel cut across, like Landolt C (broken wheel), is shown to the child and the child is asked to identify the one with the broken wheel (Fig. 2.8).

The car represents on seven pairs of cards designed to use at 10 feet, providing Snellen's equivalents from 20/20 to 20/100 (shown in Fig. 2.8) presented in a forced choice paradigm without the need for verbal responses. The visual acuity tester holds up one pair of cards at a time and asks the child to point towards the car with the broken wheels. The child should correctly score four out of four responses and then, the next smaller set of cards is used until the child can no longer consistently identify the car with broken wheels.

Advantages include:
- The child has to simply locate the broken wheel and need not to identify the direction of the opening.
- The broken wheel and Snellen tests are highly correlated and that acuities measured with this test is equivalent to Snellen chart with a certainty of 94%, if using four-of-four criterion.

3. Illiterate E-cutout test. This test is useful in children between 2½ and 3 years of age. The child is given a cutout of an E and asked to match this E with isolated Es of varying sizes. The first trial is not always successful. The mother may

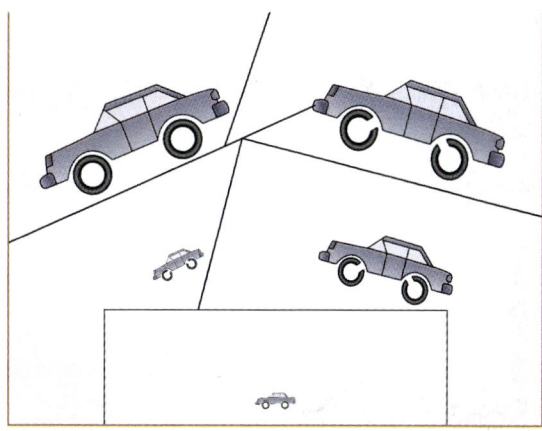

Fig. 2.8: *Broken wheel test.*

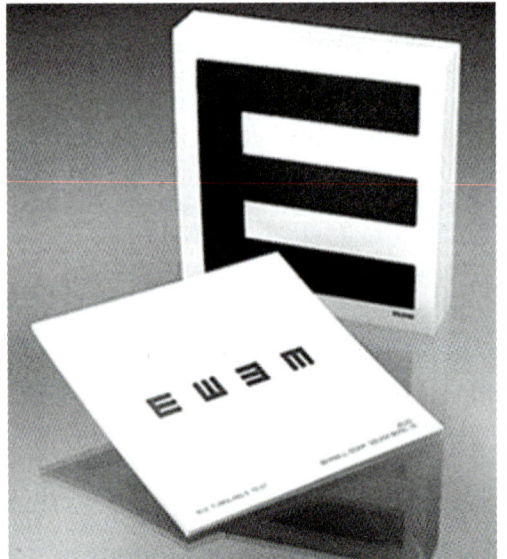

Fig. 2.9: *Tumbling E-pad test. Printed with large 20/200 E on one side and a series of five 20/20 tumbling Es on the other—calibrated to a 20 feet distance.*

be instructed to teach E-game at home. When the child starts understanding the orientation of E, a visual acuity chart consisting of Es oriented in various directions may be used.

4. Tumbling E-pad test. It consists of different sizes of E in one of the four positions (right, left, upward and downward) on a dice (Fig. 2.9). Basically, it is similar to E-cutout test.

5. Isolated hand-figure test. Sjögren has replaced the E with the isolated figure of a hand, and in some children it works better than Es.

6. Sheridan–Gardiner HOTV test is another test similar to E-cutout test (Fig. 2.10). This is an initiative test, used to test vision in the age group

of 2–5 years. The child is handed a card with HOTV and is asked to match the letters on the chart. Snellen's equivalent of 6/6–6/60 can be estimated using this method.

7. Pictorial vision charts. When the child is able to verbalize, visual acuity chart showing pictures, rather than symbols, may be used. Many such charts have been devised, and one should be chosen that presents pictures of objects with which the child is likely to be familiar. Pictorial vision charts include Kay picture test, Allen cards test, Lae symbols test and BUST.

- *Allen cards test* (Fig. 2.11). In this test, seven optotypes are presented to the child for recognition at a test distance of 15 feet (20/40) at 3 years of age and 20 feet (20/30) at 4 years of age.
- *Kay pictures* (Fig. 2.12) is another picture optotype developed to assess visual acuity in

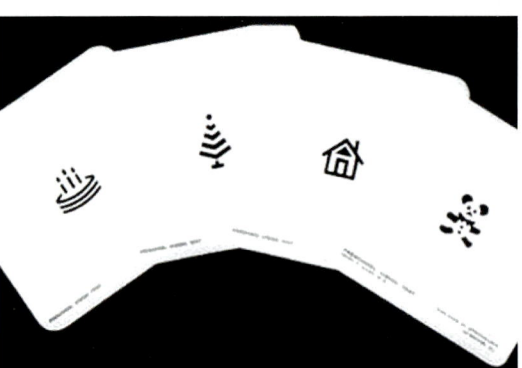

Fig. 2.11: *Allen cards test.*

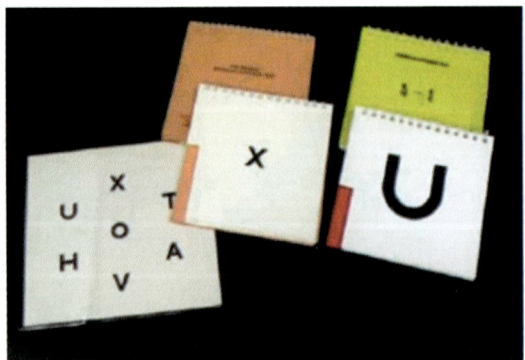

Fig. 2.10: *Sheridan–Gardiner single letter optotypes.*

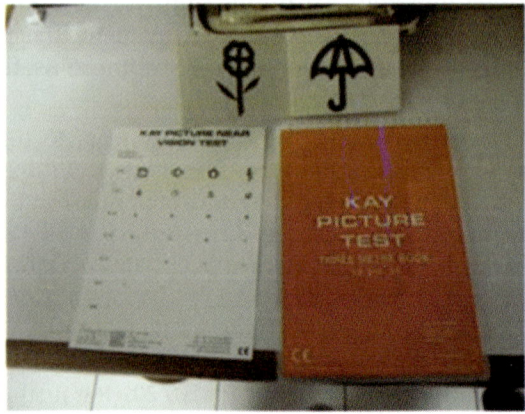

Fig. 2.12: *Kay picture test.*

young children at distance as well as at near. The figures are child friendly with matching cards for children who cannot speak. The individual elements subtend a visual angle of 1 minute of arc and the total figure subtends 10 minutes of arc at the eye. The available test booklets are for 6 m and 3 m distance. The 3 m booklet used for younger children who will not be attentive at 6 m. Near point cards are also available to assess near visual acuity.

- *Lea symbols test* (Fig. 2.13) was developed by Dr Lea Hyvärinen, a Finnish paediatric ophthalmologist, who developed a vast array of testing devices that have been standardized using four pictures—circle, square, house and apple. Lea numbers were developed in 1993 and calibrated in 1994. These optotypes can be presented as single characters, as a wall chart at a distance of 10 to 20 feet. They can be presented on a video display terminal screen or in the form of a flip book. With the Landolt C type being the reference optotype since 1988, earlier to which Snellen E chart was the reference optotype, the size of the 1.0 (20/20,6/6) optotypes was reduced from 7.5 to 6.84 minutes of arc.

  Lea symbols now have two important basic features of good optotypes that they blur equally and are calibrated against the Landolt C. This is a good way of testing individuals who do not use the western alphabet. Hence, it eliminates the problem with language barriers.

- *BUST is* another picture test designed to test visual acuity of children with vision impairment and developmental handicaps. BUST is an acronym for the Swedish words for 'visual acuity and picture perception test'. The range of visual acuity for distance acuity

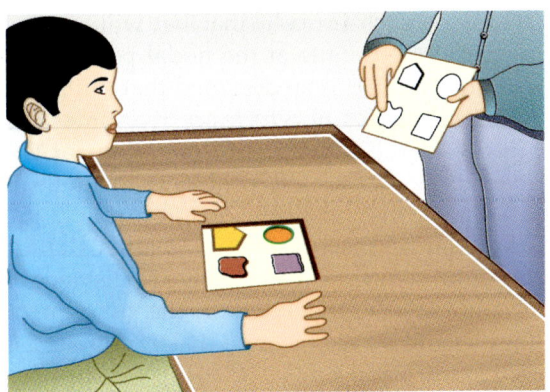

Fig. 2.14: *Light home picture cards.*

measurement values goes from 0.02 to 1.6 (20/1000 to 20/10).

7. Boek candy bead test. The child is asked to match beads at 40 cm. Snellen's visual acuity equivalent of 20/200 is estimated by this method.

8. Light home picture cards. A chart containing an apple, a house and an umbrella (Fig. 2.14), arranged in Snellen's equivalents of 20/200–20/10 is used, and the child is asked to identify the pictures along the lines. The test is carried out at 10 feet.

MEASUREMENT OF VISUAL ACUITY IN SCHOOL CHILDREN (ABOVE 5 YEARS) AND ADULTS

- *Snellen's visual acuity charts* are most commonly employed in this age group. Illiterates E charts and Landolt's C charts are used as alternative to Snellen's test types.
- *LogMAR charts* enable a more accurate estimate of acuity as compared to other charts. Because of high accuracy, these are the most commonly used charts in research settings/clinical trials.

1. Snellen's test types

The distant central visual acuity is usually tested by Snellen's test types. The fact that two distant points can be visible as separate only when they subtend an angle of 1 minute at the nodal point of the eye forms the basis of Snellen's test types. It consists of a series of black capital letters on a white board, arranged in lines, each progressively diminishing in size. The lines comprising the

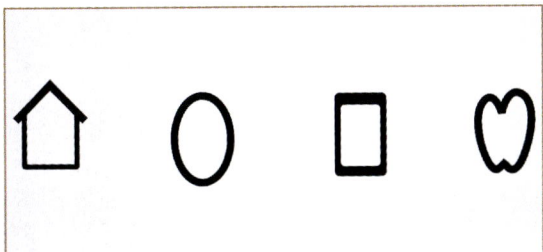

Fig. 2.13: *Lea symbols test.*

letters have such a breadth that they will subtend an angle of 1 minute at the nodal point. Each letter of the chart is so designed that it fits in a square, the sides of which are five times the breadth of the constituent lines. Thus at the given distance, each letter subtends an angle of 5 minutes at the nodal point of the eye (Fig. 2.15). The letter of the top line of Snellen's chart (Fig. 2.16) should be read clearly at a distance of 60 m. Similarly, the letters in the subsequent lines should be read from a distance of 36, 24, 18, 12, 9, 6, 5 and 4 m.

Landolt's test types. It is similar to Snellen's test types except that in it instead of the letter the broken circles are used. Each broken ring subtends an angle of 5 minutes at the nodal point and is constructed similar to letter of Snellen's test types (Fig. 2.17).

With Snellen's letters, the end point consists of letter recognition; with Landolt's rings, it consists of the detection of the orientation of the break in the circle. Each method has advantages and disadvantages. Letter targets represent a practical visual test. However, the ability to recognize the target is influenced by literacy and past experience, even if the targets are somewhat blurred. Landolt's rings were designed to eliminate these factors and present a more objective test. However, since the gap can be placed in only four positions (up, down, left and right), guessing becomes an important factor. Also letter tests remain much less confusing for the patient and the examiner, since the identification of letters is both immediate and unequivocal.

Procedure of testing. For testing distant visual acuity, the patient is seated at a distance of 6 m from the Snellen's chart, so that the rays of light are practically parallel and the patient exerts

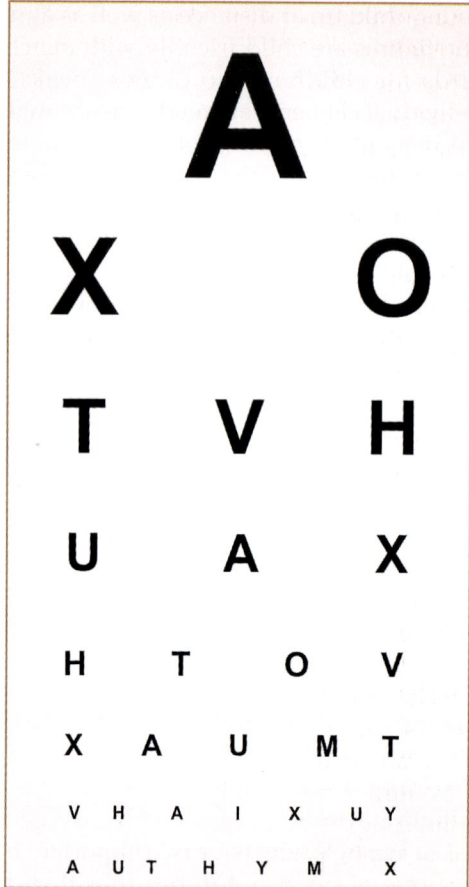

Fig. 2.16: *Snellen's test types.*

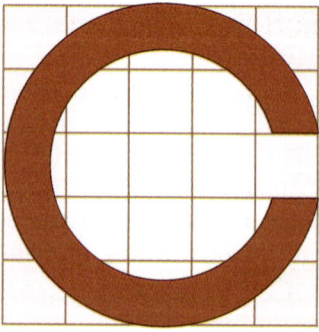

Fig. 2.17: *Construction of Landolt's visual acuity target.*

minimal accommodation. The chart should be properly illuminated (not less than 20 foot-candle). The patient is asked to read the chart with each eye separately and the visual acuity is recorded as a fraction, the numerator being the distance of the patient from the letters and

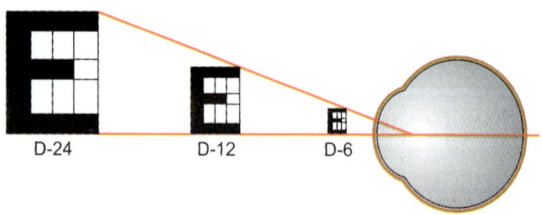

D-24   D-12   D-6

Fig. 2.15: *Principle of Snellen's test types.*

the denominator being the smallest letters accurately read.

When the patient is able to read up to 6 m line, the visual acuity is recorded as 6/6, which is normal. Similarly, depending upon the smallest line that the patient can read from the distance of 6 m, his or her vision is recorded as 6/9, 6/12, 6/18, 6/24, 6/36 and 6/60. If one cannot see the top line from 6 m, he or she is asked to slowly walk towards the chart till one can read the top line. Depending upon the distance at which one can read the top line, the vision is recorded as 5/60, 4/60, 3/60, 2/60 and 1/60.

If the patient is unable to read the top line even from 1 m, he or she is asked to count fingers (CF) of the examiner. His or her vision is recorded as CF-39, CF-29, CF-19 or CF close to face, depending upon the distance at which the patient is able to count fingers. When the patient fails to count fingers, the examiner moves his or her hand close to the patient's face. If one can appreciate the hand movements (HM), visual acuity is recorded as HM positive. When the patient cannot distinguish the hand movements, the examiner notes whether the patient can perceive light (PL) or not. If yes, vision is recorded as PL positive and if not it is recorded as PL negative.

2. LogMAR visual acuity charts

LogMAR stands for **Log**arithm of the **M**inimum **A**ngle of **R**esolution. A LogMAR chart comprises rows of letters and has equal number of letters in each line (Fig 2.18). It is used at a distance of

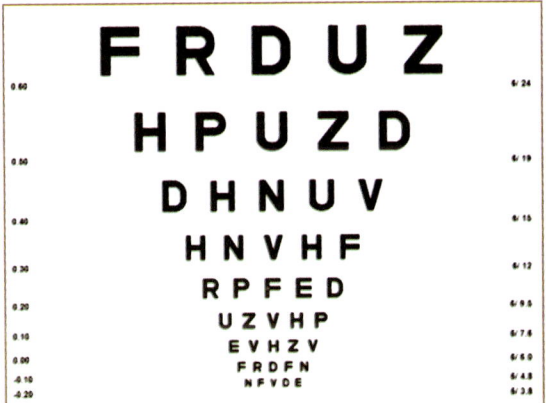

Fig. 2.18: *LogMAR visual acuity chart.*

4 meters. It is designed to enable a more accurate estimate of acuity as compared to other charts (e.g. the Snellen chart), for this reason, it is recommended in research settings.

An observer who can resolve details as small as 1 minute of visual angle scores LogMAR 0, since the base-10 logarithm of 1 is 0; an observer who can resolve details as small as 2 minutes of visual angle (i.e. reduced acuity) scores LogMAR 0.3, since the base-10 logarithm of 2 is 0.3; and so on.

Visual acuity equivalents in different notations

Table 2.4 indicates different ways for specifying visual acuity levels, viz. Minimal angle of resolution (MAR), Snellen's acuity, efficiency rating, Snellen's fraction (that is the reciprocal of the MAR) and the logarithm of Snellen's fraction.

MEASUREMENT OF VISUAL ACUITY FOR NEAR

Near vision is tested by asking the patient to read a near vision chart which consists of a series of different sizes of 'printer types' arranged in decreasing order and marked accordingly.

Near vision charts

Commonly used near-vision charts are as follows:

1. Jaeger's chart. Jaeger, in 1867, devised the near vision chart that consisted of the ordinary printers' fonts of varying sizes used at that time. Printers' fonts have changed considerably since then; however, it is now a general custom to use various sizes of modern fonts that approximate Jaeger's original choice. In this chart, prints are marked from 1 to 7 and accordingly patient's acuity is labelled as J1–J7, depending upon the print one can read.

2. Roman test types. The Jaeger's charts made from the modern fonts deviate considerably from the original standard, but they are probably sufficiently accurate for all practical purposes. However, to overcome this theoretical problem, the Faculty of Ophthalmologists of Great Britain in 1952 devised another near vision chart. It consists of 'Times Roman' type fonts with standard spacing (Fig. 2.19). According to

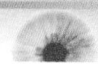

Table 2.4 *Visual acuity equivalents in different notations*

MAR or minimum angle of resolution (minutes of arc)	Snellen's visual acuity ft	m	Snell-Sterling visual efficiency (%)	Loss of central vision (%)	Snellen's fraction acuity relative 20/20	LogMAR acuity relative to
0.5	20/10	6/3	109	0	2.0	0.3
0.75	20/15	6/4.5	104	0	1.33	0.1
1.00	20/20	6/6	100	0	1.0	0
1.25	20/25	6/7.5	96	4	0.8	−0.1
1.5	20/30	6/9	91	9	0.67	−0.18
2.0	20/40	6/12	84	16	0.5	−0.3
2.5	20/50	6/15	76	24	0.4	−0.4
3.0	20/60	6/18	70	30	0.33	−0.5
4.0	20/80	6/24	58	40	0.25	−0.6
5.0	20/100	6/30	49	50	0.2	−0.7
6.0	20/120	6/36	41	60	0.17	−0.78
7.5	20/150	6/45	31	70	0.133	−0.88
10.0	20/200	6/60	20	80	0.10	−1.0
20.0	20/400	6/120	3	90	0.05	−1.3

this chart, the near vision is recorded as N5, N6, N8, N10, N12, N18, N36 and N48.

3. Snellen's near vision test types. Snellen introduced the so-called 'Snellen's equivalent for near vision' on the same principles as his distant types. The graded thickness of the letters of different lines is about 1/17th of the distant vision chart letters. In this event, the letters equivalent to 6/6 line subtend an angle of 5 minutes at an average reading distance (35 cm/ 14 inch).

The unusual configuration of letters of this chart, however, cannot be constructed from the available printers' fonts. It can only be reproduced by a photographic reduction of the standard Snellen's distant vision test types to approximately 1/17th of their normal size. Further, such a test has never become popular. The graded sizes of pleasing types of passages from literature, the reading of which helps in the interpretation, are habitually employed.

4. Lea near vision cards. This test assesses a child's functional vision at near distances. It can also be used to familiarize child with testing procedure before introducing a distance test. It consists of cards measuring 8" × 10" (20.3 × 25.4 cm) which contain proportionally spaced (logMAR) lines on one side and more tightly-spaced symbols on the opposite side. Line sizes range from 20/400 to 20/10 (6/120 to 6/3) equivalent, 0.05 to 2.00. Response key is printed on test card. Testing distance is about 16 inches/ 40 cm.

Procedure of testing

For testing the near vision, the patient is seated in a chair and asked to read the near vision chart kept at a distance of 25–35 cm, with a good illumination thrown over his or her left shoulder. Each eye should be tested separately. The near vision is recorded as the smallest type that can be read comfortably by the patient. A note of the approximate distance at which the near vision chart is held should also be made. Thus near vision (NV) is recorded as:

• NV 5 J_1 at 30 cm (in Jaeger's notation)
• NV 5 N_5 at 30 cm (in Faculty's notation)

N 36	tiger	
N 18	decade employ	
N 12	heater endear abide	theft defect
N 10	heaven prank carrier	mirror party switch
N 8	noble vision chief	receive hinder elusive
N 6	throw supreme worthy	porter table symbol

Fig. 2.19: *Near vision chart.*

Near vision equivalents in different notations

These are shown in Table 2.5.

CONTRAST SENSITIVITY

INTRODUCTION

Contrast sensitivity is the ability to perceive slight changes in luminance between regions that are not separated by definite borders and is just as important as the ability to perceive sharp outlines of relatively small objects. It is only the latter ability that is tested by means of the Snellen's test types. In many diseases, loss of contrast sensitivity is more important and disturbing for the patient than is the loss of visual acuity. Further, contrast sensitivity may be impaired even in the presence of normal visual acuity.

TYPES OF CONTRAST SENSITIVITY

1. Spatial contrast sensitivity

Spatial contrast sensitivity refers to detection of striped patterns at various levels of contrast and spatial frequencies. In its measurement, patient is presented with sine wave gratings of parallel light and dark bands (Arden gratings) and is asked to tell the minimum contrast at which the bars can be seen at each frequency. The width of the bars is defined as spatial frequency which expresses the number of pairs of dark and light bars subtending an angle of 18 at the eye. A high spatial frequency implies narrow bars, whereas a low spatial frequency indicates wide bars.

Table 2.5 *Equivalent visual acuity notations for near*								
Visual angle (minutes)	*Snellen equivalent*	*American Medical Association notation*	*Decimal notation*	*Jaeger notation*	*Faculty's Roman test types notation*	*Metre notation (m)*	*Central visual efficiency for near (%)*	*Vision loss (%)*
5.00	20/20	14/14	1.00	J1	N5	0.37	100	0
6.25	20/25	14/17	0.80	J1	N6	0.43	100	0
7.50	20/30	14/21	0.66	J2	N8	0.50	95	5
10.00	20/40	14/28	0.50	J4	N10	0.75	90	10
12.50	20/50	14/35	0.40	J6	N12	0.87	50	50
15.00	20/60	14/42	0.33	J8	N14	1.00	40	60
20.00	20/80	14/56	0.25	J10	N18	1.50	20	80
25.00	20/100	14/70	0.20	J1	N24	1.75	15	85
50.00	20/200	14/140	0.10	J17	N36	3.50	2	98

2. Temporal contrast sensitivity

Here the contrast sensitivity function is generated for time-related (temporal) processing in the visual system by presenting a uniform target field modulated sinusoidal in time, rather than as a function of spatial position.

Both temporal and spatial contrast sensitivity testing yield significantly more complete and systematic data on the status of visual performance than the conventional tests.

▇ MEASUREMENT OF CONTRAST SENSITIVITY

When a subject is presented with the grating frequencies and contrast below which resolution is impossible, it indicates the threshold level; and the reciprocal of this contrast threshold gives the contrast sensitivity.

Contrast sensitivity is measured as $(L_{max}$ 2 $L_{min})/(L_{max}$ 1 $L_{min})$, where L is the luminance recorded by photocells scanning across the gratings.

VARIABLES IN THE MEASUREMENT

There are three variables in the measurement of contrast sensitivity:

1. *Average amount of light reflected* depends on illumination of paper and darkness of ink.
2. *Degree of blackness* in relation to the white background, i.e. contrast.
3. *Distance between the grating periods* or cycles per degree of visual angle.

METHODS OF MEASUREMENT

Various methods have been developed to measure contrast sensitivity. Bodis-Wollner, introducing contrast sensitivity measurement in clinical practice, suggested the name *visuogram*, analogue to an *audiogram*, to describe a patient's 'contrast sensitivity curve'. The deficits were expressed in terms of decibels, and three types of deficits were described:

1. *High-frequency type* characterized by increasing loss at high frequency.
2. *A level-loss type* characterized by a similar loss for all spatial frequencies.
3. *A selective-loss type* characterized by deficits of spatial frequencies in a narrow band.

In general, the methods recommended to measure contrast sensitivity include: simple plates, cathode ray tube display on a screen, letter acuity charts, laser interferometer (LI) which produces grating on the retina, visual field testing using low contrast rings on stimuli, pattern discrimination test, prototype for forced choice printed test, visually evoked cortical potentials to checkerboard pattern reversal dependent contrast threshold measurement, two-alternative forced choice test and many more.

Some of the simple, inexpensive but reliable methods of measuring contrast sensitivity are described in brief in the following text.

1. Arden gratings. Arden, in 1978, introduced a booklet containing seven plates: one *screening plate* (No. 1) and six *diagnostic plates* (No. 2–7). The contrast changes from top to bottom and covers a range of approximately 1.76 log units. The plates are studied at 57 cm, with spatial frequency increasing from 0.2 cycles/degree to 6.4 cycles/degree, each being double the frequency of the previous one. A score of 1–20 is assigned to each plate, depending upon the amount of plate uncovered. Sum of six plates with an upper limit of 82 was established for normal subjects together with an interocular difference of less than 12.

2. Cambridge low-contrast gratings. Cambridge low-contrast gratings consist of a *set of ten plates* containing gratings in a spiral bound booklet. To perform the test, the booklet is hung on a wall at a distance of 6 m. The pages are presented in pairs, one above the other. One page in each pair contains gratings and the other is blank (Fig. 2.20), but the pages have the same mean reflectance. The subject is simply required to choose which page, top or bottom, contains the gratings. The pages are shown in order of descending contrast and are stopped when the first error is made. Four descending series are shown separately to each eye. When no error is made at plate 10, then a score of 11 is given. Depending upon the total score of the patient from four series, the contrast sensitivity is noted from the conversion table (Fig. 2.21).

two triplets in each line (Fig. 2.22A). The contrast decreases from one triplet to the next. The log contrast sensitivity varies from 0.00 to 2.25.

To perform the test, the chart is hung on the wall, so that its centre is approximately at the level of the subject's eye. The chart is illuminated as uniformly as possible, so that the luminance of the white areas is between the acceptable range of 60 and 120 cd/m, which corresponds

Fig. 2.20: *Cambridge low-contrast gratings.*

Fig. 2.21: *Cambridge low-contrast gratings score sheet and conversion table.*

3. Pelli-Robson contrast sensitivity chart. This chart consists of letters that subtend an angle of 38 at a distance of 1 m. The chart is printed on both the sides. The two sides have different letter sequence but are otherwise identical. The letters on chart are organized as triplets, there being

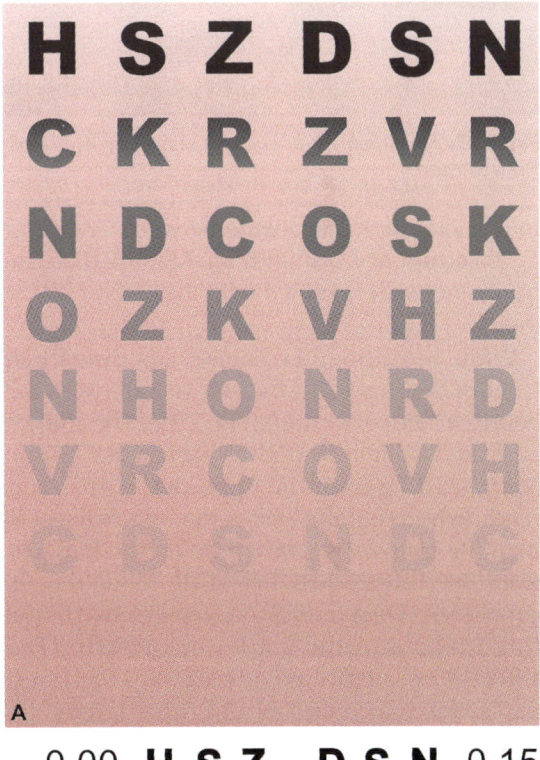

Fig. 2.22: *Pelli-Robson contrast sensitivity chart. (A) Photograph; (B) Log contrast sensitivity score of each triplet.*

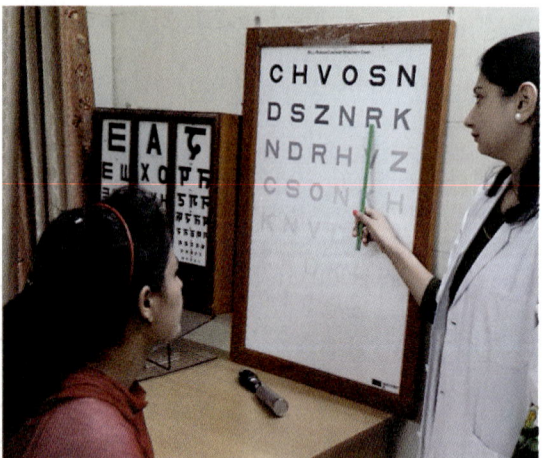

Fig. 2.23: *Measurement of contrast sensitivity with Pelli-Robson chart.*

to a photographic exposure between 1/15 and 1/30 second at f/5.6 with an ASA of 100. The luminance is determined with the help of a light meter.

While recording, the subject sits directly in front of the chart at a distance of 1 m (with the best distance correction) (Fig. 2.23). The subject is made to name or outline each letter on the chart, starting from the upper left corner and reading horizontally across the line. Subject is made to guess, even when he or she believes that the letters are invisible. The test is concluded when the subject guesses two of the three letters of the triplet incorrectly. The subject's sensitivity is indicated by the finest triplet for which two of the three letters are named correctly.

4. The Vistech chart. This chart consists of sine wave gratings and is used at a distance of 3 m from the subject. In this test, contrast is assessed at several spatial frequencies (distance of the separation of the grating bars) and the subject has to identify the orientation of the grating, i.e. whether vertical or 158 clockwise, or anticlockwise.

5. Vector vision chart. Vector vision CSV 1000 (USA) chart test frequency of 3,6,12 and 18 cpd.

6. Fact CS chart. The fact CS chart tests for 1.5, 3, 6, 12 and 18 cpd.

TESTS FOR COLOUR VISION

It is useful to group these tests into several different categories based on design. Pseudoisochromatic plates, arrangement tests, anomaloscopes, and lanterns represent the most widely used designs. Different tests are appropriate for different circumstances (Table 2.6).

PLATE TESTS

J. Stilling first introduced pseudoisochromatic designs in 1873. Today, they are the most commonly used screening tests for colour deficiency in clinical practice. These tests are inexpensive, durable, and readily available. Most tests provide very efficient (90–95%) screening of congenital red-green defects. On the other hand, the tests have distinct limitations. They must be administered under the standard viewing conditions for which they were designed. They are not effective in grading the severity of the colour defect and thus tell us limited information about the extent or type of deficiency. In short, plate tests are best used as screening tools.

Plate tests come in several forms; however, the principle of construction is the same. Ishihara test is the prototype of this category. The test consists of a series of cards on which a figure is printed in multiple colours against a multicoloured back-

Table 2.6 *Categories of colour vision tests*		
Test type	*Function*	*Example*
Screening tests	Quick diagnosis	Pseudoisochromatic plates, e.g. Ishihara test
Grading tests	Assess severity of the defect	FM 100-hue test
Diagnostic tests	Precisely classify a defect	Anomaloscope
Vocational tests	Simulate environment encountered on the job	Lantern test

ground (Fig. 2.24). The figure is recognizable to normal trichromats, but camouaged to those with colour defects. The figure used in the test is usually an easily identifiable number, letter, or shape. Figures and background are drawn in dots. The size of the dots used in plate design can be varied or uniform; however, the only difference between the figure and the background is the colour. Saturation and lightness are accounted for, such that detection of the figure in ways other than hue is unlikely.

Ishihara test

The Ishihara test is published in a full 38-plate edition, an abridged 24-plate edition and a 14-plate edition for quick screening. Scoring instructions for the Ishihara plates accompany each test. In the 38-plate edition, for example, a normal score permits four or fewer errors. In the 24-plate edition, two errors or less are considered normal. The 16-plate edition also puts two errors or less in the normal range. It does not matter which edition is used because the fail criterion is three or five errors and total number of errors has no diagnostic significance. The Ishihara can be used in children as young as 5 years. The colour differences between the figure and the background are chosen to separate normal trichromats from mild anomalous trichromats. If the differences in colour are too large, anomalous trichromats will be able to identify

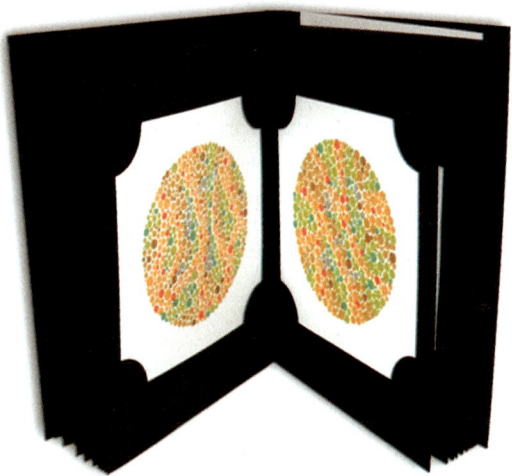

Fig. 2.24: *Ishihara's pseudoisochromatic plates.*

the hidden figure. Small differences may cause normal trichromats to fail some screening plates.

How to test colour vision by Ishihara chart

- Room should be adequately lit by daylight.
- Nature of the test should be explained to the patient.
- Full refractive correction is worn.
- It is preferable to do the test before pupillary dilatation.
- One eye is first occluded and the other eye is tested.
- The plates are kept at a distance of 75 cm from the subject with the plane of the paper at right angle to the line of vision.
- The standard time taken to answer each plate is 3–5 seconds.

Interpretation of Ishihara chart test

Interpretation of Ishihara chart, consisting of 25 plates, is summarised in Table 2.7.

ARRANGEMENT TESTS

Modern arrangement tests were first put into popular use in the 1940s and 1950s by Dean Farnsworth. Farnsworth originally designed the Farnsworth-Munsell 100-hue test (FM 100-hue test) and the Farnsworth Dichotomous test for colour blindness (Farnsworth Panel D-15). The principle of design for these tests is coloured caps of fixed chroma and value selected from the hue circle. The patient is asked to arrange randomly placed caps in what he/she perceives to be a natural order. The colour differences between adjacent caps on the FM 100-hue test were designed to be very small. Good colour vision as well as chromatic discrimination ability is needed to perform well on this test. Farnsworth Panel D-15 was designed to have larger colour differences, but, unlike the FM 100-hue test, only one box containing 15 caps is presented to the patient.

ANOMALOSCOPES

An anomaloscope is an instrument that uses the principle of colour matching to test colour vision. It serves as a clinical standard for

Table 2.7 *Intepertation of Ishihara chart test*

Plate number	Normal	Points with redgreen defects		Inference
1	12	12		Both subjects with normal and defective colour vision read plate 1 as 12.
2	8	3		
3	6	5		
4	29	17		Subjects with red-green defects read these plates as those in abnormal column. Totally colour blind are unable to read.
5	57	35		
6	5	2		
7	3	5		
8	15	17		Majority of subjects with colour vision deficiency read these plates incorrectly
9	74	21		
10	2	X		
11	6	X		Subjects with normal colour vision do not see any number. Those with redgreen deficiency read the numbers given in the abnnormal column
12	97	X		
13	45	X		
14	5	X		
15	7	X		Subjects with protanopia read these plates as given in abnormal column (1), those with deutranomaly read them as given in column (2).
16	16	X		
17	73	X		
18	X	5		
19	X	2		
20	X	45		
21	X	73		
		Protan	Deutran	
22	26	6	2	
23	42	2	4	
24	35	5	3	
25	96	6	9	

diagnosing and classifying congenital colour deficiency. The use and maintenance of an anomaloscope can be challenging and requires the expertise of a trained technician. For this reason, anomaloscopes are not used as frequently as other clinical tests.

The Nagel (model I) anomaloscope is the most common and accurate of these and uses the Rayleigh equation to diagnose red-green colour vision defects. The subject views a circular field through a telescopic barrel. This field is divided into two parts, each of which is filled with light of different spectral wavelengths. The lower half of the field is filled with spectral yellow at 589 nm. According to the Rayleigh match, the subject should be able to match the 'colour' of the upper to the lower field by adjusting the mixture of red and green light. The luminance

knob is particularly useful in distinguishing deutan from protan defects. The subject is asked to comment on whether the upper and lower fields are the same colour. Normal and dichromatic individuals will accept this as a normal or near-normal match. Deuteranomalous trichromats will state that the upper field is too red and protanomalous trichromats will state that the upper field is too green. Scoring of an anomaloscope examination begins by recording the values at which a match was made.

LANTERN TESTS

Lantern tests are simple devices geared towards measuring a subject's competency to perform a specific task, namely recognize coloured light signals. Lanterns are used in the maritime, air, and railway industries to screen employees. The subject is asked to name the colours of the light signals that are presented to him. Two types of lanterns exist: those that present single colours and those that present pairs of lights together. The speed and sequence of colour presentation is important to the efficacy of the test. Individuals with defective colour vision make characteristic mistakes in naming the colours presented to them; how ever, most lantern tests are not meant to screen or categorize colour defectives for clinical purposes.

BIBLIOGRAPHY

1. Alpern M. Accommodation. In Davson H (Ed): The Eye, Vol 3. Muscular Mechanisms. New York, Academic Press, 1962, pp 191–229.
2. Arden GB, Jacobson JJ. A simple grating test for contrast sensitivity. Preliminary results indicate value in screening for glaucoma. Invest Ophthalmol Visual Sci 1978;17:23–32.
3. Arden GB. Testing contrast sensitivity in clinical practice. Clin Vis Sci 1988;2(3):213–24.
4. Arden GB. Visual loss in patients with normal visual acuity. Trans Ophthalmol Soc UK 1978; 98:219–23.
5. Arundale K. An investigation into variation of contrast sensitivity with age and ocular patho- logy. Br J Ophthalmol 1978;62:213–5.
6. Bahrick HP, Bahrick PO, Wittlinger RP. Fifty years of memory for names and faces: a cross- sectional approach. J Exp Psychol Gen 1975;104: 54–75.
7. Barlett NR. Thresholds as dependent on some energy relations and characteristics of the subject. In: Graham CH(ed). Vision and Visual Perception. New York, Wiley, 1965, pp 154–84.
8. Berlyne DE. The influence of the albedo and complexity of stimuli on visual functions in the human infant. Bt J Psychol 1958;49–315.
9. Bodis Wollner L. Visual acuity and contrast sensitivity in patients with cerebral lesions. Science 1972;178:769–71.
10. Brown JL, Black JE. Critical duration for resolution of acuity targets. Vision Res 1976;16: 309–15.
11. Brown JL, Mueller CG. Brightness discrimina- tion and brightness contrast. In: Graham CH (Ed). Vision and Visual Perception. Wiley, New York, 1965, pp 208–50.
12. Butler T, Westheimer G. Interference with stereo- scopic acuity: spatial, temporal and disparity tuning, Vision Res 1978;18:1387.
13. Campbell FW, Green DG. Optical and retinal factors affecting visual acuity. J Physiol 1965; 181:576–93.
14. Campbell FW, Robson JG. Application of Fourier analysis to the visibility of gratings. J Physiol 1968;197:551–6.
15. Dala Sala S, Bertoni G, Somazzi L. Impaired contrast sensitivity in diabetic patients with and without retinopathy. A new technique for rapid assessment. Br J Ophthalmol 1985;69: 136–42.
16. Ditchburn RW, Ginsborg BL. Vision with a stabilised retinal image, Nature 1952;170:36–37.
17. Dobson V, Teller D. Visual acuity in human infants: a review and comparison of behavioral and electro-physiological sutdies, Vision Res 1978;18:1469.
18. Dobson V, Teller D, Lee CP, Wade B. A behavio- ral method for efficient screening of visual acuity in young infants. I. Preliminary laboratory development. Invest. Ophthalmol Vis Sci 1978; 17:1142.
19. Drum B, et al. Pattern discrimination perimetry. A new concept in visual field testing. Doc Ophthalmol Proc Ser 1987;49:433.
20. Emsley HH. Irregular astigmatism of the eye. Effect of correcting lenses, Trans Opt Soc Lond 1925;27:28.
21. Fantz R. Pattern vision in young infants, Psychol, Rec 1958;8:43.
22. Flom MC, Weymouth FW, Kahneman D. Visual resolution and contour interaction. J Opt Soc Am 1963;53:1026.
23. Hartridge H. The visual perception of fine detail. Philos Trans R Soc Lond (Biol Sci) 1947;232; 519–671.
24. Hecht S, Mintz EV. The visibility of single lines at various illuminations and the retinal basis of visual resolution. J Gen Physiol 1939;22: 593–612.
25. Hecht S, Ross S, Mueller CG. The visibility of lines and squares at high brightnesses. J Opt Soc Am 1947;37:500–7.
26. Hecht S. Vision. II. The nature of the photo- receptor process. In: Murchison C (Ed). A Hand- book of General Experimental Psychology, Worcester MA, Clark University Press, 1934; 704–828.
27. Howe JW, Mitchell KW, Mahabateswara M, Abdel-Katek MN. Visual evoked potential

latency and contrast sensitivity in patients with posterior chamber intraocular lens implants, Br J Ophthalmol 1986;70:890–4.

28. Hoyt CS, Nickel BL, Billson FA. Ophthalmological examination of the infant: developmental aspect, Surv Ophthalmol 1982;26:177.

29. L Schade O. Optical and photoelectric analogue of eye. J Opt Soc Am 1956;46:721–39.

30. Leibowitz H: The effect of pupil size on visual acuity for photometrically equated test fields at various levels of luminance, J Opt Soc Am 1952; 42:416.

31. Lempert P, Hopcroft M, Lempert Y. Evaluation of posterior subcapsular cataracts with spatial contrast acuity. Ophthalmology 1987;94(S): 14–8.

32. Lythgoe RJ. The measurement of visual acuity. Med Res Council Sp Rep Ser, No. 173, 1932.

33. Marg E, Freeman DN, Peltzman P, Goldstein P. Visual acuity development in human infants: evoked potential measurements. Invest. Ophthalmol 1976;15:150.

34. Mayer L, Fulton A, Rodier D. Grating and recognition acuities of pediatric patients, Ophthalmology 1984;91:947.

35. Pelli DG, Robson JG, Wilkin AJ. The design of a new letter chart for measuring contrast sensitivity. Clin Vis Sci 1988;2(3):187–99.

36. Pirenne MH, Marriott FHC, O'Doherty EF. Individual differences in night-vision efficiency. Med Res Council Sp Rep Ser, No 294, 1957.

37. Regan D, Neima D. Low contrast letter charts as a test of visual function. Ophthalmology 1983;90:1192.

38. Riggs LA, Ratliff F, Cornsweet JC, Cornsweet EF. The disappearance of steadily fixated visual test objects. F. opt. Soc. Amer. 1953;43,495–501.

39. Riggs LA. Visual acuity. In Graham CH (Ed). Vision and Visual Perception. New York, Wiley, 1965, pp 321–49.

40. Rodieck RW. The Vertebrate Retina. San Francisco, WH Freeman and Co, 1973.

41. Shlaer S. The relation between visual acuity and illumination. J Gen Physiol 21:165–88, 1937.

42. Skalka WH. Effect of age on Arden grating acuity. Br J Ophthalmol 1980;84:21–3.

43. Sokol S. Measurement of infant visual acuity from pattern reversal evoked potentials, Vision Res. 1978;18:33.

44. Teller DY, Movshon JA. Visual development, Vision Res. 1986;26:1483.

45. Teller DY. The forced choice preferential looking procedure. A psychophysical technique for use with human infants, infant Behav Dev 1979; 2:135.

46. Tomlinson E, Martinez D. The measurement of visual acuity: comparison of Teller acuity cards with Snellen and MBL results, Am. Orthopt. J. 1988;38:130.

47. Vaegan F, Halliday BL. A forced choice test improves clinical contrast sensitivity testing. Br J Ophthalmol 1982;66:477–91.

48. Weale RA. The Aging Eye. London, Leis, 1963.

49. Westheimer G, Hauske G. Temporal and spatial interference with vernier acuity, Vision Res. 1975;15:1137.

50. Westheimer G, McKee SP. Visual acuity in the presence of retinal-image motion, J Opt Soc Am 65:847, 1975.

51. Wilcox WW, Purdy DM. Visual acuity and its physiological basis. Br J Psychol 1933;23: 233–61.

52. Wilkins AJ, Delia SS, Somazzi L, Smith N. Age related norms for the Cambridge low contrast gratings, including details concerning their design and use. Clin Vision Sci 1988;2(3): 201–12.

53. Wolf E, Gardiner JS. Studies on the scatter of light in the dioptic media of the eye as a basis of visual glare. Arch Ophthalmol 1965;74: 338–45.

54. Woodson WE. Human Engineering Guide for Equipment Designs. Los Angeles, University of California Press, 1954.

55. Wulfing EA. Uber den Kleinsten Gesichts-winkel. Z Biol 1892;29:199.

56. Yamazaki H, Adachi-Usami E, Chiba J. Contrast thresholds of diabetic patients determined by VECP and psychophysical measurements. Acta Ophthalmol 1982;60:386–92.

Slit-lamp Biomicroscopy

Chapter Outline

INTRODUCTION
- Historical landmarks

PARTS OF SLIT-LAMP
- Observation system
- Illumination system
- Mechanical support system

TECHNIQUE OF BIOMICROSCOPY

Slit-lamp biomicroscopy routine

Methods of illumination
- Diffuse illumination

- Direct focal illumination
- Indirect illumination
- Retroillumination
- Specular reflection
- Sclerotic scatter
- Oscillating illumination of Koeppe

ACCESSORY DEVICES
- For specialized examinations

HAND-HELD SLIT-LAMP
- Uses

INTRODUCTION

Slit-lamp is the most important piece of equipment in the present day ophthalmologist's armamentarium. Modern slit-lamp with its auxiliary devices not only provides magnified views of every part of the eye from cornea to retina, but also allows quantitative measurements (intraocular pressure, endothelial cell counts, pupil size, corneal thickness, anterior chamber depth, etc.) and photography of every part for documentation.

The term slit-lamp is basically a misnomer, since slit is only one of the various other diaphragmatic openings present in the instrument. Therefore, Mawas in 1925 introduced the term *biomicroscopy* and defined it as examination of the living eye by means of a corneal microscope and a slit-lamp.

HISTORICAL LANDMARKS IN THE DEVELOPMENT AND EVOLUTION OF SLIT-LAMP

These can be summarized as:

- *Purkinje,* in 1823, attempted to develop a type of slit-lamp by using one hand-held lamp to magnify an another hand-held lens to focus strong oblique illumination. However, it was not until almost 100 years later that a version of the slit-lamp appeared that is recognizable today.

- *De Wecker,* in 1863, devised a portable *ophthalmomicroscope* that combined a small monocular microscope which rested against the face of the patient with an attached condenser lens. It lacked stereoscopic view.

- *Albert* and *Grœnough,* in 1891, developed a binocular microscope which provided stereoscopic view.

- *Czapski*, in 1897, modified the binocular corneal microscope, which is still found in many modern slit-lamps.
- *Gullstrand*, in 1911, introduced the illumination system which had for the first time a slit-diaphragm in it. Therefore, Gullstrand is credited with the invention of the slit-lamp.
- *Henker*, in 1916, developed the prototype of the modern biomicroscopy by combining the Gullstrand's slit-illumination system with the Czapski's binocular corneal microscope.
- *Hans Goldmann*, in 1933, improvised the biomicroscope in which all the vertical and horizontal adjustments for both the lamp and the slit-beam were placed on a single mechanical stage. The slit-lamp designed by Goldman was marketed in 1937 as the *Haag–Streit model 360 slit-lamp*.
- *Littmann*, in 1950, introduced the new optical principle for the biomicroscope. He incorporated the rotatory magnification changer based on the principle of Galilean telescope. The slit-lamp designed by Littmann is the forerunner of the current Zeiss slit-lamp series.
- *Modern slit-lamps* have achieved a very high degree of refinement.

PARTS OF A SLIT-LAMP

A slit-lamp (Fig. 3.1) is composed of three basic parts:
1. Observation system (microscope)
2. Illumination system
3. Mechanical support system

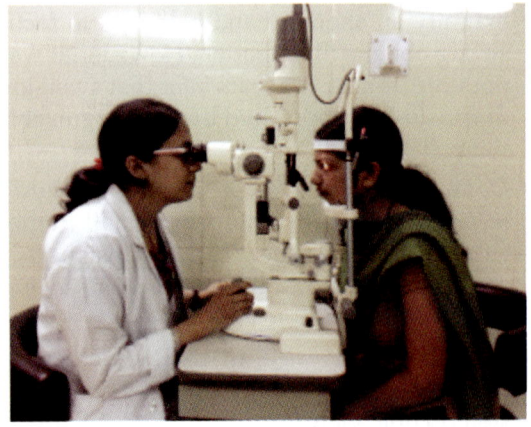

Fig. 3.1: *A slit-lamp.*

1. OBSERVATION SYSTEM (MICROSCOPE)

The observation system (Fig. 3.2) is essentially a compound microscope which is composed of two optical elements, an objective and an eyepiece. It presents to the observer an enlarged image of a near object. The slit-lamp microscope is designed to have a long working distance, i.e. the distance between the microscope's objective and the patient's eye.

- Objective lens consists of two planoconvex lenses with their convexities put together, providing a composite power of 122 D.
- Eyepiece has a lens of 110 D. To provide a good stereopsis, the tubes are converged at an angle of 10–15°.
- Prisms. To overcome the problem of inverted image produced by the compound

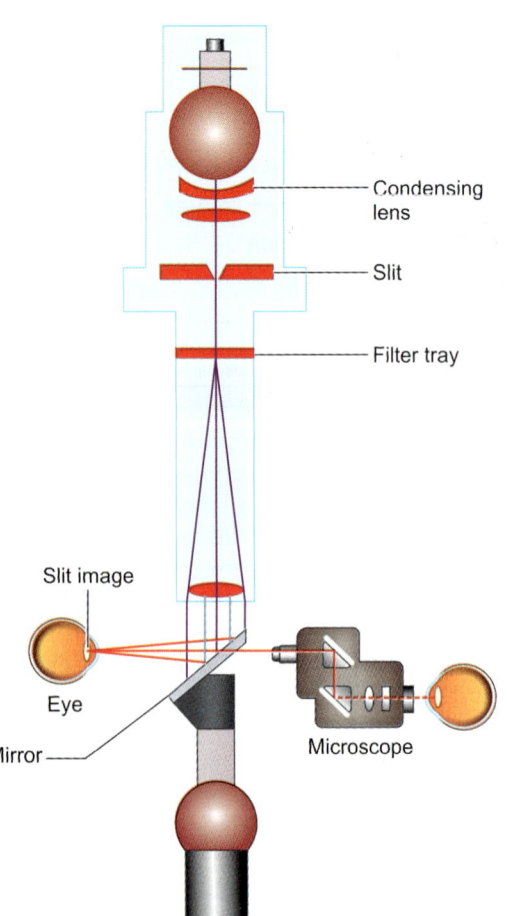

Fig. 3.2: *A cross-section of the observation system of a modern slit-lamp.*

microscope, slit-lamp microscope uses a pair of prisms between the objective and the eyepiece to reinvert the image (Fig. 3.2).

Magnification systems

Most slit-lamps provide a range of magnification from 6 to 40X. The modern slit-lamps use one of the following three systems to produce a range of magnification.

i. *Czapskiscope with rotating objectives.* This is one of the oldest and possibly still the most frequently used techniques for obtaining different magnifications. The different objectives are usually placed on a turret type of arrangement that allows them to be fairly rapidly changed during the examination.

The Haag–Streit model, the Bausch and Lomb and the Thorpe are the examples of the slit-lamps using this system.

ii. *The Littmann–Galilean telescope principle.* The Galilean magnification changer (G), as developed by Littmann (1950), is a completely separate optical system that sits neatly between the objective and eyepiece lenses and does not require either of them to change. It provides a large range of magnifications, typically five, via a turret arrangement which is completely enclosed within the microscope's body. It is called a Galilean system because it utilizes the Galilean telescopes to alter the magnification. Galilean telescopes have two optical components, a positive lens and a negative lens. It fits within the standard slit-lamp microscope along with a relay lens (R) and the prism erector (P) in the manner shown in Fig. 3.3.

The Zeiss, the Rodenstock and the American optical slit-lamps are the examples of slit-lamps using the Littmann–Galilean telescopic system.

iii. *Zoom system.* Some slit-lamps (e.g. Nikon photo slit-lamp and Zeiss-75 SL) have been produced with zoom system that allows a continuously variable degree of magnification. The Nikon slit-lamp contains the zoom system within the objective of the microscope and offers a range of magnification from 7 to 35X.

2. ILLUMINATION SYSTEM

The Gullstrand's illumination system is designed to provide a bright, evenly illuminated, finely focused adjustable slit of light at the eye. It comprises following components (Fig. 3.4):

i. *Light source.* Originally a Nernst lamp was used as a light source which was followed by Nitra lamp, arc lamp, mercury vapour lamp and finally halogen lamps. It provides an illumination of 2×10^5 to 4×10^5 lux.

ii. *Condenser lens system.* It consists of a couple of planoconvex lenses with their convex surfaces in apposition.

iii. *Slit and other diaphragms.* The height and width of the slit can be varied using two knobs provided for this purpose. In addition, there are some stenopaeic slits of 2.0 and 0.5 mm to provide conical beam of light.

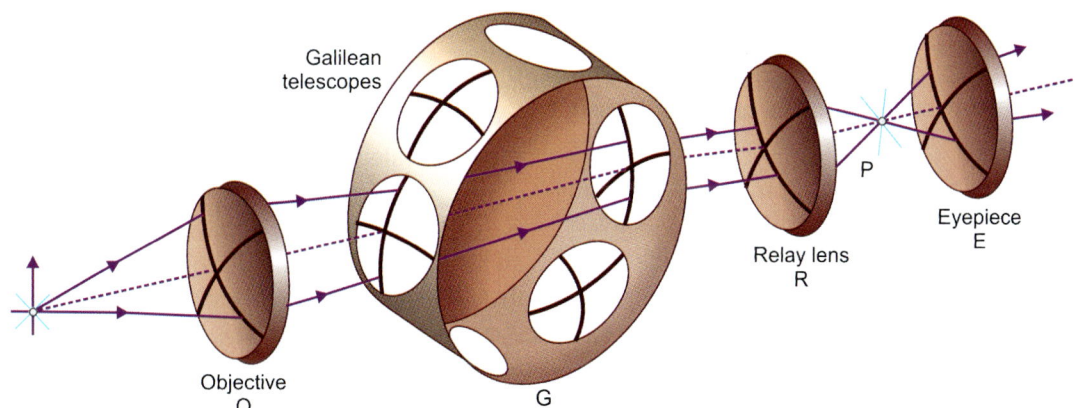

Fig. 3.3: *Galilean magnification changer (G) is placed between the slit-lamp objective (O) and the relay lens (R) which focuses the light through a prism erector (P) into the eyepiece (E).*

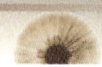

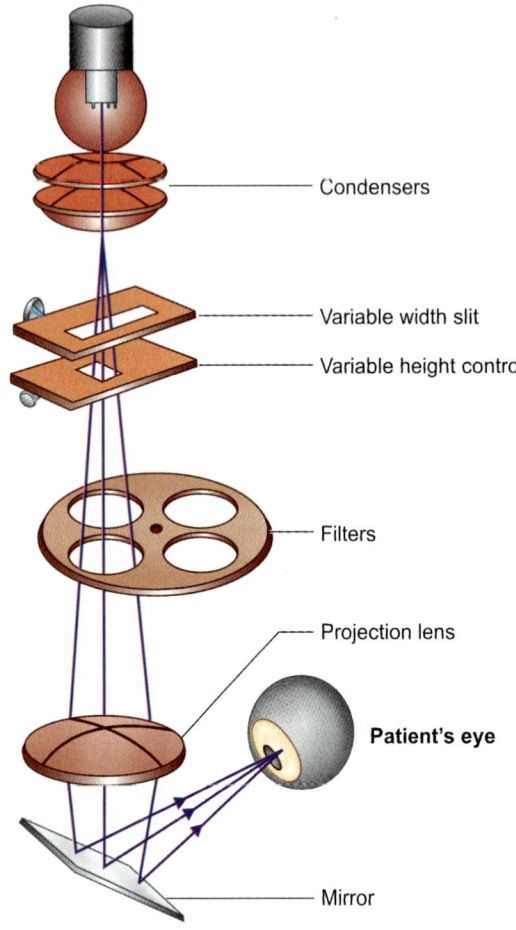

- Condensers

- Variable width slit
- Variable height control

- Filters

- Projection lens

Patient's eye

- Mirror

Fig. 3.4: *Typical slit-lamp illumination system.*

There is a facility to rotate the slit away from the vertical meridian and also the ability to tilt the projection system about a horizontal axis that is provided. These two additional degrees of freedom are included to assist in the examination of the fundus and the angle of anterior chamber.

iv. Filters. Different filters can be inserted into the illumination beam. Cobalt blue and red-free filters are provided in most of the models.

v. Projection lens. It forms an image of the slit at the eye. The diameter of the projection lens is usually fairly small. This has two advantages: first, it keeps the aberrations of the lens down, which results in a better quality image; second, it increases the depth of focus of the slit and

thereby produces a better optical section of the eye.

vi. Reflecting mirror or prism. It forms the last component of the illumination system. The illumination system of a slit-lamp has to be able to pass relatively easily from one side of the microscope to the other. To allow this, the projection system is normally arranged along a vertical axis, with either a *mirror* or *prism* finally reflecting the light along a horizontal axis. The use of a narrow prism or mirror means that when necessary, such as in examination of the fundus, the illumination axis can be made to, without obstructing the field of view, almost coincide with the viewing axis.

Optics of the illumination system

The Koeller illumination system has been adopted in slit-lamps. Optically, it is identical to that of a 35 mm slide projection with the exception that a variable aperture slit takes the place of the slit and the projection lens has a much shorter focal length. In the Koeller illumination system, as shown in Fig. 3.4, the filament of the light source is imaged by the condenser lenses at or close to the projection lens which in turn forms the image of the slit in the patient's eye.

3. MECHANICAL SUPPORT SYSTEM

Although mechanical support system is least glamorous, a brief review of the instrument's history reveals that the optical principles upon which the modern slit-lamp is based have changed little over the years, whereas the ease of examination, characteristics of all modern slit-lamps, is due to the indigenous mechanical design.

Salient features of most of the mechanical support systems are as follows:

i. Joystick arrangement. Movement of the microscope and illumination system towards or away from the eye and from side to side is usually achieved via a joystick arrangement.

ii. Up and down movement arrangement. The up and down movement is obtained via some sort of screw device that moves the whole illumination and viewing system up and down relative to the chin rest.

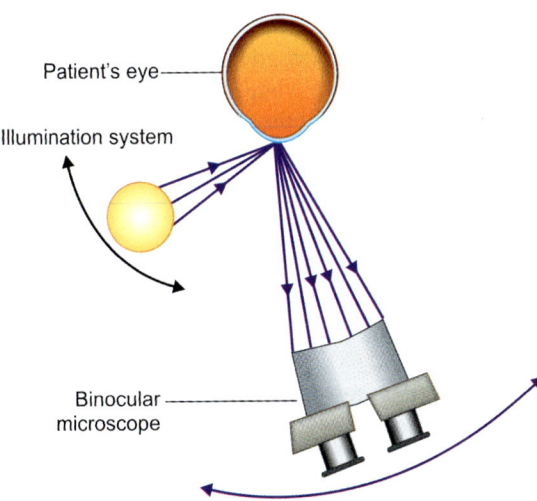

Patient's eye

Illumination system

Binocular microscope

Fig. 3.5: *Mechanical coupling of the microscope and illumination system allows their focusing on the same point.*

iii. *Patient support arrangement.* A vertically movable chin rest and the provision to adjust the height of the table has been made to accommodate the persons of all sizes.

iv. *Fixation target.* A movable fixation target greatly facilitates the examination under some conditions.

v. *Mechanical coupling.* The mechanical system not only provides a support but also a coupling of the microscope and the illumination system along a common axis of rotation that coincides their focal planes. This arrangement ensures that light falls on the point where microscope is focused. It allows either the microscope or the illumination system to be rotated around this axis without changing the focus (Fig. 3.5).

The coupling of the microscope and illumination system in this way has advantages when using the slit-lamp for routine examination of the anterior segment of the eye. However, when certain accessories, such as gonioscope or the three-mirror fundus lens, are used, this can be a disadvantage, since the slit and the microscope optics frequently do not reach a common focal point under those conditions, leaving the observer with the choice of suffering under suboptimal images or refocusing the eyepieces.

TECHNIQUE OF BIOMICROSCOPY

SLIT-LAMP BIOMICROSCOPY ROUTINE

While performing slit-lamp biomicroscopy, following routine may be adopted:

1. *Patient adjustment.* The patient should be positioned comfortably in front of the slit-lamp with his or her chin resting on the chin rest and forehead opposed to head rest (*see* Fig. 3.1).

2. *Instrument adjustment.* The height of the table housing the slit-lamp should be adjusted according to patient's height. The microscope and illumination system should be aligned with the patient's eye to be examined. Fixation target should be placed at the required position.

3. *Beginning slit-lamp examination.* Some points to be kept in mind are:

 i. Examination should be carried out in semidark room so that the examiner's eyes are partially dark-adapted to ensure sensitivity to low intensities of light.

 ii. Diffuse illumination should be used for as short a time as necessary.

 iii. There should be a minimum exposure of retina to light.

 iv. Medications like ointments and anaesthetic eyedrops produce corneal surface disturbances which can be mistaken for pathology.

 v. Low magnification should be first used to locate the pathology and higher magnification should then be used to examine it.

METHODS OF ILLUMINATION

Berliner described seven basic methods of illumination using the slit-lamp. A few guidelines for the set-up for each method of illumination are described briefly.

1. Diffuse illumination (Fig. 3.6)

The *set-up* is as given:

• Angle between microscope and illumination system should be 30–45°.

• Slit width should be widest.

• Filter to be used is diffusing filter.

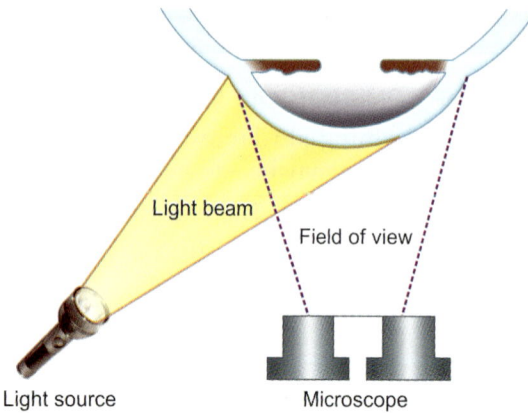

Fig. 3.6: *Set-up for diffuse illumination.*

- Magnification used is low to medium.
- Illumination should be medium to high.

Diffuse illumination is used for:
- General view of the anterior eye and the palpebral conjunctiva
- Contact lens fitting

2. Direct focal illumination. In this technique, the slit-beam is regulated until it coincides with the exact focus of the microscope (Fig. 3.7). Light is directed as a narrow slit at an oblique angle (30–45°). Heterogenous tissues like cornea and lens disperse light and become visible as bright objects against a dark background.

The direct illumination examination is carried out utilizing three slit-beam effects on the transparent structures of the eye, i.e. optical section, parallelopiped and a conical beam effect.

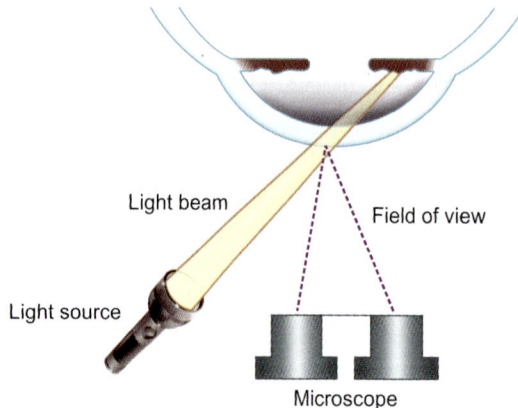

Fig. 3.7: *Set for direct illumination.*

i. *Optical section* (Fig. 3.8) is produced by a very narrow slit-beam focused obliquely. The optical section produced resembles a knife-like histological section of the tissue focused (cornea, lens and anterior part of vitreous). The whole tissue can be examined by moving the slit-beam and simultaneous focus of the microscope across the surface.

■ *Corneal optical section* (Fig. 3.9) consists of a segment of an arc with following concentric zones:
♦ Tear layer is seen as a bright *anterior most* zone.
♦ Epithelium is seen as a dark line immediately behind the tear layer.
♦ Bowman's membrane is seen as a bright line.
♦ Stroma is focused as a wider granular and greyer zone.
♦ Descemet's membrane and endothelial layers are seen as *posterior most* bright zone.

Examination of the optical section of the cornea gives useful information about:
- Changes in corneal curvature
- Changes in corneal thickness
- Depth of the corneal pathologies, e.g. location of a foreign body
- Anterior chamber angle grading by van Herrick method can be done by the use of corneal optical sections at the nasal and temporal periphery.

■ *Optical section of the lens* (Fig. 3.10) seen with slit-lamp microscope shows stratification of the lens into following layers (from front to backwards):
- Anterior capsule (Ca)
- Subcapsular clear zone (first cortical clear zone $C_1\alpha$)
- A bright narrow scattering zone of discontinuity (first zone of disjunction $C_1\beta$)
- Second cortical clear zone (C_2)
- Light scattering zone of deep cortex (C_3)
- Clear zone of deep cortex (C_4)
- Nucleus (N) which follows the clear zone of cortex represents the prenatal part of the lens. It shows further stratification with a central clear interval which has been termed the embryonic nucleus.

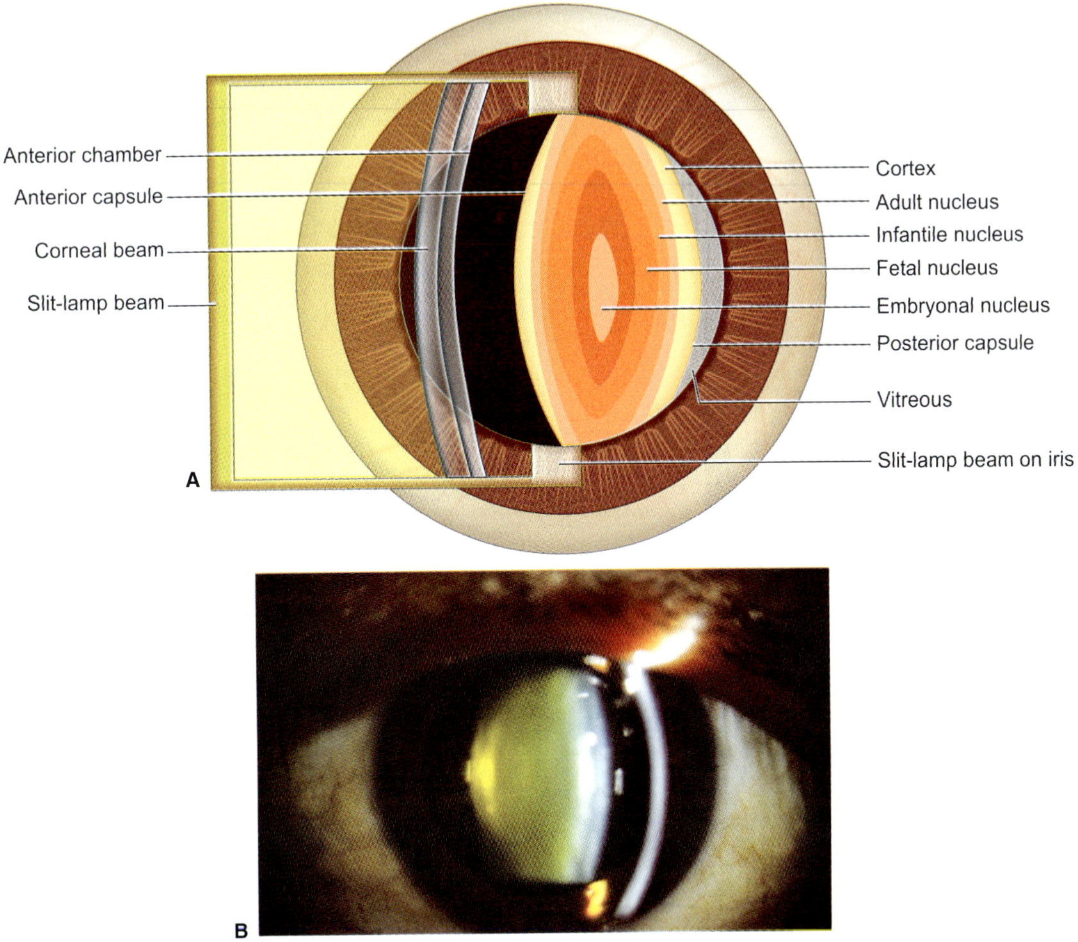

Anterior chamber

Anterior capsule

Corneal beam

Slit-lamp beam

Cortex

Adult nucleus

Infantile nucleus

Fetal nucleus

Embryonal nucleus

Posterior capsule

Vitreous

Slit-lamp beam on iris

A

B

Fig. 3.8: *Optical section of the cornea, lens and anterior vitreous seen on slit-lamp examination: (A) Diagrammatic; (B) Clinical photograph.*

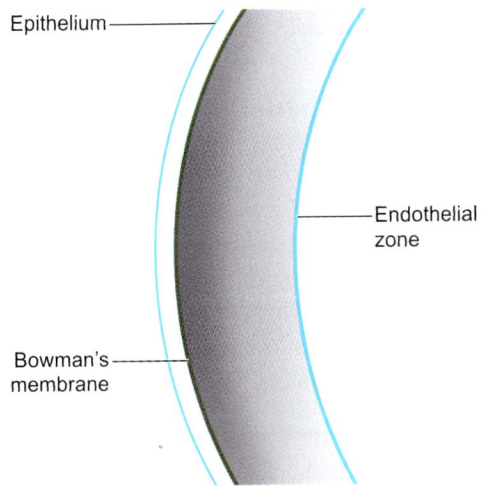

Epithelium

Endothelial zone

Bowman's membrane

Fig. 3.9: *Corneal optical section.*

The entire optical section of the lens cannot be focused in one field and thus, the microscope needs to be shifted forward to focus more posterior layer. The location and extent of lenticular opacities can be easily made in the optical section of the lens.

- *Optical section of the anterior one-third* of the vitreous can be studied with slit-lamp beam.

ii. **Parallelopiped** of the cornea (Fig. 3.11) is observed using a 2–3 mm wide focused slit. Pathologies of epithelium and stroma are better studied under this illumination. Corneal scars or infiltrates appear brighter than surroundings because they have more density. Water clefts have decreased optical density, and so appear black in optical block.

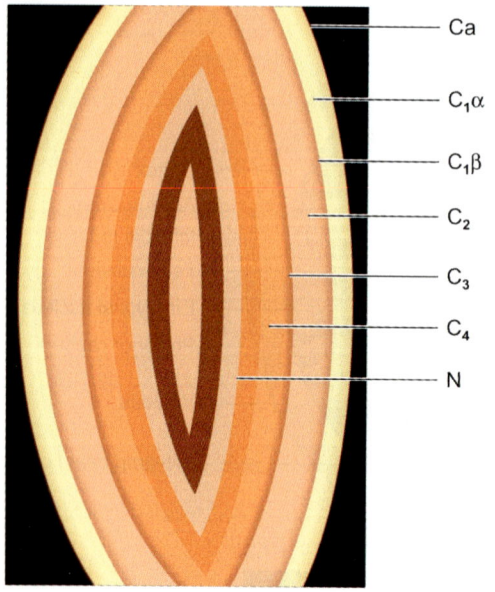

Ca

$C_1\alpha$

$C_1\beta$

C_2

C_3

C_4

N

Fig. 3.10: *Optical section of the lens.*

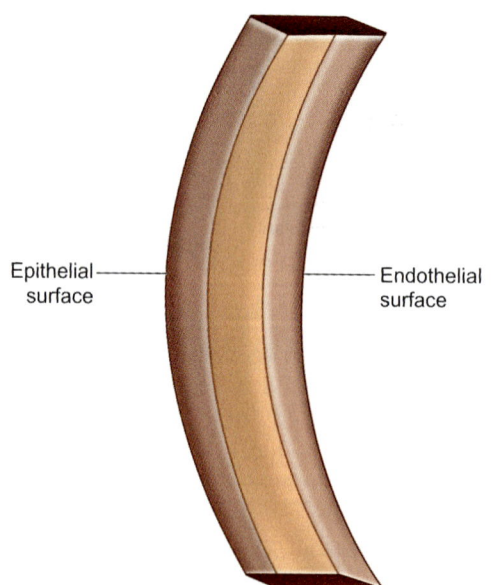

Epithelial surface

Endothelial surface

Fig. 3.11: *Parallelopiped of cornea seen on slit-lamp.*

Cells and flare in the anterior chamber can be graded by using a parallelopiped 2 mm wide 34 mm high.

iii. *Conical beam* (Fig. 3.12) is a small circular beam used to examine the presence of

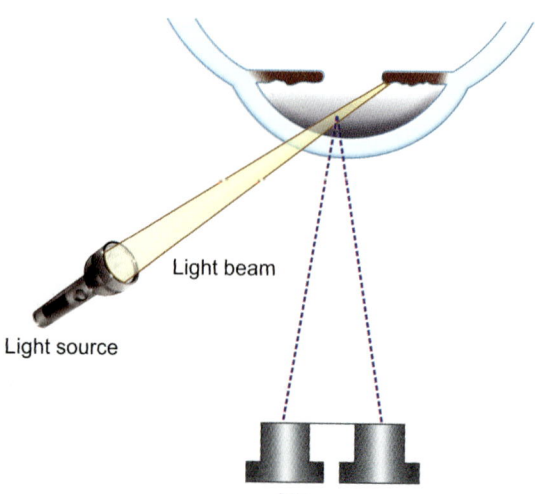

Light beam

Light source

Microscope

Fig. 3.12: *Conical beam used to examine the presence of aqueous flare.*

aqueous flare. Settings for examination of aqueous flare are as follows:

- Beam—small circular pattern
- Light source 45–60° temporally and directed into the pupil
- Biomicroscope—directly in front of the eye
- Magnification—high (16–20X)
- Focusing. Beam is focused between the cornea and anterior lens surface, and the dark zone between cornea and lens is observed. This zone is normally optically empty and appears black. Flare appears grey or milky and cells are seen as white dots. Locating the cells may be facilitated by gently oscillating the illuminator.

3. Indirect illumination. The slit-beam is focused on a position just beside the area to be examined (Fig. 3.13). The *set-up* required is as given:

- Angle between slit-lamp and microscope should be 30–45°.
- Beam width used is moderate.
- Illumination used is low, medium or high.
- Slit-lamp can be offset.

Indirect illumination is *useful* to observe:

- Corneal infiltrates
- Corneal microcysts

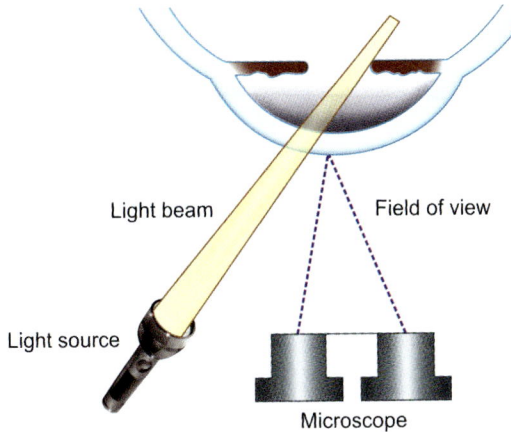

Fig. 3.13: *Set-up for indirect illumination.*

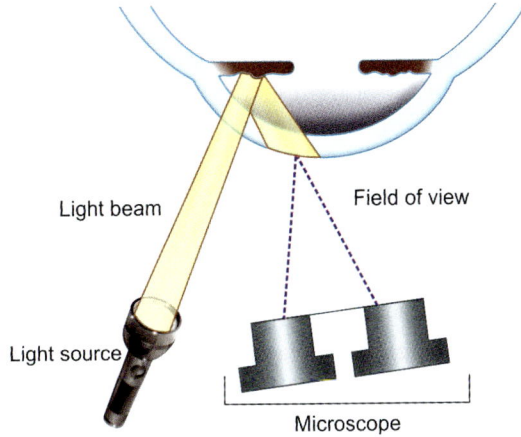

Fig. 3.14: *Set-up for retroillumination.*

- Corneal vacuoles
- Epithelial cells

4. Retroillumination. Light is reflected off the iris or fundus, while the microscope is focused on the cornea (Fig. 3.14). Graves divided retroillumination as direct and indirect, depending on the angle between observer and light.

a. *Direct:* Observer is in direct pathway of light reflected from structures. The pathology is seen against an illuminated background (Fig. 3.15).

b. *Indirect:* Observer is at right angle to the observed structure and, therefore, not in line with light, so pathology is seen against a dark, non-illuminated background (Fig. 3.16).

Based on the optical properties, Graves divided the pathologies as:

- *Obstructive.* These are opaque to light and seen as dark against a bright background, e.g. pigment or blood-filled vessel.
- *Respersive.* These scatter light but do not obstruct light completely. The pathology is seen brightly against a dark background, e.g. epithelial oedema, precipitates. Infiltrates are relucent in direct focal illumination but respersive in direct retroillumination.
- *Refractile.* These refractile pathologies distort the view of junction of illuminated and dark areas because their refractive index is different from surroundings, e.g. vacuole.

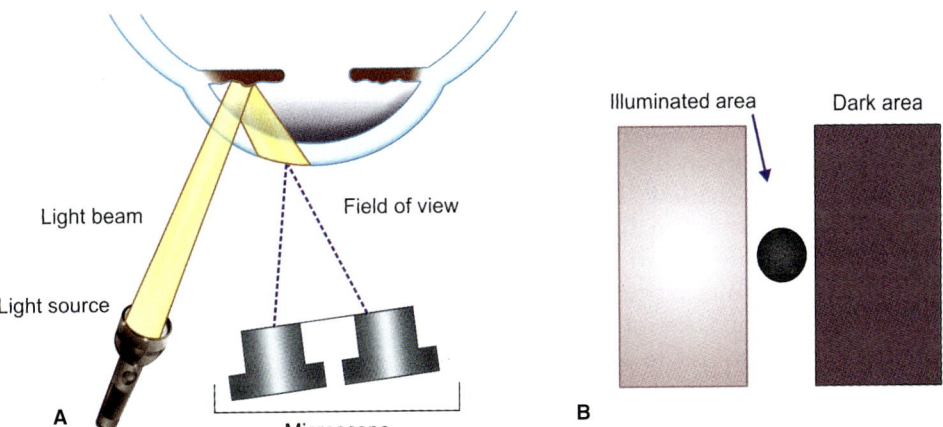

Fig. 3.15: *Direct retroillumination: (A) Cross-sectional view; (B) A keratic precipitate is seen as dark against illuminated background.*

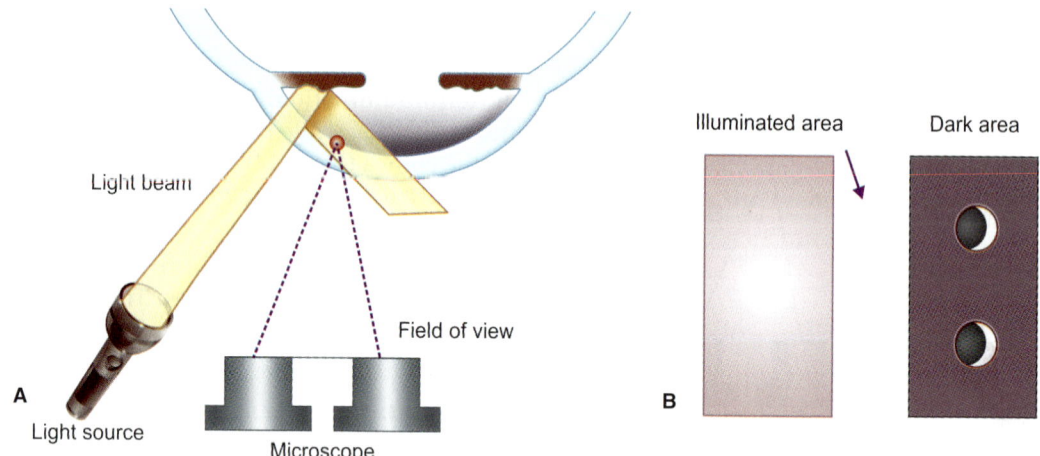

Fig. 3.16: *Indirect retroillumination: (A) Cross-sectional view; (B) A keratic precipitate seen as dark with lighted crescent on the border away from illuminated side (reversed illumination) and seen against a dark background.*

A vacuole is seen as an illuminated area bordered by dark line in direct retroillumination but in indirect retroillumination it appears as black area with a bright surface towards the illuminated area (unreversed illumination). A solid or opaque precipitate will be seen as dark area in direct retroillumination but under indirect retroillumination it will show reversed illumination; that is, its side away from the illuminated area will be bright.

Thus retroillumination can provide information regarding not only the form but also the refractive index and consistency of the pathology.

Retroillumination from the fundus. This technique is used to observe media clarities and opacities. The pupil is dilated and the slit-beam and microscope are made coaxial. The light is directed so that it strikes the fundus and creates a glow behind the opacity in the media. The media opacity creates a shadow in the glow. The microscope is then focused on the pathology directly and 10–16X magnification is used. Cornea, lens and vitreous pathologies are examined by this technique. Retroillumination of crystalline lens is required to classify and grade both cortical and posterior subcapsular cataracts using LOCS II (lens opacity classifying system II).

5. Specular reflection. Reflection of light occurs when a beam of light is incident on an optical surface, which is called *zone of discontinuity.* Such zones may be found in cornea and lens. When an observer is placed in the pathway of reflected light, a dazzling reflex will be seen which is called specular reflection. The surface from which reflection is obtained is called zone of specular reflection. Surface pathologies will scatter the light irregularly and, therefore, create dark areas in the reflex.

To get specular reflection, the patient is asked to look 30° temporally. Light beam is directed from opposite side. Optical block is focused under high magnification, 3–4 mm from limbus. Towards the side of light source, a shining reflex is seen on the cornea. When the light source is rotated still temporally, the optical block will approach the reflex. When the angle between microscope and slit-beam is about 60°, i.e. when the angle of incidence becomes equal to the angle of reflection (Fig. 3.17) at this point, dazzling reflex which is coming from tear meniscus will show the meniscus irregularities. At the same time, a deeper less luminous glow will be seen which when focused will show the endothelial mosaic. A parallelopiped beam with high illumination and high magnification is used in this technique. Similarly specular reflection from anterior and posterior capsule of lens can be

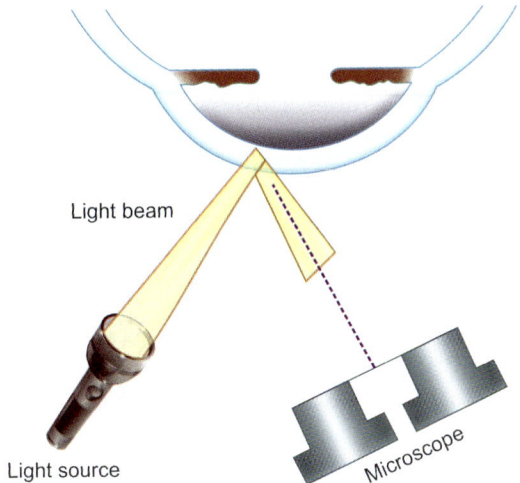

Fig. 3.17: *Set-up for specular reflection.*

obtained. Using an eyepiece reticule, endothelial cells can be measured and counted. It can also be used to study tear film details.

6. Sclerotic scatter. It is used to outline even the faintest corneal pathology. Light beam is focused at the limbus. Because of the phenomenon of total internal reflection, rays of light pass through the substance of cornea and illuminate the opposite side of limbus. If there is any pathology like corneal opacity, it becomes visible because it scatters the rays of light. A magnification of 6–10X is used and microscope is directed straight ahead (Fig. 3.18).

7. Oscillating illumination of Koeppe. In this, the slit-beam is given an oscillatory movement by which it is often possible to see minute objects or filaments especially in the aqueous which would otherwise escape detection.

ACCESSORY DEVICES

For specialized examinations with the help of a slit-lamp biomicroscope certain accessory devices that can be used with slit-lamp (78/90D examination) are given below:
- Gonioscopy
- Fundus examination with focal illumination
- Pachymetry
- Applanation tonometry
- Ophthalmodynamometry
- Slit-lamp photography
- Slit-lamp videography
- Slit-lamp as delivery system for argon, diode and YAG laser
- Laser interferometry
- Potential acuity meter test

HAND-HELD SLIT-LAMP

Hand-held slit-lamp (Fig. 3.19) is portable version of the table mounted slit-lamp which allows reasonably good examination.

Uses. It is especially suitable for:
- Bedridden patients
- Home-based examinations
- Childrens or the restless adults
- For eye camps.

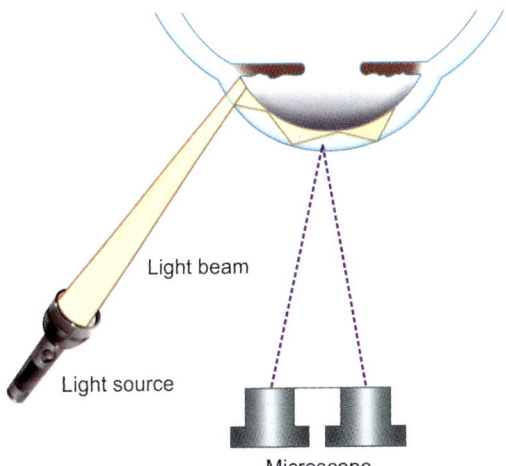

Fig. 3.18: *Set-up for sclerotic scatter.*

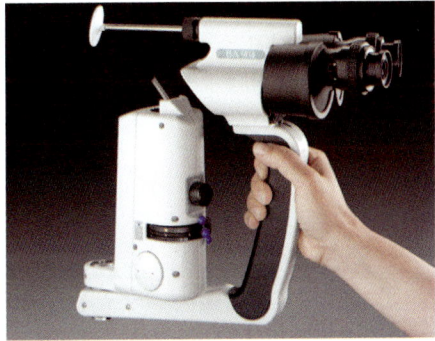

Fig. 3.19: *Hand-held slit-lamp.*

BIBLIOGRAPHY

1. Hand-Held Portable Slit Lamp from Reichert. Review of Ophthalmology 2006. www.revophth.com/index.asp?page=1_1008.htm (Accessed on September 07, 2010).

2. Knoop K, Trott A. Ophthalmologic procedures in the emergency department—Part III: Slit lamp use and foreign bodies. AcadEmerg Med 1995;2:224.

3. Koppenhöfer, Eilhard. From Lateral Illumination to Slit Lamp—An Outline of Medical History, online published 2012.

4. Schwartz Gary S. The eye exam: a complete guide, pp. 109–128 Slit Lamp Biomicroscopy, SLACK Incorporated, ISBN 978-1-55642-755-8, published 2006.

5. Slit Lamp Adapters Turn Smartphones into Clinical Cameras. Ophthalmology Web May 14, 2013. http://www.ophthalmologyweb.com/Featured-Articles/136817-Slit-Lamp-Adapters-turn-Smartphones-into-Clinical-Cameras/ (Accessed on April 05, 2017).

6. Slit-Lamp Gonioscopy. Postgraduate Medical Journal 1963;39(451):310.

7. Tate GW, Safir A. The slit lamp: History, principles, and practice. In: Clinical Opthalmology, Duane TD (Ed). Vol 1. Harper & Row, New York 1981.

8. Vivino MA, Chintalagiri S, Trus B, Datiles M. Development of a Scheimpflug slit lamp camera system for quantitative densitometric analysis, Computer Systems Laboratory, National Eye Institute, National Institutes of Health, Bethesda, MD 20892. Eye (Lond). 1993;7 (Pt 6):791–8.

Examination of Posterior Segment

Chapter Outline

INTRODUCTION

OPHTHALMOSCOPY

Distant direct ophthalmoscopy

- Procedure
- Applications

Direct ophthalmoscopy

- Optics
- Technique
- Problems
- Interpretation
- Accessory functions

Monocular indirect ophthalmoscopy

- Structural features and optics
- Indications and view of extent
- Advantages and disadvantages

Binocular indirect ophthalmoscopy

- Optics
- Practice
- Small pupil ophthalmoscopy
- Fundus drawing
- Applications, difficulties, advantages and disadvantages

BIOMICROSCOPIC EXAMINATION OF FUNDUS

Hruby lens biomicroscopy

Contact lens biomicroscopy

- Modified Koeppe lens examination
- Goldmann's three-mirror contact lens examination
- Wide-field (panfundoscopic) indirect contact

Indirect fundus biomicroscopy

- Fundus non-contact lenses
- Optics
- Technique
- Interpretation

Fundus camera

- Optical principle
- Optical system
- Modifications

Wide-Field retinal imaging systems

- Retcam II and III
- Panoret 1000AA
- Panoramic 200

LASER SCANNING IMAGING TECHNIQUES

- Scanning laser ophthalmoscopy
- Confocal scanning laser ophthalmoscopy
- Retinal thickness analyser
- Scanning laser polarimetry

INTRODUCTION

Though the conventional direct and indirect ophthalmoscopies are still the most commonly used techniques, the ophthalmic imaging technology has undergone explosive growth in the past few years. Current techniques of posterior segment evaluation and imaging have contributed significantly to the understanding of pathophysiology and treatment of a variety of posterior segment disorders. Some of the common optical instruments and techniques for posterior segment evaluation include the following:

- Ophthalmoscopy
- Slit lamp biomicroscopic examination of the fundus
- Fundus camera
- Wide-field imaging system (retinal camera)
- Scanning laser ophthalmic techniques
  - Scanning laser ophthalmoscopy (SLO)
  - CSLO or scanning laser tomography (SLT)
  - Retinal thickness analyser
  - Scanning laser polarimetry (SLP) (retinal nerve fiber analyser)
- Optical coherence tomography
- OCT ophthalmoscopy

OPHTHALMOSCOPY

Ophthalmoscopy is a clinical examination of the interior of the eye by means of an ophthalmoscope. It is primarily done to assess the state of fundus and detect the opacities of ocular media. The ophthalmoscope was invented by Babbage in 1848; however, its importance was not recognized, till it was reinvented by *von Helmholtz* in 1850. Ophthalmoscopic methods of examination in vogue are:

- Distant direct ophthalmoscopy
- Direct ophthalmoscopy
- Monocular indirect ophthalmoscopy
- Binocular indirect ophthalmoscopy.

DISTANT DIRECT OPHTHALMOSCOPY

It should be performed routinely before the direct ophthalmoscopy, as it gives a lot of useful information (vide infra). It can be performed with the help of a self-illuminated ophthalmoscope or a simple plain mirror with a hole in the center.

Procedure

The light is thrown into the patient's eye—with the patient sitting in a semidark room—from a distance of 20–25 cm, and the features of the red glow in the pupillary area are noted.

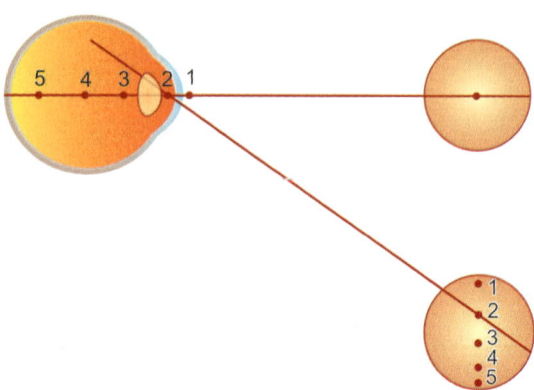

Fig. 4.1: *Parallactic displacement on distant direct ophthalmoscopy.*

Applications of distant direct ophthalmoscopy

1. *To diagnose opacities in the refractive media*. Any opacity in the refractive media is seen as a black shadow in the red glow. The exact location of the opacity can be determined by observing the parallactic displacement. For this, the patient is asked to move the eye up and down while the examiner is observing the pupillary glow. The opacities in the pupillary plane remain stationary, those in front of the pupillary plane move in the direction of the movement of the eye and those behind it will move in opposite direction (Fig. 4.1).

2. *To differentiate between a mole and a hole of the iris*. A small hole and a mole on the iris appear as a black spot on oblique illumination. On distant direct ophthalmoscopy, the mole looks black (as earlier) but a red reflex is seen through the hole in the iris.

3. *To recognize detached retina or a tumour arising from the fundus*. A greyish reflex seen on distant direct ophthalmoscopy indicates either a detached retina or a tumour arising from the fundus.

DIRECT OPHTHALMOSCOPY

It is the most commonly practised method for routine fundus examination.

OPTICS AND CHARACTERISTICS OF IMAGE

Optics

The modern direct ophthalmoscope (Fig. 4.2) works on the basic optical principle of glass plate

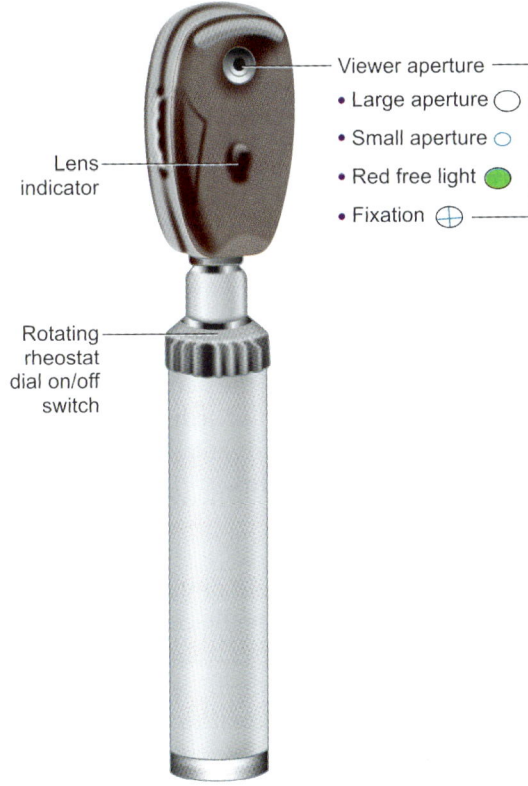

Fig. 4.2: *Direct ophthalmoscope showing viewing aperture above illuminating aperture and lens indicators.*

Viewer aperture
• Large aperture
• Small aperture
• Red free light
• Fixation

Lens indicator

Rotating rheostat dial on/off switch

A convergent beam of light is reflected into the patient's pupil (Fig. 4.3, dotted lines). The emergent rays from any point on the patient's fundus reach the observer's retina through the viewing hole in the ophthalmoscope (Fig. 4.3, continuous lines). The emergent rays from the patient's eye are parallel and brought to focus on the retina of the emmetropic observer when accommodation is relaxed.

• *In a hypermetropic patient*, the emergent ray from the illuminated area of retina will be divergent and thus can be brought to focus on the observer's retina, if the latter accommodates, or by the help of a convex lens (Fig. 4.4).

• *In a myopic patient*, the emergent rays will be convergent and thus can be brought to focus on the observer's retina by the help of a concave lens (Fig. 4.5).

Therefore, if the patient or/and the observer is/are ametropic, a correcting lens (equivalent to the sum of the patient's and observer's refractive error) must be interposed (from the system of plus and minus lenses, in-built in the modern ophthalmoscopes).

ophthalmoscope introduced by *von Helmholtz*. Optics of direct ophthalmoscopy is depicted in Fig. 4.3.

Characteristics of the image formed

In direct ophthalmoscopy, the image is erect, virtual and about 14–15 times magnified

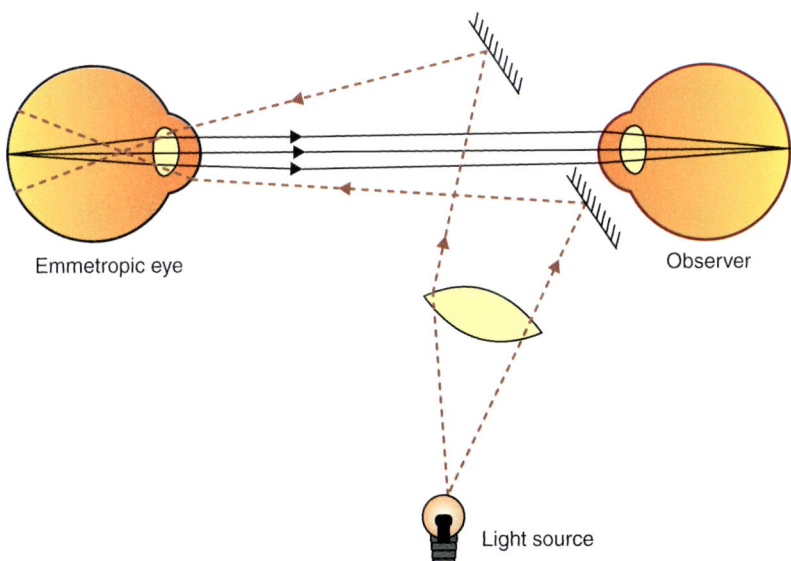

Emmetropic eye

Observer

Light source

Fig. 4.3: *Optics of direct ophthalmoscopy in an emmetropic patient.*

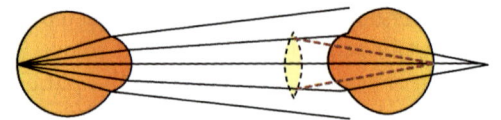

Fig. 4.4: *Optics of direct ophthalmoscopy in a hypermetropic patient.*

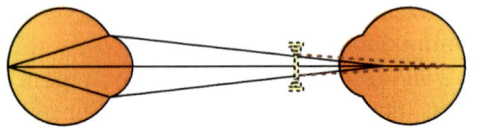

Fig. 4.5: *Optics of direct ophthalmoscopy in a myopic patient.*

(Table 4.1) in emmetropes (more in myopes and less in hypermetropes).

Magnification of the direct ophthalmoscope for an emmetropic patient viewed by an emmetropic observer is 15x. If the patient and observer have refractive errors, then the axial length and refractive power of both eyes, plus the compensating lenses of the ophthalmoscope, all influence the resultant magnification. If the patient is myopic, then the eye has plus power and the ophthalmoscope requires a minus lens for viewing a clear images. The combination results in a **Galilean telescope**, which enlarges fundus detail. The opposite effect is seen in a hyperopic eye (reverse telescope).

If neither the patient nor the observer is emmetropic, then power of a single lens in the ophthalmoscope must be equal to the mathematical sum of the patient's and the observer's refractive errors. It is important to understand that when one or both of the participants have a large refractive error or a high degree of astigmatism, it is more advantageous to use the glasses to view the fundus.

Field of view

The ophthalmoscopic field of vision (Table 4.1) is always smaller than the field of illumination in direct ophthalmoscopy. It is affected by the following factors:

• It is directly proportional to the size of the pupil of observed eye.

Table 4.1 *Magnification, field of view and characteristics of the image formed with different techniques of fundus examination*

Technique	Magnification	Field of view	Characteristics of image	Principal use
Direct ophthalmoscopy	14X	5°	Erect, virtual	Routine view of disc and surrounding area
Indirect ophthalmoscopy				
• With 114 D	4X	40°	Inverted, reversed and real	Fundus lesion inspection
• With 120 D	3X	45°	Inverted, reversed and real	Routine examination
• With 130 D	2X	50°	Inverted, reversed and real	Routine examination
Biomicroscopic examination				
• With 178 D	10X	30°	Inverted, reversed and real	Posterior pole observation
• With 190 D	7.5X	40°	Inverted, reversed and real	Posterior pole observation
• With Hruby lens	12X	10°	Erect, virtual	Optic disc and vitreous observation
• With Goldmann fundus contact lens	10X	20°	Erect, virtual	Optic disc and macula inspection
Fundus camera	2.5X	30°	Erect, virtual Photodocumentation	

- It is directly proportional to the *axial length* of the observed eye.
- It is inversely proportional to the distance between the observed and the observer's eye.
- The smaller the sight hole of the ophthalmoscope, the better the field of vision.

Technique

Direct ophthalmoscopy should be performed in a semidark room with the patient seated and looking straight ahead, while the observer standing or seated slightly over to the side of the eye to be examined (Fig. 4.6A). The patient's right eye should be examined by the observer with his or her right eye, and left with the left.

The observer should reflect beam of light from the ophthalmoscope into patient's pupil. Once the red reflex is seen, the observer should move as close to the patient's eye as possible (theoretically at the anterior focal plane of the patient's eye, i.e. 15.4 mm from the cornea).

The direct ophthalmoscope should then be focused by twirling the dial for the Reskoss disc, which has several plus- and minus-powered lasers. The optimal focusing lens on the Reskoss disc depends on the patient's refractive error, the examiner's refractive error (including unintended accommodation) and the examination distance (Table 4.2).

Once the retina is focused, the details should be examined systematically starting from disc, blood vessels, the four quadrants of the general background and the macula by utilizing the various illumination options and apertures provided in the direct ophthalmoscope (Table 4.3 and Fig. 4.6A).

Note. The problem is obtaining adequate illumination of the patient's fundus as the light source only illuminates that part of the fundus which is struck directly by light; the rest of the fundus remains dark. Therefore, the fundus can be adequately viewed only if the observed areas and the illuminated areas coincide. This can take place only if the light source and the observer's pupil are closely aligned optically (Fig. 4.6B). Most direct ophthalmoscopes (Fig. 4.2) have the

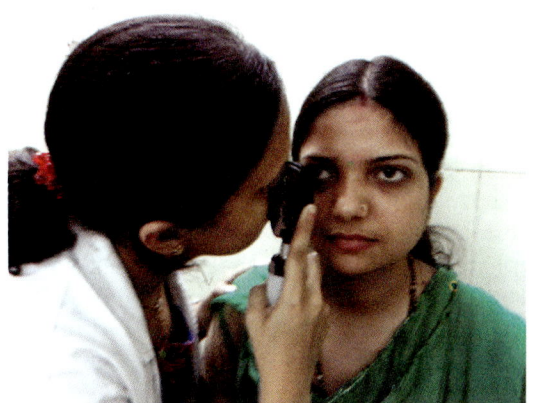

Fig. 4.6A: *Technique of direct ophthalmoscopy.*

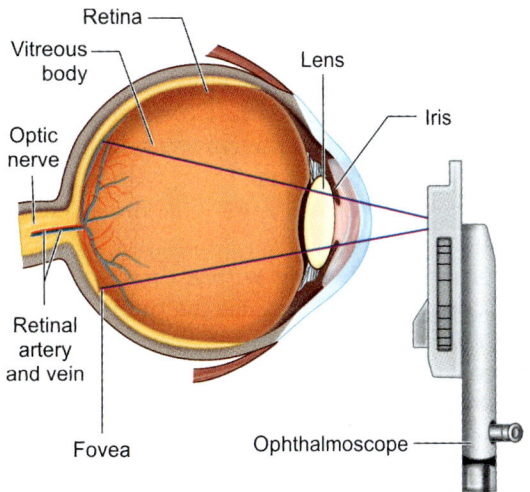

Fig. 4.6B: *The light source and the observer's pupil are closely aligned optically and that part of the fundus which is properly illuminated can be adequately viewed.*

Table 4.2 *Direct ophthalmoscope's refractive power versus patient's spherical equivalent while focusing**

Direct ophthalmoscope's refractive power	Patient's refractive error
230 D	215 D
220 D	212 D
210 D	28 D
25 D	24 D
20	2Plano
15 D	16 D
110 D	115 D

*When the examiner's eye is emmetropic or corrected and the examination distance between the ophthalmoscope and cornea is 20 mm

Table 4.3 *Various apertures and illumination options with direct ophthalmoscope*

Aperture description	Use
Large spot	For viewing through a dilated pupil
Small spot	For viewing through a small pupil
Red-free fibre	Useful in detecting changes in the nerve fibre layer and identifying microaneurysms and other vascular anomalies
Slit	For evaluating contour of retinal lesions
Reticule or grid	For measuring vessel caliber or diameter of a small retinal lesion (marked in 0.2 mm increments)
Fixation target	For testing fixation pattern (central or eccentric)
Reskoss disc	Plus and minus lenses are for focusing the retina

illuminating beam situated below the viewing aperture. Modern ophthalmoscopes have a condensing lens to intensify the light Beam and a diaphragm and projecting lens to limit the size of the light beam.

Problems faced during viewing

Unwanted reflections. To avoid both scattering and reflection of light rays into the viewing beam, both the illuminating and viewing beams must be maximally separated so that interference and hence reflections do not occur. Therefore, separation of the two beams must be maintained through the cornea and lens, yet overlap onto the retina. Thus, with a dilated pupil, reflex-free viewing is more easily obtained.

Peripheral viewing with a direct ophthalmoscope is limited because the pupil becomes too narrow for the viewing and illumination beams. The equatorial region is usually the limit in peripheral viewing with the direct ophthalmoscope. A technique to aid in peripheral viewing has to do with the change in the pupil configuration on extreme eyes gazes. When the patient looks to the right or left, the pupil is elongated vertically. In this situation the ophthalmoscope should be held vertically to

facilitate the entrance of both beams into the eye. Likewise, a horizontal elongation of the pupil results during up or down gaze, and a horizontal orientation of the scope may be helpful.

Interpretation

Generally, an ophthalmoscopic examination of the fundus starts at the optic nerve head because localization of this structure provides immediate orientation. The image is virtual and upright. The optic disc should be examined for the cup-to-disc ratio, color, clarity of margins, spontaneous venous pulsations, and any abnormalities. The tissue around the disc is studied, with emphasis placed on the blood vessels, especially the superior and inferior temporal arcades. The vessels should be evaluated for their arteriovenous ratio, color, diameter, and course. The background retinal tissue is also examined. The macula is usually examined last because of the dazzling and discomfort that is experienced by the patient. The macula should be examined for the foveal reflex, color, pigmentation, and any abnormalities.

The size of any abnormal lesion is described in terms of disc areas and distance from disc or macula is described in terms of disc diameters. For depth of the lesion a 3-D difference in focal planes for focusing the lesion in an emmetropic eye converts into a linear depth equivalent of approximately 1 mm in a phakic eye and into approximately 2 mm in an aphakic eye. This is especially useful for documenting raised lesions, e.g. disc edema.

Accessory functions of direct ophthalmoscope

Accessory functions have been built into the ophthalmoscope to widen the diagnostic capabilities.

Slit diaphragm can produce a narrow slit beam, which can be used to detect elevation or depression of retinal lesions. Here, a distortion of the beam occurs when it travels across an elevation or depression. The beam bows toward the observer on an elevated area and away from the observer in a depressed area.

Pinhole diaphragm produces a narrow beam of light that can be used to reduce reflections, which is especially helpful when viewing

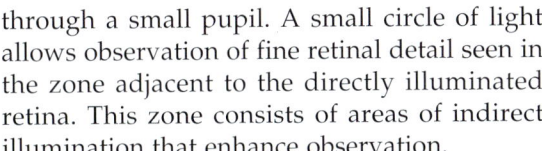

through a small pupil. A small circle of light allows observation of fine retinal detail seen in the zone adjacent to the directly illuminated retina. This zone consists of areas of indirect illumination that enhance observation.

Fixation reticle can be used to discover eccentric fixation or eccentric viewing by the patient. This may be helpful in the evaluation of strabismic patients or for measuring the size of macular lesions.

Filters of different types can be very helpful while performing ophthalmoscopy. A cobalt blue filter can be used to enhance fluorescence angiography. A red free (green) filter to absorb red light; therefore, red objects appear very dark. This is helpful when studying blood vessels and hemorrhages. Defects in the nerve fiber layer and retinal edema are more easily seen with red-free light because of shorter wavelengths that are readily scattered by superficial retinal layers.

Cross polarizing filters reduce reflection because light reflected back from the cornea is depolarized and blocked by the viewing filter, but light reflected from the retina (except for the internal limiting membranes) is polarized and remains visible. The chief drawback of polarizing filters is the substantial reduction in illumination and hence less bright view of the fundus.

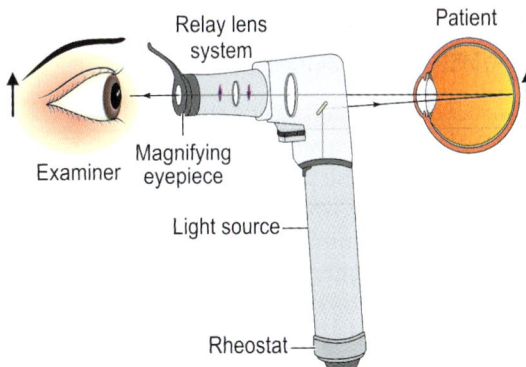

Fig. 4.7: *The optical principle of monocular indirect ophthalmoscopy, demonstrating the resultant erect magnified image.*

MONOCULAR INDIRECT OPHTHALMOSCOPY

Structural features

The monocular indirect ophthalmoscope consists of (Fig. 4.7):
- *Illumination rheostat* at its base
- *Focusing lever* for image refinement
- *Filter dial* with red-free and yellow filters
- *Forehead rest* for steady proper observer head positioning
- *Iris diaphragm lever* to adjust the illumination beam diameter.

Optics

An internal relay lens system re-inverts the initially inverted image to a real erect one, which is then magnified. This image is focusable using the focusing lever/eyepiece system (Fig. 4.7).

Indications and view of extent

Indications for use of monocular indirect ophthalmoscopy include:
- Need for an increased field of view
- Small pupils
- Uncooperative children
- Patient's intolerance of bright light of binocular indirect ophthalmoscope
- Basic fundus screening

Extent of view. Although vitreous base views are possible with monocular indirect ophthalmoscopy, its greatest effectiveness extends anteriorly to the peripheral equatorial region. The 40+ degree field of view of the monocular indirect ophthalmoscope is approximately the same as that of binocular indirect ophthalmoscope.

Advantages and disadvantages

Advantages of monocular indirect ophthalmoscopy include:
- Increased field of view similar to indirect ophthalmoscopy.
- Erect real imaging similar to direct ophthalmoscopy.

Disadvantages include:
- Lack of stereopsis
- Limited illumination
- Fixed magnification
- Fair to good resolution.

BINOCULAR INDIRECT OPHTHALMOSCOPY

Indirect ophthalmoscopy, introduced by Nagel in 1864, is now a very popular method for examination of the posterior segment. Indirect ophthalmoscopy was considered as an elementary part of examination by only the posterior segment or the retinal surgeons in yesteryears. It was the eagerness on the part of the examiner, who used only direct ophthalmoscopy, so as to come to a hasty diagnosis. He used to organize his thoughts on this cursory examination of the retina, and assumptions were made for the final diagnosis. However, in this modern era, indirect ophthalmoscopy is of great general use in ophthalmology and requires much effort and practice by the anterior as well as the posterior segment surgeons.

OPTICS OF INDIRECT OPHTHALMOSCOPY

Optical principle

The principle of indirect ophthalmoscopy is to make the eye highly myopic by placing a strong convex lens in front of patient's eye so that the emergent rays from an area of the fundus are brought to focus as a real inverted image between the lens and the observer's eye, which is then studied (Fig. 4.8A).

Optical system of binocular indirect ophthalmoscope

Optics of modern binocular indirect ophthalmoscopy is shown in Fig. 4.8B. Binocularity is achieved by reducing the observer's interpupillary distance from about 60 mm to approximately 15 mm by prisms/mirrors (Fig. 4.9). Even this artificial reduction of interpupillary distance requires larger patient's pupils for binocular viewing than those for the monocular viewing.

Field of illumination as shown in Fig. 4.10. The field of illumination is more in myopia and less in hypermetropia compared to emmetropia.

Image formation

1. *Image formation in emmetropia.* The emergent rays from the illuminated area of retina are parallel in emmetropic patients and are, therefore, brought to focus by the condensing lens at its principal focus (Fig. 4.11). Thus an inverted image of the retina is formed in the air between the condensing lens and the observer.

2. *Image formation in hypermetropia.* The emergent rays from the illuminated area of

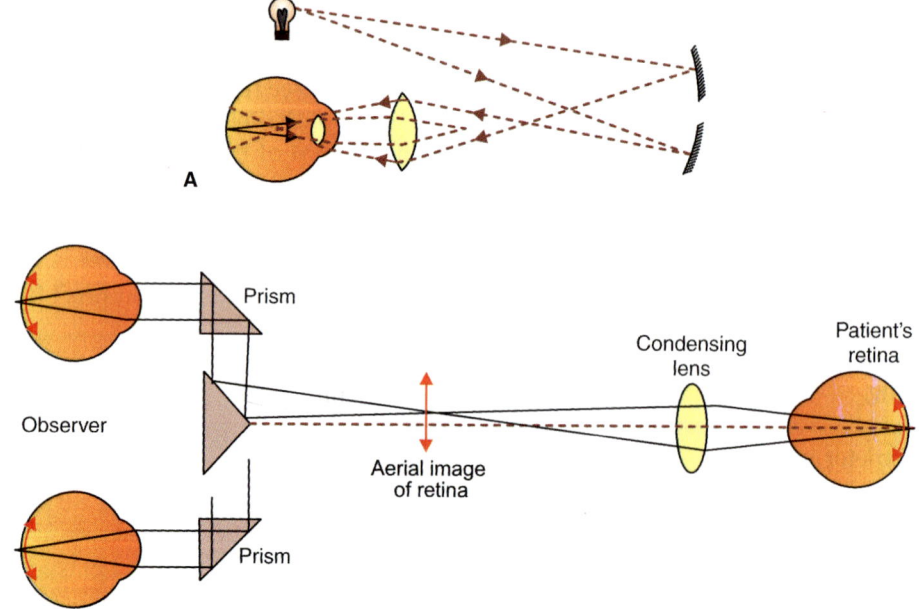

Fig. 4.8: *(A) Optics of indirect ophthalmoscopy; and (B) optical system of a modern binocular indirect ophthalmoscope.*

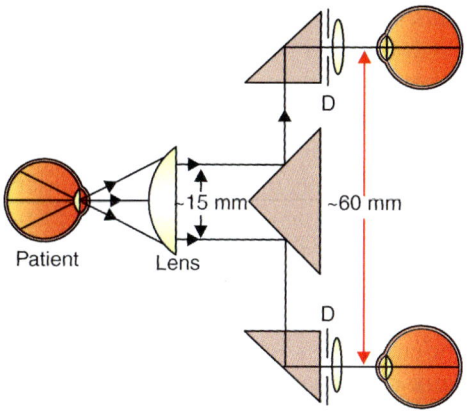

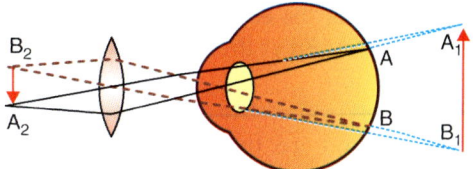

Fig. 4.12: *Image formation on indirect ophthalmoscopy in hypermetropia.*

in front of the eye. The condensing lens forms the final image A_2B_2 situated within its own focal length (Fig. 4.13).

Characteristics of the image

The image formed in indirect ophthalmoscopy is real, inverted and magnified. Magnification of image depends upon the dioptric power of the convex lens, position of the lens in relation to the eyeball and refractive state of the eyeball. About 53 magnification is obtained with a 113 D lens. With a stronger lens, image will be smaller but brighter and field of vision will be more. The important characteristics of the image formed by an indirect ophthalmoscope are as follows:

1. *Relative position of images formed in emmetropic, myopic and hypermetropic eye.* The relative positions of the images formed in emmetropic, myopic and hypermetropic eye, when the condensing lens used is situated at its own focal distance from cornea, are shown in Fig. 4.14.

Fig. 4.9: *Stereopsis is produced by the binocular indirect ophthalmoscope. Note how the two prisms widen the incoming beams so that they are incident to the eyes of the observer.*

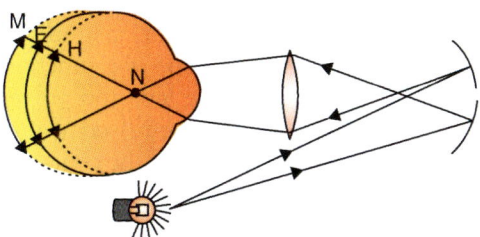

Fig. 4.10: *Field of illumination in various refractive errors.*

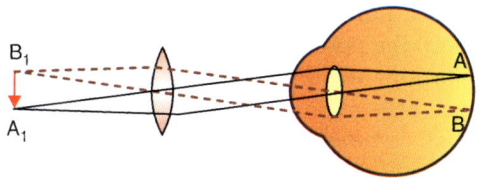

Fig. 4.11: *Image formation on indirect ophthalmoscopy in emmetropia.*

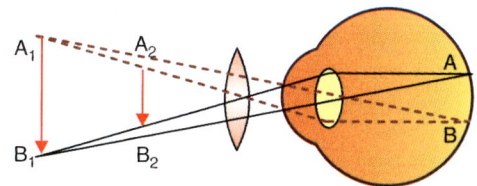

Fig. 4.13: *Image formation on indirect ophthalmoscopy in myopia.*

retina are divergent in hypermetropic patients and thus appear to come from an imaginary enlarged upright image situated behind the eye (Fig. 4.12). The condensing lens, therefore, uses this as an object and forms an inverted image of it. Since, the rays are divergent, the final image is situated in front of the principal focus.

3. *Image formation in the myopic eye.* The emergent rays from the illuminated area AB of retina in a myopic patient are convergent and, therefore, an inverted image A_1B_1 of it is formed

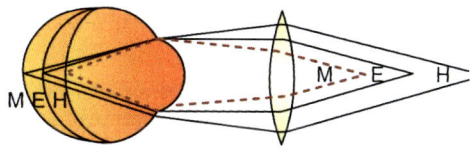

Fig. 4.14: *The relative positions of the images in indirect ophthalmoscopy in emmetropia (E), hypermetropia (H) and myopia (M).*

- *In emmetropia,* the emergent rays are parallel and thus focused at the principal focus of the lens, i.e. at E.
- *In hypermetropia,* the emergent rays are divergent and are, therefore, focused farther away from the principal focus, i.e. at H.
- *In myopia,* the emergent rays are convergent and are, therefore focused near to the lens than its principal focus, i.e. at M.

2. *Size of the image vis-a-vis refractive condition of the eye.*

i. ***In an emmetropic eye,*** the size of image always remains the same and is situated at its principal focus, because the rays emerging for such an eye are parallel (Figs 4.11 and 4.15).

ii. ***In hypermetropia,*** the size of the image will be:
- *Equal to an emmetropic eye,* if the condensing lens is held at such a distance that its principal focus (f) corresponds to the anterior focus of eye (Fig. 4.15A).
- *Larger than the emmetropic eye,* if the condensing lens is held at such a distance that its principal focus (f) is nearer than the anterior focus of the eye (F) (Fig. 4.15B).

- *Smaller than the emmetropic eye,* when the principal focus of the condensing lens (f) is farther away than the anterior focus of eye (Fig. 4.15C).

iii. ***In myopia,*** the size of image will be:
- *Equal to an emmetropic eye,* if the condensing lens is held at such a distance that its principal focus (f) corresponds to the anterior focus of eye (F) (Fig. 4.15A).
- *Smaller than the emmetropic eye,* if the condensing lens is held at such a distance that its principal focus (f) is nearer than the anterior focus of the eye (F) (Fig. 4.15B).
- *Larger than the emmetropic eye,* when the principal focus of the condensing lens (f) is farther away than the anterior focus of eye (Fig. 4.15C).

3. *Image magnification in indirect ophthalmoscopy.* Lateral (transverse, linear) magnification in an indirect ophthalmoscope is a function of the power of the condensing lens and power of the patient's eye. It may be expressed as power of the eye (60 D) to the power of the condensing lens. Therefore, a 20 D lens produces 33 lateral magnification and a 30 D lens produces 23 magnification (Table 4.1). Although the axial image remains constant in size for a given lens, if it is viewed from more than 25 cm (the reference point for the designation of magnification) the perceived magnification decreases proportionately to the viewing distance.

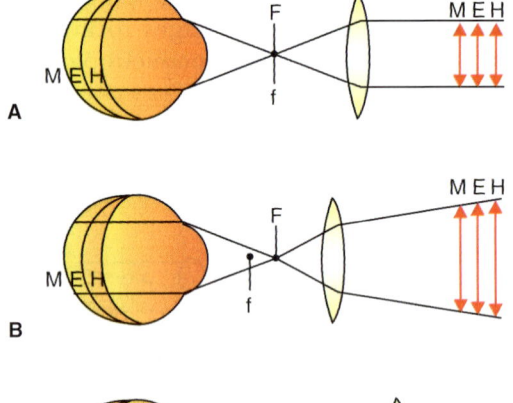

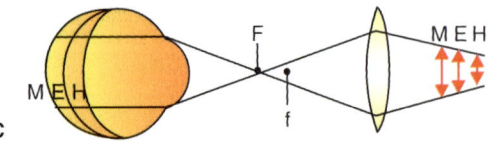

Fig. 4.15: *The size of the image in different refractive states (M: myopia; E: emmetropia; H: hypermetropia), when the condensing lens is held at such a distance that its principal focus (f): (A) Corresponds to the anterior focus of the eye (F); (B) is nearer than the anterior focus of the eye; and (C) is farther away from the anterior focus of the eye.*

Field of illumination and observation

The field of observation is always larger than the field of illumination in indirect ophthalmoscopy. The size of the pupil does not affect the size of field of observation, provided it is larger than the image of the observer's pupil formed by the condensing lens in the observed pupil.

The field of observation is in fact a function of magnification and the condensing lens diameter. An X-fold decrease in magnification equals an x^2 increase in the field of observation (Table 4.1).

Practice of indirect ophthalmoscopy

Prerequisites
- Indirect ophthalmoscope
- Dark room

- Convex lens 14 D/120 D/128 D/30 D (nowadays commonly employed lens is of 120 D)
- Pupils of the patient should be dilated.

Technique

The procedure is explained to the patient and is made to lie in the supine position, with one pillow on a bed or couch and instructed to keep both eyes open. The examiner throws the light into the patient's eye from an arm's distance (with the self-illuminated ophthalmoscope). In practice, binocular ophthalmoscope with head band or that mounted on the spectacle frame is employed most frequently (Fig. 4.16). Keeping the eyes on the reflex, the examiner then interposes the condensing lens (120 D, routinely) in the path of beam of light—close to the patient's eye and then slowly moves the lens away from the eye (towards himself or herself) until the image of the retina is clearly seen. The examiner moves around the head of the patient to examine different quadrants of the fundus. He or she has to stand opposite the clock hour position to be examined, e.g. to examine inferior quadrant (around 6 o'clock meridian) the examiner stands towards patient's head (12 o'clock meridian) and so on. By asking the patient to look in extreme gaze, and using scleral indenter, the whole peripheral retina up to ora serrata can be examined.

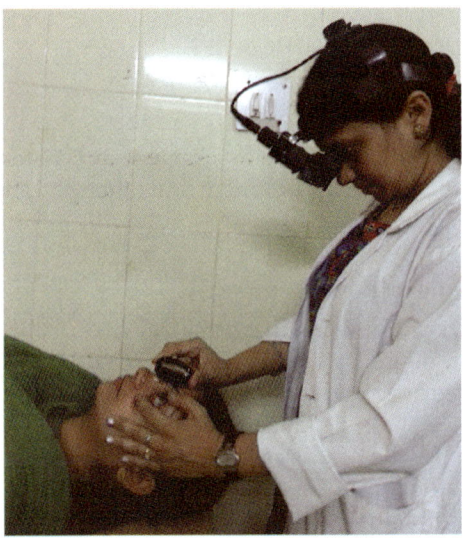

Fig. 4.16: *Technique of indirect ophthalmoscopy.*

Scleral indentation

This is done with the depressor placed on the patient's lids. This helps in making prominent the just or barely perceptible lesions. One can better appreciate the different tissue colors and densities.

- The examiner should move the scleral depressor in a direction opposite to that in which he or she wishes the depression to appear.
- The scleral depressor should be rolled gently and tangentially over the eye surface.
- The patients are most sensitive to scleral depression in superonasal quadrants.
- Sometimes a topical anaesthetic may be applied and scleral depressor is placed directly on the medial conjunctiva, causing little patient discomfort.
- The temporal part of the upper lid is sufficiently lax so that depressor can be placed inferiorly in the horizontal meridian.
- Sometimes when more posterior areas of fundus are to be examined, the examiner asks the patient to look slightly towards his or her position.

Small pupil ophthalmoscopy

In cases where the pupils do not dilate or if media opacities are enough so as to allow only few rays to enter the retina through a small clear media, small pupil ophthalmoscopy is required. Theoretically, it is possible to see the retina binocularly through 0.6 mm pupil with the 30 D lens. Indirect ophthalmoscopy can be performed through a small pupil without small pupil ophthalmoscope by using 30 D lens held as far as possible. When looking through a small pupil, it is convenient to visualize the retina, if light source is directed high in examiner's field of vision. Slight blurring can occur.

Fundus drawing

The image seen with the indirect ophthalmoscope is vertically inverted and laterally reversed; the top of the retinal chart is placed towards the foot end of the patient (i.e. upside down) (Fig. 4.17). This corresponds to the image of the fundus obtained by the examiner. The

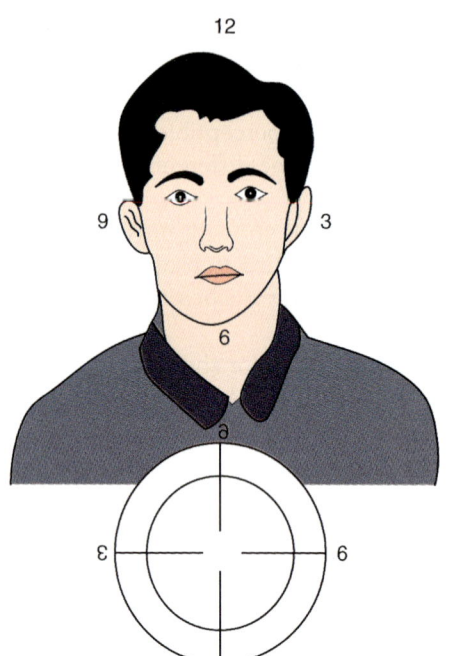

Fig. 4.17: *Position of the chart for drawing during indirect ophthalmoscopy.*

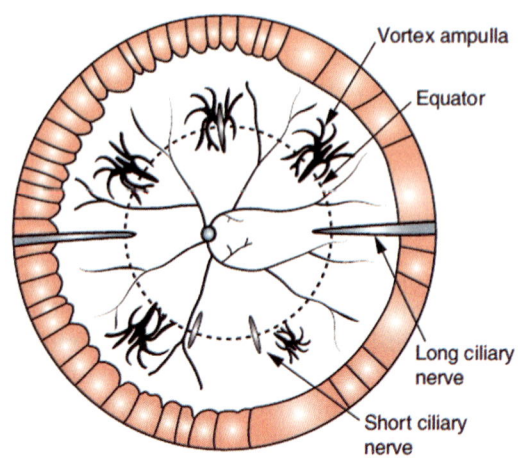

Fig. 4.18: *Normal anatomical landmarks which can be used as aids to draw the location of design seen on fundus examination.*

fundus drawing is made on a special Amsler's chart, which has 12 clock hours marked and has three concentric circles made on it. The innermost circle represents to the equator, the middle circle the ora serrata and the outermost circle the midpoint of pars plana.

Normal anatomical landmarks. For mapping of the finding, it is very useful to note the position of any lesion with respect to the *normal anatomical landmarks* on the retina (Fig. 4.18):

- *Vortex veins ampulla* are seen along the equator.
- *Long ciliary veins* may be seen at 3 o'clock and 9 o'clock positions.
- *Branching vessels* may also be used and marked to draw the pathology seen.

Symbols and colour codes used to draw the fundus, as accepted internationally (Fig. 4.19), are as below:

- *Optic disc* is always shown with red margins.
- *Arteries* are drawn as red lines.
- *Veins* are drawn as blue lines.
- *Attached retina* is shown red.

- *Thin retina* is indicated by red hatching outlines in blue.
- *Detached retina* is drawn with blue color.
- *Retinal tears* are shown as red with blue outline. Flap of the retinal tear is also drawn blue.
- *Lattice degeneration* is shown as blue hatchings outlined in blue.
- *Retinal pigment* is shown as black.
- *Retinal exudates* are shown as yellow.
- *Choroidal lesions* are depicted brown.
- *Vitreous opacities* are depicted as green.

APPLICATIONS, DIFFICULTIES, ADVANTAGES AND DISADVANTAGES

Applications

It is essential for the assessment and management of retinal detachment and other peripheral retinal lesions.

Difficulties during viewing

Reflections and light scatter are problems ophthalmoscopy, and binocular viewing requires a larger pupil than monocular viewing to meet Gullstrand's original ophthalmoscope design. Moving the beams closer together will facilitate viewing through a **small pupil** but will increase reflections and reduce stereopsis. The advantage of the indirect ophthalmoscope is the ability to

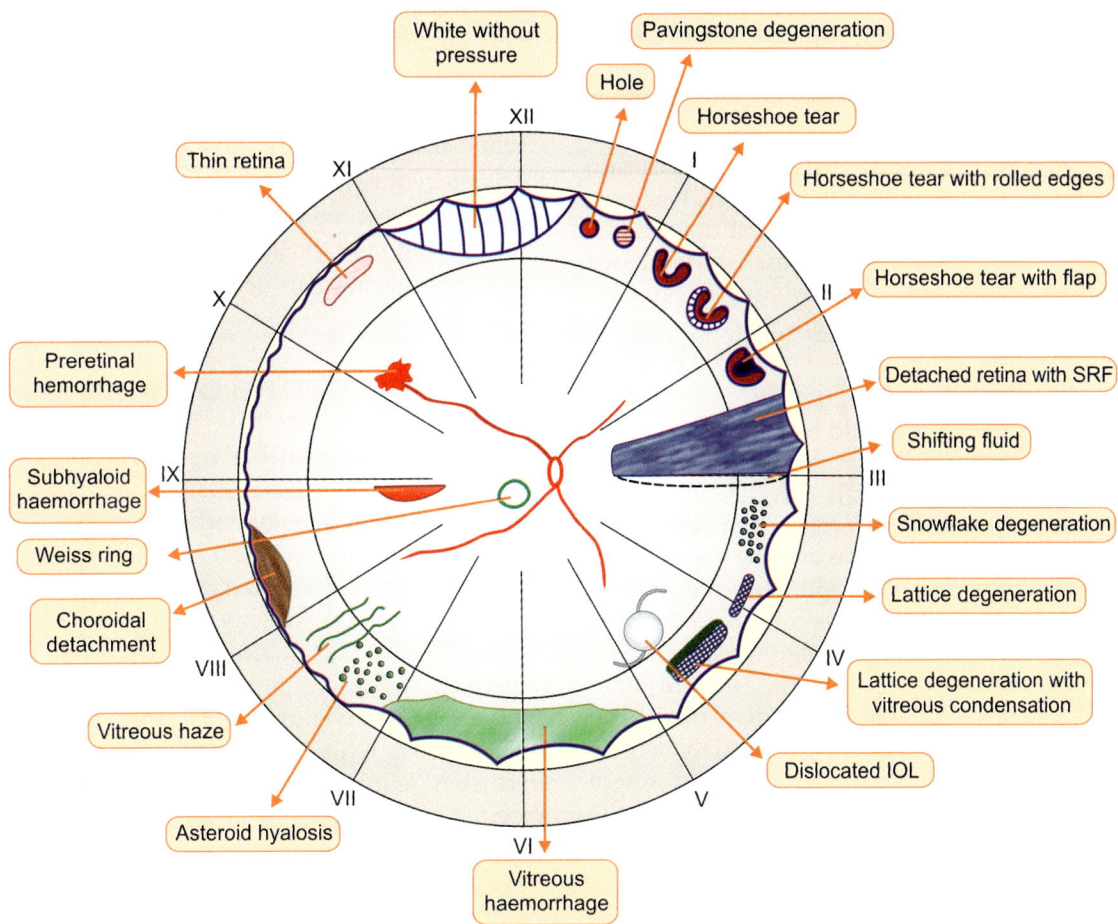

Fig. 4.19: *A sample fundus diagram showing the universal colour-coding system for a few common lesions and structures.*

change the distance between the illuminating beam and viewing beams by tilting the mirror on the scope. During indirect ophthalmoscopy, the illumination is focused in the plane of the pupil to better satisfy Gullstrand's requirements, for this will be the smallest diameter of the beam. Because a +14 D condensing lens has a longer focal length, it is held a greater distance from the eye than a +30 D lens to place the smallest diameter of the beam in the pupil.

The indirect ophthalmoscopy lens design should be to decrease **peripheral aberrations** that increase with stronger and larger lens. To overcome this problem, most condensing lenses are made of an **aspheric** design. This results in a lens with two different curves, the steeper curve on the examiner side of the lens. The illumination beam produces reflections and scatter on the condensing lens surface that can be minimized by **antireflective coatings**. If the lens is held perpendicular to the line of viewing, it produces reflections on the front and rear surfaces in the center of the lens. These reflections can be directed out of the line of light by a **slight tilt of the lens**. Observation of the reflections can be helpful for determining the **proper orientation** of the condensing lens (i.e. the steeper curvature is on the examiner's side), when facing the proper direction, the two reflections will be approximately equal in size. When opposite to this, one reflection will be significantly larger than the other. To help assist with proper orientation, modern condensing lenses have a silver or white ring painted on the edge of the lens holder's flange that faces the patient.

Excessive **lens tilt will induce astigmatic distortion** of the fundus image and should be avoided. However, this can be advantageous when viewing the peripheral fundus. By inducing astigmatism with the condensing lens at 90 degrees to the astigmatism produced during observation of the fundus periphery, it is possible to reduce peripheral optical distortions. The degree of induced astigmatism increases with greater lens tilt, and the observer can vary the tilt to obtain the clearest focus. Considerable practice is usually required before one becomes comfortable with the technique.

Peripheral viewing could be a problem. When viewing the periphery, the pupil becomes elliptical and much smaller in diameter along the short-axis. This may make it impossible to direct both viewing beams and the illumination beam into the patient's pupil. This can be remedied by tilting the observer's head 45 degrees, which may allow the illumination beam and one viewing beam to enter the pupil. This will eliminate stereopsis, but will allow a more peripheral view of the fundus. Also, it is helpful to increase the viewing distance when examining through a small pupil by moving farther away from the condensing lens; the closer one is to the pupil, the less the chances of intercepting the angle of exiting rays.

Advantages of indirect ophthalmoscopy

1. Larger field of retina is visible. There is a 10-fold increase in the area of retina visible as compared to direct ophthalmoscopy.
2. Lesser distortion of the image of the retina.
3. Easier to examine, if the patient's eye movements are present and with high spherical or astigmatic refractive errors.
4. Easy visualization of the retina anterior to the equator, where most retinal holes and degenerations exist.
5. It gives a 3-D stereoscopic view of the retina with considerable depth of focus.
6. It is useful in hazy media because of its bright light and optical property.

Disadvantages of indirect ophthalmoscopy

1. Magnification in indirect ophthalmoscopy is 5 times, whereas in direct ophthalmoscopy it is 15 times.

2. Indirect ophthalmoscopy is impossible with very small pupils.
3. The patient is usually more uncomfortable with the intense light of indirect ophthalmoscope and with scleral indentation.
4. The procedure is more cumbersome, requires extensive practice both in technique and in interpretation of the images visualized.
5. Reflex sneezing can occur on exposure to bright light.

Effect of prolonged indirect ophthalmoscopy on patient's eye

Does prolonged indirect ophthalmoscope viewing affect eyes of patient? This is a commonly asked question by the patients before repeated examinations. Many technical advances in light sources have been made in modern ophthalmoscopes. These light sources can deliver high-intensity light to the subject's eye. A study by Robertson and Erickson of prolonged indirect ophthalmoscopy on human eyes failed to reveal any long-term retinal damage. However, there were some **short-term changes** consisting of irregular bending and twisting of photoreceptor outer segment and transient corneal edema. Attempts have been made to reduce the infrared radiation through the use of fiberoptics, dichroic mirrors, and tinted condensing lenses such as the Volk yellow-tinted lenses that absorb light in both blue and infrared wavelengths.

BIOMICROSCOPIC EXAMINATION OF FUNDUS

Biomicroscopic examination of the fundus can be performed after full mydriasis, using a slit-lamp and any one of the following lenses.

1. HRUBY LENS BIOMICROSCOPY

Hruby lens (Fig. 4.20A) is a planoconcave lens with dioptric power 58.6 D which neutralizes the optical power of the normal eye (160 D) and forms a virtual, erect image of the fundus (Fig. 4.20B). This lens provides a small field with low magnification and cannot visualize the fundus beyond equator.

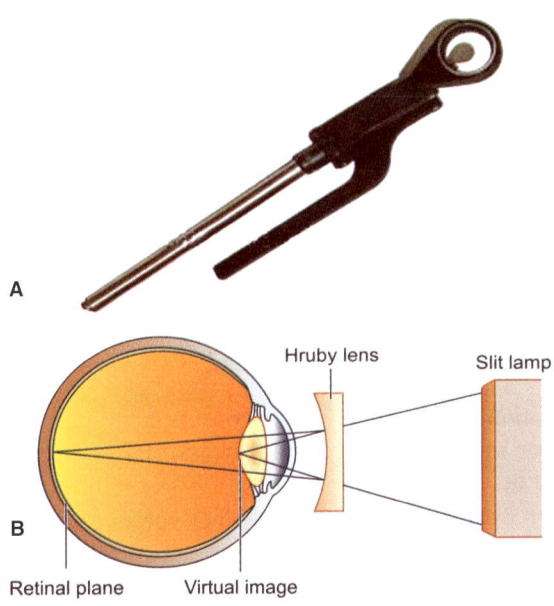

Fig. 4.20: *(A) Hruby lens; and (B) optics of Hruby lens.*

2. CONTACT LENS BIOMICROSCOPY OF FUNDUS

Contact lens biomicroscopy combines stereopsis, high illumination and high magnification with the advantages of slit-beam. Following lenses are available for contact lens biomicroscopy of the fundus.

Modified Koeppe lens examination

Modified Koeppe lens, i.e. posterior fundus contact lens (Fig. 4.21A) can be used to examine the posterior segment. It provides a virtual and erect image (Fig. 4.21B).

Goldmann's three-mirror contact lens examination

Goldmann's three-mirror contact lens (Fig. 4.21C) consists of a central contact lens and three mirrors placed in the cone, each with different angles of inclination. With this, the central as well as peripheral parts of the fundus

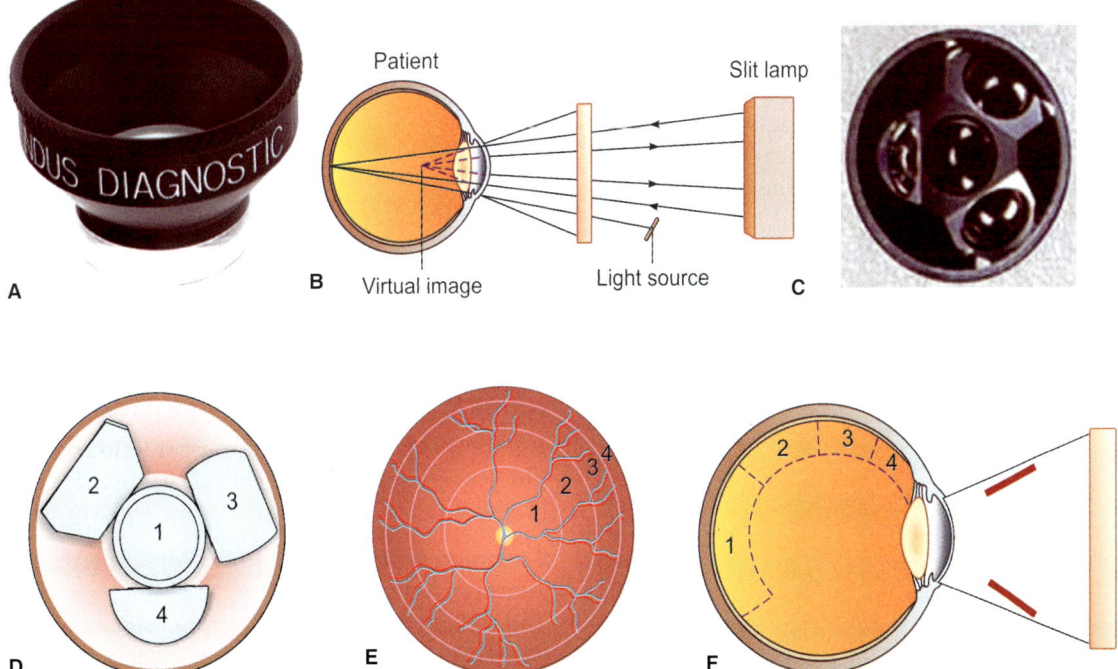

Fig. 4.21 *Contact lenses for biomicroscopy of fundus: (A) Modified Koeppe lens; (B) optics of contact lens biomicroscopy; (C) Goldmann's three-mirror contact lens; (D) front view of the Goldmann's three-mirror lens with its four optical surfaces (1, for central posterior pole; 2, for equatorial area; 3, for anterior peripheral fundus; 4, for ora serrata and pars plana); (E) diagrammatic projection of viewing range for each component of Goldmann lens; and (F) panoramic diagram of specific viewing range for each lens component.*

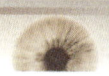

can be visualized. It also provides a virtual and erect image (Fig. 4.21B).

Technique

- Dilate the pupils as for indirect ophthalmoscopy.
- Instill topical anaesthetic drops.
- Insert coupling fluid into the cup of the contact lens, but do not overfill.
- Ask the patient to look up, insert the inferior rim of the lens into the lower fornix and press it quickly against the cornea.
- Always tilt the illumination column except when viewing the 12 o'clock position in the fundus (i.e. with the mirror at 6 o'clock).
- When viewing the different positions of the peripheral retina, rotate the axis of the beam so that it is always at right angles to the mirror.
- To visualize the entire fundus, rotate the lens for 3608 using the 59, 67 and 738 tilted mirrors to give views of the peripheral retina, the equatorial fundus and the area around the posterior pole, respectively (Fig. 4.21D to F).
- To obtain a more peripheral view of the retina, tilt the lens to the opposite side and ask the patient to move the eyes to the same side. For example, to obtain a more peripheral view of 12 o'clock position (with mirror at 6 o'clock), tilt the lens down and ask the patient to look up.
- Examine the vitreous cavity with the central lens, using a horizontal and a vertical slit-beam, and then examine the posterior pole.

Note. Since examination with contact lens biomicroscopy involves anaesthetising the cornea and a direct touch, so it is neither liked much by the patients nor by the examiners. Therefore, presently, fundus contact lenses are primarily used for therapeutic purposes (retinal photocoagulation, etc.) and not for diagnostic purposes except for certain special circumstances. Nowadays examination with fundus non-contact lenses is being preferred for diagnostic purposes.

Wide-field (panfundoscopic) indirect contact

Wide-field (panfundoscopic) indirect contact lenses with a field of view up to 1308 are available for fundus examination and for performing laser photocoagulation. The image produced by such lens is inverted.

■ 3. INDIRECT FUNDUS BIOMICROSCOPY

Indirect fundus biomicroscopy, also known as non-contact fundus biomicroscopy, has become quite popular in the last decade or so—to the extent that it has become an integral part of routine eye examination. As mentioned earlier, the non-contact lenses have replaced the contact lenses for diagnostic purposes.

Fundus non-contact lenses most commonly used for indirect slit-lamp biomicroscopy are 78 D (Fig. 4.22A) and 90 D (Fig. 4.22B), but other lenses are also available (60 D, 130 D, etc.). Almost all condensing lenses used with slit-lamp are double-aspheric lenses, so it does not matter which side is held towards the patient.

Optics of indirect fundus biomicroscopy is exactly similar to that of indirect ophthalmoscopy (*see* page 72, Fig. 4.8A). Thus, a real, inverted image is formed between the condensing lens and objective lens of slit-lamp.

Magnification provided by fundus non-contact lenses is calculated by dividing power of the eye by the power of lens. For example, 90D lens provides a magnification of 60/90 = 0.66, i.e. a minification of the image. However, the magnified image is seen because of the magnification provided by the slit-lamp. Thus, 7.5X magnification seen with 90D lens (Table 4.1) is due to 10X of slit-lamp.

Field of view. High-powered lens provides larger field of view but lesser magnification, e.g. the 190 D lens provides bigger field of view but gives lesser magnification than 178D lens (Table 4.1).

Technique of indirect fundus biomicroscopy is summarized follow (Fig. 4.22C):
Tell patient about the procedure. Make patient comfortable on slit-lamp. A quick look at anterior segment is a must before any fundus examination as it could give additional information many a times. Illumination system and microscope are preferably in click position or full alignment. Adjust slit-lamp at magnification

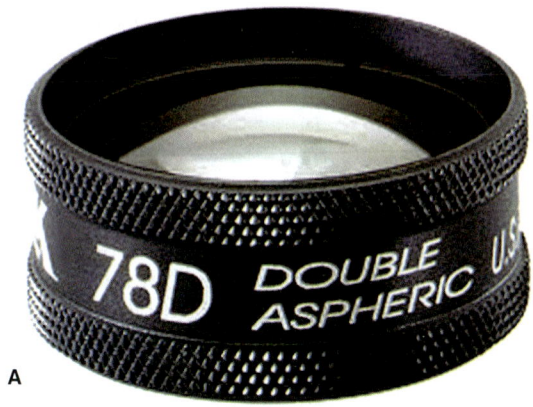

A

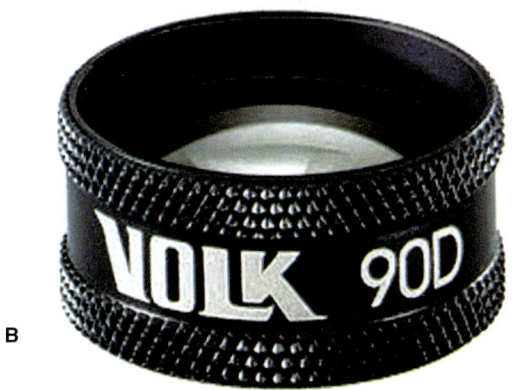

B

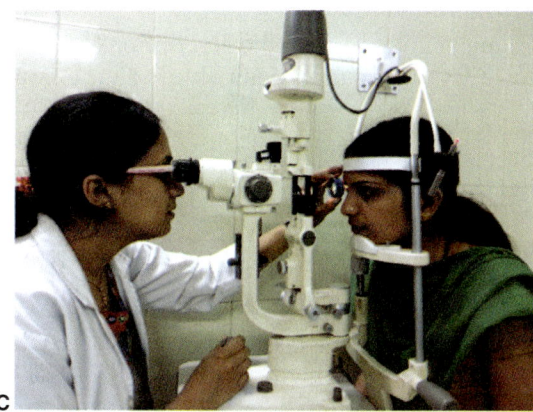

C

Fig. 4.22: *Indirect fundus biomicroscopy: (A) 78 D lens; (B) 90 D lens; and (C) technique of examination.*

stabilize the hand on the forehead band of the slit-lamp. Now pull slit-lamp backwards by approximately 2 inches. There is no correct direction for holding the lenses due to the aspheric nature of these lenses; either side can face the patient. Before seeing the retina vitreous must also be studied as important information can be got from it. Align the image in the center of the lens. As the image is inverted tell the patient to look in the direction opposite to the part of image what you want to view (Fig. 4.23).

Like slit-lamp biomicroscopy we can examine a lesion by direct illumination on the lesion, indirect illumination adjacent to lesion and retroillumination from reflected light from within the lesion. The contours of chorioretinal lesions are more apparent with narrow beam projected onto the lesion's surface. The contour of the thin slit gives us clue to elevation or depression for subtle lesions in addition to stereopsis (Fig. 4.24).

Start the fundus examination from the peripheral fundus to ensure patient cooperation. Inferior most part of lens corresponds to anterior most part of superior fundus. Hold the lens with index finger and thumb while the middle or ring finger is used to retract the upper lid. The suggested protocol for sequence of examination (1 to 7) of fundus is shown in Fig. 4.25. For documentation the easy way is to reverse the file and draw as you see.

To deal with reflection in line of sight we can tilt lens slightly, rotate lens around rotational

of 10X, low illumination and slit width of 2–3 mm. Give fixed target to the patient (e.g. examiner's ear for other eye). Focus slit-lamp on cornea, introduce the lens into the beam illuminating the patients eye by holding it in forefinger and thumb, using middle finger to widely open the upper lid of patient's eye or to

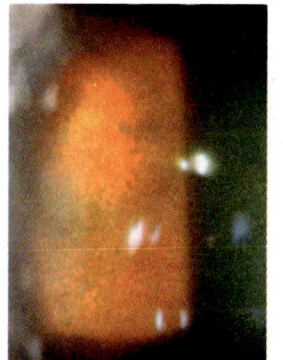

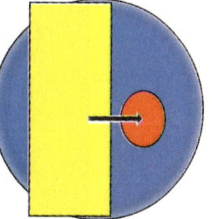

To view the disc on the right side of the examiner in this frame, we ask the patient to move the eye to the left side of the examiner ⬅

Fig. 4.23 *Align image in center of lens and to view that part of image which is not in field the patient is asked to move eye in opposite direction.*

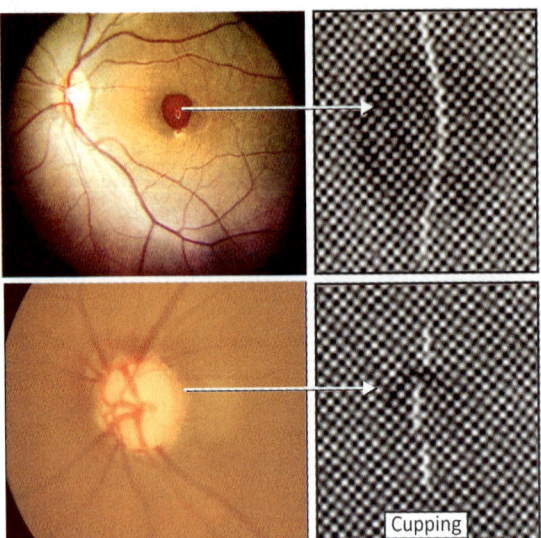

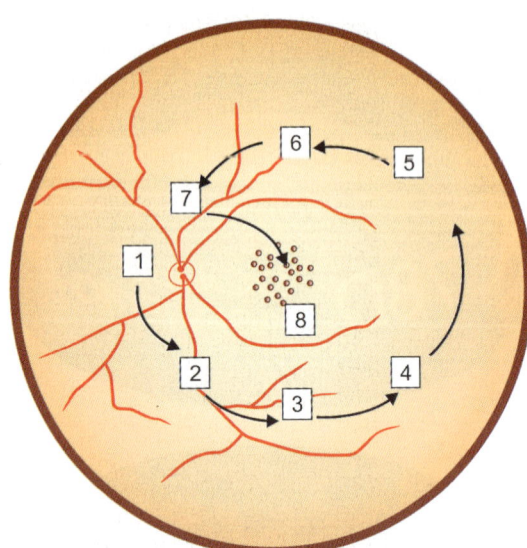

Fig. 4.24 *Kinking of narrow slit on retina helps to identify subtle contour changes in fundus.*

Fig. 4.25 *Suggested protocol for sequence of examination of fundus.*

axis, get illumination system slightly out of click position and further dilate the pupil (Fig. 4.26).

Certain tests like Watzke Allen sign are diagnostic for macular hole. We shine the slit of light on the hole and the patient sees kinking of slit or breaking of slit in center (Fig. 4.27).

The yellow tint lenses are also available and these filter the wavelengths below 480 nm, enhancing patient comfort and acceptance. The yellow tint may cause a slight colour shift in the appearance of the retina which could cause misinterpretation of optic nerve pallor and makes detection of the macular edema more difficult.

Interpretation

Of major importance is the description of fundus lesions, which includes colour, shape, size,

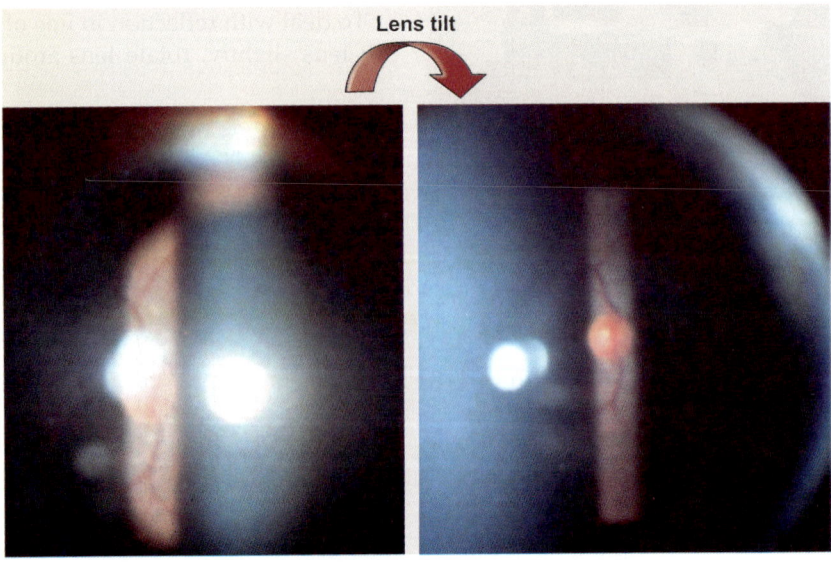

Fig. 4.26: *Demonstrating that mild lens tilt could take care of reflections causing problem in retinal examination.*

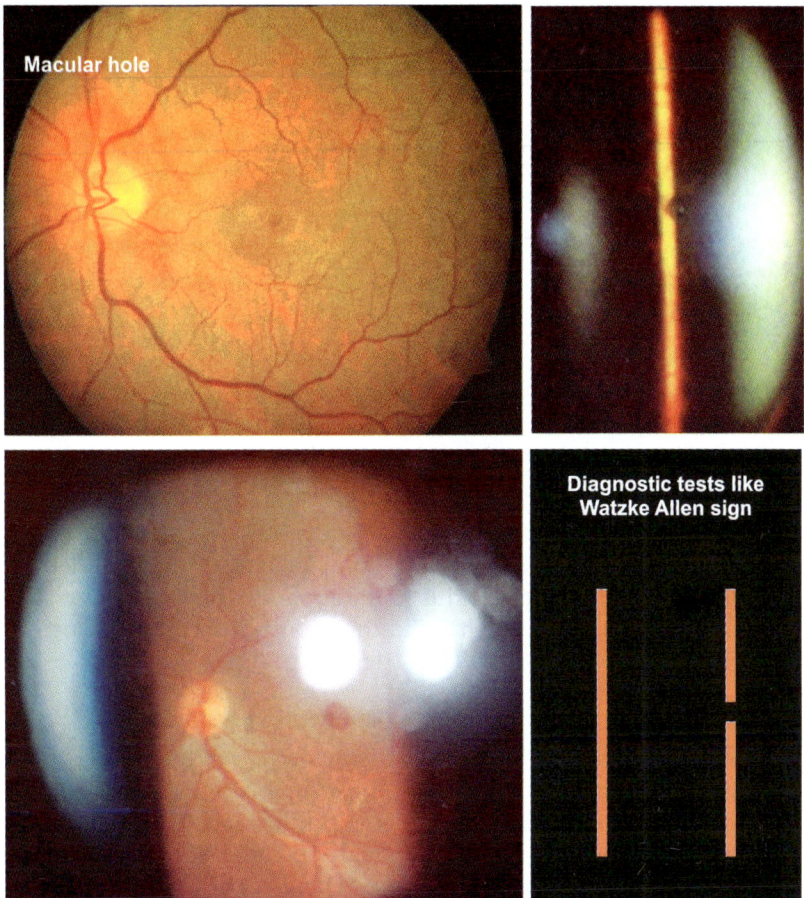

Fig. 4.27 *Watzke Allen sign in a case of macular hole could be diagnostic. The patient might identify a kink or break in continuity of the slit of light projected in the region of macular hole*

elevation, and location. Size estimation of a lesion is usually accomplished by comparing it with a structure of known dimensions, such as the optic disc.

Most fundus lesions are described relative to disc diameters (DDs) in size (e.g. a choroid nevus is "2 DDs by 3 DDs"). This is often done by viewing the optic disc first and then quickly relocating the lesion and comparing the two. Since, the horizontal diameter of a normal optic disc is 1.5 mm, it is possible to translate DDs into millimetres. For future comparison, the size of a lesion can also be compared with the reticle dimensions in direct ophthalmoscope projected on the fundus.

USES OF DIFFERENT FUNDUS EXAMINATION LENSES

Uses of different fundus examination lenses are summarised in Table 4.4.

FUNDUS CAMERA

OPTICAL PRINCIPLE

All fundus cameras are technically indirect ophthalmoscopes, and currently they are all based upon the principles of Gullstrand's ophthalmoscope. That is, the illumination and observation pathways pass through different portions of the patient's pupil to avoid reflections from the cornea and from the surfaces

Lens	To view and laser	Image	Relative mag	Spot mag	Field view
Goldman	Macula equator periphery	Virtual erect	1.00	1.08	36°
Volk area centralis	Macula equator	Real inverted	1.13	0.95	82°
Mainster standard	Macula equator	Real inverted	1.03	1.05	90°
Mainster widefield	Equator periphery	Real inverted	0.73	1.47	125°
Volk quardr Aspheric	Equator periphery	Real inverted	0.56	1.82	130°
Volk superquad	Equator periphery	Real inverted	0.56	1.92	160°
Panfundoscope	Equator periphery	Real inverted	0.76	1.41	120°

Table 4.4 *Uses of different fundus examination lenses*

of the crystalline lens. Also, an inverted aerial image of the fundus is formed within the fundus camera, and this aerial image, in turn, is reimaged onto the film plane.

OPTICAL SYSTEM

The optical system of the fundus camera thus consists of two major components: the illumination system and the observation and photography system. Each of these components occupies its own independent pathway within the apparatus and shares with the other only one common point, the front or ophthalmoscopic lens (Fig. 4.28).

Illumination system

The fundus cameras employ two light sources: a low-intensity incandescent lamp for viewing the fundus and focusing the instrument and a high-powered electronic flashtube for taking the

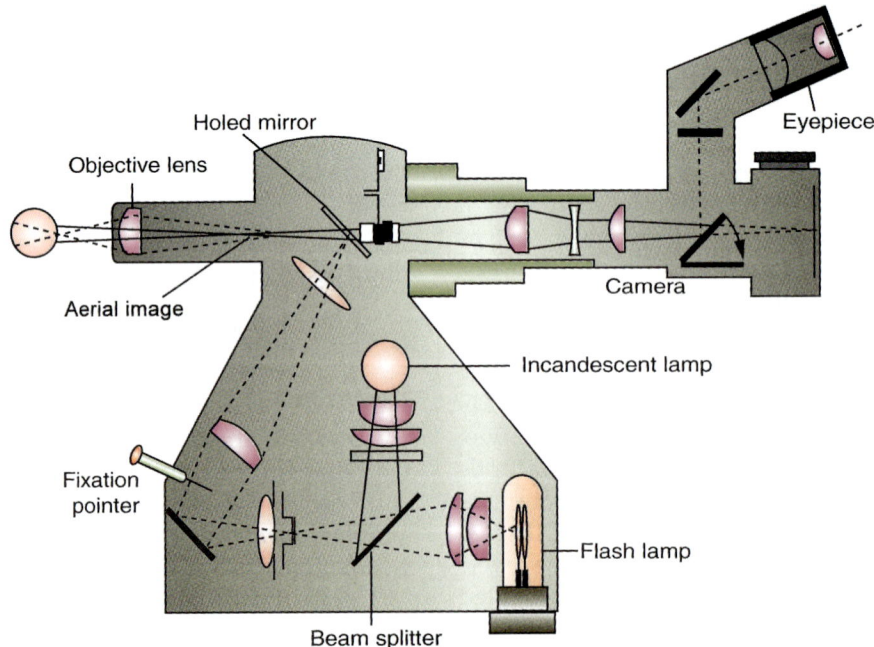

Fig. 4.28: *Schematic view of the Zeiss fundus camera to show outlines of the optical system.*

photograph. In the Zeiss fundus camera, these two light sources are optically combined through the semireflecting surface (Fig. 4.28). In most of the other commercially available fundus cameras, the incandescent lamp and electronic flashtube are mounted onto a common base, and a transillumination method is used to combine the pathway of the two lights.

From this point onwards, the light from two light sources following a common pathway passes through a diaphragm, the adjustment of which controls the size of illuminated patch upon the patient's retina. This diaphragm is imaged at the surface of a holed mirror, which is itself imaged by the ophthalmoscopic lens in the plane of the patient's pupil. These two optical elements confine the illuminating beam to an annulus (a ring of light), the width of which is controlled by the diaphragm.

Observation and photographic system

The holed mirror, which is imaged by the ophthalmoscope lens in the plane of the patient's pupil, forms the entrance pupil of the viewing system. It confines the viewing beam to central region of the pupil. It also confines the illuminating beam to an annulus that surrounds the viewing beam. The illuminating and viewing paths are, therefore, separated in the plane of the patient's pupil, thereby making the instrument reflex-free.

The ophthalmoscopic lens produces an image of the fundus between the holed mirror and the ophthalmoscopic lens. This image is viewed through the hole with a compound microscope. The objective of this microscope forms an image of the fundus, via a flip mirror, upon the ground glass screen that is placed at the focal point of the viewing eyepiece. When the photograph is taken, the flip mirror that diverts the image into the eyepiece for observation swings out of the optical pathway, thus permitting the image to be projected on to the film for photography (Fig 4.28).

The photographic component of the early instruments consisted of a small film carrier and a shutter mechanism. However, with the advent of fluorescein angiography, the simple film carrier has been replaced by a sophisticated, electronic motorized 35 mm camera system.

MODIFICATIONS IN FUNDUS CAMERA

1. *Fluorescein angiography system.* Fundus cameras have been modified for fluorescein angiography by addition of appropriate filters in the illumination and observation pathways (Fig. 4.29). Special power supplies are necessary to allow multiple exposures per second.

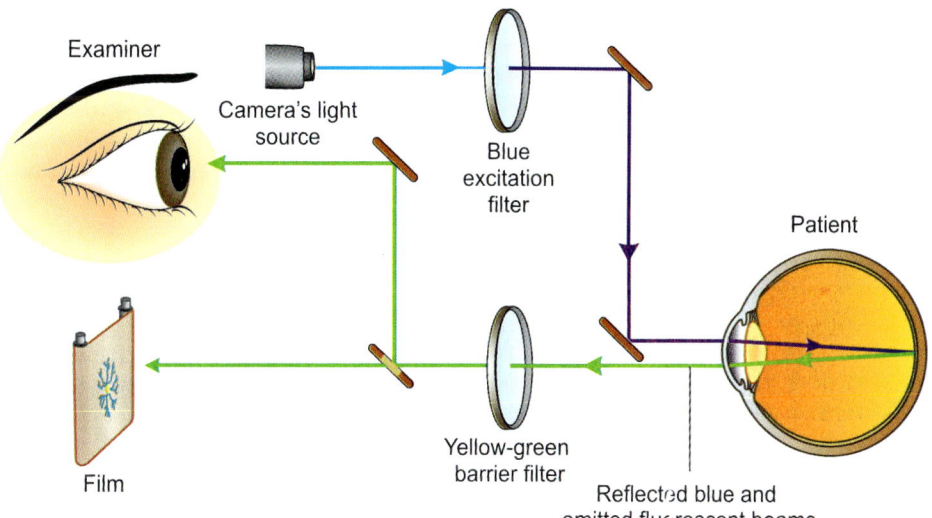

Fig. 4.29: Blue excitation filter in the fundus camera produces blue light, which excites the unbound fluorescein molecules. The reflected blue light is absorbed by the yellow-green filter allowing only the fluoresceing particles to be recorded on the film.

2. *Digital fluorescein angiography system*. Recently, digital fluorescein angiography (DFA) is being used increasingly. The DFA system uses a CCD detector in the camera in place of a film. One of the commercially available digital fluorescein angiography system manufactured is shown in Fig. 4.30.

Advantages of DFA

- The images can be instantaneously viewed on a high-resolution monitor. This allows the observer to manipulate the parameters (e.g. light intensity, centration of photography) while the study is in progress to obtain the optimum image.
- The images are recorded either on a computer hard drive or CD-ROM. The electronic recording allows immediate viewing of images and permits prompt management of the disease process.
- The angiograms can be electronically transmitted or printed form the digital data.

Disadvantage of DFA

The quality of the DFA is inferior to the film-based photographs; however, it is adequate for clinical purposes.

3. *Wide-field digital fundus fluorescein angiography* has also been introduced, specially for use in children.

4. *Non-mydriatic fundus cameras*. These use infrared light and semi-automatic or automatic focusing systems to allow fundus photography without dilating drops. The infrared light is invisible to the patient, and the pupil dilates physiologically. After alignment and focusing are completed, the white light flash is triggered, and the photograph is taken before the pupil has a chance to constrict.

5. *Wide-angle fundus cameras* up to 608 have appeared, having large diameter and aspheric objective lenses. Wide-angle photographs even up to 1488 are possible, but a contact type of objective lens and special illumination system are necessary for such photographs.

6. *Television ophthalmoscopy.* Several attempts at television ophthalmoscopy have been made, using fundus camera optics. In general, excessive illumination is required, and resolution is poor.

7. *Scanning laser ophthalmoscopy.* A promising new system is the SLO, where only a single spot of laser light is scanned over the fundus, with each point being recorded as it is illuminated. The primary advantage of this system is the extremely low level of total light required. (For details *see* page 74).

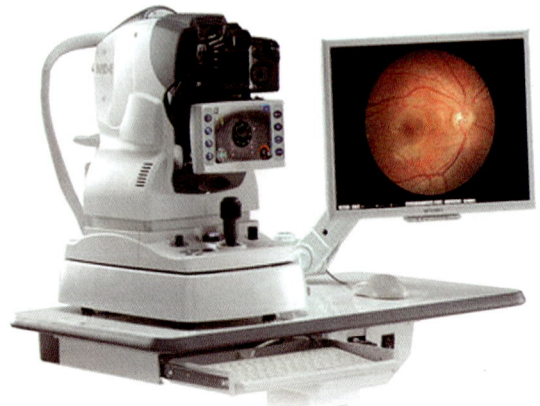

Fig. 4.30: *Digital fluorescein angiography system.*

WIDE-FIELD RETINAL IMAGING SYSTEMS

Wide-field retinal imaging systems have been developed with the capability of capturing up to 2008 field of view with one picture as compared to only 30–608 field of view with current standard fundus photography system. The salient features of the following three commercially available wide-field retinal imaging systems are described here in brief:

- Retcam II and III
- Panoret 1000AA
- Panoramic 200

RETCAM II AND III

Retcam II (Retinal camera II) is the advanced version of Retcam 120 (manufactured by Massie Research Lab., Dublin, CA).

Components of Retcam II. It is a mobile wide-field digital imaging system comprising following major components (Fig. 4.31):

- *Three-chip CCD medical grade digital video cameras* is the heart of Retcam II. It is

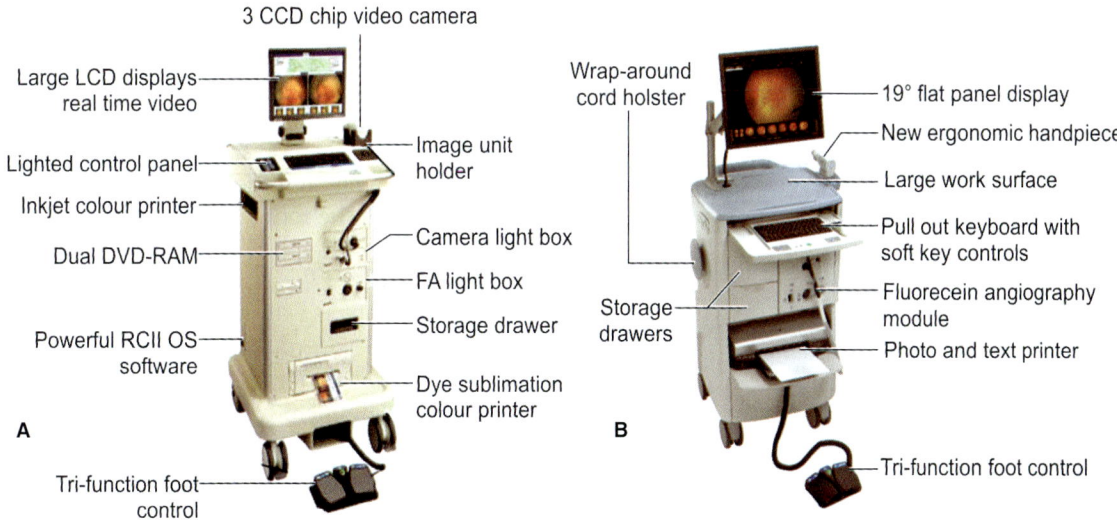

Fig. 4.31: *(A) Retcam II, the wide-field retinal imaging system; and (B) Retcam III.*

lightweight (so easy to position) and is attached to the light source and image capture unit.

- *Hand-held image capture unit* is attached with the camera by a long cable for easy patient access.
- *High-index corneal contact lenses* form the essential part of the image-capturing unit. These lenses allow capturing of oblique rays emerging from the peripheral retina. The changeable lenses (nose pieces) available to be attached to the image-capturing unit of Retcam II are as follows (Fig. 4.32):

ROP (retinopathy of prematurity) lens, for premature infants which allows 1308 field of view.

Standard children lens, a 1208 field-of-view lens for pediatric to young adult patients.

High magnification lenses, a 308 field-of-view lens for fine details.

808 *lens* for higher contrast pediatric and adult imaging.

Portrait lens or external lens for area or external imaging.

- *Image processing unit*, comprises a Windows or T computer system which gets the information from the camera. This unit is equipped with a new multipurpose software.
- *Flat LCD colour display* on 17 inch monitor allows the images to be viewed in real-time motion during acquisition.

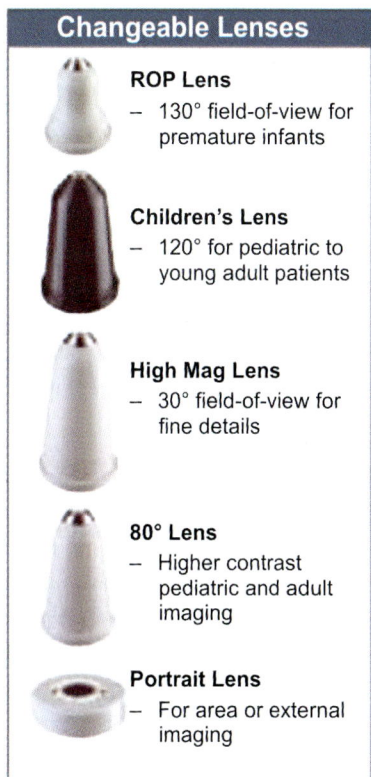

Changeable Lenses

ROP Lens
- 130° field-of-view for premature infants

Children's Lens
- 120° for pediatric to young adult patients

High Mag Lens
- 30° field-of-view for fine details

80° Lens
- Higher contrast pediatric and adult imaging

Portrait Lens
- For area or external imaging

Fig. 4.32: *Changeable high-index lens available for attaching with image-capturing unit of Retcam II.*

- *Tri-function foot control* connected to the camera controls image focus, illumination and capture.

Special features of Retcam II

- *Cone-shaped lens* provided with it is very handy to hold while scanning the retina.
- *Wide, 130 and 120°, real-time image* of the fundus is particularly useful in diagnosis and documentation of diseases such as retinoblastoma and ROP.
- *Images are stored in digital format*, thus are retrievable easily.
- *Camera has a large storage device* with good facility of transferring the images in other media like CD, USB and in other DVD device. The data can be shared with others for seeking an opinion.
- *Comprehensive database* keeps track of each imaging section for the patients, allowing for later or side by side review of the cases. This is particularly useful in assessing response to treatment as in chemoreduction for retinoblastoma and laser photocoagulation for ROP.
- *Fluorescein angiography can also be performed with it.* It is another major feature of this equipment. It is provided with a barrier filter, which helps to take the angiogram by still mode and continuous video for 20 seconds.
- In-built colour printer allows the print images and the detailed case report of the patient.

Features of Retcam III

Additional features of Retcam III (Fig. 4.31B) are summarized below.

Procedure

It involves following steps:
- *Pupils* are dilated fully.
- *Anaesthesia*. Neonates and infants can be easily examined under topical anaesthesia achieved with proparacaine eyedrops. Older children may be given short-term sedation for the procedure.
- *Separation of lids* is done with the help of a pediatric lid speculum, after placing the patient in supine position.
- *Fixation of the head* is then achieved.
- *Coupling solution* like methylcellulose gel is applied to the cornea.
- *Image capture unit* with desired lens is then positioned with gentle contact to the anterior

corneal surface. Illumination and focus are controlled by the operator with the foot switch. Often a quick scan of the entire retina can be performed in live video motion before acquisition of images. Once the desired field of view has been identified, the images can be captured with the foot switch control.

Limitations of retcam

- *Pupillary dilation* is extremely important for it, so not useful where pupillary dilation is a problem.
- *Other limitations* include need for camera lens–cornea contact, need for eyelid speculum and technical limitations of the camera.
- *Lack of stereopsis* and some loss of magnification of retinal field in exchange for a wide-angle field of view may also be seen as a limitation.
- *Cannot be used in adults* because with lens opacities that begin in adolescence and accumulate with age, the entering light is scattered more widely, causing decreased contrast sensitivity.

Advantages

- *Mobile, self-contained system* for use in nursery, ICU, operating rooms, etc.
- *Easy to use*—even technicians or nurses can operate.
- *Avoids stress and expertise* of indirect ophthalmoscopy and scleral indentation.
- *Interobserver variability* is eliminated.
- *Teaching tool for students*, and parents can be counselled.
- *Easy case management* with access to images, video clips, patient data, instant retrieval and side by side comparison.

Applications of wide-field imaging system

- *Paediatric retinal disorders* can be easily diagnosed, followed and objectively documented. Especially useful in ROP, retinoblastoma, shaken baby syndrome.
- *Pediatric anterior segment imaging*, gonioimaging for glaucomatous damage, iris lesions.
- *Fluorescein angiography* can also be performed with advances in the technique.

PANORET 1000 AA

Principle

This wide-field imaging system employs the principles of trans-scleral illumination propagated by Pomerantzeff.

Advantages

Because a trans-scleral light source provides diffuse illumination, so this system:
- Can be used in the presence of media opacities
- Can be used in cases where pupillary dilation is a problem
- Can also be used in adults
- Both fluorescein angiography and indocyanine green angiography can also be performed.

Limitations

- Patients with heavily pigmented uvea are not well-imaged.
- Since, it is introduced recently, so there is limited clinical experience with its use.

PANORAMIC 200 NON-MYDRIATIC SLO

Principle

It is a non-contact non-mydriatic system-based on the use of both a green (532 nm) and red (633 nm) laser to produce a digital image of 2000 by 2000 pixels. The resolution of image ranges from 20 to 40 m per pixel.

Applications

It is often used as a screening tool for diabetic retinopathy, age-related macular degeneration (ARMD) and glaucomatous disc changes.

Advantages

Field of view is 2008 in a single image.

Limitations

Being a table-mounted non-mobile unit, it cannot be used in small children and uncooperative patients.

LASER SCANNING IMAGING TECHNIQUES

- Scanning laser ophthalmoscopy
- Confocal scanning laser ophthalmoscopy
- Retinal thickness analyser
- Scanning laser polarimetry

SCANNING LASER OPHTHALMOSCOPY (SLO)

The scanning laser ophthalmoscopy was invented by Webb, Pomerantzeff and Hughes in 1979. The word scanning here refers to the illumination system, which samples the retina point by point rather than capturing the image as a whole, as is done with a conventional fundus camera.

Principle

The SLO operates essentially as an inverted indirect ophthalmoscope. This means that a small illumination aperture is used to illuminate the eye while a large viewing aperture collects all the light emitted by the eye (Fig. 4.33). The small aperture creates a very narrow moving beam of light which can bypass most ocular media opacities (i.e. corneal scars, cataracts, vitreous hemorrhage) to reach the surface of the retina and record its surface detail. A live video image of the retina is displayed on a computer monitor and test results are digitally recorded (Fig. 4.34).

Applications of SLO

1. *Scanning laser acuity potential test.* The letter E corresponding to different levels of visual acuity (ranging from 20/1000 to 20/60) is projected directly on the patient's retina. The examiner can direct the test letters to foveal and/or extrafoveal location within the macula and determine a subject's potential visual acuity.

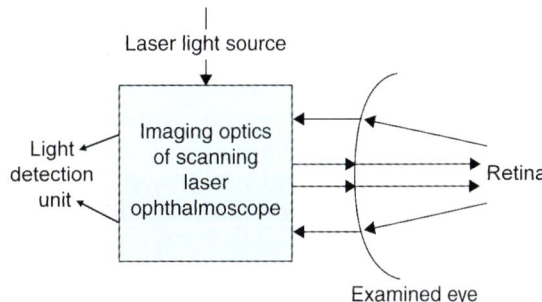

Fig. 4.33: *Optics of scanning laser ophthalmoscope as inverted indirect ophthalmoscope. Note that the light enters the eye through a small illumination aperture and the returned light is collected over a large viewing aperture.*

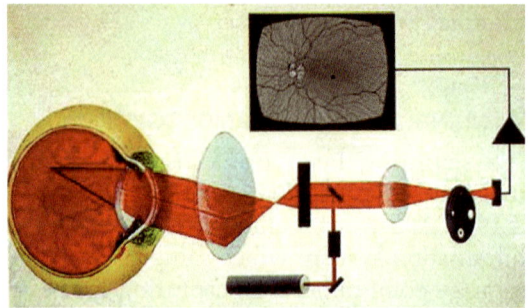

Fig. 4.34: *Optical path of recording of scanning laser ophthalmoscope (SLO).*

This may be especially helpful in individuals who have lost central fixation but who may still possess significant eccentric vision. It is also useful in separating out the component of retinal function from anterior segment contributions to overall visual dysfunction when contemplating surgical interventions.

2. *Microperimetry/scotometry.* The SLO can visualize a particular area of the retina and test its sensitivity to visual stimuli, thereby generating a map of the seeing and non-seeing areas. If central vision is lost, the patient can potentially be trained to use an adjacent retinal site to substitute for central visual function.

3. *Hi-Speed FA/ICG.* Fluorescein and indocyanine green angiography (FA/ICG) performed using the SLO is recorded at 30 images per second, producing a real-time video sequence of the ocular blood flow. The standard fundus camera sequence is limited by flash recycling to one to two frames per second, and is unreliable in its ability to document details of choroidal filling which occurs over a 1–2-second span of time.

The higher speed of image acquisition more completely captures the chorioretinal filling sequence, and can be used to accurately identify the choroidal feeder vessels of neovascular membranes. Guided by high-speed FA/ICG results, laser treatment of sight-threatening diseases like exudative ARMD can be carried out with pinpoint accuracy.

SLO versus conventional fundus camera

1. SLO samples the retina point by point while the fundus camera captures the image as a whole.

2. In SLO, a single point on retina is illuminated for less than 1,000,000th of a second while the conventional fundus camera illuminates the eye for several milliseconds during flash capture.

3. The SLO captures a temporal image while conventional fundus camera captures a spatial image.

4. In SLO, light source is always laser, so it can achieve white light imaging comparable to conventional white light fundus photography.

Advantages of SLO over conventional fundus camera

- Low light level
- Highly light efficient
- Continuous imaging
- Large depth of field
- Instantaneous image availability for review
- The high capture speed allows dynamic image studies such as blood flow
- Allows excellent imaging even in the presence of media opacities.

CONFOCAL SCANNING LASER OPHTHALMOSCOPY

The confocal scanning laser ophthalmoscopy, or CSLO, also known as scanning laser tomography, or SLT, was introduced by Webb and associates in 1987. The term *confocal* has been derived by combining the terms *conjugate* and *focal*, and it describes that the locations of the focal plane in the retina and the focal plane in the image sensor are located in conjugate positions. Confocality of the system is achieved by placing a pinhole in front of the detector, which is conjugate to the laser focus (Fig. 4.35). The size of the pinhole determines the degree of confocality, such that a small pinhole aperture will give a highly confocal image. Commercially available CSLOs include:

- Heidelberg Retina Tomography (HRT)
- Top SS

HEIDELBERG RETINA TOMOGRAPHY

Heidelberg retina tomography (HRT), the most popular instrument, is available in two models–the HRT I (introduced in November 1991) and

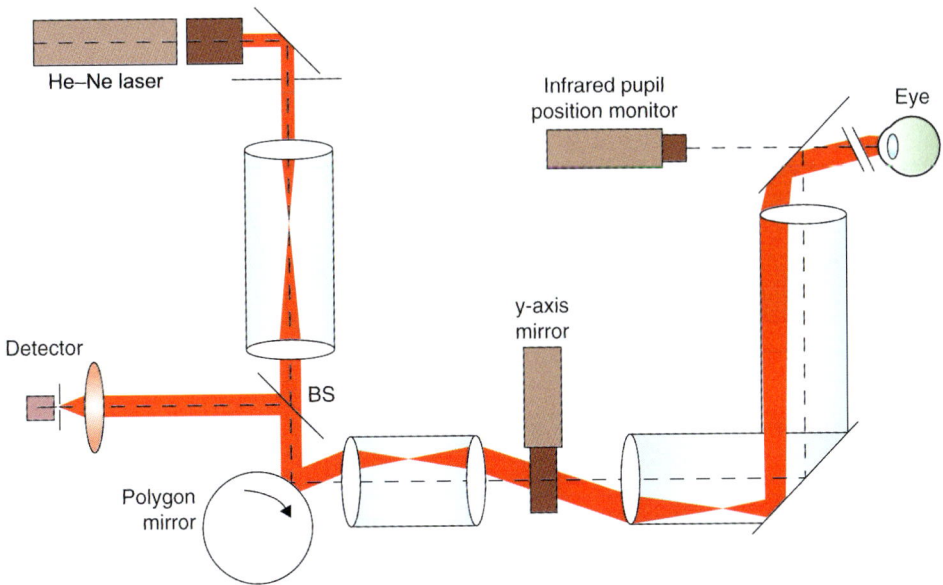

Fig. 4.35: *Optics of confocal scanning laser ophthalmoscope (CSLO).*

the HRT II C (introduced in April 1999). For both the models, the laser source is a *helium–neon diode laser* of wavelength 670 nm. The laser raster scans the x–y plane to obtain confocal optical sections of the retina. Once one plane has been scanned, the laser changes focus to scan a slightly deeper plane of the retina. This continues until a series of confocal optical sections through the depth of the fundus are obtained.

INSTRUMENT PROFILE

The instrument is small, light, portable and is table-mounted along with a notebook computer (Fig. 4.36). Press of signal button acquires optical section images within 32 milliseconds and with a repetition rate of 20 Hz two-dimensional. From the images obtained in this pre-scan of 4–6 mm depth, the software computes and automatically sets the correct location of the focal plane, the required scan depth for that eye and the proper sensitivity to obtain images with correct brightness. The Heidelberg retinal tomograph operation software automatically defines a reference plane for each individual eye. The reference plane is defined parallel to the peripapillary retinal surface and is located 50 m posteriorly to the retinal surface at the papillomacular bundle. The reason for this

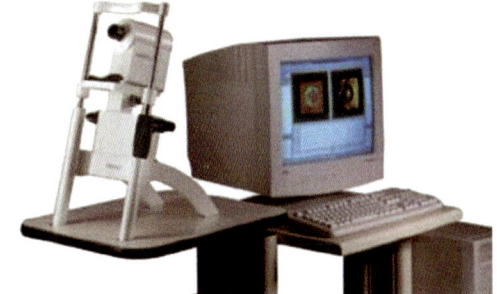

Fig. 4.36 *The Heidelberg retinal tomograph II.*

definition is that during development of glaucoma the nerve fibers at the papillomacular bundle remain intact longest and the nerve fiber layer thickness at that location is approximately 50 m. We can, therefore, assume to have a stable reference plane located just beneath the nerve fiber layer. All structures located below the reference plane are considered to be cup; all structures located above the reference plane and within the contour line are considered to be the rim.

ACQUISITION AND GENERATION OF TOPOGRAPHY IMAGE

HRT I

Image acquisition. The HRT I makes *32 scans through the retina resulting in a stack of optical*

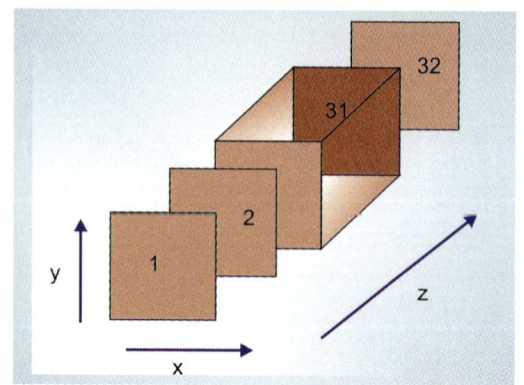

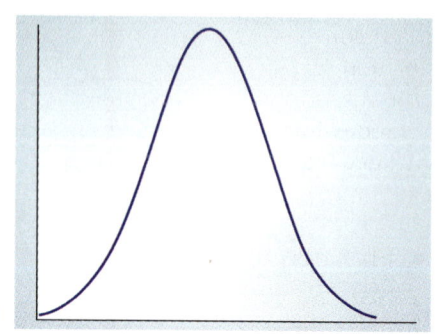

Fig. 4.37: *HRT I-image acquisition: (A) A stack of 32 image series; and (B) z-profile of pixel (x, y) in image series.*

sections which represent both an area (x–y) and depth (z) image of the retinal structure under investigation (Figs 4.37 and 4.38A). The field of view can be set to three levels—108 × 108, 158 × 158 or 208 × 208. The depth to which the laser scans varies between 0.5 and 4.0 mm in 0.5 mm steps. Thirty-two optical sections are generated at all of these depth levels, so the spacing between sections is closer at the lower depth levels and greater at the higher depth levels. The camera must be placed 15 mm from the examined eye, and the operator centers the optic disc on the monitor. The HRT I software has a quality control mechanism which informs the operator whether the image series is of good quality. Changes in focus and depth setting are advised until the series acquired is optimum. However, the operator has to examine the image series to establish whether there are any image-distorting eye movements. In such cases, the series have to be rejected. Generally, three optimum image series are obtained for each eye under examination (Fig. 4.38B). The topography images are then generated (Fig. 4.38C).

Generation of the topography image. Each confocal section of the 32-image series consists of 256 × 256 pixels. Each pixel location (x, y) has a varying brightness through the series. The distribution of reflected light intensity of each pixel through the 32 series is called the z-profile (Fig. 4.37). The z-profile is a symmetric distribution with a maximum at the location of the light-reflecting surface. By determining the position

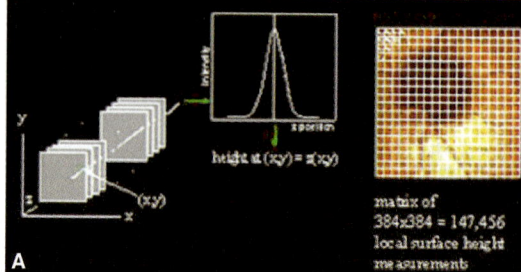

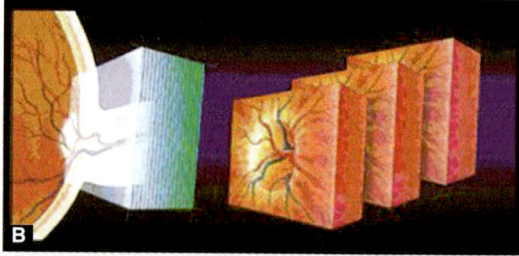

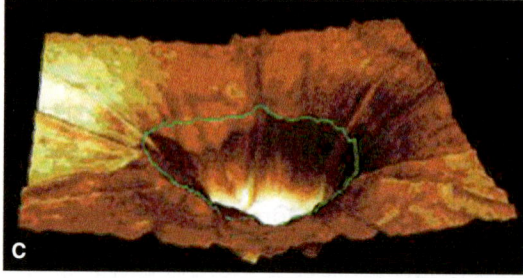

Fig. 4.38 *Principle of scanning laser tomography–concept of 3-D image composition based on 32 confocal sections: (A) A stack of 32 confocal sections (the software aligns the images but only compensates for small eye movements) the axial intensity distribution for each of the 256 × 256 pixels is plotted and the axial location of the maximum is coded into a 2-D image with 256 × 256 pixels; (B) Three separate image series acquired; and (C) 3-D image of optic nerve head.*

of the profile maximum, the height of each pixel can be determined (Fig. 4.38). The topography map is a colour-coded representation of each pixel position within the 32 series. Each of the 32 confocal sections has been designated an arbitrary red value. Section 1 is dark red, section 32 is saturated white and the sections in between decrease in redness from 1 down to 32 in equal steps.

Alongside the topography image is a reflectivity image, which gives the most visual information about the optic disc under examination similar to a fundus photo (Fig. 4.37).

HRT II

Image acquisition. The HRT II differs quite considerably from the HRT I. There is one field of view (158), and each optical section has a resolution of 384 × 384 pixels. In contrast to the HRT I, which can be used for the acquisition of both optic nerve head (ONH) and macular images, the HRT II has been designed specifically for the grabbing of ONH images alone.

In image acquisition, the operator enters the patient's details and a rough setting of the examined eye's refraction. The patient is instructed to look at an internal fixation light, which results in an automatic centration of the ONH on the monitor. The acquisition button is activated, and the CSLO proceeds with image acquisition.

An automatic pre-scan with 4–6 mm depth is performed, and from the images obtained from this pre-scan, the software computes and automatically sets the correct location of the focal plane—the required scan depth for that eye and the sensitivity to obtain images with correct brightness. Following this, the system automatically acquires three image series with the predetermined acquisition parameters. The number of image planes acquired per series depends on the required scan depth – 16 images per millimetre scan depth are acquired. There is an automatic quality control during image acquisition, and so if one or more of the acquired image series cannot be used for any reason, additional images are acquired automatically until three good quality image series have been obtained. After image acquisition, the images are

saved on the hard disc and the three topography images and the mean topography image are computed automatically.

This semi-automated image acquisition of the HRT II means that in busy practice situations, staff with minimal experience of using the instrument should be able to acquire images.

IMAGE ANALYSIS AND EXAMINATION OF RESULTS

I. SLT in glaucoma

The applications of SLT in glaucoma are:

1. *Initial examination to discriminate between the normal eyes, glaucoma suspects and glaucomatous eyes*

The printout of initial report has following details (Fig. 4.39).

Topography and reflectivity image. As described earlier (Fig. 4.37), the topography image is a colour-coded map. The red areas are on the surface and the white areas are deeper in the scan (Fig. 4.39).

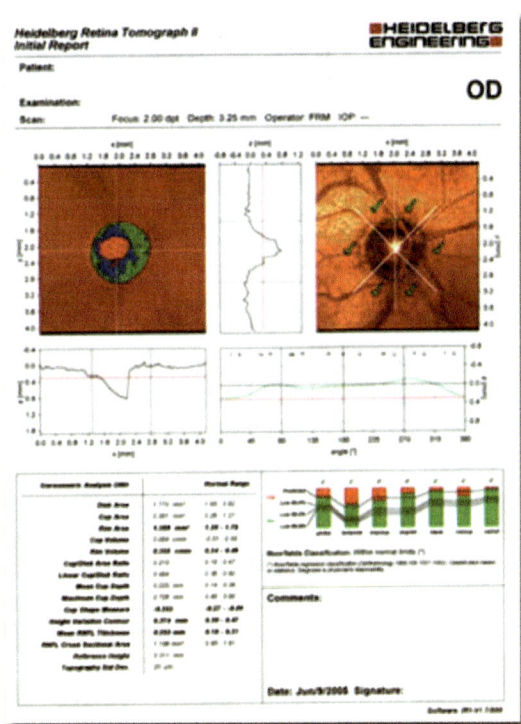

Fig. 4.39: *Initial examination report with the HRT II.*

The reflectivity image approximates a mean brightness of all images. In the reflection image, the ONH is divided into six sectors. These sectors are compared to a normal database and then classified. Moorfield's regression analysis means that the rim (green and blue) and the disc area (green, blue and red) for each sector are compared to a normal database. Depending on the patient's age and overall disc size, the eye is then statistically classified as 'within normal limit', 'borderline' or 'outside normal limit'.

Horizontal/vertical height profile, i.e. height profile along the white horizontal and the white vertical line in the tomography image. The subjacent reference line (red) indicates the location of the reference plane (separation between cup and neuroretinal rim). The two black lines perpendicular to the height profile denote the borders of the disc as defined by the contour line.

Mean height contour graph. The height difference between the reference line (red) and the height profile corresponds to the retinal nerve fiber layer (RNFL) thickness along the contour line.

Stereometric analysis of ONH. For both instruments, an operator has to define the edge of the ONH, and this is done using the mouse. Once the ONH margin, i.e. contour line which matches the inner edge of scleral ring (Elschnig's ring) has been defined, area and volumetric information about the ONH are obtained.

The result of this analysis is a set of stereometric parameters. The most important parameters are disc area, cup and rim area, cup and rim volume, and mean and maximum cup depth, a measure for the 3-D shape of the cup and for the mean thickness of the RNFL along the contour line (Fig. 4.39). Most of the stereometric parameters provided by the Heidelberg retinal tomograph change significantly with progression of glaucoma; the standard errors of the means in the visual field groups are very small, and the means differ significantly between groups. The parameters are useful, therefore, to follow the progression of the disease. But the physiologic variability of the ONH configuration is high and so are the standard deviations of the parameter values. The distributions of the parameter values of the different groups overlap each other. Hence, it is difficult (except in advanced cases) to classify an individual eye as being normal or glaucomatous, based on individual stereometric parameters.

Disc analysis with HRT II—Moorfield's analysis feature. Once the contour line has been drawn, there is the option of using the Moorfield's regression feature. This compares the optic disc imaged to a normal database and predicts the normality of the disc.

Variability in acquisition can occur due to manual contour line drawing, inter- and intratest examinations. To overcome this, Moorfield's study revealed the advantage of examining the rim area in sectors. This graphic visualizes the result of the Moorfield's regression analysis. The whole column represents the total ONH area in this specific sector. It is divided into the percentage of rim area (green) and percentage of cup area (red). The age-dependent limits of the confidence intervals are as follows:

- If the percentage of the rim is larger than or equal to the 95% limit, the respective sector is classified as 'within normal limit'.
- If the percentage of the rim is between the 95 and the 99.9% limits, the respective sector is classified as 'borderline'.
- If the percentage of the rim is lower than the 99.9% limit, the respective sector is classified as 'outside normal limit'.

2. Follow-up examination to study the progression

Glaucoma is a progressive disease, and there is significant individual variability which makes labelling an eye glaucomatous after one single test hazardous. Therefore, proven progression of the disease becomes critical to the diagnosis and management. The baseline measurements are extremely important, since those parameters alone are taken for further retesting. Therefore, the image quality (as ascertained by standard deviation) should be good and it should be ensured that ONH is centered, illumination is even, refractive error is incorporated and eye movements are minimal. It is claimed that disc changes are more frequent than field changes. Progression requires three consecutive readings (Baseline 1 three follow-up) to perform a topographic change analysis.

Topographic change analysis can be done by two methods:

i. *Change probability maps* (Fig. 4.40) are independent of the reference plane and the contour line and are calculated automatically, comparing mean topography images.

• Red signifies 'significant' depression.

• Green signifies 'significant' elevation.

• The change is calculated by local change in surface height, measured in microns, at the location selected. A height change is considered significant:

If it is repeated in at least two (better is three) consecutive follow-up examinations.

If it is region of at least 20 connected superpixels.

ii. *Parametric change* is evaluated in the follow-up diagram that plots normalized stereometric values versus time. If average normalized parametric value decreases by more than 20.05 significant in two consecutive examinations, it is deemed 'suspected' and if it appears in three consecutive examinations, it is considered 'confirmed' progression (Fig. 4.41).

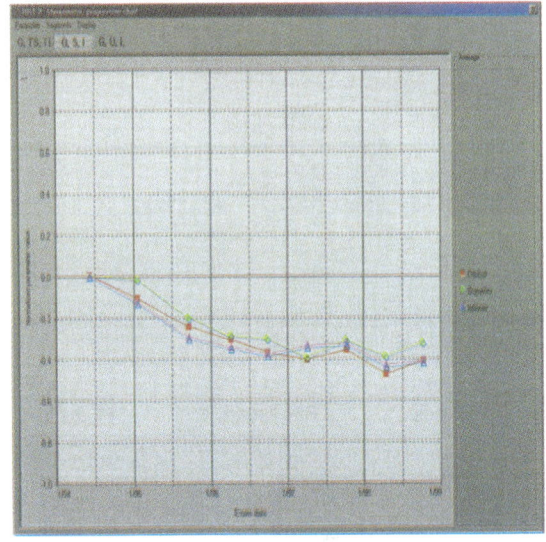

Fig. 4.41: *Parametric changes.*

Frequency of examinations. Time determines the speed of progression, and repeated examinations cannot detect disease. High-risk cases on basis of race, age, family history and raised intraocular pressure should undergo a 6 monthly examination and other patients may be followed up annually. Examinations may be done more frequently for the first 18 months in patients showing signs of clinical progression so as to start detecting statistical 'change'.

II. SLT in macular diseases

Researchers have developed a software algorithm that analyses the axial intensity distribution and computes a thickness-equivalent map of the retina. This is useful in macular pathologies such as macular edema or macular cysts. The researchers concluded that this analysis offers non-invasive, objective, topographic and reproducible index of macular retinal thickening. The scanning laser thickness analyser using HRT II uses 147, 456 points while in OCT only 600–768 points are used.

RETINAL THICKNESS ANALYSER

Retinal thickness analyser (RTA) from Talia Technology (Fig. 4.42A) is an ophthalmic imaging device for the mapping and quantitative measurement of optimal thickness and disc

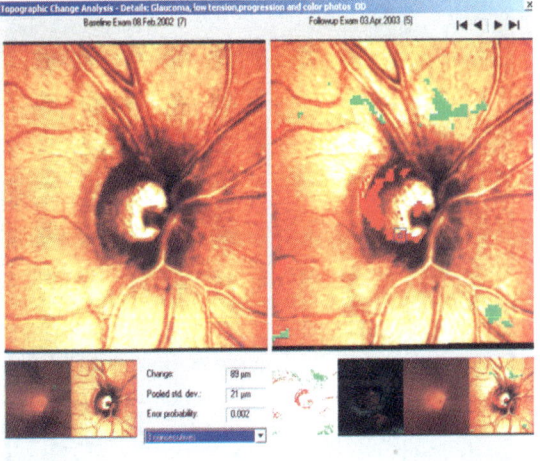

Fig. 4.40: *Change probability maps.*

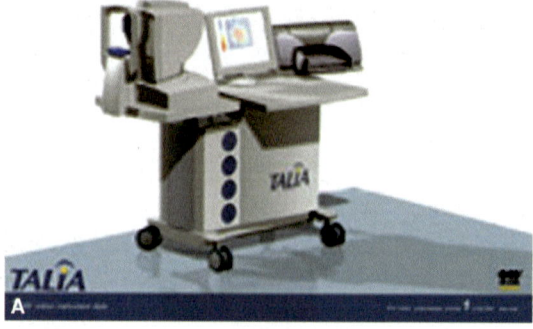

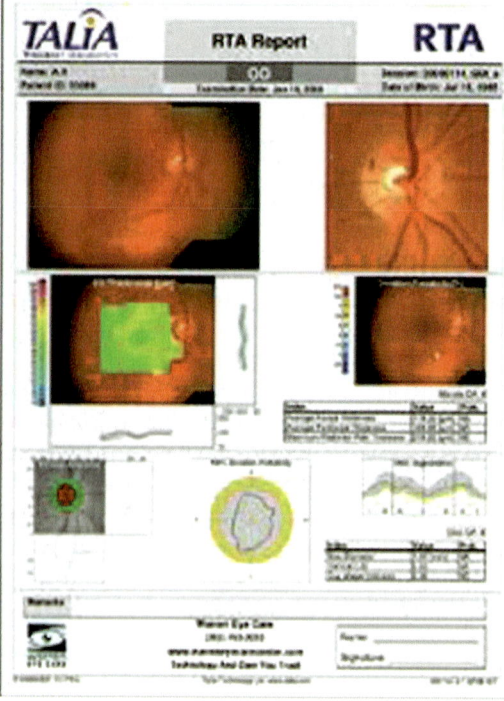

Fig. 4.42: *(A) Retinal thickness analyser (RTA); and (B) Talia, RTA report printout (Courtesy: Talia Technology).*

topography (Fig. 4.42B). It uses a computerized laser slit-lamp to measure retinal thickness at the central 208 of the macula, and overlaps a map of measurements on the patient's retinal image.

A vertical narrow green He–Ne (543.3 nm) laser slit-beam is projected at an angle on the retina while a CCD camera records the back-scattered light. Due to the oblique projection of the beam and the transparency of the retina, the backscattered light returns two peaks corresponding to the vitreoretinal and the chorio-retinal interfaces. A 3 × 3 × 3 mm scan consisting of 16 optical cross-sections is acquired within

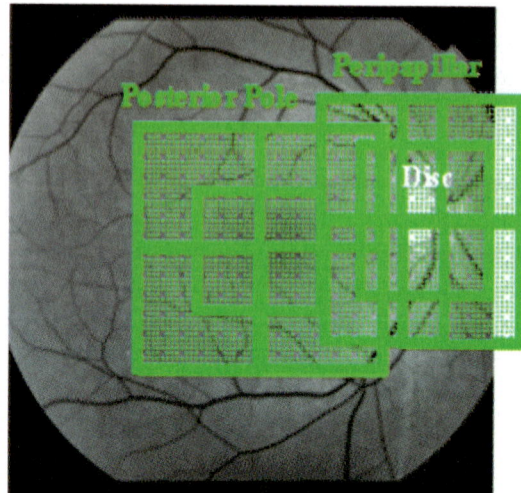

Fig. 4.43: *Thirteen RTA-scanned areas.*

0.3 seconds. Five such scans are obtained at the macula, three scans at the disc and additional five scans cover the peripapillary area (Fig. 4.43).

Clinical applications

Retinal thickness analysis

As the CCD camera records the reflected image of the retinal cross-sections, a thickness algorithm identifies the location of the anterior and posterior retinal borders (Fig. 4.44).

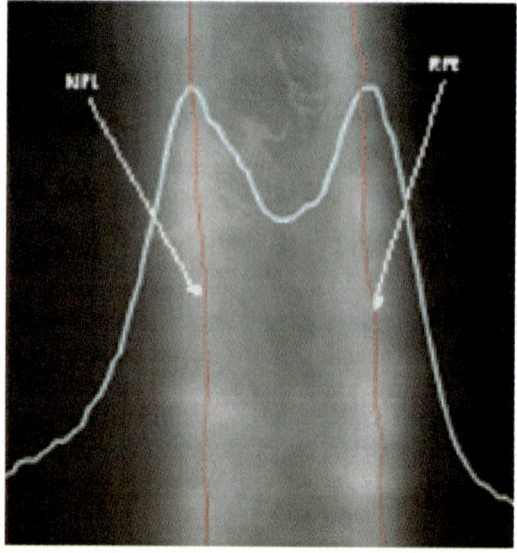

Fig. 4.44 *Light intensity profile as detected by the RTA's thickness algorithm.*

The calculated distance between the two light peaks determines the retinal thickness at a given point. The algorithm measures 16 data points on each slit, 187.5 m apart, totalling 2560 thickness measurement points.

Indications of retinal thickness analysis include:
- Diabetic macular edema
- ARMD
- Cystoid macular edema
- Macular holes
- Epiretinal membrane, etc.

ONH topography analysis

The RTA acquires three scans over the disc covering a 3 × 3 × 3 mm area. Each of the 16 slit images represents the disc topography along a vertical line. Using edge detection analysis, the topography algorithm identifies the left border of the light, corresponding to the vitreoretinal surface, and calculates the disc topography (Fig. 4.45).

In order to obtain quantitative stereometric measurements, the operator is required to draw a contour line along the disc edge. The same contour line is used in follow-up visits to ensure accurate monitoring of subtle changes. The disc

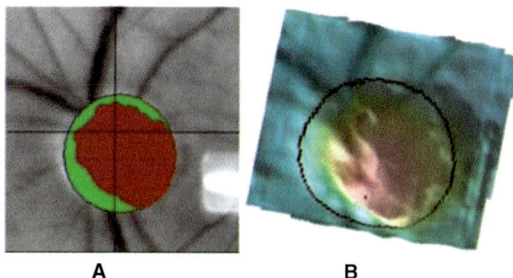

A   **B**

Fig. 4.46: *RTA—disc topography map: (A) Rim/cup area map; and (B) pseudo 3-D representation.*

topography report displays a rim/cup area map (Fig. 4.46A) and a pseudo 3-D representation of the disc topography (Fig. 4.46B).

Thus, the RTA may be used to assess the optic nerve in terms of the cup to disc (C:D) ratio as well as other ONH parameters. It is also able to monitor progression of nerve fiber layer thinning in glaucoma. Findings are presented in numerical values and may be shown in 2- or 3-D representation.

RTA: Clinical applicability in glaucoma. Early detection of glaucomatous damage is critical for successful treatment. Glaucoma is associated with ganglion cell and nerve fiber layer loss. Today we know that up to 50% of the total number of ganglion cells are located in the macula. The loss of these two layers is directly reflected in retinal thickness.

None of the other automated imaging tools has emerged as a new gold standard for early glaucoma diagnosis and monitoring. The RTA, however, in addition to imaging the optic disc cupping, identifies and quantifies the anatomical damage in the macula and the peripapillary region even before the symptoms appear.

The RTA is the only tool that provides objective assessment of all three key components of glaucoma-associated changes in the fundus of the eye: macula, peripapillary region and disc area.

Anatomy imager 3-D rendering

Recently, the RTA has incorporated an anatomy imager into the device. The anatomy imager allows 3-D rendering of retinal thickness measurements over the fundus photo captured

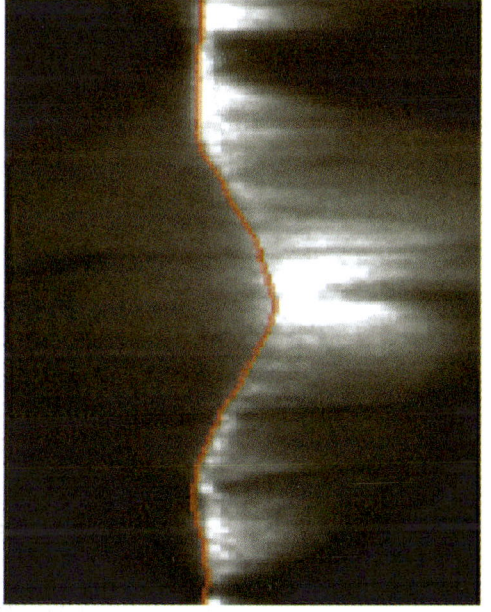

Fig. 4.45: *The vitreoretinal surface as detected by the RTA's topography algorithm.*

by the device. Alternatively, the programme allows easy importation of an external image (such as a fluorescein angiography study). The 3-D block may be rotated and cleaved as necessary to appreciate the relationship between abnormalities in retinal thickness and pathologies seen on fluorescein angiography.

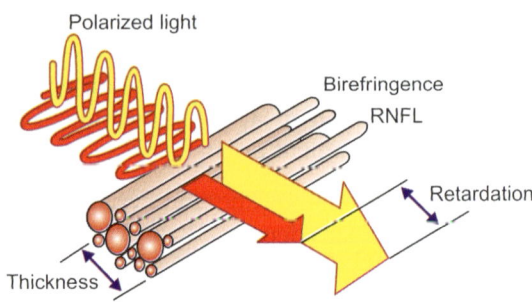

Fig. 4.47: *Optical principle of scanning laser polarimeter (SLP) (nerve fiber layer analyser).*

SCANNING LASER POLARIMETRY (SLP)

SLP provides on objective quantitative assessment of the peripapillary RNFL, and thus is also called *RNFL analyser* GDx; the commercially available RNFL analyser has two models: the GDx FCC (old model) and GDx VCC (new model). RNFL analyser with variable corneal compensation (available as GDx VCC) is the most appropriate structural test for early detection of glaucomatous damage as it quantifies the morphology of RNFL.

PRINCIPLE AND OPTICS

The RNFL analyser works on the principle of SLP. The operating principle of SLP by which it determines the RNFL thickness is the measurement of the *retardation* of a polarized laser light passing through tissues possessing the physical property of *form birefringence* (explained below).

Form birefringence refers to splitting of a light wave by a polar material into two components. These components travel at different velocities, which creates a relative *phase shift*, also termed retardation. The amount of phase shift or retardation is proportional to the thickness of polar tissue. The polar tissues are composed of parallel structures, each of which is of smaller diameter than the wavelength of the light used to image it. The RNFL behaves as a polar tissue because of the microtubules (with diameters smaller than the wavelength of light) present in the highly ordered parallel axon bundles. The greater the number of microtubules, the greater the retardation of the polarized laser light, indicating the presence of more tissue; thus giving an assessment of RNFL.

Optics. Figure 4.47 depicts the optics of SLP. The near-infrared laser light (780 nm) enters the eye at specific orientation. As the laser double passes the RNFL, it is split into two parallel rays by the birefringent microtubules (present in the axons forming RNFL). The two rays travel at different speeds, and this difference (called retardation) is measured.

Total birefringence, anterior segment birefringence and RNFL birefringence

Total birefringence—associated retardation is the sum of anterior segment birefringence (from cornea and lens) and RNFL birefringence.

RNFL birefringence can be isolated from the total birefringence by compensating for the anterior segment birefringence.

Fixed versus variable corneal compensation

- *Fixed corneal compensation (FCC)* was employed in the earlier models of nerve fiber layer analysers (e.g. GDx FCC), ensuring that all individuals had a slow axis of corneal birefringence (corneal polarization axis) 15° nasally downward with a magnitude of 60 nm (corneal polarization magnitude). However, recently it has been shown that there exists a wide variation in the axis and magnitude of corneal polarization in healthy and glaucomatous eyes.
- *Variable corneal compensation (VCC)* is required to exactly measure the RNFL birefringence. The modified version of nerve fiber layer analyser (GDx VCC) measures and individually compensates for anterior segment birefringence for each eye and thus allows the exact measurement of RNFL birefringence.

GDX VCC NERVE FIBER LAYER ANALYSER

The new modified version of nerve fiber analyser, i.e. GDx VCC (Fig. 4.48) is an SLP, which basically consists of a confocal scanning laser ophthalmoscope with an integrated ellipsometer to measure retardation.

Procedure of measurement

The measurement is performed with an undilated pupil of at least 2 mm diameter. A 780 nm infrared laser is used to scan the parapapillary area to give the RNFL measurements. Time taken is about 0.7 seconds. Total chair time is less than 3 minutes for both eyes. First the eye is imaged without compensation. The uncompensated image presents total retardation from the eye. The macular region of this image is then analysed to determine the axis and magnitude of the anterior segment birefringence. The macular region birefringence is uniform and symmetric due to radial distribution of Henle's fiber layer.

Interpretation of the GDx VCC printout

The measurements are compared with a *normative database* (from healthy volunteers of different races) to determine any significant deviations from normal limits which are flagged as abnormal with a *p* value. Most of the parameters on GDx VCC printout are calculated from the calculation circle. This is the area of 8 pixels between two concentric circles centered around the optic disc. The GDx VCC printout is interpreted as below (Fig. 4.49):

1. *Colour fundus image* is seen at the top of the printout. It is depicted as 20° × 20° image of the disc and parapapillary area (Fig. 4.49A). It is produced by more than 16,000 data points from the scanned area.

2. *Thickness (polarization) map* shows the RNFL thickness in a colour-coded format in the 20° × 20° parapapillary area as below (Fig. 4.49B):
- *Thick RNFL areas* are indicated by bright colours: yellow, orange and red.
- *Thin RNFL areas* are indicated by dark colour (dark blue, blue and green).
- *Typical normal pattern* is characterized by bright yellow and red colours (thicker areas) in the superior and inferior sectors and dark blue and green (i.e. thinner areas) in the nasal and temporal sectors.

Abnormal patterns of thickness map include:
- *Diffuse loss of RNFL* leads to its decreased thickness, seen as yellow instead of red.
- *Focal defects* are seen as concentrated dark areas.
- *Asymmetry* between superior and inferior quadrants of RNFL.
- *Asymmetry* between the RNFL of two eyes.
- *Increased thickness* of RNFL in nasal and temporal quadrants of RNFL (seen as red and yellow instead of blue).

3. *Deviation map.* It shows the location and magnitude of RNFL defects over the entire thickness map. It tells how the patient's RNFL thickness compares with values derived from the normative database in a 128 × 128 pixel (20° × 20°) region centered on the optic disc. Small colour-coded squares indicate the amount of deviation from normal at each given location and are presented over a black and white fundus image to provide a visual form of reference (Fig. 4.49C). Dark blue squares represent areas where the RNFL thickness is

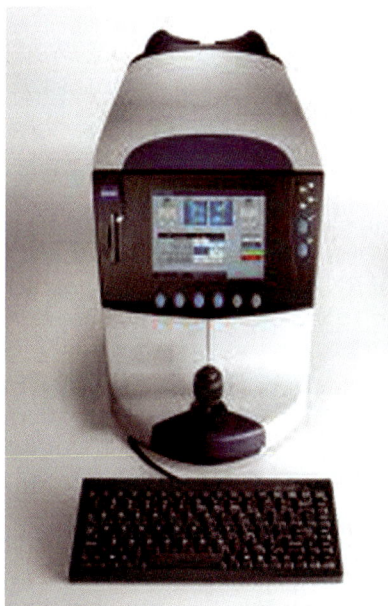

Fig. 4.48: *Commercially available nerve fiber layer analyser (GDx VCC) (Courtesy: Carl Zeiss Meditec AS).*

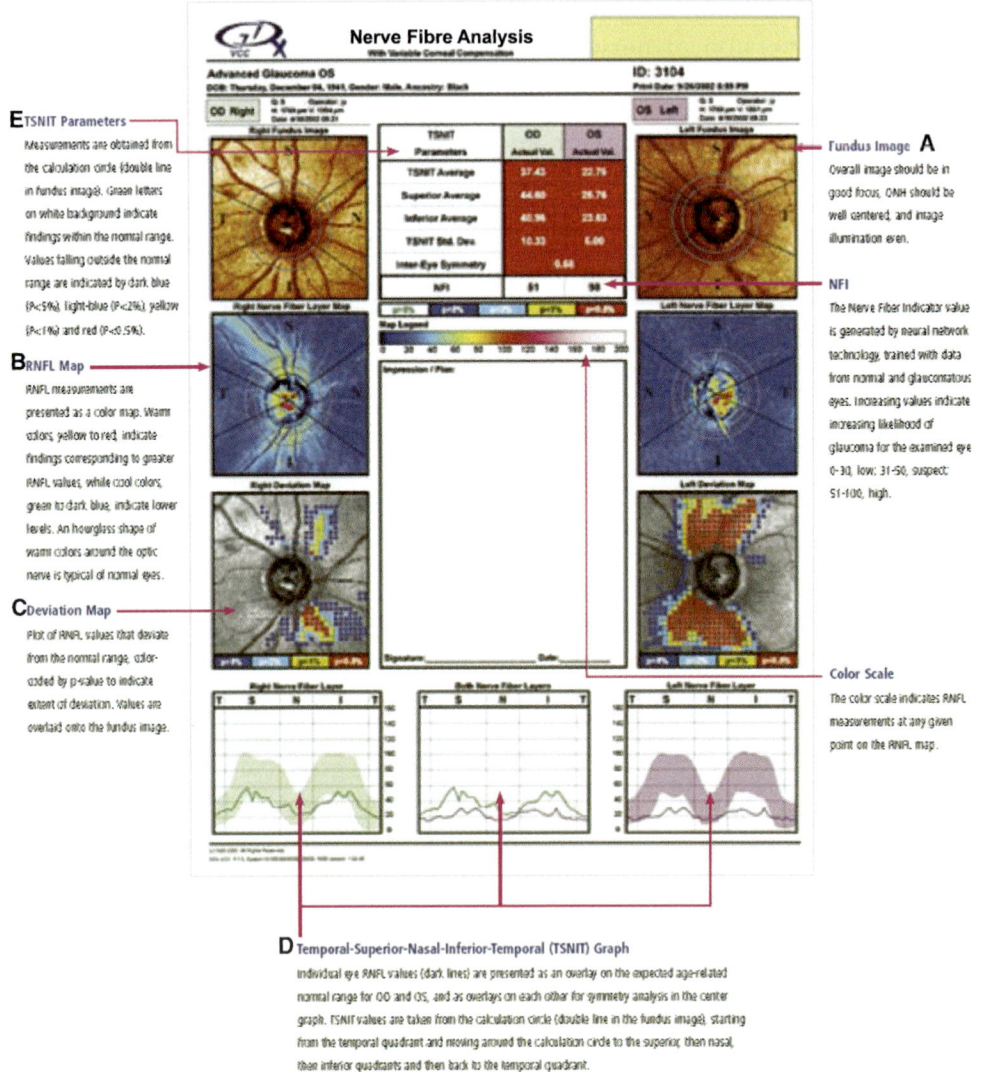

Fig. 4.49: *A representation printout of GDx VCC retinal nerve fiber layer analyser.*

below the 5th percentile of the normative database; i.e. there is only 5% probability that the RNFL thickness in this area is within the normal range. Light blue squares represent deviation below the 2% level, yellow represents deviation below 1% and red represents deviation below 0.5%. Thus, a quick look at the deviation map gives an idea of the wedge defects of RNFL and the pattern of defects.

4. *The TSNIT graphs* (Fig. 4.49D). The TSNIT, i.e. 'temporal-superior, nasal-inferior-temporal' graph displays the range and the patient's

values of RNFL thickness along the calculation ellipse in TSNIT order separately for right (OD) and left (OS) eyes.

- In a normal eye, the typical TSNIT graph shows a typical 'double-hump' pattern.
- A flat TSNIT graph indicates loss of RNFL.
- *TSNIT symmetry graph* is obtained by displaying the graphs of two eyes together. Normally, the curves from two eyes overlap. However, in glaucoma, one eye often has more advanced RNFL loss and, therefore, the two curves will have less overlap. A dip in the

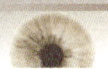

curve of one eye relative to another is indicative of RNFL loss.

TSNIT serial analysis graph and deviation from reference map for a given eye, for analysis of serial changes between visits can also be obtained from GDx VCC. This is very useful to demonstrate progression over a period of time.

5. *TSNIT parameters.* These are displayed in a table on the center of printout (Fig. 4.49E). The TSNIT parameters are summary measures based on RNFL thickness values within the calculation ellipse and include TSNIT average, superior average, inferior average, TSNIT standard deviation, intereye symmetry and the nerve fiber indicator (NFI).

- *TSNIT average* refers to average RNFL thickness around the entire calculation ellipse.
- *Superior average* is the average RNFL thickness in the superior 128 region of calculation ellipse.
- *Inferior average* is the average RNFL thickness in the inferior 1208 region of calculation ellipse.
- *TSNIT standard deviation* indicates the modulation (peak to trough difference) of the double-hump pattern. A normal eye has high and a glaucoma eye has low modulation in the double-hump pattern.
- *Intereye symmetry* measures the degree of symmetry between the right and left eyes. Normal eyes have good symmetry with values around 0.9.
- *NFI.* It is the most important parameter, since it is an indicator of the likelihood that an eye has glaucoma. NFI is generated from the patient's scanned data obtained from within and outside the calculation circle.

  The output of NFI is a single value that ranges from 1 to 100 and indicates the overall integrity of the RNFL. The higher the NFI the more likely that the patient has glaucoma. The values of NFI are generally interpreted as:
  - ♦ Normal: 1–30 (less likelihood of glaucoma)
  - ♦ Glaucoma suspect: 30–50
  - ♦ Abnormal: >50 (high likelihood of glaucoma).

Normal versus abnormal values of TSNIT parameters

Normal values of TSNIT parameters reported from Indian population are:

- TSNIT average: 54.8 ± 4.1 (45.6 – 66.8) µ
- Superior average: 66.8 ± 6.70 (55.1 – 85) µ
- Inferior average: 62.1 ± 6.6 (38.9 – 74.3) µ
- NFI: 17.2 ± 6.9 (4–35) µ

Abnormal values. Although there is no consensus on definition of abnormal scan, the following guidelines have been recommended for TSNIT average, superior average, inferior average, TSNIT standard deviation, intereye symmetry and NFI:

- Abnormal at p, <1% level
- Borderline at p, <5% level

Additional diagnostic parameters

Additional diagnostic parameters available in the machine for an extended analysis include the following:

- *Symmetry.* It is the ratio of the average of the 1500 thickest pixels each in the superior and inferior quadrants. The values closer to 1 indicate more symmetry and thus more chances of normal scan.
- *Superior ratio.* It is the ratio of superior quadrant thickness (average of 1500 thickest pixels) and temporal quadrant thickness (average of 1500 median pixels).
- *Inferior ratio.* It is the ratio of inferior quadrant thickness (average of 1500 thickest pixels) and temporal quadrant thickness (average of 1500 median pixels).
- *Superior nasal.* It is the ratio of superior quadrant thickness (average of 1500 thickest pixels) and nasal quadrant thickness (average of 1500 median pixels).
- *Maximum modulation.* It is ratio of thickest quadrant versus thinnest quadrant. Normally the maximum modulation is more than 1, since superior and inferior quadrants are thicker than nasal and temporal quadrants. Value of 1 or less indicates RNFL loss.
- *Superior maximum.* It is the average of the 1500 thickest pixels in the superior quadrant.

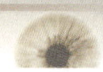

- *Inferior maximum.* It is the average of the 1500 thickest pixels in the inferior quadrant.
- *Ellipse modulation.* It is the ratio of the thickest quadrant and the thinnest quadrant within the ellipse area.
- *Ellipse average.* It is the average thickness (in microns) of RNFL in the ellipse surrounding the ONH.

Advantages and limitations of GDx VCC

Advantages of GDx VCC
- Easy to operate
- Does not require pupillary dilation
- Good reproducibility
- Does not require a reference plane
- Can detect glaucoma on the first examination
- Early detection before standard visual field
- Comparison with age-matched normative database.

Limitations of GDx VCC
- Does not measure actual RNFL thickness (inferred value).
- Low sensitivity and specificity for detection of pre-perimetric glaucoma in clinical studies.
- Does not differentiate true biological change from variability.

- Limited use in moderate and advanced glaucoma.
- No database from Indian population.
- Affected by anterior and posterior segment lesions such as:
  - Ocular surface disorders
  - Macular pathology
  - Cataract and refractive surgery
  - Refractive errors
  - Peripapillary atrophy (scleral birefringence interferes with RNFL measurement).

BIBLIOGRAPHY

1. Matthew T. Witmer, MD, Szila'rd Kiss, MD. Wide-eld Imaging of the Retina. Surv Ophthalmol 2013;58;2:143–54.

2. Rosenthal ML, Fradin S. The technique of binocular indirect ophthalmoscopy. Highlights Ophthalmol 1966;9:179–257.

3. Rubin ML. Magnification; practical instruments: the indirect ophthalmoscope. In: Optics for clinicians. 2nd edn.

4. Saine P, Tyler M. Ophthalmic Photography. A Textbook of Retinal Photography. Angiography and Electronic Imaging. Boston, MA, Twin Chimney Publishing; 1997.

Evaluation and Assessment of Traumatized Eye

Chapter Outline

INTRODUCTION
- Initial approach
- Systemic evaluation
- Initial triage

CLINICAL WORK-UP

History

Ocular Examination
- Visual function assessment
- Ocular motility
- Conjunctiva
- Cornea
- Sclera
- Anterior chamber

- Iris
- Crystalline lens
- Intraocular pressure
- Posterior segment examination

ORBITAL IMAGING
- Plain radiography
- Computed tomography
- Ultrasonography
- Magnetic resonance imaging

SURGICAL EXPLORATION AND EXAMINATION UNDER ANAESTHESIA

PATIENT COUNSELLING

INTRODUCTION

A proper evaluation of the traumatized eye is absolutely essential for appropriate and effective management of the injury. Classification of the injury and calculation of the ocular trauma score are essential aspects which should be brought into practice. It should be remembered that in case of ocular trauma, the ophthalmologist is treating the patient and not only the eye, pay attention to any systemic features, social bearing of the ocular injury and ultimately to the visual rehabilitation of the patient. Scheme of approach to a patient with ocular trauma described below is summarized in Fig. 5.1.

Initial approach. Patients usually present to the ocular emergency in a state of panic or frenzy.

The sudden threat to vision can be emotionally damning. This places upon the treating ophthalmologist an added responsibility of counselling not only the patient but also their family members. It is always advisable to maintain a confident and humane approach.

Systemic evaluation. Prior to taking history and performing a thorough examination of the eye, it is important for the attending ophthalmologist to evaluate the systemic condition of the patient. Ocular trauma can be compounded by life-threatening injuries as in cases of polytrauma commonly observed in road traffic accidents. If a systemic injury is found, its treatment will obviously take precedence over the ocular management. In these cases, the emergency team stabilizes the patient before calling in for

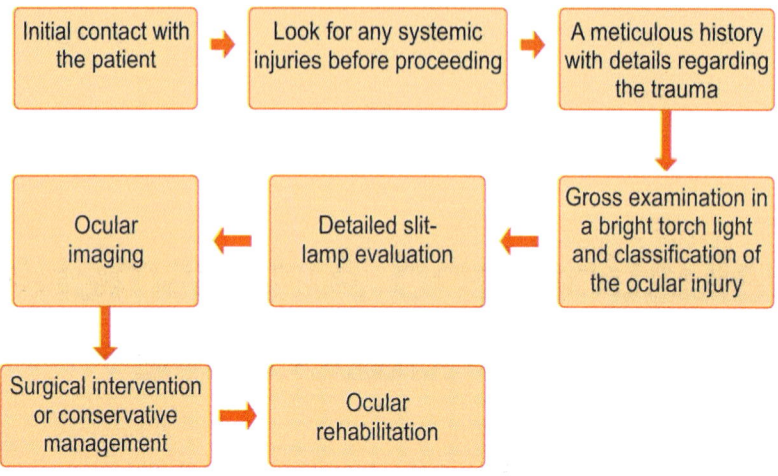

Fig. 5.1: *Scheme of approach to a patient with ocular trauma.*

an expert ophthalmic opinion. Even in cases presenting directly to the ophthalmologist, it is always better to be suspicious of occult injury to other organ systems.

Initial triage should consist of systemic evaluation of vitals, gross mental status and obvious fractures or soft tissue injuries. The patient should be referred to a trauma facility, if at any point of the examination, the following are found:

- Unstable vital parameters
- Altered mental status or an unresponsive patient
- Serious bony or soft tissue injury.

Once it is established that the systemic status is stable, the surgeon can turn attention to the ocular evaluation.

CLINICAL WORK-UP

HISTORY

The importance of a well-taken history, at the time of initial presentation, cannot be over-emphasized. Not only does this give the ophthalmologist a chance to build a rapport and earn the trust of the patient but a well-documented history is also necessary for legal proceedings. The history will guide the ophthalmologist towards the examination.

It is best to allow the patient to tell his or her version of the incident without much of an interruption. Leading questions can be asked in between to bring the patients back on track, if they ever get diverted off course. The history should highlight the following important points:

Events leading up to the injury. It is of utmost importance to elucidate the minutest detail of activity which the patient was performing at the time of sustaining the injury, e.g. whether the activity was related to sports, bow and arrow and bursting of crackers during Diwali/ Dusshera festivals, a labourer crushing stones while using a chisel and hammer, industrial or agricultural pursuits, involved in roadside accidents and finally an assault with the use of some kind of armament.

Detailed description of the mechanism of trauma to note whether:

- A high-velocity or a low-velocity trauma
- Injury with a blunt or a sharp object.

Time of the injury and time elapsed between the insult and initial presentation should be documented:

- As it decides management. A fresh open corneal wound would be dealt with urgently and more aggressively than a self-sealed corneal laceration in a quiet eye which is a week old.
- Important for medicolegal purposes.

Rural or an urban setting should be noted. The incidence of infection in cases of trauma in rural settings is higher and so is the risk of endophthalmitis.

Chemical nature of the insulting object should be noted:
- If an intraocular foreign body is suspected its nature and chemical composition must be known (iron, copper or steel)
- Any chemical agent, such as an alkali or acid, may further complicate the mechanical injury.

Prior ocular history should specifically include:
- Any history of previous ocular surgery or trauma
- Use of any ocular medications
- Prior vision of the injured eye and the un-injured eye.

Generalized medical history of any chronic systemic illness or use of any drugs or medications should be documented. It is important to note any drug allergies and status of tetanus immunization. If an open globe injury is suspected, general anaesthesia would be required and the patient should be asked about the time he last consumed solids and liquids.

OCULAR EXAMINATION

External inspection in diffuse illumination

Prior to examining the patient on the slit-lamp, a gross evaluation of the ocular condition can be made out with the help of a diffuse illumination of a pen torch.
- *Forehead and the periorbital tissues* should be inspected under bright illumination. Evaluate for the presence of any laceration, abrasion, periorbital edema and ecchymosis.
- *Look for exophthalmos*, enophthalmos or any foreign body, such as a stone present in the margins of the laceration.
- *Orbital walls* should be palpated to look for evidence of any bony discontinuity.
- *Crepitus and infraorbital hypoesthesia* may indicate an orbital fracture.

Inspection of globe

Attention should now be given to the ocular structures per se. The eyelids may be parted with the help of an eye speculum or a lid retractor in individuals wherein the periorbital oedema makes examination difficult. Inspect the globes for:
- Prolapse of intraocular contents

- Protruding foreign bodies
- Any sign of occult open globe injury (hemorrhagic chemosis, pupillary peaking).

Note. It should be kept in mind that no pressure is given on the globe lest the intraocular contents prolapse out. In cases of highly swollen lids or an uncooperative patient, the examination of the globe can be deferred till imaging is done or can be carried out under sedation.

Visual function assessment

Visual acuity. The presenting visual acuity is a crucial prognostic indicator in determining the outcome of injury. The visual acuity is measured separately for each eye. It should be preferably recorded on a standardized chart (ETDRS or Snellen). If the patients are immobilized or on a stretcher, due to systemic comorbidities, visual acuity can be assessed by asking the patient to count fingers at a specific distance. Poor vision can be recorded as either hand motions or light perception with a documentation of projection of rays. The test of light perception and projection of rays should be carried out with the brightest possible light (indirect ophthalmoscope).

Relative afferent pupillary defect. The presence or absence of RAPD is an indicator of gross visual dysfunction. The test is performed as a swinging flash-light test with a bright light source. Apparent dilation of the pupil of the eye in which light is shown points towards the presence of RAPD. It indicates an optic nerve or a severe retinal damage with a poor prognosis.

Afferent pupillary defect can also be elucidated in cases wherein the iris is injured and the pupil is not reacting. In this case rather than visualizing the direct pupillary response in each eye, only the response in the normal reacting pupil is observed. RAPD is said to be present when the pupil of the fellow eye dilates when light is moved to the injured eye.

Visual field assessment. Rapid assessment of the peripheral visual field can be carried out in the emergency setting using the confrontation test. It can give additional information about retinal or optic nerve damage.

Ocular motility assessment

- If *injury to the cranial nerves* or bony orbital margin is suspected, ocular motility must be evaluated.
- *A case of blowout fracture* with an entrapped inferior rectus muscle can be made out at this stage and treatment modified accordingly.
- However, it is not always possible to examine for motility as the patient's periorbital oedema or lack of cooperation may mask the findings.

Examination of conjunctiva

Foreign bodies or precipitates of chemicals may be lodged within the conjunctival fornices. The lids should be everted and fornices examined. Double eversion of the upper lid with a Desmarres retractor is needed to look for hidden foreign bodies in the superior fornix.

Presence of haemorrhagic chemosis should make one suspect of an underlying breach in the eyewall.

Subconjunctival haemorrhage, the posterior extent of which cannot be reached, raises the possibility of a fracture of the base of the skull.

Lacerations of the conjunctiva may be difficult to make out initially. Manipulation with a cotton swab following anaesthetic instillation can clearly delineate the edge of the laceration. A thorough search for an underlying scleral wound should be made in these cases.

Examination of cornea

Epithelial defects. Patients usually present with pain and photophobia. A drop of a topical anaesthetic helps to allay their discomfort and allows for a thorough examination at the slit-lamp. Fluorescein staining and documentation of the size of the epithelial defect is of prime importance. Look for abrasion, opacification and ulcerations.

Superficial corneal foreign body. The depth of penetration of the foreign body should be evaluated on the slit-lamp. If the entire thickness of the cornea is breached, the injury gets classified as an open globe injury. The foreign body in this case is best removed in the operation theatre. For smaller foreign bodies which are more superficial, removal on a slit-lamp with a hypodermic needle is sufficient.

Corneal wounds should be analysed whether they are full thickness or partial thickness. This can be carried out with the help of a Seidel's test. Leakage of aqueous from a full thickness breach would dilute the fluorescein dye forming a green stream (positive Seidel's test).

Examination of sclera

- A detailed examination of the sclera should be carried out to look for any breach in the eyewall. This is not always easy as the associated subconjunctival haemorrhage may prevent adequate visualization.
- If a defect in the continuity of the scleral wall is suspected and adequate visualization is not possible, a surgical exploration should be planned.

Examination of anterior chamber

Contents of anterior chamber should be analysed for the presence of any aqueous cells or flare. Traumatic iritis following the insult can lead to inflammation in the anterior chamber. RBCs may also be found in the anterior chamber with damage to the iris. Look for any retained foreign body, hyphema or hypopyon.

Depth of the anterior chamber must be noted:
Deep anterior chamber may be a sign of:
- Posterior dislocation of the lens
- Posterior scleral rupture
- Iridodialysis.

Shallow anterior chamber may be a sign of:
- Anterior dislocation of the lens
- Corneoscleral perforation
- Suprachoroidal haemorrhage
- Serous choroidal detachment.

Examination of iris

- *Iris is one of the most common sites of damage* in both open and closed globe injuries. A slit-lamp evaluation should be carried out to look for sphincter tears, iridodialysis, iridodonesis and full thickness iris defects.
- *In case of corneoscleral wounds,* the iris may be prolapsed to block the site of perforation. In

old injuries, the iris tissue may get incarcerated in the wound leading to an adherent leukoma.

Examination of crystalline lens

- A note should be made of phacodonesis, dislocation, subluxation or zonular dehiscence.
- Blunt trauma can lead to a break in the posterior capsule forming a rosette-shaped concussion cataract at the posterior subcapsular region.
- Look for the integrity of the anterior capsule. A tear in the capsule would result in anterior subcapsular opacification or in leak of cortical material into the anterior chamber and further inflammation.
- Intralenticular foreign bodies must be looked for.

Intraocular pressure measurement

- Measurement of intraocular pressure should be carried out in all cases of trauma; provided an open globe injury has been ruled out.
- Following a contusion, the intraocular pressure may rise acutely, especially if inflammation and blood is present.
- An abnormally low IOP would point towards an occult open globe injury but can also be seen with ciliary body detachment.

Examination of posterior segment

- *An in-depth analysis of the posterior segment* of the eye should be carried out after ruling out globe rupture before the media clarity is compromised.
- *90 D slit-lamp examination* should be attempted in case the media permits or else *20 D indirect ophthalmoscopy* be carried out (without indentation at this stage) in order to rule out retained intraocular foreign body, vitreous haemorrhage, retinal break (inferotemporally—direct injury) or retinal dialysis (superonasally—countrecoup injury), choroidal ruptures, macular oedema and optic nerve avulsion, etc.
- *In most cases, mydriatics* should be used to facilitate view of the retina and vitreous. It is to be borne in mind that the use of mydriatics should be properly documented so as to avoid misinterpretation of subsequent pupillary examinations. (Pupillary reflexes are also evaluated to look for evidence of neurological damage).
- *In case of open globe injuries with prolapse of uveal tissue,* it is advisable to defer the evaluation of the posterior segment to a later date after the surgical repair is completed.

ORBITAL IMAGING

It becomes necessary to bank upon imaging modalities to provide additional information whenever significant trauma is suspected to the periorbital or in cases wherein view of the posterior segment is compromised (corneal decompensation, traumatic hyphema). In cases of open globe injury, some form of an imaging investigation should be ordered to look for a retained intraocular foreign body.

PLAIN RADIOGRAPHY

- With the advent of CT scan, the dependency on plain X-ray radiography has diminished. However, if a CT scan is not available, an X-ray of the orbit can also serve as a useful tool in evaluating bony trauma (Fig. 5.2) or an intraocular foreign body (Fig. 5.3).
- In addition to the advantage of diminished exposure to radiation as compared to CT, plain X-ray orbit will save the practicing

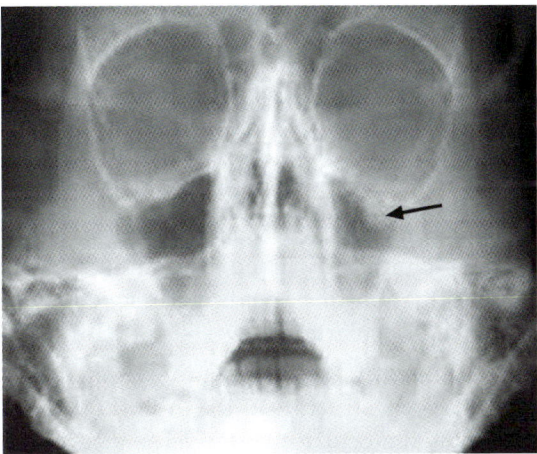

Fig. 5.2: *Plain X-ray orbit (AP view) showing herniated orbital contents (arrow) with blowout fracture.*

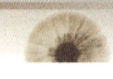

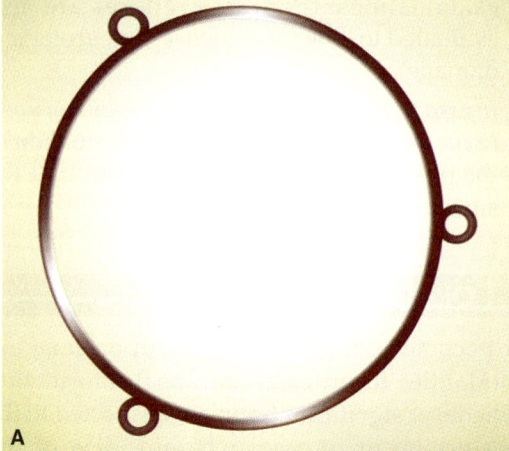

A

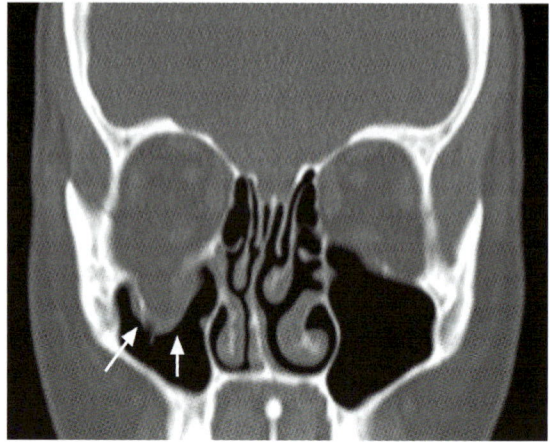

Fig. 5.4: *CT scan of orbit: Axial view depicting fracture floor of the orbit with herniation of the orbital contents*

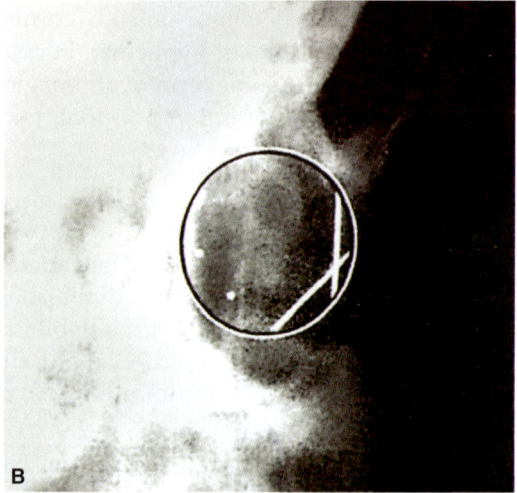

B

Fig. 5.3: *Limbal ring method of localizing RIOFB: (A) Limbal ring; (B) X-ray orbit lateral view with limbal ring.*

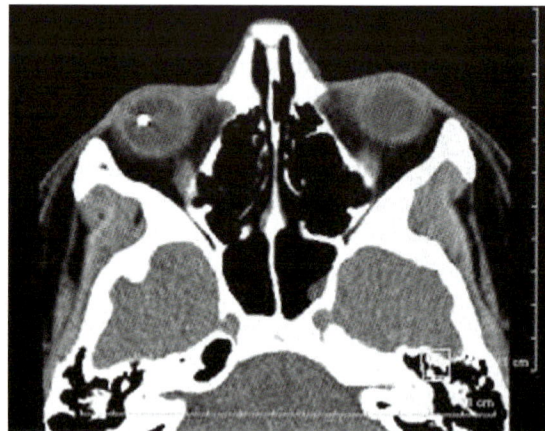

Fig. 5.5: *CT scan of the orbit depicting intraocular foreign body.*

ophthalmologist from the risk of Consumer Protection Act (CPA) and must be ordered even with the slightest suspicion of retained intraocular foreign body (RIOFB).

COMPUTED TOMOGRAPHY

- *CT scan has replaced X-ray radiography* as the most commonly used and most useful investigation in patients with severe peri-orbital or ocular trauma.
- *Coronal and axial scans* provide a detailed view of the bony structure of the orbit (Fig. 5.4) as well as the ocular anatomy. The size, shape and location of a foreign body can be easily demarcated with a CT scan (Fig. 5.5).

- Being readily available in the emergency setting, CT scan unlike ultrasonography *can be carried out even in patients with open globe injuries.*
- *Radiologist should be advised to use thinner cuts (1–2 mm) so as to better delineate the ocular anatomy.*
- *Common CT scan findings* that are suggestive of open globe injuries are:
  - ♦ Deformity of the globe
  - ♦ Intraocular foreign body
  - ♦ Intraocular air
  - ♦ Intraocular haemorrhage.
- *Sensitivity and specificity of CT scan* in determining open globe injury are 56–68% and 79–100%, respectively.

ULTRASONOGRAPHY

- *Utilizes high frequency sound waves* to delineate ocular structures in real time.
- *Ultrasonography requires a direct contact* with the lids and in cases of open globe injuries is contraindicated till the injury is repaired. In these cases, USG can be carried out in the operating room after repair with the patient under general anaesthesia.
- *B-scan ultrasonography helps to realize posterior segment pathology,* if the view of the fundus is compromised. It is useful in detecting (Fig. 5.6):
  - ◆ Retinal detachment (Fig. 5.6A)
  - ◆ Choroidal detachment (serous or haemorrhagic) (Fig. 5.6B)
  - ◆ Vitreous haemorrhage (Fig. 5.6C)
  - ◆ Posterior vitreous detachment
  - ◆ Intraocular foreign bodies (radiolucent and radio-opaque) (Fig. 5.6D)
  - ◆ Posterior breaks in the continuity of the eyewall (perforation *vs* penetrating injury).

MAGNETIC RESONANCE IMAGING

Role of an MRI in the setting of ocular trauma is limited by its availability and longer image acquisition times. Furthermore, it cannot be used if a metallic intraocular foreign body (iron) is suspected or in patients on pacemakers.

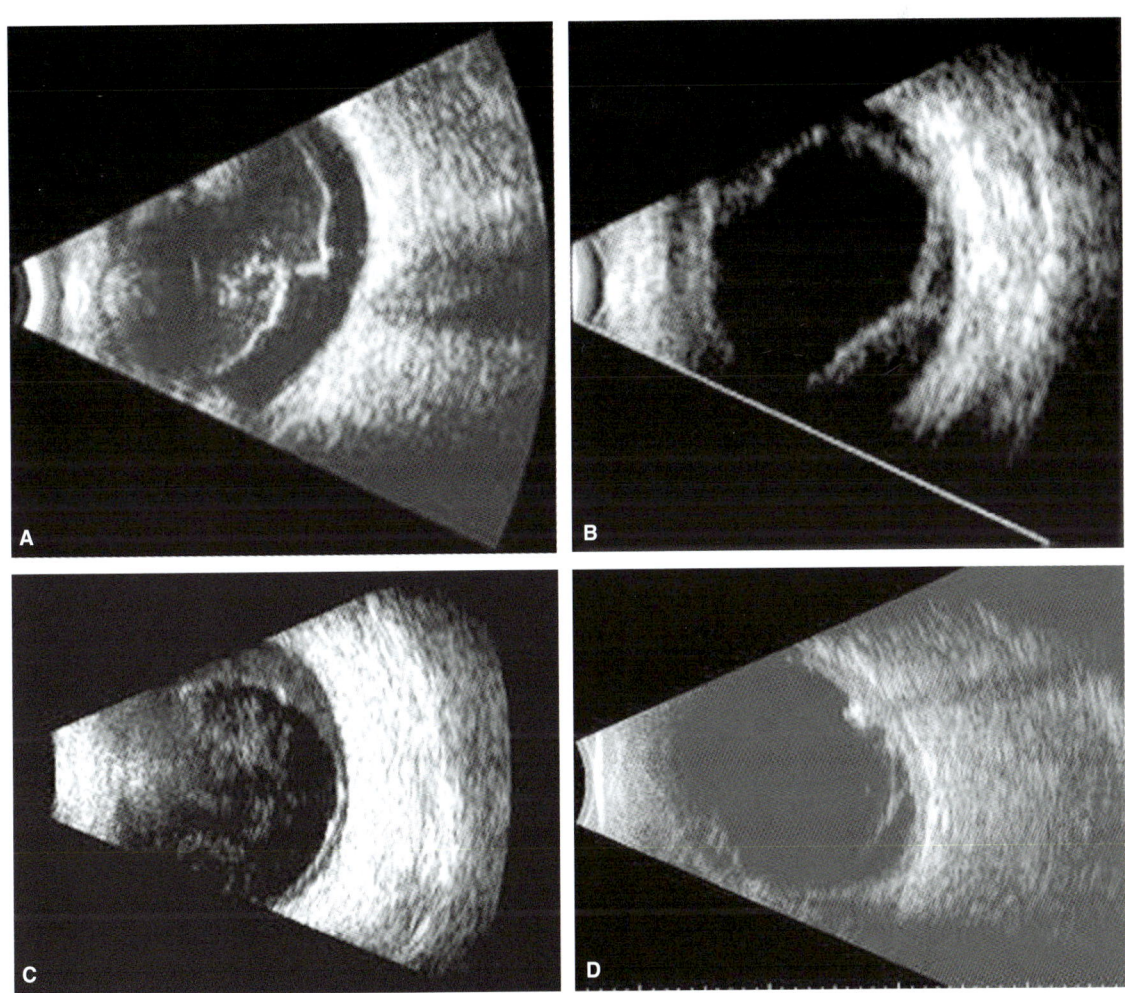

Fig. 5.6: *B scan of traumatic eyeball depicting: (A) Traumatic retinal detachment; (B) Choroidal detachment; C. Vitreous haemorrhage; (D) Intraocular foreign body.*

SURGICAL EXPLORATION AND EXAMINATION UNDER ANAESTHESIA

Indications. In cases wherein significant doubt remains about the nature of injury despite imaging modalities and examination or those cases who resist examination, a surgical exploration may be necessary for accurate diagnosis.

- *General anaesthesia* should be preferred.

- *An adequate conjunctival peritomy* should be done and the scleral shell should be evaluated under high magnification for any breach. Always remember to look at weak points on the eyewall especially at the limbus, at areas of old scars and at the insertion of extraocular muscles.

- *Cornea and anterior chamber should be examined* under high magnification. The angle can be evaluated with the help of a direct gonioscope lens.

- *Ultrasonography and indirect ophthalmoscopy* can be performed to look for posterior segment pathology.

PATIENT COUNSELLING

Last but not the least patient counselling is most important sensitive part of clinical work of eye trauma. Counselling of the patient and relatives begins at the point of initial contact in the emergency environment. This begins with initial comforting of the patient and aims to allay anxiety. The counselling must be informative, truthful, accurate and should be an ongoing process till the conclusion of treatment. This is especially important in patients who would require surgical intervention. It is true that the final visual acuity remains in doubt following ocular trauma in the initial few weeks, however, a realistic opinion about the visual prognosis can be gathered from the ocular trauma score. The patient must be encouraged not to give up hope. It is important to counsel the patient for any life adjustments that may be required.

BIBLIOGRAPHY

1. Arey ML, Mootha VV, Whittemore AR, Chason DP, Blomquist PH. Computed tomography in the diagnosis of occult open-globe injuries. Ophthalmology 2007;114:1448–52.

2. Boldt HC, Pulido JS, Blodi CF, et al. Rural endophthalmitis. Ophthalmology 1989;96:1722–6.

3. Kuhn F, Maisiak R, Mann L, Mester V, Morris R, Witherspoon CD. The Ocular Trauma Score (OTS). Ophthalmol Clin North Am 2002;15:163–5.

Examination of a Neuro-ophthalmic Case

Chapter Outline

INTRODUCTION
• Common neuro-ophthalmic manifestations

CLINICO-INVESTIGATIVE APPROACH TO A PATIENT WITH VISUAL LOSS

Visual Loss

Transient visual loss
• Terminology
• Causes
• Clinical conditions

Visual impairment
• Clinical work-up and tests
• Tests for macular pathologies
• Tests for amblyopia

Neuroimaging

Summary

CLINICO-INVESTIGATIVE APPROACH FOR A PATIENT WITH DIPLOPIA

Introduction

Causes of Diplopia
• Monocular diplopia
• Binocular diplopia

Common Lesions
• Conjugate palsies
• Internuclear ophthalmoplegia
• Skew deviation
• Convergence spasm
• Convergence insufficiency
• Divergence insufficiency

Clinical Evaluation of Diplopia

History
• Features of diplopia
• Associated symptoms
• Diurnal variation of diplopia

Examination
• General examination
• Globe, orbit and eyelid examination
• Extraocular muscle examination
• Brainstem examination
• Supranuclear pathway examination

Investigations

Treatment Modalities

INTRODUCTION

Examination of a neuro-ophthalmic case basically includes a thorough ocular, neurological and systemic clinical work-up and investigations including neuro-imaging to reach up at the proper diagnosis.

COMMON NEURO-OPHTHALMIC MANIFESTATIONS

• *Visual loss,* i.e. either transient visual loss or visual impairment due to lesions of visual pathway and or cortical centers and psychosomatic condition.
• *Diplopia,* primarily because of palsies of cranial nerves supplying various extraocular muscles.

- *Visual field defects* due to various lesions of visual pathway.
- *Deranged higher visual functions* in the form of visual-hallucinations, illusions and agnosia.
- *Papilledema* is an important neuro-ophthalmic manifestation.
- *Anomalous pupillary reflexes* make up essential clues in a neuro-ophthalmic case.

In this text examination of a neuro-ophthalmic case is discussed as:

- Clinico-investigative approach to a patient with visual loss
- Clinico-investigative approach for a patient with diplopia.

CLINICO-INVESTIGATIVE APPROACH TO A PATIENT WITH VISAUL LOSS

Visual loss can be broadly classified into
- Transient visual loss
- Visual impairment.

TRANSIENT VISUAL LOSS

Transient loss or blurring of vision in one or both eyes is not an uncommon visual complaint. The approach to such a patient is complicated by challenging differential diagnosis and over-lapping disease profiles. It is an important sign of cerebrovascular diseases in some patients and thus warrants a systematic approach in examining, investigating and treating such patients.

TERMINOLOGY

Transient visual obscuration (TVO), i.e. fleeting loss of vision lasting just a few seconds

Monocular transient visual loss includes:
- *Amaurosis Fugax,* i.e. partial or total (rare) monocular blindness lasting a few seconds to minutes.
- *Transient monocular blindness* refers to more prolonged (30 minutes to hours to days) epi-sodes of partial or total loss of monocular vision.

Binocular transient visual loss includes episodes of bilateral loss of vision lasting from 5–30 minutes and occasionally longer, involving either homonymous field, inferior or superior altitudinal fields or the central fields.

CAUSES OF TRANSIENT VISUAL LOSS (TVL)

1. Non-ischemic causes of TVL

- *Ocular surface disorders* such as dry eye, blepha-ritis (anterior or posterior) and recurrent corneal erosions
- *Corneal endothelial disorders* such as dystrophies and decompensation
- *Intermittent angle closure*
- *Uveitis*
- *Vitreous floaters*
- *Optic disc disorders* such as papilledema, papillitis, drusen and colobomas.

2. Ischemic causes of TVL

i. *Embolic diseases*
- Carotid embolic diseases, e.g. atheromas and obstruction
- Cardiac embolic diseases, e.g. valvular—rheumatic, prosthetic valves, fibrillation and myxomas
- Great vessels embolic diseases, e.g. aortic arch embolus.

ii. *Vasculitis*
- Giant cell arteritis

iii. *Hypoperfusion* as seen in:
- Carotid obstruction
- Vertebrobasilar insufficiency
- Ocular ischemic syndrome.

iv. *Vasospasm,* e.g. migraine

v. *Hyperviscosity,* e.g. polycythemia

vi. *Hypercoagulability.*

APPROACH TO A PATIENT WITH TRANSIENT VISUAL LOSS

1. History

A meticulous history is very important. It should include:

i. *Age:* In less than 50 years of age vasospasm and migraine are the commonest causes of TVL and in more than 50 years of age carotid embolic disease is a common cause.

ii. *Associated medical conditions:* To be enquired include hypertension, diabetes, coronary artery diseases and Raynaud's phenomenon.

Features of TVL:
- Monocular or Binocular TVL?
- Duration of visual loss

- Number of episodes of visual loss
- Pattern of visual loss and recovery should be noted:
  - Shade or curtain coming down and then lifting is typical of amaurosis fugax due to carotid disease.
  - Positive visual phenomenon, e.g. scintillating scotomas in migraine.
  - Transient blurring of vision with exercise and increased body temperature is typical of *Uhthoff* phenomenon seen in optic neuritis associated with multiple sclerosis.
  - Abrupt change in vision may be associated with posterior circulation ischemia.

iii. *Associated symptoms:* To be noted include headaches, weight loss, fever, scalp tenderness, loss of consciousness, diplopia, dizziness, dysarthria and focal weakness.

2. Examination and investigations in a patient with transient visual loss

In a patient with monocular visual loss
Examination tests include:
- Visual acuity
- Ocular motility in cardinal positions of gaze
- Orbital examination for proptosis. Gaze evoked blurring of vision is reported in intraconal mass lesions
- Pupillary evaluation for RAPD, and anisocoria
- Slit-lamp biomicroscopy for lids, lashes, cornea, anterior chamber (cells, flare), cataract and anterior chamber angle depth
- Applanation tonometry
- Gonioscopy to note open, closed or occludable angles
- *Fundus examination* for evalution of optic disc, retinal vessel calibre, emboli, and signs of ischemia (hemorrhages, cotton wool spots)
- *Auscultation* of carotids for bruit and cardiac murmurs
- Palpation of temporal artery
- *Pulse rate* and *blood pressure* recording.

Investigations should include:
- Complete hemogram
- Erythrocyte sedimentation rate (ESR)
- C-reactive protein (CRP)
- Coagulation profile
- Lipidogram

- Serum glucose levels
- Carotid Doppler
- Magnetic resonance imaging (MRI)
- Magnetic resonance angiography (MRA)
- Carotid angiography—Gold standard for the assessment of carotid stenosis
- Echocardiography
- ECG, Holter monitoring.

CLINICAL ENTITIES ASSOCIATED WITH TVL

Non-ischemic transient visual loss

- *Ocular surface diseases and corneal abnormalities* are one of the commonest causes of non-ischemic TVL. Patients usually complain of transient visual obscurations of vision at specific times of the day, many times a week and more so in certain seasons. Slit-lamp exam reveals abnormal tear break up time, anterior or posterior blepharitis. Patients usually respond well to warm compresses, anti-inflammatory and antibiotic therapy of short duration supplemented with tear substitutes.

- Patients with *corneal endothelial diseases and dystrophies* report episodes of blurring of vision lasting many hours usually more pronounced in the mornings. Slit-lamp exam, pachymetry and specular count are diagnostic. Hyperosmotic drops, ointments and IOP lowering drugs help in symptomatic relief. Lamellar or full thickness corneal transplants can completely cure symptoms.

- *Intermittent angle closure* is an important cause of episodes of TVL. Patients usually complain of episodes of transient blurring of vision accompanied by ocular discomfort, seeing coloured haloes and mild headaches. Slit-lamp exam to grade AC depth along with gonioscopy show occludable angles and help clinch the diagnosis. Symptoms are completely relieved by YAG peripheral iridotomy.

- *Papilledema and optic disc drusen* can be associated with episodes of transient visual obscurations or episodes of gray, black or white vision. The episodes are usually associated with changes in posture. The likely etiology for TVL in these cases is axonal compression/stasis at the elevated optic nerve head.

- *Papillitis/optic neuritis* is associated with TVS similar to cases of papilledema. The likely etiology is demyelination and inflammation of the optic nerve.

Ischemic transient visual loss

Characteristic of transient visual loss are:
- Ischemic transient visual loss occurs due to temporary interruption of the blood supply to the retina, optic nerve or retrochiasmal visual pathways in the brain.
- Patients tend to be more specific, descriptive and discrete about the pattern of visual loss and recovery—onset, duration, number of episodes, central or peripheral field involvement.

Carotid artery stenosis or occlusion is the commonest cause of ischemic TVL. Atherosclerosis is the commonest cause but other causes like Takayasu arteritis, trauma, radiation arteritis and carotid dissection should be kept in mind. Carotid related amaurosis fugax results either from emboli originating from the diseased proximal internal carotid segment to the retinal arterial circulation or from decreased blood flow to the retina. The typical features of embolic monocular TVL are sudden onset, painless, described as a shade or a curatin coming down on the field of vision which lifts and vision clears in 1–5 minutes (sometimes up to 30 minutes).

Emboli that cause TVL can often be visualized with an ophthalmoscope or slit-lamp fundus biomicroscopy (78 D, 90 D lens) and often appear distinctive, their probable site of origin can be inferred which becomes crucial directing appropriate patient evaluation.
- *Cholesterol emboli (Hollenhorst plaques)* appear as yellow-orange refractile deposits at bifurcations of vessels and are typically a sign of carotid disease.
- *Platelet fibrin emboli* are dull grey or white in colour, concave meniscus at each end, lodge along the course of vessel and are likely a result of carotid thrombosis, thrombosis associated with recent myocardial infarction or heart valves.
- *Calcium* emboli are chalky white in colour, large round or ovoid, lodge in the first or second vessel bifurcations or may overlie the optic disc. They can arise from the heart (rheumatic heart disease, calcification of mitral valve) or great vessels (calcific aortic stenosis).

Stroke and transient visual loss
- The risk of stroke from *amaurosis fugax* per annum is approximately 2% and a 1% risk of permanent visual loss.
- In patients *with carotid stenosis*, ipsilateral eye symptoms may be accompanied by those *of ipsilateral cerebral ischemia* like contralateral hemiparesis, sensory loss, language deficits and hemianopia.

Clinical work-up
- *General examination* should include pulse rate (irregular in arrhythmias, fibrillation), cardiac auscultation (murmurs) and carotid auscultation (bruit). However, presence or absence of a carotid bruit is generally not helpful for diagnosing significant carotid stenosis or predicting a carotid source of emboli.
- *Carotid ultrasound and Doppler* are effective screening tools for identification and estimation of the degree of internal carotid artery stenosis.
- *Magnetic resonance imaging–angiography* (MRA) is another non-invasive test for carotid stenosis, however, it tends to overestimate the degree of stenosis.
- *Computed tomographic angiography* (CT angio) is another screening test and can be used to confirm MRA or ultrasound findings.
- *Conventional angiography* is the gold standard test for evaluation and quantification of carotid stenosis as its specificity and sensitivity exceed those of any noninvasive tests.
- In a elderly patient if the all the general work-up including carotid tests are unrevealing then an atheroma arising from the more proximal vessels like the aorta or an acephalic migraine should be considered as possible etiologies for TVL.
- In a young patient with an unrevealing work-up, vasospasm and hypercoagulable states, due to antiphospolipid antibodies, protein C, protein S and antithrombin III levels should be considered possible causes for TVL.

Treatment

If not contraindicated, antiplatelet therapy with aspirin should be immediately started in patients with amaurosis fugax to reduce the risk of stroke. Addition of clopidogrel or anti-coagulants can also be considered in consulta-tion with an interventional cardiologist. Multiple clinical trials have established the benefit of carotid surgery for symptomatic (retinal or hemispheric TIA) carotid stenosis greater than 70%. The management of asymptomatic carotid stenosis is however extremely controversial.

■ VISUAL IMPAIRMENT

A patient presenting with diminution of vision without any evidence of structural abnormali-ties in the eye is a puzzle for an ophthalmologist. It is important to have a logical and meticulous approach to evaluate such patients so as to come to a conclusion regarding the cause of visual loss. This includes detailed history, thorough clinical examination and appropriate investigations.

■ COMMON CAUSES

Visual impairment can be broadly classified to belong to the following pathologies:
1. Refractive errors and media opacities
2. Lesions of visual pathway
   • Optic nerve lesions
   • Chiasmal lesions
   • Retrochiasmal lesions
3. Macular lesions

4. Amblyopia
5. Psychogenic/malingering

We will further see how to rule out each of them and come to a problem oriented working diagnosis. Figure 6.1 is the flow chart for assess-ment of visual impairment and segregating patients with refractive errors, media opacities.

■ CLINICAL WORK-UP AND TESTS

TESTS FOR REFRACTIVE ERRORS, MEDIA OPACITIES AND VISUAL PATHWAY LESIONS

PINHOLE TEST AND STENOPEIC SLIT TEST

As refractive errors are one of the leading causes of decreased vision they should be the first ones to be ruled out. Use of pinhole and stenopeic slit determines whether or not vision will improve with refractive correction. Improve-ment by two lines on Snellen's chart or more on looking through the pinhole or stenopeic slit makes it clear that the visual impairment is due to optical problems.

As the pinhole eliminates paraxial rays of light, minimizing blurring of the image falling on the retina, all optical defects can be neutralized to some extent with this method, not only the refractive ametropias. However, many patients, especially children and old people find it difficult to peek through the pinhole and do not give reliable responses. The method is uncertain, and improvement of less than two lines should certainly be interpreted with

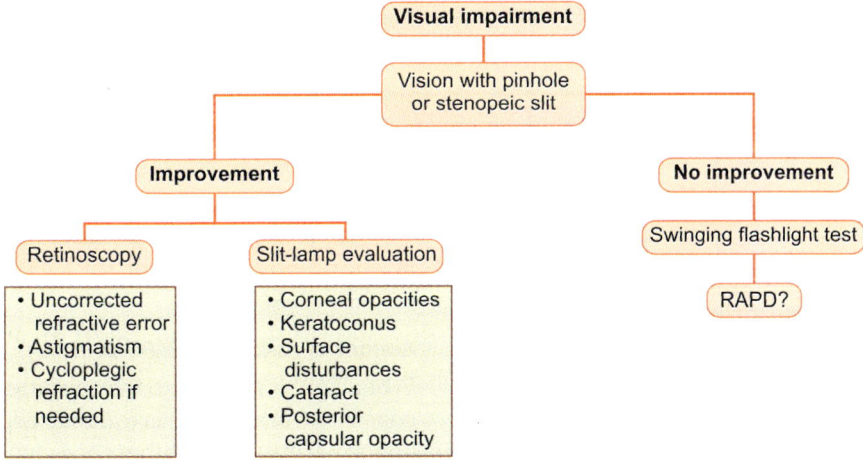

Fig. 6.1: *Flow chart for a patient with visual impairment.*

caution. Repeated subjective and cycloplegic *refraction* will usually uncover an undetected and irregular corneal astigmatism or hypermetropic error.

- Limitations of pinhole are that vision may apparently worsen in patients with central media opacities (such as posterior subcapsular cataract) and macular pathologies. Vision does not improve to 6/6 if refractive error exceeds ±4 DS.
- Detailed slit-lamp examination will reveal any obvious corneal opacities, surface irregularities, keratoconus and not to mention presence of cataract or posterior capsular opacity.
- If the vision does not improve with the pinhole, the next step will be checking the pupils for relative afferent pupillary defect.

SWINGING FLASHLIGHT TEST

This is performed to detect the presence of relative afferent pupillary defect (RAPD).

Remember: Relative = compared to the other eye, and Afferent = problem in the afferent pathway.

The main use of RAPD is in evaluating a patient who has decreased vision in one eye and normal vision in the other. If it is present, there is lesion in one of the eyes, or asymmetric optic nerve or retinal lesion. If it is not present, retina or optic nerve of both eyes are normal or symmetrically involved. But brisk pupillary reaction to light definitely rules out optic nerve pathology.

Technique of swinging flashlight test

The swinging flashlight test is performed as follows:

- *Patient is seated* in a dimly lit room and asked to fixate at a distant target. This provides maximum relaxation of the iris sphincter muscle.
- *Torchlight is shone* into one eye. The light should be directed from below so that it does not act like a near target and induce miosis associated with accommodation. It should be shone into the eye for about 2–3 seconds.
- *Pupillary reaction is observed* and the light is quickly moved across the bridge of the nose and directed into the opposite eye. If the light

is moved too slowly; the pupil is seen to constrict when finally the light falls on it and thus gives a false impression of a normal reaction.

- *Pupillary reaction of the other eye is observed* and compared in amplitude and speed to the first eye.
- *The light should be moved across one eye to the other* briskly and rhythmically at least 5 times. This is important to be sure that any papillary dilatation on one side is not just the sphincter movement due to physiological pupillary unrest. The light should be bright, but not so bright that it makes the patient photophobic.
- *RAPD can be identified even in cases where the reaction of both pupils cannot be studied,* for example, single eyed individuals, patients in whom one pupil is distorted, non-dilating and fixed or constricted due to neurological disease, iris trauma or synechiae.

Observations

While performing the swinging flashlight test, we observe the pupil that is being illuminated. But the opposite pupil also reacts in an identical manner. Thus, in these cases the examiner must observe only the reactive pupil. If the abnormal eye is the eye with the fixed pupil, then the normal eye will react briskly when the light is shone into it and will dilate when the light is shone into the opposite eye. On the other hand, if the eye with the apparently normal pupil is the affected eye, then its pupil will dilate when the light is shone onto it and constrict when the light is directed on the other eye (with the fixed pupil).

Normal response (RAPD absent)

When light is shone into one eye, the pupil constricts. When it is transferred to the other eye, its pupil is either already constricted (due to consensual reflex) or constricts further. When it is shone back into the first eye, the same response takes place.

Abnormal response (RAPD present)

When light is shone into the normal eye, its pupil constricts. When light is transferred to the other abnormal eye, it will either consistently constrict more weakly compared to the normal eye; or does not react; or actually dilates on light stimulation (phenomenon called pupillary escape); RAPD is said to be present. At this point the other eye's pupil will also be dilated.

Presence of RAPD means that cause of visual loss is unilateral or asymmetric bilateral retinopathy or neuropathy.

- Interpretation of presence of RAPD is shown in Fig. 6.2.
- On dilated fundus examination, a retinopathy severe enough to cause RAPD will be easily appreciated.
- However, optic neuropathy may be present in the absence of any fundus abnormalities.

Retinal pathologies capable of causing RAPD are:
- Central retinal artery occlusion
- Central retinal vein occlusion
- Total retinal detachment.

These will have substantial changes in the fundus and a careful dilated fundus examination can help differentiated them from neuro-ophthalmological disease.

If RAPD is absent, visual loss in these cases may be due to:
- Macular pathologies
- Amblyopia
- Psychogenic causes/malingering.

Use of neutral density filters

The neutral density filters are available ranging from 0.3 to 2 log units; in steps of 0.3 log units. Neutral density filters can be used for:
- *Quantifying the RAPD.* The neutral density filters are placed in front of the normal eye.

The density of the filter that neutralizes the RAPD is the measure of the defect.
- *Unequivocal findings.* The neutral density filters are successively placed in front of either eye. If RAPD is present in an eye it becomes more obvious when the filter is placed in front of that eye. If it is absent, when the filter is placed in front of one eye the pupil will dilate on shining light onto it; and this will repeat when the filter is shifted to the other eye, i.e. there will be an 'Artificially created RAPD'.

Grading of RAPD

Grade I. A weak initial constriction and greater re-dilatation

Grade II. Initial stall and greater re-dilatation

Grade III. Immediate pupillary dilatation

Grade IV. Immediate pupillary dilatation following prolonged illumination of the good eye for 6 seconds

Grade V. Immediate pupillary dilatation with no secondary constriction.

Note: As mentioned before, the presence of a relative afferent papillary defect almost always confirms a neuro-ophthalmological cause, but the absence of it does not rule out the same. So either ways, we must go ahead with further optic nerve function tests which complement our findings and which assume special importance in case of unequivocal results or if pupil cannot be examined.

OPTIC NERVE HEAD EXAMINATION

A meticulous optic nerve head examination using slit-lamp biomicroscope and high power

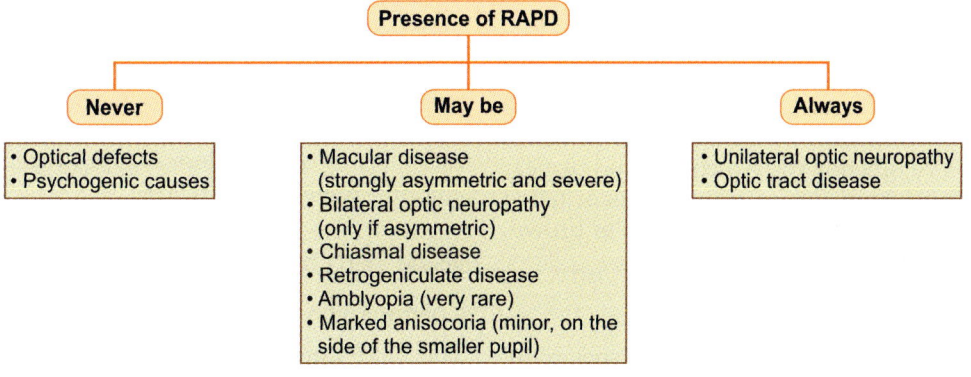

Fig. 6.2: *Interpretation of presence of RAPD.*

lenses like 78 D or 90 D gives valuable information about the acuteness of the condition and to some extent the etiology.

COLOUR VISION TESTING

Testing the colour vision helps to differentiate optic nerve pathology from other pathologies. Usually in day-to-day clinical practice, Ishihara pseudoisochromatic tests plates are used. Inability of indentifying a number at all is considered as defective colour vision. The D 15 colour vision test is based on a set of coloured plates or disks which have to be arranged in the correct order. Tests like Farnsworth-Munsell 100 hue test and Hardy-Rand-Ritter (HRR) charts are more detailed tests which include various colours which have a very subtle difference of hue which the patient has to compare and obtain the nearest match. Though these tests can identify very early or fine changes, they are very time consuming and very difficult to carry out in day-to-day busy clinics.

To determine whether the colour vision deficit is due to optic nerve involvement we need to note if:
- There is relevant history (acquired loss of colour vision)
- Colour vision worse in dim light
- Preferential inability to discriminate between red and green colours (in macular abnormalities there will be preferential loss of ability to differentiate blue and yellow colours).

Colour saturation

To patients with optic nerve disease colours appear less bright, faded (desaturated) or darker in the affected eye than the normal eye. To check for this, a red stimulus (brightly coloured stimulus preferred) is presented to each eye in succession and patient is asked if to one eye the colour appears 'brighter' or 'richer' than the other. If the patient clearly says yes it is taken as a positive response. To the eye with defective optic nerve function the red colour may appear as a faded colour such as orange, pink or faded red (indicating decreased saturation) or brown, gray (indicating decreased brightness).

BRIGHTNESS COMPARISON TEST

This test detects decreased brightness sensitivity in the affected eye if any. Bright torchlight is shone into each of the eyes and patient is asked which appears brighter. Taking the brighter one as 100% patient is asked to compare it with the other eye and determine how much is the decrease in the brightness perception in the other eye. This test is slightly more sensitive than the RAPD and may help detect an early defect.

CONTRAST SENSITIVITY TESTS

Visual acuity determines the smallest spatial detail that can be resolved for a high contrast stimulus, whereas measurement of contrast sensitivity checks the responses of visual system to different sizes and contrasts. These tests are thus useful adjuncts to reveal the deficit in patients with normal visual acuity but who may have a visual pathway lesion.

- It is usually determined by measuring the contrast thresholds for sinusoidal gratings, an alternating pattern of light and dark bars, the luminance of which varies sinusoidally in a direction perpendicular to the orientation of the grating. The size of the grating is specified according to the spatial frequency which is the number of cycles of the grating pattern (i.e. the pair of dark and light bars) per degree of visual angle. The contrast sensitivity function measures between 3 and 10 spatial frequencies from 0.5 to 30 cycles per degree.
- Other tests available to measure the contrast sensitivity are Pelli-Robson contrast sensitivity chart, Vistech contrast sensitivity chart and a low contrast version of the Bailey-Lovie visual acuity chart. These charts make use of contrast letters to measure contrast sensitivity. However, whether these tests are superior to the ones using sinusoidal gratings to measure contrast sensitivity is controversial.

Note. One must note that sensitivity losses have little specificity for differential diagnosis purposes. Similar patterns of loss can be obtained by a wide variety of conditions and at the same time many types of disorders can produce similar amounts of visual acuity loss.

VISUAL FIELD TESTING

Confrontation test

The next step is to determine any defect or decreased sensitivity in the visual fields. This

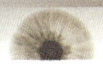

can be done in the OPD performing the confrontation test which is done as follows:

1. **Patient should be comfortably seated.** The clinician is seated about 1 meter in front of and at the level of the patient, who is asked to fixate on the bridge of the examiner's nose. While testing patient's right eye, his left eye should be occluded and the clinician's right eye should be closed.

2. **Firstly ask the patient** if he can see the examiner's full face clearly. If not, then ask him to elaborate which parts are missing or not clearly visible to him. This will tell us about any gross defects in the field of vision.

3. **Testing of single quadrants.** One or two stationary fingers are presented randomly in each quadrant of the right eye taking care that the stimulus remains well within 30 degrees of the visual field; and the patient is asked to count the fingers. Children can be asked to simulate the number of fingers seen and at the same time the examiner looks for the eye movements brought forth by the stimulus.

4. **Delineating the scotoma.** If the patient is not able to see the fingers—move the finger from the defective quadrant slowly towards the vertical meridian. Patient is asked to identify as soon as he sees the stimulus. This way we can recognize if the border of the defect is aligned to the vertical meridian. Same procedure should be repeated to if there is presence of a defect respecting the horizontal meridian.

Steps 2, 3, 4 are repeated in the left eye.

5. **Testing double quadrants.** This is performed if the patient correctly identifies stimuli in single quadrant testing but the clinician suspects presence of defect in a certain quadrant. One or two fingers of both the hands are simultaneously presented in two different quadrants and the patient is asked to count the total number of fingers seen.

6. **Brightness comparison.** If the patient responds correctly to the above tests he may be asked to compare the clarity or brightness of two fingers simultaneously presented in two different quadrants and if there is any reduction in brightness of one of them.

7. **Red desaturation test.** Two identical bright coloured objects (preferably red) are presented to the patient in two different quadrants and asked if there is any difference in the brightness of the colour in any of the quadrant. If yes, the object is moved slowly from the defective quadrant towards the vertical meridian and the patient is asked if the object becomes brighter or duller in the course. If there is marked difference, a hemianopic defect exists. Same manoeuvre is repeated with the horizontal meridian.

The confrontation test gives a rough idea about presence of any gross visual field defects. It has very less specificity and sensitivity as it depends largely on the patient's ability to understand how to perform the test and maintain fixation. Though it should never replace formal visual field testing, it assumes importance in certain scenarios like examination of a bedridden patient where technical investigations may not be possible.

Automated visual field examination

One of the most important investigations in neuro-ophthalmology is the automated visual fields examination. Central 30 degrees of field testing in standard automated perimetric programmes is preferred.

Visual field analysis must be considered
- If RAPD is present
- If any of the adjunctive clinical tests (colour vision, colour saturation, brightness sensitivity, contrast sensitivity) are abnormal
- Optic nerve head examination shows pallor/edema/optic atrophy/glaucomatous changes.

Visual field examination helps greatly to quantify the defect and localise the lesion along the afferent visual pathway and thereby can be called an important part of visual testing.

While trying to localise the lesion we must try to differentiate between a non-hemianopic and hemianopic defect. The loss of entire hemifield is not necessary for the diagnosis of hemianopic defect, it is enough that the border of the defect is aligned to the vertical fixation meridian. If the field defect is hemianopic, it points towards the cause of an optic neuropathy or retinopathy, whereas a hemianopic defect would point to a chiasmal lesion.

TESTS FOR MACULAR PATHOLOGIES

Tests that can be used to rule out macular pathologies are as follows.

Amsler's grid test

In the standard Amsler's grid chart the patient is presented a grid of black lines on a white background and a central black dot for fixation at a reading distance. The patient must wear his refractive correction. First the patient is asked if he can see the central dot. He is then asked to mark on the chart if any of the squares seem bent or distorted or of unequal sizes; or if he is unable to see any parts of the grid. The presence of meta-morphopsia is diagnostic of macular disease, as it is caused by the separation, distortion or crowding of foveal cones by oedema, fluid or scarring.

There are other types of Amsler's grids:

- White squares on black background and central white dot
- White squares on a black background with a central white dot and diagonal white limits of his scotoma
- Red squares on a black background with a central red dot. This chart helps to diagnose optic nerve, chiasmal, or toxic amblyopia related problems.

Photostress test

Baseline visual acuity of the patient is determined. Bright light is directed into one of the eyes for ten seconds. This bleaches the photoreceptors. After ten seconds the patient's Snellen's visual acuity is recorded again. The time between bleaching and recovery to within one Snellen line of the original visual acuity is measured. If the time taken to recover is substantially greater in one eye than the other, it indicates impaired regeneration of photoreceptor pigment in the retinal pigment epithelium. However, this is a highly subjective test and can hardly be relied upon for the diagnosis.

Electroretinogram (ERG)

In the standard full field (Ganzfield) ERG the potentials are excited by short flashes of light and detected by recording electrodes contacting the anterior surface of the eye. The stimulus covers the entire retina, and the recorded responses are a summation of the electrical potentials generated by the entire retina. It thus is a mass response and will detect generalized outer retinal disease and fails to detect isolated macular or other localized pathologies. Multifocal ERG (Mf ERG) is the new specialized type of ERG which is capable of highlighting such localized pathologies.

This is useful in determining the cause of visual disabilities when there are no visible findings on ophthalmoscopy.

Fundus fluorescein angiography

This is done to identify subtle macular lesions and vascular pathologies and is capable of detecting defects in the RPE and choroid too. It occasionally spots lesions not visible even on high magnification ophthalmoscopy.

TESTS FOR AMBLYOPIA

If there is absence of retinal lesion, the visual loss can be attributed to amblyopia. Amblyopia refers to poor vision caused by abnormal visual development secondary to abnormal visual stimulation.

History of squinting or cataract in childhood or congenital ptosis which occludes the visual axis may give a clue towards the presence of amblyopia. Binocular amblyopia may be considered in the cases of children with high hypermetropia. There are no confirmatory investigations for this entity and the diagnosis of amblyopia is made when all other causes are ruled out. A few simple clinical tests may aid in the diagnosis.

Testing for 'crowding phenomenon'

An amblyopic patient when asked to read single letters, is said to have a higher visual acuity then when he is asked to read an entire line. This is called *crowding phenomenon*.

Neutral density filter test

A 2 log unit neutral density filter is used in this setting. It is placed in front of the normal eye and the visual acuity is checked. It causes a drop in the visual acuity. When the same procedure is repeated in front of the other suspected amblyopic eye, it degrades the visual acuity less.

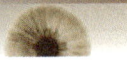

Base out prism test

This test detects the presence of a central fixation scotoma <5 degrees and is not specific for amblyopia. A 4 PD prism is placed in front of the normal eye in the base out position. The image is thus shifted temporally in that eye. There is bilateral vergence movement away from the eye behind the prism to take up fixation and similar movement of the other eye. However, since the image falls within the small scotoma the eye does not show any refixation movement. Similarly, when the prism is placed in front of this eye, there is no movement of either eye.

NEUROIMAGING

Neuroimaging is essential in certain scenarios to come to the correct diagnosis. It should be considered in cases of:

1. *Acute loss of vision*; unilateral (suspicion of haemorrhagic, ischaemic, embolic phenomenon) or bilateral (suspecting a lesion above the level of chiasma)
2. *Haemianopic field defects* on visual field analysis indicating chiasmal lesion
3. *Trauma* to rule out haemorrhage, fractures, optic nerve injury or compression
4. *Suspicion of compressive pathology.*

The choice of imaging modality depends upon the clinical diagnosis, available facilities and the cost factor. Magnetic resonance imaging (MRI) and computed tomography (CT) are the most commonly ordered investigations by a neuro-ophthalmologist.

Magnetic resonance imaging (MRI)

MRI is the investigation of choice in neuro-ophthalmology; especially for a patient with acute vision loss. It is more useful in:

- Identifying small lesions
- Identifying vascular lesions
- Characterization of lesion
- Extent and invasion of surrounding lesion
- Surgical planning if necessary.

MRI offers better delineation of soft tissues and thus an improved differentiation between retrobulbar soft tissues (fat, muscle and optic nerve), between normal components of the brain (gray and white substances) and between differing forms of pathological change (infarction, haemorrhage, inflammation, and neoplasms).

MRI with gadolinium contrast enhances the blood vessels, extraocular muscles and active lesions and is preferred in this setting.

The most important advantage of MRI scanning lies in the fact that the signal strength in the image determined by tissue-specific parameters, the T_1 and T_2 relaxation times. This produces a high-resolution image with excellent tissue identification. Normal anatomy is best demonstrated in T_1-**weighted** images, whereas T_2-**weighted** images are better for demonstrating intracranial or other pathology.

Magnetic resonance angiography (MRA) and Magnetic resonance venography (MRV) are performed when the MRI does not yield any results but there is a strong suspicion of vessel pathology.

Absolute contraindications to MRI:

- Cardiac pacemakers
- Incorporated ferromagnetic foreign bodies/implants
- Shrapnel wounds
- Aneurysm clips of uncertain origin.

Computed tomography (CT)

CT is the imaging method of choice for patients with skull/brain injuries. The presence and course of fractures in the orbit can be studied, using the windows that allow the best definition of bones' anatomy (**Bone window**). The effects of direct ocular trauma, or retrobulbar haemorrhages, are best studied when using the window settings for soft tissues (**Soft tissue window**). Thus, ophthalmic vein distension may be detected because of a traumatic carotid cavernous fistula.

In soft tissue tumours where we expect calcification or hyperostosis (like meningioma) or an orbital tumour CT scan is a better choice of investigation. Also for detection of foreign bodies CT scan is preferred as such cases are a potential contraindication for MRI.

CT with contrast is done for better visualization of blood vessels.

Contraindication of contrast: It is important to remember the contraindications for the use of contrast materials:
- Allergy to iodinated compounds
- Hyperthyroidism
- Poor renal function
- Paraproteinemia.

SUMMARY

If all the above-mentioned causes of visual loss are eliminated with the aid of clinical tests, visual field examination, neuroimaging and other diagnostic investigations; and still no cause is found; the visual loss can then be attributed to psychogenic causes.

It is often tempting enough to refer such a patient with unexplained visual loss to the neuro-ophthalmologist but what is essential is a systematic and rational approach to come to a working diagnosis and thus save the patient of anxiety, dissatisfaction and expenses.

Clinico-investigative approach to a patient with visual loss is summarized in Fig. 6.3.

CLINICO-INVESTIGATIVE APPROACH FOR A PATIENT WITH DIPLOPIA

INTRODUCTION

Diplopia essentially means double vision. Causes of diplopia range from benign and common entities such as a decompensated phoria to ominous entities such as aneurysmal third nerve palsy or sixth nerve palsy due to increased intracranial pressure. Dysfunction of the extraocular muscles may be the result of an abnormality of the muscle itself or an abnormality of the motor nerve to the muscle. The major symptom associated with this dysfunction is diplopia. Diplopia is a common presenting symptom to ophthalmologists and emergency room physicians with many potential causes that can involve many different structures. Given that the etiology of diplopia spans such a broad-spectrum, it is important to have a systematic approach in evaluating patients presenting with this symptom.

CAUSES OF DIPLOPIA

MONOCULAR DIPLOPIA

Monocular diplopia is defined as double vision that is present in the affected eye while the other eye is occluded. Monocular diplopia in nearly all circumstances is the result of local ocular aberration (defects of the cornea, iris, lens or retina). Neurologic misalignment causes binocular diplopia, whereas ocular causes such as refractive error, lead to monocular diplopia. Patients with optical causes of monocular diplopia like media opacity such as subtle changes in the optical density of anterior and

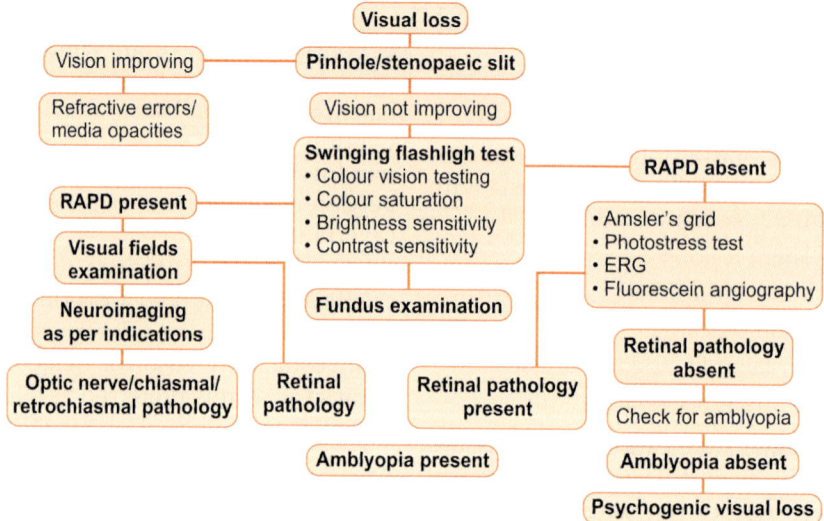

Fig. 6.3: *Summary of clinico-investigative approach to a patient with visual loss.*

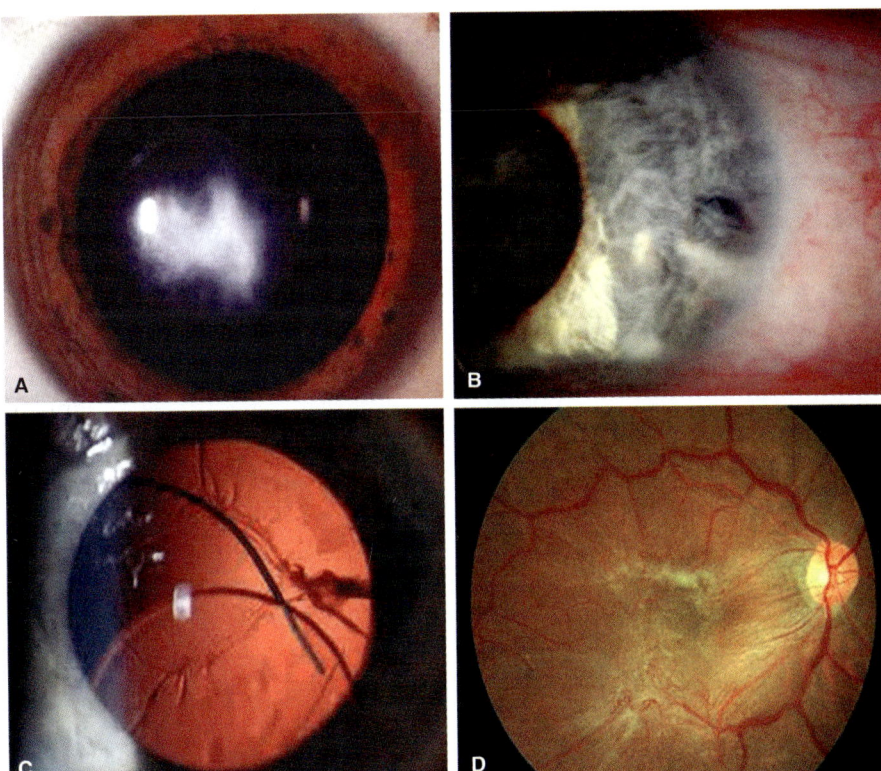

Fig. 6.4: *Common causes of monocular diplopic: (A) Corneal scar; (B) Iridotomy; (C) Subluxated IOL; (D) Macular pucker.*

posterior layers of lens in the case of incipient cataract generally describe blurring and glare and the patient may see a ghost image that is much lighter and less defined. Other causes include defects of cornea like irregular astigmatism, corneal scars (Fig. 6.4A), scars due to laser eye surgery (LASIK), iris defects (Fig. 6.4B) or in appropriately placed peripheral iridectomy, subluxated crystalline lens or IOLs (Fig. 6.4C). In all these conditions monocular diplopia resolves with pin hole. Patients with macular disorders generally describe a break, bend or distortion of the viewed edge leading to a distorted image. This type of monocular double vision generally does not improve when the object is viewed through a pinhole, in fact, vision is often worse in these cases. Common disorders of macula include choroidal neovascular membrane or an epiretinal membrane (Fig. 6.4D). The other cause of monocular diplopia which does not resolve with pinhole is central diplopia which is caused by lesion involving visual cortex and is associated with visual field defects. In this setting the patient may also complain of triple or quadruple vision.

BINOCULAR DIPLOPIA

Binocular diplopia, on the other hand, resolves with closure of either eye. From the eye to the brain, the following seven mechanisms and their associated locations should be kept in mind while gathering historical information regarding binocular diplopia:

- Orbital/ocular displacement
- Extraocular muscles restriction
- Extraocular muscles weakness
- Neuromuscular junction dysfunction
- 3rd, 4th and 6th cranial nerve dysfunction
- Cranial nerve nuclear dysfunction in brainstem
- Supranuclear dysfunctions (pathways to and between nuclei of 3rd, 4th and 6th cranial nerves).

Common causes of binocular diplopia are summarized in Table 6.1.

Table 6.1 *Common causes of binocular diplopia*	
Types of lesion	*Causes*
Orbital disorders	• Trauma • Tumour/mass • Infection
Extraocular muscle restriction	• Thyroid associated ophthalmopathy • Mass/tumour • Extraocular muscle entrapment • Injury/haematoma due to ocular surgery
Extraocular muscle weakness	• Congenital myopathies • Muscular dystrophy
Neuromuscular junction dysfunction	• Myasthenia gravis • Botulism
3rd, 4th and 6th cranial nerve dysfunction	• Ischemia • Hemorrhage • Tumour/mass • Vascular malformations • Aneurysm • Trauma • Multiple sclerosis • Meningitis
Cranial nerve nuclear dysfunction in brainstem	• Stroke • Haemorrhage • Tumour/mass • Vascular malformations
Supranuclear dysfunction	• Internuclear ophthalmoplegia • Convergence spasm • Convergence and divergence insufficiency • Pseudoabducens palsy • Skew deviation • Monocular elevator palsy

SUPRANUCLEAR PATHWAY LESIONS

GAZE PALSIES

1. *Conjugate gaze palsy.* If both eyes are equally paretic in the same direction of gaze and causes no diplopia. These are of two types:

- *Horizontal*—*conjugate* gaze palsies localize to pons or frontal cortex.

- *Vertical*—conjugate gaze palsies localize to midbrain.

2. *Disconjugate gaze palsy* results in diplopia. It is of two types:

a. *Horizontal*, e.g. internuclear ophthalmoplegia.

b. *Vertical*—skew deviation.

INTERNUCLEAR OPHTHALMOPLEGIA

Disruption of the MLF in the pons or midbrain results in an internuclear ophthalmoplegia (INO). There is adduction deficit in the eye on the same side of lesion and simultaneous nystagmus of the abducting eye in lateral gaze. The side of the adduction deficit determines the side of the INO. It is most commonly associated with multiple sclerosis and stroke.

Clinical features

The patients with INO may complain of horizontal diplopia, particularly when there is profound adduction weakness. Those patients with subtle paresis may have no symptoms or complain of blurred vision with eccentric gaze only. Since a skew deviation is frequently associated with lesions of the MLF, vertical diplopia may be another complaint. Oscillopsia may be the other symptom which may result from either the abduction nystagmus or an impaired vertical vestibular ocular reflex.

- The hallmark finding of INO is impaired adduction of the eye. Subtle cases may be evident only upon fast eye movements from midline to eccentric gaze which is known as medial rectus float. The demonstration of intact convergence in INO establishes the supranuclear localization of the medial rectus weakness and usually signifies a lesion of the MLF within the pons. In contrast patients with MLF lesions close to the third nerve nucleus may have impaired convergence. However, some patients with INO have poor convergence because of the vertical misalignment produced by the associated skew deviation. Therefore, the absence of convergence may not be a totally reliable sign to localize the lesion in a discrete part of the MLF pathway.

- The eye that is contralateral to the MLF lesion typically exhibits an abducting nystagmus in end gaze. Evidence suggests that this abducting nystagmus is an adaptive phenomenon to increase the innervation to the weak adducting eye.

- Since the otolith pathways project through the MLF, a skew deviation is commonly observed with an INO. Typically, the hypertropic eye is on the same side as the adduction weakness. There is downbeating nystagmus in the eye ipsilateral to the MLF lesion and torsional nystagmus in the contralateral eye.

- Bilateral lesions of the MLF usually produce additional eye findings, including impaired vertical pursuit and vertical gaze holding defects. Severe bilateral INOs may also result in a large angle exotropia in primary gaze in so-called WEBINO (wall eyed bilateral INO).

Diagnosis

The diagnosis of INO is usually straightforward, especially when there is impaired medial rectus dysfunction in lateral gaze with normal convergence. A unilateral INO in an older patient usually results from a brainstem infarction, while bilateral INO in a young patient typically signifies a demyelinating process such as multiple sclerosis. However, a variety of lesions may be associated with INOs including vascular malformations, tumours; head trauma, infections, vasculitides such as systemic lupus erythematosus, Behçet's disease and giant cell arteritis; nutritional disorders such as Wernicke's disease; metabolic disorders such as hepatic encephalopathy; Arnold-Chiari malformation; and degenerative conditions, progressive supranuclear palsy.

- The combination of an INO with an ipsiversive conjugate palsy is a pontine one-and-half syndrome due to simultaneous ipsilateral involvement of the PPRF and the MLF. Damage to the MLF in addition to the corticospinal tracts results in the Raymond. Cestan syndrome, characterized by an INO and contralateral hemiparesis.

SKEW DEVIATION

Skew deviation is an acquired vertical misalignment of the eyes that commonly occurs from acute brainstem dysfunction. It may also result from peripheral vestibular or cerebellar lesions. Patients may complain of binocular vertical diplopia, sometimes with a torsional component. The associated neurologic symptoms and signs often helps in differentiating skew deviation from other causes of vertical misalignment such as third and fourth nerve palsies.

Ocular tilt reaction. The combination of skew deviation with ocular torsion and a head tilt is known as the *ocular tilt reaction (OTR)*. This syndrome typically develops because of loss of otolithic input to the INC from a central lesion, which may be in the medulla, pons, or midbrain. With an ocular tilt reaction, if the head is tilted to the left, the right eye becomes hypertropic, and both eyes rotate toward the lower ear. The opposite response of the eyes occurs if the head is tilted to the right. A fourth nerve palsy is the motility disorder that may be the most difficult to distinguish from a skew deviation since both conditions may be associated with a positive head tilt or three step test. With a fourth nerve palsy, the compensatory head tilt is opposite the

side of the higher eye (similar to ocular tilt reaction), but the hypertropic eye is extorted which is opposite of the skew deviation.

Thalamic esodeviation is an acquired horizontal deviation that occurs with lesions near the junction of the diencephalon and midbrain. This disorder may be seen in younger patients with pineal tumours or craniopharyngioma or in older patients with cerebral haemorrhage.

CONVERGENCE SPASM

This condition, characterized by convergence, accommodation, bilateral papillary miosis, and pseudomyopia, may mimic bilateral sixth nerve palsies. The distinction is important because convergence spasm is almost always indicative of a functional disorder. Patients usually complain of double vision, and they often have obvious personality disorders or other hysterical symptoms. The hallmarks are pupillary constriction on attempted abduction and a variable esotropia. Other features include normal abducting saccades, intact abduction during the oculocephalic manoeuvre or testing of monocular ductions, and resolution of the myopia following cycloplegia. The miosis may resolve upon occlusion of the fellow eye by disrupting the binocular input necessary for convergence. Convergence spasm should be distinguished from convergence retraction nystagmus or pseudoabducens palsy from pretectal lesions.

CONVERGENCE INSUFFICIENCY

Patients with convergence insufficiency describe horizontal diplopia at near, typically after a period of reading. Medial rectus function is normal when ocular ductions are tested, but patients typically have an exodeviation worse at near. A common sequela of head trauma, the condition may also be seen in association with dorsal midbrain syndrome, may be a decompensation of long standing exophoria or may be idiopathic.

DIVERGENCE INSUFFICIENCY

This ocular motility deficit is characterized by acquired horizontal diplopia at distance but not near, a comitant esophoria or esotropia at distance, motor fusion at near, and full ocular

ductions without evidence of a sixth nerve palsy. Divergence insufficiency is typically benign, and affected patients are usually neurologically normal otherwise. However, since small bilateral sixth nerve palsies may mimic divergence insufficiency, elevated intracranial pressure, masses, and pontine lesions must be excluded with neuroimaging. Small vessel ischemic disease is a relatively common finding on magnetic resonance imaging studies of older patients with this condition.

- Prenuclear vertical misalignment seen in brainstem and cerebellar lesions may be comitant or incomitant with full motility but vertical misalignment decreases when patient lays supine.

CLINICAL EVALUATION OF DIPLOPIA

Diplopia may be the initial presentation of the potentially life-threatening disorder or it may be secondary to a harmless process. So, a detailed history as well as physical examination of a patient with diplopia is must to review the most common associated features that help localise the cause of diplopia.

HISTORY

The examiner should first determine whether the patient rarely sees double or has blurred vision of one eye, an overlay of the image or sees a halo surrounding the image. This information is obtained by a careful history and also we can ask the patient to draw a picture of what he sees. Once it has been confirmed that the images are truly separated, placing a cover over either eye will determine whether the diplopia is monocular or binocular.

The following questions should be kept in mind while approaching a patient with diplopia:
- Is the diplopia monocular or binocular?
- Is the onset acute or gradual?
- Is it constant or intermittent?
- Is there any variability/remission?
- Are there any associated signs and symptoms?
- History of ocular surgery/trauma?
- Any systemic diseases—Diabetes, hypertension, hyperlipidemia, hyperthyroidism, parkinsonism?

Features of diplopia

- *Onset.* Diplopia is almost always sudden in onset. The only exceptions are thyroid ophthalmopathy, divergence insufficiency and myasthenia gravis where gradual progression is seen.
- *Constant or intermittent.* We should always enquire from the patient whether the diplopia is constant or intermittent in nature. Most common causes of intermittent diplopia by far are decompensating phorias, vergence problems, accommodative spasm, headache (temporal arteritis) and myasthenia gravis. Myasthenia gravis is one condition which should be investigated in detail in a patient complaining of intermittent diplopia.
- *Separation of images.* Normally we do diplopia charting to look for separation of images. But we can always narrow down group of muscles which are affected by asking about the separation of images.
- *Horizontal separation* of two images indicates 6th nerve palsy.
- *Vertical separation* if pure can be due to 4th nerve palsy.
- *Oblique separation* of images occurs in 3rd nerve palsy.
- *Orbital processes* can cause horizontal, vertical or oblique diplopia.
- *Horizontal diplopia* worse at distance is associated with esotropia and implies lateral rectus palsy.
- If mainly at near, medial recti are implicated and is diagnosed as convergence insufficiency.
- Internuclear ophthalmoplegia and myasthenia gravis are other causes of horizontal diplopia.
- *Thyroid associated ophthalmopathy*, skew deviation and myasthenia gravis present as vertical diplopia.

Associated symptoms

Associated signs and symptoms are vital to localize the site of injury:

- Elderly patient with severe headache and isolated 3rd nerve palsy with dilated non-reacting pupil implicates a compressive injury of 3rd nerve in subarachnoid space. Most likely cause would be intracranial aneurysm of posterior communicating artery.
- Symptoms of jaw claudication, headache, scalp tenderness and arthralgias should be enquired in older patients with diplopia to rule out temporal arteritis.
- Patient should be asked about associated neurological symptoms like facial numbness or weakness, hearing loss, dysphagia, dysarthria, vertigo, incoordination or numbness or weakness of extremities to rule out brainstem injury and supranuclear pathway injuries.
- If a patient reports with eye pain and diplopia, then common causes like cellulitis, any mass lesion, inflammatory disorders like pseudotumour should be ruled out.

Diurnal variation of diplopia

Diplopia that progressively worsens throughout the day or worsens with reading is common with neuromuscular junction disorders that affect extraocular muscles like myasthenia gravis. More than 50% patients of myasthenia gravis present with ptosis and diplopia alone.

Palinopsia refers to seeing multiple images of an object immediately after turning away from the object or after the object is removed from the sight. This is known as after image or strobe effect. This condition is seen in discrete lesions with occipitoparietal or occipitotemporal cortex and homonymous visual field defects are also associated with these cortical visual illusions.

EXAMINATION

Examination of all basic visual sensory and ocular motor functions is necessary in the evaluation of diplopia.

GENERAL EXAMINATION

- In general examination of a patient note should be made of gait, physical appearance, stature, head posture, facial symmetry, moist hands or tremors on a handshake.
- Blood pressure, random blood sugar and resting pulse rate should be recorded.
- *Unaided and best corrected visual acuity followed by visual fields* to confrontation,

pupillary appearance and reaction to light and pupil response to viewing a near target should be recorded. An invaluable tool for measuring visual acuity is a hand-held pinhole device (Fig. 6.5) that allows a patient to have monocular view of an eye chart through small holes. Pinhole can eliminate refractive errors, ocular aberrations and correct monocular diplopia caused by the same. On the other hand macular disorders of the retina do not improve with pinhole.

- *An amsler grid* can be used to identify macular diseases which can be confirmed on indirect ophthalmoscopy and fundus biomicroscopy.

GLOBE, ORBIT AND EYELID EXAMINATION

- The examiner should note periorbital swelling (Fig. 6.6), forward displacement proptosis (Fig. 6.7), backward displacement enophthalmos (Fig. 6.8) or sideways displacement (dystopia) of the globe.

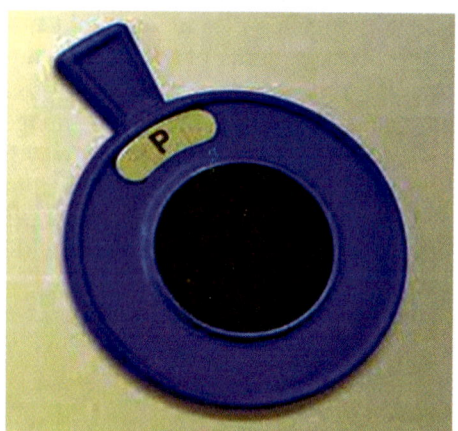

Fig. 6.5: *Pinhole.*

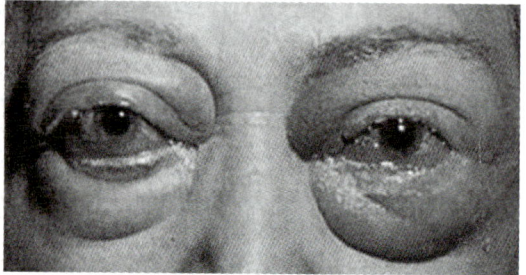

Fig. 6.6: *Periorbital swelling.*

- An exophthalmometer is used to detect and measure proptosis. Reading greater than 21 mm for either eye or a differences of more than 2 mm between each eye indicates proptosis/enophthalmos.

- *Eyelid position and function* should be examined. When the upper eyelid is above the upperborder of iris and sclera is showing, lid retraction is diagnosed and if the eyelid lags behind the eye on downward eye pursuits lid lag is present (Fig. 6.9). These two signs are commonly present in thyroid associated ophthalmopathy, whereas eyelid retraction

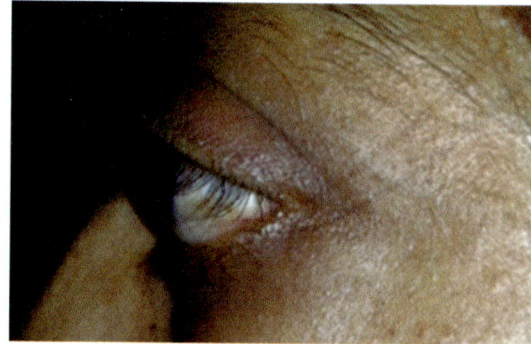

Fig. 6.7: *Proptosis.*

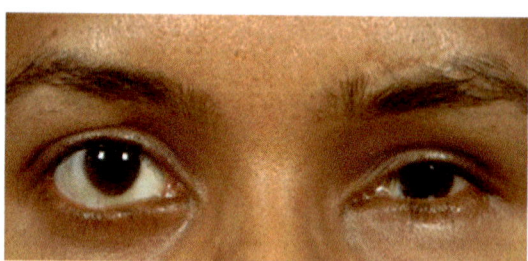

Fig. 6.8: *Enophthalmos.*

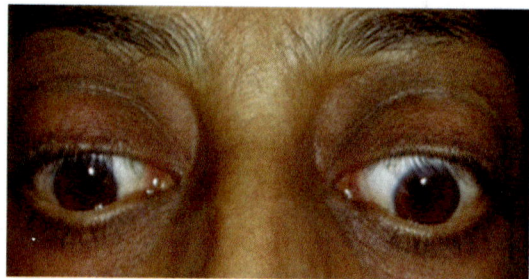

Fig. 6.9: *Lid lag.*

without lid lag is seen in dorsal midbrain disease. Ptosis is present if there is less than 4 mm between corneal light reflex and the upper eyelid with the patient fixating in primary gaze. Neurologic causes of ptosis result from dysfunction of the levator palpebrae muscle, controlled by the third cranial nerve or from dysfunction of the Müller's muscle, controlled by sympathetic innervations.

EXTRAOCULAR MUSCLE EXAMINATION

Ocular movement

The cardinal positions of gaze are examined by asking the patient to follow a target or the examiners finger held approximately 12 to 14 inches away from the patient's eyes. Ocular motility of each eye should be tested separately called ductions. Normal ductions rule out mechanical restriction of extraocular muscles but do not exclude possibility of paresis of extraocular muscles as paretic eye may move normally into the paretic field due to maximal innervation. Paresis is diagnosed by testing the versions (binocular eye movements). We should note that whether both eyes move fully and simultaneously or whether there is limitation or excessive movement of non-fixating eye. If duction/versions are limited, then one has to determine whether the limitation is caused by restrictive process, muscle weakness, neuromuscular junction dysfunction, cranial nerve palsy or supranuclear injury. Figure 6.10 shows eye movements in cardinal positions of gaze and corresponding muscles responsible for different directions of gaze.

Forced duction test

Forced duction testing is done to detect mechanical restriction. When there is an actual restriction of movement, it becomes essential to determine, whether the restriction of movement is due to the primary under action of paretic muscle or is it because of presence of contractures in the antagonist muscle. Under topical anaesthesia the eye is moved with two toothed forceps, applied to the conjunctiva near the limbus in the direction opposite that in which mechanical restriction is suspected. If no resistance is encountered then the motility defect is caused by the paralysis of muscle. If resistance is encountered mechanical restrictions do exist and contracture of muscle, conjunctiva, tenon's capsule or myositis must be considered. Restrictive diplopia, due to orbital processes such as thyroid-associated ophthalmopathy, is associated with positive forced duction testing.

Active force generation test

Active force generation test determines the active force generated by a contracting muscle and is useful in assessing the function of apparently paretic muscles. The examiner stabilizes the eye with forceps while the patient tries to move the eye in the direction of paretic muscle against this obstacle. The presence of tug on the forceps indicates that residual innervation is present and there is incomplete or partial paralysis whereas absence of tug is due to complete paralysis of muscle.

The examination of a patient with ocular misalignment involves more than the evaluation of movement of eyes. The examiner should measure ocular alignment in various directions of gaze and with a right or left head tilt.

Measurement of deviation

Methods to measure diviation include:
1. Objective method
   • Prism bar cover test.
2. Subjective methods
   • Red-green glasses
   • Maddox rod test

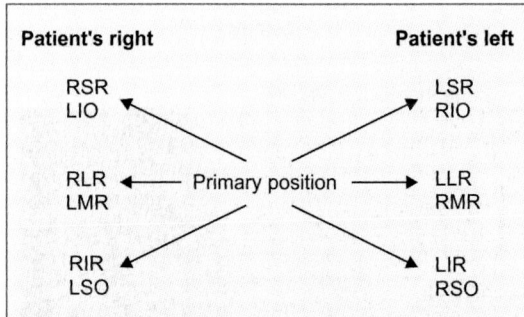

Fig. 6.10: *Eye movements in cardinal positions of gaze and corresponding muscles responsible for different directions of gaze.*

- Maddox wing test
- Hess and diplopia charting
- Lees screen test.

The motility disturbance will be obvious after inspection and testing of vergences. However, more subtle problems will require quantification of the misalignment using prism alternative cover or Maddox rod techniques.

Maddox rod test

Maddox rod can be used to determine the presence and degree of ocular misalignment. The red line is held over either the right or left eye while the patient focuses on a distant, pinpoint light source. The ridges are placed in the horizontal direction to evaluate for horizontal misalignment and in the vertical direction to evaluate for vertical misalignment. The relationship of the line to the light that the patient sees determine the type of misalignment (Fig. 6.11). The red line seen by the patient is oriented vertically, when the ridges are placed horizontally over the right/left eye and *vice versa*. The Maddox rod test is also useful in quantitating the degree of torsional misalignment.

BRAINSTEM EXAMINATION

The brainstem examination includes examination of all the cranial nerves (Fig. 6.12).

- 2nd, 3rd, 4th and 6th cranial nerve exam—visual acuity, eye movements in cardinal positions of gaze
- Facial strength and sensation
- Corneal sensations
- Masseter strength
- Hearing
- Elevation of palate and uvula
- Sternocleidomastoid and trapezius strength
- Gag reflex
- Position and strength of tongue.

SUPRANUCLEAR PATHWAY EXAMINATION

The most important examination feature of a supranuclear motility deficit is the ability to overcome the ocular motility limitation with an oculocephalic manoeuvre (oculocephalic reflex) depicted in Fig. 6.13.

In cases of supranuclear injury, the nuclei of 3rd, 4th and 6th cranial nerves are still intact and the cranial nerve fascicles are functioning normally. Therefore, stimulation of the nuclei with head movements should result in full ocular ductions.

To perform the oculocephalic reflex the patient should be instructed to fixate at a object/target 14 to 16 inches away. Then, while the patient is fixating the patient's head is tilted slowly to the

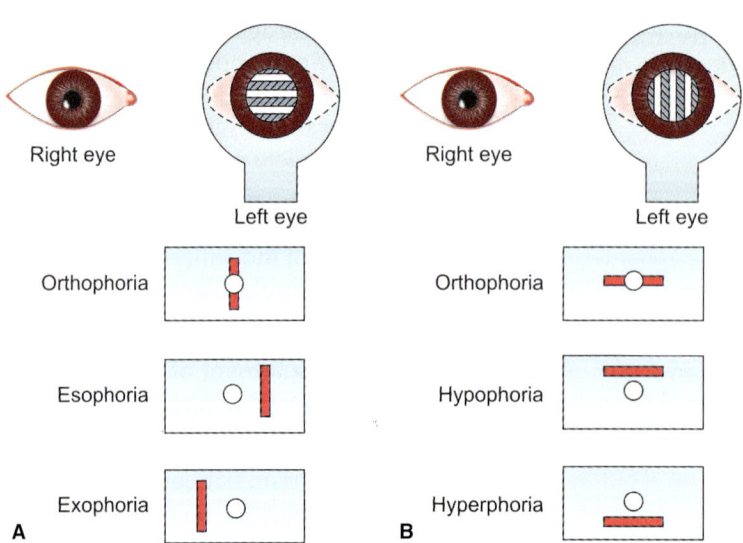

Fig. 6.11: *(A) Horizontally placed Maddox rod over left eye to detect horizontal misalignment; (B) Vertically placed Maddox rod over left eye to detect vertical misalignment.*

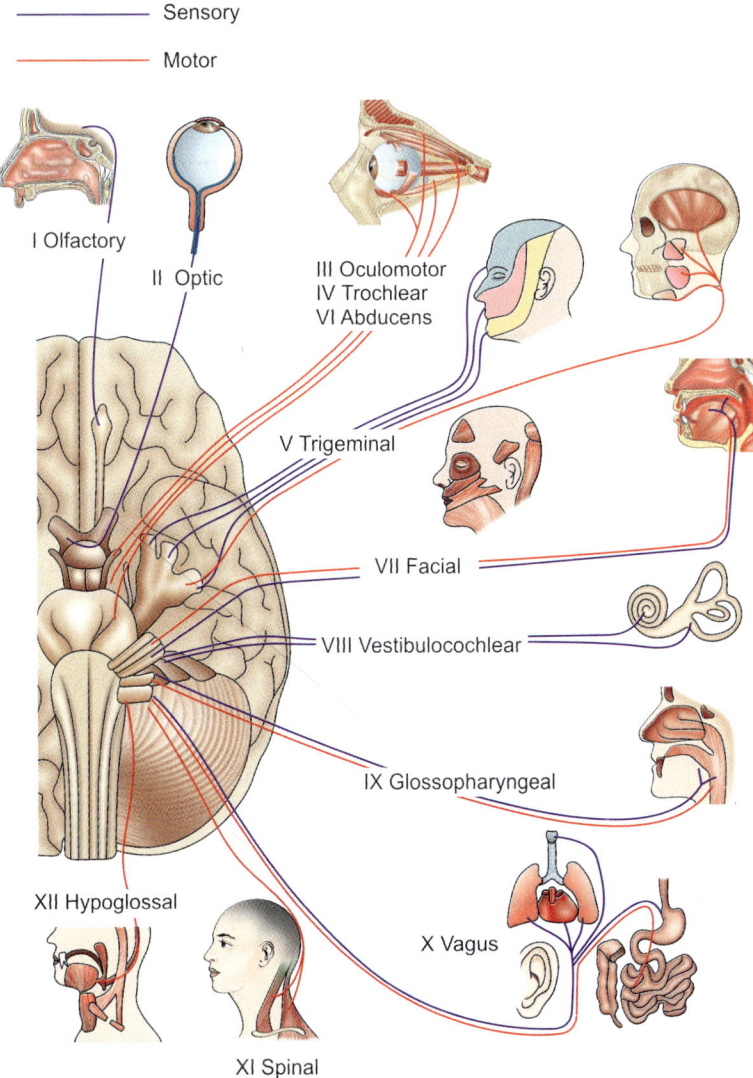

—————— Sensory

—————— Motor

I Olfactory

II Optic

III Oculomotor
IV Trochlear
VI Abducens

V Trigeminal

VII Facial

VIII Vestibulocochlear

IX Glossopharyngeal

XII Hypoglossal

X Vagus

XI Spinal

Fig. 6.12: *Cranial nerves: Origin and organs supplied.*

right/left and up/down. This head movement during fixation should overcome any limitations of ductions or versions due to supranuclear pathway dysfunction.

INVESTIGATIONS

Investigations required depend on the suspected etiology of diplopia as follows:

- **Monocular diplopia**—refraction, pinhole vision
- **Orbital disorders**—USG/CT/MRI orbit
- **Neurological causes**—CT/MRI/MRA
- **Suspected Myasthenia**—Edrophonium test

TREATMENT

The ophthalmoparesis in some of the disorders described, such as ischaemic and traumatic oculomotor palsies, will often resolve spontaneously. Other cases, such as those due to myasthenia gravis or bacterial meningitis, will improve as the underlying cause is treated.

Treatment modalities for diplopia are as under:
- *Glasses*
- *Stick-on occlusive lenses*
- *Fresnel prisms* (Fig. 6.14). Temporary Fresnel paste on prisms can be used initially followed by ground-in-prisms in chronic cases.

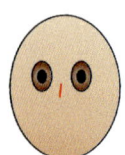

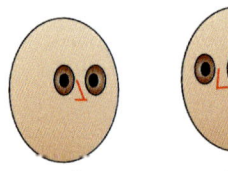

→   ←
Head turns to side, but eyes are still facing forward, or move back to midline–infact brainstem

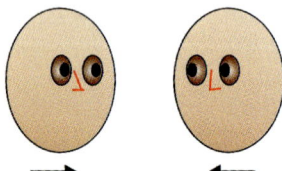

→   ←
Head turns to side, eyes turns with the head, i.e. do not correct–brainstem affected

Fig 6.13: *Demonstration of oculocephalic reflex.*

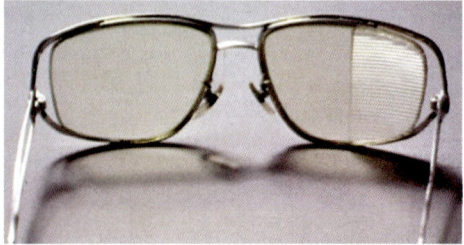

Fig. 6.14: *Stick on Fresnel prisms.*

- *Patching.* Children patched for symptomatic relief should have the patch alternated daily between eyes to prevent occlusion amblyopia.
- *Chemo-denervation.* Botox therapy (Fig. 6.15)—Botulinum toxin injections into the antagonist muscle of a paretic one, even in supranuclear disorders.
- *Immunomodulation*—steroids, immunosuppressives
- *Surgical correction of strabismus*—individuals with paresis who do not improve spontaneously, and whose condition remains stable for 6 months, are candidates for corrective eye muscle surgery.
- *Speciality consultations*—neurology, endocrinology.

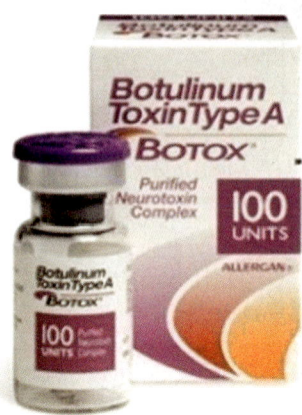

Fig. 6.15: *Botulinum toxin vial.*

BIBLIOGRAPHY

1. Burde RM. Amaurosisfugax. An overview. J Clin Neuro-ophthalmol 1989;9(3):185–9.
2. Friedman DI. Pearls: diplopia. Semin Neurol Feb 2010;30(1):54–65.
3. Lutwak N. Binocular Double Vision—A Review. American Journal of Clinical Medicine 2011;8(3): 166–9.
4. Newman NJ. Cerebrovascular disease. In Hoyt, William Graves; Miller, Neil; Newman, Nancy J.; Walsh, Frank. Walsh and Hoyt's Clinical Neuro-ophthalmology. 3 (5th ed.). Baltimore: Williams & Wilkins 1998;3420–6. ISBN 0-683-30232-9.
5. Pelak VS. Evaluation of diplopia: an anatomic and systematic approach. Clinical review article. Hospital Physician March 2004;6–25.
6. Ravits J, Seybold ME. Transient monocular visual loss from narrow-angle glaucoma. Arch. Neurol. 1984;41(9):991–3.
7. Rucker JC, Tomsak RL. Binocular diplopia. A practical approach. Neurologist 2005;11(2): 98–110.
8. Sadun AA, Currie JN, Lessell S. Transient visual obscurations with elevated optic discs. Ann. Neurol 1984;16(4):489–94.
9. Smit RL, Baarsma GS, Koudstaal PJ. The source of embolism in amaurosisfugax and retinal, 1994.
10. Torun N. A practical approach to a patient with diplopia. Journal of Experimental and Clinical Medicine 2012;28:S55–7.

Section
II

Clinical Evaluation and Investigative Techniques in Cornea

7. Clinical Evaluation and Investigations for Corneal Diseases
8. Specular Microscopy and Confocal Microscopy of Cornea
9. Corneal Pachymetry, Hysteresis and Keratometry
10. Corneal Topography and Aberrometry

Clinical Evaluation and Investigations for Corneal Diseases

Chapter Outline

CLINICAL EVALUATION

Presenting Symptoms of Corneal Diseases

Examination of Cornea

- Systematic approach for corneal examination
- Signs of common corneal diseases
- Slit-lamp Examination Technique for Cornea
- Diagnostic Dyes Used in Corneal Diseases
- Corneal drawing with colour coding

INVESTIGATIVE TECHNIQUES FOR CORNEAL DISEASES

- Pachymetry

- Keratometry
- Corneal Topography
- Confocal Microscopy
- Specular Microscopy
- Anterior Segment OCT
- Videokeratography
- Corneal Aesthesiometry

TECHNIQUES FOR MICROBIOLOGICAL AND CYTOLOGICAL EVALUATION

CORNEAL BIOPSY

CLINICAL EVALUATION

PRESENTING SYMPTOMS OF CORNEAL DISEASES

Knowledge of the clinical features is an important step in the management of corneal diseases. A proper diagnosis and treatment cannot be done without an accurate assessment of the clinical features. Common symptoms of corneal diseases are pain, decreased vision, discharge, lacrimation, redness, photophobia and blepharospasm.

PAIN

- Pain is the commonest symptom of the inflammatory lesions of the cornea due to its rich innervation.

- Pain in corneal diseases occurs due to direct stimulation of the sensory nerves in the cornea or as the consequence of inflammation or ciliary spasm.
- Direct stimulation of the corneal nerves causes pain which is severe in intensity and sharp in nature while corneal inflammation produces severe pain but of a dull aching or throbbing nature.
- The severity of pain may range from minimal discomfort to an excruciating pain.
- The type of causative organism and the depth of the ulceration influence the severity of pain. In general, superficial ulcers are more painful than deep corneal ulcers. This is due to the rich sensory nerve supply present in the superficial part of the cornea.

- A small dendrite of Herpes simplex or a Candida species cause minimal pain and may only be associated with foreign body sensation. In contrast, a patient with *Acanthamoeba keratitis* presents with an excruciating pain, during corneal epithelial involvement due to radial keratoneuritis. The pain is usually out of proportion to the objective clinical findings, the alleviation of which may require strong analgesics and narcotics.
- A sudden relief in pain, in a case of progressing corneal ulcer may be indicative of the perforation of ulcer.

DECREASED VISUAL ACUITY

- Visual loss is a common symptom in patients with corneal disease and occurs most commonly due to loss of transparency of the cornea.
- Acute loss of vision is due to acute inflammatory conditions of the cornea and is associated with other symptoms of inflammation, pain and vascular injection.
- Gradual loss of vision is more likely to be associated with a slowly evolving corneal pathology.
- Most cases of corneal ulcer report with a history of sudden decrease in vision. The extent of decrease in vision depends on the duration, severity, location of the lesion and involvement of other ocular structures.
- Central corneal ulcers, particularly those caused by organisms like *Pseudomonas, Staphylococcus aureus* and *Fusarium species* are invariably associated with significant loss of visual acuity.
- Other factors that can reduce visual acuity include the presence of an associated pupillary membrane, hypopyon, cataract, glaucoma and endophthalmitis.
- The vision may not be severely reduced in cases which have small, peripheral ulcers, such as those caused by herpes simplex and non-coagulase Staphylococcus.
- In *Acanthamoeba keratitis*, vision may not be significantly reduced during the initial stages, when the corneal epithelium alone is involved. Later, as the infection spreads deeper into the

corneal stroma, visual acuity is severely reduced.

DISCHARGE

- Almost all cases of corneal ulcers present with a complaint of discharge from the affected eye. The type of the discharge may be watery, mucoid, mucopurulent or frankly purulent.
- A watery discharge usually occurs due to a viral ulcer or a small bacterial ulcer or else it may also be due to reflex tearing.
- However, microbial keratitis caused by *Pseudomonas* and *Gonococcus species* is associated with a mucopurulent discharge.
- Corneal ulcers caused due to *Pseudomonas* are particularly associated with a greenish-yellowish discharge.
- A membranous discharge is seen with keratitis caused by *Corynebacterium diphtheria*.

LACRIMATION

Lacrimation occurs as a result of lacrimatory reflex mediated by fifth nerve (afferent) and secretomotor fibres of the seventh nerve (efferent). Fifth nerve ending in cornea are stimulated in corneal frame, inflammation and if infections.

Redness: Redness of eyes occurs due to congestion of circumcorneal vessels.

PHOTOPHOBIA

- Term applied to the discomfort experienced on the exposure to bright light due to stimulation of nerve endings.
- Severe photophobia only accompanies denudation of the epithelium, but many inflammatory diseases are accompanied by some iridocyclitis, and spasm of the sphincter of the iris and the ciliary muscle.

BLEPHAROSPASM

- It is caused by corneal irritation due to the stimulation of the terminal fibres of the corneal nerves
- This blepharospasm is not completely abolished in the dark, but is greatly diminished by thorough anaesthetisation. It is thus a reflex predominantly involving the trigeminal nerve.

EXAMINATION OF CORNEA

SYSTEMATIC APPROACH FOR CORNEAL EXAMINATION

Examination of cornea should be done under following headings: shape, size, surface, curvature, thickness, vascularisation, transparency, and sensation.

SHAPE

- The anterior surface of the normal cornea is horizontally elliptical with an average horizontal diameter of 11.7 mm and vertical diameter 11 mm.
- In hypotony the vertical diameter becomes less and the cornea looks more elliptical.
- In phthisis, the cornea looks quadrilateral in shape.
- In extreme degrees of microphthalmos the cornea becomes very small and irregular.
- Keratoglobus is an ectatic condition in which cornea becomes thin and bulges out like a globe.
- Keratoconus is an ectatic condition in which cornea becomes cone shaped.
- Cornea plana, i.e. flat curvature of cornea which may occur in patients with severe hypotony.

SIZE

The anterior surface of normal cornea is elliptical with an average horizontal diameter of 11.7 mm and vertical diameter of 11 mm. The best method to determine the corneal diameter is by corneal callipers under local anaesthesia in adults and general anaesthesia in children. Diameter should be measured both vertically and horizontally in both the eyes.

Abnormalities of corneal size can be:

Causes of decreased corneal size are: Microphthalmos, microcornea, phthisis bulbi, atrophic bulbi, and nanophthalmos.

Microcornea, when the anterior horizontal diameter is less than 10 mm. It may occur isolated or as a part of microphthalmos.

Megalocornea is labelled when the horizontal diameter is more than 13 mm. Common **causes** of increased corneal size are congenital megalocornea, buphthalmos, macrophthalmos (keratoglobus).

SURFACE

Smoothness of the corneal surface is disturbed due to abrasions, ulceration, ectatic scars and facets. Changes in smoothness of surface can be detected by slit-lamp biomicroscopy, window reflex test and Placido's disc.

Placido's keratoscopic disc is a disc painted with alternating black and white circles. It may be used to assess the smoothness and curvature of the corneal surface. Normally, on looking through the hole in the centre of disc, a uniform sharp image of the circles is seen on the cornea. Irregularities in the corneal surface cause distortion of the circles (Fig. 7.1A to C).

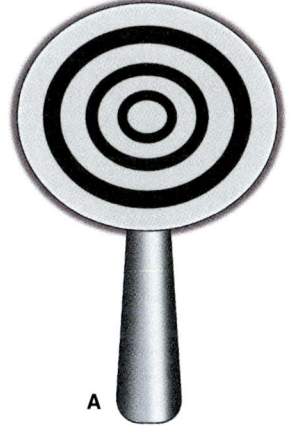
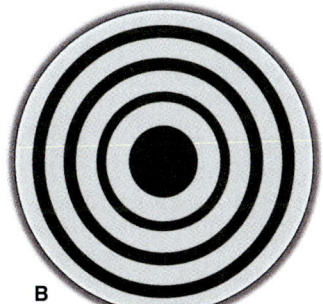
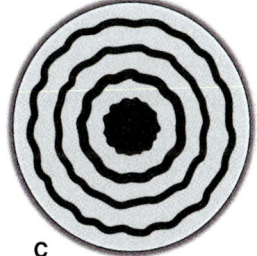

Fig. 7.1: *Placido disc (A); Placido disc reflex from normal cornea (B); Placido disc reflex from irregular corneal surface (C).*

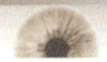

Window reflex test. Patient is seated facing a window. Image of the window formed on the normal cornea in uniform and sharp. In irregular corneal surface the image of window formed in distorted.

CURVATURE

Normally cornea is more curved than the sclera hence it bulges beyond the limbus. The average corneal curvature is 8 mm. Curvature is slightly more in the central 3 mm, which is called *the optical zone*. Curvature of the central zone is best measured by *the keratometer*, while the peripheral cornea is measured by *the photokeratoscope* and *topography*. Cornea is more curved vertically due to pressure of the lids. Increased curvature results in physiological myopic astigmatism of 0.5 D in horizontal axis. This is called with the rule astigmatism.

Corneal curvature is increased in: Keratoconus, buphthalmos, keratoglobus, and pellucid degeneration.

Corneal curvature is decreased in: Microcornea, microphthalmos, cornea plana phthisis bulbi, hypotony, perforation of globe, and postsurgical tight suture.

Corneal curvature is irregular in: Pterygium, keratoconus, keratectasia, corneal staphyloma, pellucid degeneration of cornea, ciliary staphyloma, limbal growth and postsurgical following: keratoplasty, glaucoma surgery, and retinal detachment surgery.

THICKNESS

Normal cornea does not have uniform thickness. It is thicker (0.9 mm) on the periphery and thinnest in the centre (0.6 mm). This is due to difference in corneal curvature of the two surfaces. Posterior surface is more curved than the anterior surface. Corneal thickness is measured by pachymeter. Corneal thickness is increased due to oedema of either stroma or epithelium or both.

Causes of thickened cornea are: Disciform keratitis, endothelial decompensation, epithelial oedema, corneal leucoma, and hydrops of cornea.

Causes of thin cornea are: Keratoconus, keratectasia, buphthalmos, pellucid degeneration, Mooren's ulcer, and Terrien's degeneration.

CORNEAL VASCULARIZATION

Normal cornea is avascular except for small capillary loops which are present in the periphery for about 1 mm. In pathological states, it can be invaded by vessels as a defence mechanism against the disease or injury. When vessels are present, an exact note of their position, whether superficial or deep and their distribution whether localised, general, or peripheral should be made

Superficial corneal vascularization. In it vessels are arranged usually in an arborising pattern, present below the epithelial layer and their continuity can be traced with the conjunctival vessels (Fig 7.2 A).

Deep vascularization. In it the vessels are generally derived from anterior ciliary arteries and lie in the corneal stroma. These vessels are usually straight, not anastomosing and their continuity cannot be traced beyond the limbus. Deep vessels may be arranged as terminal loops (Fig. 7.2B), brush (Fig. 7.2C), parasol, umbel (Fig. 7.2D), network or interstitial arcade.

Differences between superificial and deep vascularization of cornea are shown in Table 7.1.

Causes of superficial corneal vascularisation are: Trachoma, leprosy, phlycten, spring catarrh,

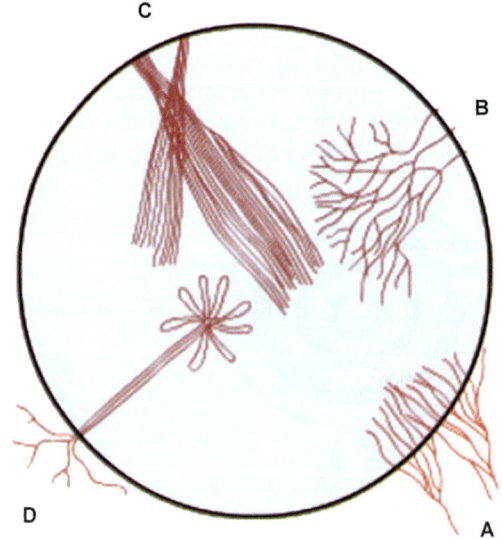

Fig. 7.2: *Corneal vascularization: (A) Superficial, (B) Deep corneal vascularisation-terminal loops, (C) Deep corneal vascularisation-brush, (D) Deep corneal vascularisation-umbel.*

Table 7.1 *Differences between superficial and deep corneal vascularization*	
Superficial corneal vascularization	**Deep corneal vascularization**
Corneal vessels can be traced over the limbus onto the conjunctiva	Corneal vessels abruptly end at the limbus
Vessels are bright red and well-defined	Vessels are ill defined and cause only a diffuse red blush
Superficial vessels branch in an arborescent manner	Deep vessels run parallel to each other in a radial fashion
Superficial vessels raise the epithelium and make the corneal surface irregular	Deep vessels do not disturb the corneal surface

riboflavin deficiency, Mooren's ulcer, indolent corneal ulcer, and vascularisation of leucoma.

Causes of deep corneal vascularisation are: Interstitial keratitis, disciform keratitis, alkali burn, and sclerosing keratitis.

Pannus

When extensive superficial vascularisation is associated with white cuff of cellular infiltration, it is termed *pannus* (Fig. 7.3). In *progressive pannus*, corneal infiltration is ahead of vessels while in *regressive pannus* it lags behind.

Causes of pannus include:
- Chlamydia inclusion conjunctivitis and trachoma
- Tight contact lens wear
- Ocular rosacea
- Phlycten
- Superior limbic keratoconjunctivitis
- Staphylococcal hypersensitivity
- Vernal keratoconjunctivitis
- Chemical burn
- Aniridia
- Leprosy.

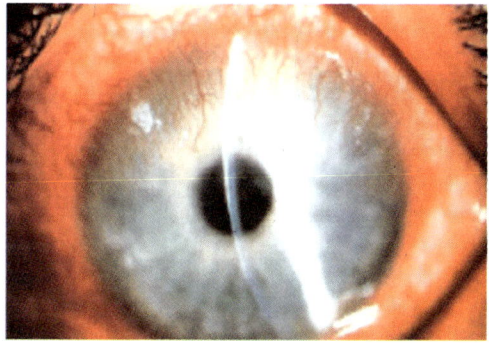

Fig. 7.3: *Pannus.*

TRANSPARENCY

To maintain its optical property cornea has to be transparent, and most of the diseases of cornea cause a loss of this transparency. Transparency of cornea is lost in corneal oedema, opacity, ulceration, dystrophies, degenerations, vascularization and due to deposits in the cornea.

Corneal opacity

Corneal opacity can be stationary or progressive. They may vary in shape, size, number and depth. They may be unilateral or bilateral. Most of the opacities are painless but some of them may be associated with pain due to non-corneal causes.

Examination for corneal opacity is best done with the help of a slit-lamp. Note the number, site, size, shape, density (nebular, macular or leucomatous) and surface of the opacity.

Position. Position of a corneal opacity is noted in relation to the limbus, pupil and meridian (face of clock).

Number. Number of corneal opacities may vary from single to multiple.

Shape. Corneal opacities may assume various shapes according to position, depth and pathology.
- *Dendritic pattern* is seen in herpes simplex and herpes zoster
- *Dome-shaped opacity* with base at the limbus, occurs following healing of phlycten
- *Tongue-shaped opacity* is produced by Sclerosing keratitis and epithelial down growth
- *Arc on the periphery* is typical of arcus senilis.

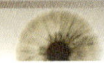

Grading of Opacity

All corneal opacities are white in colour. Their shades vary according to depth. Opacities of epithelium and superficial stroma are the faintest; those involving full thickness are the densest. Depending on the density, corneal opacity is graded as nebula, macula and leucoma.

Nebular corneal opacity. It is a faint opacity which results due to superficial scars involving Bowman's layer and superficial stroma. A thin, diffuse nebula covering the pupillary area interferes more with vision than the localised leucoma away from pupillary area (Fig. 7.4A)

Macular corneal opacity. It is a semi-dense opacity produced when scarring involves about half the corneal stroma (Fig. 7.4B)

Leucomatous corneal opacity. It is a dense white opacity which results due to scarring of more than half of the stroma (Fig. 7.4C)

Adherent leucoma. It results when healing occurs after perforation of cornea with incarceration of iris (Fig. 7.4D).

Corneal opacity at birth

Causes of corneal opacity at birth can be remembered with the pneumonic **STUMPED.**
Sclerocornea

Trauma (birth trauma)
Ulcer
Mucopolysaccharidosis
Peter's anomaly
Endothelial dystrophy, stromal dystrophy
Dermoid

Other causes are:
- Congenital glaucoma
- Interstitial keratitis
- Rubella keratitis.

CORNEAL SENSATIONS

Cornea is a highly sensitive structure. Sensitivity of the cornea is a protective mechanism. The ophthalmic branch of the fifth cranial nerve (trigeminal) carries sensory fibres for the cornea. If the cornea senses stimulation (ranging from mild irritation to intense pain), then the eyelid will close, providing protection to the cornea and distribution of tears. As the corneal sensitivity is decreased, then the blinking/ tearing mechanism will decrease, leaving the corneal epithelium exposed to dehydration. Anesthetic corneas may develop a characteristic interpalpebral horizontal band of punctate epithelial staining. Untreated, this may progress to an epithelial defect and subsequent stromal

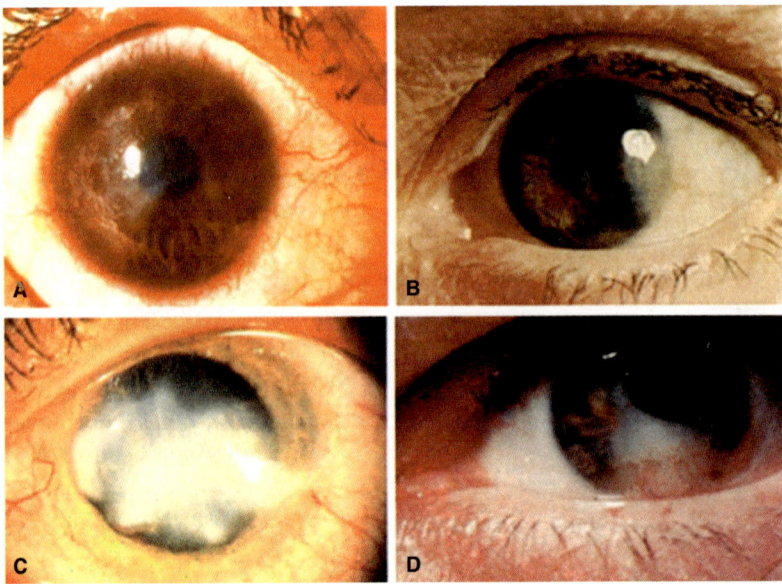

Fig. 7.4: *Corneal opacity: (A) Nebular; (B) Macular; (C) Leucomatous; (D) Adherent leucoma.*

loss (neurotrophic ulcer). Ocular sensitivity is greatest in the central cornea except in elderly patients, in whom the peripheral cornea is the most sensitive. Sensitivity drops rapidly as distance from the limbus increases. The temporal limbus is significantly more sensitive than the inferior limbus.

To test the corneal sensations, patient is asked to look ahead; the examiner touches the corneal surface with a fine twisted cotton (which is brought from the side to avoid menace reflex) and observes the blinking response (Fig. 7.5) Normally, there is a brisk reflex closure of lids. Always compare the effect with that on the opposite side. The exact quantitative measurement of the corneal sensations is made with the help of an aesthesiometer.

Causes of reduced corneal sensations

- Herpes simplex keratitis
- Herpes zoster ophthalmicus
- Hansen disease (leprosy)
- Surgical trauma (PK, LASIK, large limbal incisions, ablation of the trigeminal ganglion)
- Topical medications (anaesthetics, NSAIDs, β-blockers, and carbonic anhydrase inhibitors)
- Cocaine abuse
- Aneurysms
- Tumours (acoustic neuroma, neurofibroma, or angioma)
- Cerebrovascular events
- Multiple sclerosis
- Hereditary causes. Familial dysautonomia (Riley-Day syndrome).

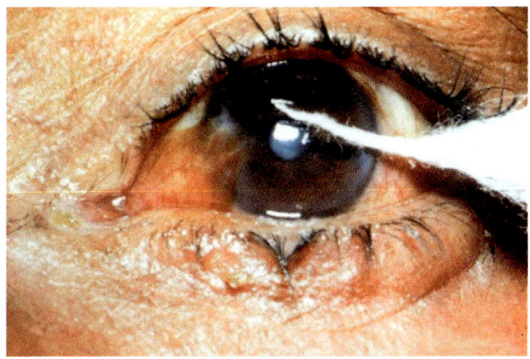

Fig. 7.5: *Testing of the corneal sensations with cotton wisp.*

SIGNS OF COMMON CORNEAL DISEASES

Superficial keratitis

Punctate epithelial keratitis (PEK). Granular, swollen epithelial cells with focal intraepithelial infiltrates. They are visible unstained but stain well with rose bengal and variably with fluorescein (Fig. 7.6).

Causes: Adenoviral, molluscum contagiosum, early herpes simplex and herpes zoster, microsporidial and systemic viral infections (e.g. measles, varicella, rubella). Thygeson superficial punctate keratitis.

Superficial punctate keratitis. Corneal epithelial defect with dot-like morphology (Fig. 7.7).

Punctate epithelial erosions (PEE): Tiny depressed grey white epithelial defects that stain brightly with fluorescein and poorly with rose bengal (Fig. 7.8).

- *Superior erosions* are caused by tarsal foreign bodies, concretions, superior limbic keratopathy, vernal catarrh, floppy eyelid syndrome and mechanically induced keratoconjunctivitis.

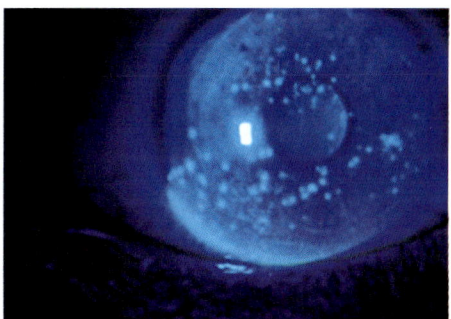

Fig. 7.6: *Punctate epithelial keratitis.*

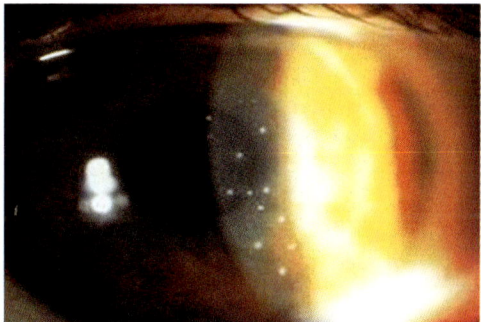

Fig. 7.7: *Superficial punctate keratitis.*

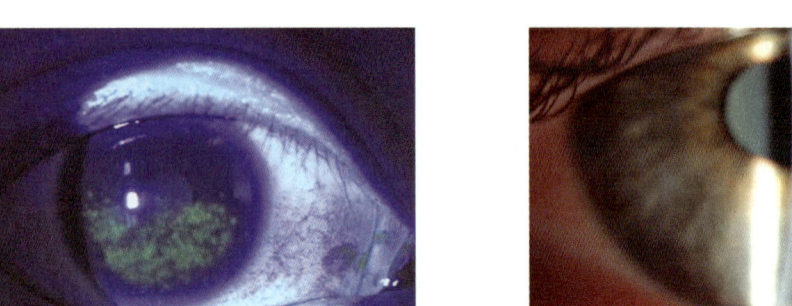

Fig. 7.8: *Punctate epithelial erosions.*

Fig. 7.10: *Punctuate subepithelial keratitis.*

- *Erosion of interpalpebral cornea* is caused by exposure to ultraviolet light, as in exposure to welding, snow blindness, and by neuro-paralytic keratitis.
- *Inferior erosions.* Chronic blepharitis, lago-phthalmos, eye drop toxicity, self-induced, aberrant eyelashes and entropion.
- *Central erosions.* Prolonged contact lens wear.
- *Diffuse erosions.* Some cases of viral and bacterial conjunctivitis, and toxicity to drops.

Subepithelial infiltrates. Tiny subsurface foci of non-staining inflammatory infiltrates (Fig 7.9).

Causes include severe or prolonged adenoviral keratoconjunctivitis, herpes zoster keratitis, adult inclusion conjunctivitis, marginal keratitis, rosacea and Thygeson superficial punctate keratitis.

Punctate subepithelial keratitis is a feature of (Fig. 7.10):
- Adenovirus
- Epstein-Barr virus infection
- Reiter disease
- Corneal graft rejection.

Corneal Ulcer

In ulcer, there is a breach in the continuity of the corneal epithelium corneal ulcers present as greyish white irregular areas surrounded by infiltration and having a margin and a floor. The ulcer stains brightly with fluorescein (Fig. 7.11) and the edges stain better than the floor.

Dendritc corneal ulcer: **Linear branch-shaped epithelial lesions** (Fig. 7.12):
- Herpes simplex dendritic ulcer (true dendrite)
- Herpes zoster

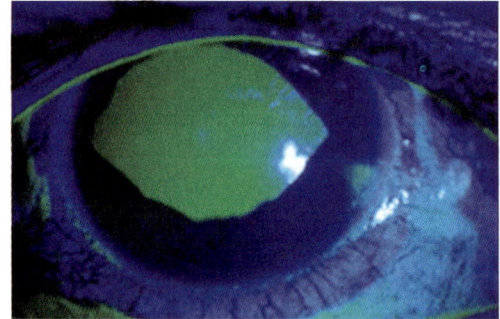

Fig. 7.11: *Corneal ulcer stained with fluorescein.*

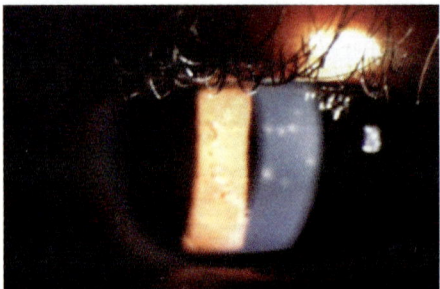

Fig. 7.9: *Subepithelial infiltrates.*

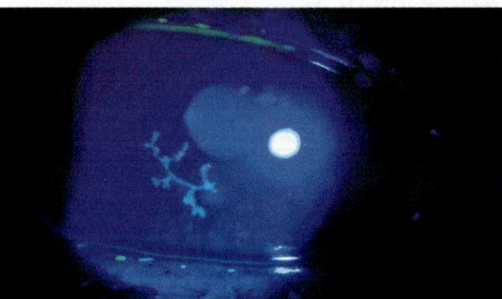

Fig. 7.12: *Corneal dendrites.*

- *Acanthamoeba*
- Epithelial rejection line
- Healing epithelial defects
- Use of soft contact lens
- Tyrosinemia II.

Corneal Oedema

- Appears like empty spaces in the epithelium that may be converted into actual bullae, which are 1–2 mm in size (Fig. 7.13).
- Bullae are vesicle-like structures laden with fluid, which on rupture produce severe pain. They are found in acute congestive glaucoma, endothelial decompensation, trauma, following IOL implantation, vitreous touching the endothelium following ICC extraction, Fuch's endothelial dystrophy, long-standing interstitial keratitis and keratoconus.

Noninflammatory stromal oedema (Fig. 7.14):
- Post cataract surgery-bullous keratopathy
- Hydrops of keratoconus/keratoglobus
- Fuch's endothelial dystrophy
- Acute angle closure glaucoma
- Corneal graft rejection
- Blunt anterior segment trauma
- Congenital hereditary endothelial dystrophy.

Corneal crystals

Aggregation of material in the corneal substance is seen in (Fig. 7.15):
- Schnyder crystalline keratopathy,
- Cystinosis
- Multiple myeloma

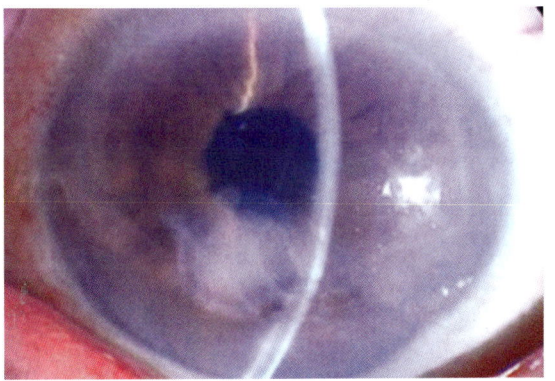

Fig. 7.13: *Corneal oedema.*

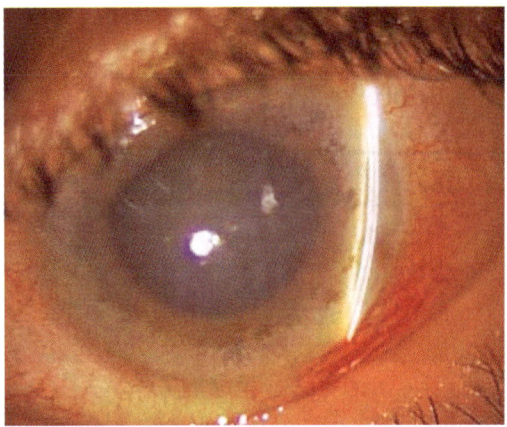

Fig. 7.14: *Noninflammatory stromal oedema.*

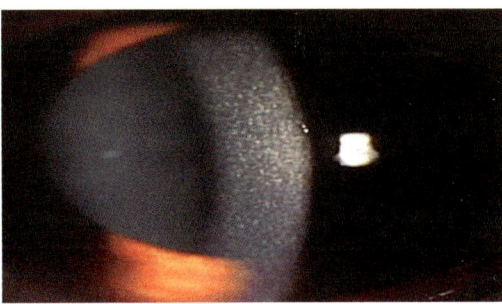

Fig. 7.15: *Corneal crystals.*

- Gout
- Uremia
- Hypergammaglobulinaemia
- Drugs (indomethacin)
- Lecithin cholesterol acyltransferase deficiency
- Tangier disease
- Chrysiasis.

Deposition of iron occurs in the intraepithelial layer

- *Rust ring.* Residual rust following metallic foreign body
- *Hudson-Stahli line.* Irregular line in inter-palpebral area in normal cornea (age related)
- *Ferry line.* Deposition of iron at advancing edge of filtering bleb
- *Stocker line.* Accumulation of iron just in front of the head of pterygium (Fig. 7.16)
- *Fleischer ring.* Circular yellow-brown ring at the base of cone in keratoconus
- *Dalgleish line.* Congenital spherocytosis.

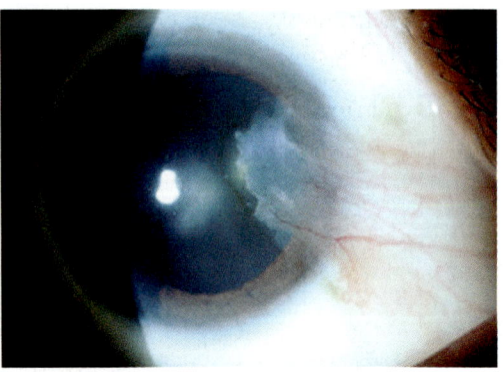

Fig. 7.16: *Stocker's line in pterygium.*

Corneal filaments

Strands of mucus admixed with epithelium, attached at one end to the corneal surface, that stain well with rose bengal (Fig. 7.17). The unattached end moves with each blink. Filaments are seen in:

- Keratoconjunctivitis sicca
- Superior limbic keratoconjunctivitis
- Recurrent erosions
- Exposure keratitis
- Eye patching.

Enlarged corneal nerves

Prominent corneal nerves are seen in (Fig. 7.18):
- Multiple endocrine neoplasia type IIb
- Keratoconus
- Neurofibromatosis type 1
- Refsum disease
- Congenital glaucoma
- Leprosy
- Primary amyloidosis
- Hereditary icthyosis

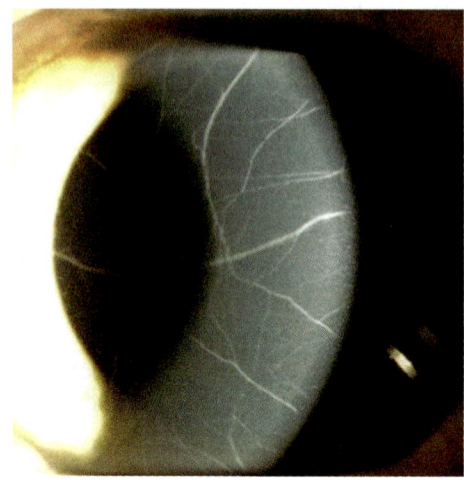

Fig. 7.18: *Enlarged corneal nerves.*

- Idiopathic
- Acanthamoeba keratitis
- Failed corneal graft.

Whorl keratopathy

Arrangement of yellow golden deposits in whorl pattern (also called Cat-Whisker's keratopathy is seen in (Fig. 7.19):
- Amiodarone
- Atovaquone
- Chloroquine
- Chlorpromazine
- Indomethacin
- Fabry disease.

Band keratopathy

Peripheral interpalpebral calcification leaving an area of clear limbus (Fig. 7.20).

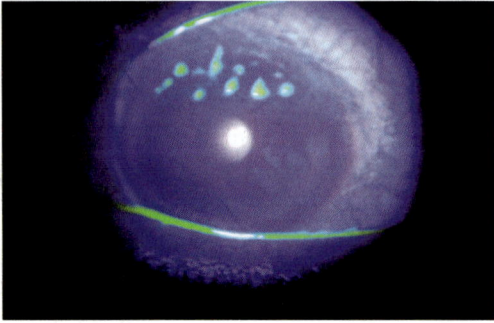

Fig. 7.17: *Corneal filaments.*

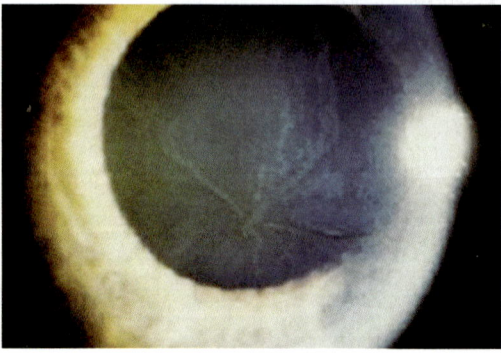

Fig. 7.19: *Whorl keratopathy.*

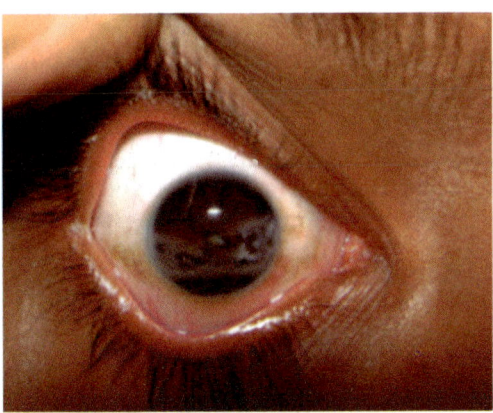

Fig. 7.20: *Band keratopathy.*

Ocular causes are:
- Chronic iridocyclitis
- Phthisis bulbi
- Silicone oil in anterior chamber.

Metabolic causes are:
- Increased calcium and phosphorous product
- Gout
- Chronic renal failure
- Hereditary icthyosis.

Nummular keratitis

Large multiple coin lesions surrounded by halo of stromal haze (Fig. 7.21)
- Herpes zoster ophthalmicus
- Epstein-Barr virus infection
- Lyme disease

- Onchocerciasis
- Brucellosis.

Interstitial keratitis (Fig. 7.22)
- Herpes simplex/herpes zoster
- Mumps
- Syphilis
- Tuberculosis
- Leprosy
- Lyme disease
- Cogan syndrome.

Encroachment from conjunctiva over cornea
- Pterygium (Fig. 7.23)
- Dermoid
- Phlyctenular keratoconjunctivitis
- Large glaucoma bleb.

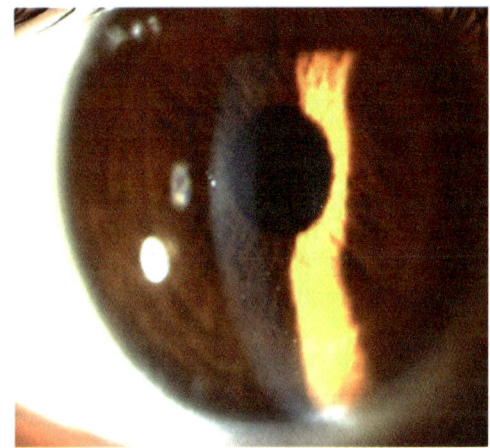

Fig. 7.22: *Interstitial keratitis.*

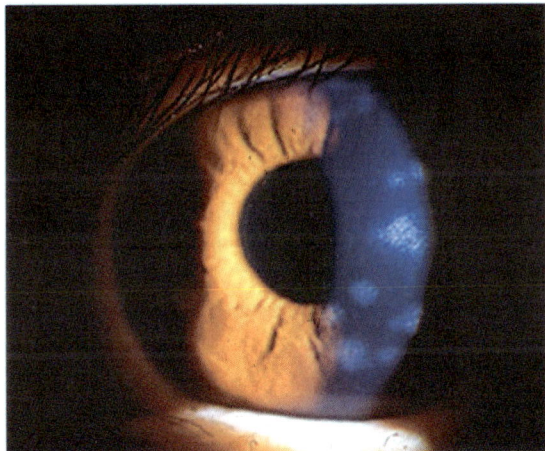

Fig. 7.21: *Nummular keratitis.*

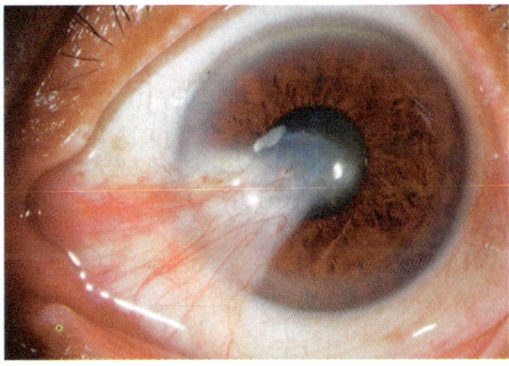

Fig. 7.23: *Pterygium.*

SLIT-LAMP EXAMINATION TECHNIQUES FOR CORNEA

Slit-lamp examination is an essential technique for examining the cornea. Normal cornea has structures which refract and scatter light. Pathological processes tend to produce irregularities which are even more obvious.

- *Direct illumination*
  - ♦ Diffuse illumination
  - ♦ Focal illumination
- *Indirect illumination*
  - ♦ Sclerotic scatter
  - ♦ Retroillumination
- *Specular reflection.*

Diffuse broad-beam illumination

The wide beam provides diffuse illumination such as would be obtained from the illumination provided by a penlight or muscle light. It is used to perform a general inspection of the anterior segment and adnexal structures under magnification (Fig. 7.24).

Applications

- Examination of sclera
- Assessment of the tear film (qualitative and quantitative)
- General observation of the surfaces of cornea and lens
- General survey of anterior segment
- Staining pattern of the ocular surface
- Assessment of contact lenses fitting.

Focal illumination

Direct focal illumination or 'slit-beam' illumination provides an optical section or parallelopiped view from light angled (not coaxial) through tissue with a bright, thin beam with lower magnification to visualize anterior chamber (AC) depth and higher magnification to visualize corneal depth and pathology (Fig. 7.25).

Applications

- To determine the depth or elevation of a defect of the cornea, conjunctiva
- To detect changes in corneal and conjunctival thickness
- To examine epithelial surface pathologies like intraepithelial cysts and bullae
- To assess depths of foreign bodies, scars and opacities.

Indirect illumination

This mode of illumination enhances contrast during visualisation of defects at various levels of the cornea. Indirect modes of illumination are retroillumination and sclerotic scatter.

Retroillumination

- It is the technique of visualizing structures against an illuminated background.
- The beam of light, directed at a location more posterior than the object of interest, is reflected

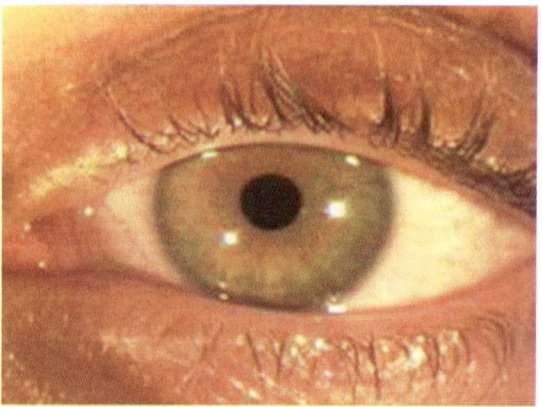

Fig. 7.24: *Diffuse broad-beam illumination.*

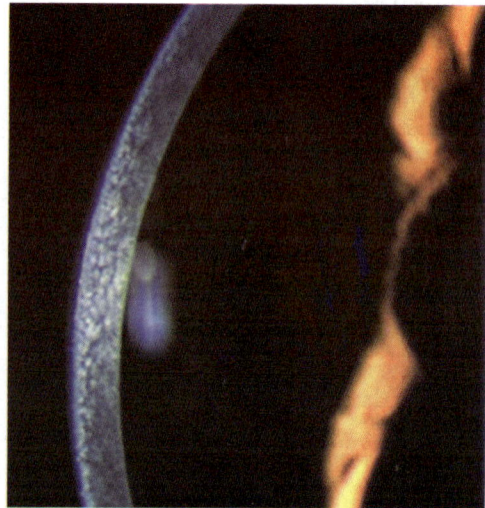

Fig. 7.25: *Focal illumination.*

and viewed in its return pathway toward the examiner.

There are two types of retroillumination:

a. *Direct retroillumination* caused by direct reflection at surfaces such as the iris, crystalline lens or the fundus (Fig. 7.26).

b. *Indirect retroillumination* caused by diffuse reflection in the medium, i.e. at all scattering media and surfaces in the anterior and posterior segments (Fig. 7.27).

The common findings include:

Cornea: Vascularizations, microcysts, vacuoles, oedema, deposits like amyloid, particles in tear film, defect or folds in the Descemet's membranes, keratic precipitates.

Sclerotic Scatter

- Sclerotic scatter is used to detect subtle epithelial or stromal irregularities (Fig. 7.28)
- It is performed by directing the light beam tangentially towards the limbus until the entire limbal circumference appears to glow.

Specular Reflection

- Specular reflection is derived from the German word Spiegel or 'mirror-like' reflection in contrast to scattered light.
- It is used to evaluate the corneal endothelium (Fig. 7.29).

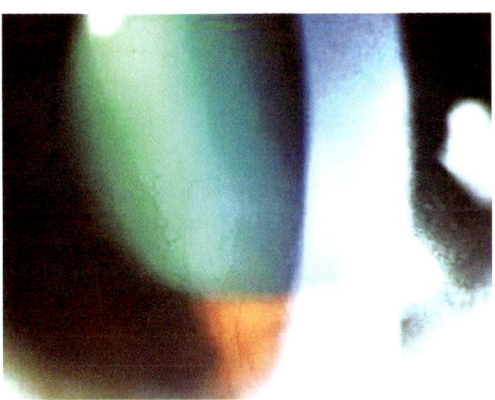

Fig. 7.26: *Direct retroillumination.*

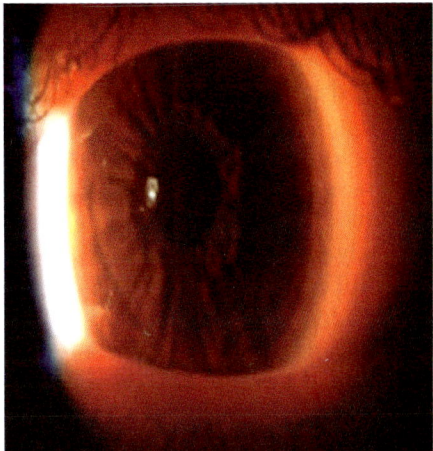

Fig. 7.28: *Sclerotic scatter.*

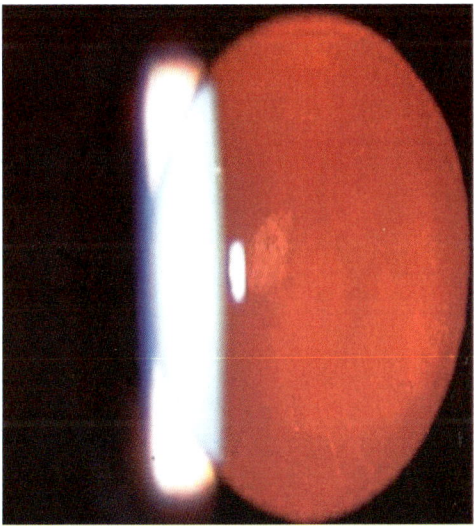

Fig. 7.27: *Indirect retroillumination.*

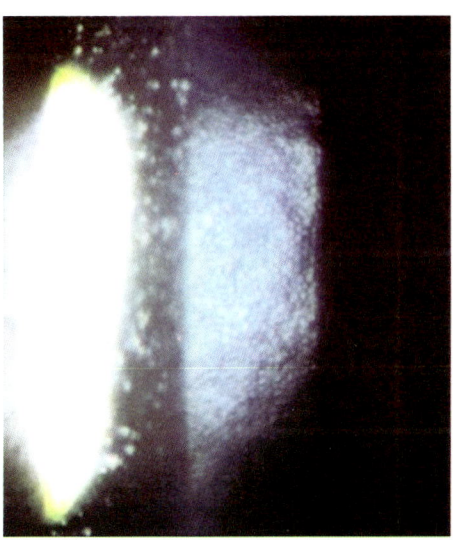

Fig. 7.29: *Specular reflection.*

- It relies on the difference in refractive indices between the two media producing reflection at the interface.

Applications
- To evaluate the endothelial cells for size and shape
- To identify the irregularities in the Descemet's membrane, e.g. guttata in early diagnosis of Fuchs' endothelial dystrophy
- Pigment deposits and keratic precipitates on the endothelium.

DIAGNOSTIC DYES USED IN CORNEAL DISEASES

FLUORESCEIN DYE
- The fluorescein molecule emits green light (520 nm) when it is excited by cobalt blue filter (490 nm).
- Nontoxic to corneal epithelium and is taken up in areas in which disruption of cell–cell junctions exist or epithelium is absent completely.
- It is useful in the documentation of corneal epithelial defects resulting from abrasion or active herpetic infection (Fig. 7.30).
- The observed patterns can often provide clues toward determining the etiology of disease. For example, exposure keratopathy typically results in fluorescein uptake in the interpalpebral space, whereas a toxic keratopathy (such as after chemical exposure) most often results in diffuse uptake across the entire cornea.

- True staining should be distinguished from pooling, in which the fluorescein collects in depressions on the ocular surface but is not taken up because of the presence of an intact epithelium.
- 'Negative' staining can also occur and refers to the pattern of fluorescein collection around elevated lesions on the surface of the eye.
- In the Seidel test, fluorescein is also used to demonstrate wound leakage by providing a fluorescent background through which streams of aqueous are revealed.

ROSE BENGAL
- Unlike fluorescein, rose bengal exhibit toxicity *in vitro*, but is considered safe for clinical applications. It is a derivative of the fluorescein molecule and stains devitalized epithelial cells and healthy epithelial cells when they are not protected by a healthy layer of mucin (Fig. 7.31).
- Accordingly, severe tear film abnormalities result in rose bengal, but not fluorescein, staining.
- The two dyes may be used consecutively to provide a more complete assessment of the integrity of the ocular surface. As with fluorescein, rose bengal comes concentrated on paper strips.
- Unlike fluorescein, however, it is nonfluorescent, and so can be viewed in direct light, and is irritating to the patient, usually requiring application of topical anaesthetic.

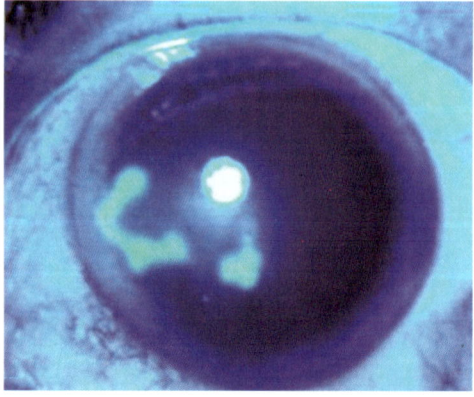

Fig. 7.30: *Fluorescein dye staining.*

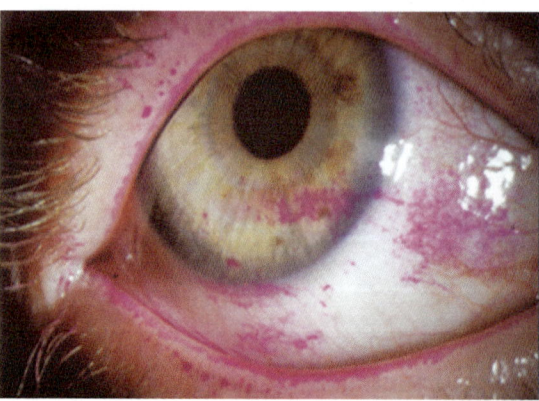

Fig. 7.31: *Rose bengal staining.*

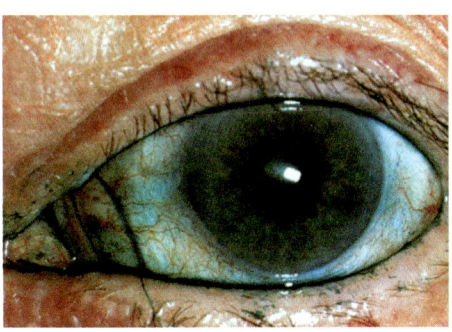

Fig. 7.32: *Lissamine green staining.*

LISSAMINE GREEN

- Lissamine green offers many of the same applications as rose bengal, and its patterns of distribution are observed and recorded with white light (Fig. 7.32).
- It similarly stains with rose bengal (dead and degenerated cells as well as disrupted cell-cell junctions) but produces much less irritation.

CORNEAL DRAWING WITH COLOUR CODING

Clinical signs should be illustrated with a colour-coded labelled diagram; including lesion dimensions is particularly useful to facilitate monitoring.

Documentation of corneal signs

Black

- Limbus
- Scars
- Degenerations/deposits/guttate
- Foreign bodies
- Sutures
- Contact lens
- Band keratopathy.

Blue

- Fine blue circles for epithelial oedema (Fig. 7.33A)
- Wavy lines to document Descemet's membrane folds (Fig. 7.33B)
- Blue shading for stromal oedema.

Brown

- Pigmentation–iron or melanin
- Pupil and iris
- Peripheral anterior synechiae.

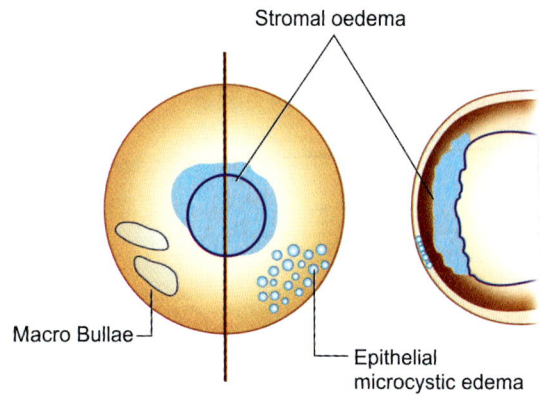

Fig. 7.33A: *Blue circles for epithelial oedema.*

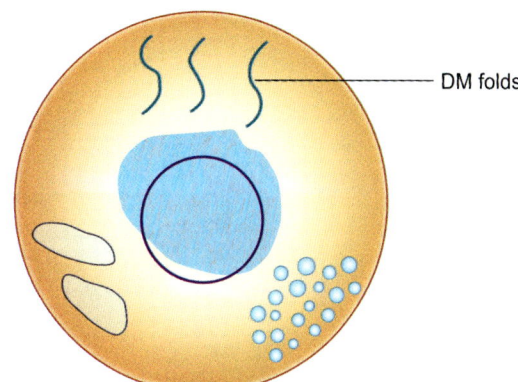

Fig. 7.33 B: *Wavy lines to document Descemet's membrane folds.*

Red

- Blood vessels are added in red. Superficial vessels are wavy lines that begin outside the limbus and deep vessels are straight lines that begin at the limbus (Fig. 7.34).

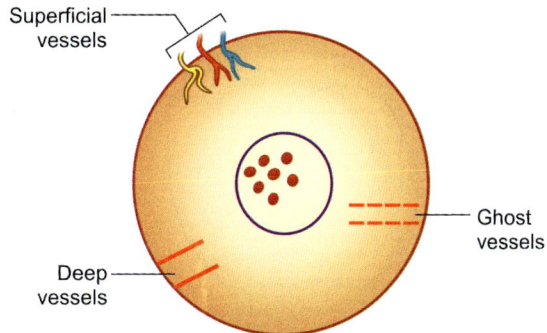

Fig. 7.34: *Red colour to document blood vessels.*

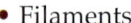

- Filaments
- Rose bengal staining
- Haemorrhages
- Hyphaema.

Yellow

- Infiltrate (Fig. 7.35)
- Hypopyon (Fig. 7.36)
- Keratic precipitates
- Nuclear sclerosis.

Green

- Fluorescein stain
- Superficial punctate keratitis (SPK)
- Epithelial defect (Fig. 7.37)
- Filaments
- Vitreous.

INVESTIGATIVE TECHNIQUES FOR CORNEAL DISEASES

PACHYMETRY

Pachymetry (Greek words: *Pachos* = thick + *metry* = to measure) is the term used for the measurement of corneal thickness (Fig. 7.38). It is an important indicator of the health status of the cornea especially of corneal endothelial pump function. It estimates the corneal barrier and endothelial pump function. It also measures the corneal rigidity and consequently has an impact on the accuracy of intraocular pressure (IOP) measurement by applanation tonometry. The normal corneal thickness varies from central to peripheral limbus. It ranges from 0.7 to 0.9 mm at the limbus and varies between

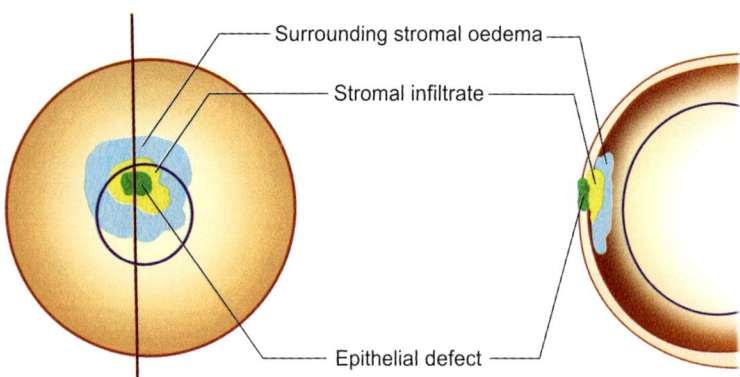

Fig. 7.35: *Yellow colour to document corneal infiltrate.*

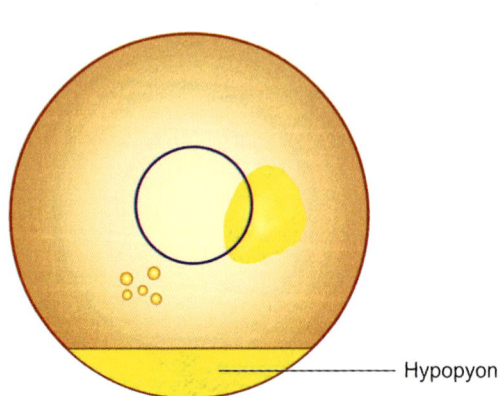

Fig. 7.36: *Yellow colour to document corneal hypopyon.*

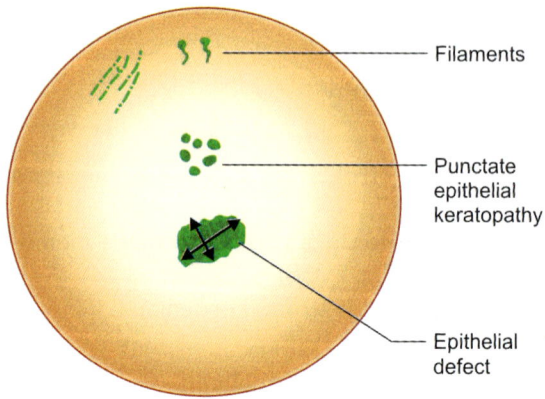

Fig. 7.37: *Green colour to document filaments and epithelial defect.*

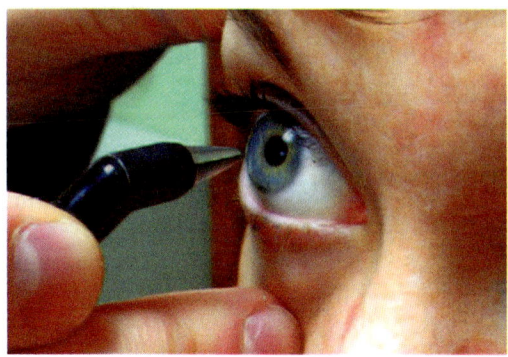

Fig. 7.38: *Corneal pachymetry.*

0.49 and 0.56 mm at the centre. The central corneal thickness (CCT) reading of 0.7 mm or more is indicative of endothelial decompensation. The mean CCT as shown by various studies is 0.51–0.52 mm. Peripheral corneal thickness is asymmetric so that temporal cornea is thinnest followed by the inferior cornea.

Applications

Corneal thickness evaluation has an important role in the following clinical situations:

Glaucoma for applying correction factor in actual intraocular pressure (IOP) determination

Congenital glaucoma to assess the amount of corneal edema.

Refractive surgeries. (a) preoperative screening, and (b) treatment plan of keratorefractive procedures like LASIK, astigmatic keratotomy, and previously even prior to radial keratotomy.

Postoperative follow-up of keratoplasty patients to determine endothelial cell function and its recovery and to become alert to early graft decompensation.

Contact lens to assess corneal edema and in orthokeratology.

Assessing the thinness of the cornea as in corneal disorders like Terrien's and Pellucid marginal degenerations, keratoconus, keratoglobus, post LASIK ectasia.

Other cases of corneal decompensation. For monitoring and evaluating corneal oedema and endothelial function as in herpetic endothelitis.

Techniques of pachymetry

Techniques for measuring CCT include optical pachymetry, ultrasound pachymetry, confocal microscopy, ultrasound biomicroscopy, optical ray path analysis or scanning slit corneal topography, and optical coherence tomography.

For further details *see* Chapter 9.

KERATOMETRY

It is also known as ophthalmometry. It is used to measure the radius of curvature of the anterior surface of the cornea (Fig. 7.39). It should be perform to know if there is any change is caused to the eye due to the fit of the contact lens. It is useful in monitoring the changes in the curvature in corneal ectatic disorders. However, unfortunately, if the curvature changes are significant, it is difficult to measure it in advance stages through keratometer. It plays a major role in calculating intraocular lens power and because of its low cost and ease of use it is widely used.

Clinical uses of keratometry

- Objective method for determining curvature of the cornea
- To estimate the amount and direction of corneal astigmatism
- The ocular biometery for the IOL power calculation

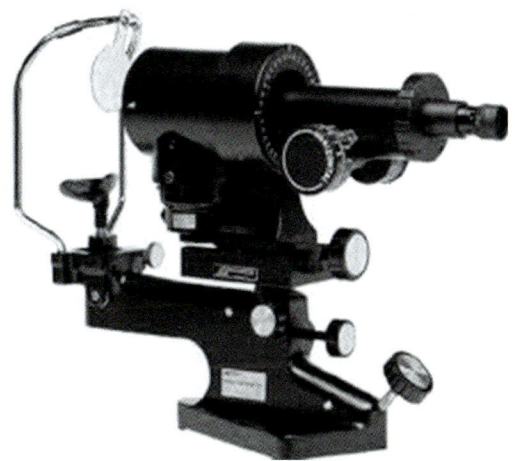

Fig. 7.39: *Keratometer (Bausch and Lomb type).*

- To monitor pre- and post-surgical astigmatism
- Differential diagnosis of axial versus refractive anisometropia
- To diagnose and monitor keratoconus and other corneal diseases
- For contact lens fitting by base curve selection
- To detect rigid gas permeable lens flexure

For details of techniques and interpretations of keratometry *see* Chapter 9.

CORNEAL TOPOGRAPHY

The cornea is the most important refractive element of the human eye, providing approximately two-thirds of its optical power (Fig. 7.40). Detailed examination of the corneal curvature is an essential part of the work-up before refractive surgery, for fitting of contact lens and for diagnosis and management of ectatic disorders. Keratometry was one of the earliest methods for measuring corneal shape. However, it gives limited information about corneal shape and appreciates only gross amount of astigmatism. These limitations led to the development of more advanced techniques for evaluating corneal shape. Three types of systems are used to measure corneal topography: Placido based, elevation based and interferometric. Recently Scheimpflug imaging has become increasingly popular.

Indications

Common indications for corneal topography in practice are:

I. *Refractive surgery patients*
   - Preoperative assessment
   - Postoperative follow-up
   - For augmentation procedures.

II. *Diagnostic indication*
   - Screening for ocular disease
   - Corneal ectasia
   - Contact lens-induced corneal warpage.

- Planning surgical incision (cataract, astigmatic keratotomy). Incision location, length, depth
- Contact lens fitting in irregular corneas
- Intraocular lens power calculation in special situations
- Management of astigmatism. Adjustment of incisions or sutures
- Keratoplasty follow-up.

For details of techniques and interpretation of corneal topography *see* Chapter 10.

CONFOCAL MICROSCOPY

Confocal microscopy is a bioimaging technique which allows noninvasive *in vivo* analysis of corneal microstructure and function (Fig. 7.41). It creates sharp images of a specimen that would otherwise appear blurred when viewed with a conventional microscope. This is achieved by excluding most of light from the specimen that is not from microscope's focal plane. It has been used to investigate numerous corneal diseases: epithelial changes, stromal degenerative or

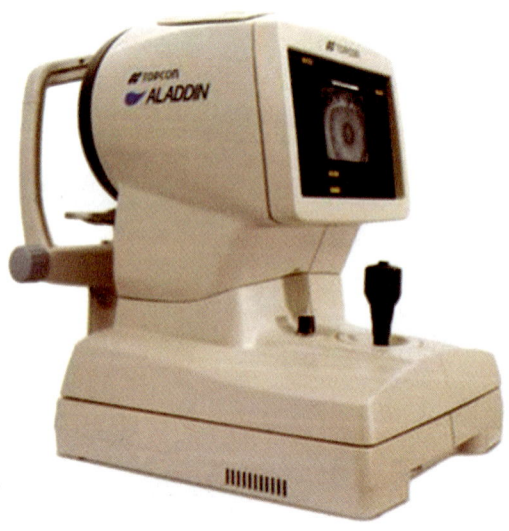

Fig. 7.40: *Corneal topographer.*

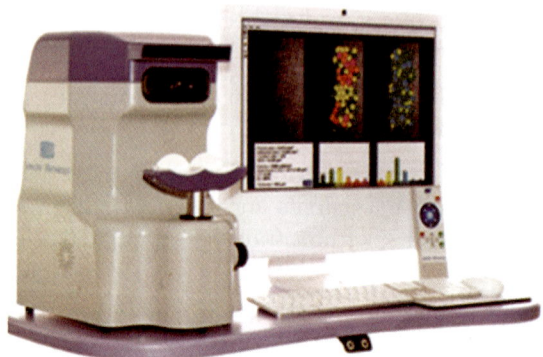

Fig. 7.41: *Confocal microscope.*

dystrophic diseases, endothelial pathologies, corneal deposits, infections and traumatic lesions.

Confocal microscopes: Prototypes

There are three different types that are used clinically in ophthalmology:
1. Tandem scanning confocal microscope
2. Slit scanning confocal microscope
3. Confocal laser scanning microscope.

Confocal microscopy of the normal human cornea

Superficial cells are seen with clear visible cell borders, bright cytoplasm and black nuclei. These cells are characteristically polygonal, usually hexagonal in shape. The intermediate layer of wing cells comprise of cells smaller than the superficial cells, with bright cell borders and dark cytoplasm. These cells are fairly uniform in size and shape. The basal epithelial cells are located just above the Bowman's membrane and are seen as a distinct mosaic with light cell boundaries. The basal epithelial cells are the smallest cells in the epithelium. The Bowman's layer appears as a homogenous acellular layer and nerve fibres of the subepithelial nerve plexus are seen as beaded nerve fibers. Keratocyte nuclei are identified as bright reflections in the stroma. The anterior stromal keratocyte nuclei are more abundant and oval compared to the posterior keratocyte nuclei which were less abundant and more oblong in shape. Endothelial cells are visible as bright cell bodies and dark cell boundaries, characteristically hexagonal in shape with fairly uniform appearance in size and shape.

Applications

- *Detection and management of infectious keratitis:* Viral, bacterial, parasitic (Acanthamoeba), and fungal.
- *Detection and management of corneal dystrophies:* Fuch's endothelial dystrophy, lattice dystrophy, epithelial basement membrane dystrophy, granular dystrophy, and corneal stem cell deficiency.
- *Monitoring contact lens induced corneal changes*

- *Pre- and post-refractive surgery assessment:* LASIK and LASEK flap evaluations and radial keratotomy
- *Monitoring corneal grafts* with the capability to distinguish between corneal oedema due to corneal graft rejection (caused by presence of inflammatory cells) and endothelial decomposition (caused by low endothelial cell counts without presence of inflammatory cells)
- *Conjunctival and limbal structures may be monitored* for cysts, inflammation and proliferation of cells. Edges of healing blebs may also be monitored
- *Endothelial cell counting capabilities.* With for a semiautomated cell count of any layer in the cornea. Monitoring of cell densities anywhere from epithelium to endothelium may be done
- *Corneal thickness/flap thickness measurement.*

For details of technique and interpretation of confocal micorscopy *see* Chapter 8.

SPECULAR MICROSCOPY

Specular microscopy is a noninvasive photographic technique that allows to visualize and analyse the corneal endothelium (Fig. 7.42).

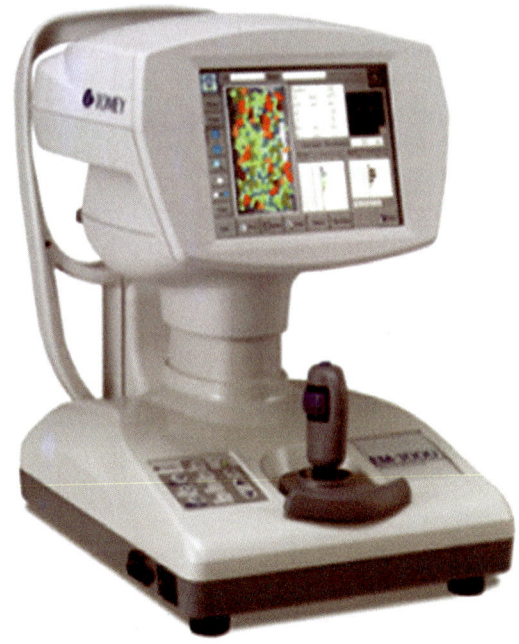

Fig. 7.42: *Specular microscope.*

Using computer-assisted morphometry, modern specular microscopes analyse the size, shape and population of the endothelial cells. The instrument projects light onto the cornea and captures the image that is reflected from the optical interface between the corneal endothelium and the aqueous humour. The reflected image is analysed by the instrument and displayed as a specular photomicrograph. In clinical practice, specular microscopy is the most accurate way to examine the corneal endothelium. The young normal corneal endothelium, as seen by specular microscopy shows a quasi-regular array of hexagonal cells, all having nearly the same size.

Analysis of specular microscopy

Quantitative analysis

Cell density. Means number of cells counted per mm square. Normal endothelial cell density decreases with age, it being 3500 cells/mm^2 in children and gradually declining to about 2000 cells/mm^2 in older eyes. An average value for adults is 2400 cells/mm^2 (1500–3500) with a mean cell size of 150–350 μm. Corneas with low cell density (fewer than 1000 cells/mm^2) might not tolerate intraocular surgery.

Coefficient of variation. The mean cell area divided by the standard deviation of mean cell area, normally less than 0.30.

Qualitative analysis

Pleomorphism means asymmetry in cell shape. **Polymegathism** means asymmetry in cell size.

Causes of polymegathism
- Long-term contact lens wear
- Postcataract surgery
- Postpenetrating keratoplasty
- Keratoconus
- Ageing
- Diabetes.

Clinical applications
- Preoperative assessment of the donor cornea
- Corneal oedema

- Corneal degenerations
- Corneal dystrophies
- Ocular inflammation
- Contact lens endotheliopathy
- Early diagnosis of Fuch's endothelial dystrophy
- Various refractive surgical procedures
- Bullous keratopathy
- Keratoconus
- Recurrent corneal erosions
- Corneal dystrophy
- Corneal ectasia
- Postcorneal transplant
- Glaucoma
- Evaluation of donor corneal endothelium and the effect of preservation (eye banking).

For details *see* Chapter 8.

ANTERIOR SEGMENT OCT

Anterior segment optical coherence tomography (ASOCT) produces high-resolution, three dimensional cross-sectional images of the anterior segment that uses low coherence interferometry to achieve axial resolution in the range of 3–20 μm (Fig. 7.43). The principle of OCT is analogous to ultrasound, but it uses light instead of sound. It is a completely non-invasive technique. As it uses interferometry for depth resolution, it can have a long working distance and a wide field of transverse scanning compared to confocal microscopy. Its applications are being expanded and now include pachymetry, corneal topography, ectatic corneal disorders, microbial keratitis, keratoplasty, corneal opacity, intrastromal corneal ring segments, anterior chamber biometry, corneal implants, anterior chamber tumours and refractive surgery.

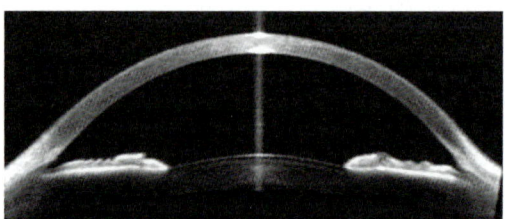

Fig. 7.43: *Anterior segment OCT.*

Applications of anterior segment optical coherence tomography

1. Measuring corneal thickness: Central corneal thickness is important for planning and performing refractive surgery, for assessing corneal diseases as well as monitoring glaucoma progression in patients with ocular hypertension and primary open-angle glaucoma.

2. Corneal topography. For details, *see* Chapter 10.

3. Ectatic corneal disorders. ASOCT is important for diagnosis and management of corneal ectatic disorders like keratoconus, Terrien marginal degeneration and pellucid marginal degeneration and their complication, especially in acute hydrops and its monitoring. Although moderate to advanced keratoconus is easily recognized by the characteristic topographic pattern and classic clinical signs, it can be difficult to distinguish subclinical forms of disease from normal corneas, because patients usually present with normal visual acuity, stable topographic patterns and minimal or no clinical signs. In these cases, OCT produces highly reliable pachymetry map, that can detect keratoconus, ectasia and corneal thinning conditions before refractive laser surgeries.

4. Microbial keratitis. OCT can also be used for corneal imaging and assessment, in conjunction with slit-lamp biomicroscopy in cases of microbial keratitis to monitor progression of the disease. OCT can be particularly useful in assessing the depth of corneal ulcers. The affected area of keratitis is represented by the OCT as higher intense regions. In deciding the response of a certain keratitis to treatment, the OCT images can be followed by examining the depth and density of these affected areas. When indicated, the area for corneal biopsy can be ascertained by identifying the densest areas of infiltration. Areas of impending perforation and severe thinning can also be imaged on ASOCT. Decision on performing either lamellar keratoplasty or full-thickness penetrating keratoplasty can be made by examining the depth of infection on the ASOCT images.

5. OCT for corneal transplantation. The anterior segment optical coherence tomography is useful in the preoperative and postoperative evaluation and management of corneal transplant patients. Recent advances in lamellar keratoplasty have made it an attractive alternative to conventional full-thickness penetrating keratoplasty (PKP). These have led to the development of customized component surgery, which involves targeted replacement of diseased corneal tissue while retaining healthy layers. Corneal surgeons have used anterior lamellar keratoplasty techniques, such as deep anterior lamellar keratoplasty (DALK), to manage conditions affecting the anterior layers. Nearly all corneal stromal can be removed with retention of Descemet's membrane and host endothelium, eliminating the risk of endothelial rejection. In endothelial keratoplasty procedures, such as Descemet's stripping endothelial keratoplasty, the AS-OCT can be used to determine donor graft thickness, graft attachment, positioning, interface issues and donor configuration. Similarly, it is useful to detect presence of a pseudo-AC following deep anterior lamellar keratoplasty in the early postoperative period.

6. Accurate measurement of opacities and rings. AS-OCT scanning allows surgeons to accurately determine the depth of corneal opacities, enabling them to choose the most appropriate treatment: excimer laser or lamellar or penetrating keratoplasty. Insertion of shallow intrastromal corneal ring segments increases the incidence of epithelial and stromal breakdown and ring extrusion. AS-OCT can assess the depth and position of intracorneal rings to determine the risk of extrusion.

7. Anterior chamber biometry. The accurate measurement of anterior chamber dimensions is important prior to implanting refractive phakic IOLs. The anterior segment optical coherence tomography produces. High-resolution images with accurate and reproducible biometry including AC depth, angle-to-angle width and iris profile, although sulcus to sulcus distance is unable to be accurately measured. This assists preoperatively in choosing the appropriate sized IOL, as well as examining the *in vivo* position of the phakic IOL, that is, its relationship to the endothelium, crystalline lens, trabecular meshwork and iris.

This is critical to avoid complications of phakic IOL insertion, such as lens endothelial touch and angle closure glaucoma. The anterior segment optical coherence tomography is able to measure these AC parameters accurately, directly and in all meridians as compared to conventional white-to-white measurements.

8. Corneal implants: The anterior segment optical coherence tomography is able to accurately determine the depth and position of intrastromal ring segments, such as intacs and kerarings. These are crescent shaped segments of polymethylmethacrylate that have been used for the treatment of post LASIK corneal ectasias, pellucid marginal degeneration and keratoconus. Implanting intacs at the proper depth is important for good visual outcome and to avoid complications, such as extrusion. Similarly, the AS-OCT can be used to image corneal inlays for the treatment of presbyopia, such as the Presbylens.

9. Anterior segment tumours: Anterior iris pathology can be imaged by AS-OCT and is able to differentiate small cystic from solid lesions. It can image small non-pigmented tumours but cannot penetrate larger tumours, pigmented tumours or tumours involving the ciliary body. Visualization of the posterior chamber is suboptimal as the infrared light is significantly attenuated by the iris pigment epithelium.

10. Laser assisted *in situ* keratomileusis and other refractive surgeries. Imaging of the corneal layers with high speed OCT provide useful information relevant to keratorefractive surgery, especially in laser *in situ* keratomileusis (LASIK). Corneal flap thickness is an important parameter in LASIK because it determines the amount of residual stroma available for ablation. By directly measuring corneal flap thickness intraoperatively, it can potentially improve the predictability of LASIK. Owing to superior resolution of morphological features, it can also be used for postoperative assessment of the anatomical correlates of the refractive outcome. It can also provide the comprehensive pachymetry map of the entire cornea and helps in the detection of normal from abnormally thin corneas in which subtractive refractive surgery like LASIK may need to be avoided.

Advantages of AS-OCT

- It is a non-contact method therefore do not cause indentation of the angle by placement of the scleral cup on the eye (which is required to maintain the water bath in UBM). Also, no possibility of corneal abrasion or punctuate epithelial erosions (possible with UBM).
- Shorter imaging time (patient set-up in UBM takes longer. Also, only one angle is imaged at a time with the UBM).
- Rapid image acquisition. Eight frames can be captured per second, allowing operator to choose the best centred image.
- Requires less expertise to perform-small learning curve for the operator.
- Target may be used to induce accommodation in the eye being imaged (this is especially useful in the evaluation of accommodative intraocular lenses).
- More comfortable for the patient, due to non-contact technique, upright position and rapid imaging acquisition.

VIDEOKERATOGRAPHY

Keratorefractive surgery has been a powerful stimulus for the development of sophisticated systems for mapping extensible corneal shape (Fig. 7.44). Videokeratography involves system for image capture, surface reconstruction and

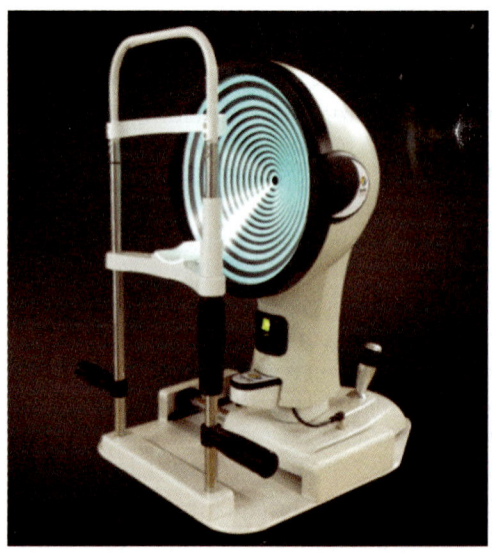

Fig. 7.44: *Videokeratography.*

data output. Image capture involves projection of an image onto the surface of the cornea and capture of the reflected image with a digital video camera. It provide both qualitative and quantitative information about the corneal surface. Surface reconstruction depends on edge detection software and algorithms for calculating corneal shape (usually expressed as dioptric power) from the image analysis. Data output can be in several forms, such as data tables, colour coded curvature maps or wire mesh models. Furthermore, developments in videokeratography have revealed considerable irregular variation within individual corneas and from one person to another. There is a degree of symmetry from one eye to the contralateral eye. Corneal topographical maps have been likened to fingerprints, there being a similarity between apparently normal corneas but also distinct differences. Corneal topography may therefore be considered as another expression of the uniqueness of the individual. Not only are maps of the corneal surface unique to the individual, they vary with time, even in people without any evidence of corneal disease. The shape determined by videokeratography is a measure of optical power, with true physical shape being inferred. In most situations, it is the corneal refractive power which is of interest and progress in videokeratography has developed parallel to keratorefractive surgery. There is a growing movement in refractive surgery which considers minor changes in corneal topography as important limitations on visual potential and amenability to surgery.

Applications for videokeratography

- To screen patients prior to refractive surgery and evaluating them after surgery
- To screen patients for irregular astigmatism, corneal warpage and keratoconus prior to refractive surgery
- To evaluate the cornea after cataract surgery and to understand patients visual complaints
- To direct management after penetrating keratoplasty
- To plan astigmatic surgery
- To fit contact lenses in patients with irregular astigmatism

- To evaluate unexplained visual loss and to determine visual complications from corneal dystrophies, scars, pterygia, recurrent erosions, and chalazia.

CORNEAL AESTHESIOMETRY

Corneal aesthesiometry is important to examine cases involving the lesions of the fifth cranial nerve, cases with ulcerative keratitis and degenerative lesions.

Quantitative methods

- Cochet-Bonnet aesthesiometer
- Noncontact air puff technique
- Larson-Millodot aesthesiometer.

Handheld aesthesiometer (Cochet-Bonnet)

- The handheld esthesiometer (Cochet-Bonnet) is a device that contains a thin, retractable, nylon monofilament that extends up to 6 cm in length (Fig. 7.45).
- Variable pressure can be applied by the device by adjusting the length. The monofilament ranges from 60 to 5 mm and as the length is decreased, the pressure increases from 11 to 200 mm/gm.
- If the filament is applied perpendicularly to the corneal surface, most patients will feel the nylon thread when it is extended to a full 6 cm.

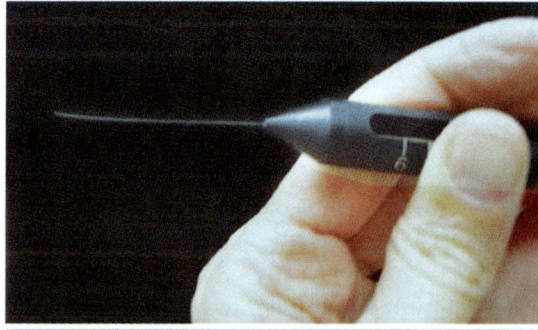
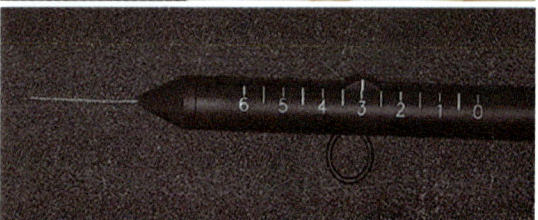

Fig. 7.45: *Cochet-Bonnet aesthesiometer.*

- If the filament has to be shortened to 4 cm or less, the corneal sensation is inferred to have decreased.
- A value below 2 cm is diagnostic of significant hypoaesthesia.

Steps for using the handheld aesthesiometer are:

- Extend the filament to full length of 6 cm
- Retract the filament incrementally in 0.5 cm steps until the patient can feel its contact
- Record the length (the shorter the length indicates decreased sensation)
- Compare the fellow cornea
- Repeat steps 1–4 in each quadrant: superior, temporal, inferior, nasal
- Sterilize the filament and retract back into the device to protect it from damage.

Limitations with this technique are that it is invasive, and can cause epithelial damage thereby producing an increased sensitivity due to the presence of free nerve endings within the corneal epithelium. Thus, the minimum stimulus is also suprathreshold and the range of stimulus intensity is limited . The bending of the thread under its own weight, particularly when the thread is long makes it difficult to make an accurate observation of the end-point. Subject apprehension also compromises the testing.

Non-contact air puff technique

- Uses controlled pulses of pressure of air to stimulate the cornea.
- It measures the corneal nerve threshold by using a composite stimulus consisting of air pressure, tear evaporation and disruption.
- An adjustable valve couples with a pressure sensor to control the output from a compressed air reservoir to within 0.01 mbar.
- The stimulus is applied to the eye through a stimulus jet comprising a brass tube of length 35 mm and diameter of 6 mm with a central 0.5 mm diameter longitudinal bore.
- The settings for stimulus duration that are available include 0.5, 0.9 and 1.5 seconds. A stimulus threshold of 0.9 mm has been recommended as standard setting presuming that a longer duration might result in corneal

drying and shorter duration might be too quick for the subject's response.
- A slit-lamp attachment enables positioning the stimulus jet close to the eye examined. A clear plastic centimeter ruler attached to the mount enables setting the testing distance at 1 cm.
- The stimulus jet is aligned to the center of the cornea.
- Testing is started with the application of suprathreshold stimulus and the patient usually responds describing it at a cold sensation or pressure type of sensation. On approaching the threshold, the stimuli may be difficult to describe.
- Measurements are made in millibars of air pressure required.

Larson-Millodot aesthesiometer

- In Larson-Millodot aesthesiometer (Fig. 7.46), the probe tip is made of fine platinum wire bent doubled so that the tip has known and reproducible dimensions.
- The probe is automatically advanced toward the eye at a constant rate upon the operator's command.
- When the cornea is touched with a force equal to the test force, the probe is retracted quickly and automatically.
- The force applied to the cornea can be set at any value within the range of this instrument and this force will not be exceeded.
- The range of settings for practical purposes is from 1 to 200 mg and any force within these limits can be set with an accuracy of ±5 mg operation.

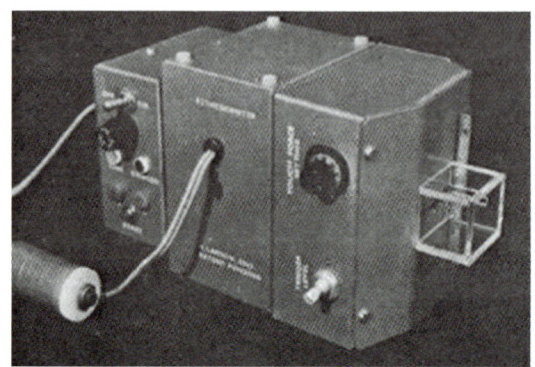

Fig. 7.46: *Larson-Millodot aesthesiometer.*

TECHNIQUES FOR MICROBIOLOGICAL AND CYTOLOGICAL EVALUATION

The key for successful treatment of microbial keratitis relies on prompt and reliable detection of the causative microorganism with timely prescription of specifically targeted effective antimicrobial agent. Figure 7.47 summarises the microbiological evaluation of corneal scraping. The culture method with or without smears for staining is the gold standard for pathogen identification. Ideally, samples should be collected prior to the start of antibiotic treatment. Treatment can be initiated based on the results of smear examination and, if required modified in accordance with the culture and sensitivity results.

Sample collection devices

- Platinum spatula
- Surgical blade no. 15
- Calcium alginate swab.

Generally, the edge of the corneal ulceration rather than the central ulcer crater is the most suitable location for scraping since viable pathogens tend to be found at this point. After scraping, staining of smeared specimen should be performed to provide an early detection of the offending organism and can guide initial antimicrobial treatment.

Laboratory methods

Laboratory method is identification of Bacteria, fungus, parasite-non viral—includes:

- Direct microscopy
- Culture and Identification
- Molecular methods.

Direct microscopy. Stains used are:

Type of stain	Organisms
Gram stain	Bacteria (mainly), fungus and *Acanthamoeba*
KOH	Fungus (mainly), *Acanthamoeba* and *Nocardia* (Fig. 7.48)
GIEMSA	Bacteria, fungi, *Chlamydiae*, *Acanthamoeba*
Acid fast	*Mycobacterium, Nocardia*
Acridine orange	Bacteria, fungi, *Acanthamoeba*
Calcoflour white	Fungus and *Acanthamoeba*

Culture and identification of pathogens

Corneal scraping with culture remains the gold standard for the diagnosis of suspected infectious keratitis. PCR may be used as a screening diagnosis test when microbial keratitis is suspected. Culture provides several key advantages including capture for organism identification and antimicrobial agent susceptibility testing.

Culture media: The standard culture media for suspected bacterial keratitis include blood agar, chocolate agar and thioglycolate broth

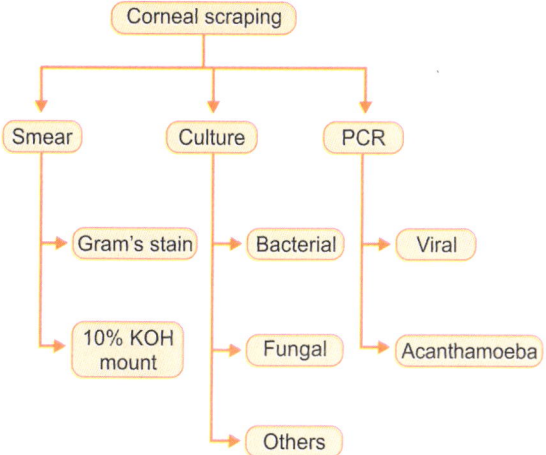

Fig. 7.47: *Microbiological evaluation of corneal scraping.*

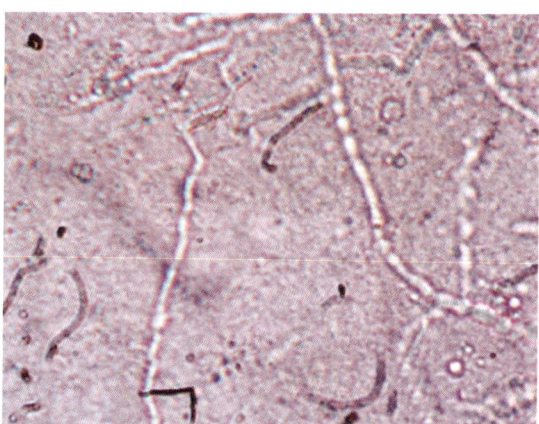

Fig. 7.48: *KOH mount showing hyphae.*

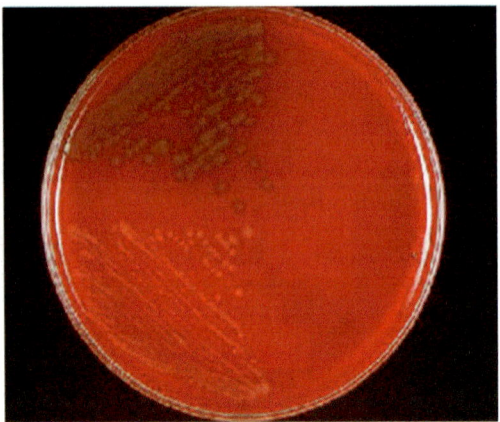

Fig. 7.49: *Blood agar culture plate.*

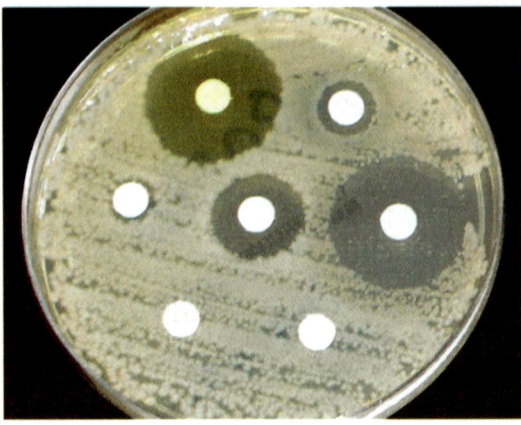

Fig. 7.50: *Antimicrobial susceptibility testing.*

(Fig. 7.49). For isolation of fungi, Sabouraud's dextrose agar (SDA) is commonly selected. Ocular specimens should be incubated in 5–7% CO_2 at 35–37°C. The incubation period varies according to each species. For aerobic bacteria, the culture media should be kept for at least 7 days before discarding.

Media	Common isolates
Blood agar	Aerobic and facultative anaerobic bacteria
Chocolate agar	Aerobic and facultative anaerobic bacteria
Thioglycollate broth	Aerobic and facultative anaerobic bacteria
SDA	Fungi
Thayer-Martin agar	Pathogenic *Neisseria*
LJ media	*Mycobacterium, Nocardia*
Brain heart infusion broth	Fungi
Non-nutrient agar	*Acanthamoeba* seeded with *E. coli*

Antimicrobial susceptibility testing

Susceptibility testing is performed to determine the most effective antimicrobial agent available. Standard disk diffusion or microdilution techniques are the preferred laboratory methods for antimicrobial susceptibility testing against bacterial ocular isolates (Fig. 7.50). Antimicrobial containing disks are placed on the agar surface inoculated with a pure culture of the organism and antimicrobial susceptibility is determined.

Viral diagnostic testing

Different used methods to identify viral pathogens consist of viral culture, microscopy, antigen detection, nucleic acid detection and serology. Viral culture followed by direct or indirect immunofluorescent antigen detection remains the gold standard of viral identification. Samples from corneal scrapings are placed on glass slides, then stained with hematoxylin and eosin. Tzanck, Giemsa, or Papanicolaou for light microscopic examination as an alternative option for possible diagnosis. The specimens for viral culture or PCR should be collected onto Dacron swabs and transported to the testing laboratory immediately. In addition, specimens should be kept moist and at 4°C during the transportation.

CORNEAL BIOPSY

Corneal biopsy is a useful procedure in the diagnosis and management of corneal inflammation, infections, degenerations, dystrophies and corneal manifestations of systemic diseases. Usually a partial thickness biopsy should be performed. Full-thickness biopsy should be reserved only for tectonic indications in advanced disease. It is indicated in cases with deep stromal abscess or in case where repeated culture shows negative reports but there is strong suspicion of infection. The cornea is anesthetized and 0.2 to 0.3 mm trephine is used to outline the area to be biopsied. Usually a depth of about 0.1 to 0.2 mm is dissected out.

The tissue is then sent for histopathological as well microbiological analysis.

Indications

Infectious corneal processes
- Deep suppurative stromal keratitis
- Keratitis with atypical presentation
- Fungal or *Acanthamoeba* keratitis that does not respond to other treatment
- Culture negative keratitis.

Neoplastic. Conjunctival neoplasms with extension through limbus onto cornea.

Techniques

- Firstly slit-lamp biomicroscopic examination should be performed. Depth of the infiltrate and overlying corneal thickness should be assessed.
- Keep the patient in supine position under operating microscope.
- Operating eye should be prepared and draped under all aseptic precautions.
- Insert the eye speculum.
- A sponge soaked in proparacaine should be placed on the limbus for 1–2 minutes so as to anaesthesise the eye.
- For a partial-thickness biopsy, trephination is performed with a small diameter punch (2–5 mm). The trephine is placed such that it includes the lesion as well as normal healthy cornea. The blade should be rotated back and forth between the thumb and forefinger.
- After trephination, careful dissection of the tissue is performed with a crescent blade, which is held flat against the cornea to prevent perforation. The corneal button must be grasped gently with the forceps to prevent crushing the tissue.

- After complete excision of the tissue, the biopsy specimen is transferred from the crescent blade to the appropriate transport media.
- Postoperatively, in the case of suspected microbial keratitis, the same antimicrobial regimen is continued.
- An antibiotic ointment may be added for comfort during the day and at night time.

Complications

Complications from biopsy include scarring, irregular astigmatism, poor or delayed healing and perforation.

BIBLIOGRAPHY

1. Basic & Clinical Science Course. External disease and cornea (2011–2012 edn.). American Academy of Ophthalmology. 2012.
2. Dua Harminder S, Faraj Lana A, Said Dalia G, Gray Trevor, Lowe James. "Human Corneal Anatomy Redefined". Ophthalmology 2013; 120(9):1778–85.
3. Facts About the Cornea and Corneal Disease". National Eye Institute. Archived from the original on 2005;03–27.
4. Huang AJW, Wichiensin P, Yang MC. Bacterial keratitis. Chapter 81. In: Krachmer JH, Mannis MH, Holland EJ: Cornea: Fundamental, Diagnosis and Management, NY, 2005;1005-33.
5. Maurice, DM. "The structure and transparency of the cornea". J Physiol 1957;136(2): 263-286.
6. Nottingham J. Practical observations on conical cornea: and on the short sight, and other defects of vision connected with it. London: J. Churchill, 1854.
7. Sachdev MS, Honavar SG, Thakar M. Diagnostic tests for corneal diseases. Indian J Ophthalmol 1994;42:89–99.

Specular Microscopy and Confocal Microscopy of Cornea

Chapter Outline

SPECULAR MICROSCOPY
- Introduction
- Optics
- Types of specular microscopes
  - Contact specular microscopes
  - Noncontact specular microscopes
- Procedure and methods of analysis
- Commercially available specular microscopes
- Clinical uses of specular microscopy

CONFOCAL MICROSCOPY OF CORNEA
- Principle
- Types of confocal microscope
- Confocal microscopy of the normal human cornea
- Confocal microscopy in corneal pathologies

OTHER CORNEAL ENDOTHELIAL SCANS
- Confoscan
- Heidelberg retinal tomograph 3

SPECULAR MICROSCOPY

INTRODUCTION

Specular microscopy is a procedure that provides the clinical and morphological study of corneal endothelial cells *in vivo* without disturbing their function. Efforts were made by Vogt, more than 75 years ago, to examine the endothelial cell morphology in the reflected light of the slit-lamp biomicroscope. However, fine rapid movements of the eye and limited magnification preclude the use of this technique for systematic studies of the endothelium. Maurice (1968) introduced the 'specular microscope' for examination of the corneal endothelial cells at high magnification (4003). This instrument used Vogt's reflection principle but separated illuminating and viewing light paths at a fixed angle in a split microscope objective. Laing (1975) adopted specular microscope for clinical use. He replaced the original

water immersion lens with a dipping case objective to applanate the cornea. Baurne et al. (1976) simplified the specular microscope for rapid endothelial examination and photography at 2003.

OPTICS

The specular microscope is a reflected light microscope which projects a slit of light on to the cornea and utilizes the light reflected from an optical interface of tissue for image formation (rather than light transmitted through the tissue sample). It is the difference in refractive indices between the endothelial cells and aqueous humour which gives rise to this specular or mirror-like reflection at the flat posterior surface. The reflected light is estimated to be about 0.02% of the incident light. Figure 8.1 shows a drawing of the optics of the visualization of the endothelial mosaic produced by slit-lamp biomicroscopy. Reflected light from the epithelium and stroma obscures the view of the endothelium

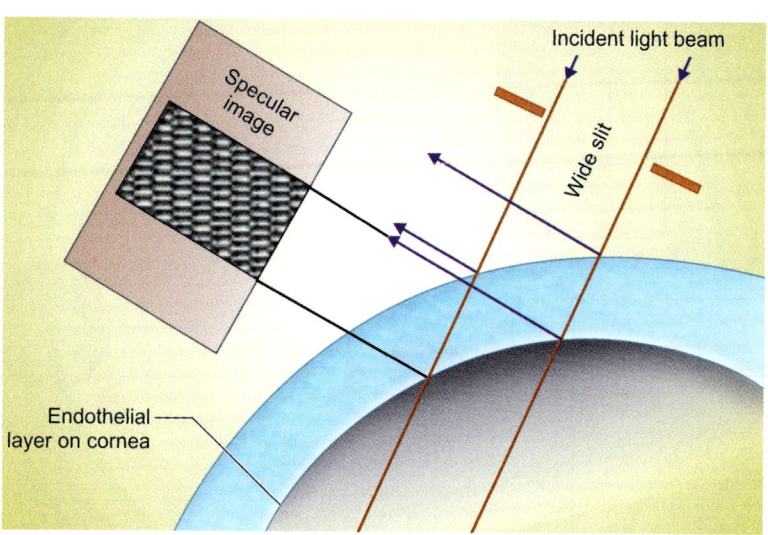

Fig. 8.1: *Schematic drawing of the endothelial layers as seen with slit-lamp microscopy. Note the wide angle between the illuminating beam and the observation path needed to remove the annoying surface reflection and stroma scatter from view of the endothelial mosaic.*

unless a narrow slit of light is used for illumination. Laing described that specular microscopy yields an image with three or four distinct zones (Fig. 8.2), depending upon the width of the illuminating slit as:

Zone 1. Epithelium/lens-coupling fluid
Zone 2. Corneal stroma
Zone 3. Corneal endothelium
Zone 4. Aqueous humour.

The boundary between endothelial region (zone 3) and aqueous region (zone 4) is almost dark and is termed the *dark boundary*. The boundary between endothelium region (zone 3)

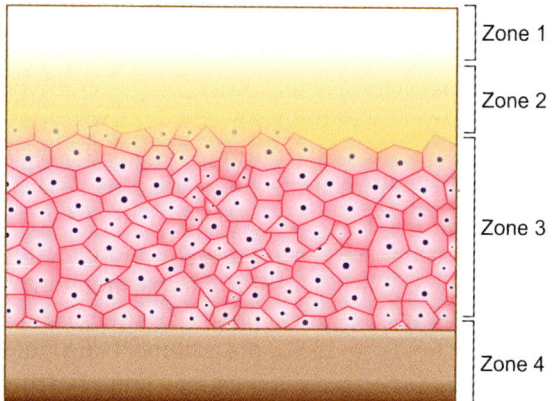

Fig. 8.2: *Specular micrograph of endothelial cells showing four distinct zones.*

and stroma (zone 2) is usually bright and is termed the *bright boundary*.

TYPES OF SPECULAR MICROSCOPES

There are two basic types of clinical specular microscopes:

1. CONTACT SPECULAR MICROSCOPES

Commercially available contact specular microscopes include:

• Keller-Konan, SP-580 (Konan Medical USA, Torrance, CA, USA)
• EM-1000 (Tomey, Erlangen, Germany).

In such types of specular microscopes, a contact lens with a coupling fluid of index of refraction similar to that of cornea is used to eliminate the corneal surface reflection. The corneal thickness in such an arrangement can be thought to also include the contact lens thickness. The reflection from the surface of contact lens replaces that of the corneal surface. However, because of the thickness of contact lens, the surface reflection is moved well over to side (Fig. 8.3).

Such specular microscopes provide good resolution and magnification. But the patients are less comfortable and there is a risk of spread of infection, if strict sterile precautions are not

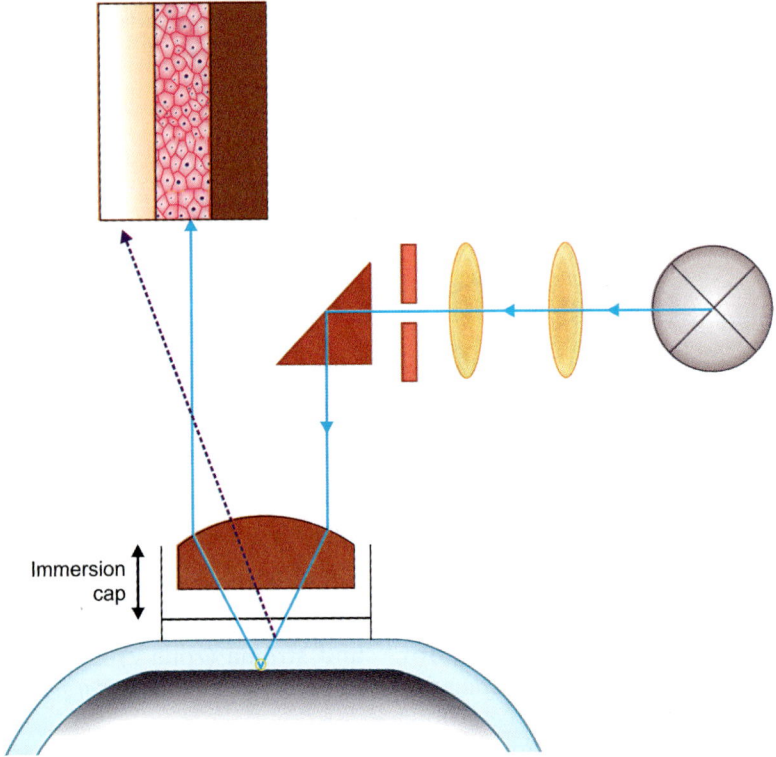

Fig. 8.3: *Optics of contact lens-assisted endothelial specular microscope.*

taken. Further, manipulating the cornea with this technique may cause *artefacts*, especially in fragile, diseased cornea.

2. NONCONTACT SPECULAR MICROSCOPES

Commercially available noncontact specular microscope includes:
- Automated SM is SP-3000p (Topcon Medical Systems Inc. Paramus, NJ, USA).

In noncontact specular microscopes, the bothersome reflection from the front corneal surface is eliminated by increasing the angle of incidence. As shown in Fig. 8.1, by increasing the angle of incidence, the anterior reflection is moved to the side, covering less of specular reflection from the endothelium. These microscopes have the advantages of greater patient tolerance and acceptability, and there is no risk of trauma to the cornea. However, a broader view is obtained at the expense of resolution and magnification due to uncontrolled eye movements.

WIDE-FIELD SPECULAR MICROSCOPES

A modification to the standard specular microscope has been described with the use of a scanning mirror. In this way, fields of 800 m in diameter have been achieved with no loss in contrast. The technique allows continuous viewing of the 800 m diameter area because of the high speed of mirror oscillation.

Advantages

The wide-field specular microscopes combine the advantages of both the above microscopes.
- Field of view is 10–15 times larger, the resolution is high and image quality is less susceptible to eye movements.
- Endothelial layer topography is more readily evaluated. The relocation of a specified region of the endothelium is relatively easy and the larger field provides more accurate cell counts.
- *Resolution of endothelium* has been further improved by the addition of highly sensitive video cameras and recording systems, as well

as a variety of optic improvements such as scanning mirror system.

- Annoying reflections from the incident light have been minimized by the improvements in optics.

PROCEDURE AND METHOD OF ANALYSIS

PROCEDURE

Currently available contact and noncontact wide-field specular microscopes are easy to use with little patient discomfort. The procedure is first explained to the patient to relieve any anxiety. The contact specular microscopy procedure is very similar to that of Goldmann applanation tonometry (Fig. 8.4A). The whole cornea should be systematically scanned to ensure complete evaluation of the endothelial mosaic–centrally, superiorly, inferiorly, nasally and temporally (Fig. 8.4B).

METHODS OF ANALYSIS

For cell analysis, a minimum of 75 cells should be counted. The early processing methods were tedious and time-consuming. The introduction of large-field microscopes has made the process a bit simplified.

Methods of endothelial cell analysis are as follows:

1. *Cell density.* The number of cells in a photographic field are counted to obtain the cell density. The cell count is calculated per square millimetre. The cell density of endothelium is around 3500 cells/mm^2 in young adults, which decreases with the advancing age (2000 cells/mm^2). There is a considerable functional reserve for the endothelium. Corneas with cell count, 1000 cells/mm^2 poorly tolerate intraocular surgery.

2. *Fixed frame analysis.* In this method, the photograph of endothelial cells is compared with the drawings of endothelial mosaic of known size.

3. *Tracing analysis.* The tracing of the individual cell outlines can be made and subsequently analysed for individual cell areas and other parameters.

4. *Analysis of digested cells.* The cells may be digested after tracing their outlines, using a digesting tablet. The analysis can then be made using a photograph—a negative image on a television screen or a videotaped recording.

5. *Computerized image analysis.* The computerized cell analysis provides the mean cell density, i.e. cells per square millimetre, and frequency distribution of the individual cell sizes, and analyses the polygonality.

QUANTITATIVE AND QUALITATIVE ANALYSIS BY SPECULAR MICROSCOPY

Calculation of cell density (quantitative analysis): To calculate the cell density, a rectangular area can be determined manually. All the cells completely within the border of the

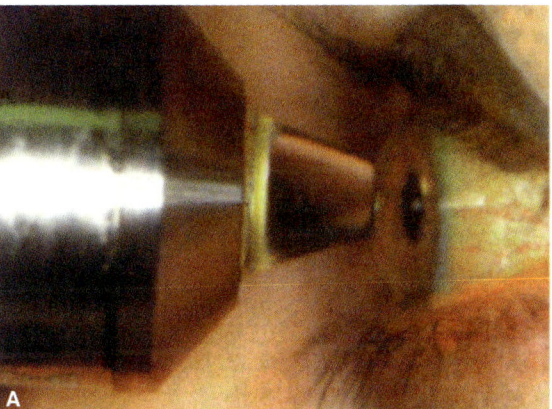
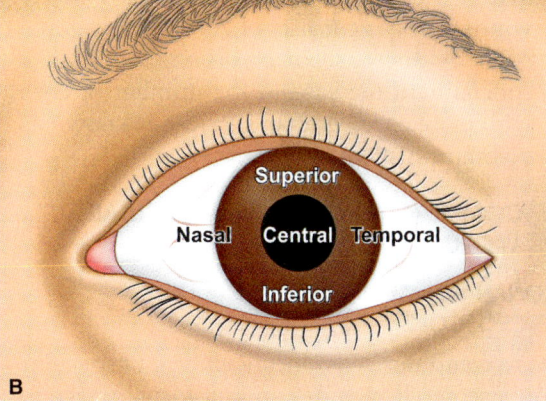

Fig. 8.4: *Procedure of specular microscopy: (A) Placement of applanation cone in the centre of cornea with the light shining through the pupil; (B) Areas of cornea for systematic scanning of endothelium.*

rectangle as well as those touching two adjacent borders are marked. However, this technique gives only the cell density in cells per square millimetre. The other method is to mark the centre of adjacent cells. This allows automated computation of the mean cell area, maximum cell area (MAX), minimum cell area (MIN), number of cells actually analysed (NUM), mean cell density (CD) and standard deviation of the mean cell area (SD).

Study of cell morphology (qualitative analysis)

Alterations in morphology—such as variations in cell size, i.e. polymegathism and cell shape, i.e. pleomorphism—and asymmetry of the cell population may be more reliable indices of endothelial stress than mean cell density alone.

- *Coefficient of variation.* The degree of uniformity of cell size is determined by measuring the areas of a population of cells and calculating the coefficient of variance, which is the standard deviation of mean cell area divided by the mean cell area, i.e. SD/AVE. The normal endothelium has a coefficient of variance of 0.25. An increase in this value means that the cell size is variable and is known as polymegathism. Cell size varies over a wide range in a number of disorders, and endothelial cells may assume shapes that are substantially different from their usual hexagonal appearance.
- *Percentage of hexagonal cells.* Cell boundaries normally intersect in a manner that results in three angles of intersection, each approximately 608. The endothelial mosaic in healthy young corneas consists of 70–80% hexagonal cells. A decrease in hexagonality with a concomitant increase in the number of cells with more or fewer than six sides is known as pleomorphism.

COMMERCIALLY AVAILABLE SPECULAR MICROSCOPES

KONAN NONCON ROBO SPECULAR MICROSCOPE

It is a computerized noncontact type of specular microscope. It includes an autofocus device to record the specular images readily. There is also an incorporated semi-automated image analyzing programme. The software programme has got two analyzing modalities for cell density and cell morphology. With Konan Noncon Roboca SP8000, it is possible (i) to calculate the individual cell area, with which the coefficient of variance can be deduced as a degree of polymegathism and (ii) to analyse the polygonality, i.e. percentage of hexagonality.

KEELER–KONAN SPECULAR MICROSCOPE

It is a contact type wide-field specular microscope. Its advantages over the noncontact type wide-field specular microscope are:

- It allows more detailed study of corneal endothelium. Different magnification cones can be used to study the endothelial morphology.
- It also allows the study of corneal epithelium, corneal stroma, the crystalline lens epithelial surface, the surface of intraocular lens (IOL) and the posterior capsule. The entire cornea can be examined by moving the cone manually over the corneal surface.

CLINICAL USES OF SPECULAR MICROSCOPY

1. Assessment of changes in the endothelium:
   - With ageing
   - Following surgical procedures such as:
     - Corneal grafting
     - Cataract surgery with or without IOL implantation
     - Newer procedures like excimer laser, LASIK, etc.
   - With associated conditions such as:
     - Glaucoma
     - Uveitis
     - Contact lens wear
     - Trauma—blunt or penetrating
   - With use of intracameral drugs, irrigating solutions and topical medications.
2. Assessment of endothelium in donor corneas and the effect of preservation.
3. Assessment of naturally occurring diseases, degenerations and dystrophies.
4. Assessment of longitudinal effect of surgical procedures.
5. Measurement of corneal thickness, i.e. pachymetry (with contact type only).

6. Assessment of the epithelium of the cornea and the crystalline lens.

CONFOCAL MICROSCOPY OF CORNEA

Clinical confocal microscopy is a new bioimaging technique which enables non-invasive analysis of corneal structure and function. Minsky described the first confocal microscope in 1957. Since then several improvisions have occurred. Bohnke and Masters (1999) have detailed the optical techniques for ocular biomicroscopy and theoretical foundations of confocal microscopy. The most modern confocal microscopes have light source focused on to a small volume within the specimen tissue, and a confocal detector is used to collect the resulting signal to produce an image with enhanced lateral and axial resolution. This new imaging paradigm and its application *in vivo* provide insight into the understanding of the structure and function of the eye.

PRINCIPLE

The principle of the confocal microscope was first described by Minsky. He proposed that both the illumination (condenser) and observation (objective) systems be focused on a single point (have common focal points); hence the name 'confocal' microscopy (Fig. 8.5). This dramatically improved the axial (z) and lateral (x, y) resolution of microscopy by eliminating out focus information, bringing lateral resolution to an order of 1–2 μm and axial resolution to 5–10 μm. This allows for possible magnification of up to 600 times, depending on the numerical aperture of the objective lens used. As the field of view of the confocal imaging systems is limited, it is necessary to rapidly scan the focal point across the sample and reconstruct the image to allow a real-time on-screen view.

TYPES OF CONFOCAL MICROSCOPE

Depending on the method of scanning, following types of confocal microscopes are known.

1. *Tandem scanning confocal microscope*. Optics of tandem scanning confocal microscope is depicted in Fig. 8.6. In it, thousands of light beams are moved over the fixed object, generating a high scan rate. These parallel beams

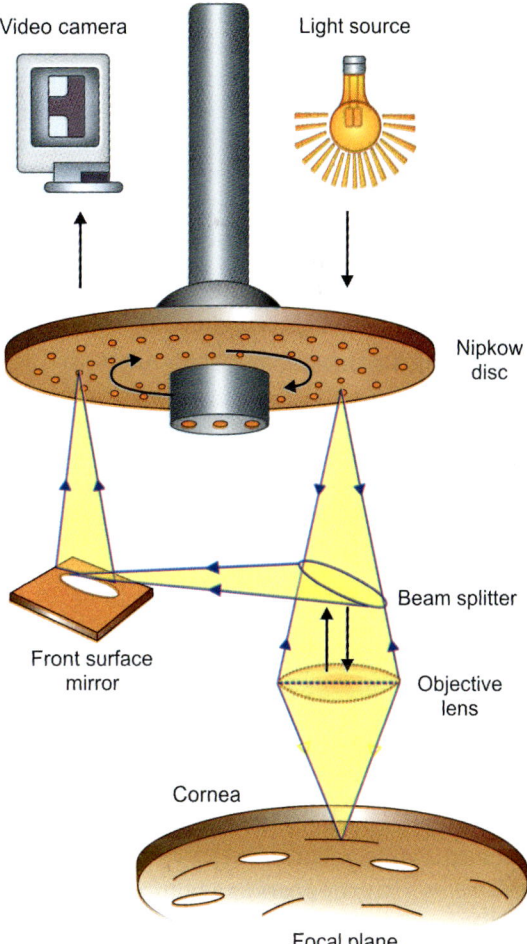

Fig. 8.6: *Optics of tandem scanning confocal microscope.*

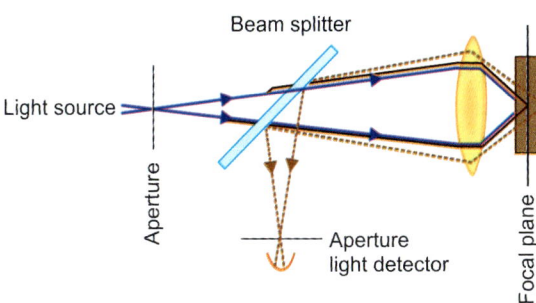

Fig. 8.5: *Diagrammatic representation of the optical principles of the confocal microscope.*

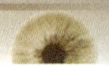

are generated by a Nipkow wheel—a disc with thousands of pinholes spinning at high-speed. These apertures are arranged in tandem, i.e. as diametrically opposed pairs. Light passes through one pinhole and is then reflected back through the corresponding pinhole situated opposite. The high-speed rotation of the disc enables the light beam to scan the full field of view many times a second, thus producing a real-time image.

2. *The scanning slit confocal microscope* uses a light source with one-dimensional spot scanning instead of two-dimensional spot scanning.

3. *The confocal laser scanning microscope* uses a laser beam and this generates a mono-chromatic, bright, intense, sharply focused and coherent light. A novel digital confocal laser scanning microscope, recently developed, is a combination of the Heidelberg retina tomo-graphy (HRT II) and the Rostock cornea module. The laser scanning microscope (LSM) has a computer-controlled hydraulic linear scanning device and a water contact objective and diode laser beam of 670 nm wavelength is used as the light source. The Rostock scanning laser confocal microscope provides reproducible images of high resolution with uniform illumination and precise depth measurements.

CONFOCAL MICROSCOPY OF THE NORMAL HUMAN CORNEA

- *Superficial epithelial cells* are seen with clear visible cell borders, bright cytoplasm and black nuclei. These cells are characteristically polygonal, usually hexagonal in shape (Fig. 8.7A).
- *Intermediate layer of wing cells* comprises cells smaller than the superficial cells, with bright cell borders and dark cytoplasm. These cells are fairly uniform in size and shape (Fig. 8.7B).
- *Basal epithelial cells* are located just above the Bowman's membrane and are seen as a distinct mosaic, with light cell boundaries. The basal epithelial cells are the smallest cells in the epithelium (Fig. 8.7C).
- *Bowman's layer* appears as a homogenous acel-lular layer and nerve fibres of the subepithelial nerve plexus are seen as beaded nerve fibres (Fig. 8.7D).

- *Keratocyte nuclei* are identified as bright reflections in the stroma. The anterior stromal keratocyte nuclei are more abundant and oval compared to the posterior keratocyte nuclei, which were less abundant and more oblong in shape (Fig. 8.7E).
- *Endothelial cells* are visible as bright cell bodies and dark cell boundaries, characteristically hexagonal in shape with fairly uniform appearance in size and shape (Fig. 8.7F).

CONFOCAL MICROSCOPY IN CORNEAL PATHOLOGIES

Confocal microscopy is useful in following corneal pathologies:

1. *Keratoconus.* The characteristic stromal changes seen are multiple 'striae' represented by thin hyporeflective lines oriented vertically, horizontally and obliquely.
2. *Corneal dystrophies,* e.g.
   - *Granular dystrophy.* Characteristic changes are highly reflective, bright, dense struc-tures in the anterior and mid-stroma.
   - *Limbus,* i.e. junction of conjunctiva and cornea is shown in Figure 8.7G.
   - *Palisades of Vogt* is shown in Figure 8.7H.
   - *Posterior polymorphous dystrophy* is characterized by multiple round vesicles at the level of Descemet's membrane and endothelium.
   - *Fuch's endothelial dystrophy.* The cornea guttata appear dark with a bright central reflex. In advanced stage, endothelial cells are seen distorted.
3. *Measurement of flap thickness in LASIK* is obtained by measuring the distance between the high reflective spike from the front surface of the cornea and the low reflective interface.
4. *Intracorneal deposits* that can be seen directly with confocal microscopy include:
   - *Exogenous deposits,* e.g. acanthamoeba cyst and ova, drug deposits (amiodarone, chloroquine), deposits after contact lens use, refractive surgery and vitreoretinal surgery using silicone oil.
   - *Endogenous deposits* as seen in Wilson's disease, hyperlipidaemia, Fabry's disease, and haemosiderosis.

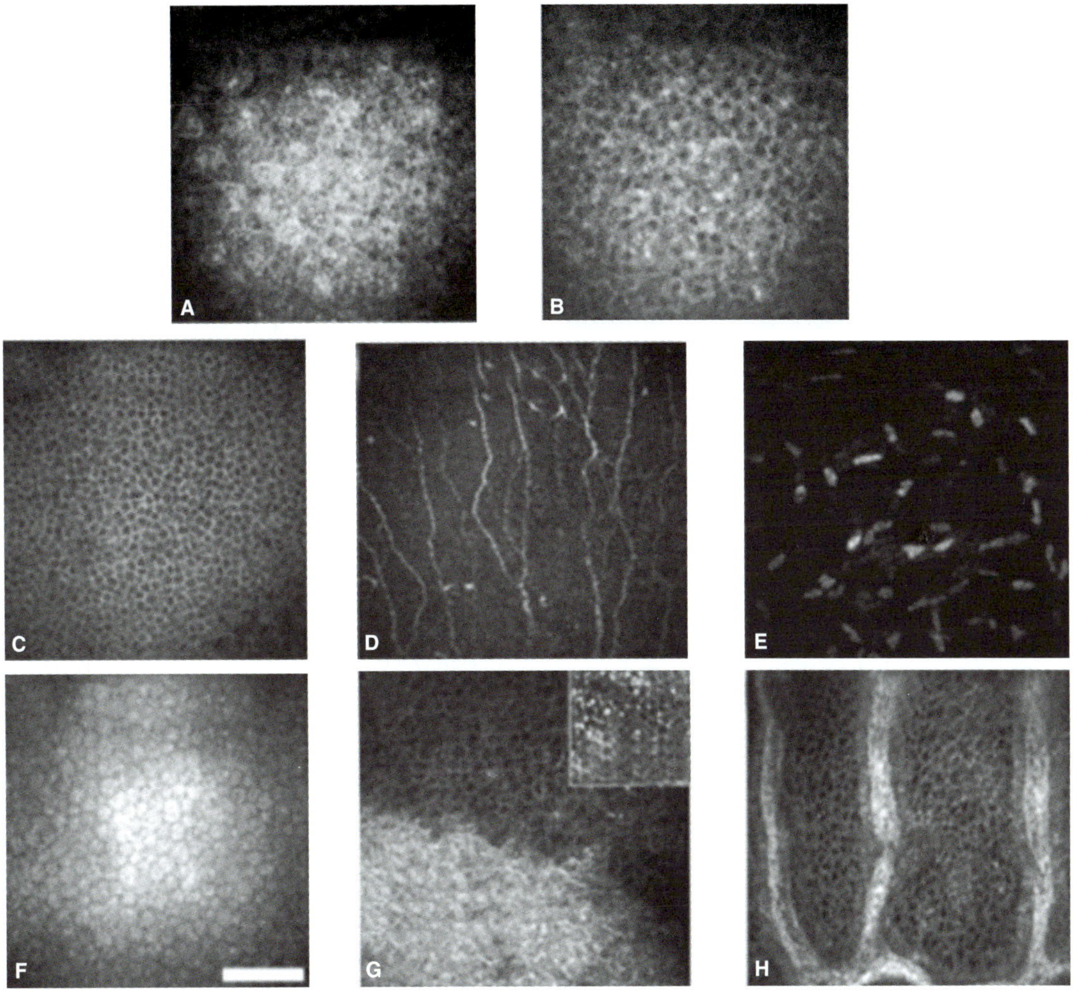

Fig. 8.7: *Confocal microscopy of normal human cornea: (A) Superficial epithelial cells are seen with prominent nuclei; (B) Wing cells; (C) Basal epithelial cells are seen as small cells with high cell density and well-demarcated cell borders; (D) Bowman's layer; (E) Mid-stroma; (F) Endothelium; (G) Limbal epithelium, i.e. junction of conjunctiva and cornea; (H) Palisades of Vogt.*

OTHER CORNEAL ENDOTHELIAL SCANS

CONFOSCAN

Confoscan 4 (Nidek, Inc) is a fully automatic, fast (takes less than 12 sec) non-contact endothelial microscope with 20X probe. It has a 5 microns accuracy in confocal pachymetry with Z-ring optics which improves the image stability. It produces high quality imaging through opacities.

HEIDELBERG RETINAL TOMOGRAPH 3 (HRT 3)

Heidelberg Retinal Tomograph 3 (HRT 3) in conjunction with Rostock Cornea Module (RCM) (Heidelberg Engineering, Germany) is a microscope which has a 1 micron resolution. It scans the entire cornea from epithelium to endothelium layer by laser. It uses 670 nm red wavelength diode laser. It offers 400 times magnification with an axial high resolution. This helps in early accurate and rapid diagnosis, expediating initiation of therapy, follow-ups and hence visual outcomes specially in *Acanthamoeba Keratitis*, in Fungal keratitis like *Aspergillus* and *Fusarium*. Confocal microscopy helps in examining flap related complications and images of the particles at the interface. It can also aid in assessment of the

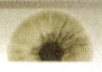

wound healing following refractive surgery. It also helps in the study of corneal nerve alterations following corneal surgery and in systemic diseases like diabetic neuropathy.

Limitation. It is difficult to visualize bacteria and viruses owing to their size less than 0.5 micron length.

BIBLIOGRAPHY

1. Amos WB, White JG. How the Confocal Laser Scanning Microscope entered Biological Research. Biology of the Cell 2003;95(6):335–42.
2. Binder PS, Akers P, Zavala EY. Endothelial cell density determined by specular microscopy and scanning electron microscopy. Ophthalmology. 1979;86:1831–47.
3. Davidovits P, Egger MD. Scanning laser microscope for biological investigations. Applied Optics. 1971;10(7):1615–9.
4. Egger MD, Petran M. New reflected-light microscope for viewing unstained brain and ganglion cells. Science 1967 July;157(786):305–7.
5. Laing RA, Oak SS, Leibowitz HM. Specialized Microscopy of the Cornea: Specular Microscopy. In: Leibowitz HM, Waring GO (Eds). Corneal

Disorders: Clinical Diagnosis and Management, 2nd ed. Philadelphia: WB Saunders Company, 1998:83–122.
6. Laing RA, Sandstrom MM, Leibowitz HM. Clinical specular microscopy. I. Optical principles. Archives of Ophthalmology. 1979; 97:1714–9.
7. McCarey BE, Edelhauser HF, Lynn MJ. Review of corneal endothelial specular microscopy for FDA clinical trials of refractive procedures, surgical devices, and new intraocular drugs and solutions. Cornea 2008 Jan;27(1):1–16.
8. Niederer RL, Perumal D, Sherwin T, McGhee CN. Age-related differences in the normal human cornea: a laser scanning in vivo confocal microscopy study. Br J Ophthalmol Sep 2007; 91(9):1165–9.
9. Patel DV, McGhee CN. Contemporary in vivo confocal microscopy of the living human cornea using white light and laser scanning techniques: a major review. Clin. Experiment. Ophthalmol 2007;35(1):71–88.
10. Sibug ME, Datiles MB, Kashima K, et al. Specular microscopy studies on the corneal endothelium after cessation of contact lens wear. Cornea 1991 Sep.;10(5):395–401.

Corneal Pachymetry, Hysteresis and Keratometry

Chapter Outline

CORNEAL PACHYMETRY

Introduction
- Methods of pachymetry

Ultrasound-Based Pachymeters
- Conventional ultrasound-based pachymeter
- Pachymetry with ultrasound biomicroscopy

Optical Pachymetry
- Slit-lamp pachymetry
- Specular microscopy pachymetry
- Pachymetry with anterior segment OCT
- Pachymetry with partial coherence interferometry

Optical Pachymetry with Corneal Topographers
- Pachymetry with orbscan II
- Pachymetry with Scheimpflug technology-based imaging

Optical Pachymetry with Ocular Response Analyser

Clinical Applications of Corneal Pachymetry
- In corneal disorders
- In glaucoma
- In refractive surgery

Factors Modifying Pachymetry

CORNEAL HYSTERESIS
- Definition and facts about corneal hysteresis
- Corneal hysteresis: Relevance in glaucoma
- Measurement of corneal hysteresis: Ocular response analyser

KERATOMETRY

Principle of Keratometry

Helmholtz Keratometry
- Optics

Bausch and Lomb Keratometer
- Principle
- Optical system and other parts
- Procedure of keratometry
- Interpretation of findings

Javal–Schiötz Keratometer
- Principle
- Optical system and other parts
- Procedure of keratometry

Surgical/Operating Keratometer
- Factors limiting accuracy

Automated Keratometer
- Advantages
- Precision
- Availability

Relationship between Radius of Curvature and Dioptric Power of Cornea
- Range of keratometer

Clinical Uses, Limitations and Sources of Error
- Clinical uses of keratometer
- Limitations of keratometry
- Sources of error in keratometry

CORNEAL PACHYMETRY

INTRODUCTION

The word 'pachos' means 'thick' in Greek. Corneal thickness measurement is necessary to evaluate the health of cornea and the endothelial pump function. It has been studied extensively in literature and finds extreme importance in today's age of keratorefractive procedures and lamellar corneal transplantation procedures. We have moved from the days of exclusive full thickness transplants to transplanting individual layers of the cornea (DSAEK, DALK, DSEK, DMEK) which rely heavily on measurement of preoperative, intraoperative and postoperative corneal thickness for preoperative decision-making and evaluating postoperative outcomes.

Normal cornea is prolate shaped with the thickness increasing form the center to the periphery. The thickness is 0.7 to 0.9 mm at the limbus and 0.49 to 0.56 mm at the center, the temporal cornea being the thinnest. Studies have shown that the corneal thickness normally increases with the age above 40.

METHODS OF PACHYMETRY

Various instruments have been devised for the measurement of corneal thickness and are referred to as 'pachymeters'. Methods of pachymetry can be divided based on the underlying technique used and based on contact versus noncontact methods.

Based on the technique, pachymetry can be divided as below:
 I. *Ultrasonic pachymetry*
  • Conventional ultrasonic pachymetry
  • Ultrasound biomicroscopy (UBM).
 II. *Optical pachymetry*
  • Slit-lamp pachymetry
  • Specular microscopy
  • Optical coherence tomography (OCT)
  • Optical low coherence interferometry
  • Confocal microscopy
  • Laser Doppler interferometry.
 III. *Optical pachymetry with corneal topographers*
  • Orbscan
  • Pentacam
  • Pachycam.

 IV. *Pachymetry with ocular response analyzer (ORA)*

Based on contact versus noncontact methods, the pachymeter can be grouped as below:
 I. *Contact methods* include:
  • Ultrasonic pachymetry
  • Optical methods such as confocal microscopy.
 II. *Noncontact method* include:
  • Optical biometry with a single Scheimpflug camera (Sirius or Pentacam)
  • Dual Scheimpflug camera (Galilei)
  • Optical coherence tomography (OCT, such as Visante)
  • Online optical coherence pachymetry (Orbscan).

Some of the modern day pachymeters are described briefly.

I. ULTRASOUND-BASED PACHYMETERS

CONVENTIONAL ULTRASOUND-BASED PACHYMETER

Ultrasound (US) pachymetry (Fig. 9.1) introduced by Henderson and Kremer in 1980, is considered to be the gold standard method for pachymetry because of a high degree of reproducibility.

Principle: The high frequency sound waves reflect from the anterior and posterior surfaces and the machine measures the time difference in transit between echoes from the transducer of the probe and the reflected signal received from the surfaces of the cornea.[1]

$$\text{Corneal thickness} = \frac{\text{Transit time} \times \text{Propagation velocity}}{2}$$

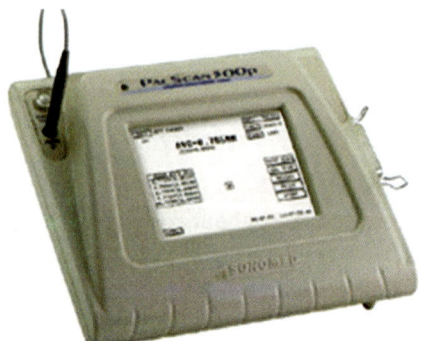

Fig. 9.1: *Ultrasonic pachymeter.*

Components

1. *Probe*. The probe handle consists of a piezo-electric crystal which vibrates at 10–20 MHz. The probe tip is narrow 2 mm in diameter to ensure a local contact on central cornea.

2. *Transducer*. The transducer sends ultrasound waves through the probe and receives echoes back form the cornea.

The exact posterior reflection point of sound may be located between Descemet's membrane and the anterior chamber. The ultrasound probe may displace the tear film 7 to 40 microns and therefore underestimate corneal epithelial thickness.

Advantages and disadvantages of ultrasound pachymetry are summarized below.

Advantages
• Fast
• Simple to use
• Minimum observer variation
• Good reproducibility
• Portable
• Intraoperative usage.

Disadvantages
• Contact method
• Need for topical anaesthesia
• Accuracy dependent on location of corneal touch
• Applanation may disturb readings
• Low resolution
• Not accurate in corneal edema
• Variability of sound velocity in wet and dry tissues.

PACHYMETRY WITH ULTRASOUND BIOMICROSCOPY (UBM)

Ultrasound biomicroscopy (UBM) is a newer technology using high frequency ultrasound to examine the anterior segment of the eye at a higher resolution. Probes may have frequencies of 35 or 50 MHz.

Advantages and disadvantages

Advantages and disadvantages of UBM Pachymetry are summarized below:

Advantages include:
• High resolution

• Useful in opaque cornea
• Separate layers of cornea discerned.

Disadvantages include:
• Coupling fluid immersion is discomforting
• Contact method
• No intraoperative usage
• No standardisation.

■ II. OPTICAL PACHYMETRY

SLIT-LAMP PACHYMETRY

Optical pachymetry using the **slit-lamp's pachymeter** attachment (Haag-Streit AG, Koenitz, Switzerland) can be done using a slit-beam projected perpendicular to the cornea.

Instrument description

Optical pachymeter is used with the slit-lamp. It hangs over the objectives of the microscope from a part attached to the microscope body. The left objective is occluded by the pachymeter while the right one has two glass plates with parallel sides placed in front of it. These plates rest one on top of the other, with the junction between them situated so as to horizontally bisect the objective. The upper plate can be rotated while the lower plate is fixed and positioned so that its faces are normal to the axis of microscope.

Optical principle

The optical pachymeter utilizes the principle of optical image doubling and is designed to measure the distance between the Purkinje-Sanson images formed by the anterior and posterior corneal surfaces, a value that represents the corneal thickness.

Optics

Working optics of the optical doubling pachymeter depicted in Fig. 9.2 is described below:
• The slit-beam (a in Fig. 9.2) illuminates the patient's cornea.
• The image is viewed through a biomicroscope, half through a glass plate orthogonal to the path of light (b in Fig. 9.2) and half through another glass plate rotated through an angle (c in Fig. 9.2).

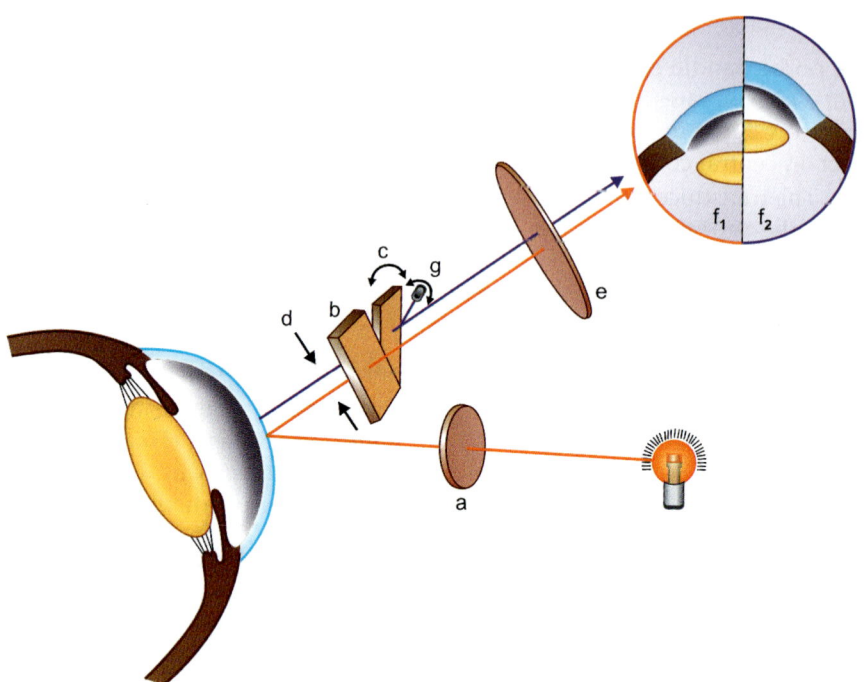

Fig. 9.2: *Optics of the optical pachymeter (for explanation see text).*

- The beam path through glass plate is displaced laterally for a distance (d in Fig. 9.2) that varies depending upon the angle of rotation.
- Through the eyepiece (e in Fig. 9.2), the observer views a split image. The half of the image (f_1 in Fig. 9.2) comes from the fixed plate and the other half (f_2 in Fig. 9.2) from the rotatable plate.

Measurement of corneal thickness

- To measure the corneal thickness (as shown in Fig. 9.3), the observer aligns the endothelial surface of one image with epithelial surface of the other image by carefully adjusting the rotatable plate (d in Fig. 9.2).
- Value of corneal thickness is read off the calibrated scale (g in Fig. 9.2).
- As the apparent thickness of the cornea varies with the angle between the slit-lamp and the microscope, it is essential to set this at some predetermined value before a measurement is made. With the Haag–Streit slit-lamp, this angle should be 40° (Fig. 9.2).
- Thickness can be read from a scale on the instrument which is graded from 0 to 1.2 mm.

- The two methods of measurement are the "just touch" method and the "overlap method" in which the outer surface of the epithelium of the top corneal section is aligned with the inner surface of the endothelium of the bottom section of the cornea.

Disadvantages of slit-lamp optical pachymeter

- Contact procedure
- Lack of repeatability
- Observer bias
- Width of slit-beam variable
- Requires a slit-lamp.

SPECULAR MICROSCOPY PACHYMETRY

Principle

Pachymetry using specular microscopy is based on the focusing of light rays on the front and back surfaces of the cornea and measures the distance between the two surfaces accordingly. Two types of specular microscopes are: noncontact and contact. Noncontact specular microscopy have been to found to give more consistent readings from operator to operator but gives a lower reading than contact methods

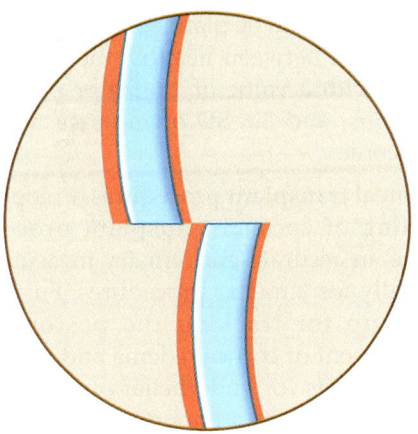

Fig. 9.3: *Showing end point of pachymetry.*

namely the ultrasound pachymetry or contact specular microscopes.

Advantages and disadvantages

Advantages include:
- Operator independent
- Noninvasive
- Measures the endothelial cell counts also.

Disadvantages include:
- Cannot differentiate central/peripheral corneal readings
- Contact method
- Less reproducible
- Can be only used in clear corneas.

PACHYMETRY WITH ANTERIOR SEGMENT OPTICAL COHERENCE TOMOGRAPHY

The OCT of the anterior segment gives high resolution images of the cornea along with colour coded maps of the corneal thickness.

Advantages of ASOCT pachymeters

- Noncontact
- Noninvasive
- Rapid acquisition
- Measures through corneal opacity
- Can measure layers of cornea separately.

PACHYMETRY WITH PARTIAL COHERENCE INTERFEROMETRY

IOL master 700 (Carl Zeiss Meditec, USA) and Lenstar (Haag-Streit) have revolutionized biometry, i.e. determination of IOL power before cataract surgery. They also measure the corneal thickness by a noncontact method from the anterior and posterior corneal surfaces. This is a rapid method, not requiring local anaesthesia as compared to ultrasonic method.

III. OPTICAL PACHYMETRY WITH CORNEAL TOPOGRAPHERS

PACHYMETRY WITH ORBSCAN II

Principle

Orbscan II (Bausch and Lomb, Rochester, New York, USA) is based on scanning optical slit technology which projects light at a 45° angle and measures the anterior corneal surface elevation/topography and pachymetry. Posterior elevation map is extrapolated from the anterior elevation map and pachymetry data by comparing them with a best fit sphere.

The whole corneal pachymetry can be mapped and the thinnest points defined in a pictorial representation.

Studies have suggested that the scanning slit observes the pachymetry from the air-tear interface of the hydrated corneal epithelium, thereby overestimating the thickness as compared to the US pachymetry with a mean difference of 28 to 54 mcm. Hence, an Acoustic factor (AF) of 0.92 has been defined to obtain values closer to the US readings. However, Orbscan II with AF of 0.92 underestimates the thickness of thin corneas of normal patients and in keratoconic eyes, post-PRK and post-LASIK eyes. AF of 0.92 has been reported to also overestimate thickness in the thickest of corneas.

Disadvantages of Orbscan II Pachymetry

- Scattering from corneal haze and interfaces may interfere with the scanning slit
- Measurements are adjusted for prolate shape of cornea only
- Motion artifacts.

PACHYMETRY WITH SCHEIMPFLUG TECHNOLOGY-BASED IMAGING

Principle

Pentacam (Oculus Optikgerate GmbH, Wetzlar, Germany) consists of an automatically rotating

Scheimpflug camera and a slit illumination system which images the entire anterior segment including the cornea, lens and the anterior chamber. 12–50 captures are made by the rotating slit with 500 true elevation points on each slit thereby calculating 2500 height values, which are then used to map a three-dimensional model of the entire anterior eye segment.

Pentacam gives the true anterior and posterior elevation maps and the entire corneal pachymetry is obtained by their difference, which is displayed in a colour map. Thinnest point is also determined.

Advantages of Pentacam pachymetry

- Noncontact
- Noninvasive
- Eye movement correction available
- High quality of images.

Disadvantages Pentacam has been of late shown to give higher readings than the US pachymeter and noncontact specular microscope. However, Pentacam has mostly been shown to be corresponding to the US values in thin corneas.

IV. PACHYMETRY WITH OCULAR RESPONSE ANALYSER

Ocular response analyser (Reichert Ophthalmic Ins., NY, USA) is a new instrument, which measures the biomechanical properties of the cornea namely corneal hysteresis (CH) along with the central thickness using an in-built 20 MHz US pachymeter.

CLINICAL APPLICATIONS OF CORNEAL PACHYMETRY

I. IN CORNEAL DISORDERS

1. Keratoconus diagnosis and management. Keratoconus (KC) is a bilateral noninflammatory progressive disease of the cornea which causes thinning and ectasia of the cornea with irregular astigmatism and cornel scarring. KC patients have both central and peripheral corneal thinning. Pentacam and other latest tomographic instruments can exactly point out the point of thinnest pachymetry based on which treatment modalities, e.g. CXL, Intrastromal ring

segments, etc. can be planned. D-vlue is used to differentiate between healthy and keratoconic corneas with a value of 1.6 SD or more being suspicious, and 2.6 SD or more as definitely keratoconic.

2. Corneal transplant procedures. Preoperative planning of corneal transplant procedures require an accurate pachymetry measurement, especially for lamellar procedures. Further, on follow-up for tracking the postoperative improvement of corneal edema and the assessment of grafts for endothelial pump function, pachymetry plays an important role.

3. Monitoring endothelial cell function. Endothelial cell loss is related to loss of maintenance of the corneal transparency and normal thickness of the cornea causing stromal edema. Cornea may be monitored for decompensation using pachymetry in postoperative cases of cataract surgery, penetrating keratoplasty, vitreoretinal surgery, etc.

II. IN GLAUCOMA

1. Glaucoma risk prediction. Ocular Hypertension Treatment Study (OHTS) group has identified thin corneas to be an independent risk factor for the development of open angle glaucoma in people with OHT and this occurrence is also affected by other parameters like age, sex and race. Increased CCT in OHT may lead to recording of a falsely high IOP whereas patients of low/normal tension glaucoma may have thin CCT leading ot falsely low IOP measurement. PITX2 mutation positive Axenfield-Reiger syndrome patients, pseudoexfoliation syndrome (PXF) cases and primary open angle glaucoma (POAG) cases may have lower pachymetry readings.

2. IOP measurement. Goldmann applanation tonometry (GAT) has been the gold standard for IOP measurement for decades now. However, Goldmann had assumed that the resistance of the cornea to indentation was compensated for the surface tension of the tear film for a corneal thickness of 520 mcm. The principle behind this is the 'Imbert-Fick's law' which assumes the cornea to be a flexible uniform sphere which is infinitely thin. Neither is the cornea regular, nor infinitely thin. Hence, measurement of IOP with indentation techniques like Goldmann Applanation Tonometry, Pneumotonometry and Non-contact tonometry (NCT) are affected by the thickness of the cornea, viz. underestimating IOP in thinner corneas and overestimating in rigid ones. A correction factor of 0.7 mcm for every 10 mm Hg increase in IOP is applied. Pneumotonometer and NCT are especially susceptible to errors more than GAT, as these procedures require indentation of a larger surface area of the cornea. Dynamic contour tonometry (DCT) is a newer modality which is very less affected by the corneal thickness changes. It measures IOP using a strain gauge which creates a tight-fitting contact on the corneal surface and hence, is not affected by the corneal biomechanical properties.

III. IN REFRACTIVE SURGERY

1. **Refractive surgery procedures.** Preoperative screening and treatment planning for hyperopia and myopia require accurate pachymetry for procedures like LASIK, PRK and SMILE. Inadequate corneal thickness may require the patient to undergo an intraocular lens implantation instead of a lamellar corneal procedure.

2. **Postrefractive ectasias.** Thinning and cornel curvatural abnormalities postrefractive surgery may be detected using the latest tomographic instruments for diagnosing postrefractive ectasias and for further management using CXL, intrastromal ring segments, PRK, etc.

FACTORS MODIFYING PACHYMETRY

1. *Age* For the majority of individuals, there is no substantial change in CCT beyond the infant years. However, some reports have found CCT to increase after 40 years of age.

2. *Sex* Inconclusive reports have been published with males having higher CCT. But generally, sex has not been found to be a modifying factor for pachymetry. Higher contact lens usage among women may falsely lead to increased CCT readings.

3. *Race* African-American persons have thinner corneas as compared to the white population. Similar trend has been observed in Asian population.

4. *Diurnal variation* Pachymetry readings have been shown to be thinnest after awakening while thickens during the overnight period. This diurnal cycle in corneal thickness could be affected in women by factors like hormonal changes along the menstrual cycle, pregnancy, or oral contraceptive pills.

5. *Contact lens usage* PMMA, hydrogel and rigid gas permeable (RGP) contact lenses affect the corneal thickness differently. The period of lens wear also becomes an important determinant. A short termedema may get resolved on prompt discontinuation of the lenses. Long-term contact lenses wearers may show thinning of the cornea. This may be related to the thinning or instability of the tear film leading to a dry eye, thereby causing increased evaporation and dessication of cornea. In refractive surgery planning, it has been advised to measure CCT after a minimum period of two weeks following contact lens wear discontinuation.

6. *Post-surgery* Almost every anterior segment surgery especially cataract surgery, penetrating keratoplasty, etc. may cause postoperative corneal edema for a week to one month, which returns to normal by 2–3 months. With modern phacoemulsification machines with improved phacodynamics and fluidics, the incidence of corneal edema and the duration of persistence of this edema has reduced.

7. *Chronic diseases* Diabetes has been associated with an increased corneal thickness. Contact lens usage or chronic diseases affecting CCT is mostly within the usual range of variance and hence they do not necessitate the routine use of CCT measurement for monitoring. However, postsurgical causes may require the same.

CORNEAL HYSTERESIS

Definition and Facts about corneal hysteresis

- **Corneal hysteresis** is a recently characterized viscoelastic property of the cornea. Cornea contains characteristics of both elastic and viscous materials. Corneal hysteresis reflects the ability of corneal tissue to absorb and dissipate energy during a bidirectional applanation process (where energy is lost as

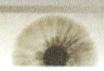

heat during the rapid loading/unloading of the cornea). In other words corneal hysteresis is a measure of the stiffness or rigidity of the cornea. To better understand corneal hysteresis, consider the memory foam material used to make pillows and mattresses. Applying pressure deforms the material, but upon releasing the pressure, the material returns to its original shape slowly (a visco-elastic response) rather than bouncing back instantly like a stretched rubber band upon release (which is a purely elastic response).

- **Corneal hysteresis is a biomechanical corneal behaviour** and not a static physical property like corneal thickness. Corneal hysteresis is lower in eyes with higher IOP and normalizes after IOP reduction. Then hysteresis is not actually an intrinsic or constant property, but a measurement characterizing how a material or system responds to the loading and unloading of an applied force.

- **Corneal hysteresis measurement is repeatable in individual eyes** and strongly correlated in right and left eyes of the same patient. Corneal hysteresis, however, differs from person to person. It is not strongly correlated with other common metrics such as corneal radius, astigmatism, spherical equivalence (SE), axial length, and IOP measured by GAT. Corneal hysteresis and central corneal thickness (CCT) are moderately correlated in normal corneas and weakly to moderately correlated in corneas with disorder. Corneal hysteresis is lower than normal in patients with corneal disorders, such as Fuchs' keratoconus, and glaucoma.

- **African-Americans have lower corneal hysteresis than Hispanics** and Whites, but it is unclear whether this is explained by the association between corneal hysteresis and CCT or intergroup differences in corneal hysteresis that are independent of CCT.

- Various investigators have found associations between corneal hysteresis and optic nerve head (ONH) morphology.

Corneal hysteresis: Relevance in glaucoma

- Several studies have compared the bio-chemical characteristics of eyes with and without glaucoma. It has been repeatedly shown that patients with glaucoma have significantly lower corneal hysteresis and CCT than individuals with normal eyes.

- Corneal hysteresis has been shown to be lower in various types of glaucomatous eyes in comparison to normal eyes; these include POAG, PACG, NTG, and pseudoexfoliative glaucoma.

- Low corneal hysteresis is associated with glaucomatous visual field and optic nerve progression.

- Low-baseline corneal hysteresis is associated with a greater magnitude of IOP reduction following various glaucoma therapies including topical prostaglandin therapy and SLT.

- Corneal hysteresis (but not CCT or IOP) was associated with overall structural glaucomatous progression seen on a retrospective study of serial fundus photographs analyzed using flicker chronoscopy. This finding indicated that corneal hysteresis is directly associated with progressive glaucomatous optic neuropathy.

- Intraocular pressure reduction leads to an increase in corneal hysteresis.

- Biomechanical properties provide valuable information about the risk of glaucoma development and progression and may predict the effectiveness of various glaucoma therapies for individual patients. Although CCT continues to be a valuable tool, clinicians should also consider incorporating hysteresis measurements into practice. In several studies comparing the two variables, corneal hysteresis was more strongly related to progression than CCT. Corneal hysteresis has been the subject of considerable research recently, and with further investigation, its clinical implications for the diagnosis and management of glaucoma will become clearer.

Measurement of corneal hysteresis: Ocular response analyser

The ocular response analyser (ORA) measures the corneal hysteresis. The ORA applies an air puff on the anterior surface of the cornea and cause the cornea to deform. It measures the intensity of the reflected infrared light from the deforming corneal surface and reports several indices for diagnosis. It measures the biomechanical properties of the cornea which is useful in comparing LASIK and surface ablation as well as to evaluate the effect of creating a flap on corneal strength. It utilizes a dynamic, bidirectional applanation process and accurately measures the IOP. It takes into account the corneal hydration, connective tissue composition and bioelasticity, and contribute to the response of the corneoscleral shell, to the force applied during the measurement of IOP. It has a built in 20 MHz ultrasound pachymeter that measures CCT.

Advantages
- It is a noncontact procedure
- Superficial anaesthesia is not required
- The technique is speedy and offers high accuracy and repeatability
- It can diagnose corneal ectasia earlier than conventional diagnostic aids.

Disadvantages
- The high cost of equipment
- The doubts in standardization and need for recurrent calibration.

KERATOMETRY

PRINCIPLE OF KERATOMETRY

Keratometry is measurement of curvature of the anterior surface of cornea across a fixed chord length, usually 2–3 mm, which lies within the optical spherical zone of the cornea.

Keratometry is based on the fact that the anterior surface of the cornea acts as a convex mirror and the size of the image formed varies with its curvature. The greater the curvature of cornea, lesser is the image size. Therefore, from the size of the image formed by the anterior surface of cornea (1st Purkinje image), the radius of curvature of cornea can be calculated as below.

In Fig. 9.4, consider an object AB that forms an image A'B' after reflection at the anterior surface of cornea. Ray AC passing towards centre of curvature C of the cornea is reflected back on itself. Ray AQ is reflected towards QS and seems to meet the ray AC at A', forming the

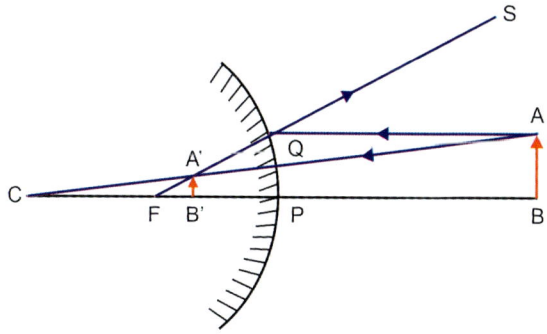

Fig. 9.4: *Principle of keratometry.*

image A'B'. Now, if the object AB is at infinity then A'B' will be very small and situated at the focus F. Therefore, B'P will be focal distance or ½ of radius of curvature of the mirror.

Thus, if $\quad AB = 0, A'B' = 1, BP = u$

and then $\quad CP = r, \dfrac{r}{2} = u\,3\dfrac{1}{0}$

or $\qquad r = \dfrac{2ul}{0}$

The distance BP denoted by u is kept constant for any instrument by using a short focus telescope in order to view the reflected image. From this it is clear that for known object size, measurements of image size will allow us to determine r, the radius of curvature.

The accurate measurement of such an image, however, raises a problem since it is impossible to immobilize the living eye completely while the image is under observation. This has been overcome by devices using the *principle of visible doubling*. In one type of instrument, the image is doubled by refraction through two rotating glass plates which are then adjusted so that the lower edge of one image coincides with the upper edge of the other. If the eye moves during the process, both the images move together, and so difficulties in adjustment are avoided. From the amount of rotation of the glass plate necessary just to double the image, its size can be calculated.

In other types of keratometers, the amount of doubling is fixed but size of external object can be varied. Helmholtz (1854) utilized this principle to devise the first keratometer. He gave the

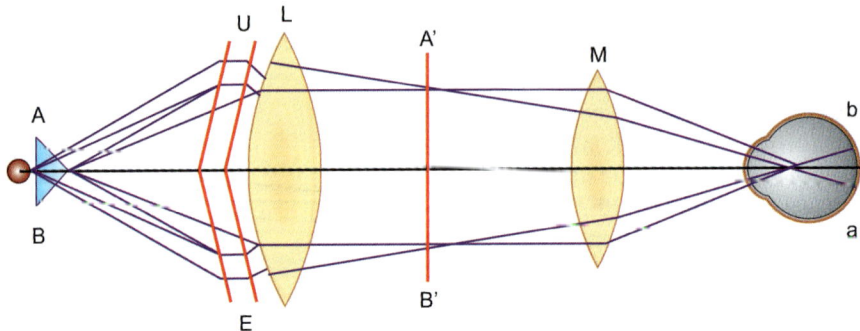

Fig. 9.5: *Optics of Helmholtz keratometer.*

name ophthalmometer to it but later on kerato-meter was found to be more appropriate term.

HELMHOLTZ KERATOMETER

Though presently not in use, the Helmholtz keratometer is described here as a tribute to the inventor. Helmholtz keratometer consists of two plates. Each plate displaces the image through half its length and the total displacement gives the size of image. The doubling of image dis-penses with the necessity of immobilizing the living eye. If the eye moves during the process, both the images move together and, therefore, difficulties in adjustment are avoided. The glass plates are of known thickness and index of refraction, placed side by side, so that each covers half of the object of a short-distance tele-scope. The axis of telescope coincides with the plane of separation of glass plates. These plates can be inclined one to the other at known angles, and the angle of incidence of light falling on them from a point in front can be varied and measured.

Optics of Helmholtz keratometer

As shown in Fig. 9.5, rays from point O meet the plates at U and E and undergo lateral dis-placement after refraction. As viewed through L, the two objects appear at A and B. The eyepiece M is so arranged that its principal focus coincides with the images A' and B' and receives parallel rays which come to the focus without accommodation on the retina at a and b. As shown in Fig. 9.6, if the position of plates is such that the two images A and B just touch at O then

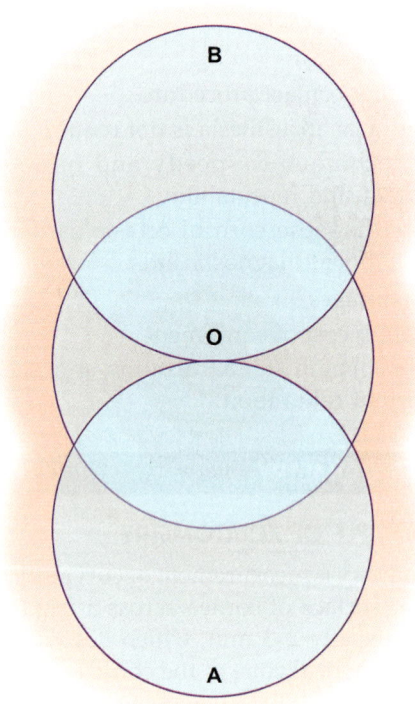

Fig. 9.6: *Measurement of the size of image in Helmholtz keratometer (observer's view).*

each plate has displaced the image through half its length and the total displacement gives the size of the image. The original instrument has undergone several modifications and nowadays several keratometers are in use.

An ideal keratometer must be able to measure the radii in various meridia about the axis of the cornea. Thus instruments are designed that can be rotated with respect to a particular axis. The objects are called mires. In order to avoid the error due to constant motion of eyes, a doubling device has been introduced.

BAUSCH AND LOMB KERATOMETER

Principle

The working of Reichert (Bausch and Lomb) keratometer (Fig. 9.7) is based on the principle of *constant object size and variable image size.*

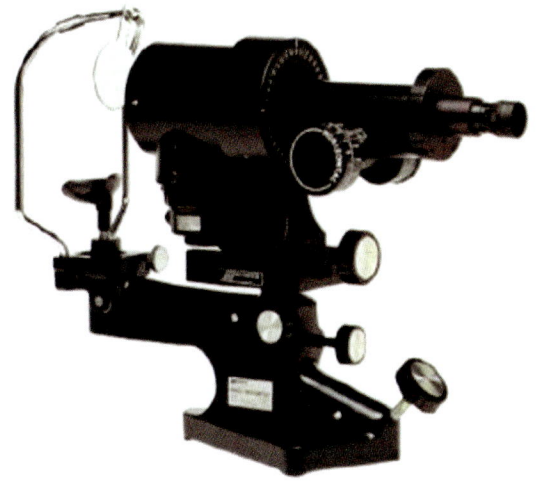

Fig. 9.7: *Bausch and Lomb keratometer.*

Optical system and other parts

The functioning of the optical system (Fig. 9.8) and the other parts of this keratometer are as below:

1. **The object** is a circular mire with two plus and two minus signs (Fig. 9.9). As shown in Fig. 9.8, a lamp illuminates the mire by means of a diagonally placed mirror. Light from the mire strikes the patient's cornea and produces a diminished image behind it. This image becomes the object for the remainder of optical system.

2. **The objective lens** focuses the light from the image of the mire (new object) along the central axis.

3. **Diaphragm and doubling prisms**. A four-aperture diaphragm is situated near the objective lens. Beyond the diaphragm are two doubling prisms, one with its base up and other with its base out. The prisms can be moved independently, parallel to the central axis of the instrument. Light passing through the left aperture of diaphragm is made to deviate above the central optical axis by a base-up prism. Light passing through the right aperture is deviated by the base-out prism, placing the second image to the right of the central axis. Light passing through upper and lower apertures does not

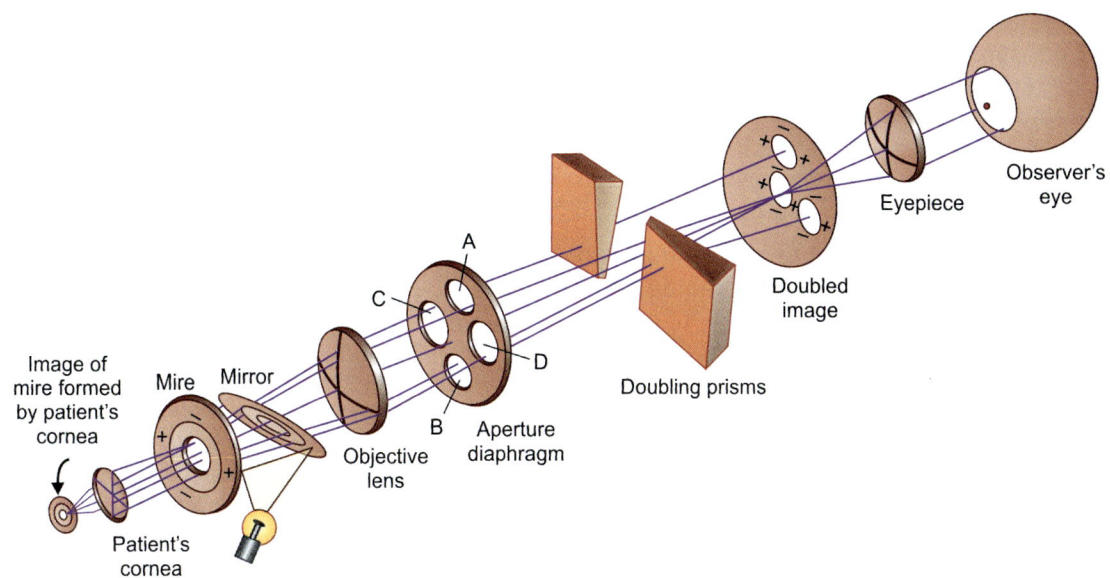

Fig. 9.8: *Optical system of Bausch and Lomb keratometer.*

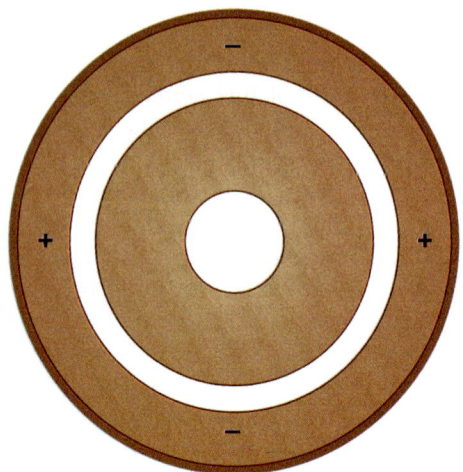

Fig. 9.9: *Configuration of the mires used in Bausch and Lomb keratometer.*

pass through either prism and an image is produced in the axis. The total area of upper and lower apertures is equal to the area of each of the other two apertures. Thus brightness of the images is equal. The upper and lower apertures also act as Scheiner's disc, doubling the central image, whenever the instrument is not focused precisely on the central mire image. So continuous monitoring of correct focus can be done. Thus, the image-doubling mechanism is unique in Bausch and Lomb keratometer, in that double images are produced side by side as well as at 90° from each other. This allows the measurement of the power of cornea in two meridia, without rotating the instrument. Therefore, it is also known as *'one-position keratometer'*. The doubling device also moves parallel to the control axis of the instrument so that the amount of separation can be raised.

4. **The eyepiece lens** enables the examiner to observe the magnified view of the doubled image.

Procedure of keratometry

1. **Instrument adjustment.** The instrument is calibrated before use. A white paper is held in front of the objective piece and a black line is focused sharply on it. The keratometer is then calibrated with steel balls. A steel ball of known radius of curvature is placed before the kerato- meter and its value is set on the scale or dial.

The mires are focused by clockwise and anti- clockwise movement of the eyepiece through trial and error. When mires are in focus, the calibration is complete.

2. **Patient adjustment.** The patient is seated in front of the instrument with chin on the chin rest and head against the head rest. The eye that is not being examined is covered with the occluder. Then, the chin is raised or lowered till the patient's pupil and the projective knob are at the same level.

3. **Focusing of mire.** After adjusting the instru- ment and the patient, the mire is focused in the centre of cornea. Figure 9.9 shows the patient's view of mire and Fig. 9.10A shows the view first seen by the examiner. Note that the central image is doubled, indicating that the instrument is not correctly focused on the corneal image of the mire.

4. **Measurement of corneal curvature.**

- *The instrument is correctly focused* on the corneal image so that central image is no longer doubled (Fig. 9.10B).

- *To measure the curvature in horizontal meridian,* the plus signs of the central and left images are superimposed using the horizontal measuring control and the reading is noted (Fig. 9.10C).

- *Then to measure the curvature in the vertical meridian,* the minus signs of the central and upper images are coincided with the help of vertical measuring control and the readings are noted (Fig. 9.10D).

- *Regular astigmatism.* For each eye the difference between horizontal and vertical dioptre readings gives the approximate amount of corneal astigmatism. Normally horizontal and vertical dioptre reading are 90° apart.

- *In the presence of oblique astigmatism,* the two plus signs will not be aligned (Fig. 9.10E). The entire instrument is then rotated till the two plus signs are aligned (Fig. 9.10F). A scale associated with the instrument rotation indicates, in degrees, one meridian of the oblique astigmatism. Corneal radius of power is then measured in this meridian and in the meridian 90° to it as described above.

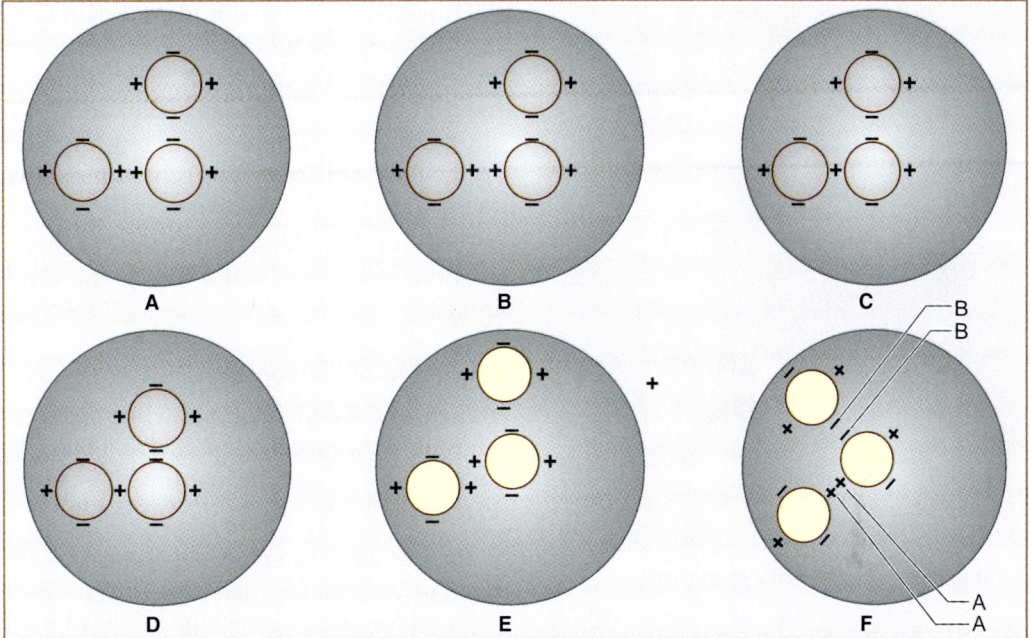

Fig. 9.10: *Examiner's view of the mires: (A) When not focussed properly; (B) Mires focussed properly but not aligned; (C) Alignment of mires when measuring horizontal meridian; (D) Vertical alignment of mires; (E) Non-aligned mires in oblique astigmatism; and (F) Alignment of plus signs in oblique astigmatism.*

Interpreting the findings

Spherical cornea is characterized by:
• No difference in the power between two principal meridia
• The mires seen as perfect sphere.

Astigmatism is characterized by:
• Difference in the power between two principal meridia
• Horizontally, oval mires are seen in with-the-rule astigmatism
• Vertically, oval mires are seen in against-the-rule astigmatism
• In oblique astigmatism, the principal meridia are between 30–60° and 120–150°.

Irregular anterior corneal surface is characterized by:
• Irregular mires
• Doubling of mires.

Keratoconus is characterized by:
• Inclination and jumping of mires is seen while attempting to adjust the mires. When an attempt is made to superimpose the plus mires, they will jump above and below each other (*pulsating mires*).
• Minification of mires is seen in advanced keratoconus (K .52 D) due to increased amount of myopia.
• Oval mires are seen due to large astigmatism.
• Irregular, wavy and distorted mires also indicate advanced keratoconus.

■ JAVAL–SCHIÖTZ KERATOMETER

Principle

The working of Javal–Schiötz keratometer (Fig. 9.11) is based on the principle of *variable object size and constant image size.*

Optical system and parts

The functioning of optical system (Fig. 9.12) and other parts of this keratometer is as below:

1. **The object** in this system consists of two mires (A and B), mounted on an arc on which they can be moved synchronously (Figs 9.12 and 9.13). Since, the two mires together form the

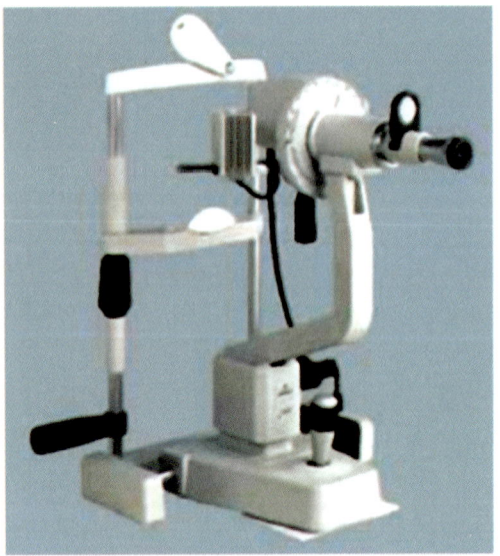

Fig. 9.11: *Javal–Schiötz keratometer.*

object, the variable size is attained by their movement.

One mire is stepped and has a green filter and other mire is rectangular and has a red filter. The mires are divided horizontally through the centre (Fig. 9.14). The mires are illuminated by small lamps. The image of these mires formed by the patient's cornea (1st Purkinje image) acts as *an object for the rest of the optical system* of the keratometer.

2. **Objective lens and doubling prism** form the *doubled image* of the new object (image of the mires formed by cornea). The doubling prism used in this instrument is a Wollaston type. It produces a fixed image doubling by the bire-fringent (double refracting) characteristic of the material of which it is made.

3. **The eyepiece lens** enables the examiner to observe the magnified view of the doubled image.

Procedure of keratometry

1. **Instrument adjustment.** A white paper is held in front of the objective piece and a black line is focused on it. Then the instrument is calibrated to make it ready for use.

2. **Patient adjustment.** The patient is seated in front of the keratometer with chin on the chin rest and forehead against the forehead rest. The chin rest is adjusted to bring the eye at the level of telescope (T) of the instrument (Fig. 9.13). The eye not being examined is covered with an occluder provided with the instrument.

3. **Adjustment of mires.** The mires are adjusted in such a way that they are focused in the centre of patient's cornea. Figure 9.14 shows the patient's view of mires and Fig. 9.15 shows the view of the doubled mire image as

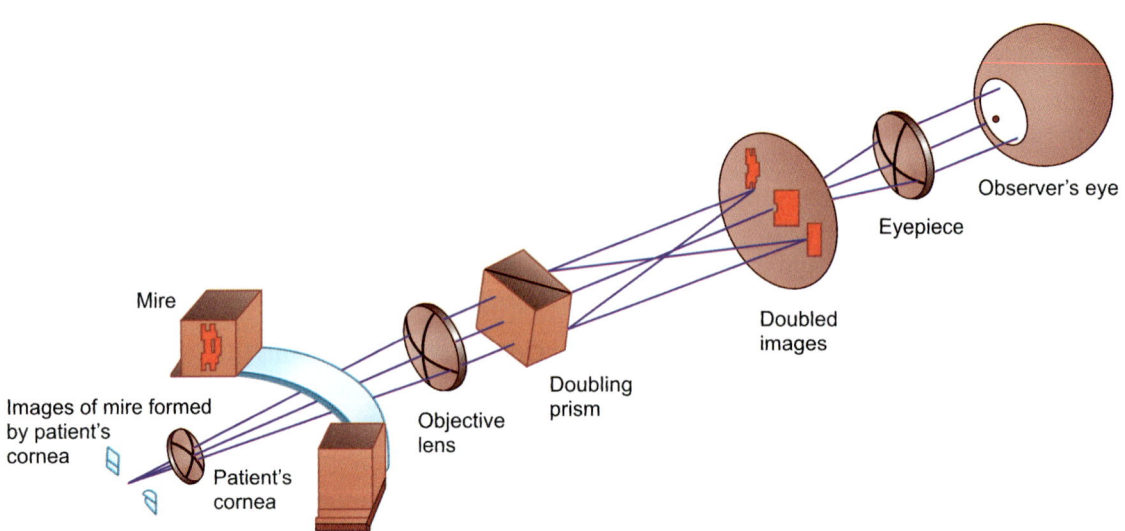

Observer's eye

Eyepiece

Doubled images

Doubling prism

Objective lens

Mire

Images of mire formed by patient's cornea

Patient's cornea

Fig. 9.12: *Optical system of Javal–Schiötz keratometer.*

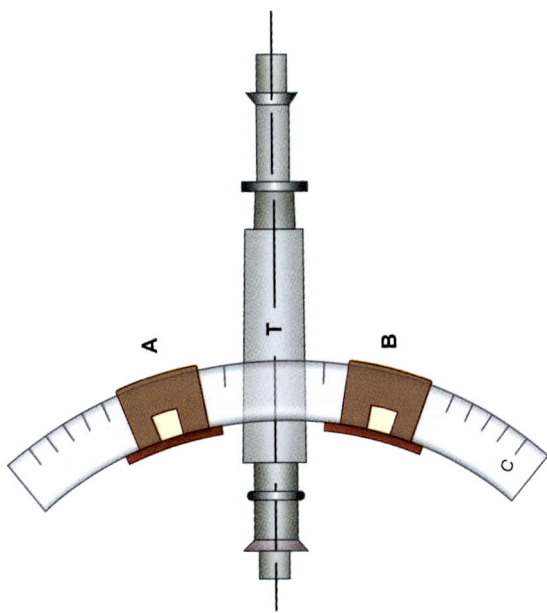

Fig. 9.13: *Basic structure of Javal–Schiötz keratometer showing placement of mires A and B on the arc.*

4. **Recording of keratometric readings.** Only the central pair of images is used when measurements are made. By changing the separation of mires, the separation of these two images can be changed. When the two control images just meet, the scales associated with the mire separation indicate the correct corneal radius and the dioptric power of the cornea.

The radius of curvature is first found in one meridian. Then the entire optical system is rotated by 90° about its central axis. The measurement of the radius of curvature in the second meridian which is perpendicular to the first one is then made in the similar way. When the corneal astigmatism is present, there may occur overlapping of the mires (Fig. 9.16) or they may move further apart. Since, the stepped mire (staircase pattern) is green and the rectangular mire is red, the area of overlap appears whitish. Each step of the mire corresponds to 1 D of corneal power and thus, the number of steps overlapped gives the approximate degree of astigmatism.

When *oblique astigmatism* is present and the mires are horizontal, the central bisecting lines of the images are not aligned (Fig. 9.17A). In such cases, the instrument is rotated until the control lines are aligned (Fig. 9.17B). A scale associated with the instrument rotation indicates, in degrees, one meridian of the oblique astigmatism. Corneal radius or power is then measured in this meridian and also in the meridian 90° to it as usual.

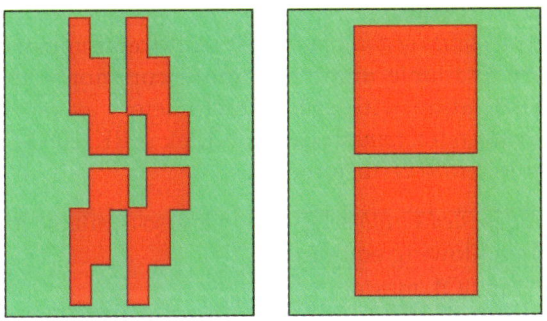

Fig. 9.14: *Patient's view of the mires.*

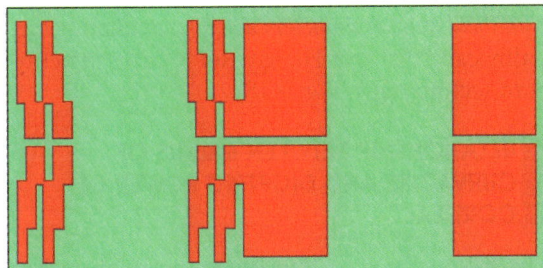

Fig. 9.15: *Examiner's view of doubled mire image.*

seen by the examiner through the instrument's eyepiece.

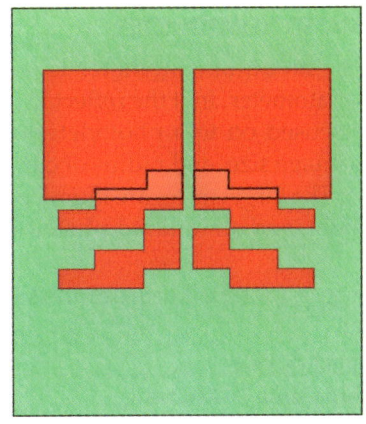

Fig. 9.16: *Overlapping of mires in corneal astigmatism.*

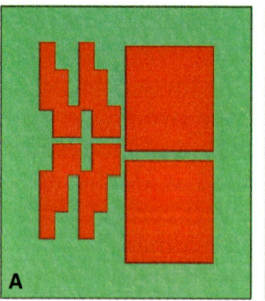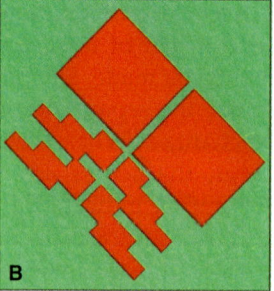

Fig. 9.17: Appearance of images in oblique astigmatism when mires are horizontal before, (A) and after alignment, (B).

SURGICAL/OPERATING KERATOMETER

The surgical keratometer is attached to the operating microscope. It is helpful in monitoring the astigmatism during corneal/limbal surgery.

Factors limiting accuracy

The accuracy of surgical keratometer is limited due to following factors:

- Difficulty in aligning the patient's visual axis and the keratometer's optical axis.
- Keratometers are calibrated for a fixed distance from the anterior cornea. The different microscope objective lenses result in different focal lengths and, therefore, different working distance.
- Air in the anterior chamber results in a second target reflection.
- External pressure on the globe results in a change in the corneal curvature.

AUTOMATED KERATOMETER

Essentially, an autokeratometer is similar to manual keratometer. In it the reflected image of target is focused on to a photodetector which measures image size, and radius of curvature is computed. The target mires are illuminated with infrared light, and an infrared photodetector is used.

Advantages of autokeratometers are the following:

- A compact device
- Very short-time consuming
- Comparatively easy to operate.

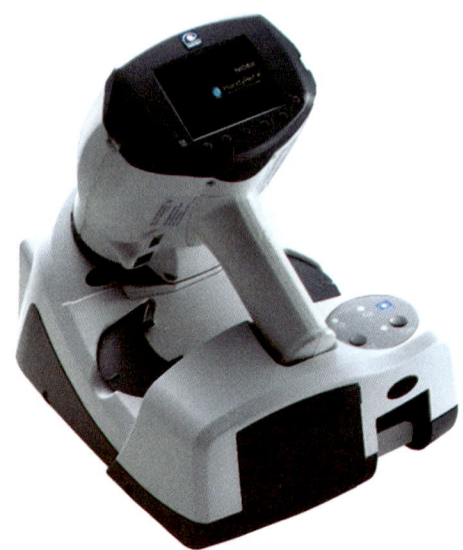

Fig. 9.18: *Handheld autokeratometer.*

Precision of autokeratometry. Almost all the studies have found exceptionally high precision with autokeratometry.

Availability of autokeratometer. Autokeratometers are available alone and more commonly in association with autorefractometers as *autokerato-refractometer*s (e.g. Nidek ARK 2000-S autokerato-refractometer).

Automated keratometry option is also available in the following equipment:

- The IOL master
- Pentacam
- Orbscan
- Corneal topographer.

Handheld autokeratometers are also available, e.g. palmscan 2000 and Handy Ref K (uses synchro scan technology) (Fig. 9.18).

RELATIONSHIP BETWEEN RADIUS OF CURVATURE AND DIOPTRIC POWER OF CORNEA

The following equation gives the relationship between radius of curvature and dioptric power of the cornea:

$$Da = \frac{n-1}{r}$$

where D is dioptric power of the cornea, n is the index of refraction of the cornea and r is the radius of cornea in metres.

Since, the invention of ophthalmometer by Helmholtz, the index of refraction of the cornea has been taken 1.3375 for calibrating the instrument. Therefore,

$$r = \frac{1.3375 - 1}{D} \text{ m}$$

or

$$r = \frac{337.5 - 1}{D} \text{ mm}$$

Usually, the keratometers are calibrated both for radius of curvature and corresponding dioptres. Otherwise, the conversion can also be made by using the above described equation. For a ready reference, conversion table is also available.

Range of keratometer is 36–52 D (6.5–9.38 mm). Its lower limit can be extended up to 30 D (5.6 mm) and upper limit up to 61 D (10.9 mm) by interposing a lens of –1.0 D and 11.25 D, respectively, in front of the objective of telescope.

CLINICAL USES, LIMITATIONS AND SOURCES OF ERROR

CLINICAL USES OF KERATOMETER

The various uses of keratometer in day-to-day ophthalmic practice are as follows:

1. It helps in measurement of *corneal astigmatic error*.
2. It helps to estimate the radius of curvature of the anterior surface of cornea. So, it is of great use in *contact lens fitting*.
3. Keratometer is used to monitor the shape of the cornea in keratoconus and keratoglobus.
4. We may be able *to assess the refractive error* in cases with hazy media (rough estimate on the basis that the normal measurement is 43.5 D– comparison of the two eyes in these cases is useful).
5. Keratometry has gained a special place in *IOL (intraocular lens) power calculation*. The K readings are taken with the help of keratometer and along with axial length, these are utilized to calculate IOL power in SRK (Sanders, Retzlaff and Kraff) formula for IOL power calculation.

6. It is used to monitor pre- and post-surgical astigmatism.
7. It is used for differential diagnosis of axial versus curvatural an isometropia.
8. It is used to detect rigid gas-permeable lens flexure.

LIMITATIONS OF KERATOMETRY

1. The measurements of keratometer are based on a false assumption that the cornea is a symmetrical spherical or spherocylindrical structure, with two principal meridia separated from each other by 90°, whereas the cornea in reality is aspheric.
2. It measures the refractive status of a very small central area of cornea (3–4 mm), ignoring the peripheral corneal zones.
3. It loses its accuracy when measuring very flat (<40 D) or very steep (>50 D) cornea.
4. Finally, small corneal irregularities would preclude the use of keratometer due to irregular astigmatism.
5. Assumed index of refraction in radius to dioptre conversion.
6. One-position instruments assume regular astigmatism.
7. Distance to focal point is approximated by distance to image.
8. The use of para-axial optics to calculate surface power.
9. It cannot describe corneal asphericity.

SOURCES OF ERROR IN KERATOMETRY

- Improper calibration
- Faulty positioning of the patient
- Improper fixation by the patient
- Accommodative fluctuation by examiner
- Localized corneal distortion
- Excessive tearing
- Abnormal lid position
- Improper focusing of the corneal image.

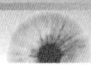

BIBLIOGRAPHY

1. Armitage BS, Schoessler JP. Overnight corneal swelling response in adapted and unadapted extended wear patients. Am J Optom Physiol Opt 1988;65:155–61.
2. Brautaset RL, Nilsson M, et al. Central and peripheral corneal thinning in keratoconus. Cornea 2013;32;257–61.
3. Cheng AC, Tang E, et al. Correction factor in Orbscan II in the assessment of corneal pachy-metry. 2006;25(10):1158–61.
4. Correia FF, Ramos I, et al. Topometric and tomo-graphic indices for the diagnosis of kerato-conus. Int J of KeratoconusEctatic Corneal Dis 2012;1:92–9.
5. Cox I, Ames K. Effect of eye patching on the overnight corneal swelling response with rigid contact lenses. Optom Vis Sci 1989;66:207–8.
6. Douthwaite W, Pardhan S. Comparison of a videokeratoscope and an autokeratometer as predictors of the optimum back surface curves of rigid corneal contact lenses. Ophthalmic Physiol Opt. 1997 Sep;17(5):409–13.
7. Elliott DB. Clinical Procedures in Primary Eye Care (3rd edn.). Edinburgh/New York: Butterworth-Heinemann Ltd 2007;pp 85–90.
8. Friling R, Weinberger D, Kremer I, Avisar R, Sirota L, Snir M. Keratometry measurements in preterm and full term newborn infants. Br J Ophthalmol 2004;88(1)8–10.
9. Fujioka M, Nakamura M, et al. Comparison of Pentacam Scheimpflug camera with ultrasound pachymetry and noncontact specular micro-scopy in measuring central corneal thickness. Curr Eye Res 2007;32:89–94.
10. Gutmark R, Guyton DL. Origins of the Kerato-meter and its Evolving Role in Ophthalmology. Survey of Ophthalmology 2010;55(5):481–97.
11. Haque S, Simpson T, et al. Corneal and epithelial thickness in keratoconus: a comparison of ultra-sonic pachymetry, Orbscan II, and optical coherence tomography. J Refract Surg 2006;22(5): 486–93.
12. Hashemi H, Roshani M, et al. Effect of corneal thickness on the agreement between ultrasound and Orbscan II pachymetry. J Cataract Refract Surg 2007;33(10):1694–1700.
13. Hoffer KJ. Biometry of 7,500 cataractous eyes. Am J Ophthalmol 1980;90(3):360–8.
14. Javaloy J, Vidal MT, et al. Comparison of four corneal pachymetry techniques in corneal refrac-tive surgery. J Refract Surg 2004;20,29–34.
15. Khoramnia R, Rabsilber TM, et al. Central and peripheral pachymetry measurements according to age using the Pentacam rotating Scheimp-flug camera. J Cataract Refract Surg 2007;33: 830–6.
16. Lass JH, Gal RL, et al. Cornea Donor Study Investigator Group. Ophthalmology, 2008; 115(4):627–32.
17. Lei Y, Zheng X, et al. Effects of long-term soft contact lens wear on the corneal thickness and corneal epithelial thickness of myopic subjects. Mol Med Rep 2015;11(3):2020–6.
18. Mandell RB, Fatt I. Thinning of the human cornea on awakening. Nature 1965;208:292–3.
19. Mehrdad Mohammadpour, et al. Central Corneal Thickness Measurement Using Ultra-sonic Pachymetry, Rotating Scheimpflug Camera, and Scanning-slit Topography Exclu-sively in Thin Non-keratoconic Corneas. J Oph-thalmic Vis Res 2016;11(3):245–51.
20. Noonan CP, Rao GP, Kaye SB, Green JR, Chandna A. Validation of a handheld automated keratometer in adults. J Cataract Refract Surg 1998;24(3):411–4.
21. Polse KA. Changes in corneal hydration after discontinuing contact lens wear. Am J Optom Arch Am Acad Optom. 1972;49:511–6.
22. Saleh Al-Ageel, et al. Comparison of central corneal thickness measurements by Pentacam, noncontact specular microscope, and ultrasound pachymetry in normal and post-LASIK eyes. Saudi J Ophthalmol 2009;23(3-4):181–7.
23. Sophia Y Wang, et al. The impact of central corneal thickness on the risk for glaucoma in a large multiethnic population. J Glaucoma. 2014; 23(9):606–12.
24. Suzuki S, Oshika T, et al. Corneal thickness measurements: scanning-slit corneal topography and noncontact specular microscopy versus ultrasonic pachymetry. J Cataract Refract Surg 2003;29(7):1313–8.
25. Tam ES, Rootman DS. Comparison of central corneal thickness measurements by specular microscopy, ultrasound pachymetry, and ultra-sound biomicroscopy. J Cataract Refract Surg 2003;29,179–84.
26. Trivedi RH, Wilson ME, Peterseim MM, Lal G. Axial length and keratometry in eyes with pediatric cataract. Annual American Society of Cataract and Refractive Surgeons Symposium on Cataract, IOL, and Refractive Surgery San Francisco, CA 2003 April;12–6.

Corneal Topography and Aberrometry

Chapter Outline

CORNEAL TOPOGRAPHY

General Considerations
- Working principles
- Commonly used topography/tomography systems

Placido-Disc-Based Corneal Topography Systems
- Placido-disc principle
- Basic unit
- Limitations of Placido-disc-based topography systems
- Commercially available systems
- Display of topographic data

Slit-Scanning Corneal Topography Systems
- Orbscan III

Scheimpflug Imaging Based Corneal Topography Systems
- Pentacam

OCT Based Corneal Topography

Very High Frequency Ultrasound Corneal Tomography Systems

Digital Rastersterography Based Topography Systems
- PAR CTS

Laser Holographic Interferometry Based Topography Systems
- Class II unit

Clinical Applications and Limitations of Corneal Topography Systems
- Clinical applications
- Limitations

ABERROMETRY AND WAVEFRONT TECHNOLOGY

Aberrations
- Ray aberrationsvs wave aberrations
- Zernick's polynomials and Zernick's terms

Ocular Wavefront
- Total ocular wavefront
- Corneal wavefront

Wavefront Aberrometry
- Hartmann–Shack aberrometry
- Tscherning aberroscope
- Ray-tracing aberrometry
- Intraoperative, real-time wavefront guided aberrometry
- Clinical applications of aberromtry

CORNEAL TOPOGRAPHY

GENERAL CONSIDERATIONS

Corneal topography refers to study of shape of corneal surface. The term corneal topography system (CTS), or videokeratography, implies computerized, video-assisted technique that provides detailed information about the shape of the corneal surface.

Present day technologies allow three-dimensional evaluation with cross-sectional images and are thus referred to as *corneal tomography systems.*

WORKING PRINCIPLES

Present day available corneal topography and tomography systems are based on one or combination of more than one below given working principles:

- Placido-disc principle-based corneal topography/tomography systems
- Slit-scanning principle corneal tomography system (e.g. Orbscan III)
- Scheimpflug imaging principle-based systems (e.g. Pentacam, Sirius, Galilie)
- High speed anterior segment optical coherence tomography (AS-OCT)
- Digital raster stereography-based topography systems
- Laser halographic interferometry-based topography systems
- Very high frequency (VHF) ultrasound-based system.

COMMONLY USED TOPOGRAPHY/TOMOGRAPHY SYSTEMS

Commonly used corneal topography systems and aberrometry systems are listed in Table 10.1.

Table 10.1 *Commonly used topography system and aberrometry system*	
A. CORNEAL TOPOGRAPHY AND TOMOGRAPHY SYSTEMS	
I. Placido-Disc-Based System	
1. EyeSys Desktop (*EyeSys Vision, Inc., US*)	Placido–ring/cone
2. Tomey TMS-4M (*Tomey Corp, Japan*)	Placido-disc-based
3. CA-200F Corneal Analyzer (*Topcon Medical Systems, Inc., Japan*)	Placido-disc-based topography system (with 24 rings measuring over 10,000 data points and eight blue led lights for fluorescein images to aid in contact lens simulation)
4. AstraMax (*Laser Sight Technology Florial*)	Placido disc based, 3D corneal topography
II. Scheimpflug Rotating Imaging-based Systems	
1. Pentacam AXL (*Oculus, Germany*)	Dual Scheimpflug and Placido-disc imaging
2. Oculyzer (*Wavelight AG, Germany*)	Dual Scheimpflug and Placido-disc imaging
3. Preciso (*iVIS Technologies, Taranto, Italy*)	Dual Scheimpflug and Placido-disc imaging
4. Galilei G6 (*Zeimer, Switzerland*)	Dual Scheimpflug and Placido-disc imaging
5. TMS-5 (*Tomey Corp, Japan*)	Dual Scheimpflug and Placido-disc imaging
6. Sirius (*CSO, Italy*)	Dual Scheimpflug and Placido-disc imaging
III. Horizontal Slit Scan-based System	
1. OrbscanIIIz* (*Bausch & Lomb, Rochester, New York*)	Dual Horizontal Slit Scan and Placido-disc Imaging
IV. Rasterstereography-based System	
1. PAR Corneal Topography System (*CTS; Par Vision Systems Corp., New Hartford, NY*)	Elevation-based systems which projects a grid on to the corneal surface after instillation of fluorescein. Distortions in grid patterns are analyzed to determine corneal elevation-based on camera and grid projection angles (Rasterstereography)
V. Very High Frequency (VHF) Ultrasound-based System	
1. Artemis 3 (*ARC Scan, Colorado*)	I. ARC Scanning with very high frequency ultrasound

Contd...

Table 10.1 *Commonly used topography system and aberrometry system (Contd...)*

VI. Optical Coherence Tomography-based Systems

1. Visante Omni (*Carl Zeiss Meditec, Germany*)	II. Rotating optical coherence tomography and placido-disc imaging
2. SS1000 Casia (*Tomey Corp, Japan*)	III. Rotating optical coherence tomography
1. RTVue-100 (*Optovue, Inc. Fremont, CA*)	Spectral Domain Optical Coherence Tomography guided corneal power measurement (both anterior and posterior curvatures)
2. IOL Master 700 (*Carl Zeiss Meditec, Germany*)	Swept Source OCT Technology with 32-Marker Placido pattern
3. 3D OCT-2000 (5) (*Topcon Medical systems*)	Spectral Domain OCT
4. Cirrus HD-OCT 5000 (2) (*Carl Zeiss Meditec, Germany*)	Spectral Domain OCT, Confocal scanning laser Ophthalmoscope (CSLO)

B. CORNEAL TOPOGRAPHERS WITH ABERROMETERS

1. KR-1W Wavefront Analyzer (*Topcon Medical Systems*) 2. i-Trace (*Tracey Technologies, Houston*)	• Hartmann-Shack Aberrometry • Near-infrared corneal topography • Ray Tracing Aberrometery • Placido-disc corneal topography (sequentially projects 256 near-infrared laser beams into the eye to measure forward aberrations, processing data point-by-point)
3. Atlas 9000 Corneal Topography System (*Carl Zeiss Meditec, Germany*)	• Placido-disc topography (22 Ring) • Patented "Cone Of Focus" alignment system • Ray-Tracing Aberrometry
4. OPD-Scan III (*Nidek, Gamagori, Japan*)	• Placido-disc topography (33 Blue mires) • Dynamic Skiascopy for Aberrometry
5. Wavelight Allegro Oculyzer II (*Alcon, US*)	• Rotating 3D Scheimpflug imaging topography • Tscherning principle Aberrometry
6. Cassini TCA (*i-Optics, USA*)	• Placido-disc Corneal Topography • Ray Tracing Aberrometry systems
7. Discovery (*Innovative visual systems, US*)	• Placido-disc Corneal Topography, and • Hartmann-Shack principle

C. ABERROMETERS

1. Zywave® II Wavefront Aberrometer (*Bausch & Lomb*)	• Hartmann-Shack principle
2. WASCA Analyzer/Aberrometer (*Carl Zeiss Meditec, Germany*)	• Hartmann-Shack principle
3. LadarWave (*Alcon, US*)	• Hartmann-Shack principle
4. Visx Waves can Wavefront Aberrometer (*Abbott Medical Optics, Inc. (AMO), US*)	• Hartmann-Shack principle
5. Wavelight Allegro Analyzer (*Alcon, US*)	Tscherning principle
6. Optiwave Refractive Analysis® (ORA) System (*Wavetec, US*)	Infrared Light and Talbot-Moiré Interferometry (Intraoperative Wavefront Aberrometer)
7. HolosIntraop Wavefront Aberrometer (*Clarity Medical Systems, Inc., US*)	Continuous real time intraoperative Wavefront Aberrometer

PLACIDO-DISC-BASED CORNEAL TOPOGRAPHY SYSTEMS

Placido-disc corneal topography systems were originally limited to evaluation of the anterior corneal surface. Presently many of the pacido-disc based systems include the imaging of back surface of cornea and direct evaluation of elevational changes of both anterior and posterior corneal surfaces, enabling point-to-point pachymetry. In other words, the corneal topography system, now can be called *corneal tomographs*, as they allow three-dimensional evaluation of corneal tissue. This technique has an excellent accuracy and reproducibility. Most corneal topographers evaluate 8000–10,000 specific points across the entire corneal surface.

PLACIDO-DISC-PRINCIPLE

Placido-disc-based corneal topography systems work on the reflection principle. The anterior surface of the cornea acts like a convex mirror and hence, the size of the image formed by it is determined by its curvature. A steeply curved cornea will produce a smaller image while a flatter cornea will produce a larger image of the same object situated at the same distance from the cornea. These devices thus measure the slope and compute the curvature. They have different projection devices that use lighted circular rings of varying sizes and numbers, these rings are reflected by convex cornea and through an opening in the centre of the target , the images are obtained by an acquisition camera.

BASIC UNIT OF CORNEAL TOPOGRAPY SYSTEMS

The basic unit of a corneal topographic/tomographic system thus primarily consists of:

- A projection device,
- Acquisition device (video camera), and
- Analtical device (a digital computer attached with a slit-lamp chin rest.)

1. Projection device

These systems imply Placido-disc-based projection device. Historically, the Placido-disc-based systems were the first to be developed and thus are the most widely used and understood. Most Placido-disc-based systems project around 8–32 concentric rings on the cornea. The rings are numbered from inside out. A specified ring in different instruments may cover different areas. Therefore, it is important to mention the diameter of the projected ring along with the number. The virtual images of these reflected rings are located anterior to the iris.

2. Video camera

The reflected images of rings projected on to the cornea are captured on charge-coupled device (CCD) camera for Video-keratoscope. The image accuracy and precision are— images of rings are digitized and algorithms are used to determine the radius of curvature of innermost ring. Once this is determined then the distance of next ring from this is calculated and used to determine curvature of this ring and so on till peripheral ring is achieved. The cornea between rings is not imaged and no actual data for these points and the apex of cornea which is inside innermost ring is also not measured.

- Dioptric power is calculated from curvature using the formula:

$$\text{Dioptric power} = \frac{\text{refractive index of cornea–refractive index of air}}{\text{radius of curvature in metres}}$$

- Measured radius of curvature is of anterior corneal surface, so provides power of anterior surface while cannot measure the true power of posterior corneal surface.

3. Computer

The video camera is hooked up to a computer that generates a 'topographic map' of corneal curvature based on the measured distance between the rings reflected from the cornea. The accuracy of corneal curvature data processing depends a lot on the software-editing features. After analysis, the graphic picture of the patients' topography is displayed in various forms.

LIMITATIONS OF PLACIDO-DISC-BASED TOPOGRAPHY SYSTEMS

Limitations of Placido-disc-based topography systems include the following:

- There is *a lack of standardization between instruments*; it depends on reference axis, alignment, and focus. The corneal apex is the point of maximum curvature on the cornea, whereas the vertex is the point nearest to the camera of the Placido instrument located on the corneal topographer axis (CT axis). Before acquisition, the topographer aligns this axis normal to the cornea. This is possible only in ideal scenario but in patients with positive angle kappa the line of sight does not pass through apex of cornea and the reflected image appears displaced and is shown as asymmetric bowtie in otherwise normal cornea. The effect of decentration is nullified to an extent in elevation based devices.

- *The elevation maps* are derived in Placido devices by using angle of reflection and by making mathematical assumptions, so cannot be as accurate as true elevation maps of slit scan Scheimpflug devices.
- *Intraobserver and interobserver* variability errors, alignment errors, focussing errors or errors of calibration
- *Central regions* require a higher degree of subpixel resolution in order to detect a 0.25-D change than do peripheral region
- *Difficulties in determination of the power and location* of the steepest meridian when using artificial tears in postpenetrating keratoplasty eyes.

COMMERCIALLY AVAILABLE PLACIDO-DISC TOPOGRAPHY SYSTEMS

Commercially available corneal topography systems based on Pacido-disc principle are listed in Table 10.1. Cardinal features of the some of presently available systems are described briefly.

1. EyeSys Desktop

EyeSys Desktop (Fig. 10.1B) from EyeSys Vision, Inc., US is a 25-ring videokeratoscopic device with USB 2 connectivity with fast image processing time of 3 seconds and colour-coded contour map plots in addition to a host of other presentation schemes including customized packages. It analyses 9000 data points. The software with the system takes the Stiles–Crawford effect into consideration and allows display of relative brightness of light entering the pupil. This results in more practically useful information. It utilises the technology of EyeSys 2000 corneal analysis system.

EyeVista is the portable available model with similar functions, with which patients confined to a bed or wheelchair can easily be examined and supine patients can be mapped in the operating room under a surgical microscope.

2. TMS–4 Topographic Modelling System

The TMS–4 Topographic Modelling System from Computed Anatomy, Inc. through Tomey Technology, Inc., Cambridge, utilizes 31 projected rings providing 7000 data points. The corneal coverage is 0.02–11.00 mm with an accuracy of 0.10 D. It has a patented laser alignment system for accurate alignment and an exclusive refractive surgery planning programme.

3. AstraMax

AstraMax is a Placido-disc corneal tomography system manufactured by LaserSight Technologies, Inc., Winter Park, Florida (Fig. 10.1C). AstraMax is a new generation 3-D corneal topography with enhanced resolution ideally suited for custom cornea-based treatment. AstraMax

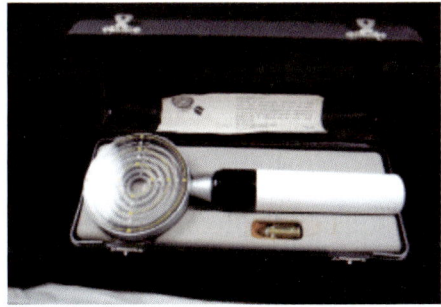 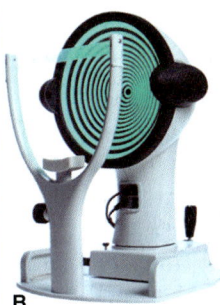 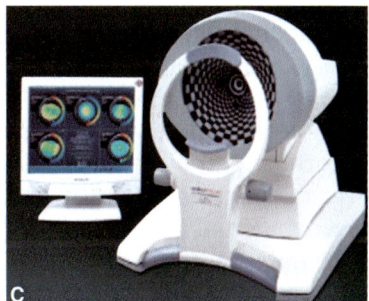

Fig. 10.1: *(A) Placido-disc keratoscope (Keeler's); (B) Corneal topography system: EyeSys Desktop (EyeSys Vision, Inc.) (C) Corneal tomography system (AstraMax).*

is a three-camera imaging system that uses stereo ray tracing for high-precision, patient-specific corneal measurements. Patented polar grid yields critical measurements to measure complex corneal shapes. High-definition graphics provide eye simulations and 3-D surface modelling.

4. Atlas 9000 corneal topography system

Working principles of Atlas 9000 Corneal Topography System(*Carl Ziess, Germany*) include;

- *Ray tracing technology* to displays higher-order corneal aberrations.
- *Placido-disc technology* with *Cone-of-Focus* alignment system. It has *nonvisible Placido ring illumination* which is comfortable for even the most light-sensitive patients. The 22-ring Placido-disc is optimized to avoid ring cross-over, which allows reliable results for a wide range of patients.

Applications. This system, based on Corneal Wavefront Analysis, is a diagnostic instrument that measures the curvature of the cornea and produces topographical images. It supports many important optometric applications, including contact lens fitting, pathology detection and management and selection of aspheric IOLs.

5. OPD scan III

The OPD III (*Nidek, Japan*) is five-in-one refractive work station which combines:

- *Wavefront aberrometry* gives assessment of visual acuity and quality of vision in addition to traditional refraction and keratometry. Simulation of retinal contrast sensitivity and visual acuity charts enable objective quantification of visual clarity.
- *Corneal topography* provides intuitive maps and numerical data for the corneal surface and provides neural network assisted detection of corneal pathology such as keratoconus suspect, keratoconus and pellucid marginal degeneration.
- *Auto refractometer* provides exceptionally accurate refractions for various pupil diameters including refractions under photopic and mesopic conditions, critical for

proper assessment of both refractive surgery patients and common refractive problems.

- *Auto keratometer* provides conventional keratometry and novel corneal surface descriptors such as APP (Average Pupil Power) and ECCP (Effective Central Corneal Power) which aid in the calculation of the correct IOL power for postoperative corneas.
- *Pupillometry* measures photopic and mesopic pupil diameters. Pupil images reveal the shape of photopic and mesopic pupils, which can alter refraction and important surgical data. Identification of the first Purkinje Image (corneal light reflex) and pupil center are provided. The distance between these two landmarks is calculated to assist in centration during refractive surgery and to assess IOL centration.

6. Cassini TCA

Cassini total corneal astigmatism (TCA) (*I-optics, USA*) uses multicoloured LED point-to-point ray tracing to provide a GPS-like analysis of the cornea along with high-resolution images utilized for surgical guidance. There is a total of 679 LEDs; 224 red, 224 green, 224 yellow and seven white. The unique measuring principle enables highly accurate and repeatable measurements of the total corneal astigmatism. Cassini TCA measures the posterior cornea using second Purkinje reflections and provides a total corneal astigmatism measurement. The multicoloured LED coverage is equal across the entire cornea, leaving no space for central scotoma. The accurate axis and magnitude of astigmatism play a vital part in the correct selection and positioning of a toric IOL.

DISPLAY OF PLACIDO-DISC-BASED CORNEAL TOPOGRAPHIC SYSTEM DATA

The corneal topographic data analysed by the computers can be displayed in the following formats:

A. Numerical power plots
B. Keratometry view
C. Photokeratoscopic view
D. Profile view
E. Colour-coded topographic maps.

The most useful form of data presentation is a colour-coded corneal contour map, which will be discussed in detail.

A. NUMERICAL POWER PLOTS

In numerical power plots, the corneal curvature of specific areas is shown in dioptre values (Fig. 10.2). The data are displayed in 10 concentric circular zones with 1 mm interval between each. The numerical values are displayed in colour, which are in agreement with the colour scale being used. The display also shows the average dioptric value of each of the 10 concentric circular zones individually along with the average overall corneal curvature.

B. KERATOMETRIC VIEW

Keratometric view (Fig. 10.3) depicts the keratometric reading in two principal meridia (K_1 and K_2) in three different zones simultaneously. The three zones measured are *central* 3 mm zone (as in a conventional keratometry), *intermediate* 3–5 mm zone and *peripheral* 5–7 mm zone.

It is an important map for assessing the skewing of semi-meridia. The more the keratometric readings in principal meridia deviate from being perpendicular to each other, the more irregular or non-orthogonal corneal astigmatism exists.

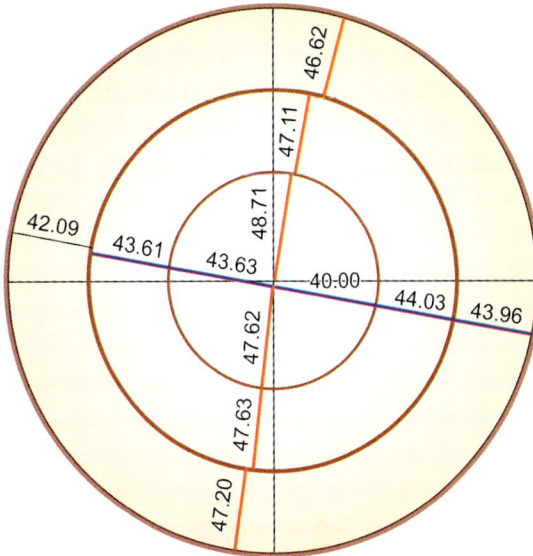

Fig. 10.3: *Keratometric view of the data (Courtesy: Dr Rajib Mukherjee).*

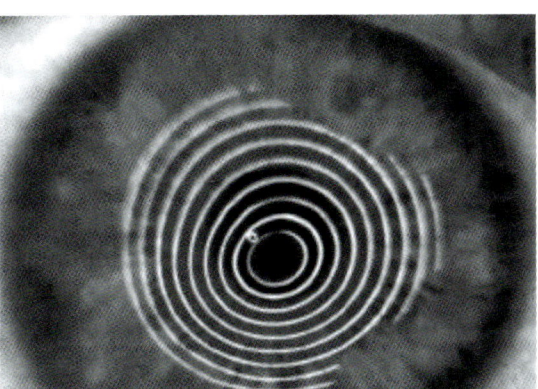

Fig. 10.4: *Photokeratoscopic view showing egging of mires in a patient with keratoconus (Courtesy: Dr Rajib Mukherjee).*

C. PHOTOKERATOSCOPIC VIEW

Photokeratoscopic view (Fig. 10.4) depicts the actual black and white photograph of the Placido rings captured by the video camera. This view helps in confirming the proper patient fixation and in identifying the eye captured. The reflected rings on the cornea are situated more towards the limbus on one side than the other, and on the nasal side the distance between the rings is comparatively narrower.

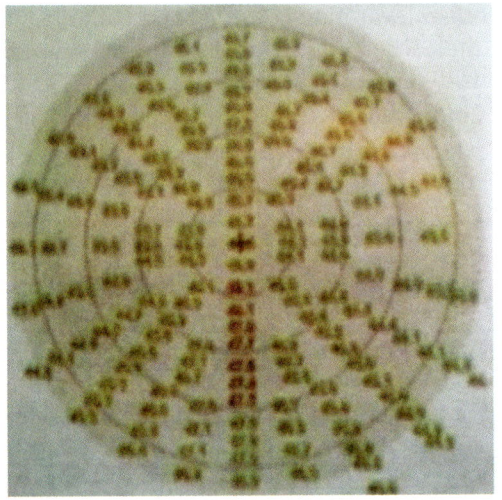

Fig. 10.2: *Numerical power plot (Courtesy: Dr Rajib Mukherjee).*

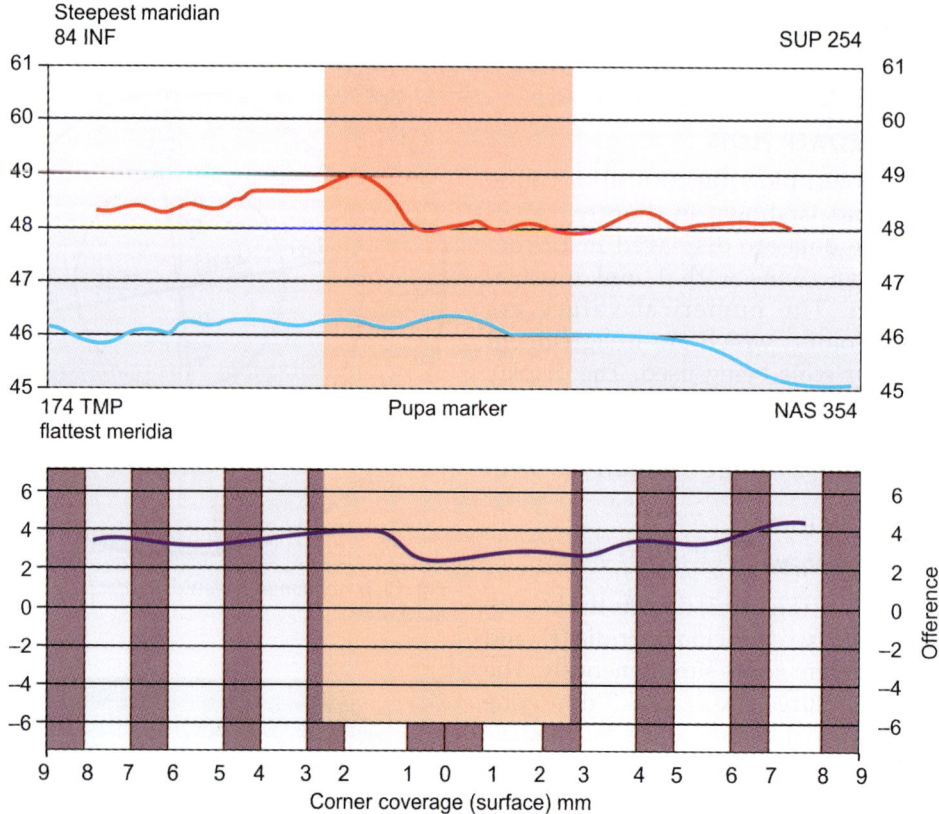

Fig. 10.5: *Profile view (Courtesy: Dr Rajib Mukherjee).*

D. PAR CTS PROFILE VIEW

The profile view (Fig. 10.5) shows the graphical plotting along the X Y axis of the steepest and the flat test meridia of the cornea and the difference between the two in dioptres. The display button shows the astigmatic difference (difference plot, Ddelta map) between the flat and steep meridia. A grey zone in this difference plot denotes the pupillary area. In a symmetrical eye, the tracing across this grey band is a straight line. In the presence of astigmatism, an apparent slag is seen. This slag increases, with the asymetricity of cornea.

E. COLOUR-CODED TOPOGRAPHIC MAP

Colour-coded contour maps of the cornea are the most useful and most commonly used display formation.

Interpretation of a colour map

While interpreting colour-coded contour maps of the cornea, following parameters should be considered:

1. Colour codes. These are used as follows:
- *Hot colours*, i.e. red and its various hues represent the steep portions of cornea.
- *Cool colours*, i.e. blue and its various hues represent the flat portions of cornea.
- So the colours red–orange–yellow–green–purple–blue denote progressively lessening refractive power.

The colour intensity is relative, meaning that an area of 45 D is less red as compared to an area of 46 D.

2. The scale used. It is very important to know the scale used before interpreting a colour map. The two apparently similar maps may in fact show markedly different cornea depending upon the scale used. The commonly used scales are absolute and normalized scales:

Absolute scale. In it, each colour represents a 1.5 D interval between 35 and 50 D, whereas above and below this range, colours represent 5 D intervals. This scale is useful in routine practice (e.g. preoperative screening).

- *Disadvantage* of absolute scale is that it does not show subtle changes of curvature and thus can miss subtle local changes (e.g. early keratoconus).

    Normalized scale. In it, the cornea is divided into 11 equal colours spanning that eye's total dioptric power. In this scale, more minute topographic details within an individual cornea are appreciated.

- *Advantage* of normalized scale is that it shows more detailed description of the surface than the absolute scale.

- *Disadvantage* of normalized scale is that the colours of two different maps cannot be compared directly and have to be interpreted based on the keratometric values from their different colour scales.

    Note: Figure 10.6 shows a corneal topography map with different scales. Many workers feel that the absolute scale is easier to read and the normalized scale magnifies clinically insignificant information.

3. *Quantitative indices*. As part of the display, quantitative indices are also generated to give extra information. These include the following:

- Predicted visual acuity based on corneal shape
- Simulated keratometric readings (Sim K)
- Mean keratometry reading
- Surface regularity index (corenal irregularity measurement)
- Surface asymmetry index (shape factor SF)
- Point spread function (PSF)

i. *Simulated keratometric readings.* These characterize corneal curvatures in the central 3 mm area. The steep simulated K reading is the steepest meridian of the cornea in central 3 mm area. The flat test Sim K reading is the flat test meridian of the cornea and is, by definition, 90° apart.

ii. *Surface asymmetry index.* The index of asphericity indicates how much the curvature changes upon movement from the centre to the periphery of the cornea. A normal cornea is prolate (i.e. becomes flatter towards the periphery) and has the asphericity Q of –0.26. A prolate surface has negative Q value and an oblate surface has positive Q value. Most myopic laser vision corrections change the anterior corneal surface from prolate to oblate. A negative SF usually indicates a post-refractive surgery eye with the centre flatter than the periphery. The SFs (e^2) for the general population are as follows:

- Normal 0.13 to 0.35
- Borderline 0.02 to 0.12 and 0.36 to 0.46
- Abnormal -1.0 to 0.01 and 0.47 to 1.0

iii. *Surface regularity index/corneal irregularity measurement (CIM).* It is a number or index which represents the irregularity of the corneal surface. The higher the irregularity index, the more difficult it is to fit the corneal surface with a contact lens. It often can predict irregular astigmatism or visual distortions. Higher CIM values indicate that ocular pathology such as keratoconus or other pathological cases is more probable. The general population exhibits the following distribution ranges:

- Normal 0.03 to 0.68 µm
- Borderline 0.69 to 1.0 µm
- Abnormal 1.1 to 5.0 µm

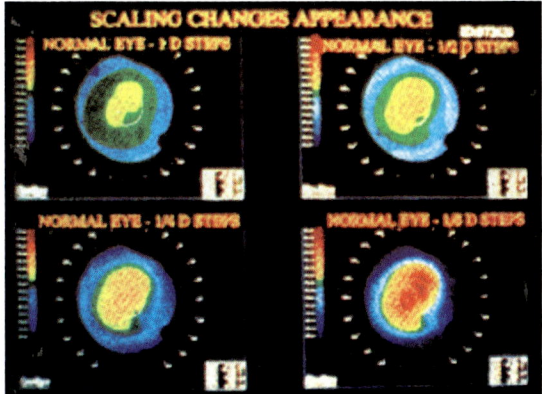

Fig. 10.6: *Scaling change showing apparently different maps of the same cornea (Courtesy: Dr Rajib Mukherjee).*

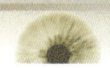

iv. *Mean Toric Keratometry*. The mean toric keratometry (TKM) indices use elevation data to compare the toric reference to the actual cornea. The mean apical curvature value helps select the best toric fit using a sphero-cylinder design. This provides the most accurate toric representation of a patient's cornea. Human TKM ranges are as follows:

- Normal 43.10 to 45.90 diopters
- Borderline 41.80 to 43.00 diopters and 46.00 to 47.20 diopters
- Abnormal 36.00 diopters to 41.70 diopters and 47.3 diopters to 60.0 diopters

Pathfinder Corneal Analysis. The Atlas Corneal Topographer (Carl Zeiss Meditec, Inc.) uses special software that combines the above indices (CIM, SF and TKM) to determine the probability of irregular corneas. This helps practitioners qualitatively and quantitatively, measure the probability of keratoconus. The Pathfinder Corneal Analysis also helps determine whether a GP or soft toric lens fits poorly on the cornea or should be replaced with a different base curve. It also helps when fitting GP lenses. New keratoconus fitting philosophies use a lens-to-cornea relationship with less central bearing. Trend with Time or Stars technology can monitor corneal disease and determine how corneal shape responds with new contact lens designs.

Corneal topographic patterns in normal corneas

The normal cornea flattens progressively from the centre to the periphery by 2–4 D, with the nasal area flattening more than the temporal area. The topographic pattern of the two corneas of an individual often shows mirror-image symmetry, and small variations in patterns are unique for the individual.

Depending upon the corneal curvature, Rabinowitz et al. in 1996 described 10 different corneal topographic patterns in normal eyes as seen on colour-coded absolute scale maps (Fig. 10.7). These can be grouped as follows (figures in the parentheses indicate approximate distribution of keratographic patterns):

Regular pattern (Fig. 10.7)
- Round (23%)
- Oval (21%)

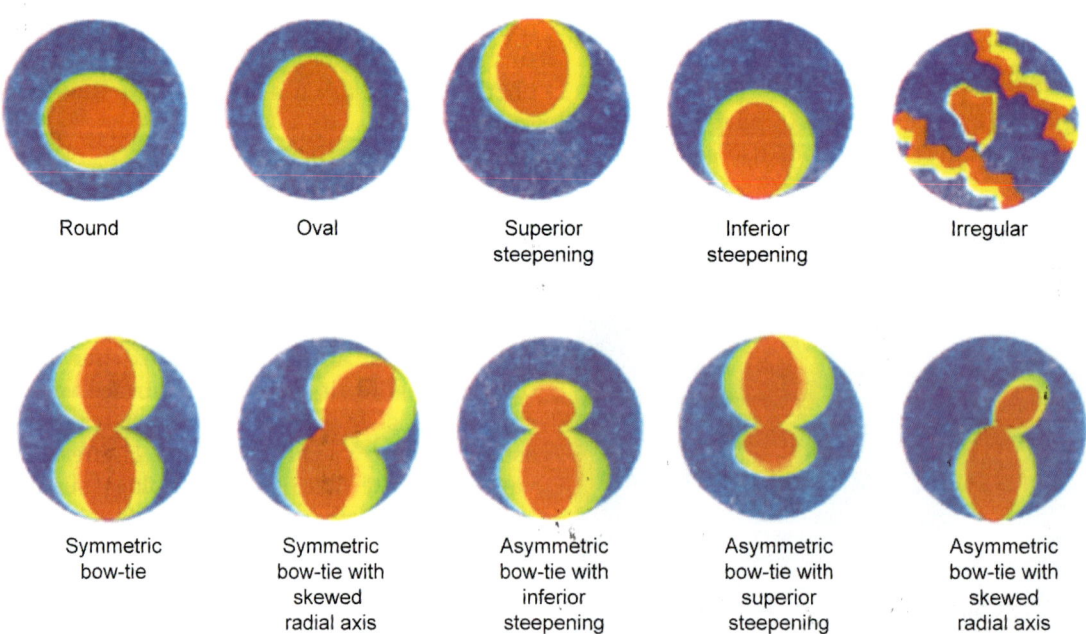

Fig. 10.7: *Corneal topographic pattern seen on colour-coded maps in absolute scale (Rabinowitz et al. 1996; Courtesy: Dr Rajib Mukherjee).*

- Steepening:
  - Superior steepening
  - Inferior steepening

Astigmatic patterns (Fig. 10.7)
- *Symmetrical and orthogonal*, i.e. bow-tie effect (18%)
  Symmetrical bow-tie with non-skewed axis
  Symmetrical bow-tie with skewed radial axis
- *Asymmetrical and orthogonal* (31%)
  Asymmetric bow-tie with superior steepening
  Asymmetric bow-tie with inferior steepening
  Asymmetric bow-tie with skewed radial axis
- *Irregular*, i.e. no pattern and non-orthogonal (7%)

Formats for display of data on colour maps

Various formats used for display of data on colour-coded maps are as follows:

1. Corneal power map (sagittal or axial)

The corneal power map (Fig. 10.8) is 24-colour representation of dioptric power at various points on the cornea. The radius of curvature is measured 360 times for each Placido ring image from centre to vertex. The sagittal algorithm averages the data points from first to the next ring and so on. Due to common reference axis, small irregularities may not be visible or smoothened out. They are spherically based and assume that centre of rotation of best fit sphere lies on optical axis. The axial map is more commonly used to produce a good estimate of overall corneal shape, which appears smooth with little noise as it provides average of adjacent curvature values.

2. Tangential map

The tangential map (Fig. 10.9) gives better geographical representation of the cornea as compared to the axial/sagittal corneal map. In it, tangents are projected outwards from the centre vertex 360°. Ring curvature is measured along the tangent (ring intersection). This is also known as *instantaneous curvature map*. This is the best indicator of corneal shape but is a poor indicator of corneal power. Therefore, tangential reading must never be used for calculating K values. This map is a very useful tool for accurate diagnosis of corneal ectatic conditions like keratoconus and also accentuates focal abnormalities as more sensitive.

3. Elevation map

Elevation is not measured directly by Placido-based topographers, but certain assumptions allow the construction of elevation maps. Elevation of a point on the corneal surface displays the height of the point on the corneal surface relative to a spherical reference surface. The reference surface in most instruments was

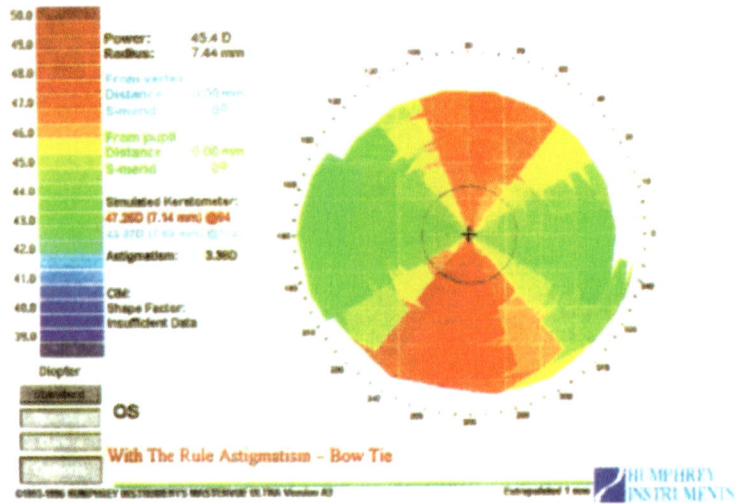

Fig. 10.8: *Corneal power map showing symmetrical 'bow-tie pattern' in a patient having with-the-rule astigmatism (Courtesy: Dr Rajib Mukherjee).*

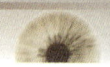

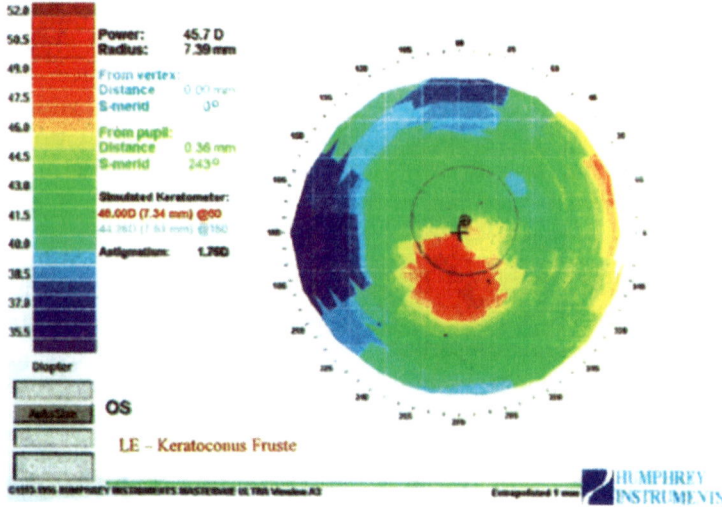

Fig. 10.9: *Tangential map showing inferior steepening in a patient with keratoconus left eye (Courtesy: Dr Rajib Mukherjee).*

chosen to be a sphere. Best mathematical approximation of the actual corneal surface, called best-fit sphere, is calculated by instrument software for every elevation map separately. The same surface may appear different when mapped against different reference surfaces. Consequently, it is difficult to compare directly two elevation maps that likely have slightly different best-fit spheres as reference values, and comparison only can be intuitive. The elevation map (Fig. 10.10) helps in distinguishing localized elevations (steep because of projection) from otherwise steep corneal area. The interpretation

can be confusing, but it is important to remember that 'Red is Raised (steep)' and 'Blue is Below (flat)'. The hotter colours show areas that are elevated above the reference sphere and cooler colours represent the areas that are depressed under the reference sphere. The elevation measurements are simply difference measurements.

In laser refractive surgery, the refractive power is changed by removing tissue from the corneal surface, and elevation data appear more relevant for calculation of ablation depth and optical zones.

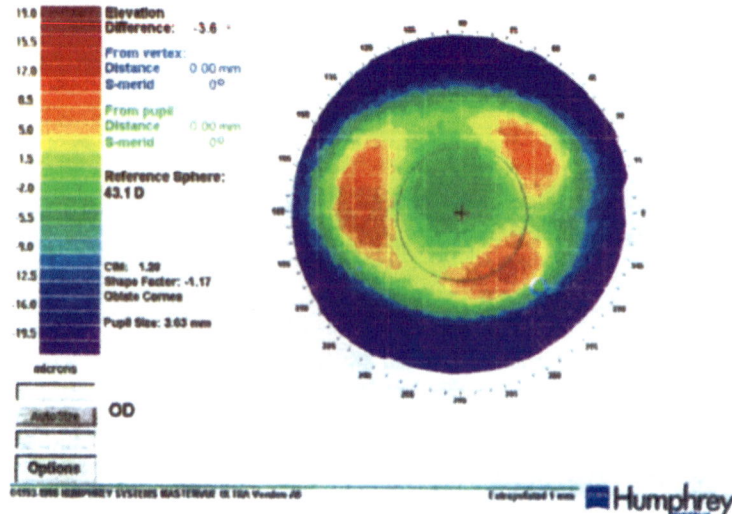

Fig. 10.10: *Elevation map of a post-radial keratotomy (post-RK) patient (Courtesy: Dr Rajib Mukherjee).*

4. Refractive power map

The refractive power map (Fig. 10.11) modified the standard map, taking into account the effects of spherical aberrations. It illustrates how the corneal curvature refracts light in true dioptres of power and not curvature. It uses ray tracings and Snellen's law of optics to perform the calculations.

In it, the spherical cornea has cooler colours in the centre with increasing hotter colours extending out to the periphery (Fig. 10.11). Thus, in true sense, the refractive map should be called the *asphericity map* of the cornea. This map is very useful for determining the optical zone for rigid gas-permeable lenses and also in performing refractive corneal surgery.

5. Irregularity map

The irregularity map (Fig. 10.12) shows areas on cornea that are hot in colour. It displays the distortion of cornea using previous elevation map results with toric reference instead of a

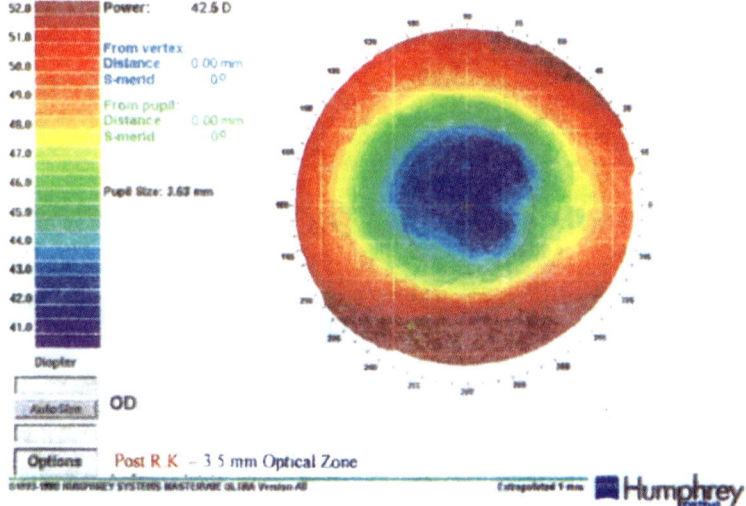

Fig. 10.11: *Refractive power map of a post-RK patient (Courtesy: Dr Rajib Mukherjee).*

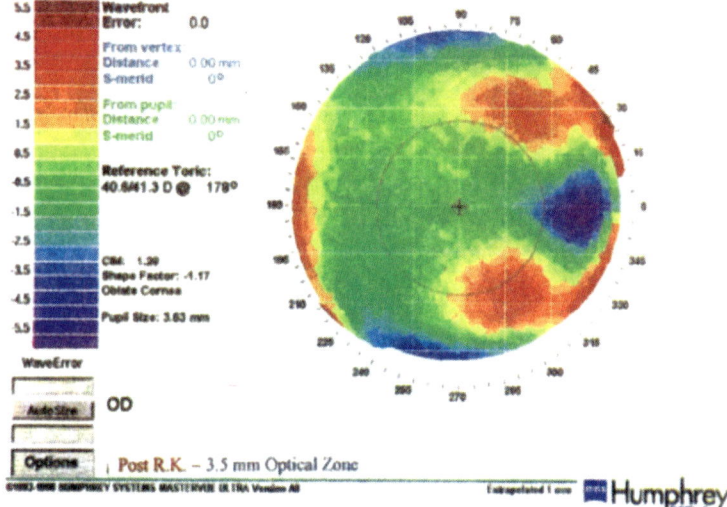

Fig. 10.12: *Irregularity map of a post-RK patient (Courtesy: Dr Rajib Mukherjee).*

reference sphere. The hotter colours represent the higher value of distortion measured in units of wavefront error. The wavefront number can be translated to dioptre of distorted power, known as *spectacle blur*. This map allows the surgeon to quickly assert, if the cornea is causing poor visual acuity. If there is a significant hot colour within the pupil zone, the acuity will be compromised.

6. Trend and time display

In this, changes occurring in topography with time (postoperatively) can be displayed in chronological order (Fig. 10.13).

7. Difference display map

Difference display map (Fig 10.14) exhibits the comparative difference in two given topographic maps.

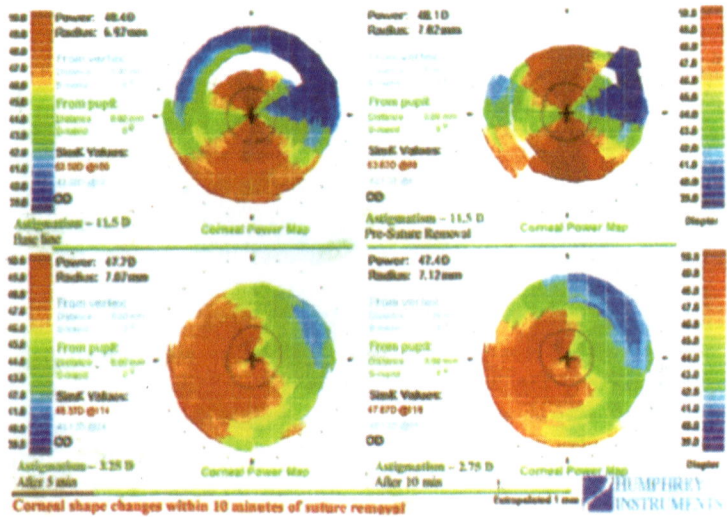

Fig. 10.13: *Trend with time display (Courtesy: Dr Rajib Mukherjee).*

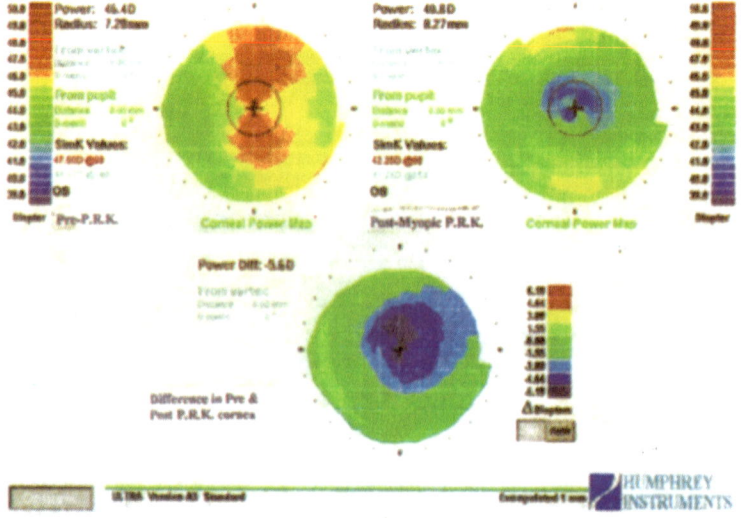

Fig. 10.14: *Difference display map (Courtesy: Dr Rajib Mukherjee).*

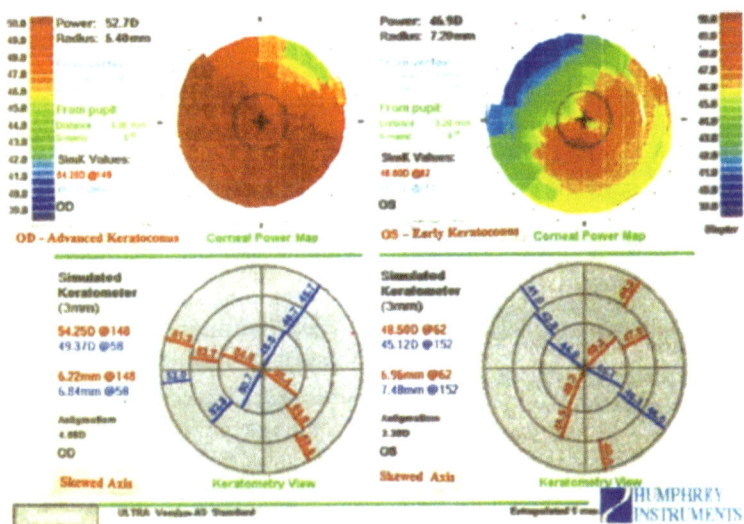

Fig. 10.15: *Right eye/left eye (OD/OS) compare map (Courtesy: Dr Rajib Mukherjee).*

8. Right eye/left eye (OD/OS) compare map
(Fig. 10.15)

Allows comparison of both eyes simultaneously.

SLIT-SCANNING CORNEAL TOMOGRAPHY SYSTEM

Working principle. Slit-imaging' tomography system uses scanning slits that step over the corneal surface to acquire topographic information. This is similar to a slit-lamp in principle. In this principle, an edge point on the corneal surface is triangulated by mathematically intersecting the diffuse reflected edge ray of the camera with the calibrated slit beam surface. Two slits are used, positioned at 45° angles to the right and left of the instrument axis. Twenty slit images are captured from each direction with overlap in a 7 mm diameter central area. Total corneal coverage is up to 10 mm, depending on the individual corneal shape. All images are captured within approximately 1.5 seconds.

In addition to the digital capture of the anterior surface of the cornea, this system is also capable of directly measuring the posterior surface. Thus corneal thickness (defined by the distance between anterior and posterior surface) can be instantly measured at any point on the cornea.

Commercially available system, based on this principle, the Orbscan listed in Table 10.1 is described here.

ORBSCAN III

Orbscan, introduced in 1995, which was later improved in 1999 to Orbscan II and now in 2014 to Orbscan III (Fig. 10.16). It combines the advantages of slit-scanning technology with an advanced Placido-disc system, i.e. it is actually a hybrid system consisting of a projective (slit-

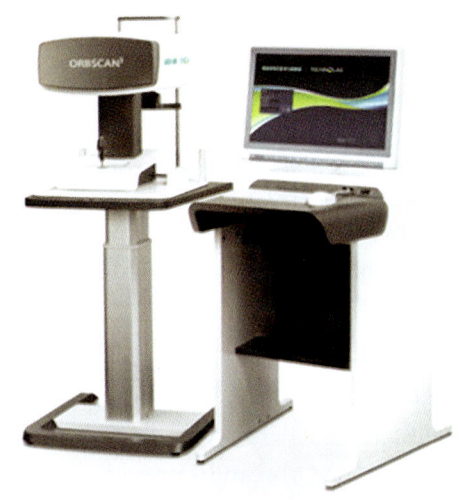

Fig. 10.16: *Orbscan III.*

scanning) and reflective (Placido-disc) technique.

The Orbscan III system uses the principle of projection. Forty scanning slit beams (20 from the left and 20 from the right with up to 240 data points per slit) are used to scan the cornea from limbus to limbus and to measure independently the x, y and z locations of several thousand points on each surface. Orbscan III acquires over 23000 data points as compared to 9000 data points Orbscan II in 1.5 seconds to meticulously map the entire corneal surface (11 mm). The images captured are then used to construct the anterior corneal surface, posterior corneal surface, and anterior iris (white to white diameter) and anterior lens surfaces. Data regarding the corneal pachymetry and anterior chamber depth are also displayed. It also provides pre- and post-operative difference map. The advantage of this system is that slit scan imaging is not dependent on spherical assumption. Eye tracking is used to reduce data error resulting from eye movement.

TOPOGRAPHY MAPS WITH ORBSCAN

The computer calculates a hypothetical sphere that matches as close as possible to the actual corneal shape being measured. This is called the best fit sphere (BFS). It then compares the real surface to the hypothetical sphere, showing areas 'above' the surface of the sphere in warm colours, and areas 'below' the surface in cool colours (Fig. 10.17).

Green is 'sea level' (match with a sphere that best matches the cornea). Warmer colours are above 'sea level'. Cooler colours are below 'sea level'. The normal cornea is prolate, meaning that meridional curvature decreases from centre to periphery. The result is a *central hill of warm colour*. Immediately surrounding the central hill is an annular sea of *cool colours* where the cornea dips below the reference surface. In the far periphery, the prolate cornea again rises above the reference surface, producing *peripheral highlands*.

Functions: The Orbscan III provides:
- Anterior and posterior corneal elevation and curvature

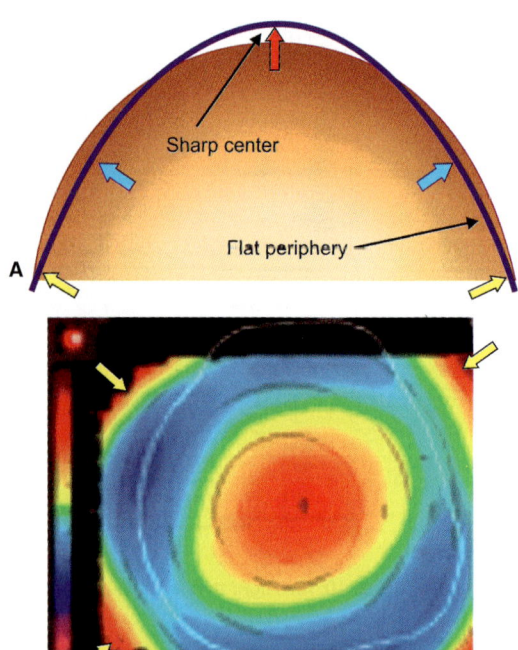

Fig. 10.17: *Orbscan elevation maps: (A) In prolate cornea; (B) In a cylindrical cornea.*

- Full corneal pachymetry
- White to white diameter
- Pre- and post-operative difference maps

Quad map

Quad map refers to the typical Orbscan map which comprises following four different maps, each portraying different information about cornea (Fig 10.18):
- Anterior elevation map (anterior float),
- Posterior elevation map (posterior float),
- Curvature map (axial keratometry map), and
- Pachymetry map.

Anterior elevation map and posterior elevation map

Anterior elevation map, also known as anterior float, and posterior elevation map, also known as posterior float are shown in the top left hand map and top right hand map, respectively, in Fig. 10.18.

As mentioned earlier, slit-scanning provides elevation data, and this can also create a 3D interpretation of the cornea. A 3D interpretation of both elevation maps can be seen in Fig. 10.18.

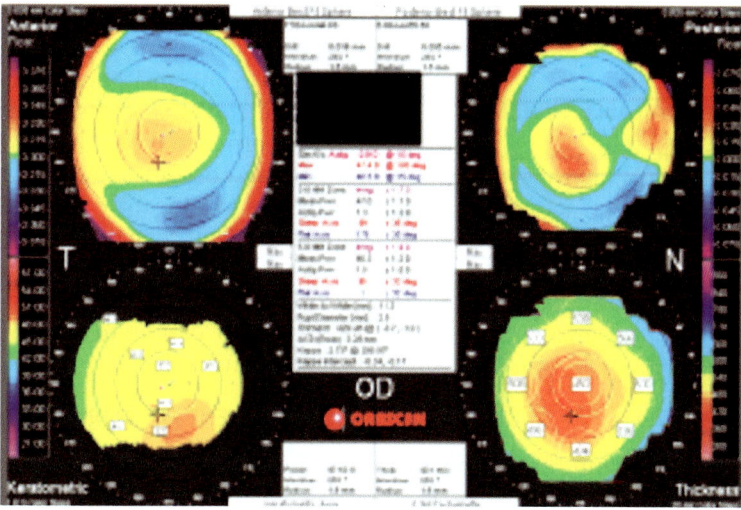

Fig. 10.18: *Orbscan: Quad map.*

The meshwork effect indicates how the cornea would appear, if it were entirely spherical and is referred to as the reference sphere. This elevation data can be interpreted usefully in a number of ways.

Curvature map (axial keratometry map)

The axial keratometry map is based on Placido technology. This is similar to maps produced from the majority of commercially available topography systems, and provides detailed keratometric information across the diameter of the cornea.

For LASIK surgery, this information is important for a number of reasons. The 'K' readings are important, because limits of 'K' readings are between certain values; the cornea must be neither too steep nor too flat. It is difficult for the microkeratome (blade designed for flap cutting), to create a good quality corneal flap in LASIK, if either of these extremes is the case, as this can lead to surgical flap complications.

In addition, 'K' readings of more than 48D are an indication of potential keratoconus, particularly where there is decentred inferonasally. Details of the 'K' readings can be found in the stats and data information in the centre of the quad map.

Pachymetry map

This is map four of our quad map in Fig. 10.18. Traditionally, pachymetry has been measured using ultrasound, which provides a reading of corneal thickness from Bowman's membrane to Descemet's membrane. Through slit-scanning technology, Orbscan provides us with a pachymetry reading from the *precorneal tear film to the endothelium,* therefore, slightly thicker readings can be expected. The Orbscan can, however, be calibrated to take this into consideration when comparing readings. The true advantage of the pachymetry map is that it *provides us with thickness information across the cornea from limbus to limbus, not just* in single points as with ultrasound. This once again gives the opportunity to detect areas of weakness, thinning or scarring. Auffarth et al state that the relationship between the highest point on anterior and posterior elevation maps, and the thinnest point (shown by a yellow dot) is an indicator of keratoconus.

SCHEIMPFLUG IMAGING BASED CORNEAL TOPOGRAPHY SYSTEMS

WORKING PRINCIPLE

Scheimpflug imaging is based on a geometric rule that describes the orientation of the plane of focus of an optical system when the lens plane is not parallel to image plane. In this scenario, an oblique tangent can be drawn from the image, object and lens planes and the point

of intersection is scheimpflug point, where image is in best focus.

COMMERCIALLY AVAILABLE SYSTEMS

Commercially available systems based on the principle are depicted in Table 10.1. Commonly used Scheimpflug imaging-based systems include:

- Pentacam,
- Galilei, and
- Sirius.

PENTACAM

Pentacam, a popular system=based on this principle can obtain 50 images in less than 2 seconds. Each image has 500 true elevation points for a total of 25000 true elevation points for surface of cornea. The pentacam has 2 cameras , one is for detection and measurement of pupil, helps in fixation and orientation. The second camera is used for visualization of anterior segment. Pentacam is able to image both anterior and posterior surface of cornea.

Latest version, Pentacam AXL (oculus optikgerate, Wetzlan, Germany) is the upgraded Pentacam HR, with axial length measurement which allows surgeons, in addition to other features, to make IOL calculations.

CLINICAL APPLICATIONS OF PENTACAM CORNEAL TOPOGRAPHY

- Measurement of corneal shape,
- Measurement of corneal thickness (pachymetry), including relative pachymetry maps.
- Measurement of corneal power.
  - Corneal elevation maps
  - Corneal curvature maps
  - Keratoconus screening
  - Preoperative screening before refractive surgery
  - Corneal wavefront analysis

MEASUREMENT OF CORNEAL SHAPE

Topography includes making a map that describes the elevations and depressions on the surfaces of the cornea similar to the way that a topographic map illustrates the mountains and valleys on a geographic terrain (Fig. 10.19). With the Pentacam, topographic analysis of the corneal front and back surfaces is based on the true elevation measurement from one side of the cornea to the other (limbus to limbus). In addition to the larger area, the Pentacam provides significantly more accurate elevation measurements than other machines. In addition, other Placido-disc-based topographic devices must infer elevation from curvature data. Such inferences can lead to improper medical conclusions.

MEASUREMENT OF CORNEAL THICKNESS (PACHYMETRY)

One of the most important measurements about the cornea besides its shape is the true thickness. Because the Pentacam provides highly accurate information about both the front and back surfaces of the cornea, it is possible to generate 25,000 data points that describe the true thickness of the cornea across its entire breadth and width (Fig. 10.20). This is the ideal as even manual ultrasound pachymetry can only image one single data point making it nearly impossible to provide the amount of thickness detail that can be obtained with the Pentacam.

- *Corneal thickness* is calculated from the top of the epithelium to the anterior surface of the endothelium, excluding the tear film. It is displayed as a color image over its entire area from limbus to limbus.
- The software allows for IOP modification taking into consideration the corneal thickness. This feature is of immense importance for obtaining IOP in post-refractive surgery patients as well as ocular hypertension and glaucoma screening.
- Important parameters like thickness in the center of the pupil, apical corneal thickness and the thinnest location are provided. The distance and position of the thinnest point relative to the apex of the cornea are also available which are useful for early detection of keratoconus.
- *Anterior chamber analysis* includes a calculation of the chamber angle, chamber volume and chamber height and a manual measuring function at any location in the anterior chamber of the eye.

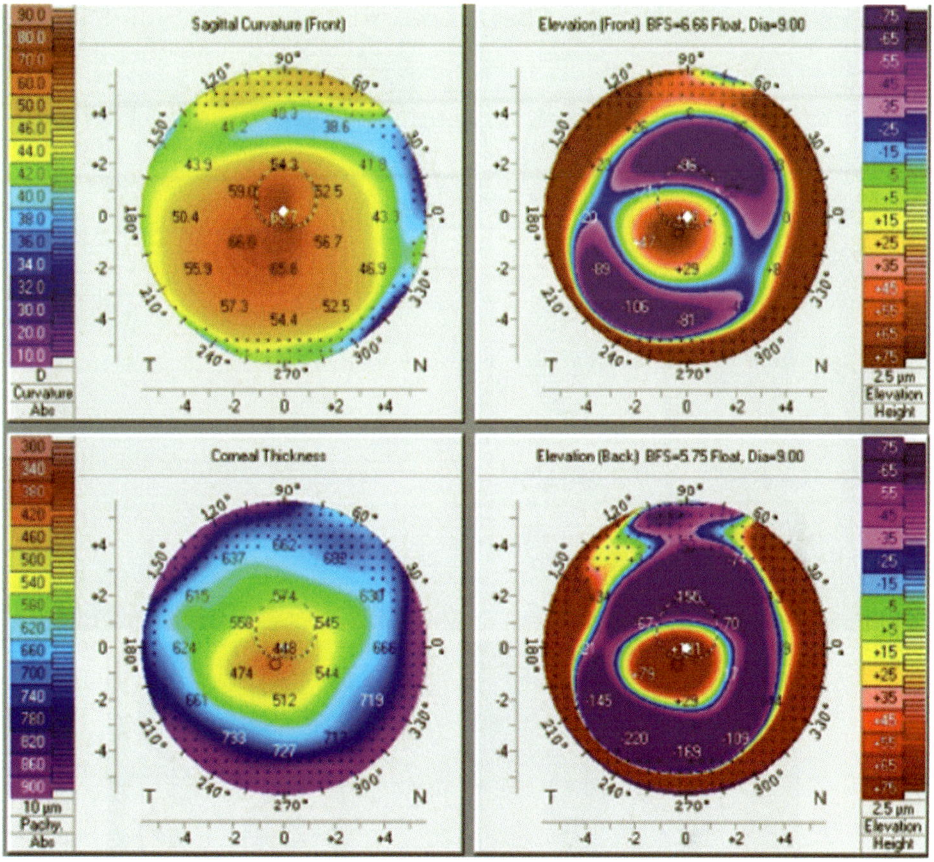

Fig. 10.19: *Pentacam: Corneal topography.*

- *It has availability of 2 map and 4 map comparisons and numerical analysis of anterior segment progression* which is useful to compare preoperative and postoperative results in refractive surgeries and also see the long-term progression follow-up in patients undergoing collagen crosslinking.

- The *corneal thickness spatial profile and percentage thickness increase graphs* describe the annular pachymetric increase from the thinnest point. These graphs are available on the Pentacam and have been successfully used.

- *Pachymetric progression indices (PPI)* are calculated for all hemimeridia over the entire 360° of the cornea, so that the average of all meridians (PPI-Ave) and the *meridian with maximal (PPI Max) pachymetric increase* are noted.

- *Ambrosio's relational thickness (ART) is calculated as the ratio between the thinnest point and*

PPI. The "ART" concept combines thinnest with the pachymetric distribution, which facilitates the identification of an abnormal cornea despite its thinnest value. The Ambrósio Relational Thickness (ART) is calculated for the average and maximal progression indices (ART-Ave and ART-Max). The best cut-offs for the diagnosis of keratoconus are 339 for ART-Max and 427 μm for ART-Ave. For detecting ectasia susceptibility, we use 391 μm for ART-Max and 512 μm for ART-Ave. Practically, it is best not to perform LASIK, if ART-Max is lower than 400 μm

- *Belin/Ambrósio Display (BAD)* considers the deviations of normality values for different parameters, so that a value of zero represents the average of the normal population and one represents the value is one SD toward the disease (ectasia) value. A final 'D' is

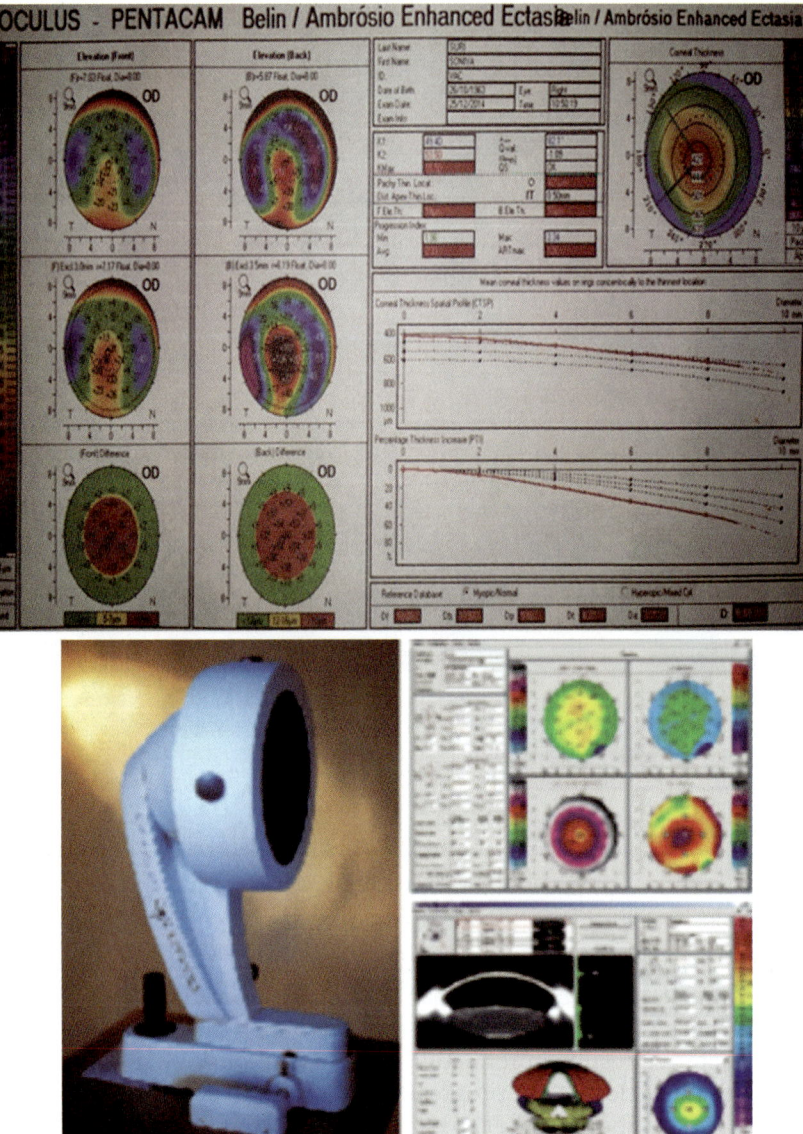

Fig. 10.20: *Pentacam analysis including pachymetry.*

calculated based on a regression analysis that weights differently the parameters.

♦ *Belin/Ambrósio Display (BAD) II* software package features an enhanced reference surface that excludes the 3.5 to 4 mm area centred on the thinnest part of the cornea in order to eliminate the ectatic regions or "mountains". The goal of the BAD was to combine elevation based and pachymetric corneal evaluation in one comprehensive display to give the clinician a global view of the tomographic structure of the cornea.

MEASUREMENT OF CORNEAL POWER

Scheimplug imaging can also be used to measure corneal power, which is of interest to surgeons performing cataract surgery. This application is especially useful in patients following excimer keratorefractive surgery, in which the relationship between the anterior and posterior surfaces is altered yielding inaccurate keratometry readings required for intraocular lens (IOL) calculation. For example, following myopic LASIK, an overestimation of keratometry readings causes an underestimation of IOL power resulting in hyperopic outcomes. Conversely, following hyperopic PRK, an underestimation of the keratometry readings causes an overestimation of the IOL power resulting in myopic outcomes.

Keratoconus screening

Pentacam is the only technology which gives the direct measurement of elevation data and hence detection of keratoconus. There is an in-built keratoconus screening software which also helps in grading of keratoconus (KK1-4).

Preoperative screening before refractive surgery

Pentacam has facility for preoperative screening before refractive surgery to exclude ectasia and formefruste. Diagnostic criteria for detecting Formefruste based on magnitude of elevation maps put forth by Michel W. Belin is as follows:

- Normal values for anterior elevation are differences less than +12 µm
  - Between +12 and +15 µm are suspicious
  - Greater than +15 µm indicate keratoconus.
- Normal values for posterior elevation are approximately 5 µm higher than those for anterior elevation.

Corneal wavefront analysis

The anterior and posterior corneal surface is described separately by Zernike polynomials based on the measured elevation data. Together the corneal wavefront analysis and keratoconus detection improve the preoperative screening for patients who are interested in refractive surgery as well as the postoperative progression control.

ADVANTAGES OF PENTACAM

Advantages of pentacam as corneal topographer include:

- Higher resolution of central cornea
- Measure surface irregularities-keratoconus
- Calculate pachymetry from limbus to limbus
- Wavefront analysis to detect higher porder aberrations.

OCULAR COHERENCE TOMOGRAPHY-BASED CORNEAL TOMOGRAPHY

Ocular coherence tomography (OCT) of the cornea is an optical method of cross-sectional scanning based on reection and scattering of light from the structures within the cornea. *Optical interferometry* is *used to generate a log rectivity prole*. Each peak of the prole corresponds to specic layers of the cornea. Low coherence interferometry achieves axial resolutions from 3 to 20 µm using a noncontact technique. A large area can be imaged in a single scan, and the images have been used to identify the thickness of the corneal epithelium, LASIK flap, intra-corneal ring segment depth, and three-dimensional structure of the cornea under normal or pathologic conditions with precision. A sample image is shown in Fig. 10.21A.

COMMERCIALLY AVAILABLE OCT SYSTEMS

Commercially available OCT systems for corneal tomography includes (Table 10.1):

- *VisanteOmni* (Carl Zeiss Meditec, Germany). It is based on rotating optical coherence tomography and Placido-disc imaging.
- *SS1000 Casia* (Tomey Corp, Japan). It is based on rotating optical coherence tomography.
- *RTVue-100* (Optovue, Fremont, USA). It is based on spectral Domain Optical Coherence Tomography guided corneal power measurement (both anterior and posterior curvatures).
- *IOL Master 700* (Carl Zeiss Meditec, Germany). It is based on swept Source OCT Technology with 32-Marker Placido pattern.

VERY HIGH FREQUENCY ULTRASOUND CORNEAL TOMOGRAPHY SYSTEM

Artemis 3 imaging machine (Arescan, Morrison, Colorado) is a very high frequency (VHF) ultrasound biomicroscope which allows corneal tomographic study. VHF ultrasound scans a series of meridia in an arc motion matched to

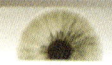

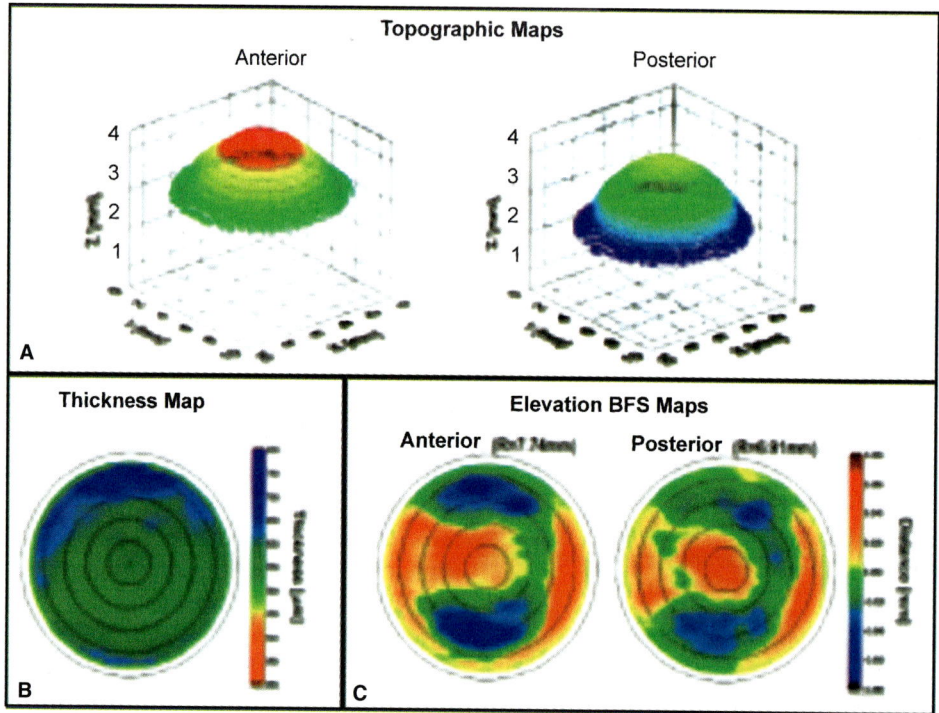

Fig. 10.21: *Corneal topography with anterior segment OCT.*

the curvature of the cornea. This allows measurement of the thickness of individual corneal layers over an 8–10 μm zone in three dimensions, as seen in Fig. 10.21B. This technology can produce topographic maps of the individual corneal layers, such as the epithelium, and the stroma. It has been reported that the topographic information can guide free cap replacement based on epithelial irregularities. This system has been shown to measure flap thickness with high reproducibility.

DIGITAL RASTERSTEREOGRAPHY-BASED TOPOGRAPHY SYSTEMS

Rasterstereography-based CTS uses a calibrated grid which is projected o to the corneal surface and the diffuse reflection is recorded at two separate known angles. Commercially available *PAR CTS* is based on this technology.

PAR CTS

The PAR CTS from PAR Microsystems Inc., PAR Vision Systems Corp., New Hartford, New York,

uses close range photogrammetry (rasterphotogrammetry) to measure and produce a corneal topographic map. A grid pattern of horizontal and vertical lines spaced 0.2 mm apart is used.

Corneal rasterphotogrammetry involves imaging of a projected grid on to the cornea. A modified operating room microscope or slit-lamp, as described by Warnick et al. can be utilized. PAR Technology (New Hartford, New York) records video images of the projected grid to give a corneal topography map. Sodium fluorescein is added to the tear film and is excited by blue light which causes a grid pattern to become visible on the cornea. This is then imaged by the camera and analysed by a digital image processor using algorithms to give information about corneal topography. The accuracy of the system is 0.3 D for a diameter of 7 mm. The contour plots of the cornea appear like keratographs, but actually each line is an isopter, representing areas of equal height on the corneal surface. The advantage of this system over the keratoscopic one is that it includes information across the whole of the cornea and even includes part of the sclera. Furthermore, the projected nature of the test does not allow interference due to corneal surface or stromal defects.

Note. This system is not much in use presently.

 LASER HALOGRAPHIC INTERFEROMETRY-BASED TOPOGRAPHY SYSTEMS

Working principle. Laser halographic interfero-metry-based CTS relies on sophisticated optical techniques of *'light wave interference' fringes as projection device.* The commercially available CTS, the Corneal Lens Analysis System II (CLAS II) unit, is based on this technique.

CLAS II UNIT

It is a non-Placido-disc-based CTS machine which is based on the technology of laser holographic interferometry. The CLAS II applies three-dimensional imaging to the analysis of corneal surface changes. The object and reference beams are not split. Instead they oscillate at the same frequency and remain in phase with each other, thus minimizing the effects of vibration. The CLAS II analyses optical aberrations from reflecting surface by measuring the optical path difference (OPD). This is a measurement of the different path that light takes when it is reflected from a surface.

Note. This system is not much in use presently.

CLINICAL APPLICATIONS AND LIMITATIONS OF CORNEAL TOPOGRAPHY SYSTEMS

CLINICAL APPLICATIONS

1. Role in early diagnosis of corneal diseases

Computer-assisted videokeratography is helpful in diagnosing following conditions in early stages, i.e. before they could have been diagnosed otherwise:

- Keratoconus
- Epithelial dystrophies and other epitheliopathies
- Terrien's marginal degeneration
- Pellucid marginal degeneration.

2. Topography and contact lenses

- Corneal topographic analysis helps in giving a comfortable fit in routine contact lens practice, particularly in rigid contact lens fitting, thus providing maximum possible visual correction.
- It is of unquestioned help in contact lens fitting of difficult cases such as:
  - Postkeratoplasty
  - Keratoconus
  - Postradial keratotomy
  Other conditions with irregular astigmatism.
- It also helps in early diagnosis of contact-lens-induced changes in cornea like central irregular astigmatism, corneal warpage and loss of radial symmetry. These changes are usually reversible.
- The practitioner and contact lens manufacturer can use corneal topography to verify contact lens specifications, however, complex they may be.

3. Topography in keratoconus

- One of the most useful applications of corneal topography is the *detection of keratoconus* before the appearance of slit-lamp findings.
- Topography has helped a lot in *understanding the features of keratoconus.* Before the introduction of this technique, keratoconus was described as having two basic shapes: oral and nipple type. Videokeratography has demonstrated that corneal shape is more complex than was previously described.
- Classically, keratoconus is depicted as a localized area of increased surface power, surrounded by concentric zones of decreased surface power (Fig. 10.22). The area of steepening may occur anywhere on the cornea. Most frequently, initial involvement is seen in inferotemporal quadrant with superior half of the cornea remaining normal at this stage. Thereafter, the steepening spreads nasally, and then eventually to the superotemporal cornea. The superonasal cornea is the last part to be affected.
- *Contact lens fitting in keratoconus,* which otherwise is very difficult, is facilitated by topography studies.

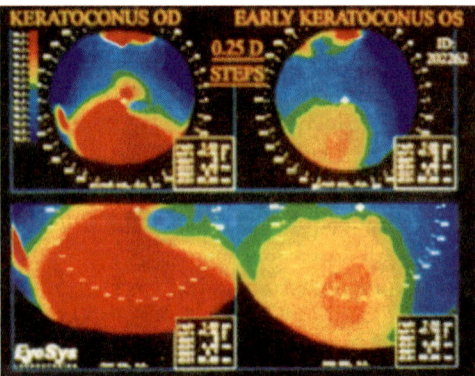

Fig. 10.22: *Corneal topography colour map in a patient with bilateral keratoconus.*

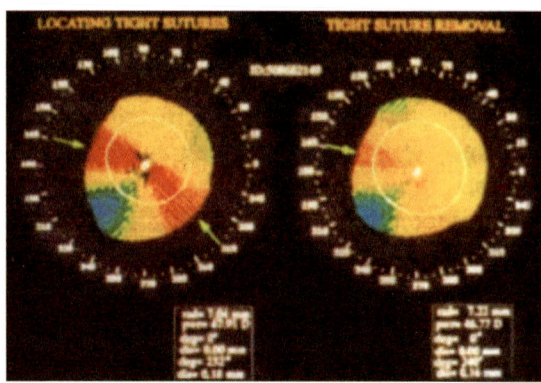

Fig. 10.23: *Corneal topography colour map in a patient with postpenetrating keratoplasty (tight suture at 1658).*

- Videographic analysis of family members of patients with keratoconus has demonstrated a mild form of disease without any overt clinical signs. This was called *formefruste* by Amsler.

4. Topography in RK

- The role of corneal topography in RK is in evaluating the cornea pre- and postoperatively, i.e. to understand better the mechanics of surgery and, therefore, to further improve the predictability of the procedure in future. *Preoperative topography* reveals that corneas with same central curvature given by keratometer may have markedly different shapes, i.e. prolate, oblate and spherical. *Postoperative topography* reveals flattening of the entire cornea with only relative peripheral steepening.
- *Repeat RK surgery*, when required, can be better planned with the help of colour-coded maps.
- *Contact lens fitting post-RK* can be a problem wherein the keratometric methods would lead to a very flat fit based on central corneal curvature measurements. Corneal topographic methods of contact lens fitting allow peripheral corneal topography evaluation and thus, the prescription of a steeper lens based on these curvatures.

5. Role of topography in postkeratoplasty astigmatism

- *Removal of tight sutures* for control of post-penetrating keratoplasty (PK) astigmatism has

been facilitated by the advent of corneal topography (Fig. 10.23).
- *Corneal relaxing incisions* when required to manage post-PK astigmatism are better planned with topographic evaluation. After the advent of topography, the relaxing incision is placed at the steepest corneal meridian at the steepest point and not at the graft–host interface as was advocated earlier.
- If topography reveals excessive corneal flattening due to wound gap (diagnosed by the typical tear drop formation on videokeratographic image), then wound revision and wedge resection may be indicated instead of relaxing incision 90°away.
- *Post-PK contact lens fitting* by corneal topographic analysis has shown better results as compared to lens selection based on keratometric finding.

6. Role of topography in PRK and LASIK

Corneal topography is virtually indispensable for performing photorefractive keratectomy (PRK) and laser-assisted *in situ* keratomileusis (LASIK). Keratorefractive surgery in general has been made more predictable with the use of corneal topography.

- Videokeratography is not only essential for screening candidates for these procedures, but it also provides important information about the quality of ablation zone, the diameter of the ablated zone, centration of the ablation and the stability of topographic alterations.

- Differential topographic maps are used to give the desired dioptric change in the corneal power.
- *Decentration of the ablation* zone detected on postoperative topography might explain post-operative halo or glare effect.
- *Irregular ablation zones* (as is seen in central islands) often explain decreased visual acuity and decreased quality of vision after these procedures. Recognition of these abnormal zones has resulted in modification of the procedures to prevent their occurrence.

7. Other applications of topography

- *IOL power calculation* can be done more accurately by employing the corneal topography to measure the necessary K value, instead of using the conventional keratometer.
- *Laser pachymetry* for corneal thickness is possible with *corneal modelling systems*, using a dual beam scanning laser slit-lamp.
- *Corneal topographic analysis* can be stored to show the pre- and postoperative conditions for self-study and patient satisfaction purposes.

LIMITATIONS

Though quite useful and advanced, computerized corneal topography does have some limitations:

1. *Algorithms for power calculation* are based on spherical optical systems, which may lead to qualitative and quantitative erroneous interpretations as the normal cornea is aspheric.
2. The *correlation between corneal curvature and power* (as shown by colour-coded maps) is valid for spheres and elliptical surfaces as long as there are no areas of abrupt transition in corneal curvature. If abrupt transition exists, software directly showing the surface elevation is more accurate than one that back calculates it from dioptric files. In fact, manufacturers have been advised to display colour curvature maps instead of colour dioptric maps.
3. *Data is averaged across meridia*, thus tending to magnify the 'blend' zones rather than show the sharp boundaries, if present, e.g. in pre- and postoperative PRK patients.

4. *The formulae employed* for power calculation are centred on the corneal apex and not on the more relevant line of sight.
5. *Central corneal power is interpolated* from central rings and it may give overestimations in cases of oblate corneas.
6. The *keratometric index of refraction (1.3375)* usually employed underestimates the changes in corneal power after procedures like PRK, as the actual index of refraction of the cornea is 1.376.
7. Videokeratography maps after an unsuccessful PRK may not show a change in corneal topography based on corneal surface, although a change in corneal thickness has taken place.
8. Placido-disc-based computerized videokeratographic instruments have *problems of critical focus* and inability to measure highly irregular corneas.

ABERROMETRY AND WAVEFRONT TECHNOLOGY

ABERRATIONS

Although the human eye is an optical marvel, yet it suffers many deviations from being an ideal optical system. All forms of deviations (refractive errors) are basically aberrations. Aberrations can be grouped as below:

I. *Lower order aberrations* include myopia, hypermetropia and regular astigmatism. These aberrations can be understood without sophisticated analytical methods and surgically can be treated by conventional LASIK. LOA constitute 85% of aberrations. There are three types of LOA:

- Tilt of prism
- Defocus
- Astigmatic aberration

II. *Higher order aberrations* are subtle deviations from the ideal optical system. These constitute 5% of aberrations of the eye and include spherical aberrations, chromatic aberrations, coma, decentring, oblique aberration and centring.

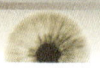

The higher order aberrations do not lend themselves to easy solutions. Thus, the higher order aberrations limit the potential visual acuity of the eye. It is a well-known fact that the retina has a much higher resolving power and a much better potential visual acuity of about 6/2–6/1.5, but this is greatly reduced by diffraction of light and the aberrations of the eye.

RAY ABERRATIONS VERSUS WAVE ABERRATIONS

There are two ways to analyse aberrations: ray aberrations and wave aberrations.

RAY ABERRATIONS

Ray aberrometry is based on Snell's law. Ideally, all rays from a single object point converge to a single image point. This ideal is never achieved in practice due to aberrations. In ray aberrometry, an imaginary plane is located near the desired image point and the intersection of each ray with the plane is plotted as a spot diagram (Fig. 10.24). Usually spot diagrams are generated for several planes in front of, at and behind the image, yielding a set of through focus spot diagrams. The advantage of the spot diagram is that it gives an immediate visual representation of the total amount of aberration present and the image quality. However, spot diagrams are more difficult to interpret when several aberrations are present, as is usually the case in most optical systems, including the eye. Therefore, in practice, ray aberrometry is not much popular.

WAVE ABERRATIONS

Wavefront refers to any isochronic surface associated with a specific object point. The term

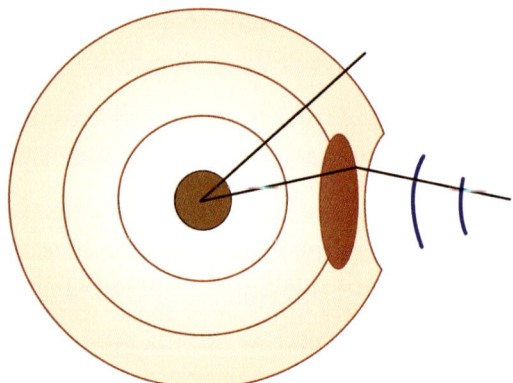

Fig. 10.25: *Diagrammatic depiction of wavefront associated with only one object point. Note that all light from a single object point reaches the wavefront simultaneously. Also note that rays are perpendicular to the wavefront.*

isochronic means equal time. Thus, the amount of time required for light to travel from a specified object point to the wavefront is equal for all rays (Fig. 10.25). Note that wavefront is associated with only one object point. Wavefront and rays are two different but closely related ways of representing how light propagates through an optical system. In fact the rays are perpendicular to the wavefront. Thus, given the shape of the wavefront, the direction of any light ray can be calculated. Conversely, from the direction of light rays, the shape of wavefront can be calculated.

Wave aberrations. In a perfect optical system, there are no distortions induced by the lens system. The ideal wavefront of the perfect optical system thus has spherical shape. The wavefront aberration refers to the OPD between the actual image wavefront and the ideal spherical wavefront. Since the wavefront aberration is the difference between two surfaces, therefore, its surface is usually shaped somewhat like a potato chip.

ZERNIKE'S POLYNOMIALS AND ZERNICK'S TERMS

The monochromatic aberrations are defined and quantified in terms of what are known as Zernick's polynomials (ZPs), consisting of Zernick's terms (ZT) and associated spot diagrams.

Using the wavefront sensor method, the aberrations up to 10th order of ZP have been

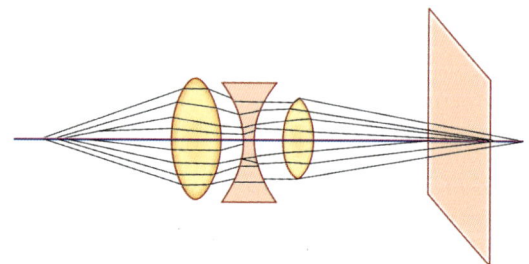

Fig. 10.24: *Ray aberrations and formation of spot diagram in relation to an imaginary plane located near the desired image point.*

determined. However, for 3 mm pupils, aberrations up to 4th order of ZP are important and the aberrations beyond 4th order are small and have minimal effect on image quality. For 7.3 mm large pupils, the 5th to 8th order aberrations have substantial contribution to the deterioration of image quality. Zernicke coefficient is an expression of the amount of each individual aberration. Equations are used to calculate ZC for each polynomials.

The most important and commonly encountered 1st to 4th orders of ZP consist of 14 Zernick's terms (ZT).

Zero to 5th order ZPs are as below (Fig. 10.26):
- *0 order ZP* is also called *piston error*. It consists of the term ZT 0. It has no clinical equivalent and is not significant.
- *1st order ZP* is also called *tilt*. The clinical equivalent is prism and it consists of terms ZT 1 and 2.
- *2nd order ZP*. It corresponds to classical *spherocylindrical correction of refractive errors* and consists of ZT 3.4 and 5. ZT 4 equals *spherical correction* that corrects the optical aberration of *defocus*. ZT 3–5 equals *astigmatism*.

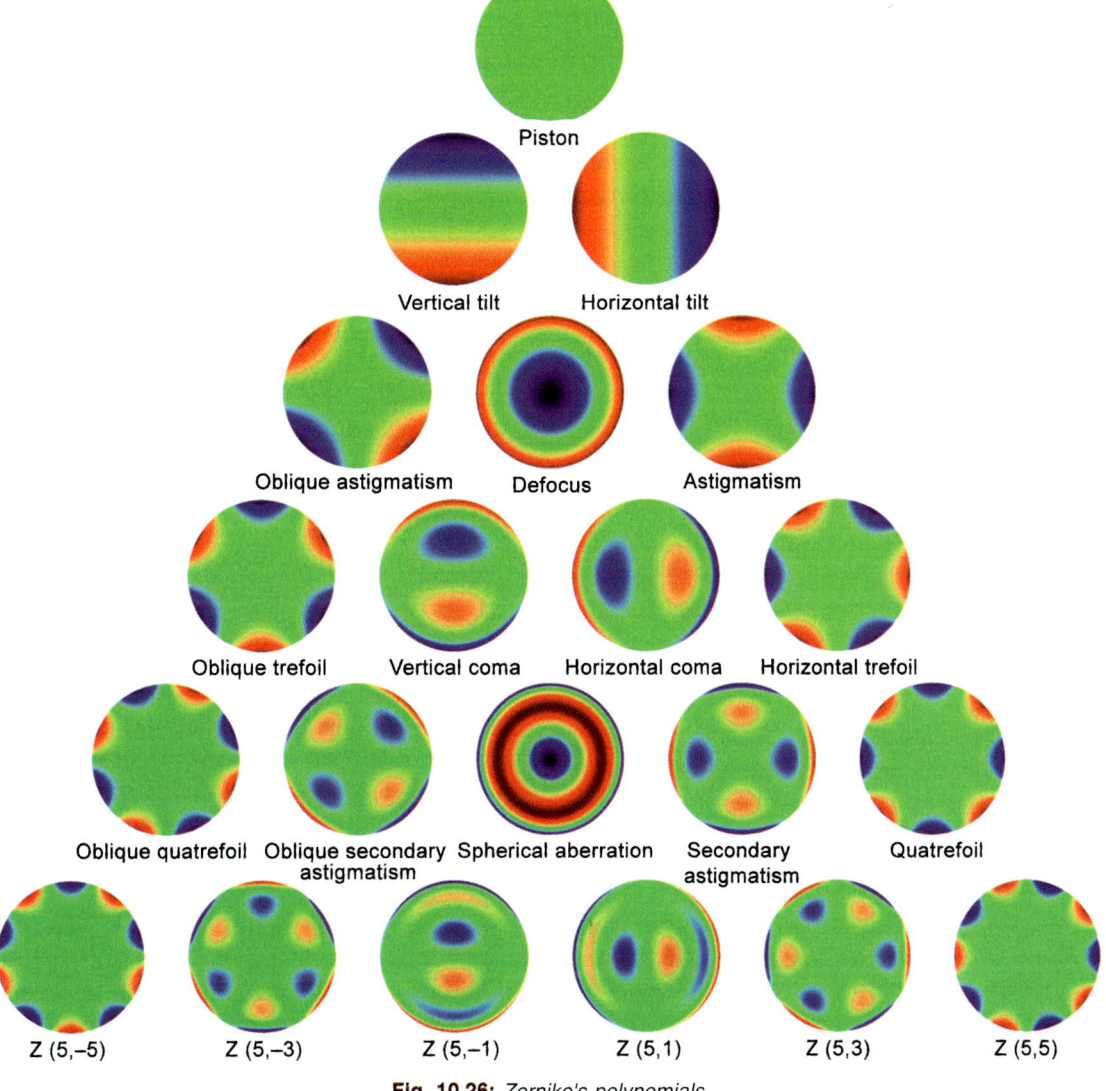

Fig. 10.26: *Zernike's polynomials.*

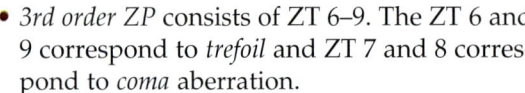

- *3rd order ZP* consists of ZT 6–9. The ZT 6 and 9 correspond to *trefoil* and ZT 7 and 8 correspond to *coma* aberration.
- *4th order ZP* consists of ZT 10–14. ZT 10 and 14 correspond to *quadrapoil* and ZT 11, 12 and 13 correspond to *spherical aberrations.*
- *5th order ZP* consists of ZT 15–20 and corresponds to *secondary coma.*

Note. In normal human eyes of young patients, the contribution to higher order aberrations is as below:

- 3rd order ZP – 40%
- 4th order ZP – 25%
- 5th and 6th order ZP – 30%

OCULAR WAVEFRONT

A wavefront is the locus of points characterized by propagation of position of the same phase: a propagation of a line in 1D, a curve in 2D or a surface for a wave in 3D. The understanding of the optical quality of the eye is becoming more accurate with the ability to precisely measure the lower and higher order wave aberrations using ocular wavefront sensing techniques. Reliable measurements of the ocular wave aberration also make it possible to correct these aberrations to improve visual performance.

TOTAL OCULAR WAVEFRONT VERSUS CORNEAL WAVEFRONT

The total ocular wavefrontis equal to corneal wavefront plus internal wavefront. Thus, the corneal wavefront is one of the components of the *total ocular wavefront* which can be calculated from the corneal topographic height data, using an algorithm. An algorithm is the calculous procedure used to reconstruct corneal geometry from the calculation of the position of points on the corneal surface relative to axis or a reference sphere.

OPTICAL PATH DIFFERENCE

Optical path difference (OPD) refers to the difference between the corneal wavefront and an ideal wavefront. It is similar to the spherical offset which is the height difference between the cornea and a sphere. The OPD forms the basis of corneal wavefront theories.

In ray tracing, the Snell's law is applied to the corneal surface to calculate OPD. Rays are traced from the fovea out of the eye. In the time, a ray travels 3 μm in the cornea, it travels for 4 μm in air. Thus, the *rule of 3*, i.e. every 3 μm of distortion from the ideal shape of the cornea will produce a 11 μm difference in the OPD map and a –1 μm difference in the wavefront error map.

CORNEAL WAVEFRONT MAP

Corneal wavefront map created from the corneal topography can be fitted with a ZP decomposition in the same way that total ocular wavefront is measured by aberrometry and fitted with the same polynomial decomposition. Further, the corneal wavefront map can be broken down into and viewed as:

- Zernike's coefficient
- PSF
- Simulated vision chart
- Modulation transfer function (like contrast sensitivity)
- A street where the patient can see a street scene simulated pre- and post-operatively. This is particularly important for the patients undergoing treatment on highly aberrated corneas to realize the meaning of wavefront and how it adds sharpness to the vision.

FACTORS AFFECTING TOTAL OCULAR WAVEFRONT

Total aberrations of the eye as measures by wavefront analyses are affected by following factors:

1. Age. Total ocular wavefront varies with age, as the aberrations increase with age due to change in both crystalline lens and the cornea. Note that the aberrations of cornea and crystalline lens neutralize each other in the young people. With the increase in age, this balance is lost and thus aberrations of the eye are increased.

2. Size of pupil. The total ocular wavefront map obtained with Hartmann-Shack sensor depends upon the size of the pupil. The pupil becomes small in size with age, which may somewhat offset the increase in aberration occurring with increase in age.

Therefore, the increase in total ocular wavefront aberration with dilatation of the pupil is more significant in the elderly. Aberrations, particularly coma, depend greatly on pupil centration. The change in pupil size with change in illumination due to effect of mydriatics/miotics shifts the pupil centration and thus changes the aberrations.

3. *Accommodation*. Due to changes in the shape, position and alignment of the lens with respect to pupil and cornea during accommodation, there occurs change in the wavefront aberrations.

4. *Chromatic aberration*. Presently used aberrometers are laser based, which can measure aberrations at only one wavelength. Thus, the chromatic aberration, one of the eye's major optical defects, is not measured by the clinically used aberrometers.

5. *Tear film*. Any local change in the tear film affects the ocular aberrations. Such an effect is more prominent in individuals with tear film anomalies, specially the dry eye.

6. *Misalignment of the eyes* during wavefront aberrometry affects the accuracy of measurement. Alignment of the eyes is especially critical for higher order aberrations.

7. *Refractive errors*, especially when large, affect the measurement of higher order aberrations. This is because the lower order aberrations affect the image quality much more than the higher order aberrations.

Note. It is important to note that corneal wavefront in contrast to total ocular wavefront is:

- Relatively stable over time and allows serial measurement
- Not affected by pupil diameter
- Not affected by accommodation.

MEASUREMENT UNIT OF ABERRATIONS

Measurement unit of aberrations is microns, which is a point-wise measure of the amount of light that is advanced or retarded with reference to a plane. The integrated or total amount of distortion from a reference surface is measured with root means square (RMS), commonly used mathematical method for reporting distortions.

- RMSg (gross): has to be correlated with manifest refraction.
- RMSh (higher): > 0.2 µ needs to be evaluated.
- RMSg lower order + higher order aberrations.

WAVEFRONT ABERROMETRY

Aberrometry refers to analysis of optical aberrations. The analysis of higher order aberrations including irregular astigmatism requires advanced technology. Until recently, there was no need to analyse these defects in detail. However, recently aberrometry has become clinically important, since the progress in imaging and refractive surgery may allow the correction of certain aberrations.

Wavefront aberrometry or the so-called wavefront technology is more popular in clinical practice and is in many ways easier than the ray aberrometry. Wavefront aberrometry refers to measurement of aberrations in the optical system of the eye by wavefront analysis. All methods of measuring the aberrations of the human eye evaluate how the light that enters the eye is modified. With each of these approaches, light is imaged on to the retina, and either the image position on the retina or the wavefront as it emerges from the eye is measured.

Commercially available aberrometers, listed in Table 10.1, can be classified into following types and according to operating principle:

  I. Backward/outgoing projection type
    - Hartmann-Shack aberrometry
  II. Forward/ingoing projection tyoe
    - Tscherning aberroscope
    - Ray-tracing aberrometry.

1. HARTMANN-SHACK ABERROMETRY

Hartmann–Shack style aberrometers are currently the most commonly used. In such devices, a single laser beam is projected as a spot on the retina (Fig. 10.27A) and the reflected bundle of rays passes through the optical system of the eye. It is then picked up by an array of small lenslets, which focus these rays into spots on an array of a CCD camera, very much like the compound eye of an insect (Fig. 10.27B). Then the mosaic of spots is used to define the wavefront and analyse its

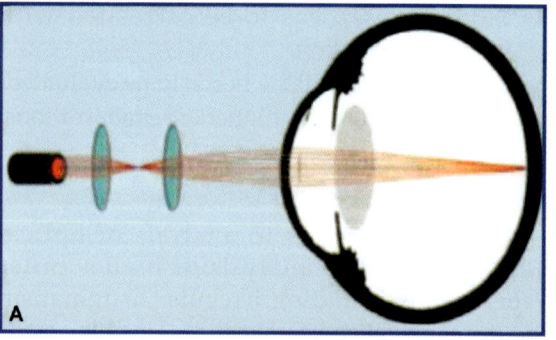 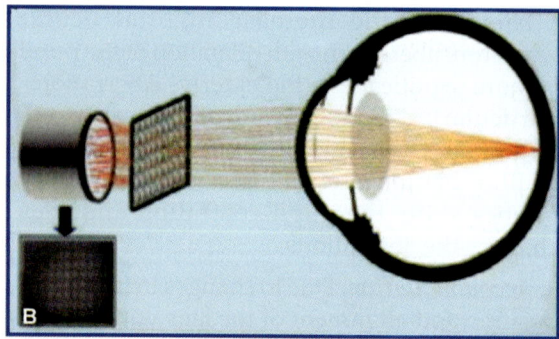

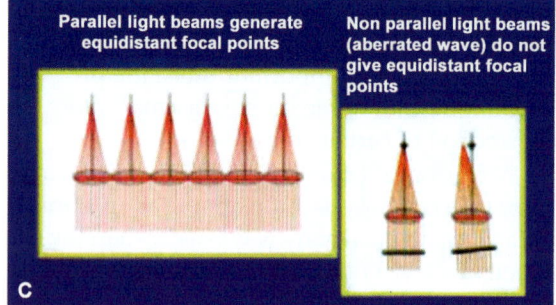 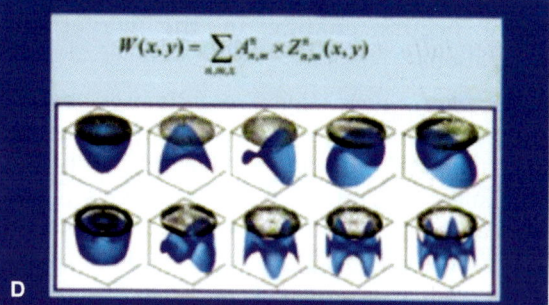

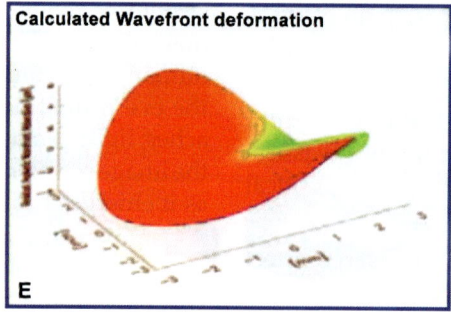

Fig. 10.27: *Optics of wavefront aberrometer: (A) A narrow laser beam is focused to the retina to generate a point source; (B) Array of small lenses focusing the outcoming light ray from the retina on the charge-coupled device camera; (C) D etermination of the wavefront deformation by analyzing the direction of the light ray; (D) Various shapes of wavefronts represented as a sum of Zernick's polynomials; (E) Wavefront pattern of astigmatism polynomials.*

deformation (Fig. 10.27C). The position, the pattern and the PSF of each spot are then analysed and a colour-coded picture of the wavefront is generated by the aberrometer. The shape of the wavefront is represented as a sum of ZPs, each describing a certain deformation (Fig. 10.27D). As an example, the wavefront pattern for astigmatism is shown in Fig. 10.27E.

Commercially available aberrometers based on Hartmann-Shack principle include:
- LASAR wave, (Alcon)
- Zywave 3, as part of Zyoptix Diofnest work station 3, i.e. ZDW³ (Bausch and Lomb)

- Waves can wavefront system (VISX)
- Corneal Wavefront Analyser (Schwind Eyetech Solution)
  - Waves can wavefront system (AMO)
  - Wavelight Oculyzer II (ALCON)
  - Alleye Oculyzer.

2. TSCHERNING ABERROSCOPE

Tscherning aberroscope is basically an ingoing retinal imaging aberrometer. In it, a bundle of equidistant light rays is shone on cornea, which is imaged on the retina. A low-light CCD camera linked to a computer is used to analyse the pattern of spots observed on the retina by a method similar to indirect ophthalmoscopy.

Retinal pattern observed is as below:
- *In a theoretically aberration-free eye*, the retinal pattern consists of equidistant spots corresponding to the incident pattern.
- *In a normal eye*, in clinical practice, the retinal pattern observed is distorted due to the presence of aberrations. The CCD measures the deviation of each spot from the ideal equidistant position.

Commercially available aberrometer based on Tscherning principle includes:
- Allergreto (from wavelight).

3. RAY-TRACING ABERROMETRY

In this system, pattern of one ray, rather than all rays at the same time, is analysed. In fact, a point incident on the retina and the location of its conjugate focus is analysed with reference to the ideal conjugate focus point. This decreases the chance of crossing the rays in highly aberrated eyes. The wavefront map is calculated from the many such points measured separately. The total time of scanning is 10–40 milliseconds.

Commercially available device based on Ray-tracing principle is:
- NIDEK OPD Scan III (from Nidek)
- i-Trace (Tracy Technologies, USA).

iTRACE SYSTEM

The iTrace system (Tracey Technologies, Houston, Tx) is a combination of ray tracing aberrometry and Placido's disk corneal topography to measure the total aberrations of the eye. It is a serial, double pass and forward projection type retinal image aberrometer. A topographer is added in the same unit as the aberrometer to measure the corneal aberrations.

Principle of iTrace

- Ray-tracing aberrometry measures forward aberrations of the light going through the eye. So, it is more physiological as the natural trajectory of the light is being analyzed.
- The iTrace uses this principle of Ray Tracing where a sequential series of infrared beams on the order of 100 microns and a 785 nm wavelength each is projected into the entrance pupil parallel to the eye's line of sight. In Fig. 10.28, a diagram of the ray-tracing

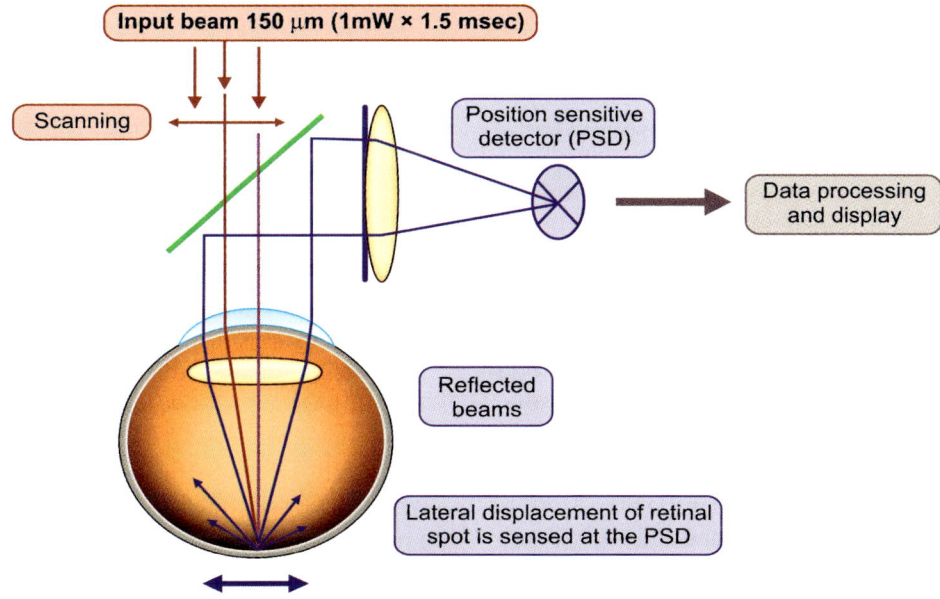

Fig. 10.28: *Diagram of the ray-tracing technique.*

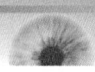

technique is shown. It measures the exact location where the laser beam reaches the retina by means of the retroreflected light captured by reference lineal sensors X, Y. Local aberrations in the path of the laser beam through the cornea and the internal structures cause a shift in the location on the retina.

- This process continues until 64 laser beams have been projected through the entrance pupil 4 times each (256 points) at high speed (approximately 250 milliseconds). Each of these points represents the entrance of parallel light rays into the eye, which become refracted by the eye's optical power and eventually focus on the retina. All 256 points would be concentrated at a single point in the center of the macula in an emmetropic eye and reconstruction of the real wavefront error is done.

Data Analysis

1. Wavefront analysis
2. Topographic analysis

I. Wavefront analysis (WF)

This depends upon the concept of retinal spot diagram (RSD), which consists of a set of points projected through the pupil onto the retina. RSD is used to obtain Modulation Transfer Function (MTF) and Point Spread Function (PSF).

PSF shows the image obtained in the retina when the patient sees a point source of light. A sharper and smaller PSF is considered to be better. The MTF is a measure of the transfer of modulation (or contrast) from the subject to the image by an optical system at different spatial frequencies. It measures how accurately it reproduces (or transfers) detail from the object to the image produced by the lens.

Basic data graphs

Basic data graphs include:

1. *Wavefront verification display* shows the RSD with the horizontal and vertical point profile.
2. *Wavefront map* [total and higher order aberrations (HOA)] is a colour coded map with warm colours showing that the wavefront is in front of the reference plane and cool colours showing retardation.
3. *The Root Mean Square (RMS),* measures the magnitude of aberrations.

4. Total refractive and HOA refractive maps
5. PSF total and HOA PSF
6. Snellen letter total and HOA
7. *Zernike polynomials bar graph,* showing the total, corneal and internal aberrations.

Uses of aberration analysis

1. *In case of high total aberrations,* it helps to decide whether the refractive procedure would be better in cornea or lens.
2. *Before and after cataract surgery* the analysis helps to study the induced or compensated aberrations by the IOL.
3. It also helps to identify which type of IOL will be suitable and to analyze different types of IOL.
4. The contribution of an opacified lens in total ocular aberrations can be measured.
5. *Measurement of angle alpha and angle kappa* to plan for premium IOL's.
6. To evaluate the corneal and total astigmatism.

II. Corneal Topographic analysis (CT)

This is based on a Placido disk format named Vista, which covers up to 10 mm of peripheral cornea. This provides:

1. Standard keratometric readings
2. Refractive power of cornea in central 3 mm
3. Corneal index: Inferorsuperior index (I-S)
4. Topographic maps, such as:
   - Standard axial map
   - Tangential curvature map
   - Refractive map
   - Elevation map
   - Corneal wavefront map.

Advantages of ray tracing aberrometry

1. It allows sequential capture of data and there is no confusion since each point is processed separately and sequentially.
2. The pattern of laser beams projected adapts to the pupil size.
3. High accuracy and resolution since each point is measured separately using linear detectors.
4. The x-y scanner can be programmed to analyze any other rectilinear or polar pattern.
5. iTrace is less susceptible to eye motion and tear film artifacts.

INTRAOPERATIVE, REAL-TIME WAVEFRONT GUIDED ABERROMETRY

These aberrometers have been evolved recently to refine the outcome of laser vision correction and cataract surgery by providing greater diagnostic refractive precision. This core technology, referred to as HOLOS (Clarity Medical Systems, Inc., Pleasanton, CA) is a novel technique for dynamically achieving accurate wavefront images or refractive profiles for real time, refinement during surgery.

OPERATING PRINCIPLE

- The aberrometer use Talbot Moire's interferometry based on two transmission grids spaced a specific distance apart and rotated relative to each other. The spectacle correction in a aberrated ocular wavefront is determined by using fourier transfer calculation and is represented in the resulting interferogram.

- *Light source (collimated) used is the 830 nm superluminescent diode*, which is launched into the eye and focused on the retina to create the returned wavefront. The collected data on the magnitude and location of the offset error by the quad detector is correlated with the refractive error of the eye. The sequential wavefront aberrometer achieves real-time, high-resolution sampling mainly by the speed at which the mirror rotates and the number and position of samples synchronized to pulses of the light source per revolution (Fig. 10.29).
- *The refractive outcome of the real-time sampling* is seen in an image overlaying a live eye image as viewed through the microscope and is presented as both qualitatively and quantitatively.
- *The qualitative data is seen* as a circle for spherical error, a thin ellipse for astigmatism and a dot for emmetropia.
- *The quantitative data is displayed* as sphere, cylinder and axis at the bottom of the screen.

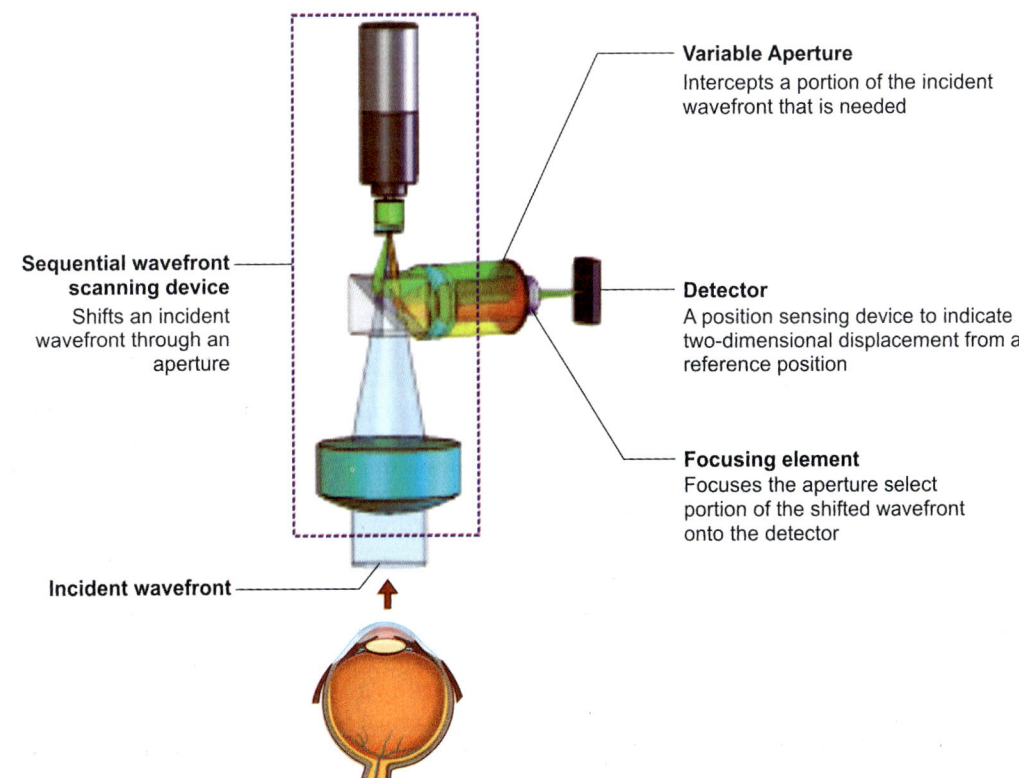

Variable Aperture
Intercepts a portion of the incident wavefront that is needed

Sequential wavefront scanning device
Shifts an incident wavefront through an aperture

Detector
A position sensing device to indicate two-dimensional displacement from a reference position

Focusing element
Focuses the aperture select portion of the shifted wavefront onto the detector

Incident wavefront

Fig. 10.29: *Working principle of intraoperative wavefront aberrometry.*

CLINICAL APPLICATIONS AND ADVANTAGES

- Identification of the astigmatic axis during surgery instead of the preoperative markings, which can save, time
- The potential to manage the LRI's by guiding their placement location and using real time feedback to titrate their length until neutralization
- The real time refraction can also guide the toric IOL rotation until neutralization
- The added size and dimensions do not change the surgeon's working distance
- Provides high quality data regardless of the microscope or room illumination
- Does not lengthen the surgical time
- The real time refractive data is integrated with the surgical video obtained.

CLINICAL APPLICATIONS OF ABERROMETRY

1. *Wavefront guided refractive surgery* has become very popular now a days.
2. *Role in early diagnosis of keratoconus.* Wavefront technology is an excellent adjunct to topography in the diagnosis of an early keratoconus. A topographic map showing slight inferior steepening accompanied by significant coma on wavefront analysis could be a cause for great concern. Preliminary research indicates that using a combination of inferior/superior value (derived from topography) and vertical coma (derived from wavefront) best separates early keratoconus from normal.

   Increase of ocular HOA in keratoconic eyes results from an increase in corneal HOA. Coma like aberrations are dominant compared with spherical like aberrations in keratoconic eyes. Wavefront analysis will enable us not only to evaluate the quality of vision but also to differentiate keratoconic eyes from normal eyes by analysing characteristics of HOA. Typically, it may show increased values of Zernike's coefficient – C_7 and C_8.

3. *Wavefront guided LASIK enhancement.* Corneal wavefront guided enhancements in patients with night vision symptoms and high positive spherical aberrations after myopic laser refractive surgery is effective in improving night vision symptoms, reducing corneal spherical aberrations and decreasing asphericity of cornea.

4. *Intraoperative real time wavefront guided aberrometry* quite useful and becoming popular.

BIBLIOGRAPHY

1. Alpins Noel JK, Ong G Stamatelatos. New method of quantifying corneal topographic astigmatism that corresponds with manifest refractive cylinder. Journal of Cataract and Refractive Surgery 2012;38(11):1978–88.
2. Aristodemou P, Knox Cartwright NE, Sparrow JM, Johnston RL. Formula choice: Hoffer Q, Holladay 1, or SRK/T and refractive outcomes in 8108 eyes after cataract surgery with biometry by partial coherence interferometry. J Cataract Refract Surg 2011;37:63–71.
3. Busin M, Wilmanns I, Spitznas M. Automated corneal topography: computerized analysis of photokeratoscope images. Graefes Arch Clin Exp Ophthalmol 1989;227(3):230–6.
4. Byun YS, Chung SH, Park YG, Joo CK. Posterior Corneal Curvature Assessment after Epi-LASIK for Myopia: Comparison of Orbscan II and Pentacam Imaging. Korean J Ophthalmol 2012; 26(1):6–9.
5. Fung, MW, et al. "Corneal Topography and Imaging" (2015). Medscape website. Updated 17 March 2016. Accessed 6 May 2017.
6. Karnowski K, Kaluzny BJ, Szkulmowski M, Gora M, Wojtkowski M. Corneal topography with high-speed swept source OCT in clinical examination. Biomed Opt Express. 2011Sep 1.2(9): 2709–20.
7. Liu Z, Huang AJ, Pflugfelder SC. Evaluation of corneal thickness and topography in normal eyes using the Orbscan corneal topography system. Br J Ophthalmol. 1999 Jul.;83(7):774–8.
8. Unterhorst HA, Rubin A. Ocular aberrations and wavefront aberrometry: A review. Afr Vision Eye Health 2015;74(1), Art. #21, 6 pages.
9. Wiley WF, Bafna S. Intra-operative aberrometry guided cataract surgery. International Ophthalmology Clinics 2011;51(2):119–29.
10. Yesilirmak N, Palioura S, Culbertson W, Yoo SH, Donaldson K. Intraoperative wavefront aberrometry for toric intraocular lens placement in eyes with a history of refractive surgery. Journal of Refractive Surgery 2016;32(1):69–70.

Section

III

Clinical Evaluation and Investigative Techniques in Glaucoma

11. Clinical Evaluation of Glaucoma: An Overview
12. Tonometry
13. Gonioscopy
14. Evaluation of Optic Nerve Head
15. Imaging in Glaucoma
16. Perimetry and Other Psychophysical Tests in Glaucoma

11

Clinical Evaluation of Glaucoma: An Overview

Chapter Outline

INTRODUCTION
- Goals of clinical evaluation
- Outlines of clinical evaluation

HISTORY TAKING
- Demographic data
- Chief presenting complaints and history of present illness
- History of past medical illness
- History of drug intake
- History of past ocular complaints
- Family history
- Social history

GENERAL PHYSICAL AND SYSTEMIC EXAMINATIONS

COMPREHENSIVE OCULAR EXAMINATION AND SPECIFIC TESTS FOR GLAUCOMA
Comprehensive Ocular Examination
- Testing of visual acuity and refraction
- Slit-lamp biomicroscopy

Specific tests for glaucoma
- Tonometry
- Gonioscopy
- Optic nerve head evaluation
- Visual field examination
- Optic nerve blood flow
- Electrophysiological tests
- Genetic testing in glaucoma

SUMMARY

INTRODUCTION

GOALS OF CLINICAL EVALUATION

Goals of clinical evaluation during the initial assessment are to know:

- *Glaucoma is present or not*, or is likely to develop (assessment of risk factors)
- *Type of glaucoma*, when present
- *Severity of glaucoma* mild, moderate or severe
- *Underlying mechanism of damage*—intraocular pressure (IOP) or non-IOP factors
- *Planning a strategy for management* and to identify suitable form of treatment.

OUTLINES OF CLINICAL EVALUATION

Clinical evaluation of glaucoma patients, like any other disease, involves:
A. *History taking* in a meticulous and thorough manner
B. *General physical and systemic examinations* relevant to glaucoma
C. *Ocular examination* in a comprehensive way
D. *Specific investigations* meant for a case of glaucoma.

HISTORY TAKING

The importance of painstaking meticulous history cannot be overemphasized. The

complete history taking should be structured as:

- Demographic data
- Chief presenting complaints and history of present illness
- History of past medical illness
- History of drug intake
- History of past ocular complaints
- Family history
- Social history.

I. DEMOGRAPHIC DATA

Demographic data should include patient's name, age, sex, occupation and religion.

Name and address are primarily required for patient's identification and also prove useful for demographic research.

Age and sex. Primary open-angle glaucoma (POAG) usually affects about 1 in 100 of the general population (of either sex) above the age of 40 years. Primary angle-closure glaucoma (PACG) usually presents between 50 and 60 years. It occurs more commonly in females than males in a ratio of 4 : 1.

Ethnicity. The ratio of POAG versus PACG reported for different ethnic groups is as below:

Ethnic group	POAG : PACG
Europian, African and Hispanics	5 : 1
Indian	1 : 1
Urban Chinese	1 : 2
Mongolian	1 : 3

Religion. Recording the religion helps in knowing the aptitude and practices prevalent in different communities.

II. CHIEF PRESENTING COMPLAINTS AND HISTORY OF PRESENT ILLNESS

Primary open-angle glaucoma (POAG)

Presenting symptoms. The disease is insidious and usually asymptomatic. Mild symptoms experienced by the patients include:
- Mild headache and eyeache.
- Difficulty in reading (patients usually give history of frequent change in near vision glasses).

- Occasionally, an observant patient may notice a defect in the visual field (scotoma).
- In late stages, patient may complain of delayed dark adaptation.

Primary angle-closure disease

Chronic PACD (asymptomatic) is more common than acute PACD (symptomatic) (3 : 1; meaning thereby that most patients do not know they have disease justifying need for glaucoma screening. Presenting symptoms of PACD, depending upon the clinical stage are summarized below.

Primary angle-closure glaucoma suspect (PACGS)/latent glaucoma. Patient does not present in this stage as there are no symptoms. PACGS is diagnosed:
- On routine slit-lamp examination in patients presenting with some other eye disease
- In fellow eye of the patients presenting with subacute or acute angle closure.

Primary angle-closure. Primary angle-closure (PAC) may manifest as subacute or acute PAC.

Subacute PAC/intermittent glaucoma. Patient presents with transient blurring of vision, coloured haloes around the light due to corneal oedema and mild headache. These symptoms are due to transient rise in intraocular pressure (IOP) and occur in intermittent attacks at irregular intervals. The attacks are usually precipitated by overwork in the evening, anxiety and fatigue.

Acute PAC (old name: acute angle-closure glaucoma). Patient presents with an attack of sudden onset of very severe pain in the eye which radiates along the branches of fifth nerve. Frequently, there is history of associated nausea, vomiting and prostrations. There is history of rapidly progressive loss of vision, redness, photophobia and watering. About 5% patients give history of typical previous intermittent attacks.

Primary angle-closure glaucoma (PACG). PACG may present as chronic congestive PACG or chronic non-congestive PACG.

Chronic congestive PACG. Patients have dull and constant pain in the eye along with marked diminution of vision. Patients usually give history of preceding attack of acute congestive glaucoma or repeated attacks of intermittent glaucoma.

Chronic non-congestive PACG. Typically presents as POAG except that the chamber is shallow and gonioscopy shows narrow angles with synechiae.

Absolute glaucoma. Such patients present with:
- Pain in the eye which is severe and irritating
- Constant headache
- Watering and redness of the eye
- Complete loss of vision (no perception of light).

  This stage results, if the chronic phase is left untreated.

Secondary glaucoma

Secondary glaucoma may present as acute or chronic disease. History should be taken to rule out the common causes, such as:
- *Uveitis,* acute or chronic
- *Steroids administration*—topical or systemic for a prolonged time
- *Ocular ischaemic diseases,* such as CRVO, proliferative diabetic retinopathy, Eales' disease, which can cause neovascular glaucoma
- *Ocular trauma* including trivial trauma in the past
- *Cataract,* may be complicated by either phacomorphic or phacolytic glaucoma.

History from a diagnosed patient of glaucoma under treatment

History taken from a diagnosed patient of glaucoma under treatment should include:
- Type of glaucoma diagnosed
- Date of diagnosis of glaucoma
- Highest IOP recording
- Glaucoma therapy taken in the past and currently being used should be recorded with specific dates
- History of adverse reactions to glaucoma agents used should be recorded in detail
- Any history of laser therapy and intraocular surgery.

Note. It will be prudent to obtain past medical records including previous visual field charts and optic disc photographs.

III. HISTORY OF PAST MEDICAL ILLNESS

Medical history relevant for glaucoma cases, which need to be ascertained is summarized below:

Respiratory diseases, such as asthma, chronic obstructive lung diseases associated with hyperresponsive airway and/or reduced lung capacity are contraindications for β-blockers.

Cardiovascular diseases, which need to be probed in a patient with glaucoma are:
- *History of past haemodynamic crisis* (e.g. postpartum haemorrhage, ruptured abdominal aneurysms, severe bleeding loss with trauma) may be responsible for optic disc pallor and cupping that mimics glaucoma but is not progressive.
- *Cardiac arrhythmias,* e.g. heart blocks, are contraindications for use of topical β-blockers and β-agonists.
- *Systemic hypertension,* when overtreated may worsen glaucoma risk and progression. Further systemic β-blocker may mask elevated IOP.
- *Vasospastic disorders,* e.g. migraine, Raynaud's syndrome may be associated with an increased incidence and severity of glaucoma, specially normal tension glaucoma (NTG).

Endocrinal disorders having relevance in glaucoma patients are:
- *Diabetes* may be associated with POAG and may be responsible for neovascular glaucoma in patients with diabetic eye diseases.
- *Thyrotoxicosis* is not the cause of rise in IOP but the prevalence of POAG is more in patients suffering from Graves' ophthalmic disease than the normal. Secondary glaucoma can also occur in thyroid ophthalmopathy.
- *Pituitary tumours* may be responsible for the optic disc pallor mimicking glaucoma.

Central nerve system (CNS) disorders
- Previous head injury, cerebrovascular accidents (CVA) and pituitary lesions may be responsible for the optic disc pallor and/or visual field defects.

- *Carotid-cavernous fistula* and intracranial arteriovenous malformations may cause elevated episcleral venous pressure and secondary glaucoma.
- *Early dementia* may affect compliance, understanding and insight into the disease.

Musculoskeletal diseases, such as osteoarthritis or rheumatoid arthritis may affect the ability to administer the eyedrops.

Urogenital problems, such as urinary stones, may limit use of systemic carbonic anhydrase inhibitors (CAIs).

Pregnancy and lactation may render all interventions hazardous.

IV. HISTORY OF DRUG INTAKE

Certain drugs being used by the patients presently or used in the past may have influence on glaucoma:

- *Steroids* used by any route, as also mentioned earlier, may be associated with steroid-induced glaucoma. *Note.* Steroid may be found in some traditional medicine especially being used by quacks.
- *Antiglaucoma drugs,* after prolonged use, may increase chances of trabeculectomy failure.
- *Anticholinergics/tricyclic* antidepressant drugs can cause angle-closure glaucoma.
- *Anticonvulsants (vigabatrin)* are reported to cause nasal peripheral field loss without disc changes.
- *Systemic beta blocker* and calcium channel blockers may interact with topical beta blockers.

V. HISTORY OF PAST OCULAR COMPLAINTS

A probe into history of past illness should be made to know:

- *Frequent change of glasses may be seen.* Myopes are at higher risk for POAG and hypermetropes are at higher risk for PACD.
- *History of similar complaints in the past* may be present in recurrent conditions, such as intermittent attacks of primary angle-closure glaucoma, recurrent attacks of glauco-matocyclitic crisis, inflammatory glaucoma especially associated with viral keratouveitis.
- *History of similar complaints in other eye* may be present in patients with primary angle-closure disease.
- *History of trauma to eye in the past* may be present in patients with angle recession glaucoma, cyclodialysis cleft.
- *History of ocular diseases in the past* which may or treatment of which may cause secondary glaucoma, such as uveitis; use of steroids for VKC, intraocular surgery; ocular ischaemic diseases, e.g. CRVO, Eale's disease, proliferative diabetic retinopathy.
- *History of systemic diseases in the past* which may cause secondary glaucoma includes epidemic dropsy, tuberculosis, syphilis, etc.

VI. FAMILY HISTORY

- *Several genes* [e.g. TIGR/MYOC (myocillin), OPTN (optineurin)] and modes of inheritance have been implicated in the development of POAG, juvenile and developmental forms of glaucoma.
- *Family history of glaucoma when positive* should be aimed at knowing the age of diagnosis, presentation, systemic association, progression, and visual status of the affected relative. It is unequivocal that positive family history is *an important risk factor* for the POAG, with greater risk being first degree relatives of glaucoma.
- *Examination of the patient's relative can* also provide important information regarding the appearance of the optic nerve, in particular the cup-to-disc ratio, which has been shown to be inherited.

VII. SOCIAL HISTORY

Social history helps to reveal a patient's ability to understand and successfully manage the challenge of a chronic disease, e.g.

- How regularly the patient can attend for follow-up?
- Can the patient afford and comply with treatment?
- How the glaucoma will affect the patient's work/family?

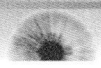

GENERAL PHYSICAL AND SYSTEMIC EXAMINATIONS

General physical and systemic examinations should be carried out in each case of glaucoma. The conditions relevant to management of glaucoma are summarized in medical history (see page 55).

COMPREHENSIVE OCULAR EXAMINATION AND SPECIFIC TESTS FOR GLAUCOMA

COMPREHENSIVE OCULAR EXAMINATION

A thorough ocular examination in a suspected case of glaucoma should include:
- Testing of visual acuity and refraction
- Slit-lamp biomicroscopy

TESTING OF VISUAL ACUITY AND REFRACTION

Visual acuity should be tested both for far and near. Refraction should be carried out to record the best corrected visual acuity as baseline evaluation.

SLIT-LAMP BIOMICROSCOPY

A thorough and meticulous ocular examination should be carried with slit-lamp biomicroscopy. Special attention should be given to the signs of primary as well as secondary glaucoma:

1. Conjunctival signs

- *Episcleral congestion* may occur due to elevated episcleral venous pressure
- *Ciliary flush* may occur due to congestion of deep conjunctival vessels in acute congestive glaucoma
- *Conjunctival filtration blebs* may be noted in old operated cases of glaucoma.

2. Corneal signs

- *Oedema* with epithelial vesicles may be noted in acute rise of IOP
- *Krukenberg's spindle* and pigment on corneal endothelium is seen in pigment dispersion syndrome.

- *Keratic precipitates* (KPs) may be seen in inflammatory glaucoma.
- *Fuch's corneal dystrophy* may be associated with POAG.
- *Corneal diameter* is increased in buphthalmos.
- *Breaks in Descemet's membrane* (Haab's striae) is a sign of buphthalmos.
- *Central corneal thickness (CCT)* lower than normal is being considered an important risk factor for conversion from ocular hypertension to glaucoma. CCT should be measured in every glaucoma and glaucoma suspect patient. Average CCT lies between 520 and 580 mm. Thinner cornea gives false low reading of IOP on Goldman applanation tonometry (GAT) and conversely thicker cornea gives false high reading of IOP.

3. Anterior chamber signs

- *Peripheral anterior chamber depth* (van Herring's technique) is shallow in primary angle-closure disease.
- *Aqueous flare and cells* may be seen in acute primary angle closure and in inflammatory glaucoma.
- *Lens proteins* in the anterior chamber (post-cataract surgery or following ocular trauma) may cause lens particle glaucoma.
- *Hyphaema* is a cause of haemorrhagic glaucoma.

4. Iris signs

- *Iris atrophy patch* may be seen of exfoliative glaucoma, old attack of acute PAC.
- *Dilated and congested iris vessels* may be seen in acute PAC.
- *Rubeosis iridis* is a sign of neovascular glaucoma.
- *Posterior synechiae may be seen in post-inflammatory glaucoma.*
- *Transillumination defect* may be seen is iridocorneal endothelial syndrome.

5. Pupillary signs

- *Mid-dilated, vertically oval and poorly reactive pupil* is seen post an angle-closure attack.
- *Relative afferent pupillary defect (RAPD)* may be seen in glaucomatous optic neuropathy.

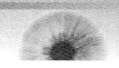

- *Mildly dilated round pupil* with sluggish reaction may be seen in advanced POAG.

6. Lens signs

- Pseudoexfoliative material (exfoliative glaucoma)
- Glaukomflecken (post-angle-closure attack)
- Swollen intumescent lens may cause phacomorphic glaucoma
- Phacodonesis may be seen in glaucoma due to subluxation and phacolytic glaucoma.

SPECIFIC TESTS FOR GLAUCOMA

Specific tests for glaucoma patients should include:

- Tonometry
- Gonioscopy
- Optic nerve head evaluation
- Visual field testing and other psychophysical tests
- Optic nerve blood flow
- Electrophysiological tests
- Genetic testing.

Specific tests for glaucoma patients are deliberated in detail in the coming text and just mentioned briefly here.

1. TONOMETRY

- Tonometry needs to be performed on each follow-up visit, since IOP is the only modifiable risk factor for glaucoma.
- Till date the preferred method is Goldmann-style Applanation Tonometry (GAT). Tonopen may be used, if GAT is increased by taking multiple measurement and averaging the results.
- Central corneal thickness (CCT) need to be considered with GAT in patients with ocular hypertension and glaucoma. Although available formulae to correct IOP based on CCT do not improve prediction of glaucoma development, it is important to account for a thin cornea.
- For details of tonometry, *see* Chapter 12.

2. GONIOSCOPY

- Gonioscopy, visualization of the angle of anterior chamber with the help of a gonioscope is essential to classify glaucoma into open-angle glaucoma and angle-closure glaucoma based on the configuration of the angle.
- Small indentation gonioscopy (e.g. Zeiss 4 mirror).
- Initially the gonioscopy need to be performed in each case of glaucoma and then regularly on each follow-up in angle-closure patients.
- The ideal testing conditions include dim room illumination, minimal intensity of the slit-lamp illumination, a low slit-beam height such that light does not impinge on the pupil and no pressure on the eye with the gonioscope. Then, wait for 30–45 seconds for the pupil to dilate before deciding, if the angle is open.
- Gonioscopy is useful in dividing angle-closure patient into:
  - Primary angle-closure suspects (PACS)
  - Primary angle-closure (PAC)
  - Primary angle-closure glaucoma (PACG)
- For details of gonioscopy, *see* Chapter 13.
- Additional diagnostic tools, such as anterior segment optical coherence tomography (OCT) and ultrasound biomicroscopy (UBM) can be supplementary, but are not necessary in routine evaluation of glaucoma suspects.

3. OPTIC NERVE HEAD EVALUATION

Optic disc changes, usually observed on routine fundus examination, provide an important clue for suspecting POAG.

- Optic nerve head changes are typically progressive, asymmetric and present a variety of characteristic clinical patterns. It is important to measure the size of the optic disc.
- Special attention should be paid to the shape and contour of neuroretinal rim. Localized narrowing of the inferior or superior rim that does not extend to the rim should arouse suspicion. If the rim extends to the edge of the disc for a clock hour, it is called a notch, typical of glaucomatous damage.
- Pallor of the rim outside the area of loss or out of proportion to the 'cupping' is suggestive of other neurological causes.
- Peripapillary choroidal atrophy is a soft sign of glaucomatous damage. It is significant, if associated with other signs, or if it increases in size.

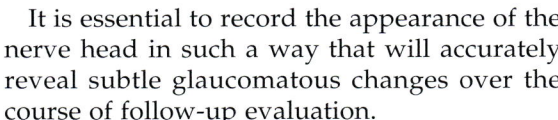

It is essential to record the appearance of the nerve head in such a way that will accurately reveal subtle glaucomatous changes over the course of follow-up evaluation.

Examination techniques. Careful assessment of disc changes can be made by direct ophthalmoscopy, slit-lamp biomicroscopy using a +90/78/60 D lens, Hruby lens or Goldmann contact lens and indirect ophthalmoscopy.

Recording and documentation techniques include:
- Serial drawings
- Photography and photogrammetry
- Structural changes, such as nerve fibre layer loss and rim notches often precede perimetric loss and can be measured in glaucoma suspects to determine initial risk and appropriate follow-up. Confocal scanning laser tomography (CSLT), i.e. Heidelberg retinal tomograph (HRT) is an accurate and sensitive method for this purpose.
- Other advanced imaging techniques include optical coherence tomography (OCT) and scanning laser polarimetry, i.e. nerve fibre analyser (NFA).

Glaucomatous changes in the optic disc can be described as early changes, advanced changes and glaucomatous optic atrophy.

For detail of optic nerve head evaluation, *see* Chapters 14 and 15.

4. VISUAL FIELD EXAMINATION
- Visual field defects in glaucoma are initially observed in Bjerrum's area (10–30° from fixation point) and correlate well with optic disc changes.
- Visual field examination defines state of the optic nerve function and defines visual impairment.
- Visual fields must never be interpreted in isolation. The field should be correlated with structural changes in the optic disc and NFL.

- Many options exist today for testing visual field function/sensitivity. Automated visual field tests (using Humphrey Field Analyser/Octopus) are more commonly used.
- Visual field examination should be performed when glaucoma is suspect. In cases of glaucoma, on therapy the follow-up visual field testing should be performed as per recommended guidelines.

Psychophysical tests other than visual fields include:
- Colour vision testing
- High pass resolution perimetry
- Motion detection perimetry

New techniques of perimetry, like blue on yellow and FDT may help in detecting glaucoma damage earlier than standard white on white perimetry.

5. OPTIC NERVE BLOOD FLOW
Assessment (using devices, such as HRF—Heidelberg retina flowmeter) has gained importance in recent years especially in patients with normotensive glaucoma.

6. ELECTROPHYSIOLOGICAL TESTS
Such as multiple visual evoked potential, multifocal ERG are also recommended for early detection of glaucoma.

7. GENETIC TESTING IN GLAUCOMA
It is also gaining importance. It is recommended that genetic testing can help to customize the glaucoma treatment protocols which is called *personalised medicine.*

Therefore, it is recommended to perform a comprehensive eye examination for every patient with the objective of detecting this potentially sight-threatening disease, glaucoma.

SUMMARY OF GLAUCOMA EVALUATION

Figure 11.1 summarizes the work-up for a glaucoma suspect.

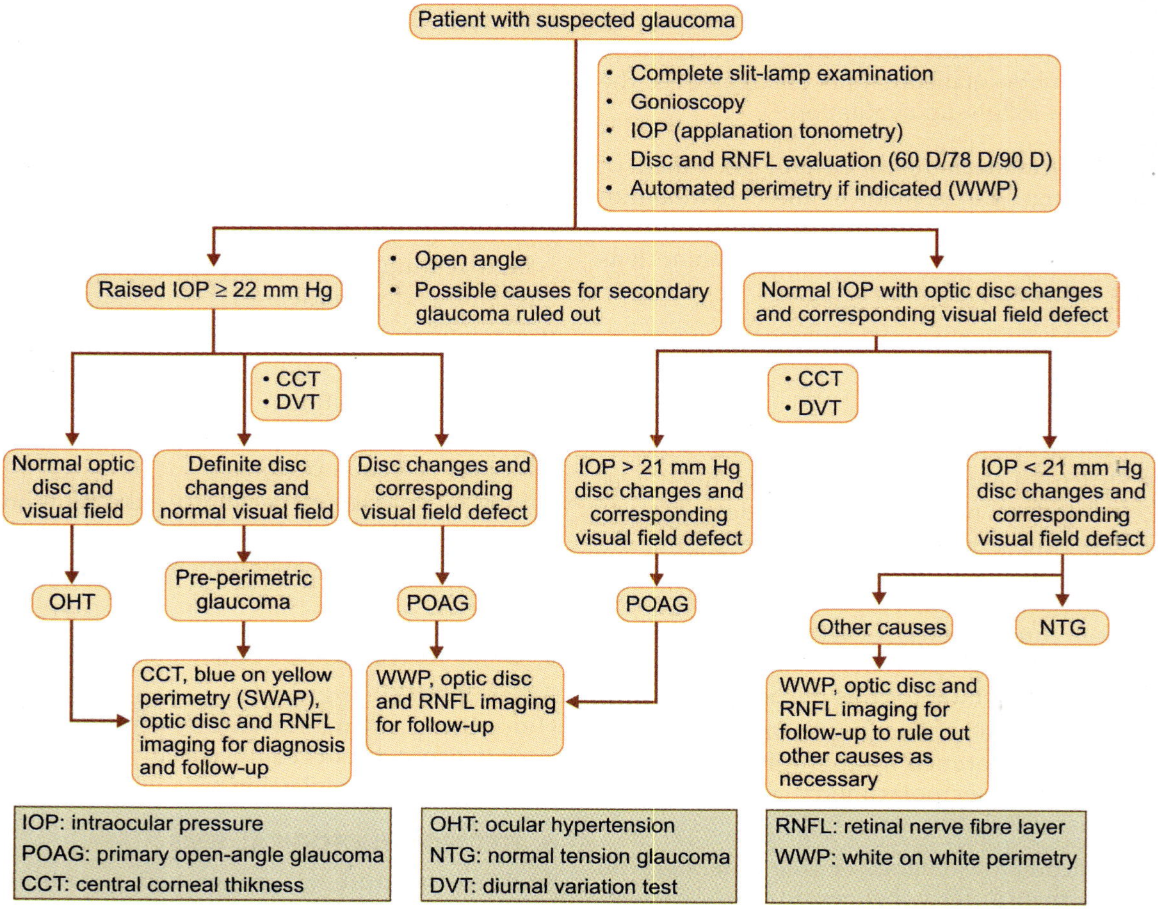

Patient with suspected glaucoma

- Complete slit-lamp examination
- Gonioscopy
- IOP (applanation tonometry)
- Disc and RNFL evaluation (60 D/78 D/90 D)
- Automated perimetry if indicated (WWP)

Raised IOP ≥ 22 mm Hg

- Open angle
- Possible causes for secondary glaucoma ruled out

Normal IOP with optic disc changes and corresponding visual field defect

- CCT
- DVT

- CCT
- DVT

Normal optic disc and visual field

Definite disc changes and normal visual field

Disc changes and corresponding visual field defect

IOP > 21 mm Hg disc changes and corresponding visual field defect

IOP < 21 mm Hg disc changes and corresponding visual field defect

OHT

Pre-perimetric glaucoma

POAG

POAG

Other causes

NTG

CCT, blue on yellow perimetry (SWAP), optic disc and RNFL imaging for diagnosis and follow-up

WWP, optic disc and RNFL imaging for follow-up

WWP, optic disc and RNFL imaging for follow-up to rule out other causes as necessary

IOP: intraocular pressure	OHT: ocular hypertension	RNFL: retinal nerve fibre layer
POAG: primary open-angle glaucoma	NTG: normal tension glaucoma	WWP: white on white perimetry
CCT: central corneal thikness	DVT: diurnal variation test	

Fig. 11.1: *Flow chart for work-up for a patient with ocular hypertension and glaucoma suspect.*

BIBLIOGRAPHY

1. Jonas JB, Budde WM, Panda-Jonas S. Ophthalmoscopic evaluation of the optic nerve head. Surv Ophthalmol 1999;43:293–320.

2. Sommer A. Glaucoma risk factors observed in the Baltimore Eye Survey. Curr Opin Ophthalmol 1996;7:93–8.

3. Thomas R, Parikh RS. How to assess a patient for glaucoma. Community Eye Health 2006;19:36–7.

Tonometry

Chapter Outline

INTRODUCTION
- Manometry
- Tonometry

INDENTATION TONOMETRY
Basic concept and theory
Schiötz tonometer
- Principle
- Technique
- Conversion of scale reading to baseline IOP
- Errors of indentation tonometers
- Electronic Schiötz tonometer

APPLANATION TONOMETRY
Variable area (fixed force) applanation tonometers
- Maklakov tonometer
- Other variable area applanation tonometers

Variable force (fixed area) applanation tonometers
- Goldmann applanation tonometer
  - Principle

- Technique
- Sources of error
- Effect of central corneal thickness
- Hand-held Goldmann type tonometers
- Mackey-Marg tonometer
- Tono-Pen
- Pneumotonometer

MISCELLANEOUS ADVANCEMENT IN TONOMETERS
- Pascal dynamic contour tonometer
- Diatom transpalpebral tonometer
- Reichert's ocular response analyser
- Icare or rebound tonometer
- SmartLens
- Preview—pressure phosphene tonometer
- Implantable IOP sensors

TONOMETRY IN SPECIAL SITUATIONS

OCULAR RIGIDITY

INTRODUCTION

MANOMETRY

Manometry is the only direct measure of IOP. In this method, a needle is introduced either into the anterior chamber or into the vitreous, which is then connected with a suitable mercury or water manometer to measure the IOP (Fig. 12.1).

Disadvantages
- Not a practical method for routine in human beings.
- Needs general anaesthesia which has its other effects on the IOP.
- Introduction of the needle produces breakdown of blood–aqueous barrier and release of prostaglandins which alter the IOP.

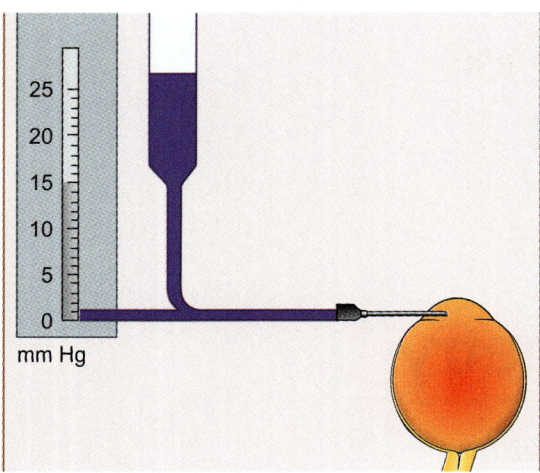

Fig. 12.1: *Manometry.*

Uses. Manometer is of the greatest and perhaps of the only use for a continuous measurements overtime and recording the changes in IOP induced by physiological and pharmacological manipulations in the experiment research work on animal eyes.

TONOMETRY

Tonometry is an indirect method of measuring the intraocular pressure (IOP) with the help of specially designed instruments known as tonometers. Tonometry has been over 180 years long journey. In late 19th century, Donders designed the first instrument which displaced intraocular fluid by contact with the sclea. The first commonly used mechanical tonometer designed by Schiötz in early 1990's soon became the new gold standard.

All clinical tonometers measure the IOP by relating a deformation of the globe to the force responsible for the deformation. They are broadly of two types, differing according to the shape of the deformation (Fig. 12.2): the indentation or impression tonometers (truncated cone) and the applanation tonometers (simple flattening).

INDENTATION (IMPRESSION) TONOMETRY

Indentation (impression) tonometry is based on the fundamental fact that a plunger will indent

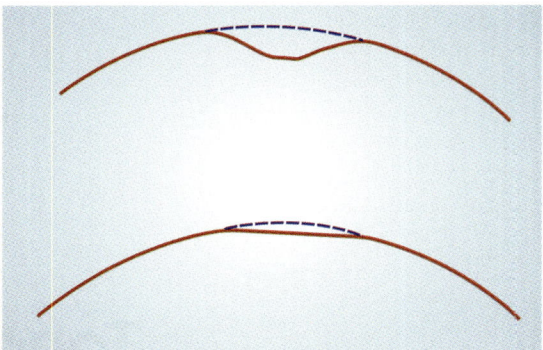

Fig. 12.2: *Corneal deformation created by (A) indentation tonometers (a truncated cone); and (B) applanation tonometers (simple flattening).*

soft eye more than a hard eye. The indentation tonometer in current use is that of Schiötz who devised it in 1905 and continued to refine it through 1927. Because of its simplicity, reliability, low price and relative accuracy, it is the most widely used tonometer in the world.

BASIC CONCEPT AND THEORY OF INDENTATION TONOMETRY

As the tonometer is placed on the cornea (Fig. 12.3), the different forces come into play:

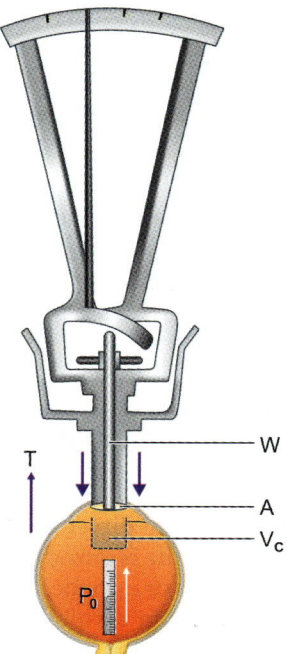

Fig. 12.3: *Basic principle of indentation tonometry.*

W, the weight of the tonometer, acts over an area A and indents the cornea displacing a volume V_c. The tensile force T set up in the outer coats of the eye at everywhere tangentially to the corneal surface, with a component opposing W, so that an additional force T is added to the original baseline or resting intraocular pressure (P_0) which is artificially raised to a new value (P_t). Thus, the scale reading of the tonometer actually measures the artificially raised IOP (P_t) (Fig. 12.3).

SCHIÖTZ TONOMETER

A Schiötz tonometer consists of the following parts (Fig. 12.4):
- *Handle* for holding the instrument in vertical position on the cornea
- *Footplate* which rests on the cornea
- *Plunger* which moves freely within a shaft in the footplate
- A bent *lever* whose short arm rests on the upper end of the plunger and a long arm which acts as a pointer needle. The degree to which the plunger indents the cornea is indicated by the movement of this needle on a scale
- *Weights:* 5.5 g weight is permanently fixed to the plunger, which can be increased by extra weight to 7.5, 10 and 15 g.

Technique of Schiötz tonometry

After anaesthetising the cornea with 2–4% topical xylocaine, patient is made to lie supine on a couch and instructed to fix at a target on the ceiling. The examiner separates the lids with left hand and gently rests the footplate of the tonometer vertically on the centre of cornea. The reading on scale is recorded as soon as the needle becomes steady (Fig. 12.5).

It is customary to start with 5.5 g weight. However, if the scale reading is less than 3, additional weight should be added to the plunger to make it 7.5 g or 10 g as indicated; since with Schiötz tonometer the greatest accuracy is attained when the deflection of the lever is between 3 and 4.

Conversion of scale reading to baseline IOP

The conversion of P_t (pressure with the tonometer on the eye) to P_0 (baseline/resting intraocular pressure) is obtained from the conversion tables developed by Friedenwald.

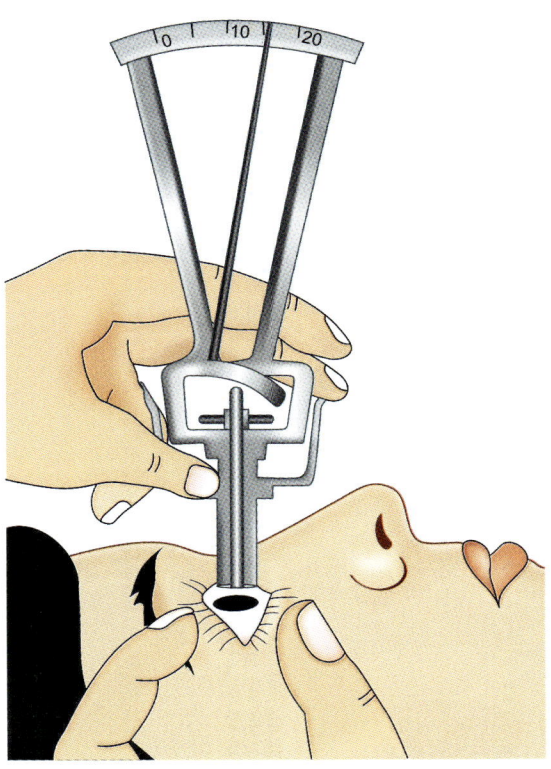

Fig. 12.5: *Technique of Schiötz tonometry.*

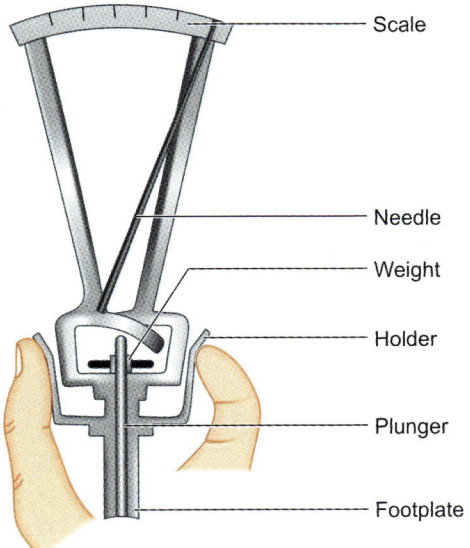

Scale

Needle

Weight

Holder

Plunger

Footplate

Fig. 12.4: *Schiötz tonometer.*

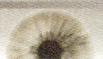

The calibration was carried by experiments in cadaveric eyes connected with a manometer through a cannula. The scale readings of the tonometer with different weights were recorded for different levels of IOP set in the manometer. The observations were plotted on a semilog scale, which serve as Friedenwald nomogram (Fig. 12.6). The original conversion tables, referred to as the 1948 tables were calculated using an average K of 0.0245. Friedenwald later revised the average K to a value of 0.0215, on which he based a new set of table known as Friedenwald Table (1955) (Table 12.1). Subsequent studies indicate that the 1948 tables agree more closely with measurements by Goldmann applanation tonometry.

Errors of indentation tonometry

1. *Errors inherent in the instrument.* These may be in the form of difference in the weight of different parts of the tonometer, difference in the size and shape and curvature of the footplate, friction arising in the working of plunger and differences in the smoothness of

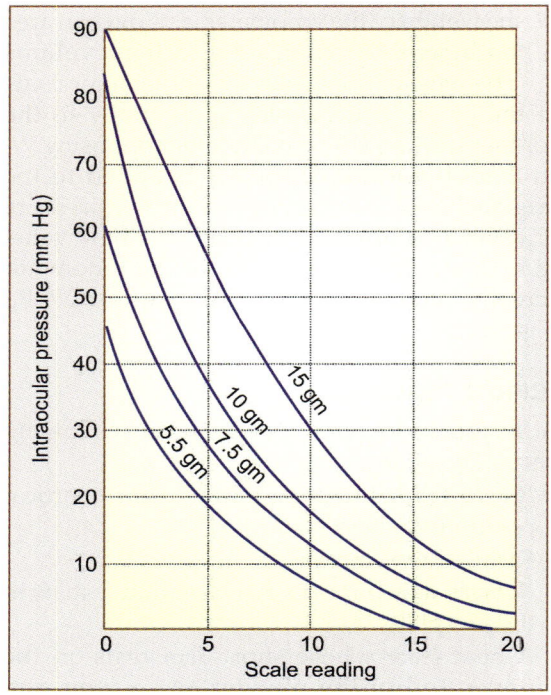

Fig. 12.6: *Friedenwald 1955 nomogram for Schiötz tonometer.*

Table 12.1. *Friedenwald (1955) Table for Schiötz tonometry*

| Schiötz scale reading | IOP (mm Hg) with different plunger body weights | | | |
	5.5 g	7.5 g	10 g	15 g
3.0	24.4	35.8	50.6	81.8
3.5	22.4	33.0	46.9	76.2
4.0	20.6	30.4	43.4	71.0
4.5	18.9	28.0	40.2	66.2
5.0	17.3	25.8	37.2	61.8
5.5	15.9	23.8	34.4	57.6
4.0	20.6	30.4	43.4	71.0
4.5	18.9	28.0	40.2	66.2
5.0	17.3	25.8	37.2	61.8
5.5	15.9	23.8	34.4	57.6
6.0	14.6	21.9	31.8	53.6
6.5	13.4	20.1	29.4	49.9
7.0	12.2	18.5	27.2	46.5
7.5	11.2	17.0	25.1	43.2
8.0	10.2	15.6	23.1	40.2
8.5	9.4	14.3	21.3	38.1
9.0	8.5	13.1	19.6	34.6
9.5	7.8	12.0	18.0	32.0
10.0	7.1	10.9	16.5	29.6

gliding movement of the pointer on the scale. The American Academy of Ophthalmology and Otolaryngology has established a committee on tonometer standardization, which has got rigid criteria for Schiötz tonometers.

2. *Errors due to contraction of extraocular muscles.* When a tonometer is placed on the eye, always there occurs some reflex contraction of the extraocular muscles, which tends to increase the intraocular pressure.

3. *Errors due to accommodation.* When the tonometer is brought near to the eye, there is a tendency to look at the tonometer and thus inadvertently accommodation comes into play. The contraction of ciliary muscle in accommodation also increases the facility of aqueous outflow by pulling on the trabeculae and thus causes some lowering of IOP.

4. *Errors due to ocular rigidity.* Conversion tables of Schiötz tonometer are based on an average coefficient of ocular rigidity (K). However, the ocular rigidity may differ significantly in certain eyes and thus false values of IOP are obtained. Thus, the deduction of IOP from tonometric readings will be higher in an eye with a higher ocular rigidity and lower in an eye with an abnormal low ocular rigidity. Factors affecting ocular rigidity are described in the section of ocular rigidity.

5. *Errors due to variation in corneal curvature and thickness.* Either a steeper or thicker cornea will cause a greater displacement of fluid during indentation tonometry which leads to a falsely high IOP readings. Thus, errors may arise in cases of microphthalmos, buphthalmos, and high myopia and corneal scars.

6. *Errors in scale reading.* An error of one scale reading on either side may occur during observations. Thus, an actual IOP of 17.3 mm Hg (scale reading 5) may be noted as 14.6 mm Hg (scale reading 6) or 20.6 mm Hg (scale reading 4).

7. *Blood volume alteration.* The variable expulsion of intraocular blood during indentation tonometry may also influence the IOP measurement.

8. *Moses effect.* At low scale readings, the cornea may mould into the space between the plunger and hole, pushing the plunger up and leading to falsely high pressure readings.

9. *Repeated measurements* lower the IOP.

Conclusion. Thus, from the above, it is quite clear that the results of indentation tonometry are never absolutely accurate. An error to the tune of ± 2 mm Hg in normal range of IOP and of ± 4 mm Hg in higher range of IOP has been reported.

Sterilization of Schiötz tonometer

Dissemble between each use and the barrel is cleaned with two pipe cleaners, the first soaked in alcohol and the second dry. The footplate is cleaned with alcohol swab. All surfaces must be dried before reassembling.

Electronic Schiötz tonometer

It provides a continuous recording of IOP that is used for tonography. The scale is also magnified which makes it easier to detect small changes in IOP. It is limited to experimental studies in the present era.

APPLANATION TONOMETRY

The concept of applanation tonometry is based on *Imbert-Fick law* which states that the pressure inside a sphere (P) is equal to the force (W) required to flatten its surface divided by the area of flattening (A), i.e. P = W/A (Fig. 12.7).

Therefore, one can determine the pressure by measuring either the force necessary to flatten a fixed area or by measuring the area flattened by a fixed force. Applanation tonometers have been designed using both the principles.

I. VARIABLE AREA (FIXED FORCE) APPLANATION TONOMETERS

This type of tonometer measures the area of the cornea that is flattened by a known force.

Maklakov tonometer

Introduced in 1885, it consisted of a dumb-bell-shaped metal cylinder with flat end plates of polished glass on either end with diameter of 10 mm. A set of four such instruments was available, weighing 5, 7.5, 10 and 15 g.

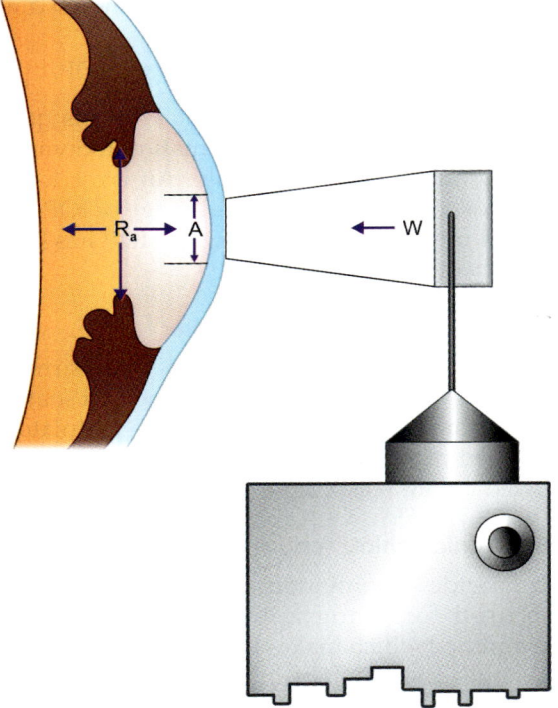

Fig. 12.7: *Imbert-Fick law: W = PA; Modified Imbert-Fick law: W + S = PA1 + B.*

Technique

A thin coat of the dye is smeared on the anaesthetised cornea with the patient supine, the flat bottom of the tonometer allowed to rest on the cornea. In this way, the dye from the flattened part of cornea is transferred to the tonometer bottom, which allows the measurement of the area flattened by a fixed force. The IOP is then read from the conversion tables.

Presently, this tonometer is not much popular.

Other variable area applanation tonometers

Other variable area applanation tonometers developed are:
- *Applanometer:* Ceramic end plates
- *Tonomat:* Disposable end plates
- *Halberg tonometer:* Transparent end plate for direct reading
- *Barraquer tonometer:* Plastic tonometer for use in operating room

- *Ocular tension indicator:* Uses Goldmann prisms and standard weight, for screening (measures above or below 21 mm Hg)
- *Glaucotest:* Screening tonometer with multiple end plates for selecting different cut-off pressures.

II. VARIABLE FORCE (FIXED AREA) APPLANATION TONOMETERS

This type of tonometer measures the force that is required to applanate a standard area of the corneal surface.

Fick in 1888 devised the first fixed area applanation tonometer. However, it was Goldmann who in 1954 modernized this concept and developed a tonometer which has revolutionized the use of applanation tonometry all over the world. This method of tonometry is far more accurate than indentation tonometry since in this technique a very tiny area of the cornea is applanated so the ocular rigidity does not interfere with the readings.

Some of the fixed area applanation tonometers are described below:

Goldmann applanation tonometer (GAT)

Currently, Goldmann applanation tonometer (GAT) is the most popular and accurate tonometer. It is mounted on the end of a lever hinged on a standard slit-lamp.

Technique

After anaesthetising the cornea with a drop of 2% xylocaine and staining the tear film with fluorescein, patient is made to sit in front of a slit-lamp. The cornea and biprisms are illuminated with cobalt blue light from the slit-lamp. The examiner views through the centre of a plastic biprism, which is used to applanate the cornea. Biprism is then advanced until it just touches the apex of cornea (Fig. 12.8). At this point, two fluorescent semicircles are viewed through the prism. Then, the applanation force against cornea is adjusted until the inner edges of the two semicircles just touch (Fig. 12.9). This is the end point. The prisms are calibrated in such a way that inner margins of semicircles touch when 3.06 mm of cornea is applanated. The intraocular pressure is determined by

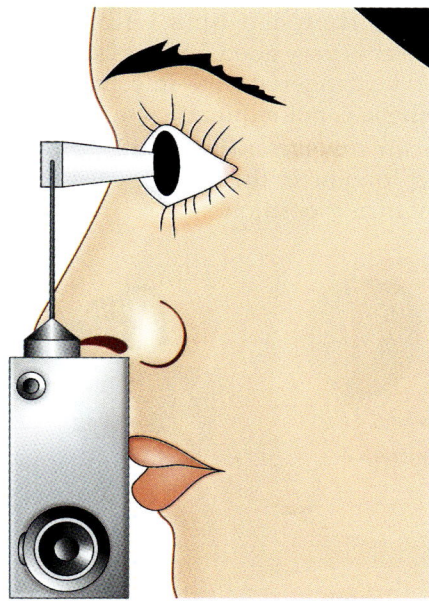

Fig. 12.8: *Technique of applanation tonometry.*

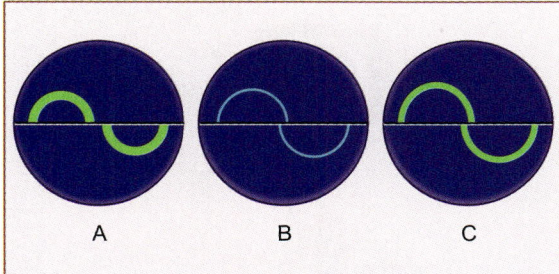

Fig. 12.9: *Goldmann applanation mires showing end point of applanation tonometry: (A) too small mires; (B) too large mires; (C) end point.*

multiplying the dial reading with ten to obtain IOP in mm Hg.

Sources of error

1. *Fluorescein concentration* affects the thickness of the mires leading to overestimation (with thick mires) or underestimation (with thin mires) of IOP.

2. *Inappropriate vertical alignment* gives higher IOP readings.

3. *Central corneal thickness.* There is underestimation of IOP in thin corneas and overestimation in thick corneas.

4. *Corneal curvature.* For every 3D increase in corneal curvature, IOP rises approximately by 1 mm Hg as more fluid is displaced under steeper corneas causing increase in ocular rigidity.

5. *Corneal astigmatism.* With the rule (WTR) astigmatism underestimates while against the rule (ATR) astigmatism overestimates the IOP. To minimize this, tonometer biprism should be rotated so that axis of least corneal curvature is opposite the red mark on the biprism. This results in a separation of 43° and an applanation of an area of approximately 7.35 mm^2. The other method is to obtain measurements in both vertical and horizontal meridians and average these readings.

6. *Irregular corneal surface* leads to distortion of mires.

Effect of central corneal thickness

Variations in central corneal thickness (CCT) change the resistance of the cornea to indentation so that this is no longer balanced entirely by the tear film surface tension thus affecting the accuracy of IOP measurement. A thinner cornea (physiological variation, pathological or post-PRK/LASIK) would require less force to applanate it, leading to underestimation of IOP and *vice versa*.

Goldmann applanation tonometer was designed to give accurate reading when the CCT was 520 μ. There occurs a change in applanation readings of 0.7 mm Hg per 10 μ. Thus, a correction factor, as described by Dredsner (Table 12.2), is required to get accurate IOP levels with applanation tonometry.

Sterilization

Methods used to sterilize applanation tonometer biprisms include:

- Soaking applanation tip for 5–15 minutes in diluted sodium hypochlorite, hydrogen peroxide 3% or isopropyl alcohol 70%, or by wiping with alcohol, hydrogen peroxide, povidone iodine or 1 : 1000 merthiolate are some easy and handy methods to sterilize the biprism of applanation tonometer.
- Ten minutes of rinsing in running tap water.
- Soap and water wash.

Table 12.2 *Dredsner correction table for IOP measured using GAT*

Corneal thickness (in µ)	Correction factor (in mm Hg)
460–485	+3
486–512	+2
513–536	+1
537–562	0
563–587	–1
588–612	–2
613–637	–3
638–662	–4
663–687	–5

- Disposable film covers for tips
- Exposure to UV light.

Hand-held Goldmann type tonometers

I. *Contact type*

1. *Perkin's applanation tonometer* (Fig. 12.10). It is a hand-held tonometer utilizing the same biprism as in the Goldmann applanation tonometer. It is small, easy to carry and does not require slit-lamp. The light source is powered by a battery and the force is varied manually. A counterbalance makes it possible to use the instrument in either the vertical or horizontal position. It is not used commonly now.

2. *Draeger applanation tonometer.* Similar to the Perkin's tonometer, but uses a different biprism and has an electric motor that varies the force.

II. *Non-contact type*

1. *Air-puff tonometer* (Fig. 12.11). It is a non-contact tonometer. In this, central part of cornea is flattened by a jet of air. This tonometer is very good for mass screening as there is no danger of cross-infection and local anaesthetic is not required.

2. *Pulse air tonometer* (Fig. 12.12). It is a non-contact tonometer that can be used with the patient in any position.

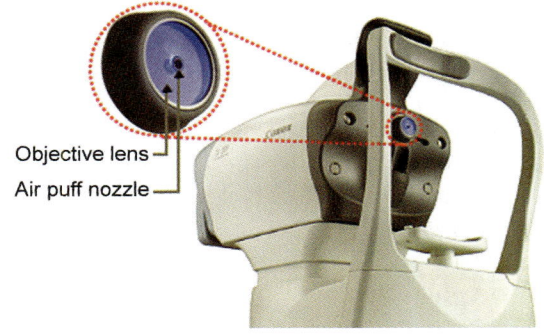

Objective lens
Air puff nozzle

Fig. 12.11: *Air-puff tonometer.*

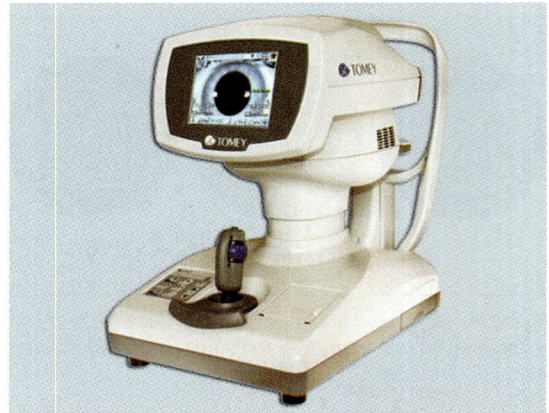

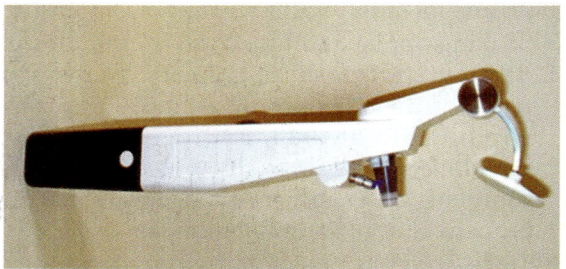

Fig. 12.10: *Perkin's hand-held applanation tonometer.*

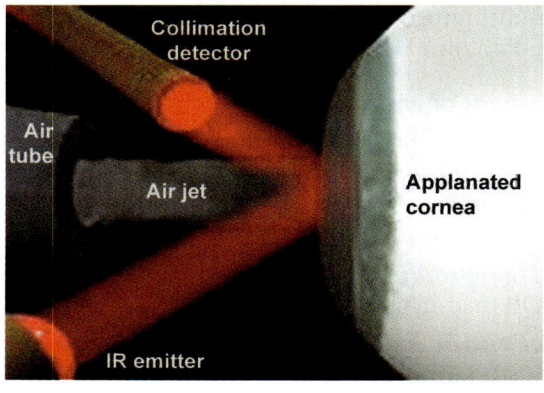

Collimation detector

Air tube

Air jet

Applanated cornea

IR emitter

Fig. 12.12: *Pulse air tonometer.*

MacKay-Marg tonometer

The original MacKay-Marg tonometer (MMT), which is no longer available, consisted of a 1.5 mm diameter plunger affixed to a rigid spring that extends 10 microns beyond the plane of surrounding rubber sleeve. Movement of the plunger is electronically monitored by a transducer and recorded on a moving paper strip. When the tonometer is placed on the cornea, the tracing that represents the force applied to the plunger begins to rise.

- *At 1.5 mm area of corneal applanation*, tracing reaches a peak and the force applied is equal to sum of IOP and force required to deform the cornea.
- *At 3 mm flattening,* force required to deform cornea is transferred from plunger to surrounding sleeve, creating a dip in tracing corresponding to IOP.
- *More than 3 mm* of area gives artificial elevation of IOP.

It is most accurate in eyes with scarred, edematous and irregular corneas.

Other MacKay-Marg type tonometers

1. *Tono-Pen* (Fig. 12.13). It is the most commonly used MacKay-Marg type tonometer today. It is a hand-held instrument with a strain gauge that creates an electrical signal as the footplate flattens the cornea. A built-in single-chip microprocessor senses the proper force curves and averages 4 to 10 readings to give a final digital readout. It also provides the percentage of variability between the lowest and highest acceptable readings from 5 to 20%.

2. *Pneumotonometer* (Fig. 12.14). In this, the cornea is applanated by touching its apex by a silastic diaphragm covering the sensing nozzle (which is connected to a central chamber containing pressurised air). There is a pneumatic-to-electronic transducer present which converts the air pressure to a recording on a paper-strip, from where IOP is read. It gives significantly higher IOP estimates.

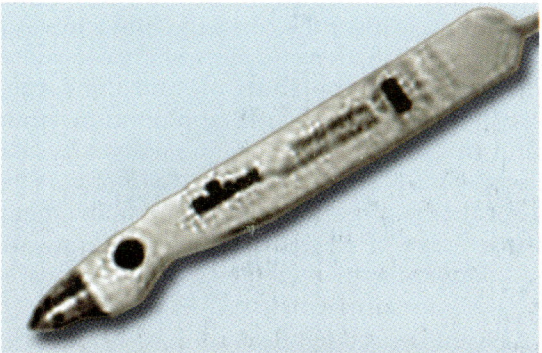
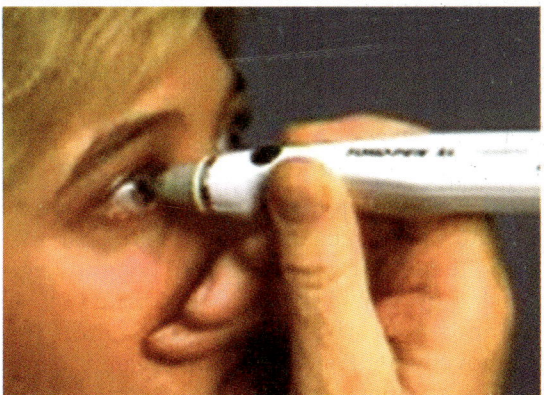

Fig. 12.13: *Tono-Pen.*

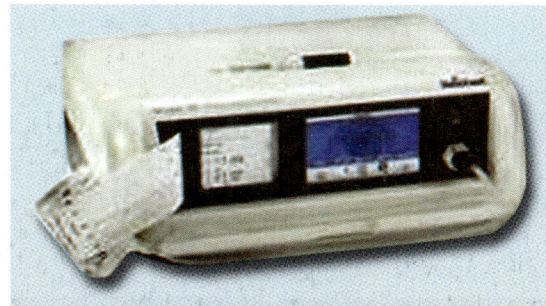
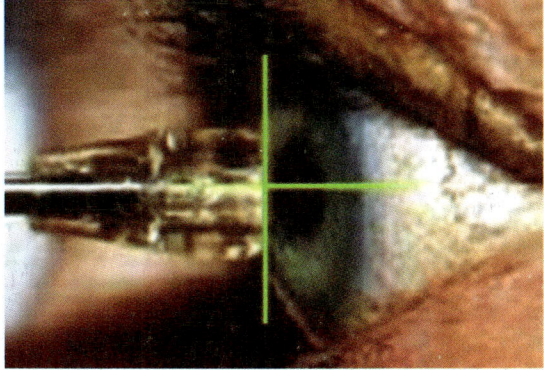

Fig. 12.14 *Pneumotonometer.*

MISCELLANEOUS ADVANCEMENTS IN TONOMETERS

Pascal dynamic contour tonometer

It is a newer applanation tonometer (Fig. 12.15) that uses principle of contour-matching to measure IOP instead of applanation to eliminate the systemic errors inherent in previous tonometers.

It uses a miniature pressure sensor embedded within a tonometer tip contour-matched to the shape of the cornea. The tonometer tip rests on the cornea with a constant appositional force of one gram. When the sensor is subjected to a change in pressure, the electrical resistance is altered and the Pascal's computer calculates a change in pressure in concordance with the change in resistance.

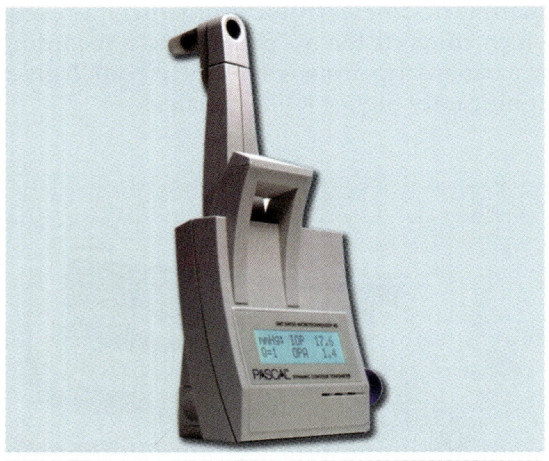

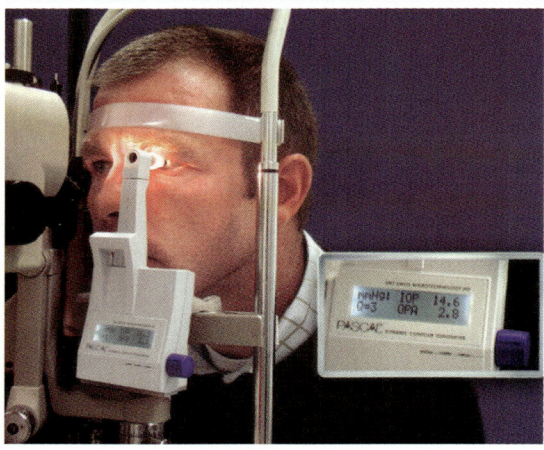

Fig. 12.15: *Pascal dynamic contour tonometer.*

It repeatedly samples IOP 100 times per second in addition to ocular pulse amplitude and the systemic pulse rate and provides a digital output of the IOP and a graphic output of the ocular pressure pulse. A complete measurement cycle requires about eight seconds of contact time. Audio feedback helps the clinician to ensure proper contact with the cornea.

Diatom transpalpebral tonometer

It is a hand-held device using a free falling thin rod on the stretched upper eyelid. It is based on processing the rod acceleration time resulting from its free fall from the constant height and the interaction with eye through the eyelid.

It requires no contact with the cornea, therefore, sterilization of the device and anaesthesia are not required. It is of use especially in children, those with corneal pathology, or those who have had corneal surgery.

Reichert's ocular response analyser

It measures corneal hysteresis. A short 20 ms air impulse causes the cornea to move inward, through applanation and into a slight concavity. Then the air pump shuts off and the cornea moves through a second applanation while returning back to its baseline convexity. An electro-optical collimation detector monitors the corneal curvature throughout the movement. The average of pressure values at the inward and outward applanation event times provides the IOP measurement.

Less influenced by the corneal resistance and thickness, it is useful in post-LASIK IOP measurement.

The IOP value is a calculated value and not the true IOP, therefore, prone for errors.

Icare or rebound tonometer

Icare or rebound tonometer (Fig. 12.15) consists of a pair of coils coaxial with the probe shaft, a solenoid coil and a sensing coil. A lightweight probe is propelled towards the cornea by the solenoid and the sensing coil monitors the movement. The speed immediately before impact, the deceleration during impact and the ratio of these parameters are correlated to the IOP.

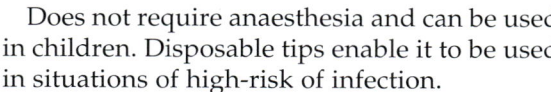

Does not require anaesthesia and can be used in children. Disposable tips enable it to be used in situations of high-risk of infection.

It tends to overestimate IOP compared to GAT.

SmartLens

It has a contact lens that incorporates an electronic pressure sensor, which is able to measure IOP and ocular pulse amplitude continuously by applanation of the central cornea. There is a Myler membrane covered hole at the centre of the lens. The cavity behind the membrane is filled with silicone oil and is connected with a piezoelectric pressure transducer. The measurement of IOP is achieved by the transmission of pressure through the oil to the transducer when the applanation membrane is displaced during its contact with the cornea.

It is being used mainly in experimental studies.

Preview—pressure phosphene tonometer

It is a patient self-monitoring device that utilizes a psychophysical technique based on entopic phenomenon of pressure phosphenes.

Implantable IOP sensors

- *IOP-IOL probe.* A sensor incorporated in the haptics of an IOL for continuous monitoring of IOP.
- *Contact lens sensor.* It correlates the spherical deformation of eyeball with the changes in IOP.
- *Choroid-IOP sensor.* Sensor lies in contact with choroid.

TONOMETRY IN SPECIAL SITUATIONS

Tonometry on irregular corneas

Pneumatic tonometers provide the most accurate result in eyes with diseased or irregular corneas. There is overestimation of IOP with Tono-Pen in such patients.

Tonometry over soft contact lens

Pneumotonometer and Tono-Pen measure IOP through bandage contact lenses with reasonable accuracy.

Tonometry in presence of intraocular gases

In eyes after pars plana vitrectomy and gas fluid exchange, there occurs alteration in scleral rigidity rendering indentation tonometry unsatisfactory. Pneumatic tonometers underestimate Goldmann IOP measurement. Tono-Pen measurements are comparable.

Tonometry in shallow anterior chamber

There is much variability in IOP measurements with GAT, pneumotonometer and Tono-Pen.

Tonometry in eyes with keratoprosthesis

Due to rigid surface of keratoprosthesis, it is impossible to measure IOP with indentation or applanation tonometers. Digital IOP assessment is the only applicable method in such eyes.

OCULAR RIGIDITY

Ocular or scleral rigidity is an expression of the stretchability of the eye in response to an increase in the intraocular pressure. The stretchability of any substance depends upon its inherent elasticity plus its thickness and a time-dependent variable called viscoelasticity. Viscoelasticity refers to the change in elasticity that occur overtime. Like most viscoelastic systems, the sclera will stretch proportionately more with initial elevations of intraocular pressure, and as the pressure increases, the resistance to further stretching also increases. Therefore, small increase in the intraocular volume at a low pressure causes a small increase in IOP, wherein similar small volume changes at high IOP will cause a much large increase in IOP. This property of sclera, labelled as ocular rigidity, seems an unfortunate term because most persons associate the word rigidity with resistance to bending rather than resistance to stretching. Therefore, the term scleral distensibility would be preferable to scleral rigidity.

FACTORS AFFECTING OCULAR RIGIDITY

Friedenwald denoted the coefficient of scleral rigidity by the word 'E'. He calculated it on cadaveric eyes and found the average value of 'E' to be 0.0215. The Schiötz scale reading intraocular pressure (P_0) conversion table of

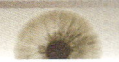

Friedenwald has been calibrated using average value of ocular rigidity coefficient, assuming that it should work in most of the individuals. But, in practice, variation of ocular rigidity above or below the average value is not so uncommon among different patients. Thus, a high ocular rigidity will cause a falsely high IOP and a low 'E' value will lead to a falsely low reading.

However, in clinical practice, ocular rigidity measurements for individual patients are not made as often as they should be; this introduces significant errors and makes dependence on the scleral rigidity hazardous.

Conditions influencing ocular rigidity

1. Refractive errors. Higher values are reported in hypermetropes and lower than the normal in myopes.

2. Elevated IOP. E-value is decreased with increase in the IOP; this may explain the lower 'E' during water drinking provocative test.

However, in long-standing glaucoma, 'E' has been found to be increased.

3. Drugs. Miotics, especially strong cholinesterase inhibitors, are said to reduce 'E'. Vasodilation may also diminish 'E', while vasoconstriction causes an increase.

4. Surgery. Ocular rigidity is reduced following retinal detachment surgery, or the intravitreal injection of compressible gas leading to a falsely low IOP estimation with indentation tonometry.

5. Age. Reports vary widely regarding the correlation of 'E' value and advancing age.

DETERMINATION OF OCULAR RIGIDITY

The technique of determining ocular rigidity is based on Friedenwald's concept of differential tonometry. To determine ocular rigidity, tonometric readings are obtained with any two weights (say 5.5 and 10 g). (A more accurate method is to use the applanation tonometry value as P_0 and one Schiötz reading.) The

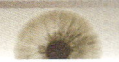

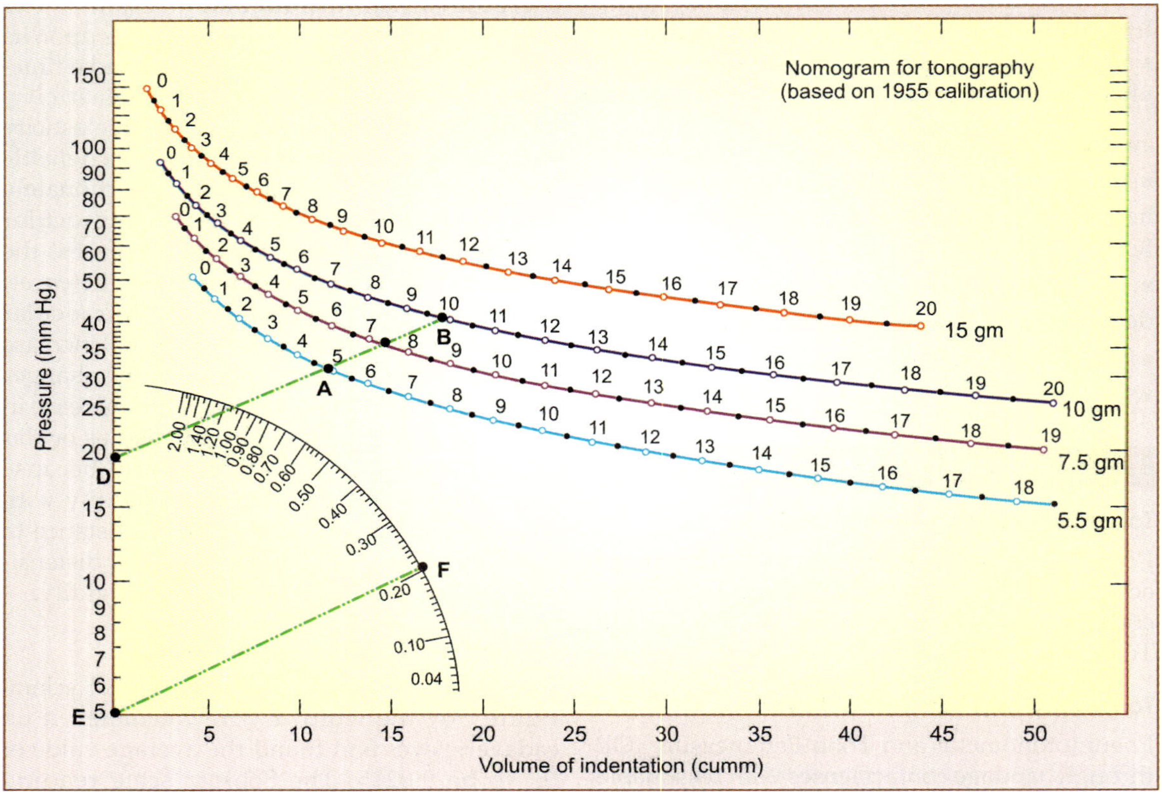

Fig. 12.16: *Scleral rigidity from Friedenwald nomogram (for details see text).*

intraocular pressure in an eye with average normal ocular rigidity will be the same whatever weight is used. But if the rigidity is high then the 10 g weight will show a higher TOP and if the rigidity is low, the IOP with 10 g will be lower than that determined by 5.5 g weight.

In cases with abnormal ocular rigidity, a correction for it has to be done using the Friedenwald nomogram (Fig. 12.16), which consists of the following:

- There are four slanting curves showing scale readings with 5.5, 7.5, 10 and 15 g weights.
- The ordinate (left margin) of the nomogram shows the IOP in mm Hg.
- The abscissa (lower margin) of the nomogram shows the value of indentation in cu mm.
- The semicircular scale at the lower left hand corner shows the coefficient of ocular rigidity.

How to use Friedenwald nomogram

Plot the result of differential tonometry on the nomogram. In Fig. 12.16, the point A represents the scale reading with 5.5 and B with 10 g weight during differential tonometry. The line joining A and B if extended to the left intersects the ordinate (left margin) at the point D which shows the actual value of intraocular pressure (P_0). Draw another line EF extended through lower left hand corner and parallel to the line DAB. Read scleral rigidity where the line EF crosses the semicircular scale. Normal average coefficient of ocular rigidity is 0.0215.

BIBLIOGRAPHY

1. Comparison of intraocular pressure measured by Pascal dynamic contour tonometry and Goldmann applanation tonometry. Eye 2006; 20:191–8.
2. Development of a completely encapsulated intraocular pressure sensor. Ophthalmic Res 2000;32(6):278–84.
3. Effect of corneal parameters on measurements using the pulsatile ocular blood flow tonograph and Goldmann applanation tonometer. Br J Ophthalmol 2004;88(4):518–22.
4. First steps toward invasive intraocular pressure monitoring with a sensing contact lens. Invest Ophthalmol Vis Sci 2004;45(9):3113–7.

Gonioscopy

Chapter Outline

PRINCIPLE AND INDICATIONS
Principle
Indications
• Diagnostic
• Therapeutic
TECHNIQUES OF GONIOSCOPY
Direct gonioscopy
• Procedure
• Advantages and disadvantages
Indirect gonioscopy
• Commercially available gonioprism
• Procedure

Functional techniques
• Advantages and disadvantages
GONIOSCOPIC VIEW AND GRADING OF ANGLE
• Gonioscopic view of angle structures
• Grading system for the angle
• Biometric gonioscopy
CLINICAL USES AND LIMITATIONS
• Clinical uses
• Critical questions to be answered during gonio-scopy
• Limitations and artefacts

PRINCIPLE AND INDICATIONS

The term gonioscopy, derived from the Greek words gō′nē (angle) and ōs′k-pē (view), was coined by Trantas in 1907. It is a clinical technique that is used to examine structures in the anterior chamber angle. Gonioscopic assessment is essential for diagnosing the type of glaucoma and for planning the appropriate therapy. In fact, without reasonable proficiency in the technique of gonioscopy, anybody should be able to manage glaucomas.

PRINCIPLE OF GONIOSCOPY

A direct view of the angle of anterior chamber is not normally possible with the slit-lamp because of overhanging opaque scleral shelf and the fact that light which emanates from the angle is reflected back into the eye by the cornea owing to phenomenon of total internal reflection.

The total internal reflection at the cornea occurs because the angle of incidence of the rays from the anterior chamber angle structures is greater than the critical angle of the cornea–air interface, which is approximately 46° (Fig. 13.1). The solution to this problem is to eliminate cornea optically. Gonioscopic contact lenses where refractive index is similar to that of cornea eliminate the optical effect of the front corneal surface. Therefore, light rays from the anterior chamber angle enter the contact lens and are made to pass through the new contact lens–air interface by one of the following two basic designs:

1. Direct gonioscopes. In these, the curve of the contact lens (goniolens) is such that the critical

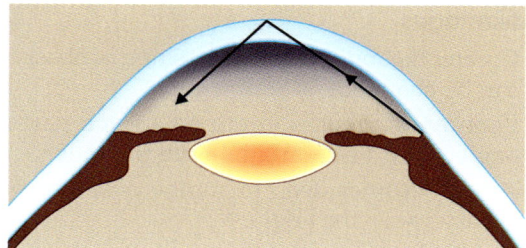

Fig. 13.1: *The angle of incidence of light rays originating from the angle structures is greater than the critical angle of the cornea–air interface, resulting in total internal reflection.*

angle is not reached and the light rays are refracted at the contact lens–air interface (Fig. 13.2).

2. Indirect gonioscopes. In these, the light rays are reflected by a mirror in the contact lens (gonioprism) and leave the lens nearly at right angle to the contact lens–air interface (Fig. 13.3).

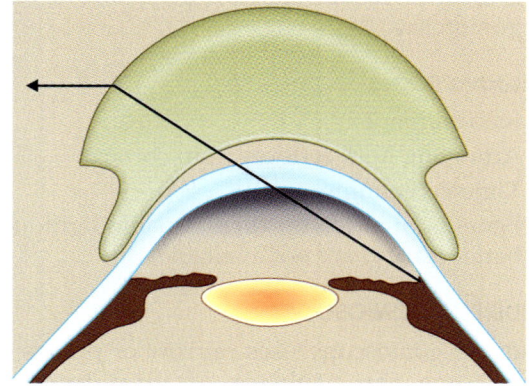

Fig. 13.2: *Schematic drawing of optics of a direct gonioscope.*

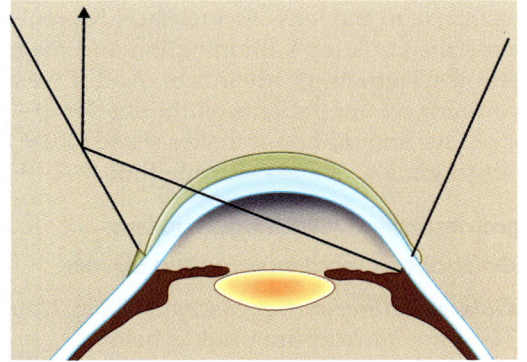

Fig. 13.3: *Schematic drawing of optics of an indirect gonioscope.*

INDICATIONS

Diagnosis and management of glaucoma essentially needs good gonioscopic knowledge. It helps in viewing the trabecular meshwork and determining the cause for elevated intraocular pressure. The indications of gonioscopy can be divided into diagnostic and therapeutic ones.

Diagnostic indications

- Classification of glaucoma—open angle or closed angle
- Assessment of the anterior chamber angle recess and risk of angle-closure
- Identification of plateau iris
- Look for presence and extent of neovascularization of angle
- Assessment of abnormal angle pigmentation
- Identification of the abnormal pigmentation in pigmentary glaucoma
- Visualization of pseudoexfoliative material in the angle
- Look for post-traumatic angle recession, cyclodialysis
- Rule out foreign body in the angle after open-globe injury
- Neoplastic invasion into angle structures (ciliary body tumour)
- Diagnosis of blood in the Schlemm's canal (raised EVP)
- Look for Copper deposition on Descemet's membrane (KF ring)
- Evaluation of trabeculectomy fistula
- Visualization of glaucoma drainage devices
- Diagnosing anterior insertion of iris in developmental glaucoma
- Visualization of congenital anomalies—aniridia, iris processes.

Therapeutic indications

- Laser trabeculoplasty/goniophotocoagulation
- Goniotomy/gonioplasty/trabectome surgery
- Reopening of a blocked trabeculectomy opening
- Nd:YAG laser after deep sclerectomy
- Laser of suture tied around tube of a glaucoma drainage device

- Indentation gonioscopy to break an acute attack of angle-closure
- Insertion of microsurgical implants into Schlemm's canal.

TECHNIQUES OF GONIOSCOPY

As mentioned earlier, gonioscopy is of two types:
1. Direct gonioscopy
2. Indirect gonioscopy

DIRECT GONIOSCOPY

It is performed with a steep convex lens, which permits light from the angle to exit the eye closer to the perpendicular at the lens–air interface. These lenses are used with a portable slit-lamp or an operating microscope. Direct gonioscopy is useful but fairly impractical for routine use. Various types of direct goniolenses are given:

- *Koeppe goniolens* is the most commonly used for diagnostic direct gonioscopy.
- *Huskins-Barkan's lens* is a prototype surgical goniolens used for goniotomy.
- *Swan Jacob's lens* is also used for surgical purpose.
- *Richardson-Shaffer's goniolens* is basically a small Koeppe lens used for infants.
- *Worth goniolens.* It anchors to cornea by partial vacuum.
- *Sieback goniolens.* It is a tiny goniolens which floats on the cornea.

Procedure

Cornea is first anaesthetised with 4% xylocaine instilled topically. The ideal position for direct gonioscopy is the patient lying supine with the examiner sitting on the side of the eye to be examined. With the patient looking up, lower lip of goniolens is inserted below the lower lid. Now the patient is asked to look down and upper lip is placed beneath upper eyelid. Now with patient's head turned towards the examiner, the nasal lip of goniolens is slightly raised and normal saline drops are used for irrigation. This way all the air bubbles also rise on the top and are removed. Now gonioscopy is performed with the patient looking to the ceiling. A systematic approach is to be followed: Nasal angle—superotemporal than inferior angle.

Advantages

- Greater flexibility because position of observer can be changed.
- Panoramic view is obtained so one part of angle could be compared with the other.
- Angle becomes deep in supine position so it is easy to see the angle.
- Detailed examination of minor structures is possible because the observer can change his or her height to look deeper into anterior chamber.
- Causes lesser distortion of anterior chamber.
- Can be used in sedated/anaesthetised patients as in infants.
- Provides a straight view rather than inverted view.
- Using two lenses, both eyes can be examined simultaneously.
- Can be used for surgical procedures, like goniotomy.

Disadvantages

- Inconvenient
- Annoying light reflexes from cornea
- Time-consuming
- Benefits of slit-lamp (like variable light and better clarity) are not available.

INDIRECT GONIOSCOPY

Indirect gonioscopy uses mirrors or prisms to overcome the problem of total internal reflection. Gonioprisms have an angled mirror through which light rays from anterior chamber angle are reflected so that they emerge perpendicular to the lens–air interface. Moreover, it uses the slit-lamp's illumination and magnification system to its advantage. And if we are examining all our patients on the slit-lamp—as indeed we should be—it makes sense to use an indirect gonioscope at the same time.

Commercially available gonioprisms

I. Gonioprisms requiring coupling agents

1. *Goldmann three-mirror gonioprism* (Fig. 13.4A). The three mirrors are used as below:
   - *Mirror having inclination of 59° and domed upper border is used for gonioscopy.*

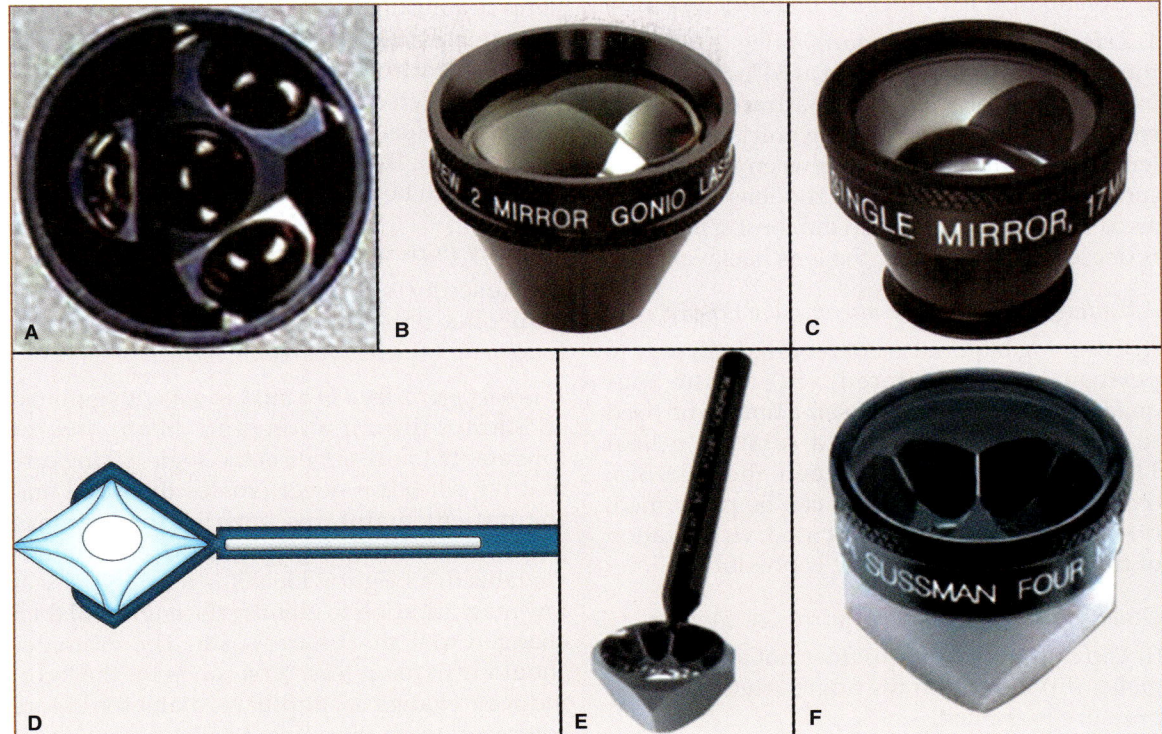

Fig. 13.4: *Various types of gonioscopes: (A) Goldmann three-mirror gonioprism; (B) Goldmann two-mirror gonioprism; (C) Goldmann single-mirror gonioprism; (D) Zeiss four-mirror gonioprism; (E) Posner gonioprism; (F) Sussman lens.*

Goldmann goniomirror has broad area of contact (approximately 12 mm) with cornea and under pressure may artificially close the angle.
- *Mirror inclined at 67° is used to examine pars plana area of ciliary body.*
- *Mirror having inclination of 73° is used to examine ora serrata area of the peripheral fundus.*

2. *Goldmann two-mirror gonioprism* (Fig. 13.4B). Both the mirrors are inclined at 62°. It needs to be rotated once to examine the whole angle.

3. *Goldmann single-mirror gonioprism* (Fig. 13.4C). The mirror is inclined at 62°. It is a prototype diagnostic gonioprism. It is to be rotated three times to examine the whole angle.

Advantages of Goldmann gonioprisms
(i) Easy to use, (ii) excellent view, (iii) stabilizes the globe and, therefore, can be used in argon

laser trabeculoplasty, (iv) peripheral retina can be seen, (v) Goldmann two-mirror gives best *in situ* view of the angle.

Disadvantages of Goldmann gonioprisms
(i) Curvature of lens is more than that of cornea so a coupling material is required. It blurs vision and fundus; therefore, field charting, direct and indirect ophthalmoscopy cannot be done immediately after its use. (ii) Only one mirror is there for gonioscopy so it needs to be rotated by 360°. (iii) It cannot be used for indentation gonioscopy. (iv) Broad area of contact with cornea is there in case of Goldmann three-mirror and underpressure, it can lead to artefactual closure of angle.

4. *Allen Thorpe gonioprism*. It has got four prisms instead of mirrors and allows examination of the whole angle without rotating the prisms.

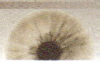

II. Gonioprisms not requiring coupling agents

1. Zeiss four-mirror gonioprism (Fig. 13.4D) has four identical mirrors angled at 64° which allow examination of the four quadrants without rotation of the lens. By turning only 11° through lens, the smaller areas in between the mirrors can be visualized. Because the lens has small area (9 mm) of contact with the cornea, the angle is deepened by pushing the lens backwards.

Advantages of Zeiss four-mirror gonioprism

(i) Coupling material is not required, (ii) easy to perform when mastered, (iii) all the four quadrants are visible at the same time so no need to rotate the gonioprism; a rotation of just 11° covers the area between the mirrors, (iv) indentation gonioscopy can be performed, (v) as coupling material is not used, visualization of fundus and photography is possible.

Disadvantages of Zeiss four-mirror gonioprism

(i) Difficult to master, (ii) does not stabilize the globe, (iii) may open the angle artefactually, if pressure is applied.

2. Posner gonioprism (Fig. 13.4E). It is similar to Zeiss gonioprism but is made of plastic instead of glass and also has fixed rather than detachable handle.

3. Sussman lens (Fig. 13.4F). It is also similar to Zeiss lens except that it has no handle.

4. Tokel gonioprism. It is a single-mirror gonioprism and has got a wider field of view.

Procedures of indirect gonioscopy

(1) The eye is anaesthetised with the topical anaesthetic agent. Coupling fluid is poured into the well of the gonioscope. (2) The patient who is sitting on the slit-lamp is asked to look down. (3) The thumb of one hand is used to retract the upper lid. (4) The lower edge of the gonioscope is placed on the lower lid and the gonioscope is tipped onto the cornea in one smooth manoeuvre. In the event of difficulty in keeping the gonioscope in place, a solution like hydroxy-propyl methylcellulose 2.5% may be used. This is thick and a little messy, so once one is more experienced, one can use the less viscous hydroxypropyl methylcellulose 0.7%. (5) Slit-

lamp beam is focused on the mirror that shows the angle diametrically opposite to it. Image in indirect goniomirrors is inverted, but not laterally reversed. Three types of illuminations are used: diffuse, sclerotic scatter and direct focal illumination. By using all these, various subtle findings can be elicited.

Essential steps of gonioscopy

Gonioscopy should be performed for all glaucoma patients at diagnosis and during follow-up (at least yearly).

It is best performed in a dark room with minimal slit-lamp illumination and beam height (preferably 1 mm) aimed at the angle, taking care that the slit-beam never crosses the pupil and the patient maintains gaze in the primary position. If the angle structures are not visualized, a bright wide slit is used initially at low magnification to identify the angle and then changed to a short narrow slit. The examiner should wait for at least 60 seconds for the light-induced change in pupillary diameter before commenting on the angle detail.

Identifying the corneal wedge (Fig. 13.5) is the key step in defining the angle structures. By using a thin slit of light inclined 15–20° from the angle of the oculars and sharp focus, projected onto the iridocorneal angle, two light reflections are noted, one from the external surface of the cornea and the other from the internal surface of the cornea. These two reflections meet at the end of Descemet's membrane, the beginning of Schwalbe's line. At this landmark, the external and internal reflections of the three-dimensional parallele-piped of light merge into a two-dimensional single line with a brighter luminance, which extends in a perpendicular direction across the trabecular meshwork. However, identifying the corneal wedge may be difficult in some cases. By gently sliding the gonioscopy lens in the direction of the mirror being used, the examiner gains a better view of the cornea and the corneal wedge. Locating the wedge is easiest in the superior and inferior angles as it is easy to generate a vertical slit. Hence, the inferior and superior angle should be viewed first and then the temporonasal angle.

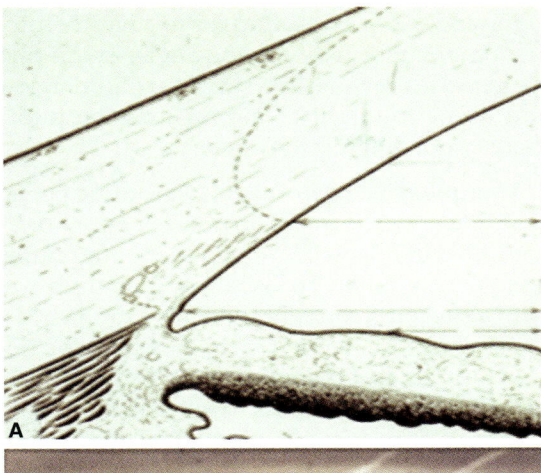

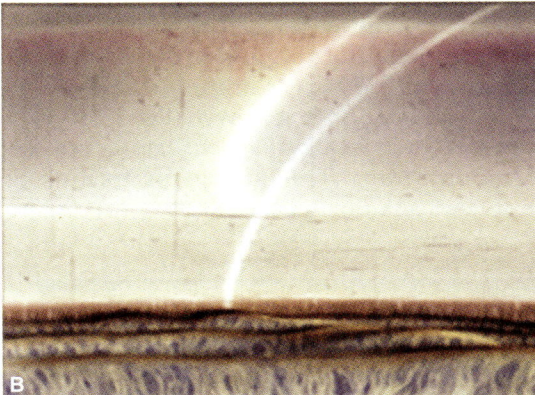

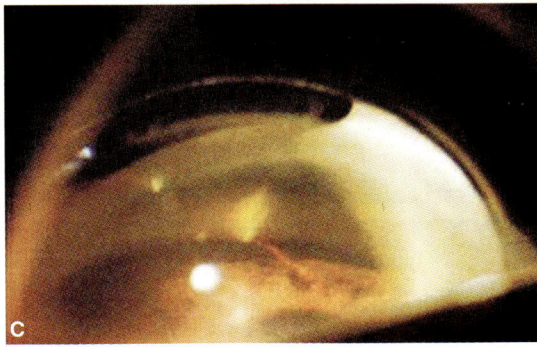

Fig. 13.5: *Corneal wedge: (A) Diagrammatic depiction; (B) as seen on the slit-lamp; and (C) as seen through the gonioscope.*

Then the observer should see if the posterior pigmented (functional) part of the trabecular meshwork is visible or not.

- *It is visible in open-angles (Fig. 13.6).*
- *If the posterior part of the trabecular meshwork is not visible, it indicates that there may be iridotrabecular contact (angle-closure, Fig. 13.7)*

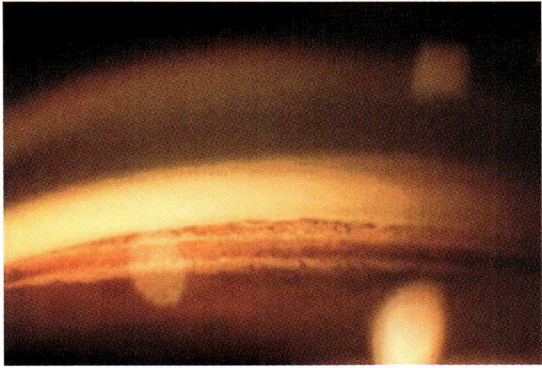

Fig. 13.6: *Open-angle with view of iris, ciliary body, scleral spur and trabecular meshwork.*

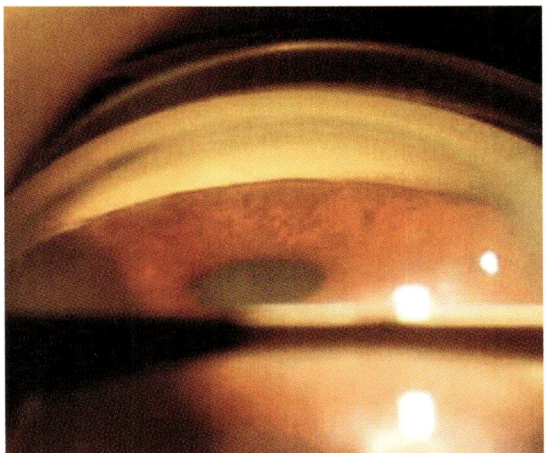

Fig. 13.7: *Closed-angle with no structure visible between iris and corneal periphery.*

and further manipulation/indentation has to be done to view the angle and distinguish between appositional versus synaechial closure.

Functional techniques of gonioscopy

Gonioscopy is performed on a patient in order to answer at least two questions:
- Is the angle occludable?
- Are there any abnormalities in the angle?
- There are other questions, such as grading, of the angle.

To answer the above questions, gonioscopy is done by three functional techniques:
- Gonioscopy *in situ*
- Manipulative gonioscopy
- Indentation gonioscopy.

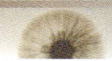

1. *Gonioscopy in situ*. To answer the first question, the testing conditions must be appropriate; what we want is an *in situ* view of the angle. The act of placing any lens on the eye disturbs the angle, but we can routinely use a two-mirror lens to obtain as much of an *in situ* view as possible. The patient is asked to look straight ahead with the lens on the eye. The room lights are then dimmed; the illumination and the height of the slit-beam are decreased so that it does not impinge on the pupil and cause pupillary constriction (with attendant arte-factual opening of the angle). The angle is then observed *in situ* to assess its occludability.

When no angle structure is directly visible on routine gonioscopy *in situ*, the closure of the angle can be due to three reasons:

a. Optical or apparent closure (due to steep iris configuration)

b. Appositional closure

c. Synaechial closure.

Having assessed occludability, we look for any other abnormality in the angle. To do this, we increase the room and slit-lamp illumination, and allow the light to impinge on the pupil, thereby opening up the angle.

2. *Manipulative gonioscopy*. On routine gonio-scopy *in situ*, the angle structures may not be identified in eyes with a steep iris configuration and a narrow angle. To visualize the angle in eyes with a steep iris configuration, the examiner has to use a special manoeuvre to look over the iris. This technique of manipulating the goniolens to visualize over a steep iris (over the hill view) is known as dynamic or manipulative gonioscopy. This can be achieved in Goldmann type of lenses by simply asking the patient to look in the direction of the mirror or moving the mirror towards the angle being viewed (Fig. 13.8A to D). This procedure is called *manipulation* (as opposed to indentation). This allows us to look for peripheral anterior synaechiae.

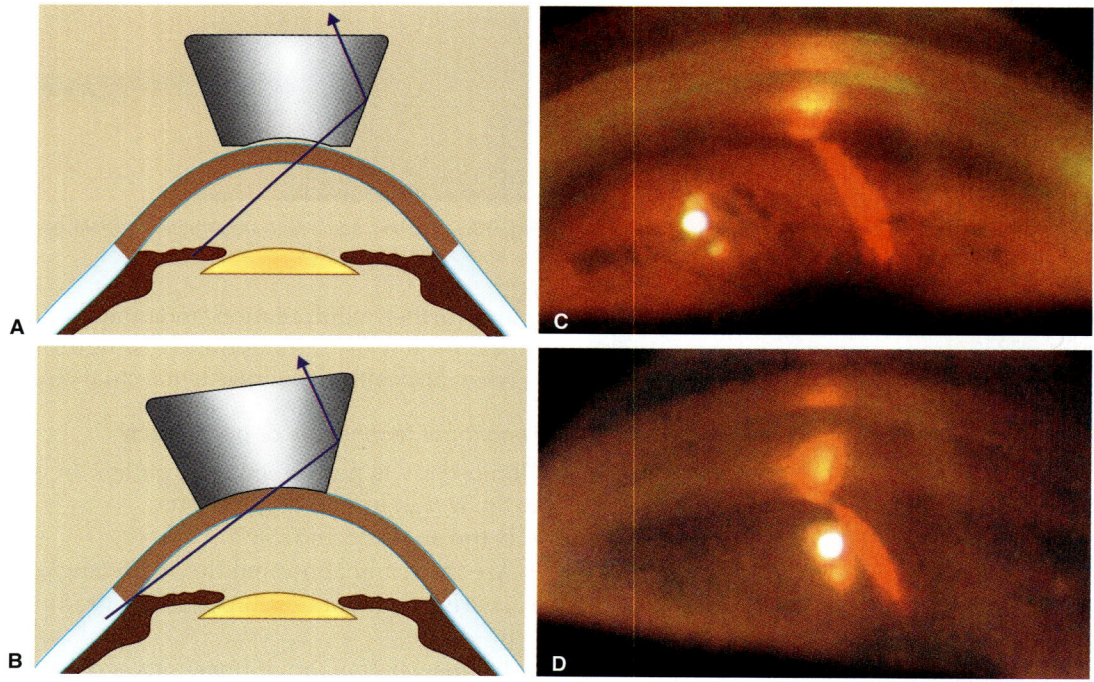

Fig. 13.8: *Gonioscopy in situ versus manipulative gonioscopy in steep iris configuration: (A) Schematic diagram to show how steep iris does not allow view of the angle on gonioscopy in situ; and (B) gonioscopy view, shows narrow-angle recess; (C) Schematic diagram to show how manipulation of the gonioscope allows the view of angle recess; and (D) the gonioscopic view shows open-angle recess.*

3. *Indentation gonioscopy.* If manipulation does not reveal the angle, it can be achieved by *indentation* using an indentation lens. Sussman four-mirror lens is preferred for indentation, since it is held in the hand while Zeiss four-mirror and Posner lenses have to be held by handle. Indentation gonioscopy requires more of patient's cooperation. The indentation lens has to be continuously held just in opposition to the cornea without any pressure. It helps us to differentiate between angle closure due to synaechiae from appositional closure. Indentation deepens appositionally closed angle because of aqueous being pushed in the angle (Fig. 13.9).

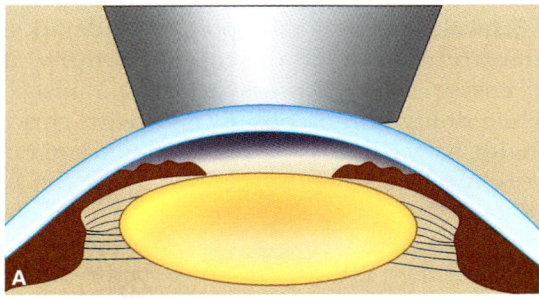
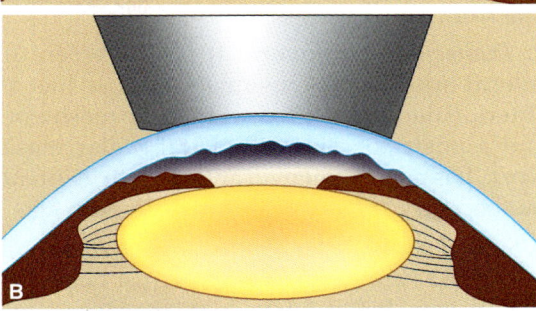
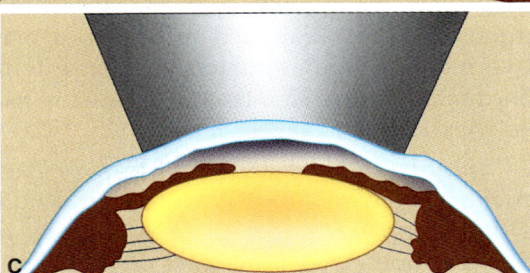

Fig. 13.9: *Schematic diagram to depict how indentation opens the angle recess: (A) Closed angle without indentation; (B) On indentation, the aqueous is pushed into the angle and the angle recess is opened in oppositional closure; (C) In synaechial angle closure, the angle recess is not opened on indentation.*

Besides specific indentation lenses, Goldmann two-mirror lens can also be used. Another reason for using Goldmann two-mirror lens is that it is about half the price of an indentation lens. Although it would be nice to have both, but if one can afford only one lens, one can certainly manage very well with a two-mirror lens alone, which is useful 95% of the time.

Advantages and disadvantages of indirect gonioscopy

Advantages
- Easier to learn
- Faster to perform
- Requires less instrumentation and space
- Slit-lamp provides better optics and lighting
- Corneal wedge can be used to localize angle structures
- Indentation gonioscopy can also be done
- Magnified stereoscopic view of optic disc can also be obtained.

Disadvantages
- Comparison is not possible
- Limited positioning of light rays
- Difficult to perform in horizontal meridian
- Mirror image seen, so confusing
- Excessive pressure may open or close the angle artefactually
- Exaggerates the degree of angle closure.

DISINFECTION OF GONIOSCOPIC LENSES

The American Academy of Ophthalmology issued guidelines for cleaning gonioscopic lens—keeping in mind the presence of HIV and other infectious agents in tears:
- After removing the lens from the patient's eye, it should be immediately rinsed with clean cold water. Mild soap or detergent is then used to clean the surface followed by rinsing with cold clean water and drying with a non-linting cloth.
- For disinfection, glutaraldehyde or bleaching powder is used. The lens is soaked in 2% glutaraldehyde for at least 20 minutes or a 10% bleach solution (1 part bleach to 9 parts water) for 10 minutes.
- The lens is then thoroughly rinsed with clean cold water and dried. It can also be wiped for

10 seconds with a sterile swab soaked in 70% isopropyl alcohol or cleaned with 1 : 1000 merthiolate solution.

- Sterilization follows disinfection which is achieved by ethylene oxide exposure (ETO) at 56°C (130°F) for one hour.
- Glass lenses can be autoclaved, when require.

Note. Formalin and phenol have been found to damage lenses.

GONIOSCOPIC VIEW AND GRADING OF ANGLE

GONIOSCOPIC VIEW OF ANGLE STRUCTURES

While performing gonioscopy, one can identify the structures from anterior to posterior or *vice versa*. *Angle structures* seen from anterior to posterior are (Fig. 13.10A):

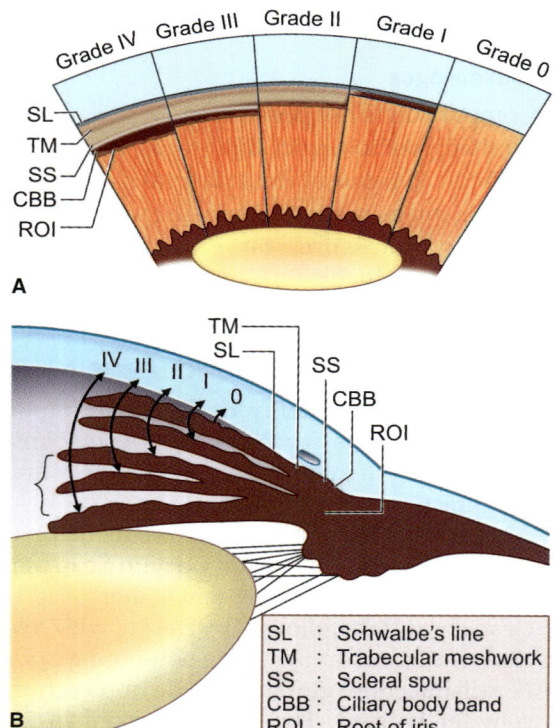

A

B

SL	:	Schwalbe's line
TM	:	Trabecular meshwork
SS	:	Scleral spur
CBB	:	Ciliary body band
ROI	:	Root of iris

Fig. 13.10: *Diagrammatic depiction of various angle structures as seen in different grades of angle width (Shaffer's grading system): (A) Diagrammatic depiction of gonioscopic view; (B) Configuration of the angle in cross-section of the anterior chamber.*

1. *Schwalbe's line.* It is the peripheral termination of the cornea where the Descemet's membrane ends. It is marked only by a slight change in colour from trabecular meshwork or by a faint white line. It can be best identified by locating the *corneal wedge.* A thin slit of light slightly inclined from the oculars is projected onto the cornea. In the angle, two separate corneal reflections are perceived; one illuminates the inner and the other illuminates outer aspect of the cornea. In addition to the inner and outer parts of the cornea, the lines also illuminate the opaque scleral face. The portion between the two lines is called the corneal wedge; the corneal wedge intersects at and identifies Schwalbe's line.

Schwalbe's line is an important landmark in identifying the gonioscopic anatomy in confusing angles. It is easy to make a mistake while doing gonioscopy in eyes with closed angles, hazy corneas and pigmentation anterior to Schwalbe's line. Such a false angle can be mistaken for an open-angle. Therefore, one should stress on identifying the Schwalbe's line first and then identifying the structures from anterior to posterior.

2. *Trabecular meshwork.* It lies between the scleral spur and Schwalbe's line. It has an anterior non-pigmented trabecular meshwork and a posterior pigmented trabecular meshwork. It is non-pigmented and smooth in infants but becomes coarse and pigmented with age.

3. *Scleral spur.* It appears as thin, white or light grey band (yellowish in elderly) just below the trabeculum. It is a fairly consistent landmark. Argon laser burns, if applied posterior to it, may have increased inflammatory response with concomitant increased intraocular pressure and peripheral anterior synaechiae.

4. *Ciliary body band.* It is light grey or dark brown, just posterior to the scleral spur. Width of the ciliary body band varies (narrow in hypermetropes, wide in myopes or aphakics).

5. *Root of iris.* Iris contour is slightly convex or flat. Colour varies in different individuals. Radial markings and crypts are present. Peripherally, concentric contraction rolls are present.

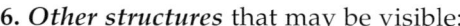

6. Other structures that may be visible:
- *Iris processes*. These are normal variants that should have disappeared in the normal course of development. They appear as fine strands extending from iris to the scleral spur. Unlike peripheral anterior synaechiae, iris processes follow the concavity of the angle, do not inhibit the movement of iris during indentation gonioscopy and do not obstruct the flow of aqueous.
- *Blood vessels*. Blood vessels may be present normally and are branches of the major circle of iris. Unlike neovascularization, they are either arranged radially or form loops.
- *Schlemm's canal*. It lies deep in the posterior portion of trabecular meshwork and, therefore, is not visible generally. It can be made visible by filling it with blood. This could be done either by compressing ipsilateral jugular vein or by pressure from Goldmann's lens.

GRADING SYSTEMS FOR THE ANGLE OF ANTERIOR CHAMBER

Several grading systems have been devised to quantify the findings and for future reference:

I. Scheie's grading

Scheie gave his gonioscopic classification of the anterior chamber angle, based on the extent of visible angle structures as:
- *Wide open*. All structures visible.
- *Grade I narrow*. Hard to see over iris root into recess.
- *Grade II narrow*. Ciliary body band obscured.
- *Grade III narrow*. Posterior trabeculum obscured.

- *Grade IV narrow* (closed). Only Schwalbe's line visible.

II. Shaffer's grading

In this system, an estimation of the angle width is achieved by observing the amount of separation between the two imaginary lines, constructed tangential to the inner surface of the trabeculum and the anterior iris surface. This grading system also provides a method of comparing the widths of the different chamber angles. The system assigns a numerical grade (0–4) to each angle with associated anatomical description, the angle width in degrees and implied clinical interpretation is as below (Table 13.1 and Fig. 13.10).

1. *Grade IV* (35–45°) is the widest angle characteristic of myopia and aphakia in which the ciliary body can be visualized with ease. It is incapable of closure.
2. *Grade III* (20–35°) is an open angle in which at least the scleral spur can be identified. It is incapable of closure.
3. *Grade II* (20°) is a moderately narrow angle in which only the trabeculum can be identified. Angle closure is possible but unlikely.
4. *Grade I* (10°) is a very narrow angle in which only Schwalbe's line and perhaps also the top of the trabeculum can be identified. Angle closure is not inevitable, although the risk is high.
5. *A slit angle* is one in which there is no obvious iridocorneal contact but no angle structures can be identified. This angle has the greatest danger of imminent closure.

Grade	Angle width	Configuration closure	Chances on gonioscopy	Structures visible
Table 13.1 *Shaffer's system of grading the angle width*				
IV	35–45°	Wide open	Nil	From Schwalbe's line to ciliary body
III	20–35°	Open angle	Nil	From Schwalbe's line to scleral spur
II	20°	Moderately narrow	Possible	From Schwalbe's line to trabecular meshwork
I	10°	Very narrow	High	Schwalbe's line only
0	0°	Closed	Closed	None of the angle structures visible

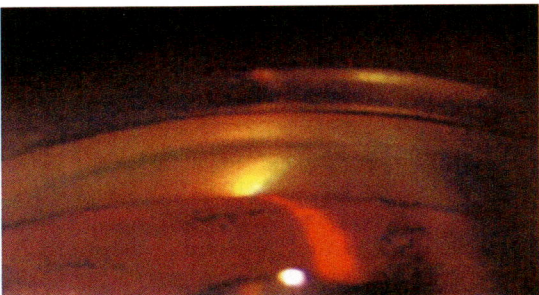

Fig. 13.11: *Gonioscopic photograph revealing grade 0—angle closure.*

6. *Grade 0* (0°) is a closed angle resulting from iridocorneal contact; it is recognized by the inability to identify the apex of the corneal wedge (Fig. 13.11).

III. RP Centre gonioscopic grading

It has been described by Dr Rajendra Prasad Centre for Ophthalmic Sciences, AIIMS, New Delhi, and is based on indirect gonioscopic findings. There is a good interobserver agreement of this system.

Grade 0: No dipping of the beam

Grade 1: Dipping of the beam

Grade 2: Schwalbe's line and anterior one-third of the trabecular meshwork visualized

Grade 3: Middle one-third of trabecular meshwork visualized

Grade 4: Posterior one-third of trabecular meshwork visualized

Grade 5: Scleral spur visualized

Grade 6: Ciliary body band visualized

Note. Grade 3 and less are considered narrow. Grade 2 and less are considered closed. The above classification can easily be modified to state the structures seen. This has the advantage that it does not have to be committed to memory; the angle is graded according to the structure seen without converting it into a numerical representation, thus decreasing the chance of interobserver variability.

IV. Modified gonioscopic grading

N: No dipping of the beam

D: Dipping of the beam

SL: Schwalbe's line and anterior one-third of trabecular meshwork seen

TM: Middle one-third of trabecular meshwork visualized

SC: Posterior one-third of trabecular meshwork (location of Schlemm's canal) visualized

SS: Scleral spur visualized

CB: Ciliary body band visualized

Whatever the classification used (or not used), in addition to the grading, the ophthalmologist should make a forced choice decision as to whether the angles are occludable or not, based on the type of entry into the angle (narrow or wide) and the angle structures visible.

SCHEMATIC DRAWING OF GONIOSCOPIC FINDINGS

Gonioscopy involves various systems of classifying the anterior chamber angle but they stop short of giving information about other pathologies seen. Becker came out with a scheme of representing the gonioscopic findings which involves (Fig. 13.12):

• Drawing a dark circle, depicting scleral spur

• Drawing three lighter circles outside that for the trabecular meshwork

• Drawing three circles inside it, depicting various levels of insertion of the iris

• Drawing the pupil in the centre

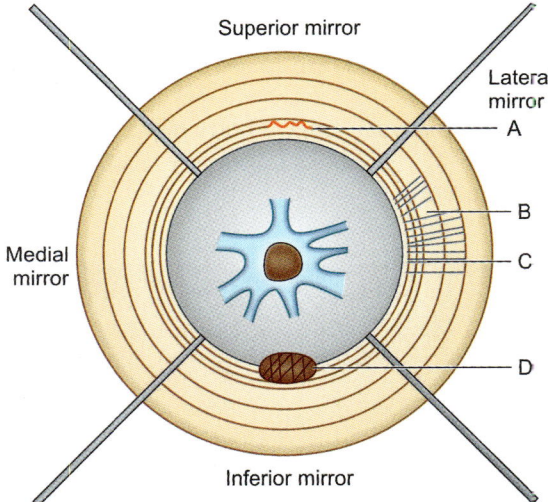

Fig. 13.12: *Schematic drawing of gonioscopic findings: (A) neovascularization; (B) peripheral anterior synaechiae; (C) level of insertion of iris; (D) peripheral iridectomy.*

Table 13.2 *Colour codes for gonioscopic findings*

Findings	Colour
Iris	Drawn in colour of the eye, e.g. blue and brown
Iris pathology, e.g.	
Iridectomy	Black, cross-hatched
Blood vessels	Red
Synaechiae	Orange
Membranes	Yellow
Pigment	Black
Depigmentation	Purple
Angle recession	Brown, cross-hatched

• Each eye is examined quadrant-wise—going clockwise, starting from the inferior angle because it usually is the widest and helps in orientation. Colour coding of findings simplifies the interpretation and provides all the information at one glance. For colour coding of gonioscopic findings, refer to Table 13.2.

Gonioscopic findings could be simplified to drawing only three circles as shown in Fig. 13.13.

These methods of standardized representation reduce the need for writing down every finding.

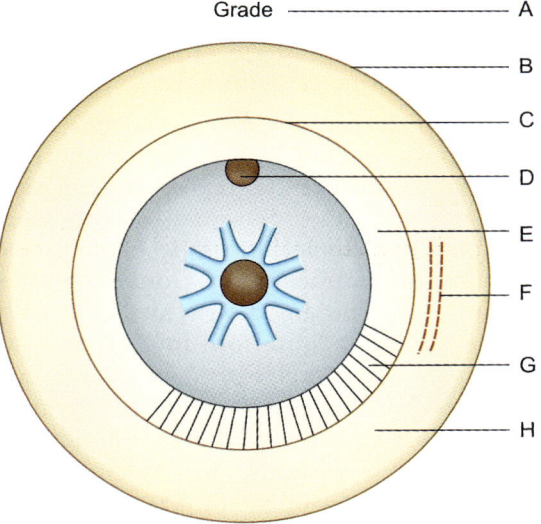

Grade ———————————— A
———————— B
————— C
————— D
———— E
——— F
——— G
——— H

Grade

Fig. 13.13: *Modified method of representing gonioscopic findings: (A) grading of angle; (B) Schwalbe's line; (C) scleral spur; (D) peripheral iridectomy; (E) angle recess; (F) position of Schlemm's canal; (G) peripheral anterior synaechiae; (H) trabecular meshwork.*

They also help in better communication of facts between ophthalmologists. They also make follow-up quicker because the ophthalmologist does not have to refer to voluminous notes each time the patient comes for follow-up.

BIOMETRIC GONIOSCOPY

This is a new method for objective measurement of the anterior chamber angle, proposed by Congdon, et al. *Ophthalmology* 1999;106:2161–67. In this method, gonioscopic measurements are performed with the help of a special reticule. The anterior chamber angle is viewed under the following conditions on a Haag-Streit 900 BM slit-lamp: Ambient lighting from a small side lamp is used to provide only an indirect illumination with a total magnification of 16°, power of 6 W, middle filter setting and a slit-lamp beam of 4 mm length and 1 mm width. The reticule is mounted on a slit-lamp 10° ocular and ruled in 0.1 mm units, which is used to measure the distance between the insertion of the iris and the Schwalbe's line. Measurements are recorded separately in the superior, inferior, nasal and temporal quadrants. If the angle is closed, a measurement of 0 is recorded while an occludable angle is defined as one with an average measurement of 0.25 mm or less for the four quadrants.

This method correlates well with other measures of the anterior chamber angle like conventional gonioscopy and Scheimpflug photography, shows a much higher degree of interobserver reliability than conventional gonioscopy and can be readily learned and performed by an inexperienced observer. Hence, it offers a definite advantage over conventional gonioscopy, which is purely a subjective technique and has a long learning curve.

CLINICAL USES AND LIMITATIONS

CLINICAL USES OF GONIOSCOPY

Some of the many uses of gonioscopy are listed below:

• *To make the crucial differentiation* between primary open-angle glaucoma and primary angle-closure glaucoma.

- *To diagnose and provide a prognosis* for the congenital glaucomas.
- *To diagnose secondary glaucomas*, especially subtle angle recession, uveitic glaucoma and that due to early neovascularization, and iridocorneal endothelial syndromes. The black pigment balls are quite characteristic of the resolved hyphaema. This sign may be the only indicator of past trauma.
- *To diagnose conditions, like tumours* of the anterior segment, ciliary body cysts, intra-ocular foreign body and for early detection of Kayser-Fleischer ring.
- *To diagnose unusual causes of glaucoma*, e.g. a haptic of a posterior chamber lens protruding through the peripheral iridectomy and resting in the angle of anterior chamber. The resultant pseudophakic pigmentary glaucoma can only be diagnosed by gonioscopy.
- *Gonioscopy for treatment*. To perform argon laser trabeculoplasty, laser iridoplasty, laser cyclophotocoagulation. Gonioscopy is also necessary for follow-up on patients who have undergone peripheral iridotomy, trabeculectomy. It now becomes obvious that in addition to the patient care and academic purposes, learning gonioscopy has the potential to more than pay for the cost of gonioscopes.
- *Indentation gonioscopy can be used to break* an attack of acute angle-closure glaucoma.

CRITICAL QUESTIONS TO BE ANSWERED DURING GONIOSCOPY

1. *What are the angle structures visible?* The angle configuration depends on the posterior most angle structure visible in primary position without manipulation. If you are able to see the scleral spur in such circumstance, then angle is considered to be open.

2. *Does the iris touch the trabecular meshwork?* Irido-trabecular contact can be in the form of appositional/synaechial contact. Peripheral anterior synaechiae (Fig. 13.14) represent non-reversible contact. If peripheral anterior synaechiae are present, the extent of same should be specified to know its effect on the trabecular outflow.

3. *Is there evidence of previous irido-TM contact?* Coarse and blotchy pigment clumps

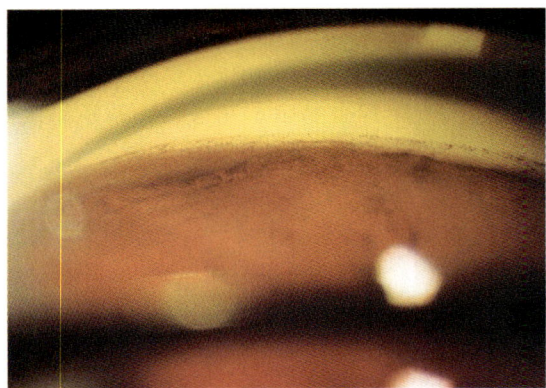

Fig. 13.14: *Peripheral anterior synaechiae.*

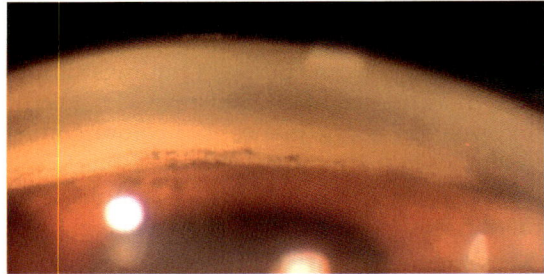

Fig. 13.15: *Pigment clumps in angle forming pseudo-trabecular meshwork in angle-closure glaucoma.*

(Fig. 13.15) in the angle are suggestive of previous irido-trabecular contact.

4. *Is iridotrabecular contact—reversible?* Iridotrabecular contact can be synaechial or appositional. Indentation gonioscopy with Zeiss type lenses (Posner, Sussman) is the 'Gold Standard' for detecting angle closure and differentiating appositional from synaechial closure. When no angle structure is directly visible before indentation, four things can happen on indentation (Fig. 13.16A to D).

- The iris moves peripherally backwards, assumes a concave configuration and the angle recess widens. This represents an appositional closure with a suspicion of a relative pupillary block.
- The iris moves peripherally backwards, but the periphery of the iris bulges out and does not assume a concave configuration. This represents an anteriorly displaced ciliary body and iris root, typically seen in plateau iris.

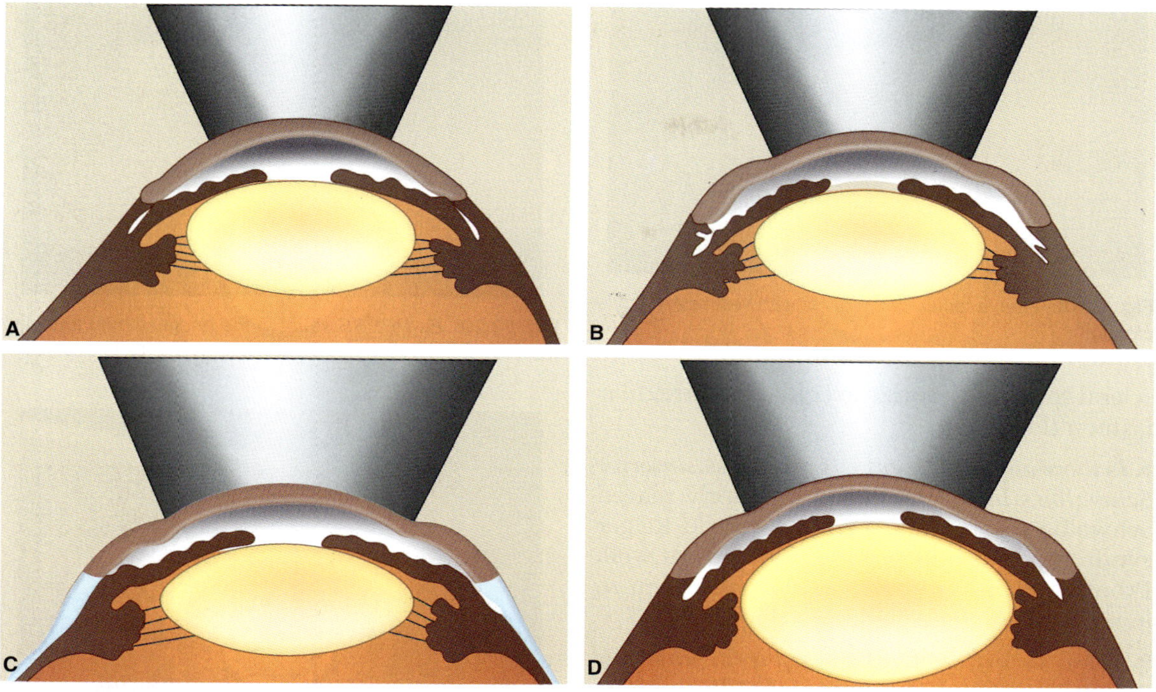

Fig. 13.16: *Indentation gonioscopy: (A) In an apparently closed angle; (B) Angle opens up in a case with appositional closure; (C) Indentation reveals synaechial closure; (D) Thick lens does not allow the chamber to deepen or the iris to move backwards.*

- The angle widens but iris strands remain attached to the outer wall of the angle. This represents organic synaechial closure of the angle.
- The iris moves only slightly and evenly backward, but retains a convex profile. This can occur due to an anteriorly displaced lens or a large diameter (thick) lens.

5. *What is the amount of angle pigmentation?*
Pigmentation in the angle can be in terms of:
- Pigmentation of trabecular meshwork—mild, moderate or heavy (Fig. 13.17)
- Pigmentation clumps as in uveitic, post-traumatic glaucomas
- Abnormal pigmentation anterior to trabecular meshwork
- Coarse, blotchy pigments in angle-closure glaucoma.

6. *What is the type of iris configuration and angle recess?* Iris configuration can vary from convex, regular to concave. Angle recess is the

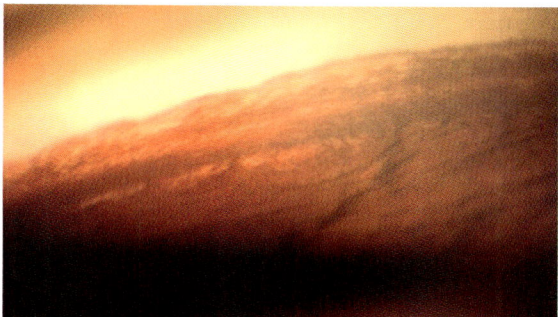

Fig. 13.17: *Dense and even angle pigmentation in pigment dispersion syndrome.*

angle between a line tangential to the trabecular meshwork and a line tangential to the iris surface about one-third from periphery. It is usually narrow than 20° in angle-closure glaucoma.

7. *Is there any new vessels crossing scleral spur?*
Angle neovascularization iris (NVI) is characterized by single vascular trunks which cross the

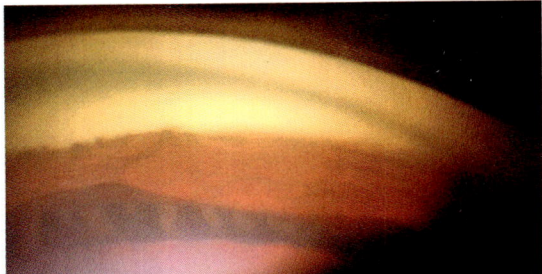

Fig. 13.18: *Neovascularization of iris with secondary angle closure.*

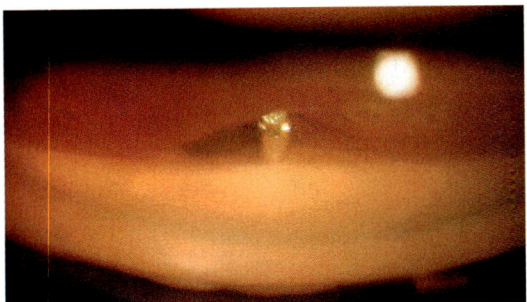

Fig. 13.20: *Ex PRESS shunt in the angle with tip touching the iris.*

scleral spur and arborize irregularly in irregular fashion (Fig. 13.18).

8. Is there any prominent iris processes, anterior Schwalbe's line? Prominent, anteriorly placed Schwalbe's line can be seen in Axenfeld-Reiger syndrome. It can be a normal variant as well. Prominent iris processes are usually seen in juvenile open-angle glaucoma (Fig. 13.19).

9. How to differentiate peripheral anterior synaechiae from iris processes? Peripheral anterior synaechiae are broader, irregular, tent-shaped and bridge the recess instead of following it. They obscure the underlying angle details and are associated with anterior pigmentation. Iris processes, instead, are brown, lacy, finger-like fine extensions of the peripheral iris which follow the angle concavity.

10. Patency of trabeculectomy ostium, view new microimplants? Gonioscopy can be used to assess the fistula created during filtering glaucoma surgery and it can also aid in visualizing new microimplants, such as Ex PRESS shunt (Fig. 13.20).

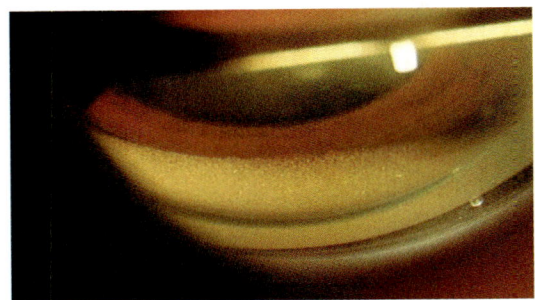

Fig. 13.21: *Silicone oil globules in post-vitrectomy glaucoma.*

11. What do I see in post-vitrectomy secondary glaucoma patients? Emulsified oil globules can be seen with increased pigmentation of angle in such patients (Fig. 13.21).

12. What should be seen in post-traumatic patients? Gonioscopy is a must in unilateral glaucoma patients and it can show: Hyphaema (Fig. 13.22), synaechiae, increased pigmentation, cyclodialysis (Fig. 13.23), iridodialysis, angle recession (Fig. 13.24) and fibrosis of angle.

LIMITATIONS AND ARTEFACTS

Limitations of gonioscopy

- Gonioscopy is a contact investigation which causes discomfort to the patient.
- It can transmit a conjunctival infection to the patient.
- Gonioscopy should not be performed in suspected open-globe injury or early in the course of closed-globe injury with hyphaema as pressure can precipitate re-bleed.

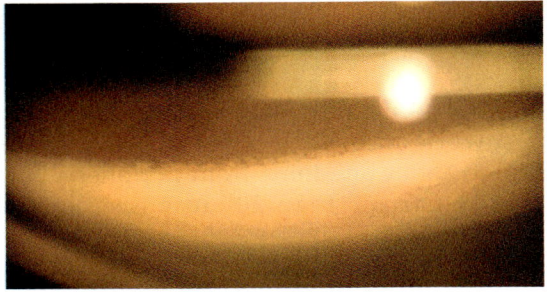

Fig. 13.19: *Prominent iris processes.*

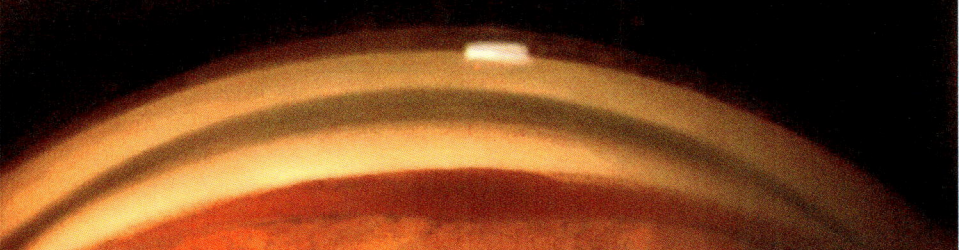

Fig. 13.22: *Post-traumatic hyphaema.*

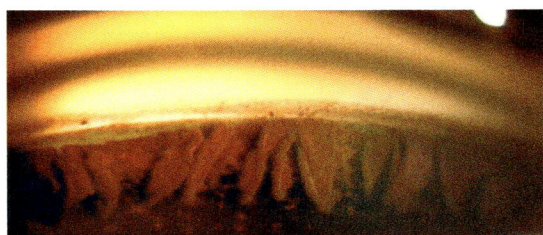

Fig. 13.23: *Cyclodialysis cleft with ciliary processes visible in a closed-globe injury with disinjection of iris from ciliary body.*

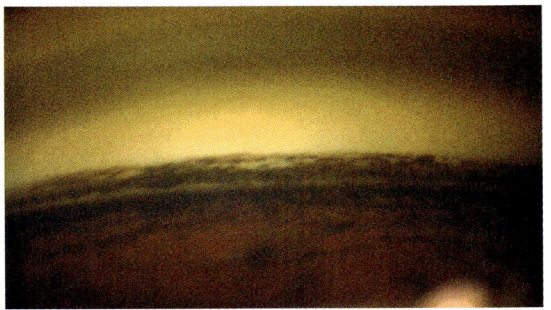

Fig. 13.24: *Angle recession.*

- Gonioscopy is difficult in cases of acute angle closure with corneal oedema and eyes with corneal opacification.
- Excessive pressure while using Goldmann type of lens may artefactually close the angles and while using corneal type of gonioscopes it may give an open-angle appearance in narrow recess angle configuration.
- Use of slit-lamp illumination while doing gonioscopy leads to pupillary constriction and opens up/changes the angle configuration.

- Gonioscopy cannot objectively quantitate the angle parameters and there is a wide inter-observer variability.
- Gonioscopy is not useful to identify pathologies behind the iris.
- Indentation gonioscopy can lead to formation of corneal folds, distorting the view of angle structures and may cause corneal epithelial injury.
- It has a long learning curve requiring regular practice on a large number of patients.

Artefacts

- Excessive pressure artefactually opens an angle while using Goldmann's four-mirror or closes the angle while using Goldmann's single-mirror.
- Residues on lens because of oily secretion or methylcellulose may give rise to artefacts.
- Mirror in Goldmann's goniomirrors is closer to the centre of cornea; therefore, angle recess is better seen, which could give erroneous impression of open angle in case of narrow angle glaucoma.

BIBLIOGRAPHY

1. Fisch BM. Gonioscopy and the Glaucomas. Boston: Butterworth-Heineman, 1993.
2. Gonioscopy: A text and atlas. Tanuj Dada. Jaypee Publications, 2014.
3. Gorin G, Posner A. Slit Lamp Gonioscopy. Baltimore: Williams & Wilkins Company, 1967.
4. Kanski JJ, McAllister JA. Glaucoma: A Color Manual of Diagnosis and Treatment. Oxford: Butterworth-Heineman, 1989.

5. Prokopich CL, Flanagan JG. Gonioscopy: evaluation of the anterior chamber angle. Part 1. Ophthal. Physiol. Opt 1996;16(2):S39–42.

6. Rubin ML. Optics for Clinicians, 2nd edition. Gainsesville, FL. Triad Scientific Publishing, 1974;56.

7. Salzmann M. Die Ophthalmoskopie der Kammerbucht. Z Augenheilk 1914;31:1.

8. Trantas AL. 'Ophthalmoscopie de l' angleirido-corneen (gonioscopie). Conclusions a entirer pour la nature du canal de Schlemm Arch Ophthalmol (Paris) 1918;36:257.

9. Vargas E, Drance SM. Anterior chamber depth in angle closure glaucoma: Clinical methods of depth determination in people with and without the disease. Arch Ophthalmol 1973;90(6): 438–45.

Evaluation of Optic Nerve Head

Chapter Outline

INTRODUCTION
• Techniques for disc evaluation

OPTIC DISC CHANGES IN GLAUCOMA
Intrapapillary changes
• Optic disc size
• Optic disc shape
• Neuroretinal rim shape
• Cup–disc ratio
• Position of central retinal vessels and branches

Peripapillary disc changes
• Optic disc haemorrhages
• Nerve fibre layer defects

• Diameter of retinal arterioles
• Peripapillary choroidal atrophy

Diagnostic clues

PATTERNS OF OPTIC DISC CHANGES AND SUBTYPES OF GLAUCOMATOUS DISCS
• Focal glaucomatous optic disc
• Myopic glaucomatous optic disc
• Senile sclerotic optic disc
• Concentrically enlarging optic discs

DIFFERENTIAL DIAGNOSIS AND CONCLUSION
• Differential diagnosis of optic disc cupping
• Conclusion

INTRODUCTION

Glaucoma is defined as a chronic optic neuropathy, typically causing structural damage in the optic disc, usually accompanied by or leading to corresponding functional changes in the visual field. Though intraocular pressure (IOP) assessment and perimetry aid in diagnosis of glaucoma, individually neither of these are enough by themselves. Raised intraocular pressure (IOP) is the only treatable causal risk factor for glaucoma but neither sufficient nor necessary for the diagnosis.

Damage to the RGC axons within the lamina cribrosa is the central pathophysiology underlying visual loss due to glaucoma. Despite the availability of sophisticated imaging devices, clinical optic disc evaluation has proved to be indispensable in clinical practice and has been shown to be valuable for evaluating change. Glaucoma diagnosis is essentially diagnosing glaucomatous optic neuropathy (GON).

An estimated 12 million people are affected by glaucoma in India, the majority of whom (90%) are undiagnosed. By 2020, this number is expected to be 16 million. The major element of glaucoma strategy is case detection, i.e. to at least detect and manage the 'obvious' and clear-cut glaucoma cases with established functional loss. To achieve this, a clinician must be proficient at examining the optic nerve head and be able to diagnose even subtle changes, ranging from early changes to glaucomatous optic atrophy.

TECHNIQUES FOR DISC EVALUATION

Glaucoma affects the surface contour of the optic nerve head. Surface changes are best appreciated with a stereoscopic view. Therefore, the initial examination, and follow-up examination for surface changes, should be made through the pupil when it is at least 4 mm in diameter. Interim examination, for disc haemorrhages, can also be performed through an undilated pupil. Stereoscopic examination of the posterior pole is best performed with the following techniques:

I. Indirect fundus-lens technique. With enough magnification at the slit-lamp, the 60 D, 78 D and 90 D fundus lenses provide high magnification stereoscopic view and have an advantage in identifying many subtle alterations in the ONH, such as discrepancies between the cup size based on colour criteria and contour criteria.

A +90 D lens provides a wide field of view but less magnification in comparison to a +60 D, which provides a narrower field of view but × 1.15 magnification. It is this magnification and depth of field that makes the +60 D lens an excellent choice for examining the optic disc. A +78 D lens lies between these lenses with properties of both.

II. Direct fundus-lens technique involves examination with central part of Goldmann and Zeiss four-mirror at the slit-lamp. The direct fundus lens examination is very useful for ONH and retinal nerve fibre layer (RNFL) examination and can give additional information, such as RNFL defects and disc haemorrhages. Three-dimensional information using parallax movements is possible.

OPTIC DISC CHANGES IN GLAUCOMA

Evaluation of glaucomatous optic disc changes requires assessment and understanding of the morphology and pathology affecting the optic nerve head. Normally, the size and location of optic cup and pallor are the same. However, this is not always the case, especially in disease states. Thus, these two parameters should not be thought of as being synonymous.

- Neural rim is the tissue between the cup and disc margins and it represents the location of the bulk of the axons. Normally, it is seen as orange-red colour because of the associated capillaries.

- *Retinal vessels* ride up the nasal wall of the cup, often kinking at the cup margin before crossing the neural rim to the retina.

Complete optic nerve head evaluation includes eight intrapapillary and four peripapillary features (Table 14.1).

INTRAPAPILLARY CHANGES

Optic disc size

• *Optic disc size is independent* of age after first decade and refractive error less than ± 5.0 D provides only little variation in size estimation.

• *Normally mean area* of the optic nerve head ranges from 2.1 to 2.8 mm².

• *Estimation of optic nerve head size can be done by direct ophthalmoscope*. 5 degree aperture of the Welch Allyn direct ophthalmoscope in an emmetropic eye equals and area of 1.7 mm² thereby providing rough estimation of optic nerve head size.

• *Another method to evaluate the disc* is by direct measurement of horizontal and vertical diameters of the optic nerve head on slit-lamp and the obtained values are corrected with a correction on 1.26 (diameter × 1.26).

• *Optic disc diameter* (mm) = (X/H) × D × C
    X = height of beam as measured by the millimetre rule (mm)

| Table 14.1 *Intrapapillary and peripapillary features for glaucomatous disc evaluation* ||
8 Intrapapillary features	4 Peripapillary features
2 aspects of optic disc: Size; shape	Optic disc haemorrhage
2 aspects of NRR: Size; shape	RNFL assessment
3 aspects of cup: Size; shape; C/D ratio	Arteriolar diameter
Position of central retinal vascular trunk	Parapapillary choroidal atrophy

H = height setting on the beam height indicator when checking with the millimetre rule (mm)

D = diameter of disc as measured by the beam height indicator (mm)

C = correction factor based on high plus lens power

■ *Corrective factor for different lenses* are for Volk 90.0 D × 1.5, 78 D × 1.3, 60 D × 1.

■ *Optic disc size correlates with* a variety of morphological and clinical features.

■ *Small discs* are associated with small cups (Fig. 14.1), ONH drusen, pseudopapilloedema, and non-arteritic anterior ischaemic optic neuropathy.

■ *Intermediate disc* size is associated with arteritic anterior ischaemic optic neuropathy, central retinal vein occlusion, and the most common forms of glaucoma—POAG, juvenile open-angle glaucoma, age-related ('senile sclerotic') open-angle glaucoma, and pseudo-exfoliation glaucoma.

■ *Large discs* have a greater neuroretinal rim area more axonal fibres, larger size and number of laminar pores thereby less susceptible to damage when compared to small disc and is associated with large cups (Fig. 14.2), morning glory syndrome, congenital optic nerve pit.

Optic disc shape

■ Optic disc shape is independent of age, sex, body weight, and height.

■ Normal optic disc is oval and has a vertical dimension 7–10% larger than the horizontal dimension.

■ Corneal astigmatism affects the shape of the disc as seen in high degree of astigmatism.

■ Myopia of more than 12 D is associated with increase in ovality of disc.

Neuroretinal rim shape

■ Neural retinal rim (NRR) changes in glaucoma is what leads to subsequent changes in the cup and thereby loss of visual field.

■ Cup-to-disc ratio provides only an indirect assessment of the amount of neural tissue in the optic nerve head and thereby may be misleading, because a larger diameter of the nerve head may be associated with a thinner neural rim width and larger cup size despite a stable number of axons.

■ Normally, the NRR follows the ISNT rule: The neural rim of the normal optic nerve head is typically broadest in the inferior quadrant, followed by the superior and then the nasal rims, with the temporal rim being the thinnest.

■ As glaucoma progresses, the NRR is diffusely lost in all sectors. Its diminution can predict

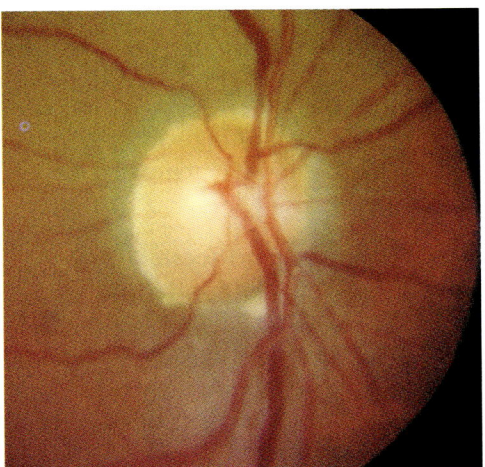

Fig. 14.1: *Small disc with small cup.*

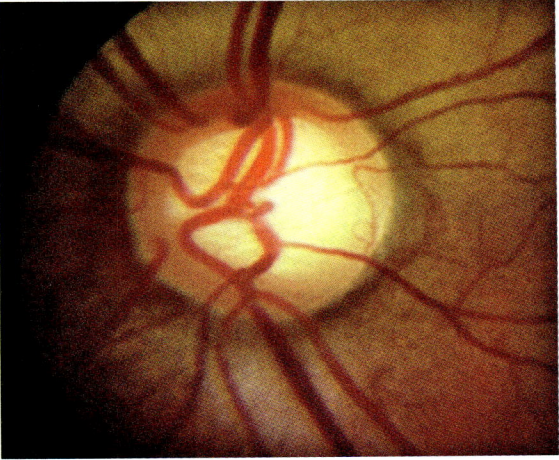

Fig. 14.2: *Large disc with large cup.*

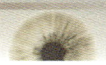

for subsequent visual field loss. Infero-temporal and superotemporal regions are the earliest to be lost, followed by the temporal sector, and lastly the nasal rim.

- NRR area is most import predictor of optic nerve head status. NRR pallor can also act indicator to identify, non-glaucomatous optic atrophy which manifests with neither with enlargement of the optic cup nor with a decrease in the NRR area—but rather with increased NRR pallor and attenuation of the peripapillary retinal vessels.

- Also of clinical interest is the observation that the sector of the NRR farthest from the central trunk of retinal vessels may be affected by rim loss earlier than other sectors.

Cup–disc ratio

- *Normally*, there is vertically oval disc and has a horizontally oval cup with cup disc ratios (CDR) larger horizontally. Seven per cent of normal people have a reversed cup disc ratio.

- *There is symmetric enlargement* of the physio-logic cup in glaucoma, but usually some portion of the rim erodes more rapidly than the rest. Figure 14.3 shows a glaucomatous disc with 0.9 cupping.

- *In myopic eyes* and discs with age-related open-angle glaucoma, the cup tends to be shallow, especially temporally.

- *Contour cup vs. colour cup.* To assess the width of the NRR, the edge of the cup has to be

clearly delineated, most people equate the central pallor of the disc, with cup, but in some glaucomatous discs, there is a discrepancy between the extent of central pallor (colour cup) and the site at which the vessels change their contour (contour cup).

- *NRR thinning* can be localized and appear as a notch, or less frequently, as a pit at the disc rim.

- *An acquired pit of the optic nerve* (APON) is a discrete, focal area of depression within the optic cup at the level of the lamina cribrosa. APONs occur more frequently unilaterally, inferotemporally in 70–80% cases (supero-temporally in rest) and in patients with normal-tension glaucoma (NTG). They often correspond to a deep, sharp-margined scotoma approaching or involving fixation.

- *When notches are present* both inferiorly and superiorly, the cup becomes vertically oval. In glaucoma, the vertical cup always enlarges faster.

- *Cup deepening is characterized by:*
  - *Overpass cupping,* i.e. blood vessel crossing over an area of NRR loss prior to sinking in and taking on the bayonet appearance
  - *Laminar dot appearance,* i.e. exposure of the lamina cribrosa.

- *Disadvantages of the CDR system* for diagnosing and quantifying glaucoma are the variation in cup sizes in the population and more importantly, the fact that the discs do not grow concentrically and eccentric cups may display localized notching. There may be significant intra- and inter-observer error in this method. Therefore, disc damage likelihood score system (Fig. 14.4) was created by Dr George Spaeth.

Disc damage likelihood score

Disc damage likelihood score (DDLS) relies on the optic nerve head as a direct indicator of disease. The DDLS is based on the radial width of the neuroretinal rim measured at its thinnest point. The unit of measurement is the rim/disc ratio—that is, the radial width of the rim compared to the diameter of the disc in the same axis.

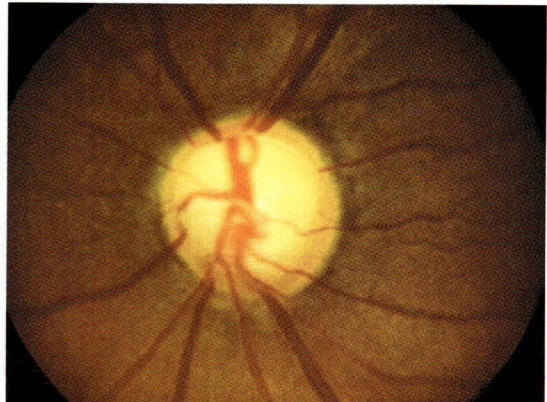

Fig. 14.3: *Advanced GON with a C : D ratio of 0.9.*

New DDLS stage	Narrowest width of rim (rim/disc ratio)			
	For small disc <1.50 mm	For average size disc 1.50–2.00 mm	For large disc >2.00 mm	Old DDLS stage
1	0.5 or more	0.4 or more	0.3 or more	0a
2	0.4 to 0.49	0.3 to 0.39	0.2 to 0.29	0b
3	0.3 to 0.39	0.2 to 0.29	0.1 to 0.19	1
4	0.2 to 0.29	0.1 to 0.19	Less than 0.1	2
5	0.1 to 0.19	Less than 0.1	0 for less than 45°	3
6	Less than 0.1	0 for less than 45°	0 for 46° to 90°	4
7	0 for less than 45°	0 for 46° to 90°	0 for 91° to 180°	5
8	0 for 46° to 90°	0 for 91° to 180°	0 for 181° to 270°	6
9	0 for 91° to 180°	0 for 181° to 270°	0 for more than 270°	7a
10	0 for more than 180°	0 for more than 270°		7b

Fig. 14.4: *Disc damage likelihood score.*

When there is no rim remaining the rim/disc ratio is 0. The circumferential extent of rim absence (0 rim/disc ratio) is measured in degrees. Caution must be taken to differentiate the actual absence of rim from sloping of the rim, e.g. can occur temporally in some patients with myopia. A sloping rim is not an absent rim. Because rim width is a function of disc size, disc size must be evaluated before attributing a DDLS stage. This is done with a 60 D or a 90 D lens with appropriate corrective factors. Because the scale divides glaucomatous progression into 10 stages, it is better able to monitor disease progression than methods with fewer stages, such as the algorithm described by Hodapp-Parrish-Anderson.

Position of central retinal vessels and branches

- Rim sector farthest from the major trunk of the central retinal vessels is susceptible to damage.
- Normally, the retinal vessels pass perpendicularly through the disc tissue to reach the retina. These vessels travel vertically along the cup wall and then horizontally on the retinal surface, the change in course is seen as a bend in the vessel.

- Outward shifting of the bend is associated with thinning of neuroretinal rim. They tend to get nasalised as the glaucomatous changes advance. In early stages, there orientation is vertical bearing of circumlinear vessels common in glaucomatous cups. It may be seen normally as well.

PERIPAPILLARY DISC CHANGES

With the advancement of glaucoma, the following changes occur in the juxtapapillary region: Optic disc haemorrhage, changes in the RNFL; variations in the diameter of retinal arterioles; and patterns of peripapillary choroidal atrophy.

Optic disc haemorrhages

- Located within the neuroretinal rim the disc haemorrhages are usually flame-shaped haemorrhages but can sometimes be blot haemorrhages (Fig. 14.5).
- They are usually seen extending across the disc rim into the retina, but they may occur deep in the disc tissue. As they appear in areas of preserved NRR, they are not usually seen in advanced cases of cupping in which little rim remains.

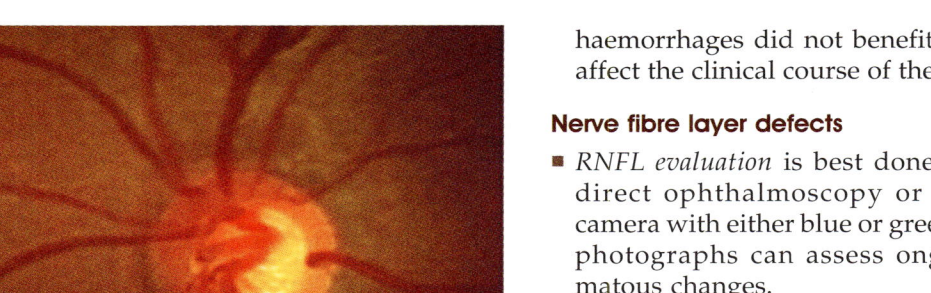

Fig. 14.5: *Optic disc haemorrhage.*

- They may last up to 35 weeks from the time of presentation.
- Non-glaucomatous factors, such as aspirin use and diabetes, are also associated with such haemorrhages.
- Normotensive glaucomas have a predilection for optic disc haemorrhage.
- They may very rarely be found in non-glaucomatous eyes (about 1%).
- *Major studies:* EMGT, OHTS, and collaborative normal tension glaucoma study (CNTGS) indicated that disc haemorrhages were strongly associated with progression.

Curiosities

- *OHTS.* Majority of eyes with disc haemorrhages have not converted to glaucoma.
- *EMGT.* While disc haemorrhages were predictive of progression, IOP-reducing treatment was unrelated to the presence or frequency of disc haemorrhages. Disc haemorrhages were equally common in both the treated and untreated groups of patients. The results may suggest that disc haemorrhages cannot be considered an indication of insufficient IOP-lowering treatment, and that glaucoma progression in eyes with disc haemorrhages cannot be totally halted by IOP reduction. The results also suggest that disc haemorrhages do not occur in all patients with glaucoma.
- *CNTGS.* While disc haemorrhages predicted progression, treating eyes with disc

haemorrhages did not benefit the patient or affect the clinical course of the disease.

Nerve fibre layer defects

- *RNFL evaluation* is best done by a red-free direct ophthalmoscopy or a wide-angle camera with either blue or green filters. Serial photographs can assess ongoing glaucomatous changes.
- *In healthy eyes*, the RNFL appears slightly opaque with radially oriented striations, which has been likened to "horsehair" (Fig. 14.6). Fibres of RNFL follow an arcuate pattern above and below the macula and are typically brighter at the superior and inferior arcuate bundles than the temporal and nasal bundles.
- *RNFL defects* usually precede the appearance of functional changes in the fields. RNFL defects can be—localized wedge defects and diffuse loss which alone or in combination of both in glaucoma patients.
- *Localized loss* is more easily and consistently recognized, but is less common. The nerve fibres are seen most easily in the retinal area adjacent to the superior and inferior temporal aspects of the disc (superior and inferior Bjerrum's area), where the RNFL is thickest, more obvious in moderately dark fundi as in young and becomes increasingly difficult to see in patients with media opacities or lighter fundus pigmentation as for older patients.

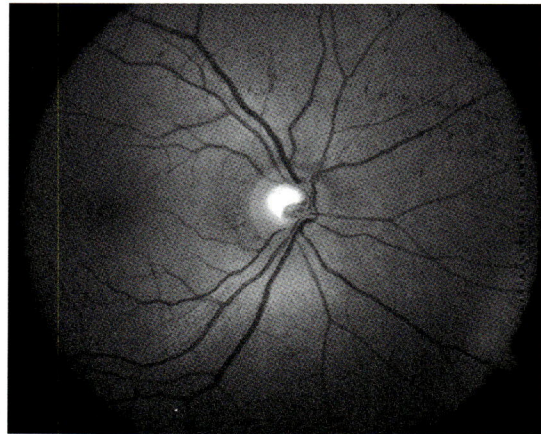

Fig. 14.6: *Red-free photograph showing radial striations of RNFL in a healthy disc.*

Localized loss may occur along with diffuse or generalized loss.

- *Diffuse loss* is more difficult to assess. In cases where RNFL is poorly visible, vessels and vascular reflexes can help differentiate a normal patient from a thinned or generally atrophic RNFL in a patient with disease. If the retinal vessel reflexes are bright and sharp and smaller branches are easily visualized, generalized atrophy may be present.

Diameter of retinal arterioles

- As disease progresses, there is progressive loss of the axonal mass and so demands for peripapillary perfusion decreases. This leads to diffuse narrowing of the retinal vessels on the ONH.
- Narrowing of the retinal vessels is a non-specific indicator of optic atrophy, seen both with descending atrophy and non-arteritic anterior ischaemic optic neuropathy. Such narrowing increases with age but is significantly pronounced in proportion to the degree of optic atrophy.

Peripapillary choroidal atrophy

Normal optic nerve head may be surrounded by zones that vary in width, circumference, and pigmentation. A scleral lip, which appears commonly as a thin, even, white rim that marks the disc margin, usually for the full 360°, represents an anterior extension of sclera between the choroid and optic nerve head. There are two zones described in conjunction with glaucoma:

Beta zone: This zone is broader, irregular and incomplete area of depigmentation.

- An area of depigmentation is caused by retraction of retinal pigment epithelium from the disc margin, with a thinning or absence of choroid next to the disc, thereby exposing underneath sclera (Fig. 14.7).
- It is commonly seen with a tilted scleral canal, as in myopia.
- When zone beta completely surrounds the ONH, it is called the *halo glaucomatous*.
- It also prognosticates the risk of glaucomatous damage in ocular hypertension.

Alpha zone. It is a peripapillary crescent of increased pigmentation that may represent a malposition of the embryonic fold with a double layer or irregularity of retinal pigment epithelium. It is located outside beta zone but may be seen adjacent to the disc, if the zone beta is absent.

DIAGNOSTIC CLUES

To summarize, clues for diagnosing glaucoma are:

- Neuroretinal rim tissue that does not respect the 'ISNT' rule

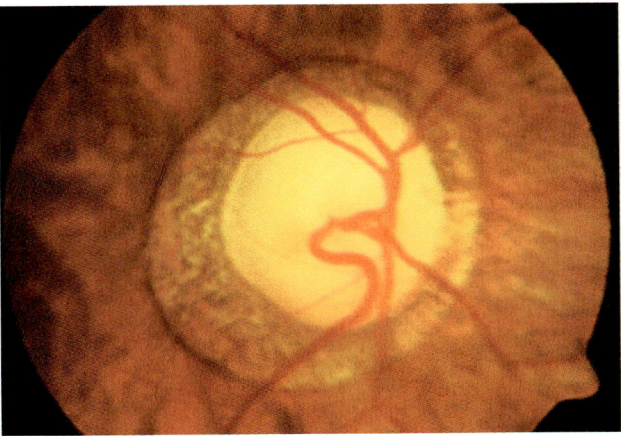
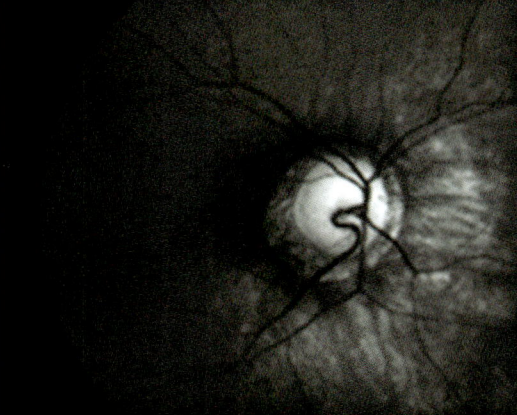

Fig. 14.7: *Glaucomatous optic discs with diffuse thinning of NRR with corresponding total atrophy of the retinal pigment epithelium and choriocapillaris, designated beta zone.*

- Associated notching of the rim, verticalization of the optic cup with baring of a circumlinear vessel
- Vessel bayoneting at the optic rim (indicating bean-pot cupping) and nasalization of vessels
- Disc haemorrhage (Drance haemorrhage) and
- Abnormally large peripapillary atrophy
- Laminar dot sign is seen in advanced glaucoma.

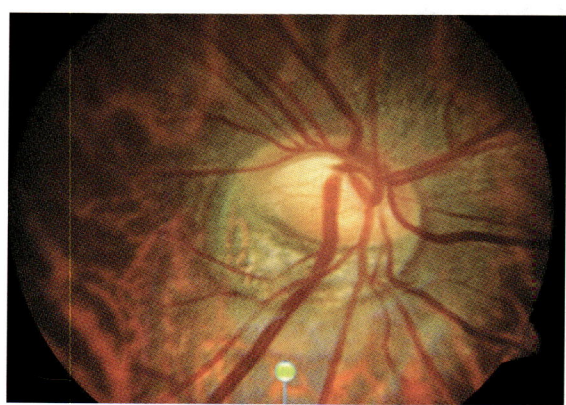

Fig. 14.9: *Myopic glaucomatous optic disc.*

PATTERNS OF OPTIC DISC CHANGES AND SUBTYPES OF GLAUCOMATOUS DISCS

Focal glaucomatous optic disc

In this, there is localized NRR loss at inferior or superior pole just temporal to midline (Fig. 14.8). Such disc changes are commonly associated with migraine and vasospasm. Clinical associations for this disc appearance include a higher frequency among women, scotomas near fixation in the superior visual field, and smaller disc size than other glaucomatous disc types. It may be associated with localized field defects with early threat to fixation.

Myopic glaucomatous optic disc

These discs tend to occur in younger male patients. Myopic glaucomatous discs are usually tilted or obliquely implanted (Fig. 14.9). It has a shallow appearance and is usually associated with the presence of temporal crescent.

Additional features of glaucomatous damage, such as notching, are often present.

Senile sclerotic (atrophic glaucomatous) optic disc

It is shallow, saucerized cup and a gently sloping NRR, variable peripapillary atrophy and peripheral visual field loss (Fig. 14.10). As the concentric cupping progresses, the neural rim may nevertheless retain a pale but almost normal colour. The clinical appreciation of such colour/cup discrepancy is important and often explains why visual field loss appears to be greater than the optic disc changes. The clinical associations for this disc appearance include a higher frequency in older patient group. Hypertension and cardiovascular disease is more common.

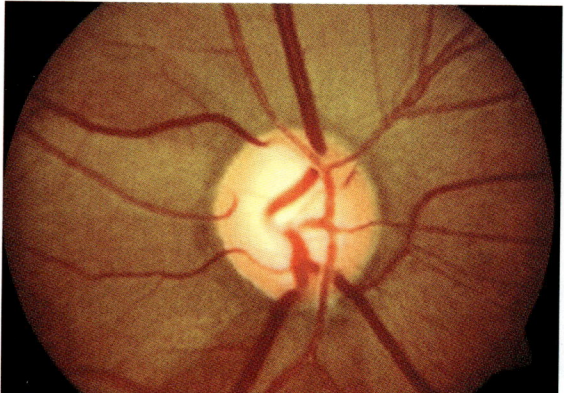

Fig. 14.8: *Focal ischaemic glaucomatous optic disc.*

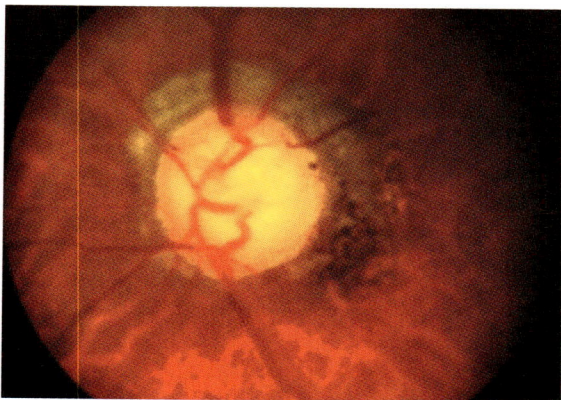

Fig. 14.10: *Senile sclerotic glaucomatous optic disc.*

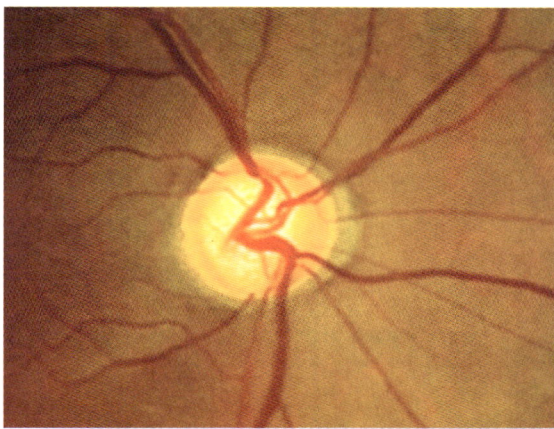

Fig. 14.11: *Concentrically enlarging optic disc.*

Concentrically enlarging optic discs

These discs have uniform NRR thinning (Fig. 14.11) and are frequently associated with diffuse visual field loss. At presentation, IOP is often significantly elevated.

DIFFERENTIAL DIAGNOSIS AND CONCLUSION

DIFFERENTIAL DIAGNOSIS OF OPTIC DISC CUPPING

Other types of optic neuropathies have been reported to cause cupping of the optic nerve, mimicking that found in glaucoma, include:

- Arteritic anterior ischaemic optic neuropathy (A-AION)
- Non-arteritic anterior ischaemic optic neuropathy (NA-AION)
- Posterior ischaemic optic neuropathy (PION)
- Intracranial tumours
- Optic neuritis
- Dominant optic atrophy
- Methanol toxicity
- Shock optic neuropathy
- Leber hereditary optic neuropathy.

CONCLUSION

Patients remain undetected till the late stages of glaucoma due to the asymptomatic nature of the disease combined with the diagnostic dilemma of glaucoma. Diagnosis of end-stage glaucoma straightforward but time delay in diagnosis makes blindness inevitable. So judicially diagnosing glaucoma in earlier stage by careful evaluation of early glaucomatous changes in the optic nerve head can alter the course of the disease and change the prognosis. It is best, if we can detect cases at a stage of early optic neuropathy and there is reasonable certainly that treating the particular patient will help prevent visual impairment due to glaucoma.

BIBLIOGRAPHY

1. Brown GC. Differential diagnosis of the glaucomatous optic disc. In: Varma R, Spaeth GL, Parker KW, editors. The optic nerve in glaucoma, Philadelphia, Lippincott-Raven, 1993.
2. Drance SM, Begg IS. Sector haemorrhage: A probable acute disc change in chronic simple glaucoma. Can J Ophthalmol 1970;5:137–41.
3. Gross PG, Drance SM. Comparison of a simple ophthalmoscopic and planimetric measurement of glaucomatous neuroretinal rim areas, J Glaucoma 1995;4:314.
4. Jonas JB, Gusek GC, Naumann GO. Optic disc, cup and neuroretinal rim size, configuration and correlations in normal eyes. Invest Ophthalmol Vis Sci 1988;29:1151.
5. Jonas JB, Fernandez MC. Shape of the neuroretinal rim and position of the central retinal vessels in glaucoma, Br J Ophthalmol 1994;78:99.
6. Papastathopoulos KI, Jonas JB. Focal narrowing of retinal arterioles in optic nerve atrophy. Ophthalmology 1995;102:1706.
7. Quigley HA, Broman AT. The number of people with glaucoma worldwide in 2010 and 2020.Br J Ophthalmol 2006;90:262–7.
8. Quigley HA, Miller NR, George T. Clinical evaluation of nerve fiber layer atrophy as an indicator of glaucomatous optic nerve damage: Arch Ophthalmol 1980;98:1564.
9. Schwartz B. Optic disc changes in ocular hypertension. Surv Ophthalmol 1980;25:148–54.
10. Schwartz B, Reinstein NM, Lieberman DM. Pallor of the optic disc: Quantitative photographic evaluation. Arch Ophthalmol 1973;89:278–86.
11. Tsai CS, Ritch R, Shin DH, et al. Age-related decline of disc rim area in visually normal subjects. Ophthalmology 1992;99:29–35.
12. Varma R, et al. Positional changes in the vasculature of the optic disc in glaucoma. Am J Ophthalmol 1987;104:457.

Imaging in Glaucoma

Chapter Outline

INTRODUCTION

POSTERIOR SEGMENT OPTICAL COHERENCE TOMOGRAPHY IN GLAUCOMA

Time domain (stratus) OCT scan of posterior segment in glaucoma
• Indications
• Screening protocols
• Glaucoma analysis protocols
• Technique of Stratus OCT scanning
• RNFL scanning using Stratus® versus Cirrus™ OCT

Spectral domain (cirrus) OCT in glaucoma
• Glaucoma analysis protocol by Cirrus™
• Indications of RNFL scanning
• Case study illustrating the usefulness of OCT

CONFOCAL SCANNING LASER OPHTHALMOSCOPY
• Image acquisition
• Components of HRT report

• Evaluating scan quality
• Strengths and limitations of HRT

SCANNING LASER POLARIMETRY
• Introduction
• Image acquisition
• Component of GDx report
• Quality assesment
• Strengths and limitations

ULTRASOUND BIOMICROSCOPY
• Introduction
• Image acquisition
• Clinical applications in glaucoma
• Conclusion

ANTERIOR SEGMENT OPTICAL COHERENCE TOMOGRAPHY
• Introduction
• Applications of AS-OCT in glaucoma
• Advantages and limitations

INTRODUCTION

Establishing functional and structural damage of optic nerve head forms an integral part of glaucoma management. Perimetry is a well-established modality monitoring the functional status in patients of glaucoma. Stereometric examination of optic disc and evaluation of optic disc photograph are subjective methods of assessment of the structural status of optic disc.

In the last decade, various objective methods of *in vivo* imaging, namely time domain optical coherence tomography (TD OCT), confocal scanning laser ophthalmoscopy (CSLO), and scanning laser polarimetry (SLP), have been introduced in clinical practice. The recent development of spectral domain optical coherence tomography (SDOCT) has added another dimension of studying the ganglion cell complex. It is perceived that structural damage precedes functional damage in glaucoma. By the time white on white perimetry shows some defect, about 40–45% of ganglion cells have been damaged, hence the importance of imaging the optic disc and retinal nerve fibre layer. The technologies are new and evolving, it should be interpreted cautiously. The purpose of this section is to provide the basic understanding of these devices, so that they can be utilized appropriately in the diagnosis as well as follow-up of glaucoma patients.

POSTERIOR SEGMENT OPTICAL COHERENCE TOMOGRAPHY IN GLAUCOMA

Tomography is imaging by sectioning or 'slicing' through tissue. In ophthalmology, optical coherence tomography (OCT) represents this technique. OCT can image the anterior segment (cornea and anterior chamber) (Fig. 15.1A) and posterior segment (vitreous and retina) (Fig. 15.1B), but focussing limitations cannot effectively image both anterior and posterior chambers simultaneously.

Time domain technology was the first wave of OCT technology represented in clinical use by the Zeiss Stratus OCT. This is the proprietary design of the Carl Zeiss Company.

Spectral domain/Fourier domain is the second wave of OCT technology developed by many companies, with many spectral domain OCT machines coming on the market at about the same time.

PRINCIPLE

The principle of OCT imaging is based on the measurement of delay in back reflected light from various tissue structures. The OCT utilizes an infrared diode light source (wavelength of 830 or 1310 nm) and a Michelson-type interferometer that detects differential light back scattering from the tissue microstructures. The amplitudes and delays in tissue reflections are scanned by the reference mirror and the interferometric signal is simultaneously recorded. The OCT's false-colour images denote the regions with strongest reflection with red and white colours and the regions with weakest reflection with blue and black.

TIME DOMAIN (STRATUS) OCT SCAN OF POSTERIOR SEGMENT IN GLAUCOMA

INDICATIONS

OCT can be used for both detection and progression of glaucoma. It is particularly important in the setting of suspicious optic discs but normal visual fields which may be the stage of 'pre-perimetric glaucoma' undetected on standard achromatic perimetry.

SCREENING PROTOCOLS

The Stratus OCT enables scanning three regions for glaucoma detection—peripapillary retinal nerve fibre layer (RNFL), the macular region and the optic nerve head.

1. *RNFL measurements.* With the OCT are able to differentiate glaucomatous from normal subjects with good sensitivity and specificity. The RNFL thickness in the inferior region and the mean RNFL thickness are reported to have the best performance to discriminate healthy eyes from eyes with early to moderate glaucoma.

2. *Optic nerve head (ONH) analysis.* The utility for the topographic evaluation of the optic nerve head with the OCT for glaucoma diagnosis and monitoring still needs to be further evaluated. As the automatic algorithm for detection of the

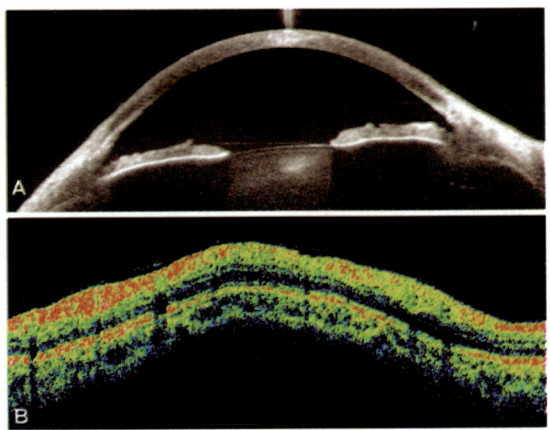

Fig. 15.1: *OCT: (A) Anterior segment; (B) Posterior segment.*

disc margin is based upon the determination of the ends of the RPE/choriocapillaris layer, it is possible that disc margin evaluation may be influenced by changes in these layers, such as in progressive peripapillary atrophy in glaucoma. Another source of error may be that the ONH measurements are obtained from six linear scans, each is composed of 128 sampling points in a radial spoke-like pattern with mathematical interpolation to fill in the gaps.

Nevertheless, recent reports have demonstrated good discriminating ability of (albeit different) ONH parameters. One study showed the rim area and horizontal integrated rim width as the best ONH parameters, while the other found the cup-disc area ratio as the best ONH discriminator.

3. Macular thickness. The mean macular thickness of glaucomatous eyes has been shown to be significantly lower than that of normal control eyes. In addition, a significant correlation between OCT macular thickness and visual field mean defect in glaucomatous eyes had been demonstrated. However, the ability of these measurements to discriminate glaucomatous form normal eyes is less than that of RNFL measurements.

GLAUCOMA ANALYSIS PROTOCOLS

Most frequently used glaucoma analysis protocols include:
- RNFL thickness (single eye)
- RNFL thickness average (OU)
- RNFL thickness serial analysis (OU)
- Optic nerve head analysis (single eye)
- Guided progression analysis.

RNFL thickness protocol

The RNFL thickness is the most frequently used scan protocol. Advantages of imaging the RNFL for glaucoma are:
- RNFL thickness is lost as the glaucomatous disease state progresses
- The status of the RNFL thickness can be followed serially from visit to visit
- RNFL thickness of the patient can be compared to the range of thickness derived from a 'normal' population.

RNFL thickness protocols include:

RNFL thickness (single eye). This is a peripapillary scan protocol (Fig. 15.2). The 3.4 mm diameter circular scan has been found to be optimum for RNFL measurement. The scan circle is centred at the optic disc. Graphs of RNFL thickness are shown along scans made around the optic disc. The normal scan appearance is of 'double hump pattern' indicative of increased RNFL thickness at superior and inferior poles.

RNFL thickness average (OU). This analysis protocol shows retinal nerve fibre thickness representing the right and left eye around the optic disc (Fig. 15.3). One map shows RNFL thickness using a colour code, and the other shows average RNFL thickness in microns. The Stratus OCT has incorporated normative age-matched RNFL thickness data. The software displays graphs that are colour-coded according to the probability of the RNFL thickness measured in the particular patient being normal when compared to age-matched controls.

RNFL thickness serial analysis (OU). This analysis protocol allows the comparison of RNFL thickness over time. It utilizes circle scans around the optic disc to analyze the changes in RNFL thickness from one exam visit to the next. The RNFL thickness graphs of up to 4 visits are superimposed on the same chart and each visit is colour-coded (Fig. 15.4).

Optic nerve head analysis (single eye). The algorithm detects and measures all features of the disc anatomy based on the anatomical markers (disc reference points) on each side of the disc where the RPE ends (Fig. 15.5).

The output chart enables measurement of the optic disc, optic cup, neuroretinal rim and cup/disc ratios using these measurements (Fig. 15.5).

Guided progression analysis. Recent introduction to the guided progression analysis (GPA) protocol, the advanced serial analysis on the Stratus OCT, has enhanced the clinicians ability to detect progression, since it compares the change detected over time to the variability of

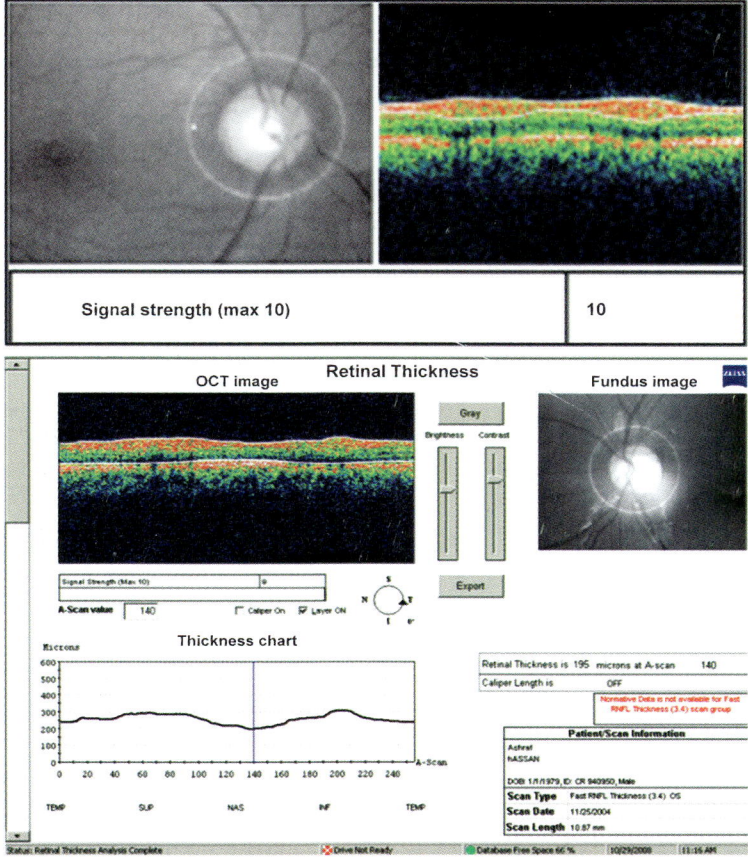

Fig. 15.2: *RNFL thickness (single eye).*

the measurements seen in a patient with glaucoma of the same stage (Fig. 15.6).

TECHNIQUE OF STRATUS OCT SCANNING

Technique of OCT scanning for different protocols includes following steps:

1. *Initial preparation.* The initial preparation for scan acquisition is common for all protocols. The patient details are entered (or selected from the patient menu, if it is a follow-up scan). The height of the Stratus OCT desktop and chin-rest is adjusted to bring the forehead-rest level with the patient's forehead. The height of the chin cup is so adjusted so that the eyes align with the alignment markers on the side of the patient head mount.

2. *Scan acquisition.* From the main window (Fig. 15.7), the glaucoma tab (A) is selected. This would open up a window with the glaucoma protocols (B) displayed. The desired scan protocol is selected by 'double clicking' on it.

This activates the scan acquisition window (Fig. 15.8), from which video and scan parameters can be adjusted from a single interface, enabling the acquisition of high quality scans.

In this window, the scan image is seen on the left of the screen (A), and the video image is seen on the right (B).

3. *Scan placement.* The scanner activates by default in the scan alignment mode, in which the scanner traces an aiming pattern which is seen on the video monitor. This is useful for scan

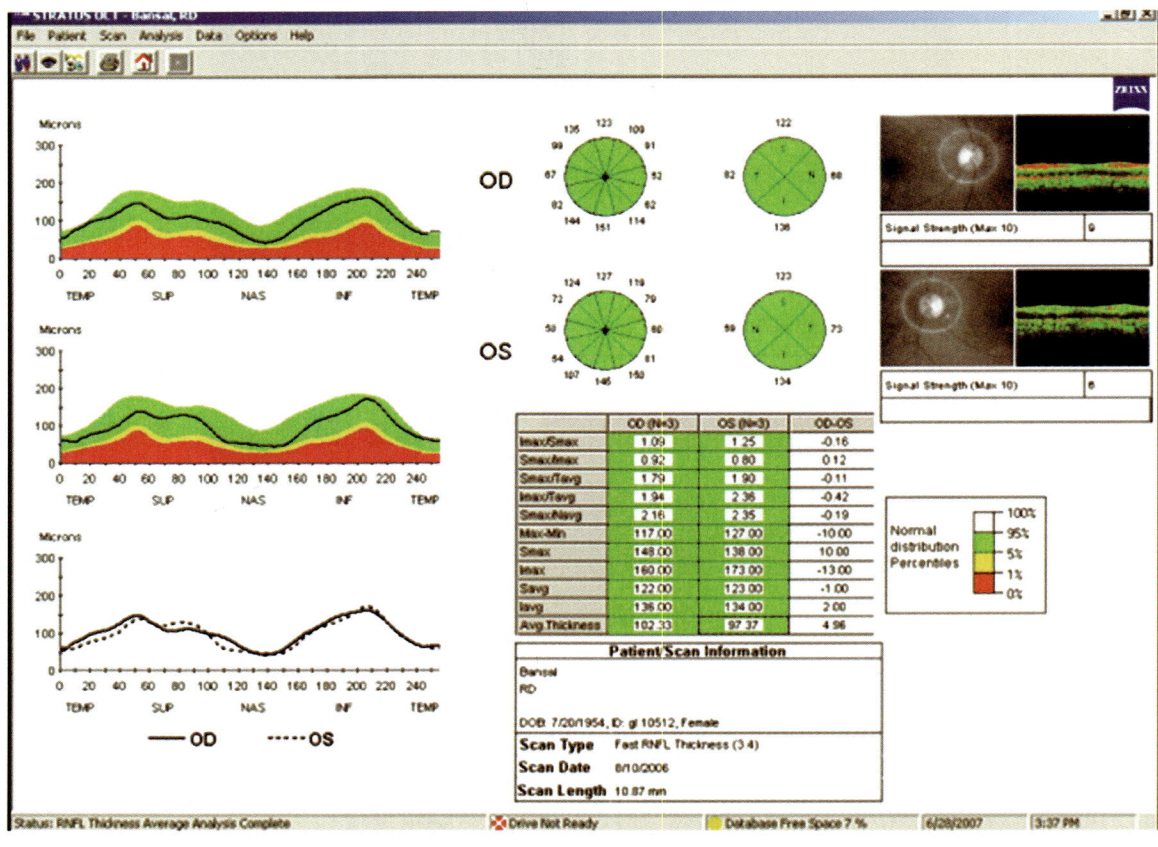

Fig. 15.3: *RNFL thickness average analysis (both eyes).*

placement on the desired position on the optic disc or retina.

- *Scan placement for RNFL protocols.* These are circle scans centred in the middle of the optic disc (Fig. 15.9A).
- *Optic nerve head protocols.* These are line scans arranged like spokes of a wheel, the centre of which should be in the middle of the optic disc (Fig. 15.9B).

Once the video image is satisfactory, and a scan image is placed satisfactorily, the scan mode button is clicked to display the scan acquisition mode. Here the scanner traces the actual scan pattern to be used more slowly. The scan is frozen with or without the flash, using the freeze with flash or freeze without flash buttons. If the quality of the scan image frozen on screen is satisfactory, it is saved using the save button. (If not entirely satisfied, one can

click the cancel button and return to the scan acquisition mode to acquire another scan.)

LIMITATIONS OF TIME DOMAIN TECHNOLOGY WHEN USED FOR RNFL THICKNESS ANALYSIS

Three major sources of error while using the Stratus OCT for RNFL thickness measurement are: motion artifacts, failure to identify the upper and lower borders of the RNFL on low signal to noise ratio scans, and lack of registration.

1. *Motion artifacts.* OCT scan acquisition takes just short of 2 seconds because the reference arm is moving. It is difficult for an eye with good fixation to remain motionless for this time. In eyes with decreased vision due to pathology, eye movement increases dramatically due to which the eye continues to move even after the operator centres the scan circle. This results in a decentred scan (Fig. 15.10).

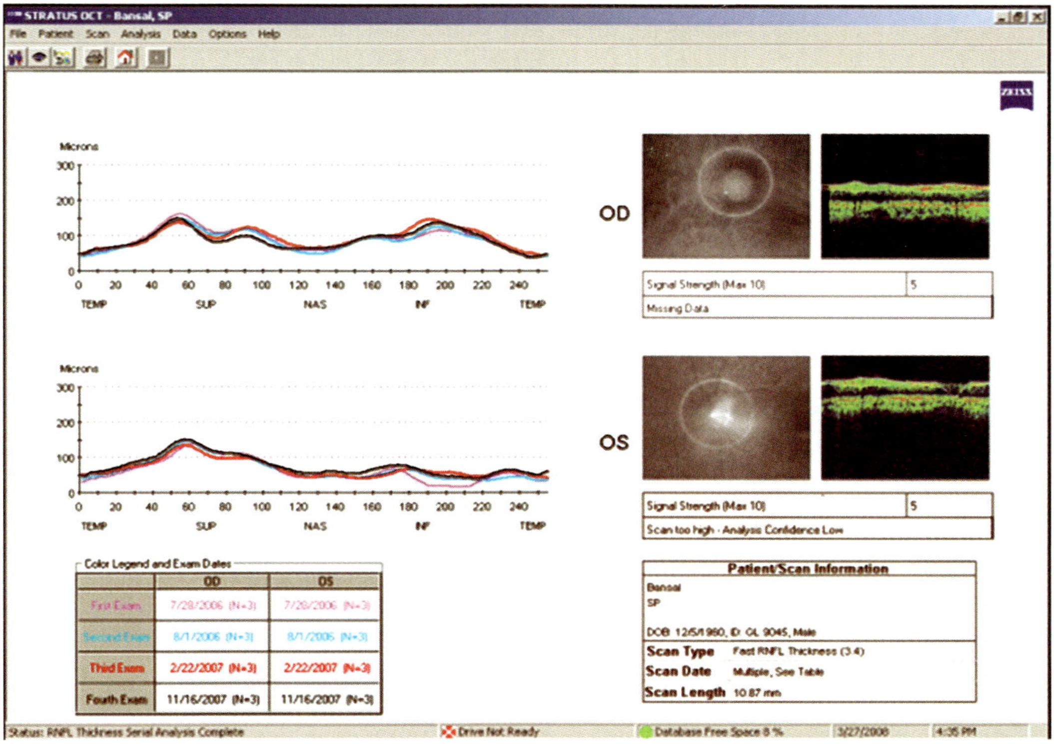

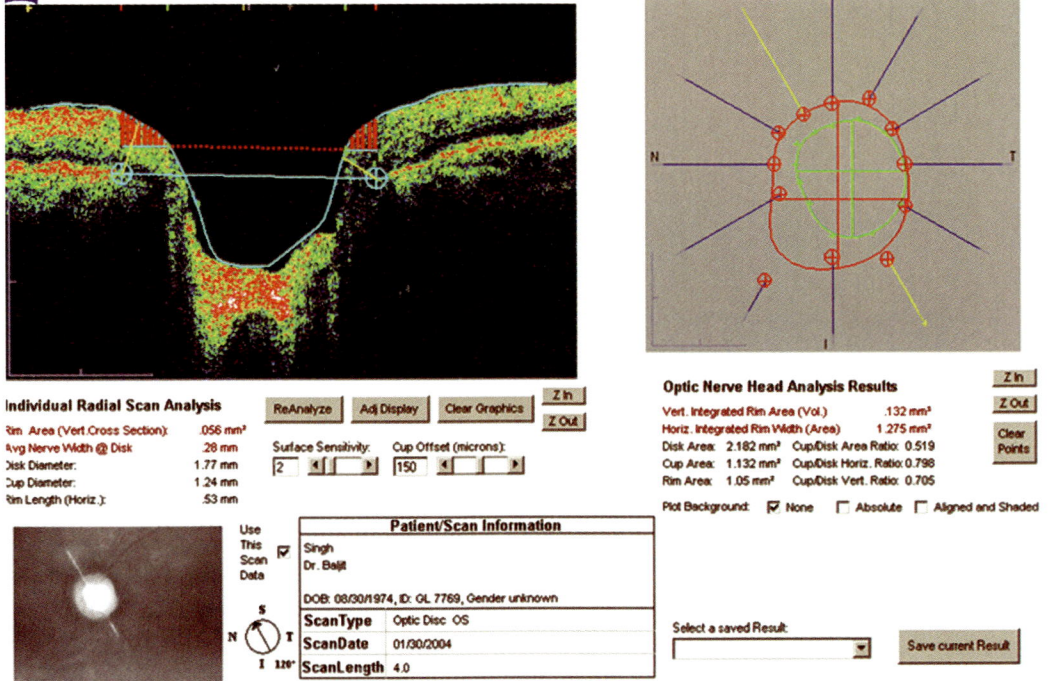

Fig. 15.4: *RNFL thickness serial analysis.*

Fig. 15.5: *Optic nerve head analysis (single eye).*

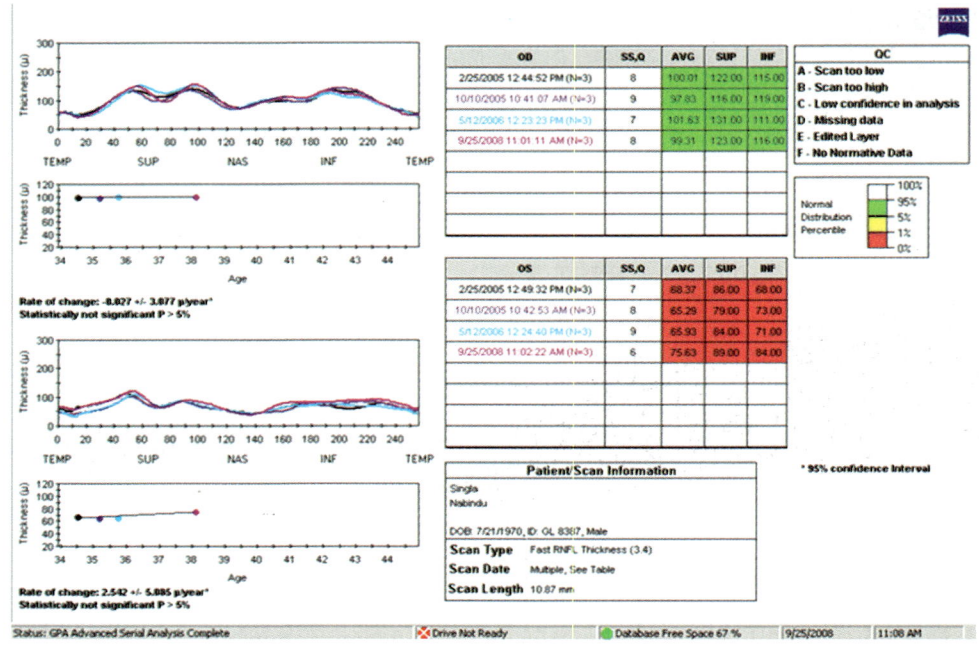

Fig. 15.6: *GPA advanced serial analysis.*

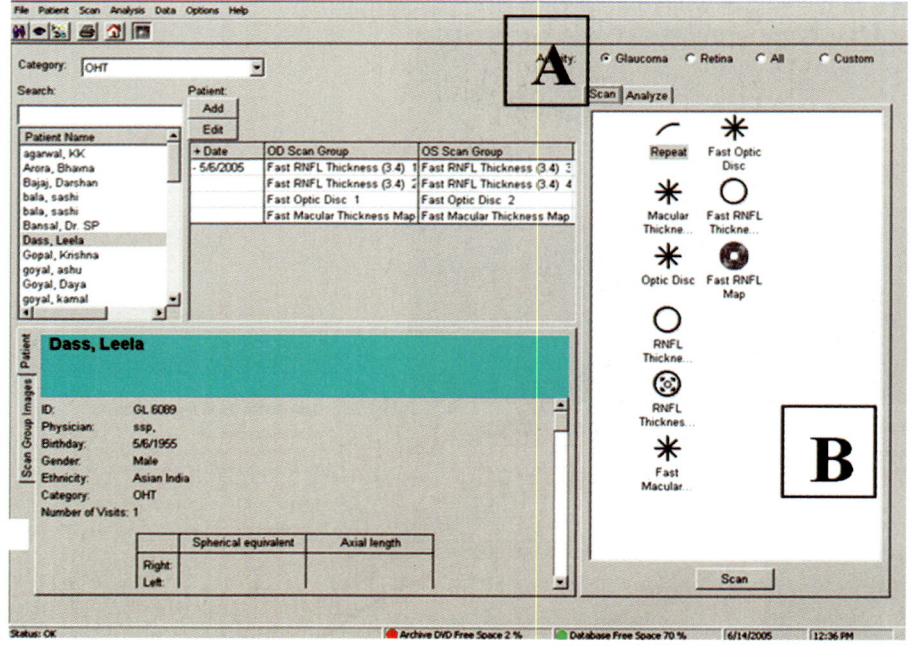

Fig. 15.7: *Main window.*

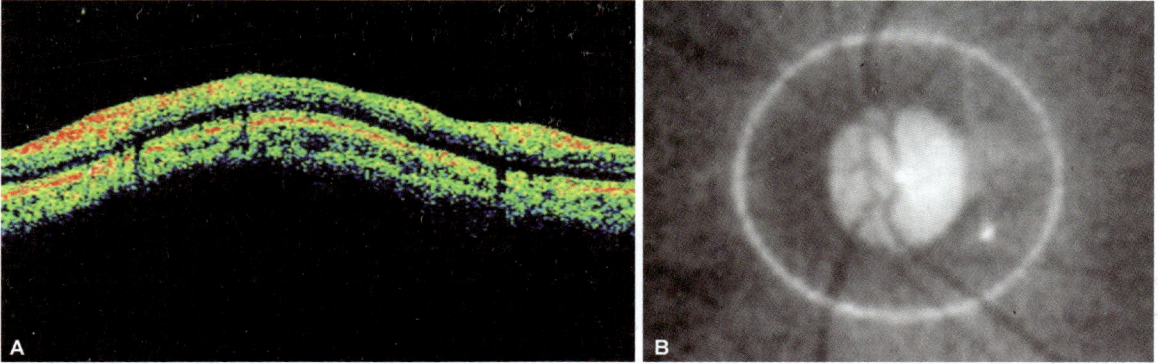

Fig. 15.8: *Scan acquisition window.*

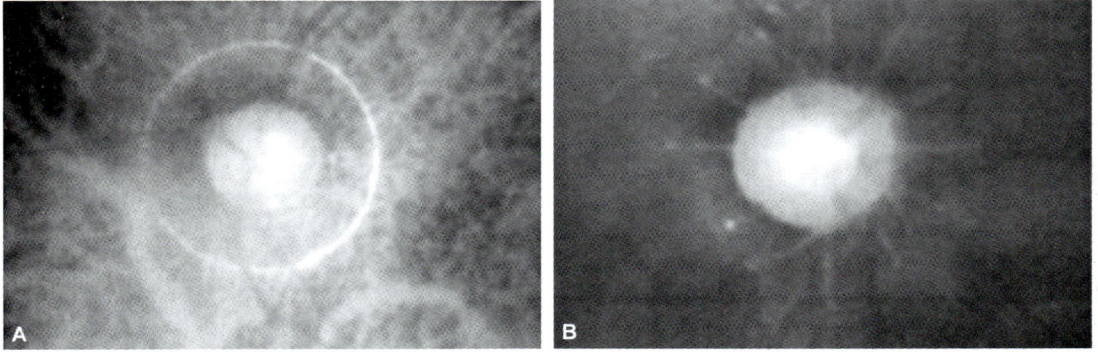

Fig. 15.9: *(A) RNFL scan placement around optic disc; (B) ONH scan placement on optic disc.*

2. *Failure to identify the borders of the RNFL on low signal to noise ratio (SNR) scans.* Boundaries of RNFL are identifiable because they are more highly reflective than the bordering structures (Fig. 15.11). RNFL thickness is measured as the vertical distance between the two lines. There are measurement errors when the software fails to identify the upper and lower boundaries accurately. A poor scan may be due to optical opacities or operator error (Fig. 15.12). There is reduced signal-to-noise ratio and this prevents the software from making a proper identification and tracing.

3. *Lack of registration.* When performing serial scans over time, it is important to scan in the exact same position around the optic nerve head. With the Zeiss Stratus OCT 3, it is difficult to register the scanning circle with anatomical landmarks in order to keep the positioning the same.

Theoretically, one can use a 'landmark' (Fig. 15.13) to mark a certain characteristic, such as a bend in the blood vessel, but practically the operator must be relied upon to centre the circle visually as best as he or she can.

RNFL SCANNING USING STRATUS® VERSUS CIRRUS™ OCT

Table 15.1 and Fig. 15.14 sum-up the RNFL scanning using Stratus® versus Cirrus™ OCT machine.

SPECTRAL DOMAIN OCT IN GLAUCOMA

Glaucoma analysis protocol by Cirrus™

The scan protocol used is the optic disc cube 200 × 200. It generates a cube of data through a 6 mm square grid. The machine acquires a series of 200 horizontal scan lines each is composed of 200 A-scans. A 3.4 mm circle of RNFL thickness

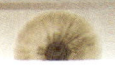

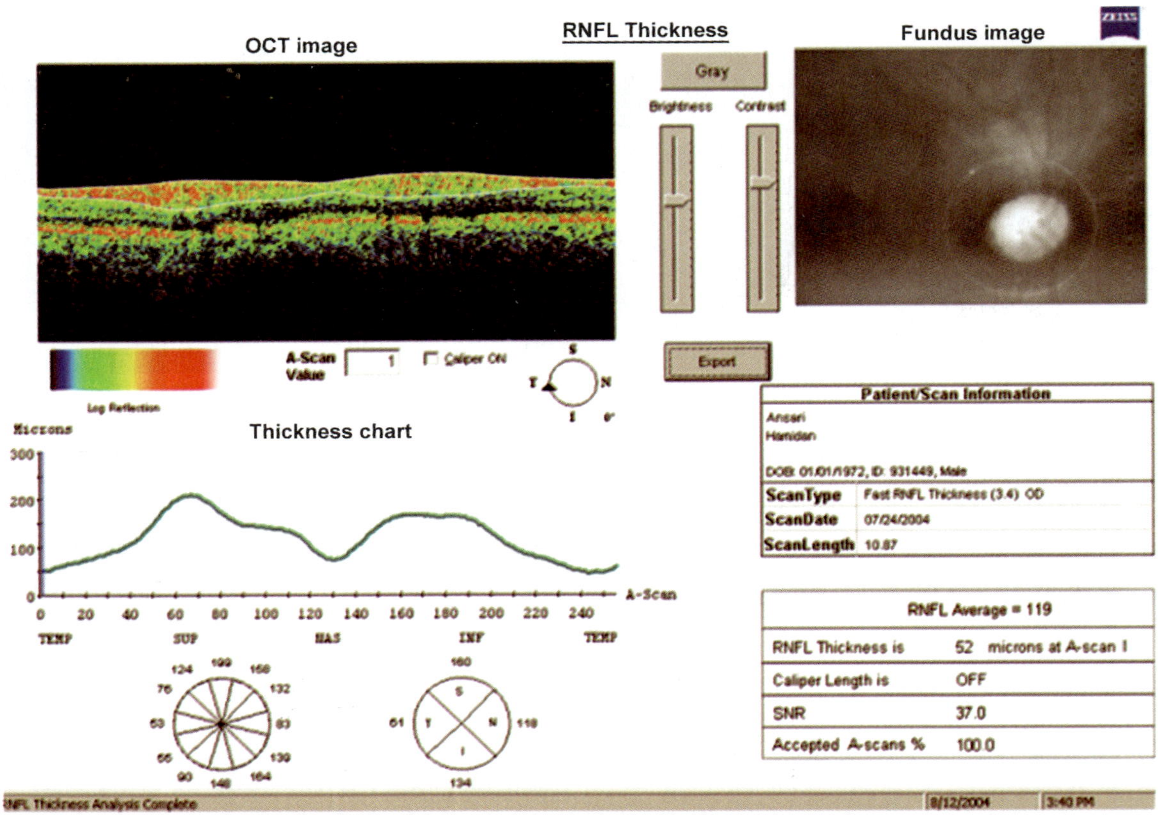

OCT image

RNFL Thickness

Fundus image

Gray

Brightness   Contrast

A-Scan Value   1   □ Caliper ON

Export

Log Reflection

Thickness chart

Microns

300

200

100

0

| 0 | 20 | 40 | 60 | 80 | 100 | 120 | 140 | 160 | 180 | 200 | 220 | 240 |

TEMP   SUP   NAS   INF   TEMP

A-Scan

Patient/Scan Information
Ansari
Hamidan
DOB: 01/01/1972, ID: 931449, Male

ScanType	Fast RNFL Thickness (3.4) OD
ScanDate	07/24/2004
ScanLength	10.87

RNFL Average = 119	
RNFL Thickness is	52 microns at A-scan I
Caliper Length is	OFF
SNR	37.0
Accepted A-scans %	100.0

RNFL Thickness Analysis Complete

8/12/2004   3:40 PM

Fig. 15.10: *Decentred scan.*

Table 15.1 *Sum-up of RNFL scanning using the Stratus® and Cirrus™ OCT*

	Stratus®	Cirrus™
Scan protocol	Fast RNFL	Optic disc scan (200 × 200)
Scans	256 scans × 3 circles	512 scans extracted circle × 1
Laser source wavelength	820 nm	840 nm
A-scan speed	400 per sec	27,000 per sec
Axial resolution	8–10 microns	5 microns (better coherence)
Transverse resolution	20 microns	15 microns

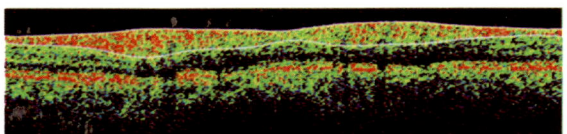

Fig. 15.11: *Good SNR scan with RNFL boundaries clearly visible.*

extracted in this cube (Fig. 15.15). It comprises 512 axial scans—equal to that of a regular Stratus RNFL scan.

Indications of RNFL scanning by spectral domain OCT for glaucoma

It is useful as a baseline and follow-up tool for objective RNFL assessment in ocular hypertensives (OHT) and glaucoma suspects with discs suspicious for glaucoma. In patients with glaucoma, it can be used as an adjunct to visual fields when it is very difficult to assess progression. It may also be useful in glaucoma

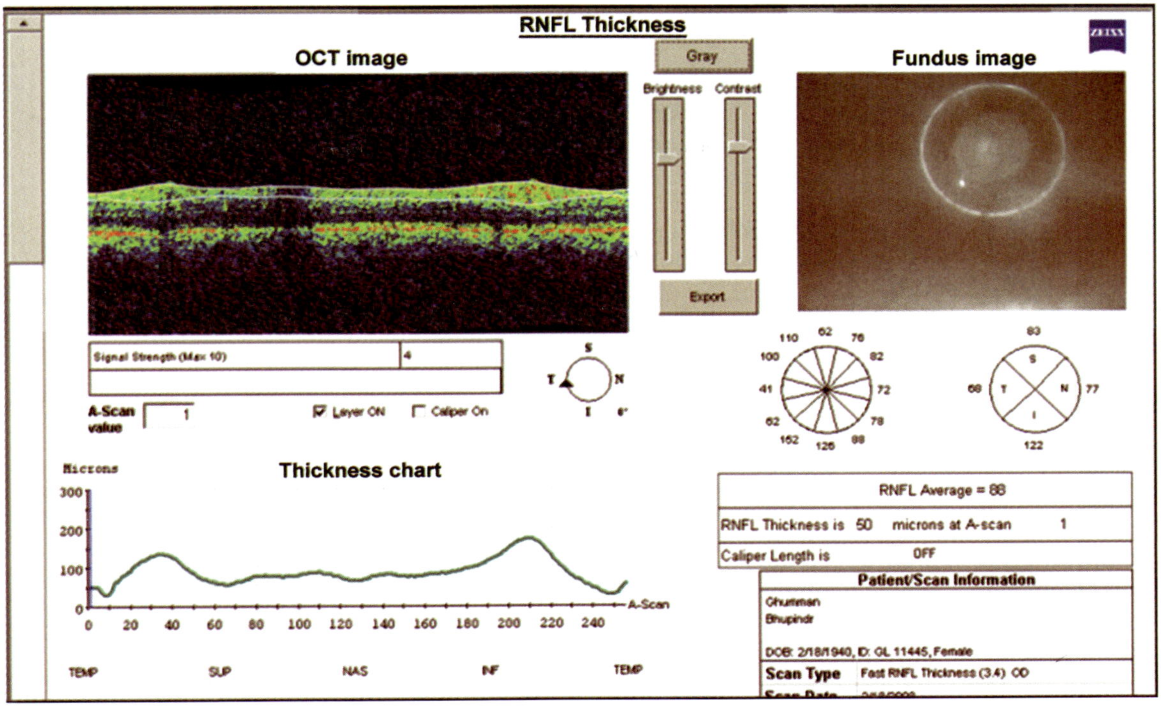

RNFL Thickness

OCT image | Gray | Fundus image

Brightness Contrast

Export

Signal Strength (Max 10) | 4

A-Scan value | 1 | ☑ Layer ON | ☐ Caliper On

Microns | **Thickness chart**

RNFL Average = 88

RNFL Thickness is 50 microns at A-scan 1

Caliper Length is OFF

Patient/Scan Information

Ghurman Bhupindr

DOB: 2/18/1940, ID: GL 11445, Female

Scan Type | Fast RNFL Thickness (3.4) OD

Fig. 15.12: *Poor SNR scan with RNFL boundaries not visualized, resulting in erroneous thin RNFL measurement visible.*

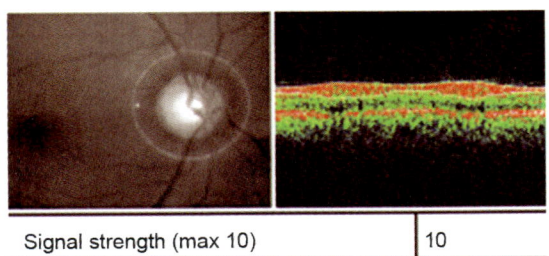

Signal strength (max 10) | 10

Fig. 15.13: *White dot as landmark to mark seen circle position.*

patients with macular pathology and poor fixation where visual fields may not be possible.

Case study illustrating the usefulness of the OCT

A 50-year-old male with asymmetric primary open-angle glaucoma had his IOP controlled on medication. The right eye was normal. The left eye had glaucomatous optic neuropathy with corresponding visual field (VF) defects. The optic disc appearance and IOP remained stable over 3 years (Fig. 15.16).

The visual fields showed progression in the left eye and a nasal step in the right eye (Fig. 15.17).

The glaucoma progression analysis on the Humphrey's visual field analyzer showed up the MD slope as significant (Fig. 15.18). It showed 3 contiguous points deterioration from baseline at 5% significance on 2 consecutive tests, resulting in the GPA being flagged as possible progression.

The dilemma was that the optic disc looked stable. The IOP was 14 mm Hg on treatment.

The guided progression analysis on Stratus OCT showed stable RNFL thickness during this time period (Fig. 15.19).

The visual fields were repeated. This time they were better. The flag 'possible progression' disappeared on subsequent field tests and the MD slope also reverted to 'non-significant' (Fig. 15.20).

The OCT in this case was a useful adjunct as an objective assessment of RNFL thickness which helped guide the decision towards

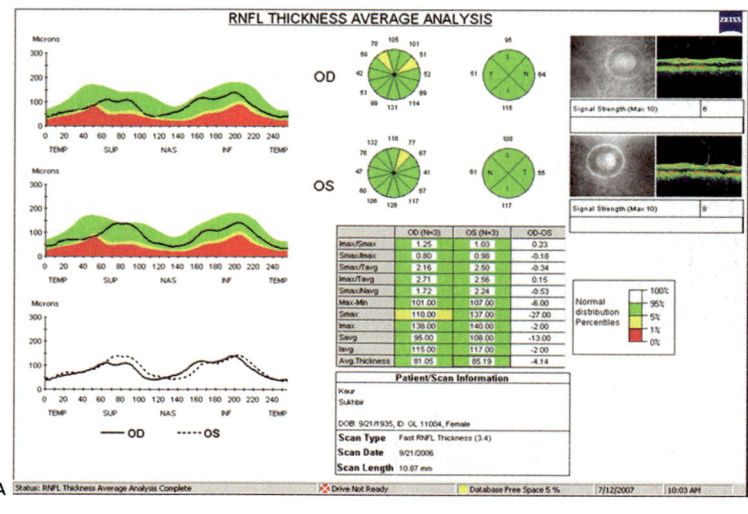

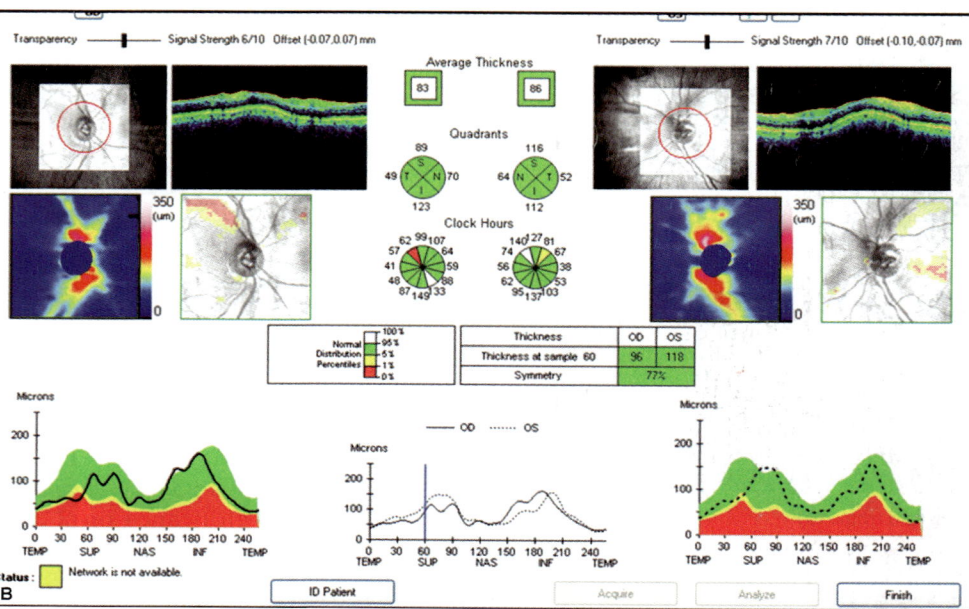

Fig. 15.14: *Patient with superotemporal RNFL defect imaged with the Stratus OCT (A); and Cirrus OCT (B).*

observation rather than relying upon progression in a functional test like the visual field evaluation.

PITFALLS WITH OCT

Apart from being a useful adjunct in the diagnosis and follow-up of glaucoma, it is worthwhile to remember that the OCT after all is a machine and cannot replace a good clinical exam. An abnormal OCT does not mean

glaucoma, just as much as a normal OCT does not mean absence of disease.

The following examples will illustrate how the OCT can be misleading.

1. Abnormal OCT not glaucoma by default

If one just looks at the optic discs (Fig. 15.21) and OCT images (Fig. 15.22) of this 64-year-old woman, one would be justified in making a diagnosis of glaucoma in the right eye.

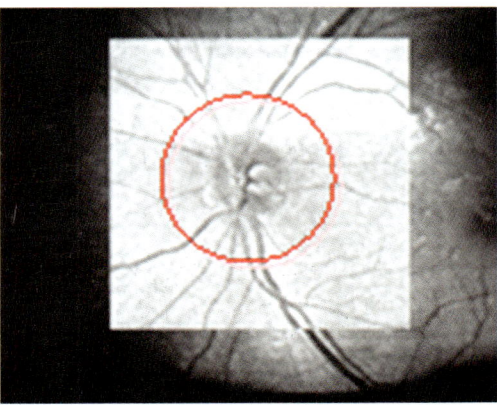

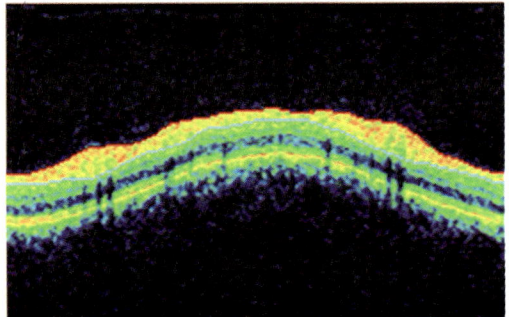

Fig. 15.15: *Optic disc cube 200 × 200.*

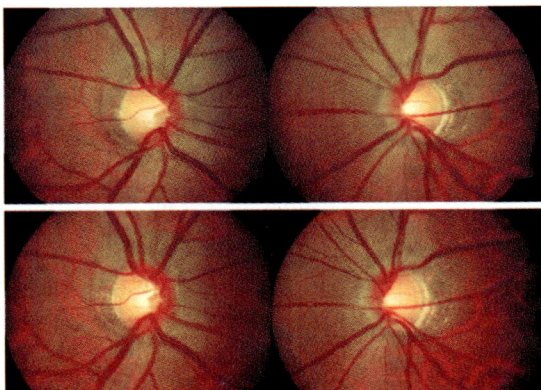

Fig. 15.16: *Serial optic disc photographs.*

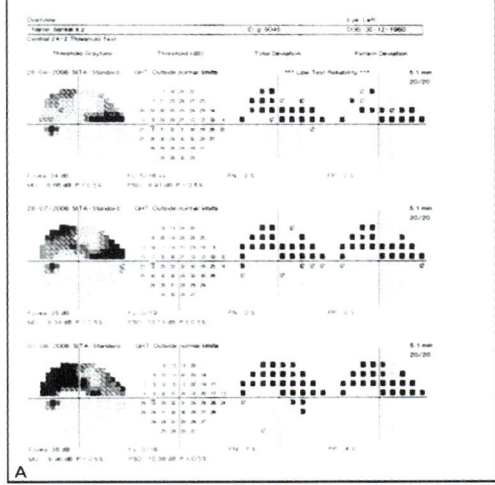

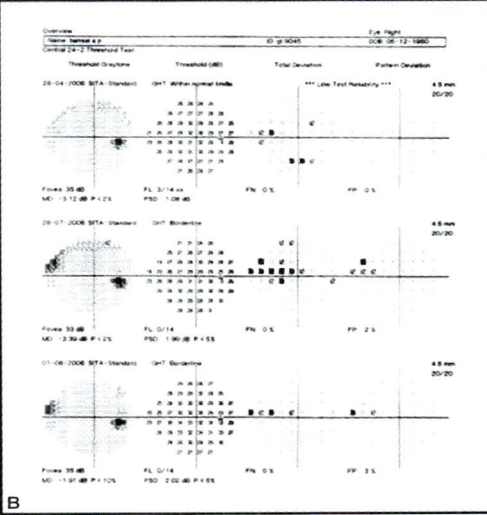

Fig. 15.17: *Visual field progression in left eye (A); and a nasal step in right eye (B).*

There is superior neuroretinal rim thinning clinically. The OCT shows flattening of the normal RNFL hump superiorly and corresponding loss of rim in the optic disc cross-sectional scan images.

However, clinical examination reveals a relative afferent pupillary defect in the right eye, and a large scar of trauma to the right side of the head (Fig. 15.23). This makes a diagnosis of traumatic optic neuropathy which has resulted in RNFL loss. Any RNFL loss would show up as an abnormality on the OCT, but it does not necessarily mean that it is due to glaucoma.

2. Normal OCT does not rule out glaucoma

This 60-year-old woman presented with complaints of intermittent headache. The IOP was 16 and 18 mm Hg. The right eye optic disc was normal, while the left eye showed an infero-temporal notch with disc haemorrhage (Fig. 15.24) and RNFL defect.

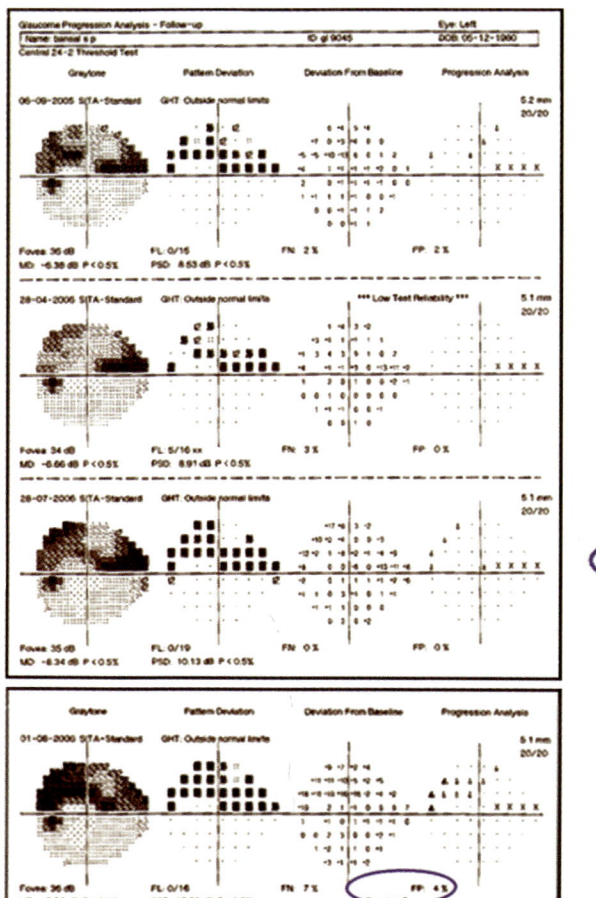

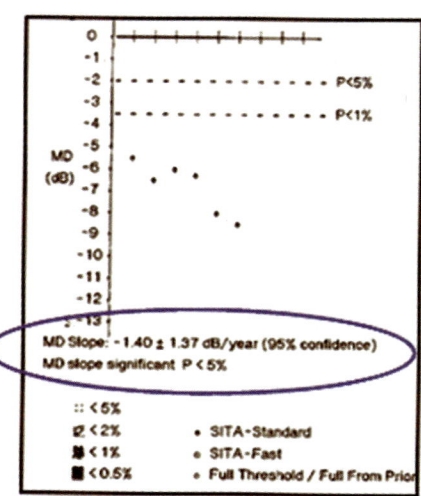

Fig. 15.18: *Significant MD slope on glaucoma progression analysis (GPA).*

There were corresponding visual field defects in the left eye (Fig. 15.25).

Despite clinically fulfilling a diagnosis of glaucoma, all RNFL measurements on the OCT were flagged green and looked normal (Fig. 15.26).

Conclusion

OCT is a very useful adjunct in glaucoma management and probably has a greater role in objectively following up patients. The new generation spectral domain OCT looks like having overcome some of the limitations of the older time-domain technology. Nevertheless, as for any other investigative modality, it is never to be used in isolation without understanding the clinical setting in which the test was performed.

CONFOCAL SCANNING LASER OPHTHALMOSCOPY

The confocal scanning laser ophthalmoscopy (CSLO) commercially available for optic disc imaging is the Heidelberg retina tomograph (HRT), whose latest version is HRT III (Fig. 15.27). The data of older versions (HRT and HRT II) are compatible with HRT III and are transferable.

IMAGE ACQUISITION

It uses a focused diode laser beam of 670 micron to scan over the area of the fundus to be imaged. A pinhole, or confocal aperture, is placed in front of the photo detector to eliminate scattered light. The aperture is conjugate to the laser focus, and

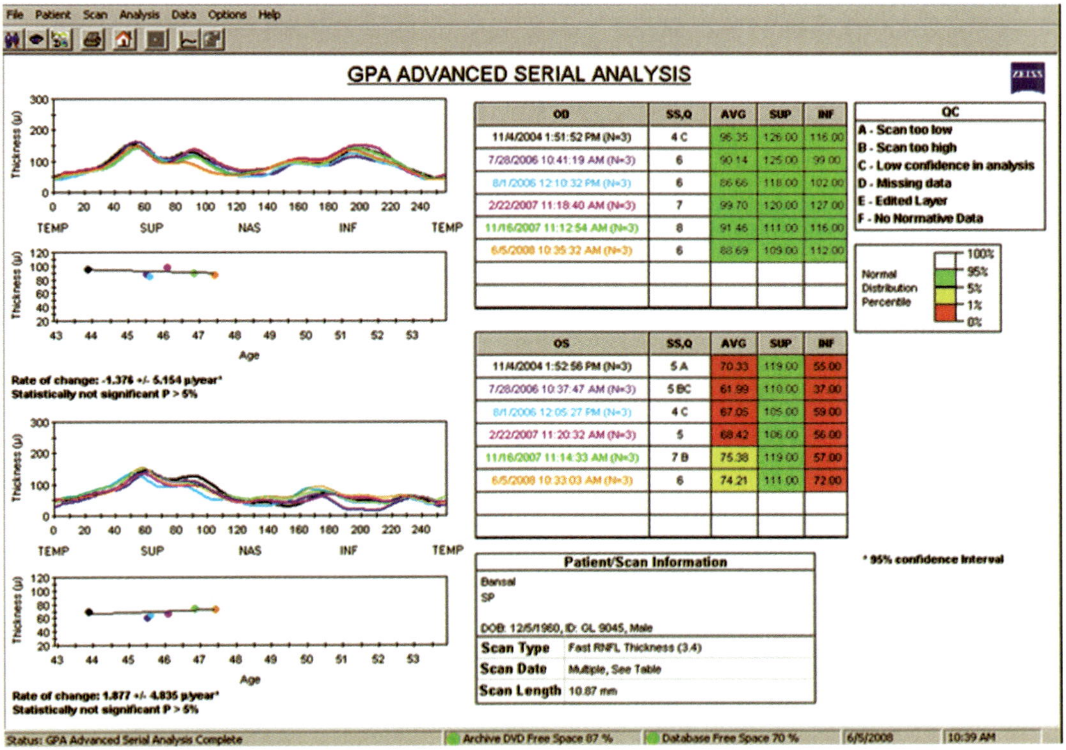

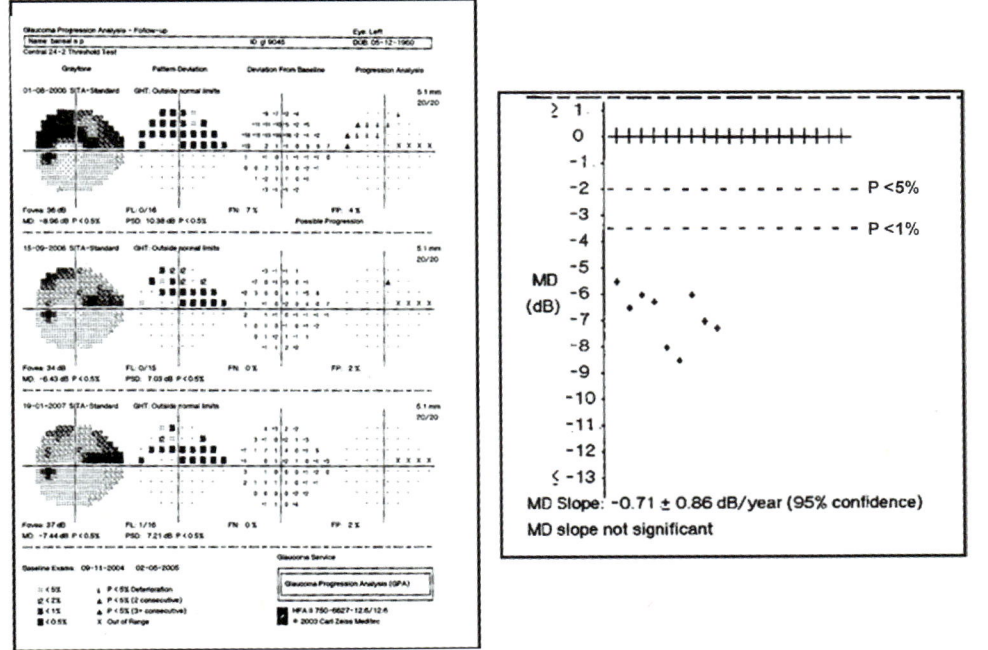

Fig. 15.19: *GPA on OCT showing no change in RNFL thickness.*

Fig. 15.20: *MD slope after repeat visual fields.*

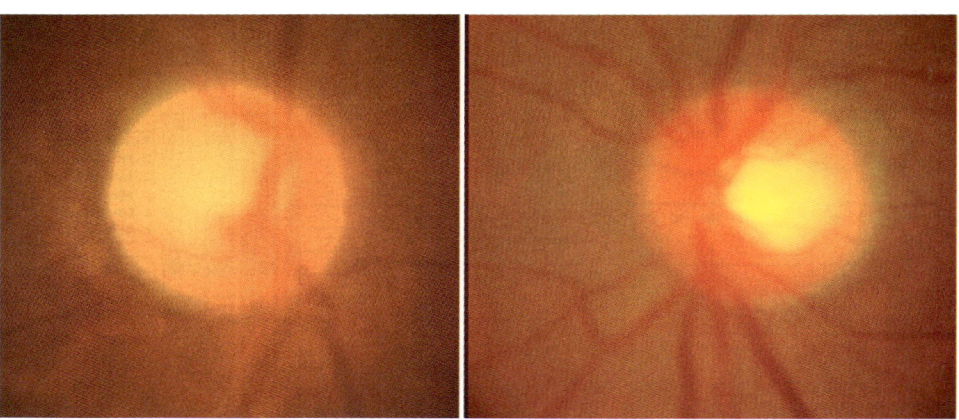

Fig. 15.21: *Optic disc photographs suggestive of glaucoma.*

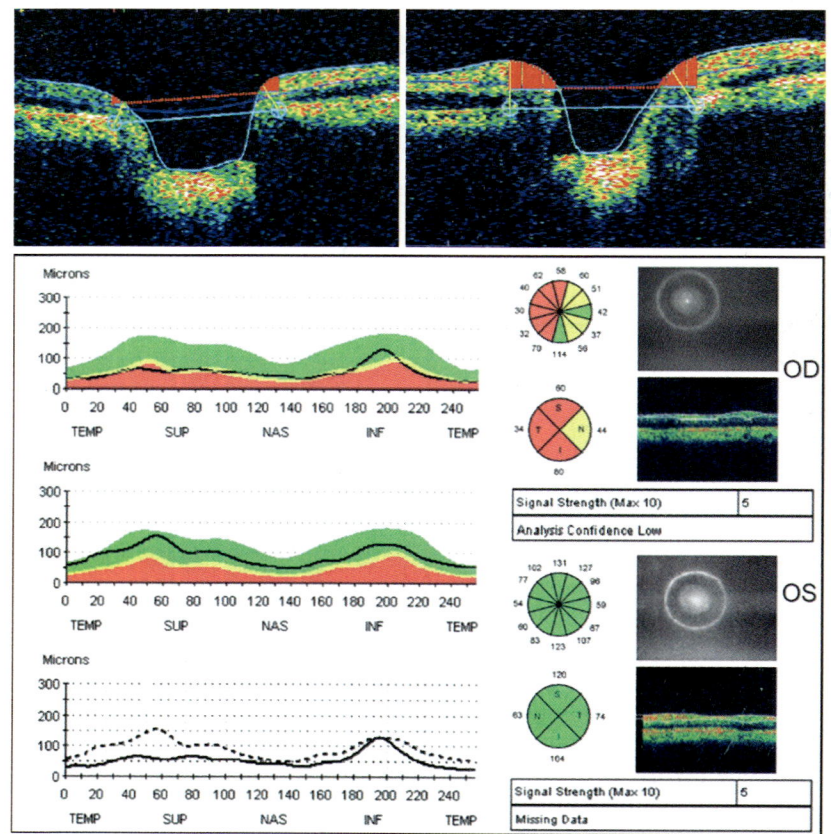

Fig. 15.22: *ONH and RNFL thickness on OCT of the same patient whose optic disc photographs are shown in Fig. 15.21.*

the resulting image is said to be 'confocal'. This allows much higher axial and lateral resolution than that achieved with conventional light microscopy, such as with a fundus camera. Volume of tissue from which reflected light at that instant is accepted by the confocal aperture

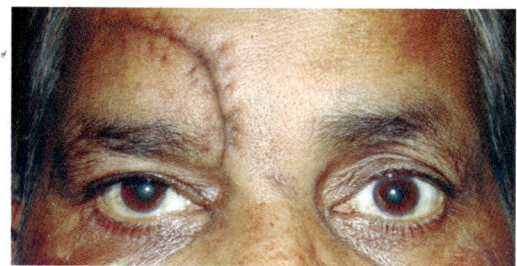

Fig. 15.23: *Large scar of trauma to right side of the head of a patient with traumatic optic neuropathy whose fundus photographs (Fig. 15.21) and OCT findings (Fig. 15.22) are suggestive of glaucoma.*

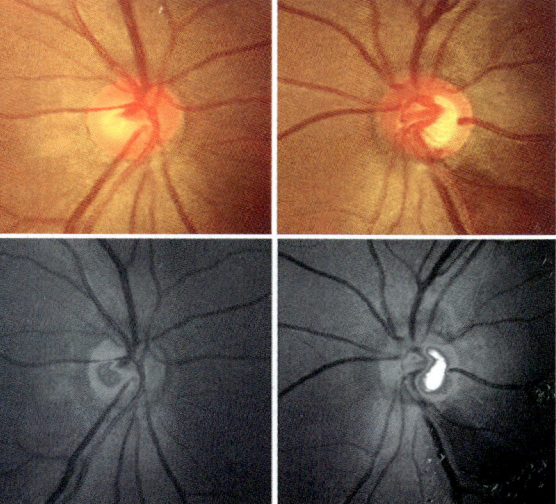

Fig. 15.24: *Optic discs of the patient.*

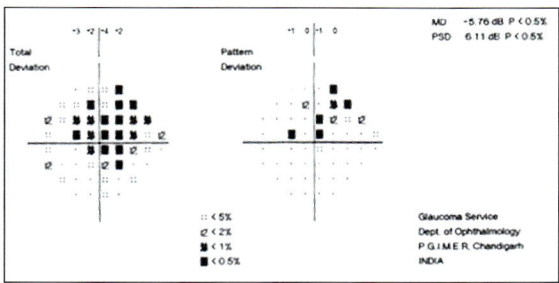

Fig. 15.25: *Visual field defect.*

is called a voxel, the size of voxel is inversely proportional to resolution of the image. It acquires high resolution images, both perpendicular to the optic axis (x- and y-axis) and along the optic axis (z-axis). Oscillating mirrors in the

HRT device redirect the laser beam to the x- and y-axis, along a plane of focus that is perpendicular to the optic axis (z-axis). A bi-dimensional image ($15 \times 15°$) is obtained at each focal plane. As the device changes the focal plane, other bi-dimensional images of the optic nerve are obtained. Each one represents an optical section of the optic nerve. A total of 64 sections, each done with 1/16 mm of depth interval, are obtained and used to create a three-dimensional image of the optic nerve. These 64 sections are equivalent to a depth of 4 mm.

Once the image is taken, the operator delineates the optic nerve contour line over the reflectance or topography image. The operator places points at the external edge of the disc border and the machine draws a 'best-fit' ellipse linking these points together. Heidelberg retina tomography proceeds to define the 'reference plane' based on the disc contour drawn by the operator.

The reference plane is located 50 microns posterior to the mean height along a 6° arc of the contour line at the temporal inferior sector. Structures above the reference plane and within the contour line are considered to be rim. Anything below the reference plane is considered cup. Computation of stereometric parameters, classification of the eye and comparison to previous examinations are then done by the HRT. Classification of the eye is done with Moorefield's regression analysis or other discriminating method in HRT II, or with neural network analysis in HRT III.

The latest software available, HRT III, can provide ONH stereometric analysis without manual delineation of the disc margin by the operator. After a three-dimensional model of the ONH is constructed, five optic nerve parameters are calculated and then analyzed with an artificial intelligence classifier, the relevance vector machine (RVM). From this analysis, a glaucoma probability score (GPS) is created. Adjustments are made to the parameters to account for differences in age and disc size by both versions of HRT. However, HRT III is equipped with a larger and more diverse normative database than its predecessor. There are several printout formats currently

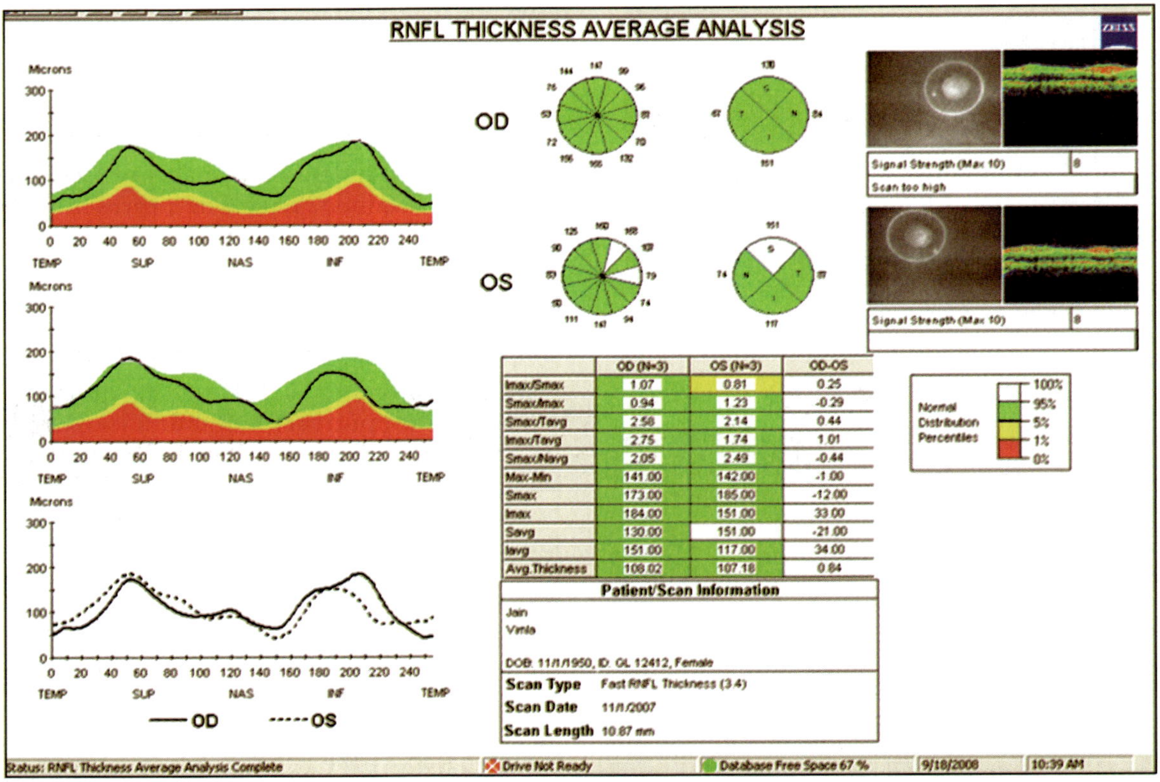

RNFL THICKNESS AVERAGE ANALYSIS

OD

OS

| Signal Strength (Max 10) | 8 |
| Scan too high | |

| Signal Strength (Max 10) | 8 |

	OD (N=3)	OS (N=3)	OD-OS
Imax/Smax	1.07	0.81	0.25
Smax/Imax	0.94	1.23	-0.29
Smax/Tavg	2.58	2.14	0.44
Imax/Tavg	2.75	1.74	1.01
Smax/Navg	2.05	2.49	-0.44
Max-Min	141.00	142.00	-1.00
Smax	173.00	185.00	-12.00
Imax	184.00	151.00	33.00
Savg	130.00	151.00	-21.00
Iavg	151.00	117.00	34.00
Avg.Thickness	108.02	107.18	0.84

Normal Distribution Percentiles
- 100%
- 95%
- 5%
- 1%
- 0%

Patient/Scan Information	
Jain	
Vimla	
DOB: 11/1/1950, ID: GL 12412, Female	
Scan Type	Fast RNFL Thickness (3.4)
Scan Date	11/1/2007
Scan Length	10.87 mm

— OD ·····OS

Status: RNFL Thickness Average Analysis Complete | Drive Not Ready | Database Free Space 67 % | 9/18/2008 | 10:39 AM

Fig. 15.26: *Normal RNFL thickness on OCT in a patient whose optic discs (Fig. 15.24) and visual field defect (Fig. 15.25) are suggestive of glaucoma.*

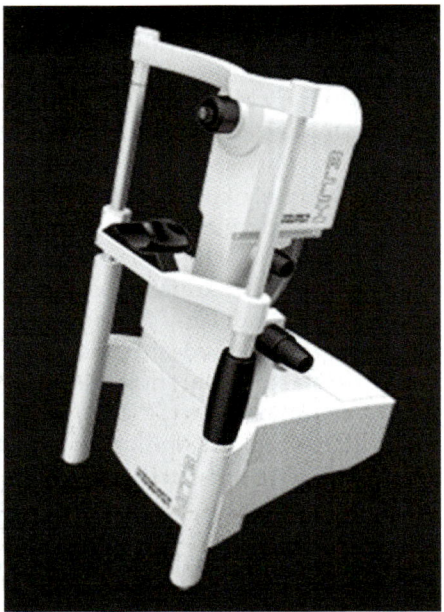

Fig. 15.27: *HRT III (Courtesy: Heidelberg Engineering).*

available: Initial report, follow-up report and 'OU report,' among others. Discussed below are the different components of HRT printout.

COMPONENTS OF HRT REPORT

Interpretation of HRT III report printout (Fig. 15.28) is as below:

1. *Patient data.* Name, sex, date of birth, patient ID, and date of exam are provided here.

2. *Topography image.* This is the colour-coded representation of disc. Darker colour represents superficial areas while lighter colour represents deeper areas. Colours, like green and blue, indicate neuroretinal rim tissue (above the reference plane) while red indicates the cup (area below the reference plane). Blue indicates sloping rim.

3. *Reflectance image.* It is also a colour represen-tation image where brighter areas representing highest reflectance, like the cup and is similar

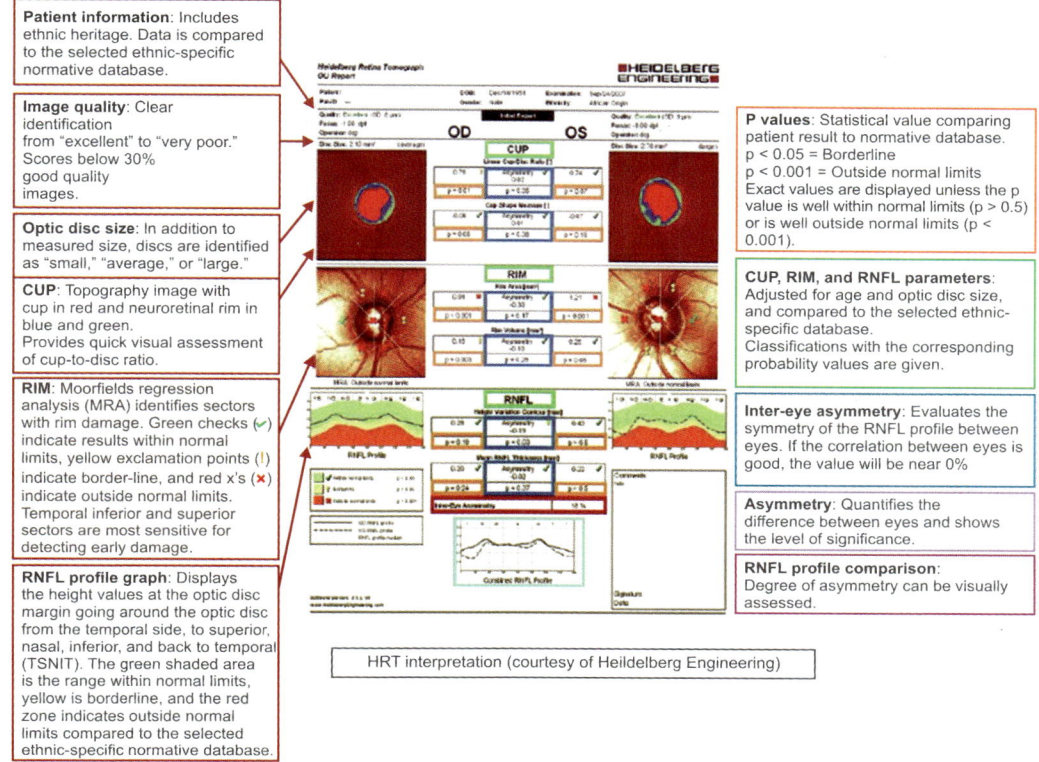

Patient information: Includes ethnic heritage. Data is compared to the selected ethnic-specific normative database.

Image quality: Clear identification from "excellent" to "very poor." Scores below 30% good quality images.

Optic disc size: In addition to measured size, discs are identified as "small," "average," or "large."

CUP: Topography image with cup in red and neuroretinal rim in blue and green. Provides quick visual assessment of cup-to-disc ratio.

RIM: Moorfields regression analysis (MRA) identifies sectors with rim damage. Green checks (✔) indicate results within normal limits, yellow exclamation points (!) indicate border-line, and red x's (✖) indicate outside normal limits. Temporal inferior and superior sectors are most sensitive for detecting early damage.

RNFL profile graph: Displays the height values at the optic disc margin going around the optic disc from the temporal side, to superior, nasal, inferior, and back to temporal (TSNIT). The green shaded area is the range within normal limits, yellow is borderline, and the red zone indicates outside normal limits compared to the selected ethnic-specific normative database.

P values: Statistical value comparing patient result to normative database. p < 0.05 = Borderline p < 0.001 = Outside normal limits Exact values are displayed unless the p value is well within normal limits (p > 0.5) or is well outside normal limits (p < 0.001).

CUP, RIM, and RNFL parameters: Adjusted for age and optic disc size, and compared to the selected ethnic-specific database. Classifications with the corresponding probability values are given.

Inter-eye asymmetry: Evaluates the symmetry of the RNFL profile between eyes. If the correlation between eyes is good, the value will be near 0%

Asymmetry: Quantifies the difference between eyes and shows the level of significance.

RNFL profile comparison: Degree of asymmetry can be visually assessed.

Fig. 15.28: *Interpretation of HRT III printout (Courtesy: Heidelberg Engineering).*

to a photograph. The reflectance image is overlaid with Moorfields analysis.

4. *Retinal surface height variation graph.* It consists of green and red lines where green line representing the retinal height and a red line representing the reference. It graphically represents the retinal height along the contour line and of the thickness of the nerve fibre layer. It appears as 'double hump' where hills or 'humps' correspond to the superior and inferior nerve fibre layers, which are normally thicker than the rest of the areas. Left to right the graph depicts: the thicknesses of the temporal (T); temporal-superior (TS); nasal-superior (NS); nasal (N); nasal-inferior (NI); temporal-inferior (TI); and temporal (T) sectors.

5. *Vertical and horizontal interactive analysis.* It depicts optic nerve retinal surface height in horizontal and vertical cross-sections. A non-smooth or jagged trace represents a better quality scan. Observation of the trace can provide information of the disc steepness, presence of sloping, etc.

6. *Stereometric analysis.* HRT II provides a list of 14 nerve parameters. They are: disc, cup and rim area, cup and rim volume, cup/disc area ratio, linear cup/disc ratio, mean cup depth, maximum cup depth, cup shape measure, height variation contour, mean retinal nerve fibre layer (RNFL) thickness, RNFL cross-sectional area and reference height. To the right of the stereometric parameters, a column specifies ± one standard deviation from the mean of the normative database for each of the parameters. HRT III only provides values for 6 stereometric parameters in the 'OU printout'. These are: cup/disc area ratio, cup shape measure, rim area and volume, height variation contour and mean RNFL thickness. Each value is designated as within normal limits, borderline or outside normal limits after comparing to the normative database.

7. *Moorfields regression analysis (MRA)*. The MRA is based on a normative database of 112 Caucasian subjects with refractive error ± 6D and disc size within the range of 1.2–2.8 mm. The ratio values of these subjects represents the value obtained in 50% of the normal subjects studied. In this way, outside normal limits (red x) represents the rim area of any segment (global assessment or any of the 6 sectors) is below the 99.9% prediction interval, that is, 99.9% of 'normals' have a higher rim area/disc area value than that of the nerve being classified as outside normal limits (ONL). Borderline (yellow checkmark) represents the rim area between the 95 and 99.9% prediction lines. Green checkmark (within normal limits) appears when rim areas fall above the 95% prediction level.

The Moorfields analysis graph is shown in the printout, indicating the predicted intervals on which the nerve classification is based. Green colour represents the rim and red represents the cup. Seven different columns representing all sectors are shown and classified as within normal limits (WNL), borderline (BL) or ONL. Moorfields classification is shown over the reflectance image as a green checkmark, yellow exclamation point, or a red 'x'. The Moorfields classification of the nerve is written at the bottom of the graph. Disc is classified on the basis of the worst classified sector in Moorfields regression. Moorfields regression analysis can discriminate glaucomatous nerves from normals with 84.3% sensitivity and 96.3% specificity. It tends to overestimate rim area in small optic nerves and to underestimate rim area in large nerves. So on either extreme of disc size range, care should be taken when analyzing these scans.

8. *Glaucoma probability score (GPS)*. A new addition in the HRT III generation allows calculation of the GPS. A three-dimensional model of the ONH and peripapillary RNFL is constructed by using five parameters: cup size, cup depth, rim steepness, and horizontal and vertical RNFL. The complete three-dimensional model is then subjected to analysis by an artificial intelligence classifier, the relevance vector machine (RVM), that compares it to a predetermined normal and glaucoma model and then derives the probability of glaucoma for the scanned eye:

- Probability <28% is within normal limits (WNL)
- Probability between 28 and 64% in borderline (BL)
- Probability >64% is outside normal limits (ONL).

EVALUATING SCAN QUALITY

The value of any data lies on identification of good quality scan. Good quality indicators are even luminance and sharp borders of the topography and reflectance images, as well as good centration of the disc. The standard deviation (SD) measures, variability of the same pixel values among three different scans. The average light intensity for each point is what is used for the RNFL height measurement. The manufacturer has suggested not analyzing scans with an SD value greater than 40. It is important to point out that SD should not be the only parameter to use when assessing quality. A poor quality scan can still have a low SD value, if there is small or no variability among the three scans. The manufacturer's classification of scans by SD values is:

- 10: Excellent
- 11–20: Very good
- 21–30: Good
- 31–40: Acceptable
- 41–50: Poor
- 50: Very poor.

Looking at cross-sections can also help determine the degree of noise in the obtained images. The contour cross-sectional trace should be soft and not 'jagged'.

STRENGTHS AND LIMITATIONS OF HRT

HRT machines have stood the test of time and HRT III machine (the latest version) is backward compatible. The data from the previous models can be transferred to the newer models so that the progression over time can be evaluated. The most important aspect of the structural imaging systems. The sensitivity and specificity for both MRA and GPS are in the same range of around 83% sensitivity and 87% specificity. However,

both the systems of analysis are dependent on the disc size for sensitivity and specificity. Small discs show lower sensitivity and higher specificity as compared to larger discs which show higher sensitivity and lower specificity. The measurements are based on the contour line and standard reference plane. It is considered as a major limitation. Some of the eyes show variable HRT measurements based on intraocular pressure, is another limitation. We should remember that we should never rely too much on the diagnostic abilities of these devices and only judicious use should be incorporated in the management of glaucoma.

Progression analysis

In the printout of progression analysis, the top row is topography image and the second row is the corresponding reflectance image of the serial scans performed on different dates. The follow-up reflectance images show superimposed red areas (significantly depressed from baseline) and green areas (significantly elevated from baseline). When at least four scans have been performed on one patient, an additional third row significance map appears, which starts flagging significance level, if the same area is showing similar change in at least three consecutive scans. This gives a fairly good idea about progression based on event-based analysis.

Tread analysis

This has multiple stereometric parameters. When multiple tests have been performed, all stereometric parameters combined can be studied either globally or sector-wise. Similarly, any isolated stereometric parameter also can be studied either globally or in a particular sector. The starting point on trend line is 0 and if it moves downward and reaches up to 1.0, it is a definitive trend of deterioration.

HRT SCANS OF NORMAL AND GLAUCOMATOUS DISCS

Figures 15.29 to 15.32 show representative cases with normal disc, early, moderate and advanced glaucomatous changes, respectively.

SCANNING LASER POLARIMETRY (GDx)

INTRODUCTION

Scanning laser polarimetry is used to measure peripapillary RNFL thickness. The principle utilized in this technology is of birefringence. Birefringent intraocular tissues are the cornea, lens and the retina. In the retina, microtubules in retinal ganglion cell axons which are arranged parallel cause change in the polarization of light passing through them. This change in the polarization of light is known as retardation, and this can be measured. The retardation caused by the RNFL is linearly related to the thickness of RNFL. Glaucoma Diagnostics (GDx Carl Zeiss Meditec; Jena, Germany, and Dublin, California) (Fig. 15.33) utilize this technology. Different birefringence patterns are detected when the RNFL is healthy versus atrophied from glaucoma.

IMAGE ACQUISITION

This device also uses a polarized diode laser (780 nm) to fixed scan circle of 3.2 mm diameter centred on the optic disc. Images with abnormal definition of the blood vessel borders or the optic nerve indicate eye movement leads to erroneous acquisition. Data acquired from the scanned area are displayed as a 256 × 256 pixel colour-coded grid which displays a 'heat map' of RNFL thickness, with hotter colours representing greater retardation that is thicker RNFL values. In a normal RNFL thickness map, bright yellow and red indicates thicker RNFL and is seen in the superior and inferior sectors, while green and blue indicates thinner RNFL and is seen in the nasal and temporal sectors. A statistical deviation map and a TSINT graph are included in the printout.

The new generation has the GDx variable corneal compensator (GDx VCC) and GDx enhanced corneal compensator (ECC). GDx VCC provides individual customized compensation of anterior segment birefringence using retardation measurements obtained from the macula.

GDx ECC performed significantly better than GDx VCC in glaucoma detection in patients with more severe atypical retardation patterns.

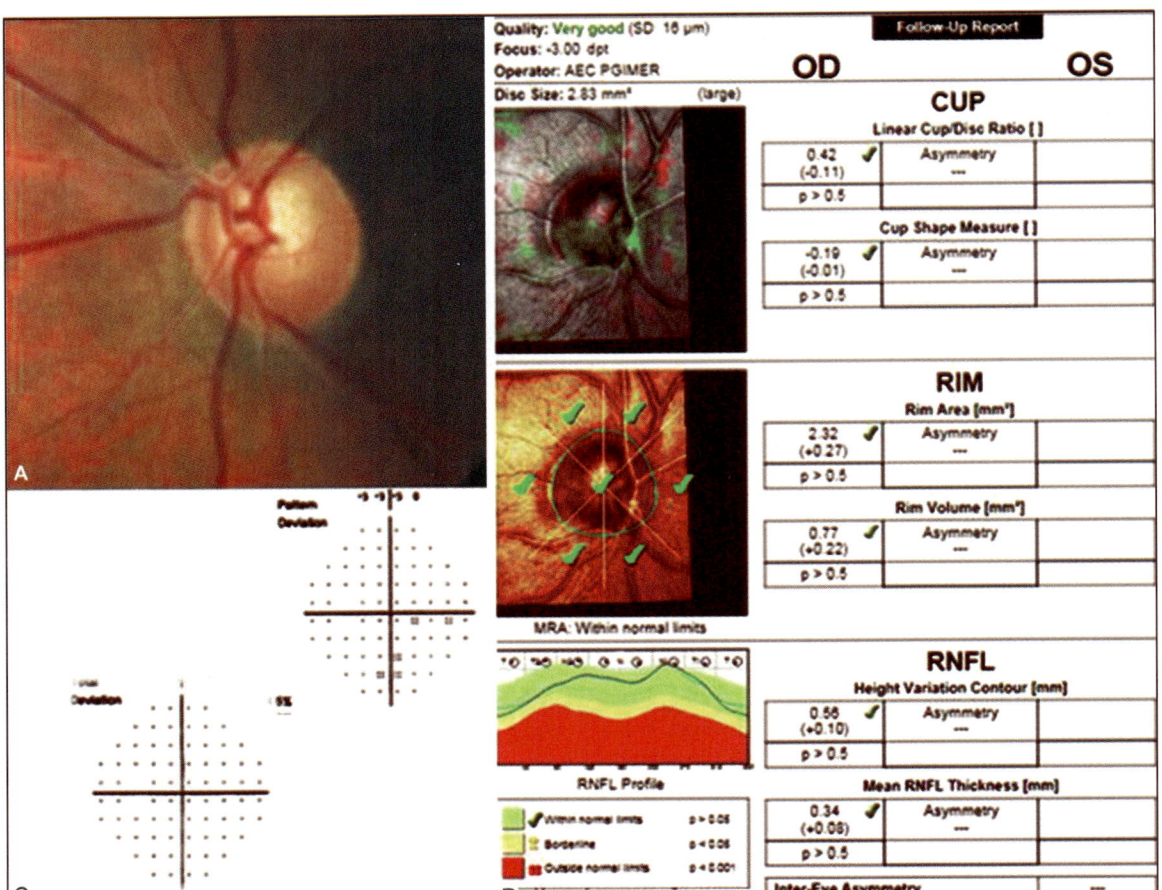

Fig. 15.29: *Normal disc: (A) Colour photograph of a right optic nerve; (B) Corresponding image from an HRT II showing thinning of RNFL. Red colour shows areas of neuroretinal rim thickness less than normative database; (C) Field changes correlating disc changes on total and pattern deviation plot.*

It is based on the form birefringence shown by Henle's fibre layer of fovea as it is known to be uniform (form birefringence is an optical property where light refracts differently in perpendicular planes due to the molecular organization of a material). Scanning laser polarimetry of the macula without VCC gives rise to a non-uniform pattern at the fovea due to birefringence of the cornea. It is seen as hourglass pattern and it indicates the axis and magnitude of the uncorrected cornea birefringence.

COMPONENTS OF THE GDx REPORT

1. *Patient data.* It consists of patient's name, date of birth, gender and ethnicity which are given at the top of the printout.

2. *Quality score.* An ideal quality score ranges from 7 to 10.

3. *Reflectivity image.* It is located at the top of the report display. It is a image of the posterior pole that measures 20° × 20°. 16000 or more data points are acquired to construct this image. This image provides information about the quality of the scan. The ellipse is centred over the ONH in this image. The ellipse size is defaulted to a small setting can be changed by changing the calculation circle thereby changing the size of the ellipse. The calculation circle is the area located between the two concentric circles, one which measures the temporal-superior-nasal-inferior-temporal (TSNIT) and other that measures nerve fibre indicator (NFI) parameters. One can measure beyond a large peripapillary

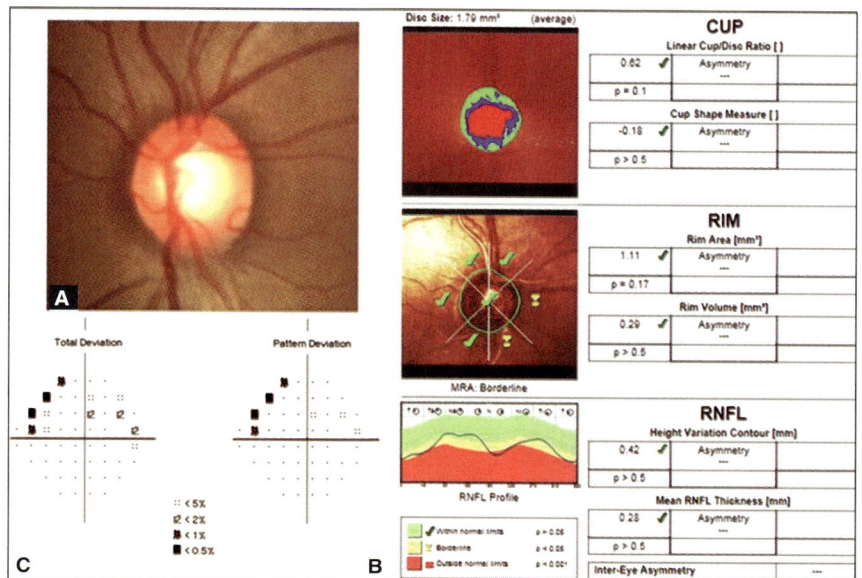

Fig. 15.30: *Early glaucomatous change: (A) Colour photograph of a right optic nerve; (B) Corresponding image from an HRT II showing thinning of RNFL. Red colour shows areas of neuroretinal rim thickness less than normative database; (C) Field changes correlating disc changes on total and pattern deviation plot.*

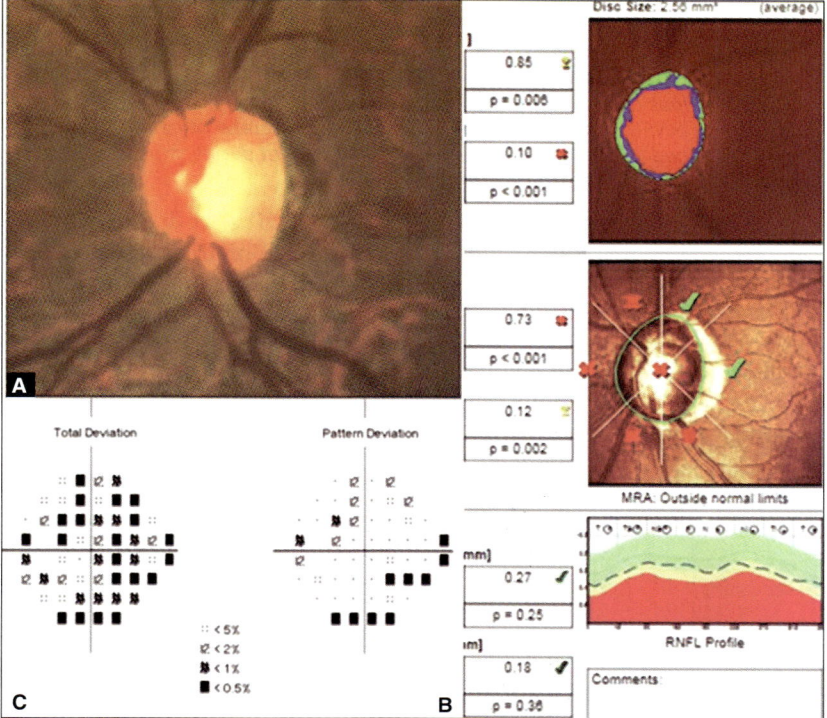

Fig. 15.31: *Moderate glaucomatous change: (A) Colour photograph of a right optic nerve; (B) Corresponding image from an HRT II showing thinning of RNFL. Red colour shows areas of neuroretinal rim thickness less than normative database; (C) Field changes correlating disc changes on total and pattern deviation plot.*

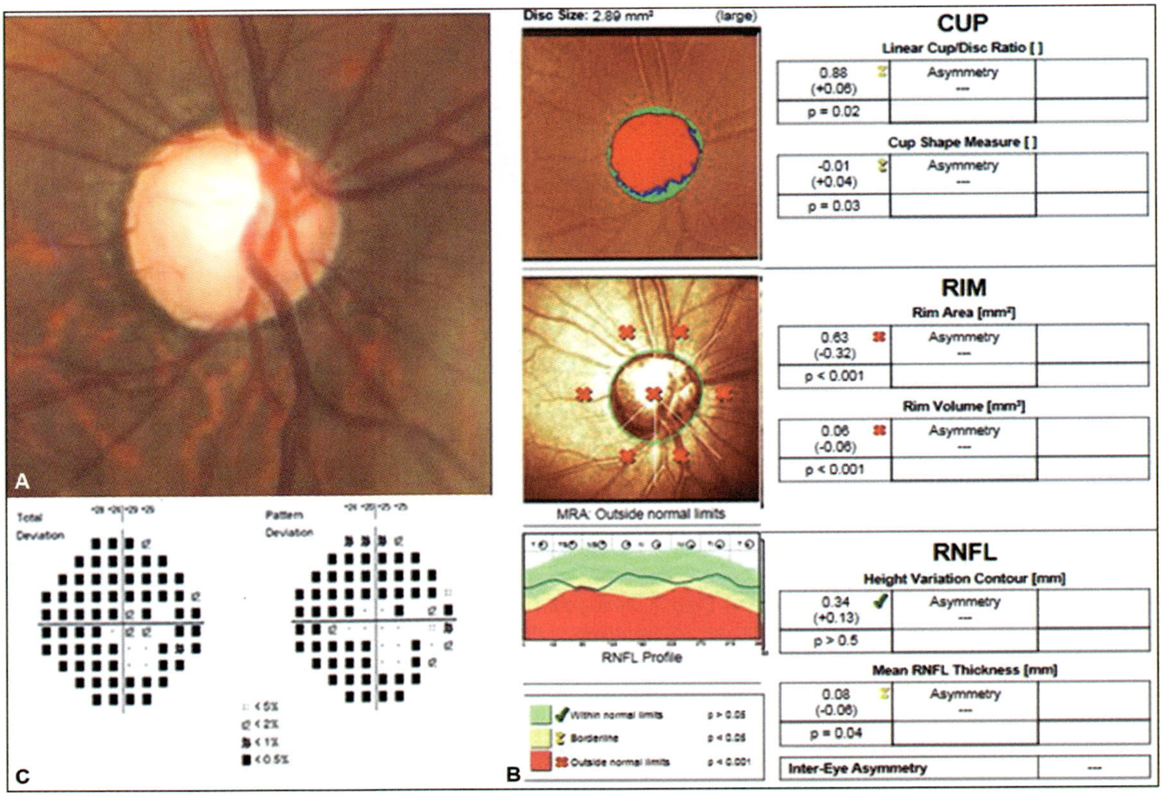

Disc Size: 2.89 mm²	(large)			

CUP

Linear Cup/Disc Ratio [ ]

0.88	⚡	Asymmetry
(+0.06)		---
p = 0.02		

Cup Shape Measure [ ]

-0.01	⚡	Asymmetry
(+0.04)		---
p = 0.03		

RIM

Rim Area [mm²]

0.63	✖	Asymmetry
(-0.32)		---
p < 0.001		

Rim Volume [mm³]

0.06	✖	Asymmetry
(-0.06)		---
p < 0.001		

MRA: Outside normal limits

RNFL Profile

✓ Within normal limits	p > 0.05
⚡ Borderline	p < 0.05
✖ Outside normal limits	p < 0.001

RNFL

Height Variation Contour [mm]

0.34	✓	Asymmetry
(+0.13)		---
p > 0.5		

Mean RNFL Thickness [mm]

0.08	⚡	Asymmetry
(-0.06)		---
p = 0.04		

Inter-Eye Asymmetry	---

Total Deviation   Pattern Deviation

≤ 5%
< 2%
< 1%
< 0.5%

Fig. 15.32: *Advance glaucomatous damage: (A) Colour photograph of a right optic nerve; (B) Corresponding image from an HRT II showing thinning of RNFL in all quadrants. Red colour shows areas of neuroretinal rim thickness less than normative database; (C) Advanced visual field changes on total and pattern deviation plot.*

atrophy area by resizing the calculation circle and ellipse.

4. *RNFL thickness map or retardation image.* This is a colour-coded map depicting the different thicknesses of peripapillary RNFL. Hot colours, like red and yellow, mean high retardation or thicker RNFL and cool colours, like blue and green, mean low retardation or thinner areas. A typical scan is of a vertical bow-tie pattern that is the one with thicker RNFL superiorly and inferiorly.

5. *TSNIT graph or (RNFL profile plots).* Located at the bottom of the report display. It measures RNFL thickness values around the measurement annulus in relation to the normal range of thickness values (normative data of over 500 eyes). This graph demonstrates the patient's RNFL thickness as a black line drawn over a shaded area of normality. The green and purple shaded areas indicate the normal range of values for the left and right eyes, respectively.

6. *TSNIT symmetry graph.* This graph with right and left eye plots superimposed on each other.

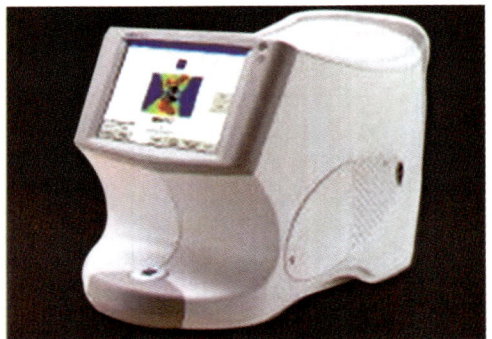

Fig. 15.33: *GDx PRO (Courtesy: Carl Zeiss Inc.).*

7. TSNIT comparison graph and serial analysis graph. It compares two or more scans of the same eye obtained on different visits of the patient. They are not a part of the regular printout.

8. Deviation from normal map. This map compares RNFL thickness of patient the values derived from the normative database. Colour-coded squares are used to indicate the amount of deviation from normal at each given location. A colour legend defining statistical significance of deviation from normal is seen at the bottom.

9. TSNIT parameters. These are computed automatically from the calculation circle data and are compared to the normative database. They are also colour-coded on the basis of different p values. The parameters are: TSNIT average (average thickness values within the calculation circle), superior average (average of pixels in superior 120° of the calculation circle), inferior average (same as above, but along the inferior 120° of the calculation circle), TSNIT standard deviation and inter-eye asymmetry. Inter-eye symmetry values near 1.0 represent good symmetry, and values near 0 represent poor symmetry. A GDx VCC scan may be considered abnormal, if the TSNIT average, superior average, inferior average, TSNIT standard deviation, and inter-eye symmetry have p <1%. A GDx VCC scan may be considered borderline, if these same parameters fall outside normal at the p <5% level.

10. Nerve fibre indicator (NFI). The NFI is an indicator of the likelihood that an eye has glaucoma. It is a proprietary value, consensus regarding the definition of an abnormal scan has not been established. Data within and outside the calculation circle are used to generate the NFI value. It ranges from 0 to 100. The higher NFI reflects towards patient being glaucomatous.

GDx offers the following as a guideline on the NFI interpretation:
- <30: Low likelihood of glaucoma
- 30–50: Glaucoma suspect
- >50: High likelihood of glaucoma.

Recently, software has been introduced in the GDx VCC to assess serial images for the identification of progression (GDx Review with Guided Progression Analysis (GPA)™, Carl Zeiss Meditec, Dublin, CA, USA). The analysis software requires an external computer linked to the GDx VCC. To assess and confirm RNFL progression requires detection of change on three consecutive follow-up images which is compared to an average of two high quality baseline scans. Three algorithms are used to evaluate statistically significant progression and changes are colour-coded: Red demonstrates likely reduction in RNFL thickness, yellow indicates possible reduction, and purple indicates possible increase in RNFL thickness. Narrow focal RNFL change may be detected using the image progression map.

QUALITY ASSESSMENT

Proper focusing and illumination of the retinal area being scanned is necessary.

The ONH must be inside a black square when scan is being acquired. Motion artifacts may occur, if the eye moves too much, and that can decrease the quality of the scan. These are sometimes noticed as black rectangles at the edges of the scans or lines along the vessels. The ellipse must be centred over the ONH. Centration is usually more important than adequate size. A typical scan identified by the thicker bundles along the vertical axis, where the RNFL is thicker (vertical bow-tie). An atypical scan is one where the overall thickness is increased, where the thickness axis is tilted or where the thickness is along radial lines through the periphery of the scan. An objective way to evaluate atypical scans is with a support vector machine, which assigns a typical scan score.

STRENGTHS AND LIMITATIONS

GDx allows for rapid and simple imaging of peripapillary RNFL. Good interactive features to assess for quality of the image are included in the software. Pupillary dilation is not required. Macular pathology was a hindrance in assessing the GDx VCC but now alternative strategies for corneal compensation in eyes with macular pathology have been described. In general, the reported sensitivity and specificity of scanning laser polarimetry to detect glaucoma is above 80%.

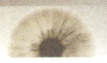

Figures 15.34 to 15.37 show representative cases with normal disc, early, moderate and advanced glaucomatous changes, respectively on HRT, OCT and perimetry.

ULTRASOUND BIOMICROSCOPY

INTRODUCTION

Ultrasound biomicroscopy (UBM) is an imaging technique that uses high frequency ultrasound to produce images of the eye at near microscopic resolution.

Ultrasound biomicroscopy was introduced in the late 1980s by Pavlin et al. It was originally designed to have a field of view of 2 × 2 mm and a frequency of 100 Mega Hertz (MHz). With it the first views of enucleated eyes were obtained. Details of the angle of the eye, the cornea, the sclera, the iris and the ciliary body were visualized with impressive clarity. However, despite good resolution, there was the

drawback of non-appreciation of deeper structures. To overcome this problem, the next design incorporated transducers ranging from 50–80 MHz with a field of view of 4 × 4 mm. This proved to be a useful compromise that allowed important structures of the anterior segment to be well-visualized.

The UBM was brought into clinical use in 1990 using a water bath. Scanning was performed by placing the probe close to the area of interest and observing the resulting image on the screen. Fine movement of the probe was performed manually with reference to the screen image.

Today, the UBM is an important adjunct in the diagnosis and management of conditions involving the anterior segment of the eye usually not visualized through established clinical methods or conventional ophthalmic ultrasound. In addition, ultrasound biomicroscopy also provides a view of subsurface structures in their normal relationships without the distortion

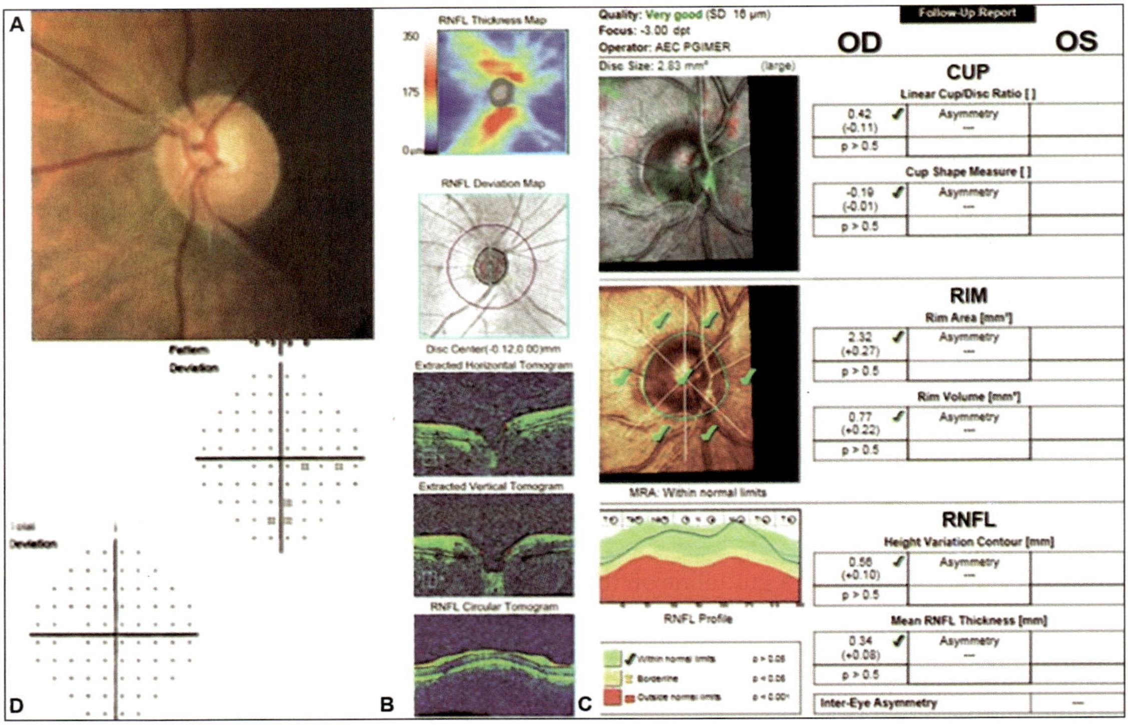

Fig. 15.34: *Normal disc: (A) Colour photograph of optic nerve; (B) OCT shows healthy RNFL; (C) Corresponding image from an HRT II correlating OCT finding; (D) Normal field changes on perimetry.*

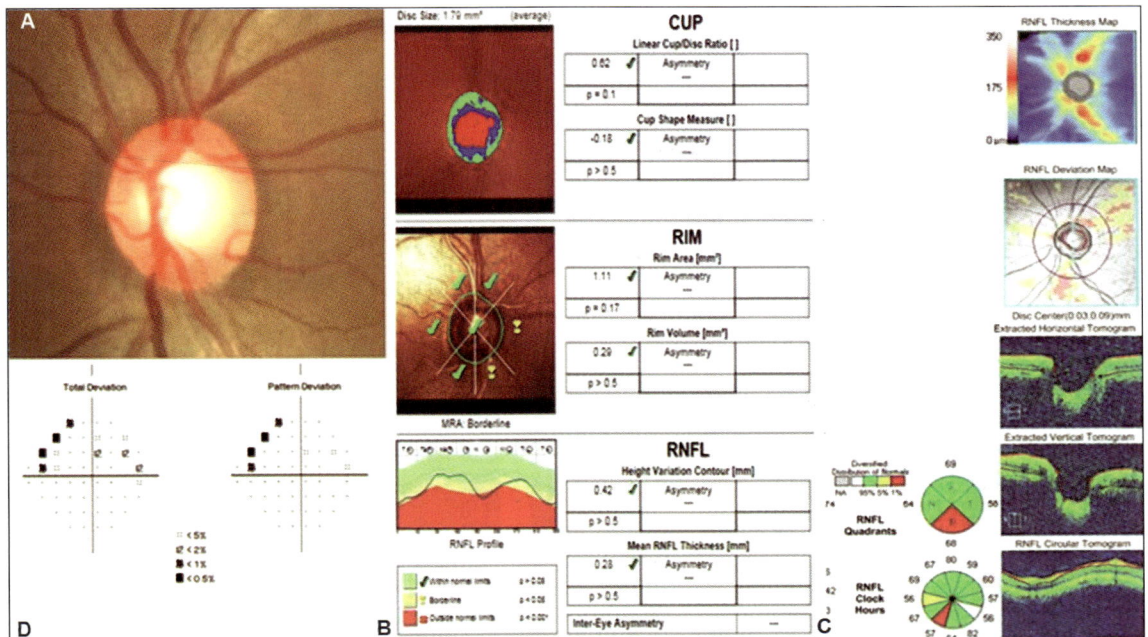

Fig. 15.35: *Early glaucomatous change: (A) Colour photograph of optic nerve showing slight inferior thinning of NRR; (B) HRT II MRA showing; (C) Correlating RNFL thinning on OCT; (D) superior field changes on perimetry.*

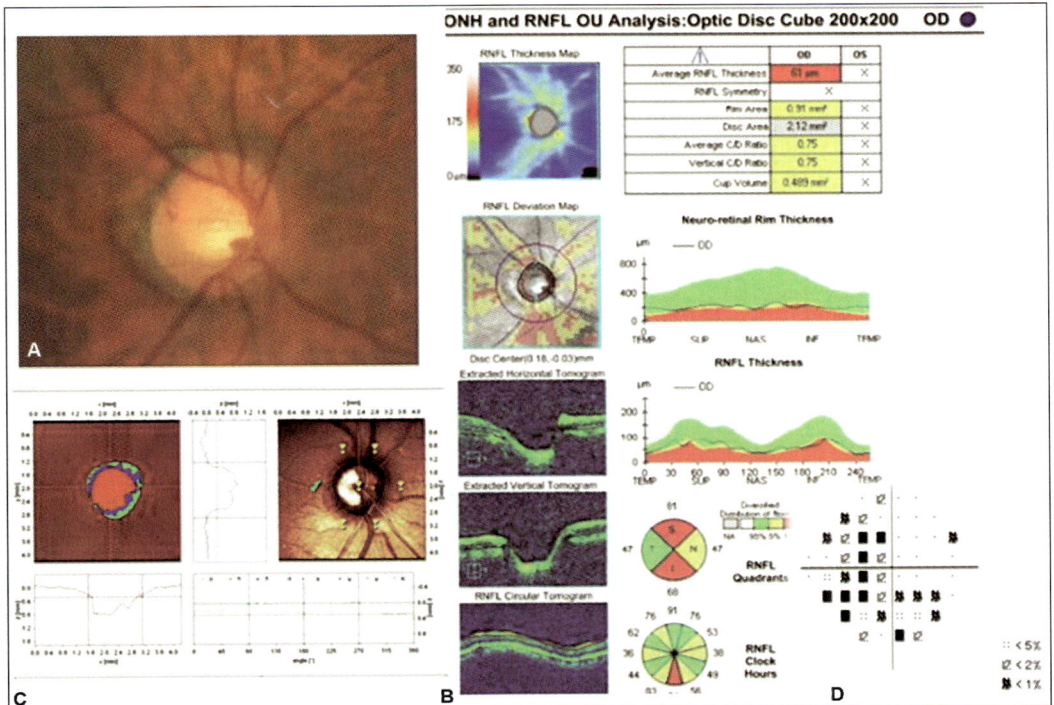

Fig. 15.36: *Moderate glaucomatous damage: (A) Colour photograph of optic nerve showing NRR loss superiorly, inferiorly and nasally; (B) Correlating RNFL loss on OCT; (C) Corresponding image from an HRT II showing borderline thinning in all quadrants except in temporal quadrant; (D) Associated field changes on perimetry.*

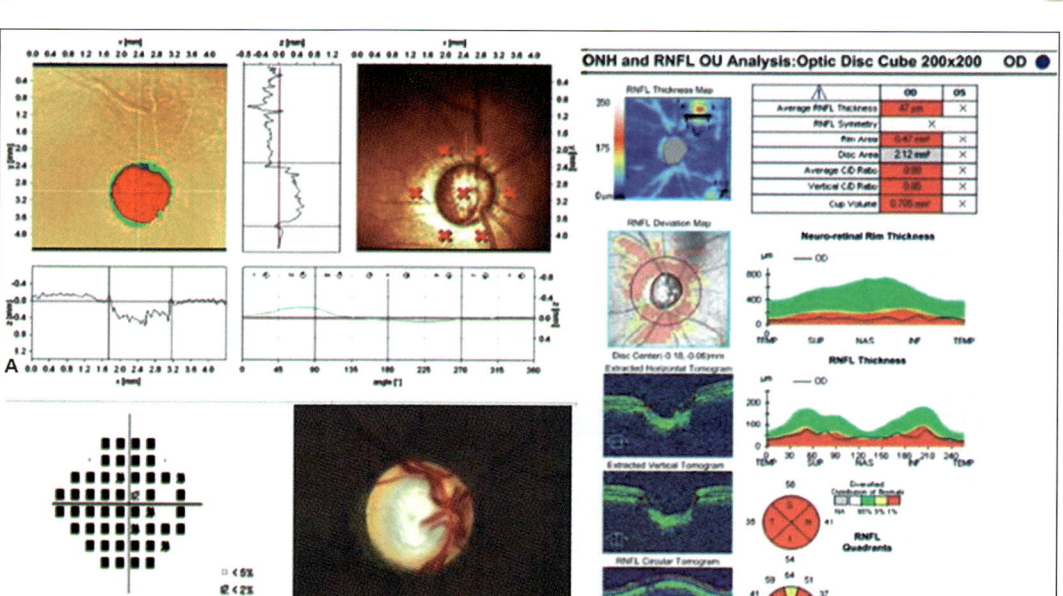

Fig. 15.37: *Advance glaucomatous changes: (A) HRT II MRA showing thinning of RNFL in all quadrants; (B) Correlating RNFL loss as seen on OCT; (C) Advanced visual field changes seen on perimetry; (D) Colour photograph of glaucomatous optic nerve head showing advanced loss of neuroretinal rim.*

that occurs with preparation of histological specimens. It has also enhanced our knowledge regarding specific glaucoma types, such as angle closure glaucoma which may be caused by pupillary block or plateau iris syndrome, pigmentary glaucoma, lens-induced angle closure, iris cysts and tumours, ciliary body rotation due to effusion, and malignant glaucoma.

The present UBM machines typically have high frequency transducers (50–100 MHz), providing a lateral resolution of 50 μ and axial resolution of 25 μ. The tissue penetration is 4–5 mm.

IMAGE ACQUISITION

Images are acquired with the patient lying supine. Room illumination, fixation, and accommodative effort affect anterior segment anatomy and should be held constant, particularly when quantitative information is being gathered.

In the paradigm instruments UBM, the probe is suspended from a gantry arm to minimize motion artifacts (Figs 15.38 and 15.39). In the OTI

(Ophthalmic Technologies, Toronto, Canada) device, the probe is small and light enough not to require a suspension arm (Fig. 15.39).

Scanning is performed with the patient in the supine position under topical anesthesia. The room illumination and fixation is to be kept constant to prevent changes in accommodation and pupil size to any measurements being taken.

A plastic eye cup of the appropriate size (usually 20.0 mm) is inserted between the lids,

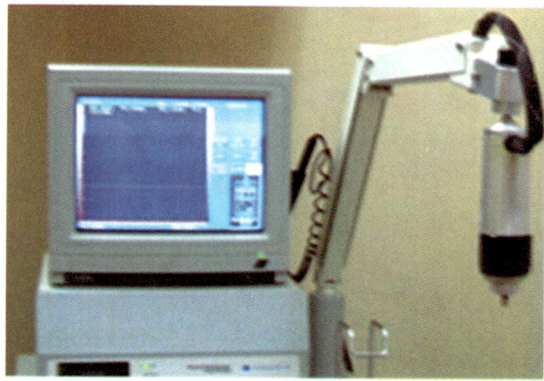

Fig. 15.38: *Paradigm P45 UBM machine.*

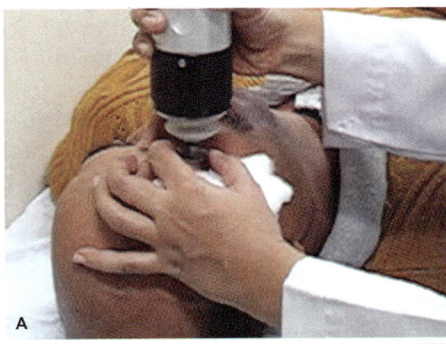

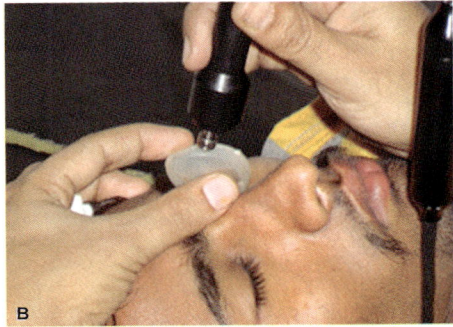

Fig. 15.39: *(A) Left: probe in position using paradigm UBM machine; (B) Right: probe in place using the OTI UBM machine.*

holding methylcellulose or normal saline coupling medium (Fig. 15.39). Usually scanning is performed in radial cuts in the area of interest. This may be uncomfortable and may potentially distort the eye anatomy and angle configuration. The procedure is minimally invasive and may make it impractical for many clinical situations, such as perforating ocular injuries or infective corneal perforations. In addition, a highly skilled operator is needed to obtain high quality images, and the learning curve of the technique is fairly steep.

Also this is one technique where it is preferable and at times may be mandatory for the treating physician to do the procedure himself, since it is imperative to image precisely the area of interest. The high magnification renders general scanning of the eye of little use for both diagnosis and management.

CLINICAL APPLICATIONS IN GLAUCOMA

The applications of UBM in glaucoma are manifold and what follows are representative of the potential of this exciting investigative modality.

1. Trauma

Trauma can result in many derangements in the anterior segment stating from angle recession, iridodialysis, unexplained hypotony due to a cyclodialysis cleft or an occult intraocular foreign body. Many times, UBM is the only modality that is able to pick up these abnormalities (Fig. 15.40).

2. Primary angle closure

Commonly primary angle closure (PAC) occurs as a result of papillary block (Fig. 15.41). But non-pupillary block mechanisms, such as Plateau iris syndrome, can also cause PAC.

UBM helps in differentiating between the two and helps in taking the decision of an iridoplasty in case a laser iridotomy is insufficient to control the disease (Fig. 15.42).

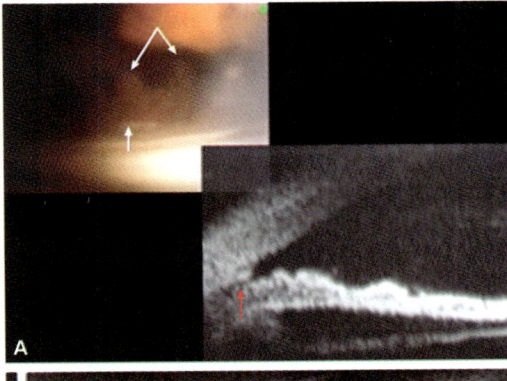

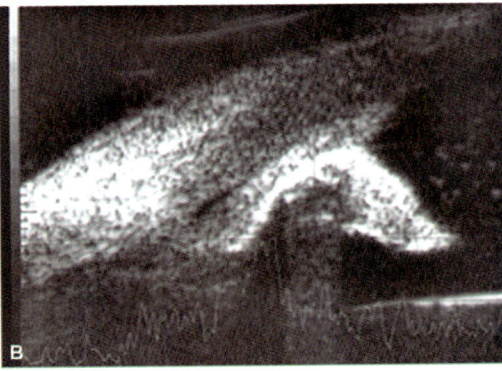

Fig. 15.40: *UBM showing: (A) Small cyclodialysis cleft; (B) Occult foreign body embedded in the posterior iris stroma. Note the back shadowing from foreign body (reproduced with permission from Kaushik S, Pandav SS. Ultrasound Biomicroscopy in glaucoma. In: Recent Advances in Ophthalmology. Nema HV, Ed. Delhi: Jaypee Highlight Medical Publishers Ltd. 2010: 98–110).*

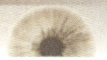

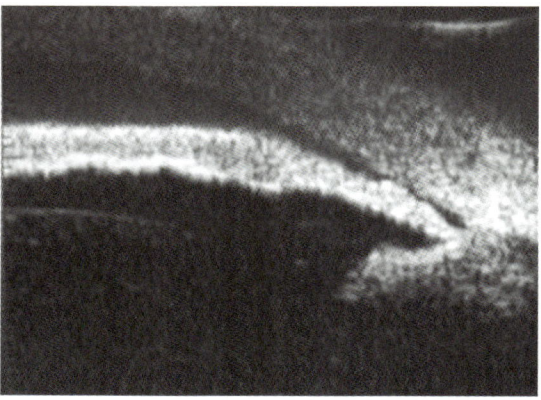

Fig. 15.41: *Pupillary block angle-closure. Note the wide ciliary sulcus and convex configuration of iris forming a bombe-like pattern and closing the angle.*

3. Iris/ciliary body cysts

Sometimes iris or ciliary body cysts may close the angle in what can be termed a "pseudo-plateau iris" configuration. On gonioscopy, where is a trademark "bumpy" appearance of the preripheral iris and the UBM demonstrates the underlying cause (Fig. 15.43).

4. Pigment dispersion syndrome

UBM has helped in understanding the pathophysiology of pigment dispersion syndrome. The iris has a concave appearance, which causes the aqueous to dam anteriorly causing what is termed a "reverse papillary block". The posterior surface of the iris rubbing against the zonules causes release of pigment

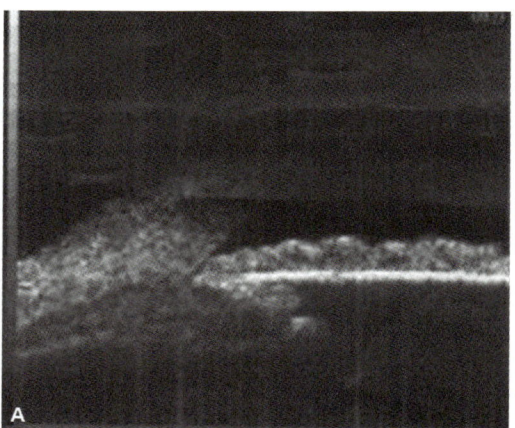

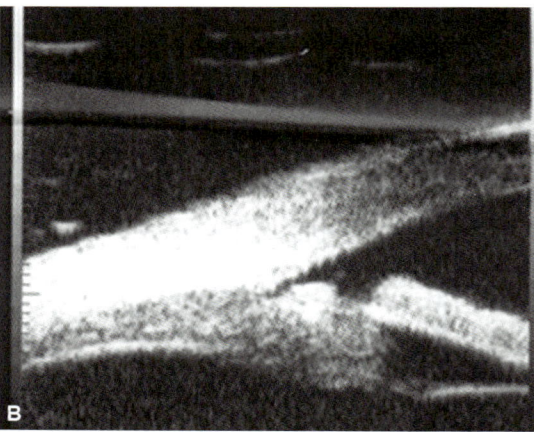

Fig. 15.42: *Plateau iris syndrome: (A) Note the ciliary processes pushing up the iris to close the angle. No ciliary sulcus is appreciable; (B) Patent laser iridotomy but angle is still closed. Prominent ciliary process is pushing up the iris and crowding the angle.*

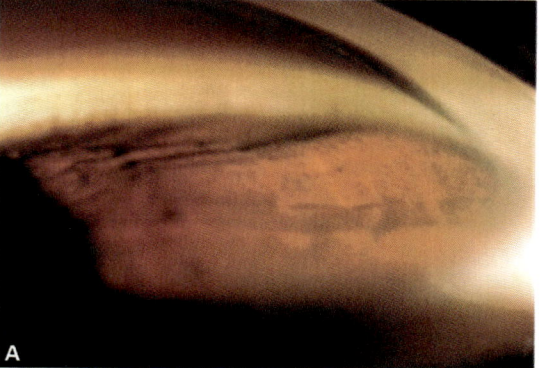

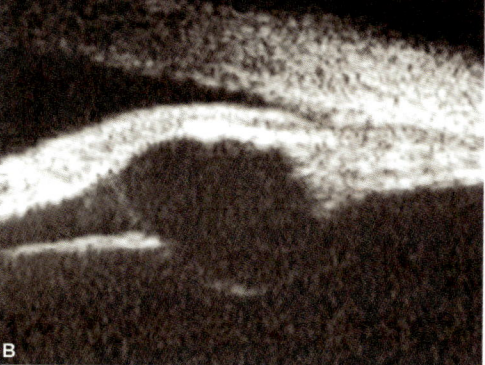

Fig. 15.43: *(A) Gonioscopy showing bumpy appearance of peripheral iris; (B) UBM picture reveals a large iridociliary cyst.*

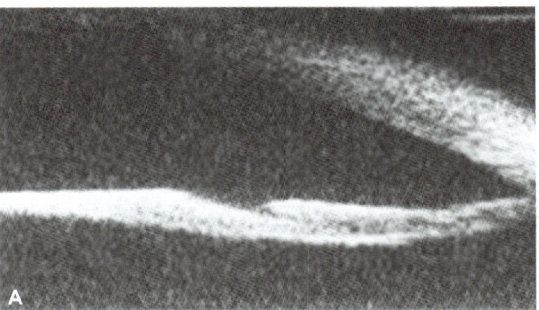 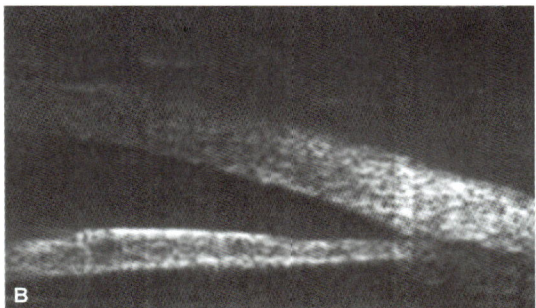

Fig. 15.44: *(A) Pigmentary glaucoma with concave iris configuration; (B) Same iris after laser iridotomy. Note the straightening of the iris.*

throughout the anterior segment. Laser irido-tomy is beneficial in many cases (Fig. 15.44).

5. Pseudoexfoliation with angle-closure

Though pseudoexfoliation is usually associated with an open-angle secondary glaucoma, it is not uncommon to see pseudoexfoliation with angle-closure also. In such cases, it is very important to carefully look at the anterior chamber depth and examine the lens for phacodonesis. The zonules in this condition are weak and many times may be broken leading to the lens becoming more spherical and causing a secondary angle-closure (Fig. 15.45).

6. Imaging failed trabeculectomy blebs

Trabeculectomy is the gold standard for glaucoma surgery. However, failure of the bleb after an interval of apparent success is a fairly common problem. Filtration surgery failure is most commonly due to fibrosis involving episcleral–tenon–conjunctival interface. The status of filtration under the scleral flap cannot be commented upon reliably by clinical examination. Most reports of bleb needling describe disrupting the subtenon's scarred tissue without entry in the subscleral space or the eye, since it is essentially a blind procedure. However, unless there is aqueous flow under the scleral flap, disruption of episcleral-tenon scar tissue alone may not be effective. UBM is a useful tool for evaluation of the filtering bleb. It can visualize the internal sclerostomy opening, aqueous outflow route under the scleral flap and other bleb characteristics. It can also be used as a predictor for success of needling in scarred blebs (Fig. 15.46).

CONCLUSION

Ultrasound biomicroscopy technology is a very useful non-invasive quick and convenient tool in qualitative and quantitative assessment of the anterior segment. It has clarified concepts in the pathophysiology of diseases, such as pigment dispersion, plateau iris and pseudoexfoliation glaucoma. Limitations of limited resolution and poor tissue penetration remain. Future advancements including incorporation of Doppler technology may further enhance the utility of the device in quantitative assessment of the anterior segment.

Fig. 15.45: *Pseudoexfoliation glaucoma with broken zonules. Note the pseudoexfoliative material on the zonular surface giving it a granular look. Also notice the secondary angle-closure caused by forward movement of the spherical lens.*

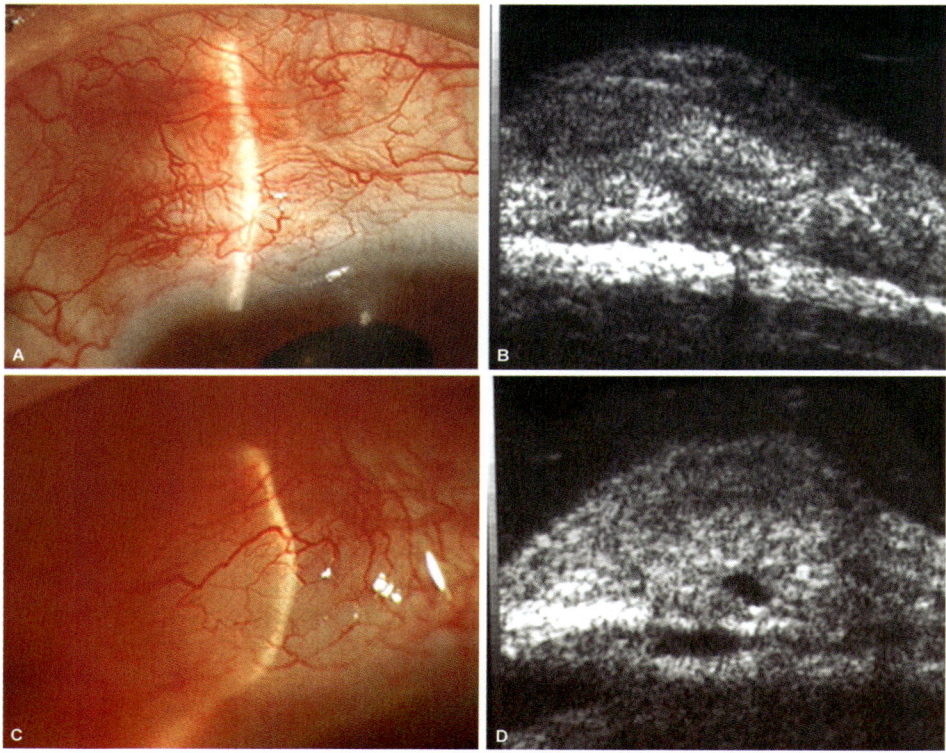

Fig. 15.46: *(A) Scarred trabeculectomy bleb; (B) UBM appearance of the same bleb showing high internal reflectivity with no aqueous spaces; (C) Same bleb after needling; (D) Note on UBM the spaces within the bleb after needling.*

ANTERIOR SEGMENT OPTICAL COHERENCE TOMOGRAPHY

INTRODUCTION

Anterior segment optical coherence tomography (ASOCT) is an imaging modality that provides both quantitative and qualitative information on the cornea, anterior chamber angle, iris and crystalline lens. Assessment of the anterior segment is an integral part of glaucoma examination. Traditionally, the anterior segment and iridocorneal angle are evaluated with the help of a slit-lamp, gonioscope and UBM. The advancement of technology, led to development of low coherence interferometry, upon which optical coherence tomography (OCT) is based. OCT provides multiple detailed cross-sectional images of the internal structures in biological tissues. Currently, two anterior segment OCT (AS-OCT) models are commercially available— the Visante OCT (Carl Zeiss Meditec, Dublin, CA, USA) and the slit-lamp OCT (SLOCT) (Heidelberg Engineering, GmbH, Dossenheim, Germany).

Ophthalmic OCT was initially developed for retinal imaging and used a near-infrared 800 nm superluminescent diode (SLD) as the light emitting source. This OCT model was subsequently applied to anterior segment imaging, capturing images of the cornea, anterior chamber angle, iris and crystalline lens.

With the improvements in speed and light penetration, the entire anterior segment can now be captured in one frame, in 0.125 seconds and in 18 μm resolution (Visante™ OCT User Manual, 2006).

APPLICATIONS OF AS-OCT IN GLAUCOMA

OCT allows fast imaging and can be used in patient who are non-compliant, younger age and in the immediate postoperative period where UBM may be difficult to perform.

1. *Anterior chamber and angle.* Gonisocopy differentiates between angle-closure and open-angle glaucoma. It is a contact based technique and has a learning curve and requires illumination. AS-OCT enables assessment of narrow or suspicious angle that may be occludable. OCT scans can be performed with light on or off and thereby give valuable information in regards to occludability of the angle. The most important parameters are the angle opening distance (AOD) and the trabecular–iris angle (TIA), angle recess area (ARA) and trabecular–iris space area (TISA). The ARA is, theoretically, a better measurement parameter than the AOD because it takes into account of the whole contour of the iris surface rather than measuring at a single point on the iris as is the case with the AOD. Other parameters assessed are anterior chamber depth (ACD). Anterior chamber volume (ACV) is another useful parameter for detecting individuals at risk of developing primary angle-closure.

2. *Imaging of filtering blebs.* The non-contact nature of OCT imaging provides a much safer approach to examine the intrableb morphology in the early postoperative period, thereby offering a unique opportunity to study the healing and remodelling process inside the blebs longitudinally. Using ASOCT, four different patterns of intrableb morphology, including diffuse filtering blebs, cystic blebs, encapsulated blebs and flattened blebs were identified and found to be closely related to slit-lamp appearance and bleb function.

3. *Trauma.* In ocular trauma and in post-operative period, AS-OCT should be kept in mind for evaluating any trauma/postoperative-associated changes in ocular anatomy, e.g. cyclodialysis cleft.

4. *Glaucoma drainage implants.* The position, patency and course of drainage tubes can be ascertained using AS-OCT. ASOCT would be especially helpful in assessing the tube inserted into the ciliary sulcus. The anatomic relationships can be assessed, as can compression of the tube at the scleral entry site.

5. *Evaluation of iris after iridotomy.* Patency in doubtful cases can be confirmed on AS-OCT.

ADVANTAGES AND LIMITATIONS OF AS-OCT

Advantages of the AS-OCT
- High speed, non-invasive
- Can image in the immediate postoperative period
- Visante OCT can give us a limbus to limbus view.

Limitations of AS-OCT
- Limited role in opaque or cloudy media
- Ciliary body, retroiridal structures not visualized.

BIBLIOGRAPHY

OPTICAL COHERENCE TOMOGRAPHY

1. Bowd C, Weinreb RN, Williams JM, et al. The retinal nerve fibre layer thickness in ocular hypertensive, normal, and glaucomatous eyes with optical coherence tomography. Arch Ophthalmol. 2000 Jan;118(1):22–6.
2. Budenz DL, Chang RT, Huang X, et al. Reproducibility of retinal nerve fibre thickness measurements using the stratus OCT in normal and glaucomatous eyes. Invest Ophthalmol Vis Sci 2005;46:2440–3.
3. Forooghian F, Cukras C, Meyerle CB, et al. Evaluation of time domain and spectral domain optical coherence tomography in the measurement of diabetic macular edema. Invest Ophthalmol Vis Sci 2008 Oct;49(10):4290–6.
4. Gyatsho J, Kaushik S, Pandav SS, et al. Retinal nerve fiber layer thickness in normal, ocular hypertensive, and glaucomatous Indian eyes. An Optical Coherence Tomography. Study J Glaucoma 008;17:122–7.
5. Lalezary M, Medeiros FA, Weinreb RN, et al. Baseline optical coherence tomography predicts the development of glaucomatous change in glaucoma suspects. Am J Ophthalmol 2006;142: 576–82.
6. Leitgeb RA, Schmetterer L, Hitzenberger CK, et al. Real-time measurement of *in vitro* flow by Fourier-domain colour Doppler optical coherence tomography. Opt Lett 2004;29:171–3.
7. Leung CK, Chan WM, Chong KK, et al. Comparative study of retinal nerve fibre layer measurement by Stratus OCT and GDx VCC. I: correlation analysis in glaucoma. Invest
8. Leung CK, Cheung CY, Weinreb RN, et al. Retinal nerve fibre layer imaging with spectral-domain

optical coherence tomography: A variability and diagnostic performance study. Ophthalmology 2010 Feb;117(2):267–74.

9. Leung CK, Cheung CY. Evaluation of retinal nerve fiber layer progression in glaucoma: A study on optical coherence tomography guided progression analysis. Invest Ophthalmol Vis Sci 2010;51:217–22.

10. Medeiros FA, Zangwill LM, Bowd C, et al. Evaluation of retinal nerve fibre layer, optic nerve head, and macular thickness measurements for glaucoma detection using optical coherence tomography. Am J Ophthalmol 2005; 139:44–55.

11. Moreno-Montanes J, Olmo N, Alvarez A, et al. Cirrus high-definition optical coherence tomography compared to stratus optical coherence tomography in glaucoma diagnosis. Invest Ophthalmol Vis Sci Sep 8, 2009.

12. Schuman JS, Pedut-Kloizman T, Hertzmark E, et al. Reproducibility of nerve fibre layer thickness measurements using optical coherence tomography. Ophthalmology 1996;103:1889–98.

13. Sony P, Sihota R, Tewari HK. Quantification of the retinal nerve fibre layer thickness in normal Indian eyes with optical coherence tomography. Indian J Ophthalmol 2004 Dec;52(4):303–9.

14. Sung KR, Kim DY, Park SB, et al. Comparison of retinal nerve fibre layer thickness measured by Cirrus HD and Stratus optical coherence tomography. Ophthalmology Jul 2009;116(7): 1264–70.

15. Vizzeri G, Weinreb RN, Gonzalez-Garcia AO. Agreement between Spectral-Domain and Time-Domain OCT for measuring RNFL thickness. Br J Ophthalmol. 2009 Jun;93(6):775–81.

16. Wollstein G, Ishikawa H, Wang J, et al. Comparison of three optical coherence tomography scanning areas for detection of glaucomatous damage. Am J Ophthalmol 2005;139:39–43.

CONFOCAL SCANNING LASER OPHTHALMOSCOPY

17. Hatch WV, et al. Interobserver agreement of Heidelberg retina tomography parameters, J Glaucoma 1999;8:232.

18. Mikelberg FS, Parfitt CM, Swindale NV. Ability of the Heidelberg retina tomograph to detect early glaucomatous visual field loss, J Glaucoma 1996;4:242.

19. Wollstein G, Garway-Heath DF, Hitchings RA. Identification of early glaucoma cases with the scanning laser ophthalmoscope, Ophthalmology 1998;105:1557.

SCANNING LASER POLARIMETRY

20. Garway-Heath, DF, Greaney MJ, et al. Correction for the erroneous compensation of anterior segment birefringence with the scanning laser polarimeter for glaucoma diagnosis. Invest Ophthalmol Vis Sci 2002;43:1465–74.

21. Huang XR, Knighton RW. Linear birefringence of the retinal nerve fibre layer measured *in vitro* with a multispectral imaging micropolarimer. J Biomed Opt 2002;7:199–204.

22. Knighton RW, Huang XR. Analytical methods for scanning laser polarimetry. Optics Express 2002;10: 1179–89.

23. Knighton RW, Huang XR. Analytical model of scanning laser polarimetry for retinal nerve fiber layer assessment. Invest Ophthalmol Vis Sci 2002; 43:383–92.

ULTRASOUND BIOMICROSCOPY

24. Dada T, Gadia R, Sharma A, et al. Ultrasound biomicroscopy in glaucoma. Surv Ophthalmol 2011 Sep-Oct;56(5):433–50.

25. Kaushik S, Ichhpujani P, Ramaswamy A, et al. Occult Intraocular Foreign Body: Ultrasound biomicroscopy holds the key. Int Ophthalmol 2008;1:71–3.

26. Kaushik S, Tiwari A, Ichhpujani P, et al. The use of Ultrasound Biomicroscopy to predict the long-term outcome of sub-tenon needle revision of failed trabeculectomy blebs: A pilot study. Eur J Ophthalmol 2011 Nov;21(6):700–7.

27. Pavlin CJ, Foster FS. Ultrasound biomicroscopy. High-frequency ultrasound imaging of the eye at microscopic resolution. Radiol Clin North Am 1998; 36:1047–58.

28. Pavlin CJ, Foster FS. Ultrasound biomicroscopy of the eye. 1st edition, New York, springer-Verlag 1995;140–54.

29. Pavlin CJ, Harasiewicz K, Sherar MD, et al. Clinical use of ultrasound biomicroscopy. Ophthalmology 1991;98:287–95.

30. Pavlin CJ. Practical application of ultrasound biomicroscopy. Can J Ophthalmol 1995;30: 225–9.

31. Sherar MD, Starkoski BG, Taylor WB, et al. A 100 MHz B-scan ultrasound back scatter microscope. Ultrasonic imaging 1989;11:95–105.

ANTERIOR SEGMENT OCT

31. Bechmann M, Thiel MJ, Neubauer AS, et al. Central corneal thickness measurement with a retinal optical coherence tomography device versus standard ultrasonic pachymetry. Cornea 2001;20:50–4.

32. Leung CK, Chan WM, Ko CY. Visualization of anterior chamber angle dynamics using optical coherence tomography. Ophthalmology 2005;112:980–4.

33. Leung CK, Yick DW, Kwong YY, et al. Analysis of bleb morphology after trabeculectomy with Visante anterior segment optical coherence tomography. Br J Ophthalmol 2007;91:340–4.

34. Leung DY, Lam DK, Yeung BY, et al. Comparison between central corneal thickness measurements by ultrasound pachymetry and optical coherence tomography. Clin Experiment Ophthalmol 2006;34:751–4.

35. Madgula IM, Kotta S. Stratus optical coherence tomogram III: A novel, reliable and accurate way to measure corneal thickness. Indian J Ophthalmol 2007;55:301–3.

36. Wirbelauer C, Scholz C, Hoerauf H, et al. Corneal optical coherence tomography before and immediately after excimer laser photorefractive keratectomy. Am J Ophthalmol 2000;130:693–9.

37. Wong AC, Wong CC, Yuen NS, et al. Correlational study of central corneal thickness measurements on Hong Kong, Chinese, using optical coherence tomography, Orbscan and ultrasound pachymetry. Eye 2002;16:715–21.

16

Perimetry and Other Psychophysical Tests in Glaucoma

Chapter Outline

PERIMETRY

Visual fields: general considerations
• Definition, limits and analogy
• Central versus peripheral fields
• Methods of assessment of visual fields

Kinetic perimetry
• Types
• Indications
• Techniques

Static perimetry
• Advantages
• Terminologies in automated perimetry
• Testing patterns and strategies

• Evaluation of HFA single field printout
• Interpretation of visual field defects
• Octopus printout
• Visual fields: frequently asked questions
• Practical pearls

OTHER PSYCHOPHYSICAL TESTS IN GLAUCOMA
• Introduction
• Anatomical basis
• Short wavelength automated perimetry
• Frequency doubling perimetry
• Motion detection perimetry
• Flicker-defined form perimetry
• High pass resolution perimetry
• Pulsar perimetry

PERIMETRY

VISUAL FIELDS: GENERAL CONSIDERATIONS

DEFINITION, LIMITS, AND ANALOGY

Definition

Visual field. Visual field refers to the sum total of visual perception for an eye fixed on a stationary object of regard with the head and body held fixed in position.

Field of gaze. The visual field is different from the 'field of gaze', in which the eye is permitted to have freedom of rotational movement while the head and body are kept in a constant position.

Field of view. Here both the eye as well as the head can be moved.

Normal limits

• The normal human visual field (Fig. 16.1A) extends to approximately 60° nasally (toward the nose, or inward) from the vertical meridian in each eye, to 100° temporally (away from the nose, or outwards) from the vertical meridian, and approximately 60° above and 75° below the horizontal meridian.

• The macula corresponds to the central 13° of the visual field; the fovea to the central 3^c.

• The normal visual field reaches 180° in the horizontal plane (160° for monocular vision) and 135° in the vertical plane.

Classic analogy

The visual field can be compared with a topographic map of an island. Traquair proposed the concept of "an island of vision surrounded by a sea of darkness". The height of the island correlates to the sensitivity of the retina. Vision perception is most sensitive at the fovea, and sensitivity decreases towards the periphery. In the 'island of vision', a deep well represents the blind spot, roughly 15° temporal to the point of fixation. The blind spot is an absolute visual field defect caused by the optic nerve head, which has no overlying retina (Fig. 16.1B).

CENTRAL VERSUS PERIPHERAL FIELDS

The visual field can be divided into central and peripheral fields:

- *Central field* includes an area from the fixation point to a circle 30° away. The central zone

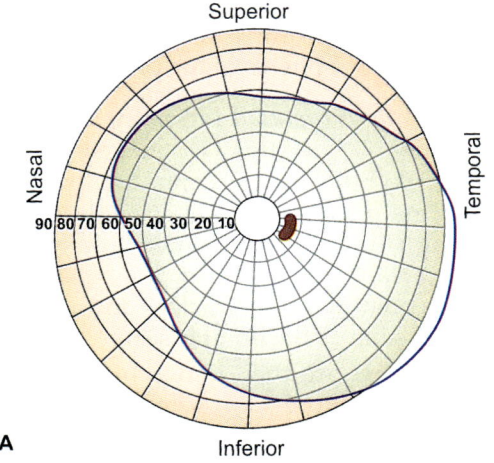

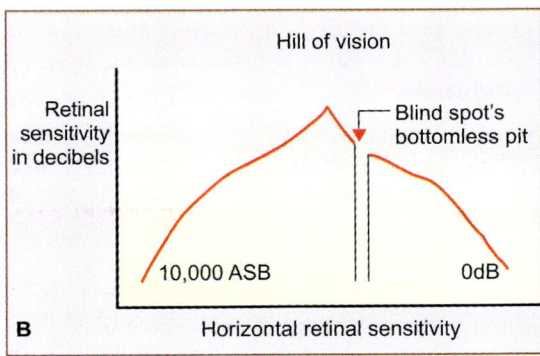

Fig. 16.1: *(A) Extent of normal visual field; (B) Traquir's normal hill of vision.*

contains physiological blind spot on the temporal side.

- *Peripheral field* of vision refers to the rest of area beyond 30° to outer extent of field of vision.
- *Isopter.* Visual field, i.e. the three-dimensional hill of vision can be divided into many isopters depending upon the perception sensitivity. Thus, each isopter can be defined as a threshold line forming points of equal sensitivity on a visual field chart.
- *Scotoma* refers to an area of loss of vision totally (absolute scotoma) or partially (relative scotoma) in the visual field.

METHODS OF ASSESSMENT OF VISUAL FIELDS

Campimetry

This refers to examination of the visual field projected onto a flat surface, e.g. on a transparent screen or flat-panel monitor. It is best suited to examination of the central visual field, up to approximately 20° of eccentricity.

Perimetry

This refers to examination of the visual field performed with a hemispherical surface onto which the visual field is projected. The standard unit of measurement in the visual field is the differential light sensitivity (DLS). Basic principle underlying all forms of perimetry is same. The eye to be examined is positioned at the geometric centre of the hemisphere, such that all points on its inner surface are equidistant from the eye. The surface is uniformly illuminated and test objects are small spots of light that are projected on top of the adapting background.

Indications for perimetry

Indications for visual field testing include visual field deficits, vision loss, headache, and neurologic deficits.

Perimetry is typically the only clinical procedure that evaluates the status of the afferent visual pathways for locations outside the macular region. It is used especially for detection of glaucoma.

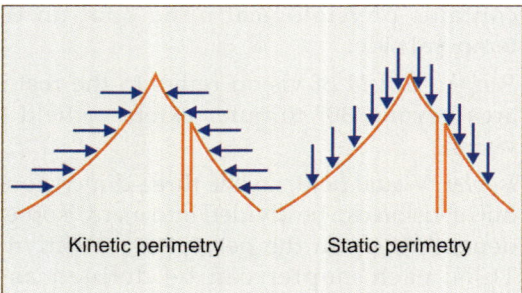

| Kinetic perimetry | Static perimetry |

Fig. 16.2 *Kinetic versus static perimetry.*

Once glaucoma has been diagnosed, it helps in the following:
- Progress of disease
- Effectiveness of treatment
- To explain visual prognosis.

Types of perimetry

Kinetic perimetry. In this form, test objects used are fixed in size and brightness. They are moved from non-seeing areas into seeing portions of the visual field, the subject is asked to respond when the object first becomes visible.

Static perimetry. In this form, stationary test objects that vary in size and brightness, but never move are employed. Brightness of the test object at a point is gradually increased till the patient responds.

Basic differences between the two forms of perimetry are enlisted in Table 16.1 and shown in Fig. 16.2.

KINETIC PERIMETRY

Kinetic perimetry is still an indispensable diagnostic method in a number of clinical situations where the periphery needs to be tested or where automated static perimetry reaches its limits.

Types of kinetic perimetry

1. *Manual kinetic perimetry*

Prototype is Goldmann perimeter. In 2007, the production of the Goldmann perimeter ceased.

2. *Semiautomated kinetic perimetry*

Prototype is Octopus 101. Strong agreement has been shown with Goldmann perimetry for type and location of defect.

3. *Automated kinetic perimetry*

Prototype is Octopus 900. The Octopus 900 provides 90° full field projection perimetry with a range of 47 decibels and capable of performing both kinetic and static perimetry programmes (Fig. 16.3).

Indications include:
- Assessment of young children
- Patients with poor vision or severely restricted visual fields
- Patients with brain injury involving the posterior hemispheres of the brain.

Techniques of automated perimetry is summarized below:
- Using the built-in telescope, the examiner tracks the patient's eye for good fixation. A moving stimulus is presented from a non-seeing area to a seeing area. It is repeated at various points around the clock and a mark is made as soon as the point is seen.
- These points are then joined by a line, an 'isopter'. The process is repeated with a point of lesser luminescence and another isopter is created. Thus, a number of isopters are plotted so the end result is a chart of the maximal peripheral vision for decreasing level of brightness.

Table 16.1 *Differences between kinetic and static perimetry*		
	Kinetic	*Static*
Stimulus presentation	From non-seeing to seeing	Can be presented from seeing to non-seeing or *vice versa*
Optimal stimulus speed	4 deg per sec	Independent of reaction time
Sensitivity for detection of shallow focal loss	Likely to be missed, especially if in periphery	More sensitive than kinetic
Time required for test	Dependent on patient reaction time	Manual static more time consuming than automated static

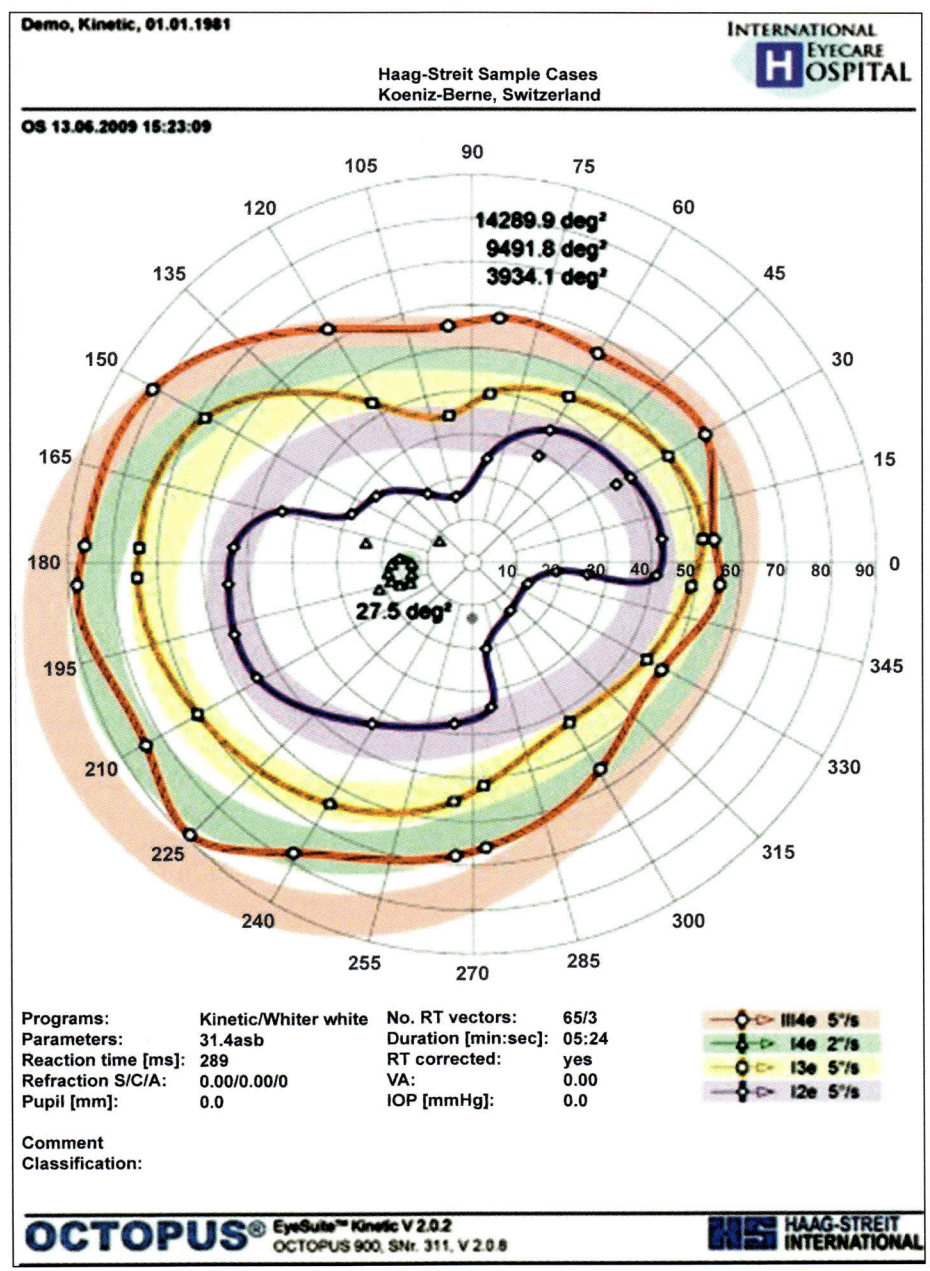

Fig. 16.3: *Octopus 900 kinetic perimetry.*

- The results differ depending on photopic, mesopic, or scotopic background luminosity.
- For current Octopus kinetic perimetry, the visual field strategy currently utilised when screening with Octopus perimeter is a 5°/sec stimulus speed for peripheral and central visual field isopters using I4e and I2e targets along with a 3°/sec stimulus speed using I4e target for blind spot mapping and further evaluation of field loss area. This is coupled

with suprathreshold static assessment within the central visual field using the I4e target.

STATIC PERIMETRY

Static perimetry requires presenting a stimulus of a constant size of varying intensity at a fixed location to determine the threshold sensitivity at that locus. This technique is performed at every designated location in a preselected area and pattern, and a map of threshold sensitivities for a given field of vision is generated.

ADVANTAGES OF AUTOMATED STATIC PERIMETRY OVER MANUAL KINETIC PERIMETRY

- Test administration is more standardized and, therefore, more reproducible.
- Less input from a technician is required, minimizing testing variability.
- Reliability is improved with automated fixation monitoring and reduced examination time for static testing compared with manual static testing.
- Patient dependability may be quantitated and statistically assessed.

AUTOMATED PERIMETRY: TERMINOLOGIES AND VARIABLES

Luminous intensity

- Current standard unit of luminous intensity is candela/m² (cd/m²).
- Unit used in HFA is apostilb (asb), which is an European unit; Apostilb (asb) is a unit of brightness per unit area and is defined as 35^{-1} candela/m².
- Americans use millilambert instead of apostilb.
- 10,000 asb = 1 lambert or 3183 cd/m².
- 1 asb is the least intense stimulus that can be seen foveally.

Concepts of luminous intensity: Log

Basic mathematics of log tables:
- $10^1 = 10$
- $10^2 = 100$
- $10^3 = 1000$
- $10^4 = 10000$
- $10^5 = 100000$

- $10^6 = 1000000$
- $10,000 \times 100 = 1,000,000$ or $10^4 \times 10^2 = 10^6$ (Note: 4 + 2 = 6)

In considerations of luminosity, log scale (geometric progression) is used because sensation relates to factors rather than addition of intensity, e.g. if a patient has failed to see a 1000 asb stimulus, increasing intensity by 1 asb will not have any meaning as the difference would be very little to appreciate. However, if it is increased by 1/10 of a log factor, it will increase illumination by 25% and 3/10 of log factor will double the intensity.

Decibel

Decibel is not a unit of luminosity. It describes retinal sensitivity, i.e. less the light required to be perceived by retina at a particular point, more is the sensitivity of retina at that point. In a normal person, it is maximum at fovea. One dB is described as one-tenth of log unit. Maximum intensity of stimulus that HFA can produce is 10000 asb. Figure of 10000 can have a maximum log of 4 ($10000 = 10^4$). Since 1 dB is 1/10 of log, maximum possible sensitivity is 40 dB which is equivalent of 1 asb which is the minimum intensity of stimulus which can be perceived by a young trained observer and thus, this 40 dB is the maximum possible foveal threshold in a HVF printout.

Automated perimeter variables

1. *Background illumination*. HFA uses 31.5 apostilb (asb) background illumination. Apostilb (asb) is a unit of brightness per unit area (and is defined as 35^{-1} candela/m²).

2. *Stimulus intensity*. HFA uses projected stimuli which can be varied in intensity over a range of more than 5% log units (51 decibels) between 0.08 and 10,000 asb. In decibel notation (dB), the value refers to retinal sensitivity rather than to stimulus intensity. Therefore, 0 dB corresponds to 10,000 asb and 51 dB to 0.08 asb (Fig. 16.4). In contrast to kinetic perimetry, the higher numbers indicate a logarithmic reduction in test object brightness, and hence greater sensitivity of vision (Fig. 16.4).

3. *Stimulus size*. HFA usually offers five sizes of stimuli corresponding to the Goldmann

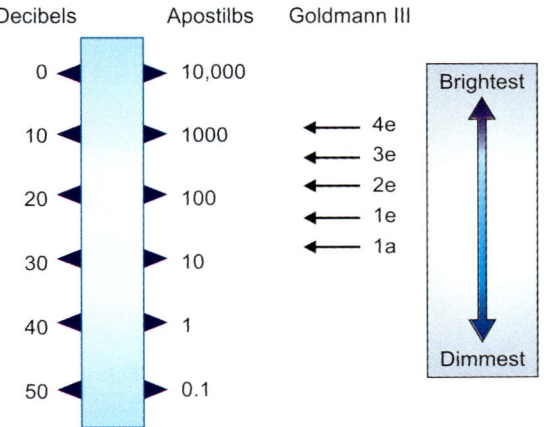

Fig. 16.4: *Stimulus intensity scales compared.*

perimeter stimuli I through V. Unless otherwise instructed, the standard target size for automated perimetry is equivalent to Goldmann size III (4 mm²) white target.

4. *Stimulus duration.* Stimulus duration should be shorter than the latency time for voluntary eye movements (about 0.25 seconds). HFA uses a stimulus duration of 0.2 sec while Octopus has 0.1 sec.

Concept of threshold, suprathreshold and infrathreshold

Threshold. Minimal intensity of light at which a stimulus is perceived by the visual system at a specific location in the field of vision. In statistical terms, it is the point on a frequency-of-seeing curve at which a stimulus is perceived 50% of the time.

Suprathreshold. Intensity of light at which stimuli are perceived greater than 95% of the time on the frequency-of-seeing curve, or any stimulus brighter than threshold.

Infrathreshold. Intensity of light at which stimuli are perceived with a frequency of less than 5%, or any stimulus weaker than threshold.

A threshold value is determined by presenting stimuli of gradually increasing and decreasing intensities, determining the dimmest stimulus presented that is seen and the brightest that is not seen, and either averaging these values or using the last seen or not-seen stimulus as the

threshold value. Threshold sensitivity may vary with retinal adaptation (background illumination), stimulus colour and size, duration of stimulus presentation, and degree of stimulus movement.

TESTING STRATEGIES AND PROGRAMMES

Testing strategies

Two basic categories of testing strategies are offered by most instruments: suprathreshold screening and threshold testing.

Suprathreshold screening

This enables rapid discovery of gross field defects. A fixed stimulus that is presumed to be threshold at approximately 30° is used for the entire test area, without adjusting for decreased sensitivity as per the normal contour of the hill of vision. The tested points are recorded as either seen or not seen.

Indications for screening include:
- *Baseline testing* for a patient before ocular or neurosurgical operative procedures
- *Routine examination* for occupational licensing
- *Localization* of a postchiasmal neuro-ophthalmologic lesion.

Threshold testing

Threshold strategies report actual retinal sensitivities at each point tested in numeric form (dB). As in the screening strategies, the sensitivities are displayed in a pattern corresponding to that employed in the test. Along with actual values, a display of differences from expected values or depth of defect may be provided. If the actual values are within 4 to 5 dB of expected values, they are considered within the limits of normal variability and may be recorded as 'normal'.

Visual threshold is the physiologic ability to detect a stimulus under defined testing conditions. The normal threshold is defined as the mean threshold in normal people in a given age group at a given location in the visual field. It is against these values that the machine compares the patient's sensitivity. Thresholds are reported in decibels in a range of 0–50. Fifty decibel (dB) is the dimmest target the perimeter can project. 0 dB is the brightest illumination the perimeter can project. The lower the decibel value the lower the sensitivity; the higher the decibel value, the higher is the sensitivity.

Threshold testing provides more precise results than suprathreshold testing and is thus preferred by most clinicians, although it takes more time and the equipment often costs more.

Common threshold testing strategies

1. Full threshold testing. This testing modality involves performing the bracketing (staircase) process at every point tested (4-2 on the Humphrey and 4-2-1 on the Octopus perimeter). A stimulus brighter than the patient's expected threshold is presented at a point. If the stimulus is seen, stimuli of successively reduced intensity are presented until the stimulus is not seen. Then stimuli of increasingly higher intensity are presented until one is seen. Most instruments use 4 dB increments until threshold is crossed for the first time. Subsequent changes in intensity are usually of 2 dB steps. A point somewhere between suprathreshold and infrathreshold is determined to be threshold for that point. Most perimeters bracket until threshold is crossed twice, from the suprathreshold and infrathreshold directions. Several points in the field are in the process of being thresholded at the same time.

2. FASTPAC is a rapid thresholding strategy in the Humphrey Field Analyzer:

• This uses a 3 dB step size and estimates the threshold after only one crossing, but thresholds the four primary seed points in a similar manner to standard full-threshold testing (Fig. 16.5).

• Half of the points start at 1 dB brighter and the other half start at 2 dB dimmer than the predicted threshold values.

• After a single crossing, the threshold is estimated. Thresholds of locations that differ from expected values by 4 dB or more are then re-estimated.

Studies have shown that FASTPAC, underestimates mean deviation and pattern standard deviation when compared with the standard algorithm.

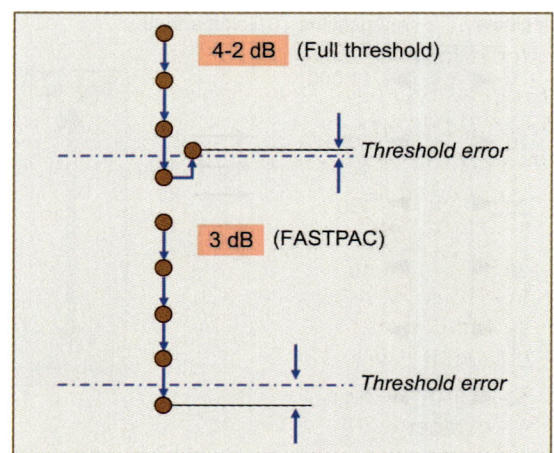

Fig. 16.5: *Bracketting in FASTPAC versus full threshold.*

3. Swedish interactive thresholding algorithm (SITA). SITA strategy uses continuous estimation of threshold values and measurement errors throughout the test, using advanced visual field models and mathematical analyses performed in real-time. Models are initially based on prior visual fields. Staircase procedures are used to alter stimulus intensities at predetermined test point locations. Test time is further reduced by eliminating catch trials to determine the frequencies of false-positive answers and by using a more effective timing algorithm. The SITA Standard and SITA Fast strategies are available as software implemented on the Humphrey Field Analyzer II.

Threshold testing is preferred over screening strategies for patients in whom a defect is likely to be present (e.g. those with optic neuritis accompanied by reduced acuity, glaucoma patients with pathologic-appearing optic discs).

Testing Programmes

Basic testing patterns are chosen depending on the area of field to be tested and the density and distribution of points within. The options for areas to be tested include the central 30°, the peripheral 30 to 60° area, full 60°, central 10°, and central 5°. Special test configurations are also available, including glaucoma patterns (central 30° plus peripheral nasal step area and temporal periphery), peripheral nasal step area,

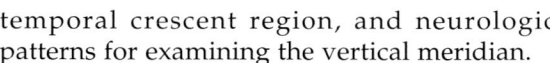

temporal crescent region, and neurologic patterns for examining the vertical meridian.

Standard test programmes used with satic threshold strategy on the Humphrey Field Analyzer can be grouped as below:

A. *Central field tests*
- Central 30–2 test
- Central 24–2 test
- Central 10–2 test
- Macular test.

B. *Peripheral field tests*
- Peripheral 30/60-1
- Peripheral 30/60–2
- Nasal step
- Temporal crescent

C. *Speciality tests*
- Neurological-20
- Neurological-50
- Central 10–12
- Macular test

D. *Custom tests.*

HFA SINGLE PRINTOUT: EVALUATION

The standard HFA printout is obtained using a software called *STATPAC printout*. For the purpose of evaluation, the Humphrey single field printout (STATPAC printout) with central 30-2 test can be studied in eight parts I to VIII as described below (Fig. 16.6).

I. Patient data and test parameters: general information

At the top of printout page (part I) are printed:
- Patient's data [name, date of birth, eye (right/ left), pupil size and visual acuity]
- Test parameters (test name, strategy, stimulus used, background).

For interpreting any field, first look at the general information for the following reasons: The data provided is about both the testing conditions and demographics. It helps to identify the patient. It is important to look at the test pattern and test strategy being used as tests using different test strategies may not be comparable.
- *Correct name and date of birth of the patient* not only identify the patient but are absolutely

essential to enable comparison with normative data for the present field and also with future fields to detect change.
- *The date and time of testing* is given on top right. It is advisable to record the date in DD/MM/ YYYY format as it is most familiar format in our country.
- *Eye being tested* should be confirmed as a wrongly entered eye would not allow fixation monitor tests and a wrong normogram for the eye would identify blind spot as scotoma.
- *Pupil size* is automatically detected in newer models. Fields may be carried out on a normal or a dilated pupil but not while it is dilating.
- *Visual acuity* of the patient and trial lens selection are given. Not using proper trial lens in cases obviously requiring the same may cause generalized depression of fields.
- *Stimulus size*, colour and background brightness should be noted as an improper stimulus size will misrepresent fields and certain STATPAC features may not be available for non-standard parameters.

  A larger stimulus size may be rquired in patients with poor vision or coloured stimuli may be used for certain retinal or optic nerve conditions.
- *Test duration*, if prolonged, indirectly indicates that the patient was taking too long as points were thresholded repeatedly which could be due to unreliable responses, fatigue or increased variability in defective fields. A SITA Standard test typically takes around 7 minutes.
- *Foveal threshold*. A look at the foveal threshold just under the test duration can yield useful information. A good foveal threshold but a poor visual acuity may indicate improper refraction while *vice versa* may indicate early foveal damage.

II. Reliability Indices

Patient reliability may be appraised by several parameters. These include the fixation losses, false-positive and -negative responses, and degree of response variability. During the examination, rest periods as well as additional

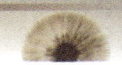

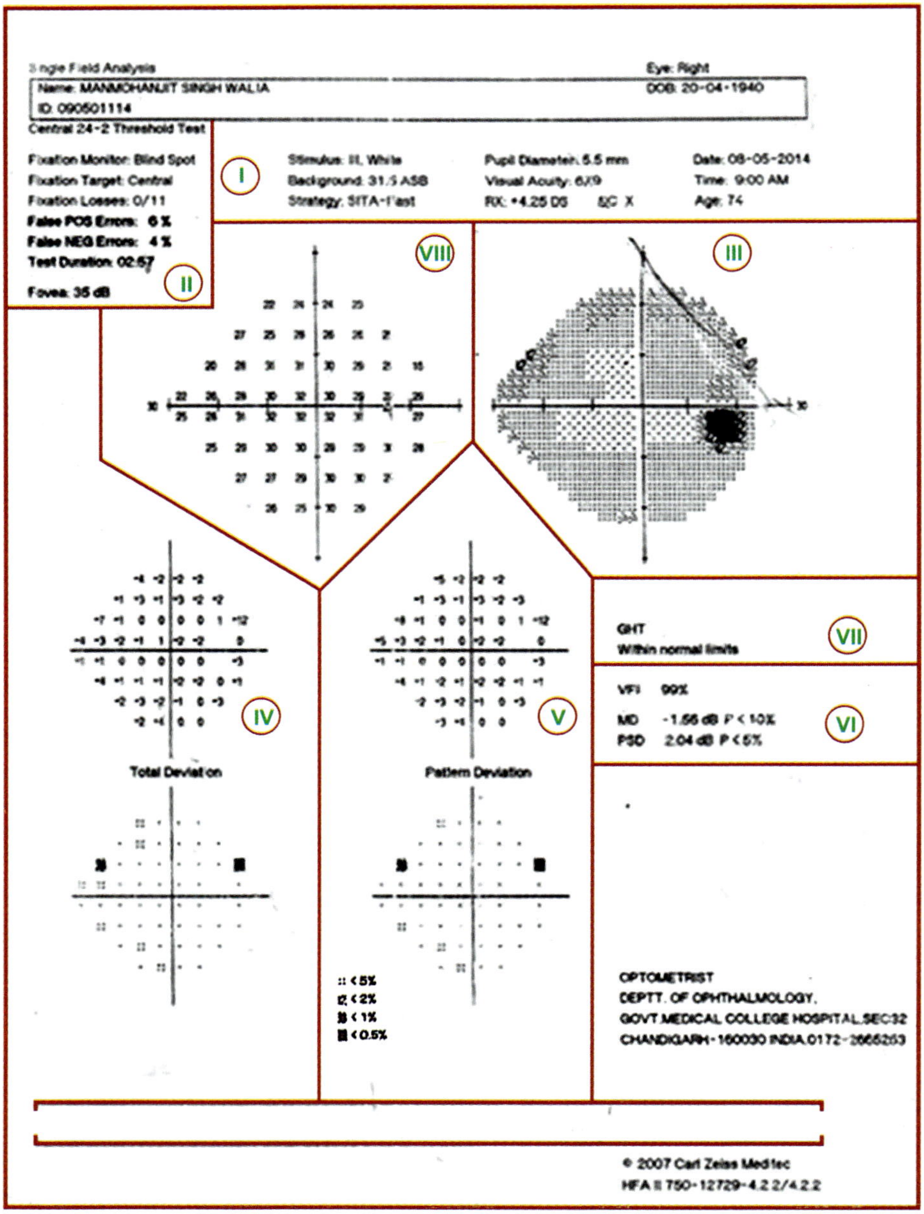

Single Field Analysis · Eye: Right

Name: MANMOHANJIT SINGH WALIA · DOB: 20-04-1940

ID: 090501114

Central 24-2 Threshold Test

Fixation Monitor: Blind Spot · Stimulus: III, White · Pupil Diameter: 5.5 mm · Date: 08-05-2014
Fixation Target: Central · Background: 31.5 ASB · Visual Acuity: 6/9 · Time: 9:00 AM
Fixation Losses: 0/11 · Strategy: SITA-Fast · RX: +4.25 DS DC X · Age: 74
False POS Errors: 6%
False NEG Errors: 4%
Test Duration: 02:57
Fovea: 35 dB

GHT
Within normal limits

VFI 99%
MD -1.56 dB P < 10%
PSD 2.04 dB P < 5%

Total Deviation

Pattern Deviation

:: < 5%
:: < 2%
:: < 1%
■ < 0.5%

OPTOMETRIST
DEPTT. OF OPHTHALMOLOGY,
GOVT. MEDICAL COLLEGE HOSPITAL, SEC-32
CHANDIGARH - 160030 INDIA. 0172-2665253

© 2007 Carl Zeiss Meditec
HFA II 750-12729-4.2.2/4.2.2

Fig. 16.6: *Normal Humphrey visual field printout.*

instructions may be needed to ensure optimal reliability. In addition, if machine-determined parameters of reliability suggest that the patient performed poorly but fixation was observed to be of good quality, the field may be of more value than would have otherwise been determined.

1. Fixation losses

Methods to monitor fixation

i. *Blind-spot monitoring technique.* It is done by repeatedly representing the stimulus to blind spot and noting the response. Fixation losses are recorded as a fraction, with the number of losses of fixation in the numerator and the number of

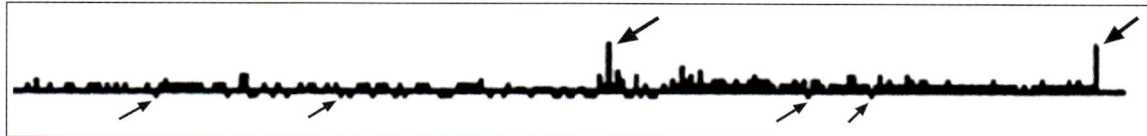

Fig. 16.7: *Gaze tracking.*

blind-spot presentations in the denominator. It is also known as Heijl-Krakau method.

ii. *Sensor monitoring.* If eye movement sensors are used, an absolute number of fixation losses is recorded.

iii. *Manual monitoring* of fixation by the examiner.

iv. *Gaze tracker.* It is printed at the bottom of the test result (Fig. 16.7)

- Upward deviation going fully up indicates 10 degrees gaze error (fixation loss).
- Downward deviation indicates blinks (wherein the tracker could not measure fixation).
- An even smooth line, with minimal excursions implies good fixation.

Reliability status

Fixation losses when exceed 20% the test results are considered unreliable. If this arbitrary cut-off point be increased to 33%, which would decrease the number of fields deemed unreliable without significantly affecting the sensitivity or specificity of the test.

Pseudofixation losses may be seen from high refractive errors due to lens-induced shift in blind spot location.

2. False-positive and negative responses

False-positive response is recorded when a patient signals that a stimulus has been seen when one has not been presented, usually in response to an audible click rather than a visual stimulus. It gives an unusually white out graph (white scotoma).

False-negative response is registered when a patient fails to respond to the presentation of a stimulus at a given location that is significantly brighter than the previously determined threshold at that point (suprathreshold). It gives a clover leaf-like pattern of graph.

Reliability status

Examinations in which false responses of greater than 33% are registered have been considered unreliable. A higher rate of false-negative responses has been shown to occur in patients with glaucomatous field loss compared with normal.

Cut-off values of reliability indices

The visual field examination is considered unreliable, if three or more of the following reliability indices have below mentioned values:

- Fixation losses $\geq$ 20%
- False-positive error $\geq$ 33%
- False-negative error $\geq$ 33%
- Short-term fluctuation $\geq$ 4.0 dB
- Total questions $\geq$ 400.

III. Grayscale

Grayscale simulation of the test data is depicted in part III of the printout (Fig. 16.6). Grayscale printout is generated by delegating different symbols to actual decibel values of threshold sensitivities, with a specific symbol representing a particular range of stimulus intensities. Darker areas indicate a lower differential light sensitivity and lighter areas indicate zones of higher sensitivity. The resultant printout assigns a retinal sensitivity to every area of field tested, but in reality only a limited number of points were actually thresholded. To allow for conti-nuity, values of presumed retinal sensitivity are interposed to unassessed area of the field. It gives only a gross assessment of the field. The darker the printout, the worse is the field. The grayscale provides the field defects at a glance. However, in general we do not make a diagnosis based on the grayscale. The main emphasis on statistical help shows in part IV to VIII of the printout (threshold values).

IV. Total deviation plots

Total deviation plots provide the deviation of patient's threshold values from that of age corrected normal data. The two total deviation plots are numeric value plot and the probability plot (grayscale symbol plot).

Numeric value plot. Simple threshold sensitivities are measured in decibels and given in the numeric plot. Values above 40 dB are generally not expected and may be indicative of a trigger happy field. The actual numeric values may not be concentrated upon for day-to-day interpretation of field but only with specific purposes. In other words, numeric value plot represents the differences in decibels. SA zero value means that the patient has the expected threshold for that age. Positive numbers reflect points that are more sensitive than average for that age; whereas negative numbers reflect points that are depressed compared with the average.

Probability plot (grayscale symbol plot). In the lower part of part IV of the printout, the total deviation plot is represented graphically. The darker the graphic representation the more significant it is.

Note. In general, the total deviation plot is an indicator of the general depression and is not capable of revealing the hidden scotomas that may be present in the overall depressed field.

V. Pattern deviation plots

The two pattern deviation plots (numeric pattern deviation plot and probability pattern deviation plot) shown in part V of the printout are similar to total deviation plots except that here STATPAC software has corrected the results for the changes caused by cataract, small pupil, etc.

VI. Global indices

Global indices are depicted in the part VI of the printout. Global indices refer to some calculations made by STATPAC software to provide overall guidelines to help the practitioner to assess the field results as a whole rather than on point-to-point basis as shown in the total deviation and pattern deviation plots.

Below mentioned four global indices are provided with the full threshold programme

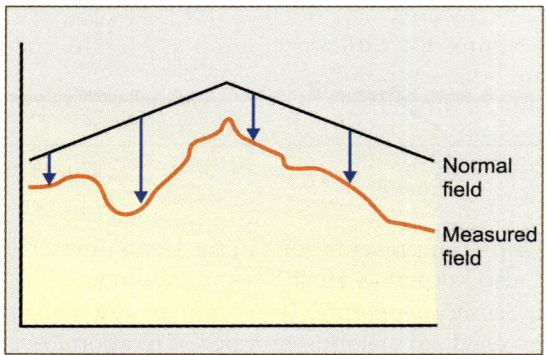

Fig. 16.8: *Total/mean deviation: Relative visual field sensitivity = Normal field sensitivity—Measured field sensitivity.*

which summarize the status of visual fields at a glance. Principally, the global indices are used to monitor progression of glaucomatous damage rather than for initial diagnosis.

1. *Total deviation or mean deviation.* The mean sensitivity is an average value of threshold sensitivity for all points tested. The mean deviation is the difference between mean sensitivity obtained and that expected (Fig. 16.8). Mean deviation should be in the range of zero in normals. It is more affected by generalized decreases in sensitivities rather than by small, localized defects but is increased in the presence of any defect. Mean sensitivity may also be decreased by media opacities, significant pupil constriction, blur, and unreliability.

2. *Pattern standard deviation.* Pattern standard deviation reflects the regional non-uniformity of a visual field, or frequency of deviation of sensitivity values after adjusting for the mean defect of the entire field (Fig. 16.9). It is a measure

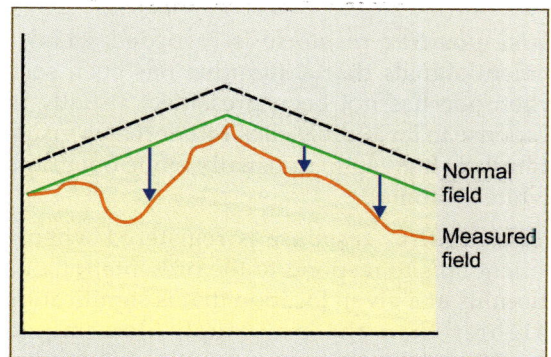

Fig. 16.9: *Pattern deviation: Individual visual field sensitivity.*

of variability within the visual field, i.e. it measures the difference between a given point and adjacent points. A high value indicates an irregularity to the expected normal hill of vision, suggesting localized defects. Therefore, a normal value is in the range of zero. A low value is also found in a field with a diffuse but regular decrease in threshold sensitivities. It actually points out towards localized field loss and is most useful in identifying early defects. It loses its advantage in marked depression.

3. Short-term fluctuation (SF). It is a measure of the variability between two different evaluations of the same 10 points in the field. It is not available with SITA strategy. A high SF means either decreased reliability or an early finding indicative of glaucoma.

4. Corrected pattern standard deviation (CPSD). It is the PSD corrected for SF. It indicates the variability between adjacent points that may be due to disease rather than due to intra-test variability.

VII. Glaucoma Hemifield Test (GHT)

Glaucoma Hemifield test compares 24-2 visual fields into 10 regions, with 5 inferior regions representing mirror images of 5 corresponding superior regions (Fig. 16.10). These clusters of points have been developed based on the anatomical distribution of the nerve fibres and are specific to the detection of glaucoma. Differences between corresponding superior

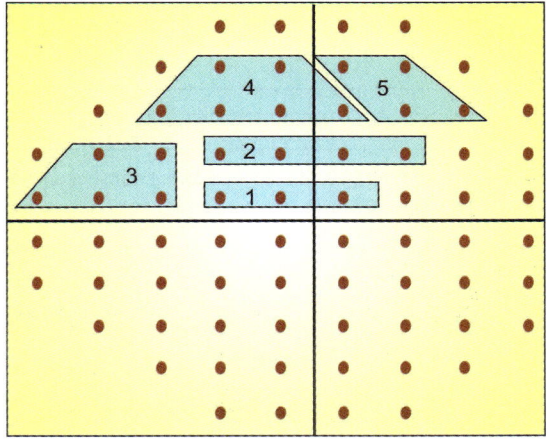

Fig. 16.10: *Glaucoma Hemifield test.*

and inferior zones are compared with the differences present in the population of normal controls. Possible test outcomes are:

Outside normal limits. The GHT outside normal limits denotes that either the values between upper and lower clusters differ to an extent found in less than 1% of the population or any one pair of clusters is depressed to an extent that would be expected in less than 0.5% of the population. In other words, the GHT is described as 'outside normal limits' when differences between a matched pair of corresponding zones exceeds the difference found in 99% of the normal population, or when both members of a pair of zones are more abnormal than 99.5% of the individuals with the normative population.

Borderline. The GHT is considered borderline when the difference between any one of the upper and lower mirror clusters is what might be expected in less than 3% of the population. In other words, the GHT is described as borderline when matched pairs of zones are abnormal at the 97th percentile within the normative database.

General reduction of sensitivity. VFs are described to have generalized reduction of sensitivity when both conditions for 'outside normal limits' are not met, and the best region of the VF is depressed to a level at the 99.5th percentile within individuals of the normative database. In other words, GHT is considered to have generalized reduction sensitivity, if the best part of field is depressed to an extent expected in less than 0.5% of the population.

Abnormally high sensitivity. The GHT is described as having abnormally high sensitivity when the overall sensitivity in the affected region of the VF is better than 99.5% of individuals within the normative population. In other words, abnormally high sensitivity is labelled when the best part of the visual field is such as would be expected in less than 0.5% of the population.

Within normal limits. VFs are described as being within normal limits when none of the above conditions are met.

VIII. Actual threshold values

Actual threshold values are shown in part VIII of the printout may be inspected for any pattern or scotoma when clinical features are suspecian and even if all the seven other parts of the printout are normal.

Scotoma by definition is the depressed part of the field as compared to the surrounding and not as compared to normal.

Sensitivity of the test is lost when the actual test threshold values are below 15 dB.

INTERPRETATION OF VISUAL FIELD DEFECTS

Systematic approach to interpretation of glaucoma field defects on HFA

In assessing a visual field, particularly that of a glaucoma patient, a systematic approach is recommended.

Step I. Evaluate the field for diffuse or generalized changes when compared to normals or previous fields. Look at the level of overall sensitivities using mean deviation values. If a reduction is noted, look for confounding factors such as media opacities, pupil diameter, or blur.

Step II. After generalized defects, look for localized defects. Look for one or several contiguous loci at which threshold sensitivity is less than that at surrounding loci. Local areas of minimally decreased sensitivity may be within normal limits (one point reduced by 5 dB). The more severely the sensitivity is reduced, the more likely the area in question is pathologic. Several adjacent points of reduction may represent a true defect and deserve careful follow-up or additional testing.

Glaucomatous defects are more likely to occur in Bjerrum's area (10 to 20°), paracentral area (within 10°), and nasal step regions. When loci of reduced sensitivity are detected in these areas, they should arouse suspicion of glaucoma.

Classify the defect as per Hodapp-Anderson-Parrish criterion (Table 16.2).

Classical examples of early visual field defect, advanced visual field defect and split fixation, are depicted in Figs 16.11 to 16.13 respectively.

Assessing the visual field progression in glaucoma

Important considerations

• Although structural damage appears first in glaucoma, evaluation of longitudinal series of visual fields to determine the progression of glaucoma remains one of the most commonly used method to detect early changes in the function and indicates worsening of disease

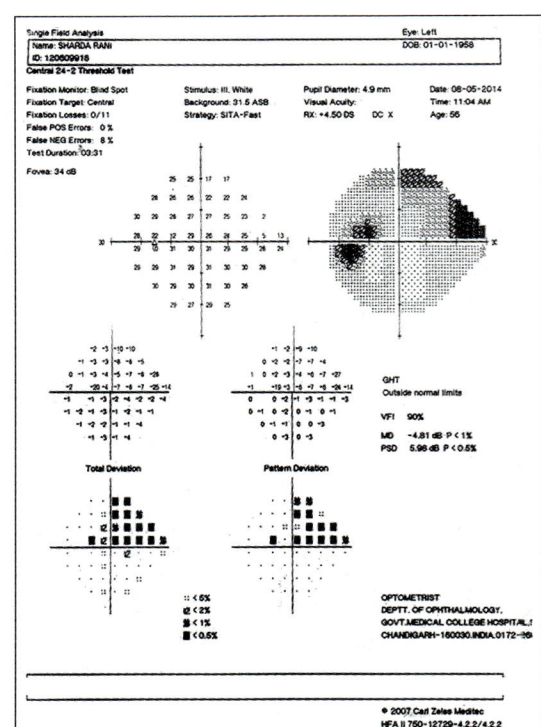

Fig. 16.11: *HVF SITA-FAST 24-2 showing early visual field defect in superior arcuate region.*

Class	MD	Pattern deviation	Significance	Sensitivity within five degrees
Early	−6.00 to −12.00 dB	<18 locations	<10 locations	No location <15 dB
Moderate	< −12.00 dB	<37 locations	<20 locations	No location at 0 dB only one horizontal Hemifield <15 dB
Severe	< −12.00 dB	>37 locations	>20 locations	Any locations at 0 dB or <15 dB

Table 16.2 *Hodapp-Anderson-Parrish criterion*

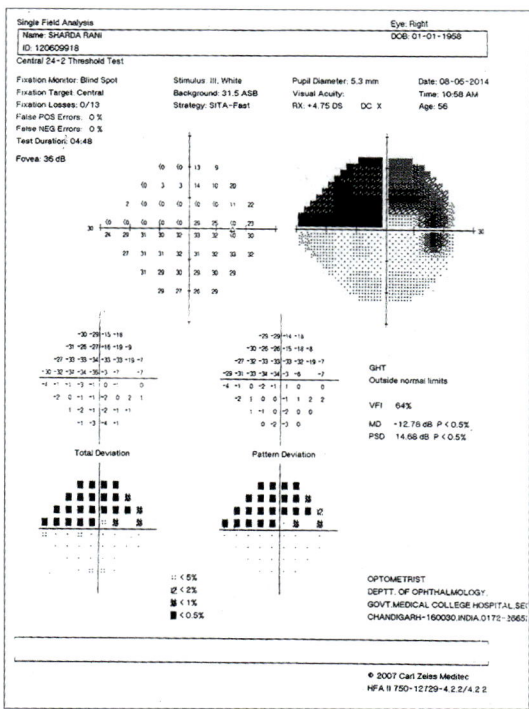

Fig. 16.12: *HVF SITA-FAST 24-2 showing advanced visual field defect involving fixation.*

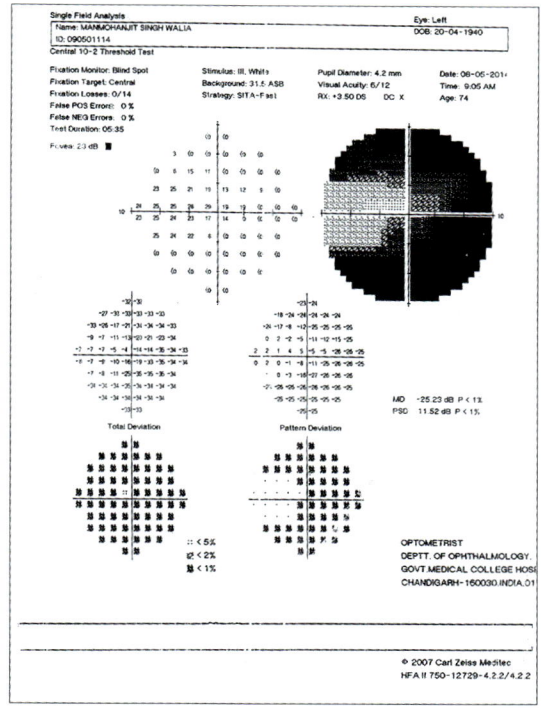

Fig. 16.13: *HVF SITA-FAST 10-2 showing split fixation.*

and an indication of intensification of treatment regime.

- The time required to detect progression and the pattern of progression are influenced by several factors including underlying rate and type of progression, degree of variability and frequency of examination.

- Whenever a change is detected in the visual fields, it is important to assess whether it is just a variability or true change from neuronal loss prior to jumping at any conclusion.

Note. Reliability indices should be regarded as the primary consideration whenever assessing the visual fields for progression.

Visual field progression: methods used for assessing

1. *Subjective judgement* by just looking at a series of visual field printouts. It is dependent upon the clinical expertise of the clinician and is reliable in expert hands.

2. *Overview printout,* in which up to 16 previously tested visual fields can be shown

in a single printout without any statistical analysis.

3. *Statistical methods* which include detecting the changes in global indices, like mean deviation. If there is stable field, mean deviation is unlikely to change. However, in cases where there is localized progression in certain parts of the field, mean deviation may not show change and thus is unreliable.

4. *Progression analysis software,* like glaucoma progression analysis (GPA) in Humphrey and peritrend in Octopus, are now being widely used. These are capable of detecting changes in a part of field and individual locations. This compares a single visual field to the results of one or two earlier tests. In other words, a follow-up examination is compared to a baseline of a single or a mean of two or more previous tests. Progression is said to have occurred, if threshold sensitivity at a particular test location changes more than the expected variability of the mean of previous tests. The glaucoma progression analysis software also classifies whether there is no progression, possible progression, or likely progression of visual field loss.

5. Visual field index (VFI) is a new measure that captures glaucoma progression. The VFI uses regression to offer a trend-based analysis of the speed by which visual field loss is occurring. The VFI generates a score from 0 (complete loss of field) to 100 (completely full field).

Note. Whenever a progression in field loss is suspected, before reaching a firm conclusion or recomending a change in therapy it is advisable to:
- Repeat the visual field examination
- Perform a coroborative optic nerve head and fundus evaluation.

Non-glaucomatous visual field defects

I. Visual field defects caused by neurological diseases, such as:
- *Optic neuritis, tobacco–alcohol amblyopia, mechanical compression of optic nerve:* Central scotoma.
- *Anterior ischaemic optic neuropathy (AION)?* Non-arteritic anterior ischaemic optic neuropathy (NAAION): Altitudinal defect (Arteritic—generally more extensive)
- *Optic nerve head oedema:* Enlargement of blind spot
- *Optic nerve head drusen:* Arcuate defect
- *Optic nerve head coloboma*
- *Thyroid ophthalmopathy:* Variable defects
- *Optic chiasma:* Variable degree of bitemporal hemianopia
- *Post-chiasmal lesions:* Variable degree of homonymous hemianopia.

II. Visual field defects caused by retinal diseases, such as:
- *Diabetic retinopathy:* Multifocal mottled
- *Retinal detachment:* Relative scotoma
- *Retinoschisis:* Absolute scotoma with sharp margins
- *Retinitis pigmentosa:* Circular defect to tunnel vision
- *Retinal vascular lesions:* Arterial absolute; venous variable
- *BRVO.* Arcuate defect
- *Field defects related to lasered retina.*

OCTOPUS PRINTOUT

Data representations in the Octopus printout are similar to those in the Humphrey printout (Fig. 16.14). Patient and examination data are at the top of the printout, followed by the value table (numeric scale) and the grayscale (which is coloured).

Numeric scale and grayscale are followed by a comparison table and a corrected comparison table (total deviation and pattern deviation). The probability plots for those tables follow.

Visual field indices (global indices) are at the bottom right hand side of the printout page.

Indices. Mean sensitivity (MS) which is the mean value of all test results, mean defect (MD) which is the same as mean deviation, lost variance (LV) which is the same as pattern standard deviation, and corrected lost variance (CLV), which is the same as corrected pattern standard deviation. The reliability factor (RF) is a score of patient's reliability (0 to 15%).

Bebie curve is a cumulative defect curve that allows ranking of VF defects (it looks only at the defects, not the field). In the presence of established glaucoma diagnosis, this is useful to monitor the progression of both overall depression and localised defects.

Staging VF testing is a useful feature. It allows collecting examination results from points considered most important for glaucoma diagnosis in the first and second stages (80% of the test). This allows printing of these results and stopping the testing process, in case of patient fatigue. In all other perimeters, the entire testing process has to be completed before printing of the results.

Octopus criteria for a visual field defect
- MD greater than 2 dB
- LV greater than 6 dB
- At least 7 points with sensitivity decreased by ≥ 5 dB, 3 of them being contagious.

Octopus versus Humphrey's field analyzer terminologies

Table 16.3 briefly compares the Octopus versus Humphrey's field analyzer terminologies.

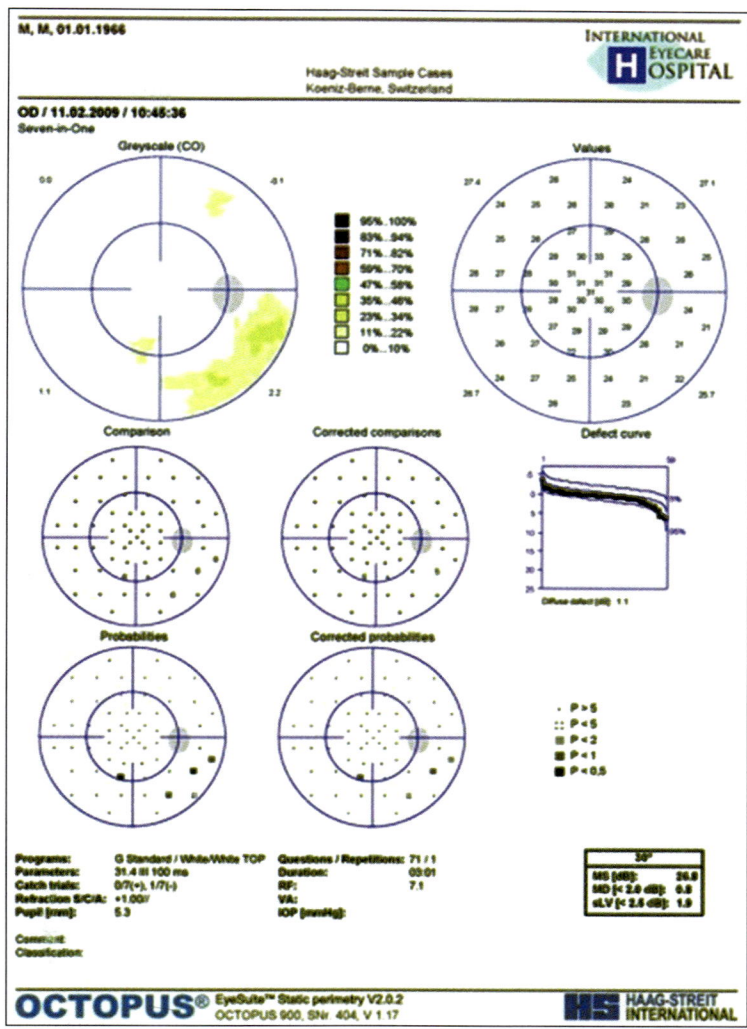

Fig. 16.14: *Octopus visual field printout (Source: www.haag-streit.com).*

VISUAL FIELDS: FREQUENTLY ASKED QUESTIONS

Why is target presentation random in automated static perimetry?

The computer allows stimuli to be presented in a pseudorandom, unpredictable fashion. Patients do not know where the next stimulus will appear, so fixation is improved, thereby increasing the reliability of the test. Random presentations also increase the speed with which perimetry can be performed by bypassing the problem of local retinal adaptation, which requires a 2-second interval between stimuli, if adjacent locations are tested.

Concept of foveal threshold?

As one ascends the hill of vision toward the fovea, the sensitivity of the retina increases, dimmer targets will become visible, and the brightness of the target at threshold will decrease. Therefore, as retinal sensitivity increases, the differential light threshold measured in apostilbs decreases (HFA: 1 apostilb = 40 dB). The decibel scale is a relative scale created by the manufacturers of automated perimeters to measure the sensitivity of the island of vision. It is an inverted logarithmic scale. Zero decibel is set as the brightest stimulus that the perimeter can produce.

Table 16.3 *Essential parameters: Humphrey's field analyzer (HFA) versus Octopus automated perimeter*

Parameter	HFA	Octopus
Testing conditions		
Bowel type	Aspherical bowl	Direct projection
Background illumination	31.5 asb	31.4 asb
Stimulus size	Goldmann size I–V	Goldmann size III and V
Stimulus duration	200 ms	100 ms
Luminance for zero dB	10,000 asb	4800 asb
Testing strategies		
	Full threshold 4-2 bracketing	Normal 4-2-1 bracketing
	SITA fast	TOP (tendency oriented perimetry)
	SITA standard	Dynamic
Test programmes	30-2 (76 points)	G1
	24-2 (54 points)	G1x (59 points)
	10-2 (68 points in 10°)	M2x (45 points in 5°)
	Macula (10 points in 5°)	
Deviation plots	Total deviation	Comparison
	Pattern deviation	Corrected comparison
Global indices	Mean deviation	Mean defect
	Pattern standard deviation	Loss variance
	Corrected pattern standard deviation	Corrected loss variance
Cluster testing in Bjerrum's area	Glaucoma Hemifield test	Defect curve (Bebie curve)
Glaucoma progression software	Glaucoma progression analysis (GPA)	Peritrend

Why is fovea most sensitive?

The highest concentration of cones is in the fovea, and most of these cones project to their own ganglion cell. This one-to-one ratio between foveal cone and ganglion cell results in maximal resolution at the fovea.

Why is background illumination of HFA 31.5 asb?

It has been taken from Goldmann's calculation which suggested that 31.5 asb is the minimum intensity for photopic recording of visual fields. This is also the level of luminance to which eye can quickly adapt, can produce most reliable and stable response properties within and between subjects.

Anderson's and Patella's criteria for perimetric diagnosis of glaucoma?

1. Three or more contiguous non-edge points depressed <5% population and at least 1 point depressed <1% population should be clustered in the arcuate area
2. PSD depressed <5% population
3. GHT-outside normal limits

Why is grayscale condemned by glaucoma specialists?

Grayscale gives gradations of darkness in fixed scale of 5 dB. Thus, a change of threshold from 21 to 22 dB will give same colour gradation as that from 16 to 24 dB. However, it has role in explaining the patient about damage and in cases with high false positive where white areas are seen. It does help us in understanding some artifacts, e.g. clover leaf pattern in a fatigued patient.

What does 24-2 mean?

A 24-2 test points 24° around the fovea. The second number refers to the testing protocol.

The HVF has historically had two main testing protocols, 1 and 2. Protocol 1 tested points directly on the horizontal and vertical axes. Protocol 2 test points on either side of the horizontal and vertical axes. Since defects found right on the line can be difficult to interpret, everyone uses 2.

Why is 24-2 better than 30-2?

Humphrey programme 24-2 eliminates the most peripheral ring of test locations from programme 30-2, except in the nasal step region, and tests only the central 24°. This test is very useful because the peripheral ring of thresholds provides the least reliable data, and testing time can be shortened.

What is VFI?

The VFI is a new global metric that represents the entire visual field as a single percentage of normal. It is based largely on the pattern deviation and weighs central points more than peripheral ones.

A full visual field has a VFI of 100% while a perimetrically-blind visual field has a VFI of 0% represents the percentage of useful vision a patient has left.

VFI takes the patient's age and the 'velocity' of the change in visual field into account. The rate of change of the VFI over time characterizes the rate of progression, while a statistical analysis of this rate generates a p-value indicating whether or not the rate of change is significantly different from zero.

Visual field requirement for driving?

'A minimum horizontal field of vision of 120° and no significant defect within 20° of fixation'.

How to interpret gaze tracker?

Upward deflection (gaze deviation); downward deflection (blink).

PRACTICAL PEARLS

- Test a patient's better-seeing eye first, especially if he or she has not undergone perimetry before.
- Foveal function should always be on. The foveal function helps clinicians to determine the etiology of visual field loss.

- Goldmann size III (about ½ degree in diameter) is generally used, but Goldmann size V (approximately 2 degrees in diameter) is available for patients with decreased visual acuity (<20/200) or other visual impairment.
- When examining the test results, you must hold the two printouts (right eye printout in your right hand facing your right eye, and left eye printout in your left hand facing your left eye), and examine them together.

OTHER PSYCHOPHYSICAL TESTS IN GLAUCOMA

INTRODUCTION

For the past several years, several different perimeters and test strategies have been developed, but none has had more studies and has been more used than standard white-on-white perimetry with the Humphrey Field Analyzer (HFA); Carl Zeiss Meditec, Dublin, CA, USA). Although SAP is still considered the gold standard, function-specific perimetry may offer advantages for early diagnosis.

Other tests have been developed in addition to traditional perimetry to detect early glaucomatous visual loss. Psychophysical tests are designed to isolate various retinal pathways. Psychophysical tests other than traditional perimetry include:

- Short wavelength automated perimetry
- Frequency doubling perimetry
- High-pass resolution (ring)
- Motion detection types of perimetry
- Pattern discrimination types of perimetry
- Contrast sensitivity (both spatial and temporal)
- Colour vision.

ANATOMICAL BASIS

At this point, it would help to understand the basic retinal anatomy and physiology. Retinal nerve fibres transmit signals from the retinal receptor cells by way of the optic nerve to the lateral geniculate body and ultimately to the visual cortex. These are broadly classified into the magnocellular (M) cells, and the parvocellular (P) cells.

P cells. The P cell pathway is responsible for high contrast, low temporal frequency (or static) stimulus detection.

M cells. The M cell pathway detects low-contrast; high temporal frequency (or motion) stimuli, and constitute approximately 10% of the total retinal nerve fibres. Non-linear M cells are a subset of the large diameter M cells, and are affected before any other cell type in glaucoma. Therefore, detection of this cell loss helps to identify RGC loss before it can be detected by traditional automated perimetry.

SHORT WAVELENGTH AUTOMATED PERIMETRY

It is also known as blue on yellow perimetry as in this blue colour stimulus is presented on a yellow background. Blue colour saturates rods and yellow colour stimulates only the short wavelength system (SWS) cones, i.e the koniocellular pathway. It uses the same testing patterns as standard white-on-white perimetry, however, it is able to detect visual field changes earlier. Additionally, the size of defect in SWAP is larger and progression typically greater than standard automated perimetry. But it is more variable and is affected by the absorption properties of crystalline lenses.

FREQUENCY DOUBLING PERIMETRY

Frequency doubling illusion. When a low spatial frequency sinusoidal grating with alternating wide light and dark bars (Fig. 16.15) undergoes

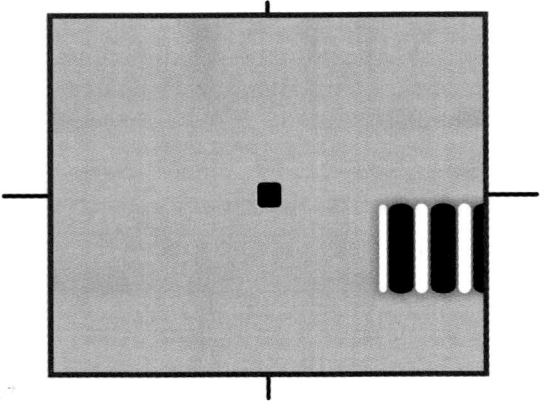

Fig. 16.15: *FDP target: Sinusoidal gratings consisting of alternate black and white bars.*

high temporal-frequency counterphase flicker, (i.e. the black and white bands reverse to become white and black, respectively in a rapid sequence) the spatial frequency of the grating appears doubled. This phenomenon is called the frequency doubling illusion.

Selective testing of the magnocellular pathway by presenting alternate grating stimuli, therefore, may help in early detection of glaucomatous cell loss.

First and second generations of FDT instruments never achieved sufficiently widespread clinical use despite confirming this technology's potential.

Newer Humphrey matrix perimeter with Welch Allyn frequency-doubling technology from Carl-Zeiss Meditec has found its foothold into clinical practice.

Matrix offers three main testing algorithms for generating visual fields. One is a screening algorithm similar to SITA-Fast where parts of the visual field are not retested. In the new testing protocol, the FDT Matrix utilizes grating targets smaller than the original FDT to enable standard 24-2 and 30-2 test patterns, which look identical to those in SAP. It also can perform central 10-degree testing, which can be used to follow a patient with advanced glaucoma. It is a portable device and particularly useful in children.

MOTION DETECTION PERIMETRY

Motion detection may be related to temporal contrast sensitivity—both seem to be modulated primarily by the M ganglion cells. Motion detection perimetry is a method that measures a subject's ability to detect a coherent shift in position of dots in a circular area against a background of non-moving dots (Fig. 16.16). Motion size threshold is the smallest detectable circular area in which the subject can detect motion. Subjects respond by touching a computer screen with a light pen where they detect motion stimuli. Their localization errors, as the number of pixels from target centre and reaction time, are then calculated.

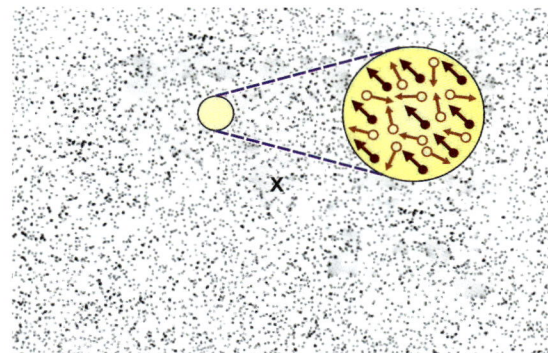

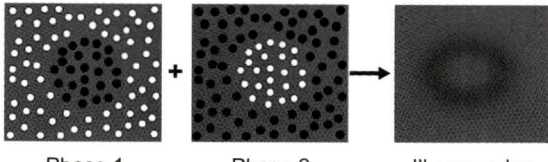

Fig. 16.17: *Phase reversal of randomly positioned black and white dots in flicker-defined form (FDF) perimetry. At high temporal frequencies, subjects cannot differentiate between the flickering dots but perceive an illusory circular edge contour.*

Fig. 16.16: *Motion perimetry video display. The small circle (left) represents a medium-sized random-dot motion perimetry target. A magnified view of the target (right) shows that 50% of the dots are moving in random directions (°) and 50% are moving coherently (•). X, fixation target.*

FLICKER-DEFINED FORM PERIMETRY

Flicker-defined form (FDF) as a testing stimulus was conceived for preferential stimulation of the magnocellular projecting retinal ganglion cells (RGCs). This psychophysical approach was thought to have advantages for the early detection of glaucoma due to theories of reduced redundancy (selective testing) and/or selective damage to the magnocellular RGCs. FDF is now thought to measure early functional changes due to impaired higher order visual mechanisms required for complex and integrated neural processing involving both temporal and spatial vision. The Heidelberg Edge Perimeter (HEP; Heidelberg Engineering) has FDF stimulus for early detection of glaucomatous visual deficits. The flickering stimulus of the HEP creates an illusionary edge contour that the patient perceives as a circle against the mean luminance background (Fig. 16.17). This process aims to facilitate better 'test/retest' reliability by diminishing the degree of variability in patients' responses.

HIGH PASS RESOLUTION PERIMETRY (HPRP)

High pass resolution perimetry uses a series of ring stimuli varying in size that are displayed on a computer monitor at various locations within the central visual field. The stimuli resemble visual acuity optotypes, such as the Landolt C and consist of a dark ring surrounding

a central circular white region (Fig. 16.18). HRP tests 50 locations inside the 30° central visual field.

The locations are distributed in a pattern reminescent of normal isopters. This is calculated to facilitate both visual recognition of common field defect patterns and statistical analysis of results. The subject is asked to press the response button each time astimulus is detected, and the programme performs a staircase procedure to increase and decrease target size until a detection threshold is achieved. Normal examination time is about 5 minutes. Being a resolution test, it is sensitive to media opacities.

Ophthimus (High Tech Vision, Malmö, Sweden) is the currently marketed high pass resolution perimeter.

PULSAR PERIMETRY

Pulsar perimetry was developed in 2000 and the Pulsar T30W test utilizes a circular sinusoidal grating pattern that examines 66 areas of the central 30 degrees VF (Fig. 16.19). The stimulus consists of a circular sinusoidal 5 degrees diameter grating pattern that is presented for 500 msec (Fig. 16.20). The stimulus undergoes a

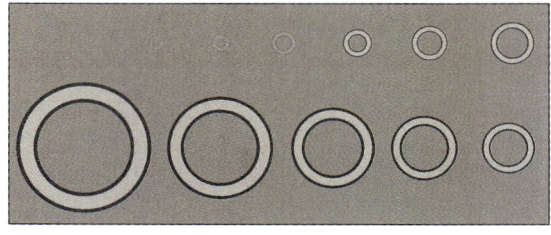

Fig. 16.18: *Ring stimuli of high pass resolution perimeter.*

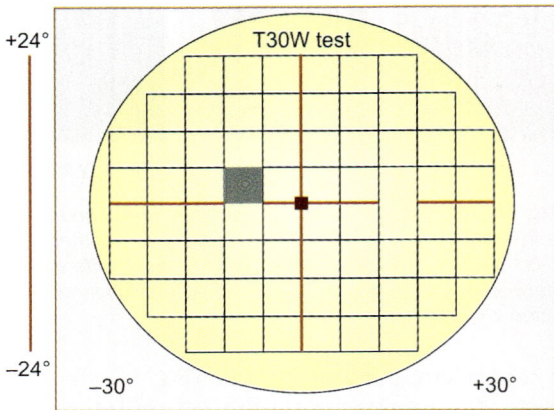

Fig. 16.19: *Size and distribution of the 66 test-areas in the central visual field in pulsar perimetry.*

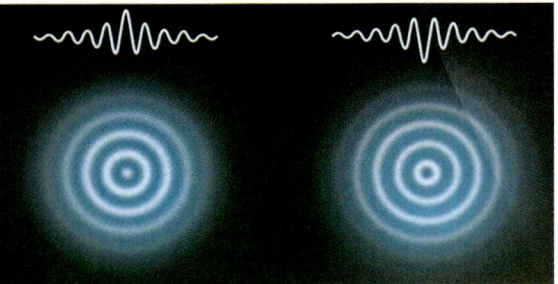

Fig. 16.20: *Pulsar stimulus.*

counterphase pulse motion at 30 Hz, in which both spatial resolution (SR, from 0.5 to 6.3 cyc/deg on a 12-step log scale) and contrast (C, from 3 to 100% on a 32-step log scale) are simultaneously modified. Threshold sensitivity based on tendency oriented perimetry (TOP) threshold strategy is expressed in spatial resolution contrast (SRC) units. Pulsar has given promising preliminary results in the early detection of glaucomatous VF damage.

Pulsar and FDT use a similar counterphase flickering grating stimulus with high temporal frequency. The testing methods differ in that FDT uses a squared test target, while the circular stimulus used in Pulsar helps to keep the same level of contrast around the edges, in order to avoid stimulation of those cells that selectively respond to a given orientation. FDT uses fixed low spatial frequency and contrast is modified, whereas the Pulsar T30W test examines the contrast sensitivity function by measuring the contrast threshold resolution at several spatial frequencies. The instruments use different threshold strategies; MOBS in FDT and TOP in Pulsar.

OCTOPUS® 600 (Haag Streit Diagnostics) is the first perimeter combining both the Pulsar method for early diagnosis and standard white-on-white perimetry in one device.

BIBLIOGRAPHY

1. Johnson CA, Adams AJ, Casson EJ, Brandt JD. Blue-on-Yellow perimetry can predict the development of glaucomatous visual field loss. Archives of Ophthalmology, 1993;111:645–50.
2. Johnson CA. Psychophysical factors that have been applied to clinical perimetry. Vision Res. 2013 Sep 20;90:25–31.
3. Johnson CA, Sample PA, Zangwill LM, Vasile CG, Cioffi GA, Liebmnn JR, Weinreb RN, Structure and function evaluation (SAFE) II. Comparison of optic disc and visual field characteristics. Am J Ophthalmol 2003;135:148–54.
4. Sample PA, Dannheim F, Artes PH, Dietzsch J, Henson D, Johnson CA, Ng M, Schiefer U, Wall M; IPS Standards Group. Imaging and Perimetry Society standards and guidelines. Optom Vis Sci. 2011 Jan;88(1):4–7.
5. Stamper RL. Psychophysical changes in glaucoma. Surv Ophthalmol. 1989;33:309–13.

Section

IV

Clinical Evaluation and Investigations in Uveitis

17. Clinical Approach to Uveitis
18. Investigations in Uveitis
19. Pathological Diagnostic Tests in Uveitis

Clinical Approach to Uveitis

Chapter Outline

INTRODUCTION
- Aims of clinical work-up

HISTORY TAKING IN UVEITIS

History of present illness
- Demographics
- Diet, domestic and personal history
- Symptoms of uveitis

Past and family history
- Past history
- Family history

SYSTEMIC WORK-UP
- Systemic history
- Systemic examination

OCULAR EXAMINATION
- Examination of lid and adnexa
- Examination of conjunctiva
- Examination of cornea
- Examination of anterior chamber
- Examination of pupil
- Examination of iris
- Examination of lens
- Evaluation of IOP
- Examination of vitreous
- Examination of fundus

FOLLOW-UP EXAMINATION

INTRODUCTION

Uveitis is a distinct ocular inflammation which encompasses a multitude of diseases. The underlying cause can be attributed to local ocular immune dysregulation, or may be part of a systemic disease. A meticulous approach to uveitis plays a pivotal role in the identification of etiology, anatomical localisation, and pathological involvement. In the diagnosis of uveitis, such as Fuchs uveitis syndrome, Vogt-Koyanagi-Harada disease, laboratory analysis can contribute little and examination can clinch the diagnosis. Besides diagnosis, a thorough clinical examination is critical to administer treatment and to judge the response in both infectious and autoimmune forms.

Aims of clinical work-up are to identify, if the uveitis is:
- Anterior, intermediate, posterior or panuveitis.
- Granulomatous or non-granulomatous
- Unilateral or bilateral
- Idiopathic, autoimmune or due to infection
- Associated with systemic disease
- Stage of the disease
- Severity if active or resolving
- Associated ocular complications.

Key to a targeted and an efficient patient evaluation is a thorough history, physical examination, and review of systems. With this information, the practitioner can generate a differential diagnosis and a subsequent strategy for laboratory evaluation and treatment. A meticulous elicitation of history of the systemic status will help direct the examination and supplement the various laboratory tests.

HISTORY TAKING IN UVEITIS

An elaborate history taking is the corner stone of the management of a case of uveitis. It has been estimated that more than 75% of diagnoses can be made on the basis of the medical history and a thorough systemic examination. Because of frequent association of uveitis with rheumatologic, infectious diseases, it is very important to look beyond the eye and to perform a thorough physical examination and to obtain a meticulous history to clinch the diagnosis.

HISTORY OF PRESENT ILLNESS

1. Demographics

Age

Age is an important factor in history taking as few conditions are known to occur more predominantly in some age group:

- *Children:* Juvenile rheumatoid arthritis, retinoblastoma, toxocariasis, masquerade syndrome
- *Young adults:* Pars planitis, multiple sclerosis, and Fuchs' heterochromic iridocyclitis
- *Middle age:* Reiter's syndrome, ankylosing spondylitis, acute multifocal posterior placoid epitheliopathy, Vogt-Koyanagi-Harada syndrome, Behçet's disease
- *Old age:* Large cell lymphoma or choroidal melanoma, endogenous endophthalmitis, masquerade syndrome.

Note. However, it should be kept in mind that certain diseases, like toxoplasmosis, sarcoidosis and tuberculosis, can be found at any age.

Gender

Uveitis associated with juvenile rheumatoid arthritis is found much more frequently in females, while uveitis associated with ankylosing spondylitis and Reiter's syndrome is usually seen in males. Most of the patients with Behçet's disease are males.

- *Male predominance:* Juvenile rheumatoid arthritis, rheumatoid arthritis
- *Female predominance:* Ankylosing spondylitis, Reiter's syndrome, Behçet's disease.

Race

Conditions, like ankylosing spondylitis, Reiter's syndrome, and other HLA-B27-associated arthritides are common in whites and sarcoidosis occurs most commonly in blacks. Vogt-Koyanagi-Harada syndromes are most prevalent in Asians. In the Mediterranean countries, Behçet's disease is more common.

- *Asians:* Behçet's disease and VKH syndrome
- *Middle Eastern population:* Behcet's disease
- *African American:* Sarcoidosis and syphilis
- *Caucasians:* HLA B27, white dot syndromes and multiple sclerosis.

Geographical location

Geographical location of the patient often helps us in diagnosis of certain conditions as few clinical entities are more commonly seen in the some specific parts of the world. For example, Behçet's disease is more common in countries situated along the old Silk Road, a trade route used for centuries by Greeks, Romans and Chinese. Reported rates of the disease is higher the countries, situated along this route and highest in two ends of the old silk road–Turkey and Japan.

• *Tuberculosis*	Developing countries
• *Histoplasmosis*	Mississippi-Ohio-Missouri river valleys
• *Coccidioidomycosis*	Southwest United States, Central and South America
• *Birdshot choroiditis*	USA
• *Lyme disease*	USA
• *Behçet's disease*	Turkey, Iraq, Saudi Arabia, Iran, Afghanistan, Pakistan, Northern Chiana, Mongolia, The Koreas and Japan

2. Diet, domestic and personal history

- *Dietary habits.* A history of the ingestion of raw or undercooked meat in toxoplasmosis. Persons who ingest unpasteurized milk are at risk of contracting tuberculosis and brucellosis
- *History of contact with pets* (cat, dogs and pigs) is important when considering a diagnosis of

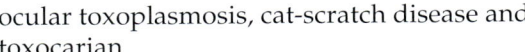

ocular toxoplasmosis, cat-scratch disease and toxocarian
- *History of exposure to sewers or rodent urine* may give us a clue for the diagnosis of leptospirosis
- *Farmers* are far more prone to develop brucellosis than the general population
- *History of sexual activity and preferences* is a must in suspected cases of human immunodeficiency virus (HIV) infection, syphilis, etc.

3. Symptoms of uveitis

The symptoms in a case of uveitis depend on various factors. These are: part of the uveal tract involved, presentation and course of the uveitic entity (acute or chronic) and onset (sudden and insidious). For example, a case of anterior uveitis can present with an acute, chronic, or recurrent form. The severity of symptoms can range from very severe symptoms in a case of sudden onset acute uveitis to nil or minimal symptoms in a case of insidious-onset chronic anterior uveitis.

Ocular pain

The pain in iridocyclitis is due to ciliary spasm. The ciliary body is innervated by the trigeminal nerve, and pain caused by irritation of the nerve endings by the product of inflammation. The pain in uveitis can be variable and mostly described as a dull aching or a throbbing pain localized to the eye. Sometimes it can be associated with referred pain which seems to radiate over a larger area served by the trigeminal nerve.

Pain in scleritis is typically dull and boring in nature, exacerbated by eye movement, is worse at night often interfering with sleep, and characteristically wakens the patient from sleep.

Photophobia

Photophobia or intolerance to bright light is often accompanied by tearing (watering) and blepharospasm. Photophobia is usually caused by ciliary muscle spasm but can also be due to pupillary muscle involvement or corneal involvement.

Redness of eye

Redness of the eye in uveitis is primarily due to ciliary injection or circumcorneal injection, or 'ciliary flush'. It is manifested by a ring of dilated or engorged episcleral vessels radiating from the limbus.

Blurred vision and floaters

Anterior uveitis. Blurred vision is usually caused by ciliary spasm or in early stage cloudy media.

Intermediate uveitis most often presents with floaters and blurred vision. Floaters occur because of shadows cast by the products of inflammation in vitreous, like vitreous cells, debris, etc. Most common cause of decreased vision in these patients is cystoid macular oedema (CME).

Posterior uveitis usually presents with decreased vision, floaters, photopsias, metamorphopsia, scotomata, nyctalopia or a combination of these. The decreased vision may be due to the primary effects of inflammation involving retina and choroid, often directly affecting macular function or due to the complications of inflammation like CME, epiretinal membrane (ERM), retinal ischaemia, and choroidal neovascular membrane (CNVM).

PAST AND FAMILY HISTORY

- Previous episodes of uveitis, and type of treatment are important in recurrent uveitis.
- Past history of trauma or surgery would be useful in lens-induced uveitis or sympathetic ophthalmitis.
- Family history of infectious diseases may be positive in patient with infectious uveitis.

SYSTEMIC WORK-UP

SYSTEMIC HISTORY

A detailed history of various systemic diseases should be taken:
- *History of tuberculosis* should be taken in patients with vasculitis, choroiditis, etc.
- *Endogenous endophthalmitis* is more common in old patients with diabetes mellitus, renal failure and with patients on immunosuppressant. It is of paramount importance to look for the evidence of septic foci, like boil, carbuncle, abscess, etc. in such patients.

Arthralgia

An elaborate history of joint pain should be taken especially in patients presenting with

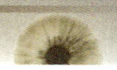

non-granulomatous uveitis. Information on type of joint involved, onset, timings and nature of the joint pain often provides useful clue to the diagnosis of a case of uveitis.

Uveitic entities with arthralgias include Behçet's disease, sarcoidosis, SLE, juvenile idiopathic arthritis (JIA), Lyme disease, syphilis, psoriatic arthritis, Reiter's syndrome, ulcerative colitis.

SYSTEMIC EXAMINATION
Skin lesions

Rashes can be seen in various conditions with uveitis. Malar butterfly rashes can be seen in patients with systemic lupus erythematosus (SLE). Thickening of skin can be seen in patients with scleroderma. Increased cutaneous sensitivity can be seen in various conditions including SLE, Behçet's disease. Acne-like eruptions are often seen in certain conditions, like Behçet's disease and it should be differentiated from similar skin lesions seen in patient on oral corticosteroid therapy.

- *Nodules.* Sarcoidosis, SLE, leprosy, Crohn disease, ulcerative colitis
- *Rash.* Syphilis, Lyme disease, Reiter's syndrome, leprosy, sarcoidosis, herpes zoster, Behçet's disease, psoriasis, SLE, Kawasaki disease
- *Erythema nodosum.* Behçet's disease, sarcoidosis, acute posterior multifocal placoid pigment epitheliopathy (APMPPE), tuberculosis
- *Vitiligo, poliosis.* Vogt-Koyanagi-Harada (VKH) syndrome
- *Keratoderma blennorrhagicum.* Reactive arthritis.

Hair loss and abnormalities

Hair loss and abnormalities may be associated with uveitis:
- *Hair loss* can be seen in patient with Vogt-Koyanagi-Harada (VKH) syndrome, SLE and syphilis
- *Abnormalities,* like poliosis, are common in VKH patients and madarosis can be seen in leprosy patients
- *Increased sensitivity to hair* is often complained by patients with VKH

Examination of ear, nose and throat

Examination of ear, nose and throat is also important. Relapsing polychondritis is a rare small-vessel vasculitis which predominantly affect cartilaginous structures of the body, such as pinna of the ear, nasal cartilage, larynx and trachea. Relapsing polychondritis should be ruled out in patients with episcleritis and scleritis. Saddle nose deformity is characterised by a loss of height of the nose, because of collapse of the nasal bridge. Saddle nose deformity in a patient of uveitis should give rise to the suspicion of conditions, like Wegener's granulomatosis, leprosy, syphilis or relapsing polychondritis.

- *Bilateral ear pinna inflammation.* Relapsing polychondritis
- *Saddle nose deformity.* Syphilis, Wegener's granulomatosis (SLE), relapsing polychondritis
- *Sinusitis.* Sarcoidosis, Wegener's granulomatosis
- *Salivary/lacrimal gland swelling.* Sarcoidosis, lymphoma
- *Lymphadenopathy.* Lymphoma, HIV.

Gastrointestinal

Oral ulcer. Aphthous ulceration can be seen in patients with Behçet's disease, reactive arthritis, SLE, herpes simplex, Reiter's syndrome, ulcerative colitis, etc.

Gastrointestinal disorders. Though uncommon, uveitis can be associated with Crohn disease, ulcerative colitis.

Central nervous system

Neurological signs are common during prodromal stage of Vogt-Koyanagi-Harada (VKH) syndrome and can include neck stiffness, headache and confusion. Patients of VKH can have auditory symptoms, like tinnitus, dysacusis (difficulty in processing details of sound due to distortion in frequency or intensity), vertigo, etc. Similarly demyelinating diseases, like multiple sclerosis should be ruled out in cases with intermediate uveitis, retinal vasculitis, etc.

- *Headaches.* Vogt-Koyanagi-Harada (VKH) syndrome, tuberculosis, herpes zoster, large cell lymphoma, cryptococcal meningitis, toxoplasmosis
- *Auditory/vestibular.* VKH disease
- *Cranial neuropathy.* Lyme disease, sarcoidosis, multiple sclerosis, syphilis, herpes simplex virus
- *Cerebral vasculitis.* Acute posterior multifocal placoid pigment epitheliopathy (APMPPE).

Pulmonary

Pulmonary involvement is common in various uveitic conditions, especially granulomatous uveitic entities. It is very important to elicit a proper history regarding symptoms, like hemoptysis, dyspnoea, cough, sputum, chest pain and fatigue.

- *Cough/breathlessness.* Tuberculosis, sarcoidosis, *Pneumocystis carinii*, Wegener's granulomatosis
- *Nodules/hilar adenopathy/infiltrates.* Ocular histoplasmosis, sarcoidosis (hilar adenopathy), malignancy, tuberculosis, *Pneumocystis carinii pneumonia.*

Genitourinary system

Examination of genitourinary system is important as many uveitic entities can have genitourinary involvement which can help one to clinch the diagnosis. However, history taking or examination of genitourinary system should be conducted tactfully so that the patient does not become embarrassed, or offended. Recurrent genital ulcer is a common feature of Behçet's disease, but urethritis is not common feature of the disease. Presence of urethritis in a uveitic patient with joint pain can give clue to the diagnosis of reactive arthritis (previously called Reiter's syndrome). Also circinate balanitis is a common feature of reactive arthritis. Circinate balanitis is a form of skin inflammation where skin around the shaft and tip (glans) of the penis become inflamed and scale.

- *Genital ulcers.* Behçet's disease, Reiter's syndrome, syphilis

- *Hematuria.* Wegener's granulomatosis, polyarteritis nodosa (PAN), systemic lupus erythematosus (SLE)
- *Circinate balanitis.* Ankylosing spondylitis, Reiter syndrome
- *Nephritis.* PAN, Wegener's granulomatosis, tubulointerstitial nephritis and uveitis (TINU).

■ OCULAR EXAMINATION

A. External examination and examination of lid and adnexa

A careful examination of lid and adnexa can provide important clue in patients with uveitis.

- *Kaposi's sarcoma* may appear as purplish-red to bright-red and highly vascular with surrounding telangiectatic vessels in upper eyelid.
- *Enlargement of the lacrimal gland* can be seen in sarcoidosis.
- *Characteristic skin lesions or scar marks* can be seen in a case herpes zoster ophthalmicus (HZO). Herpes zoster ophthalmicus is defined as herpes zoster involvement of the ophthalmic division of the fifth cranial nerve. Skin lesion at the tip, side, or root of the nose is a strong predictor of ocular inflammation and corneal denervation in HZO and is known as Hutchinson's sign. The skin rash of HZO evolves through erythema, macules, papules, and finally pustulation and crusting. Periorbital oedema and ptosis may or may not be present. It should be noted that a minority of patients in HZO can have only ophthalmic symptoms and no skin lesions with dermatomal distribution pain (zoster non-herpete).

B. Examination of conjunctiva

- *Ciliary injection should be differentiated from conjunctival hyperaemia* (Table 17.1). Conjunctival hyperactive with discharge is usually seen in conjunctivitis. It is important to note that purulent conjunctivitis can be seen in Reiter's syndrome and psoriatic arthritis.
- Ciliary injection or 'ciliary flush', is manifested by a ring of dilated episcleral vessels radiating from the limbus. It should be distinguished from the deeper and more peripheral injection

Table 17.1 *Ciliary injection versus conjunctival hyperaemia*	
Ciliary injection	*Conjunctival hyperaemia*
Engorgement of episcleral vessels	Engorgement of anterior and posterior conjunctival vessels
Bright reddish violet in colour	Bright red in colour
Radially arranged blood vessels	Irregular branching vessels
Most intense near limbus	Most intense in fornix
Blood vessels do not move with conjunctiva	Moves with conjunctiva
Blood flow is from limbus to fornix	Blood flow is from fornix to limbus

of scleritis and from the sectoral or diffuse injection of episcleritis. Also it is of paramount importance to differentiate ciliary injection of uveitis from conjunctivitis by the lack of involvement of the fornix and palpebral conjunctiva and absence of symptoms like discharge.

- *Perilimbal vitiligo* is often observed in patients with Vogt-Koyanagi-Harada syndrome and is known as *Suguira's sign.*
- *Subconjunctival haemorrhage* can be seen in patients with leptospirosis.
- *Nodules or any mass like lesion.* Nodular scleritis often associated with severe tenderness. Conjunctival nodules are often seen in patients with sarcoidosis. Sarcoid nodules are millet-shaped discrete solid nodules of variable size. They can be single or multiple.
- *The sine qua non of scleritis* is the presence of scleral oedema and congestion of the deep episcleral plexus. Slit-lamp examination using red-free light is extremely helpful in determining the pattern and depth of episcleral vascular congestion and engorgement. In scleritis, the sclera assumes a violaceous hue. It is very important to examine patients in daylight with the unaided eye to note the subtle colour differences of the vessels. Also inflamed scleral vessels have a crisscross pattern. They are adherent to the sclera and cannot be moved with a cotton-tipped applicator. Engorged scleral vessels cannot be blanched with 10% phenylephrine, whereas phenylephrine easily blanches engorged vessels in the superficial episcleral and conjunctival plexuses. A tender nodule can indicate nodular scleritis which need systemic work-up.

C. Examination of cornea

Keratic precipitates. Due to the convection current in anterior chamber, the circulating inflammatory cells can deposit in corneal endothelium which is known as keratic precipitates (KPs). KPs are normally deposited in inferior half of the cornea in base down triangle-shaped configuration (Arlt's triangle).

- *Mutton-fat or large KPs* can be seen in granulomatous uveitis
- *Fine KPs* are seen in herpetic eye diseases and in other non-granulomatous conditions
- *Stellate or star-shaped KPs* are seen in Fuch's heterochromic iridocyclitis
- *Old KPs* are pigmented, have crenate margins.

Band-shaped keratopathy. Deposition of calcium hydroxyapatite in Bowman's layer can be seen in conditions, like chronic uveitis, and juvenile idiopathic arthritis. It typically begins at the periphery of the interpalpebral region and spread centrally. If visual axis is involved, it can cause marked diminution of vision. On slit-lamp examination, small clear dot-like areas are observed giving 'Swiss cheese' appearance to band keratopathy. These clear small dot-like areas represent the location where corneal nerves penetrate Bowman's layer.

Scar or ulceration

- Cornea should be examined properly for superficial or deep scar, dendritic epithelial keratitis to detect keratouveitis.
- Stromal thinning and epithelial ulceration due to inflammation may be observed in peripheral ulcerative keratitis (PUK). PUK may also be the first sign of a systemic necrotizing vasculitis, like rheumatoid arthritis, Wegener's granulomatosis, etc.

D. Examination of anterior chamber

Cells. Cells in the aqueous humour is generally seen after inflammation of the iris and ciliary body. Cells in the anterior chamber are counted using slit-lamp with a beam of 1 x 1 mm slit and graded according the SUN working group grading scheme (Table 17.2).

Table 17.2 *SUN working group grading scheme for cells in anterior chamber*

Grade	Cells in field of 1 mm by 1 mm slit-beam
0	< 1
0.5+	1–5
1+	6–15
2+	16–25
3+	26–50
4+	> 50

- Polymorphonuclear leucocytes are the predominant cells in an acute case and in chronic cases, lymphocytes, plasma cells, monocytes and macrophages are seen.
- Larger cells are generally swollen macrophages or clumps of lymphocytes.
- Inflammatory anterior chamber cells are generally white in colour and should not be confused with pigmented cells. Pigmented cells can be iris pigments, dead erythrocytes, or macrophages filled with pigment like melanin.
- Iris pigments can be seen in the anterior chamber after dilatation and should be distinguished from cells.

Cells in aqueous humour migrate across the iris and ciliary vessels and depending on the nature and severity of inflammation, their numbers and types vary. In the aqueous, the cells are seen circulating due to the convection current.

Flare. In normal condition, aqueous humour is optically empty and if a slit-lamp beam is passed through, it cannot be seen. In case of inflammation, when breakdown of the blood–aqueous barrier occurs, there is increased protein content in the aqueous and if slit-beam is obliquely aimed across the anterior chamber, the path of the beam can be seen, which is termed flare. Flare is graded according to the scheme proposed by SUN classification (Table 17.3).

Table 17.3 *SUN working group grading scheme for anterior chamber flaire*

Grade	Description
0	None
1+	Faint
2+	Moderate (iris and lens details clear)
3+	Marked (iris and lens details hazy)
4+	Intense (fibrin or plastic aqueous)

Flare is often the first sign of uveitis and it may persist despite adequate control of inflammation.

Flare can also be measured using a laser flare photometry, which quantifies anterior chamber protein by measuring light scattering of a helium–neon laser beam in the anterior chamber.

Hypopyon. Often the inflammatory circulating cells particularly leucocytes can deposit at the bottom of the anterior chamber and can form hypopyon. Thus, it is very essential to examine the area of the inferior limbus in uveitic patient. SUN classification has recommended that presence or absence of a hypopyon should be recorded separately while documenting a case of uveitis. It should be kept in mind that hypopyon frequently occurs in patients with endophthalmitis and should always be ruled out especially in patients who had undergone recent intraocular surgery.

Causes of hypopyon
- HLA-B 27 ant uveitis
- Ankylosing spondylitis
- Behçet's disease
- Endophthalmitis
- *Drugs:* Rifabutin

Hypopyon seen in Behçet's disease is mobile and often visible only during gonioscopy (microhypopyon). *Often retained lens fragments, tumour cells can* deposit in anterior chamber and mimic hypopyon. These are known as pseudohypopyon.

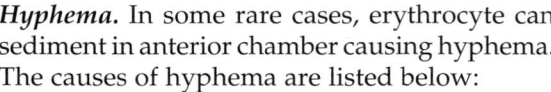

Hyphema. In some rare cases, erythrocyte can sediment in anterior chamber causing hyphema. The causes of hyphema are listed below:

Causes of hyphema
- Viral uveitis
- Trauma
- Malignancies
- Fuchs
- Chronic uveitis with rubeosis
- Any severe uveitis
- Post anterior chamber taps.

E. Examination of pupil

- *Pupillary reaction* in acute cases of iritis or iridocyclitis becomes sluggish or abolished and constriction of pupil occurs.
- *Posterior synechiae.* Often the exudates released during acute inflammation causes plastering of posterior surface of iris with anterior capsule of the lens. These irido-lenticular adhesions are known as posterior synechiae.
    - *Festooned pupil:* Due to the application of cycloplegic topicals, often some parts of the posterior synechiae dilate thus making the pupil festooned-shaped.
    - In cases of severe anterior chamber inflam-mation, the pupillary margin may become plastered to the lens capsule which is called annular or ring *synechiae or seclusio pupillae.*
    - And if the pupillary aperture is blocked by the exudates forming a membrane over it, then it is called *occlusio pupillae.*
- Similarly adhesion between iris and the cornea near the anterior chamber angle can occur due to inflammatory process and known as peripheral anterior synechiae (PAS).

Note. Posterior synechiae can lead to pupillary block glaucoma and peripheral anterior synechiae can cause secondary angle-closure glaucoma.

- *Afferent pupillary defect* is seen in patients with neuroretinitis.

F. Examination of iris

Iris pattern. In acute iritis or iridocyclitis, iris loses its normal pattern due to imbibition of inflammatory exudates in it and such iris is often called muddy iris.

Iris nodules. Accumulations of inflammatory cells in the iris or on iris surface can be clinically noted as iris nodule. Nodules seen in pupillary borders are known as Koeppe nodule and nodules on the iris surface is known as Busacca's nodule. Iris nodules are seen in granulomatous uveitis.

Heterochromia. Comparison of the colour of iris between two eyes can detect heterochromia of iris which can be either hypochromic (abnormal eye is lighter than fellow eye) as seen in Fuch's heterochromic iridocyclitis or hyperchromic (abnormal eye is darker than fellow eye) as seen in melanosis of iris.

Iris atrophy is a characteristic feature of herpetic uveitis. Herpes viruses generally produces sector iris atrophy due to a occlusive vasculitis

Causes of iris atrophy:
- Viral infections
- Anterior segment ischaemia
- Leprosy
- Syphilis
- Previous attacks of angle-closure glaucoma
- Iatrogenic (previous intraocular surgery).

Roseolae. In syphilis, dilated, hyperaemia of the iris vessels are noted which is known as roseolae.

G. Examination of lens

Posterior subcapsular cataract is a common compli-cation after long-standing uveitis as well as chronic corticosteroid therapy.

H. Intraocular pressure (IOP)

Hypotony. Patients with acute iridocyclitis have low IOP due to infiltration of the ciliary body by inflammatory cells which lead to reduction of aqueous production.

Raised IOP. Release of prostaglandin during inflammation can also cause reduction in IOP.
- Sometimes patients with uveitis can present with significant rise in IOP. Conditions like herpes simplex uveitis, herpes zoster uveitis, Posner-Schlossman syndrome, and

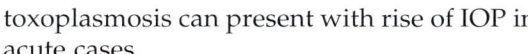

toxoplasmosis can present with rise of IOP in acute cases.

- In case of long-standing uveitis, extensive membrane formation over ciliary body or ciliary body detachment can cause ocular hypotony and eventual phthisis bulbi.

Cause of rise of intraocular pressure in uveitis:

- Clogging of trabecular meshwork with inflammatory cells
- Inflammation of trabecular meshwork fibres (trabeculitis)
- Peripheral anterior synechiae
- Pupillary block from posterior synechiae
- Corticosteroid-induced IOP rise (steroid responder).

I. Examination of vitreous

- *Cells in the anterior vitreous or retrolental space* should be looked for after pupillary dilation. Though there is no standard grading system for vitreous cells, documentation of this finding is important for follow-up of a uveitic case.
- *Vitreous should be carefully examined* with a 78/90 D and also with indirect ophthalmoscope with indentation for snowball opacities, snow-banking in pars plana region and vitreous strands.
- *For classifying vitreous haze,* SUN classification has adopted the National Eye Institute system for grading vitreous haze with the provison that the designation 'trace' be recorded as 0.5+ (Table 17.4).

J. Examination of fundus

Optic disc should be carefully examined with the help of slit-lamp biomicroscopy. Disc

Table 17.4 *SUN working group grading for vitreous haze*

Grade	Description
0	Nil
0.5+	Trace
1+	Few opacities, mild blurring
2+	Significant blurring, but still visible
3+	Optic nerve visible, no vessels visible
4+	Dense opacity obscures optic nerve head

hyperaemia, disc oedema, or optic neuritis is seen in various uveitic conditions. Glaucomatous damage to the optic disc due to secondary glaucoma, neovascularisation of the optic disc, optic disc granuloma and optic atrophy may also occur in uveitic patients.

Examination of retinal vasculature for vasculitis, vascular sheathing, and accumulation of inflammatory cells around vessels is important. Vascular sheathing is seen as white parallel lines along vessels. Sometimes inflammatory exudates are seen around the vessels in patients with sarcoidosis, known as candle-wax drippings. Also it is important to determine whether retinal veins, retinal arteries, or both are affected as it can help in differential diagnosis of the uveitic entity (Table 17.5).

Table 17.5 *Causes of involvement of retinal vessels in uveitis*

Arterial involvement (arteritis)	Venous involvement (phlebitis)
• Acute retinal necrosis • Systemic lupus erythematosus • Behçet's disease	• Sarcoidosis • Frosted branch angiitis

Patch of inflammation. Careful examination of the posterior segment can reveal inflammatory patches in the fundus. It is important to distinguish such leisons whether it involves retina or choroid or both (Table 17.6). Sometimes these lesions are associated with subretinal fluid or localized haze in vitreous.

Retinal detachment. Often a patient can present with a retinal detachment. Exudative retinal detachments can be seen in a number of ocular inflammatory diseases like VKH syndrome. One

Table 17.6 *Retinitis vs choroiditis*

Retinitis	Choroiditis
• Appears as a whitish patch	• Appears as yellowish patch
• Ill-defined margins	• Relatively well-defined margins
• Superficial	• Deeper (deep to the retinal blood vessels)

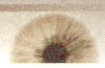

should be able to distinguish rhegmatogenous retinal detachment from such cases, which require a surgical management. Sequelae to vasculitis can lead to development of traction retinal detachment and should be dealt properly.

Macular lesions. Meticulous examination of the fovea with slit-lamp biomicroscopy often helps to identify cystoid macular oedema, choroidal neovascular membrane or sight-threatening inflammatory lesions, like serpiginous choroiditis. Cystoid macular oedema is a common in patients with uveitis which, if long-standing, can lead to formation of macular hole.

FOLLOW-UP EXAMINATION

The initial follow-up of uveitis patients should be scheduled between 1 and 7 days, depending on severity and should include visual acuity, IOP measurement, slit-lamp examination, assessment of cells and flare, indirect ophthalmoscopy and visual field examination using Amsler grid/automated perimetry. Fundus evaluation should be performed to look for complications, such as cystoid macular oedema, epiretinal membranes, macular holes, tractional bands, vitreous haemorrhage, secondary glaucoma or retinal detachment.

BIBLIOGRAPHY

1. Biswas J. Pathology of Uveitis. Afro-Asian Journal of Ophthalmology 1999;9:206–9.
2. Cunningham ET, Nozik RA. Duane's Clinical Ophthalmology. Vol. 37. Philadelphia: Lippincott-Raven; 1997. Uveitis: Diagnostic approach and ancillary analysis; pp. 1–25.
3. Cunningham ET. Jr Uveitis in children. Ocul Immunol Inflamm 2000;8:251–61.
4. Deschenes J, Murray PI, Rao NA, Nussenblatt RB. International Uveitis Study Group (IUSG): clinical classification of uveitis. Ocul Immunol Inflamm 2008;16(1):1–2.
5. Diagnosis and treatment of uveitis. WB Saunders Company, Philadelphia 2002;731–812.
6. Harper SL, Chorich LJ, Foster CS. Diagnosis of uveitis. In: Foster CS, Vitale AT, editors. Diagnosis and Treatment of Uveitis. Philadelphia: WB Saunders; 2002. pp. 79–103.
7. Inungu J, Lewis A, Mustafa Y, Wood J, O'Brien S, Verdun D. HIV Testing among Adolescents and Youth in the United States: Update from the 2009 Behavioral Risk Factor Surveillance System. Open AIDS J. 2011;5:80–5.
8. Jabs DA, Johns CJ. Ocular involvement in chronic sarcoidosis. Am J Ophthalmol 1986; 102:297.
9. Jabs DA, Nussenblatt RB, Rosenbaum JT. Standardization of Uveitis Nomenclature (SUN) Working Group: Standardization of uveitis nomenclature for reporting clinical data. Results of the first international workshop. Am J Ophthalmol 2005;140:509–16.
10. Nussenblatt RB, Palestine AG, Chan CC, Roberge F. Standardization of vitreal inflammatory activity in intermediate and posterior uveitis. Ophthalmology 1985;92(4):467–71.
11. Nussenblatt RB, Whitcup SM, Palestine AG. Examination of the patient with uveitis. Uveitis: Fundamentals and Clinical Practice, 2nd ed. St. Louis: Mosby; 1996; pp. 58–68.
12. Posterior Segment Intraocular Inflammation Guidelines. Edited by John V Forrester, Anabella Okada, David Ben Erza, Shigeaki Ohno. ISBN 90-6299-167-X
13. Rajapure V, Tirwa R, Poudyal H, Thakur N. Prevalence and risk factors associated with sexually transmitted diseases (STDs) in Sikkim. J Community Health 2013;38:156–62.
14. Rao NA, Forster DJ, Aigsburger JJ. General approach to the uveitis patient. The Uvea: Uveitis and Intraocular Neoplasms. Vol. 2. New York: Gower Medical Publishing; 1992, pp. 2.1–2.18.
15. Rathinam SR, Namperumalsamy P. Global variation and pattern changes in epidemiology of uveitis. Indian J Ophthalmol 2007;55:173–83.
16. Smith RE, Nozik RA. 2. Baltimore: Williams and Wilkins; 1986. Uveitis: Goals of Uveitis Management; A clinical approach to diagnosis and management; pp. 23–4.
17. Suttorp-Schulten Rothova A. The possible impact of uveitis in blindness: A literature survey. Br J Ophthalmology 1996; 80:844–8.
18. Yeh S, Grace A. Levy-Clarke, Nussenblatt RB. Introduction to Uveitis. Chap 90. In: Albert DM, Jakobiec FA, (Eds). Principles and Practice of Ophthalmology. Philadelphia: WB Saunders Co 2008;1:1113–23.

Investigations in Uveitis

Chapter Outline

INTRODUCTION
- Clinical workup and checklist
- List of investigations in uveitis

LABORATORY INVESTIGATIONS
- Haematological investigations
  - Routine blood investigations
  - Serological tests
- Urinalysis
- Stool examination for parasites

SKIN TESTS
- Mantoux test
- Histoplasmin skin test
- Kveim test
- Behçet's skin puncture test
- Cutaneous anergy

RADIOLOGICAL TESTS
- X-rays
- CT scan

NUCLEAR MEDICINE STUDY
- Gallium study

ANCILLARY TESTS IN UVEITIS
- Fundus autofluorescence
- Laser flare photometry and laser flare cell photometry
- Ultrasound biomicroscopy
- Fluorescein angiography
- Indocyanine green angiography
- Optical coherence tomography
- Ultrasonography
- Electrophysiological tests in uveitis

INTRODUCTION

Uveitis encompasses entities of varying duration, severity, location and above all a vast plethora of possible etiologies with quite similar and overlapping presentations. Examination of a patient with uveitis needs to be meticulous as the incidence of association with systemic disease is high.

The biggest challenge in uveitis is identification of the cause. One strategy used by nearly all clinicians is the formulation of a list of potential diagnoses and from a brief interaction with the patient, followed by a focused history and examination. Then appropriate investigations shorten the list of diagnostic possibilities.

Although a thorough clinical and systemic investigation is important. Investigations which include laboratory test, ancillary investigations like FFA, ultrasound, imaging studies like optical coherence tomography are often necessary to identify the cause of uveitis.

The list of investigations described here include a battery of tests because of its varied etiology. However, an experienced ophthalmologist soon learns to order a few investigations of considerable value which will differ in individual case depending upon the information gained from a through clinical workup.

Clinical workup and checklist

Before ordering investigations, following should be ensured:

- Uveitis oriented history
- Complete ophthalmic examination
- Identification of anatomic location
- Extent of uveitis
- Overall systemic evaluation
- Compare with clinical characteristics of known uveitic entities
- Make short list of etiological possibilities
- Order 'tailored' laboratory tests to establish/rule out such etiology.

List of Investigations in uveitis

Investigations in uveitis can be grouped as below:

- Laboratory investigations
- Skin tests
- Radiological tests
- Nuclear medicine
- Ancillary tests
- Pathological tests (described in Chapter 19).

LABORATORY INVESTIGATIONS

- *Certain uveitic entities may not require laboratory tests* like Fuchs' heterochromic iridocyclitis, uveitis due to trauma, first attack of non-granulomatous acute anterior uveitis, an unequivocal case of Vogt-Koyanagi-Harada (VKH) syndrome and sympathetic ophthalmia.
- *No standard laboratory evaluation exists* for the patients with uveitis, except in screening for syphilis and possibly sarcoidosis because both of which can present in myriad of ways.
- *Certain laboratory tests can be done in general* to all uveitis patients. These are erythrocyte sedimentation rate (ESR), total and differential white blood cell count.
- *Tailored laboratory investigations relevant to the clinical entity* in question is the right approach in identifying the etiology of a uveitic entity.

Laboratory tests can be grouped as below:

I. *Haematological investigations*
    A. *Routine blood investigations*
- TLC and DLC
- ESR
- Blood sugar.

    B. *Serological tests*
- Antibody detection in infectious uveitis
- Rheumatoid factor
- Antinuclear antibody
- Lupus anticoagulant
- Serological tests for syphilis
- Toxocara serology
- Serological tests for toxoplasmosis
- Serological tests for herpetic group of viruses
- Serological tests for HIV
- Chalamydia serology
- Borrelia titers in lyme disease
- Leptospira antibodies
- Bacterial serology
- Brucellosis antibody test.

    C. Other haematological test.
    D. Detection of major histocompatibility antigens.

II. *Urinalysis*
III. *Stool examination*

I. HAEMATOLOGICAL INVESTIGATIONS

A. ROUTINE BLOOD INVESTIGATIONS

Routine blood tests are of limited value for the diagnosis of specific causes of uveitis. However, they are important when immunosuppressants are planned for the treatment of uveitis. They also provide a baseline to note therapeutic response and drug side effects.

1. *Total and differential counts* (TLC and DLC) sometimes could give clues to the etiology of the disease like:

- *Leucocytosis,* i.e. total count can be increased in bacterial infections
- *Eosinophilia* is seen in patients with sarcoidosis and parasitic infection
- *Lymphocytosis* is seen in tuberculosis and viral infections

2. *Erythrocyte sedimentation rate (ESR)* is raised in connective tissue disorders, sarcoidosis and also in infectious conditions such as tuberculosis, syphilis, etc.

3. *Estimation of the CD4/CD8 lymphocyte ratio* is an important haematological investigation in patients with suspected HIV infection. This ratio is said to have a sensitivity of 85% but a lower specificity.

Normal CD4 and CD8 count is above 400/cumm and 200–800/cumm, respectively. The CD4/CD8 ratio is usually 2.0 and in AIDS patient becomes reversed with a value of 0.5–1.0.

4. *Blood sugar levels* should be estimated to have baseline values and to rule out diabetes mellitus.

5. *Blood uric acid* should be estimated in patients suspected of having goute.

B. SEROLOGICAL TESTS

1. Antibody detection in infectious uveitis

Detection of specific antibodies to infectious agents with the various available laboratory tests helps us to click a diagnosis of infectious organism causing uveitis. *Facts which are very important to note before going to the individual antibody detection* laboratory methods include:

- *Infants are born with* very low levels of self-synthesized serum immunoglobulins and majority of an infant's IgG has been transferred transplacentally from mother.
- *IgG synthesis* in human usually begins about 2 months of age and normal adult levels of IgG is attained during late adolescence.
- *IgM is a relatively large molecule* to cross placenta, thus detectable IgM titles at any age indicates exposure to an infectious agent.

Tests available for antibody detection include:
- *Radioimmunoassay* (RIA)
- *Enzyme-linked immunosorbent assay* (ELISA)
- *Immunofluorescent assay* (IFA) systems: Indirect variants of this test are the fluorescent treponemal antibody (FTA) test used to detect syphilis and the indirect fluorescent antibody test for toxoplasmosis.
- *Complement fixation* (CF)
- *Agglutination and flocculation tests*

- *Indirect, or passive, agglutination* is used in the latex agglutination test for Toxoplasma spp., and to detect IgM rheumatoid factor.
- *Venereal Disease Research Laboratory (VDRL)* test for syphilis is a flocculation test, which combines the features of agglutination and precipitation tests to give a visible foaming rather than clumping reaction.

2. Rheumatoid factor

Rheumatoid factor is an autoantibody directed against the Fc region of IgG. Various immuno-assays are available for detection of rheumatoid factor.

- *The classic Rose-Waaler test* is haemagglutination test for rheumatoid factor in the serum, which depends on the ability of rheumatoid factor to agglutinate sheep erythrocytes coated with anti-sheep immunoglobulin.
- *The latex agglutination test*, in which latex particles coated with human IgG aggregate in the presence of IgM rheumatoid factor, can identify only the IgM isotype of rheumatoid factor.
- *Enzyme-linked immunosorbent assay (ELISA)* can measure IgG, IgA, and IgM rheumatoid factors. Oligoarticular rheumatoid arthritis may be associated with a negative test for IgM rheumatoid factor but a positive test for IgG rheumatoid factor.

3. Antinuclear antibody

Plasma cells, the activated B cells of patients with autoimmune diseases, produce antibodies directed against their own tissues. Antinuclear antibodies (ANA) are usually autoantibodies that are reactive with antigens in the nucleoplasm. These antibodies probably occur in the circulation of all human beings, but the employed test is only considered 'positive' if they occur at titres elevated significantly above the normal serum level. This test has limited value but probably most common test ordered to rule out systemic rheumatic disease.

- The presence of antinuclear antibodies in serum often warrants the presence of systemic collagen vascular disease, however, it can be found in normal individuals also.

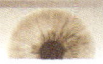

- It is a sensitive screening test for systemic lupus erythematosus.
- Antinuclear antibody is a very useful investigations for juvenile idiopathic arthritis.

4. Lupus anticoagulant

The lupus anticoagulant is an acquired serum immunoglobulin that prolongs several co-agulation measurements. Lupus anticoagulants are anti-phospholipid antibodies found in at least 10% of patients with systemic lupus erythematosus as well as in patients with infectious, drug-induced, malignant, and other autoimmune disorders, and otherwise healthy persons.

Despite the association with impaired co-agulation, thrombotic systemic and ocular disease occurs in lupus anticoagulant positive patients. Symptoms of disturbed vision may bring these patients to medical attention.

5. Tests for syphilis

Laboratory testing for syphilis is indicated in a broad variety of ocular diseases. Scrapings of mucocutaneous lesions to confirm a diagnosis of primary or secondary syphilis can be examined directly by phase-contrast or dark-field microscopy and confirmed by direct immunofluorescence, or DFATP, testing. In the absence of obvious superficial lesions, serology is required to make a diagnosis. These tests fall into two categories:

  i. Nontreponemal
 ii. Treponemal.

Nontreponemal or nonspecific antibody tests

Nontreponemal or nonspecific antibody tests measure IgM and IgG directed against a phospholipid antigen called cardiolipin, or diphosphatidylglycerol, produced coincidentally during luetic infections. These are also known as Wasserman, or reaginic, antibodies.

VDRL test is the simplest and most practical of these tests employing a slide microflocculation technique, and the RPR (rapid plasma reagin) circle card test. Positive tests are reported as the highest serum dilution producing a reaction. These nontreponemal tests are widely used for screening, as well as for quantitative assessment of treatment response. The quantitation VDRL titer is both helpful in diagnosis and in following the course of treatment. If positive, titers are low in primary syphilis, usually below 1:32, while in secondary syphilis it is virtually always greater than 1:32. A high or rising titer is essentially diagnostic of syphilis, despite the long list of diseases producing false-positive results. False-positive test results occur in 10 to 30% of the population, depending on a given laboratory's location.

The VDRL and RPR tests are, therefore, very sensitive but somewhat nonspecific. Following successful treatment of early syphilis, the titer declines approximately fourfold at 3 months, and eightfold at 6 months. Titers should be negative within 1 year of treatment of sero-positive primary syphilis, within 2 years for secondary syphilis, or within 5 years for late latent syphilis. If titers do not return to negative, persistent active infection or reinfection should be suspected, especially if the titer is greater than 1:4. If secondary syphilis is clinically suspected despite a negative nontreponemal test, a prozone phenomenon due to excess antibody might be responsible and additional dilutions should be ordered. The VDRL rises more slowly than the fluorescent treponemal antibody (FTA) test and thus may miss an early primary infec-tion. Therefore, an FTA test should be obtained whenever syphilis is clinically suspected, despite a negative VDRL test. The VDRL is the only test that can be reliably employed in evaluating cerebrospinal fluid.

Treponemal or specific tests

These include:
- *Treponema pallidum* immobilization test (TPI)
- Fluorescent treponemal antibody absorption (FTA-ABS) test
- Microhaemagglutination for *Treponema pallidum* (MHA-TP) test

In syphilis, as in all infections, it is best to use an antigen specific for the organism believed to be infecting the patient. These treponemal or specific tests measure antitreponemal IgG and remain positive throughout life; therefore, they cannot be used to distinguish between active or prior disease.

Treponema pallidum immobilization test (TPI), introduced in 1949,was the first treponemal test developed. Because of technical difficulty and poor standardization, it is rarely used now, although it has served as a valuable benchmark for the development of newer tests.

Fluorescent treponemal antibody absorption (FTA-ABS) test is an indirect immunofluorescent test found to be reactive in about 80% of patients with primary syphilis. The VDRL test is positive in only 50% of patients with primary syphilis, while both the FTA and VDRL tests are positive in all patients with secondary syphilis. The specificity of the FTA-ABS test is greatly enhanced by first absorbing the specimen with nonpathogenic treponemal strains. The FTA-ABS can be used to rule out a biologically false-positive nontreponemal test, although even this test is susceptible to false-positive reactivity, particularly in the presence of lupus erythematosus.

Microhaemagglutination with the MHA-TP test, or haemagglutination with the HATTS can also be performed for specific measurement of treponemal antibody. All of the specific treponemal tests are interpreted as reactive, borderline, or nonreactive. The automated MHA-TP is more rapid and less expensive than the FTA-ABS but may be less sensitive during primary and early secondary disease.

6. Toxocara serology

In this parasitic disease, the diagnosis does not rest on identification of the parasite. Since, the larvae do not develop into adults in humans, a stool examination would not detect any Toxocara eggs. A presumptive diagnosis rests on clinical signs, history of exposure to puppies, laboratory findings (including eosinophilia), and the detection of antibodies to Toxocara.

Antibody detection tests are the only means of confirmation of a clinical diagnosis of visceral larva migrans (VLM), ocular larva migrans (OLM), and covert toxocariasis (CT), the most common clinical syndromes associated with Toxocara infections. *Enzyme immunoassay (EIA)* currently recommended serologic test for toxocariasis with larval stage antigen extracted from embryonated eggs or released *in vitro* by cultured infective larvae. The latter, Toxocara excretory–secretory (TES) antigens, are preferable to larval extracts because they are convenient to produce and because an absorption-purification step is not required for obtaining maximum specificity. Evaluation of the true sensitivity and specificity of serologic tests for toxocariasis in human populations is not possible because of the lack of parasitologic methods to detect Toxocara parasites. These inherent problems result in underestimations of sensitivity and specificity. Evaluation of the Toxocara EIA in groups of patients with presumptive diagnoses of VLM or OLM indicated sensitivity of 78% and 73%, respectively, at a titer of >1:32. When the cut-off titer for OLM cases was lowered to 1:8, sensitivity was increased to 90%.

7. Toxoplasmosis serology

About 40% of the adult population worldwide has been exposed to toxoplasmosis, but this can be much higher in areas where hygiene is poor or raw meat is routinely ingested. Infection leads to IgA, IgG, and IgM antibody production, which despite high titers is not necessarily protective. Complement fixation, latex agglutination, indirect haemagglutination, direct and indirect IFA, immunodiffusion, ELISA tests, and the Sabin-Feldman dye test have all been employed in the quantification of anti-toxoplasma titers.

Dye test was well-documented and reliable, but it lacked standardization, required a great deal of technician time, required live Toxoplasma organisms, and was only available in a few centres.

ELISA and indirect IFA tests are now the most clinically useful. Titers may vary considerably among these tests, so laboratory methodology must be kept consistent when a suspected flare-up is evaluated by sequential serology. Nevertheless, any titer of specific anti-Toxoplasma antibody may be significant. State laboratories will often only report positive tests if a titer of greater than 1:16 is found. There have been, however, cases of pathologically proven toxoplasmic retinitis in which serum antibody levels were positive only in undiluted specimens. The initial diagnosis of ocular toxoplasmosis is usually based on the characteristic focal, necrotizing retinal lesion; positive serum antibodies are used to confirm the clinical impression.

8. Serological tests for herpetic group of viruses

Human herpetic infections result from primary inoculation or reactivation of latent neural virions and include herpes simplex virus (HSV) types 1 and 2, varicella-zoster virus (VZV), cytomegalovirus (CMV), and Epstein-Barr virus (EBV).

Acute retinal necrosis syndrome or Kirisawa's uveitis entails anterior uveitis, vitreous inflammation, and progressive necrotizing vaso-occlusive retinitis with a poor prognosis for visual recovery. The disease may be unilateral or bilateral and generally occurs in otherwise healthy patients. Retinal necrosis syndromes have been attributed to HSV-1, HSV-2, CMV and VZV infections. Significant acute anti-herpes titer elevations, if present, can be useful in the diagnosis of active retinitis, as appropriate intravenous antiviral therapy should be started immediately. If CMV infection is implicated by acute serology in a patient started on empiric acyclovir without clinical improvement, a switch to ganciclovir may be indicated; CMV is far less sensitive to acyclovir than the other herpes viruses. Convalescent serum titers are often inconclusive and arrive from the laboratory long after the retinitis has taken its toll. Aqueous antibodies to HSV-1 in acute retinal necrosis syndrome may indicate local antibody production, antibody sequestration within the eye, or damage to the blood–ocular barrier.

Anti-HSV antibody clearly does not prevent reactivation of herpes labialis, and titers will often show no increase whatsoever with recurrent oral episodes. Seroconversion in paired sera may provide evidence of a primary HSV infection. In general, significant HSV titer rises occur only with primary infections.

Serodiagnosis of VZV infection

In the serodiagnosis of VZV infection, acute and convalescent phase sera should be tested in parallel in the same run. The value of VZV serology is limited somewhat by the fact that heterotypic antibody liter rises to VZV may occur in certain patients with HSV infection who have experienced a prior infection with VZV. This is most likely a heterotypic antibody response to common antigens in the two viruses. Thus a fourfold VZV titer rise is significant only in the absence of a concomitant HSV titer rise in the same specimens. Many clinicians will order paired sample testing for HSV-1, HSV-2, VZV, and CMV herpes virus types in appropriate patients.

Serodiagnosis of CMV infection

CMV recovery from urine, throat, or other body fluids is the preferred diagnostic method for congenital infection and may be of use in ocular disease.

Serodiagnosis in infants is complicated by the presence of transplacental maternal IgG. Although there are some technical difficulties with detection of CMV-specific IgM, this test is excellent for the rapid confirmation of an acute or congenital infection. Up to 20% of patients remain persistently IgM positive, indicating a latent CMV carrier state that regularly becomes re-established in host tissue. In suspected adult disease, a fourfold titer rise indicates a recent infection, due to either reinfection or reactivation. Since CMV titers can remain elevated for extended periods, elevated but unchanged acute and convalescent titers may indicate a recent infection in which the acute specimen was obtained relatively late in the patient's illness.

CMV antibodies are not helpful in the diagnosis of retinitis in patients with acquired immuno-deficiency syndrome (AIDS), especially since the clinical picture is so typical. Furthermore, CMV antibodies are very common in patients at risk for AIDS and CMV serum titers may be negative in AIDS patients despite the presence of CMV retinopathy.

CMV-positive titers should be confirmed by culture whenever possible. In acute CMV infections, characterized by fever, thrombocytopenia, hepatosplenomegaly, pneumonitis, and lymphadenopathy, virus is recoverable from most patients' urine and from 50% of throat swabs. Isolation from buffy coat cells, spun urine, saliva, subretinal fluid, or biopsy specimens can be diagnostic. Isolation, however, does not necessarily establish CMV as the responsible organism; asymptomatic viraemia has been described, and biopsy specimens often contain other pathogens, rendering the clinical interpretation tenuous. Direct specimen examination for CMV by exfoliative cytology, histopathology, immunofluorescence, electron microscopy, or DNA hybridization techniques can also assist in the diagnosis of CMV infection. Fresh spun urine should be passed through a membrane filter, and trapped cells should be stained with hematoxylin eosin or Papanicolaou reagents. Characteristic large cells with prominent eosinophilic inclusions are seen in positive preparations. Similar cells are also rarely seen in HSV infections.

Serodiagnosis of EBV infection

EBV isolation is usually not clinically useful due to the ubiquity of EBV found in healthy persons, technical difficulties in culturing the organism, and a long incubation period.

Serologic studies are the method of choice. In primary infections with symptoms compatible with infectious mononucleosis, a positive heterophil antibody is diagnostic. This IgM antibody agglutinates sheep red blood cells but not guinea pig kidney.

A *slide spot test* is now used for screening and confirmed by the *Paul-Bunnell test*. The heterophil antibody rises rapidly, remains high, and then falls rapidly, generally after 4 weeks of illness.

9. Human immunodeficiency virus serology

Although the diagnosis of AIDS cannot be made in a person who is antibody-negative for human immunodeficiency virus (HIV), positive serology does not establish a diagnosis, as there are many healthy persons who are positive for the antibody. An *ELISA test* is available for routine documentation of HIV-specific antibodies, with informed consent required in nonmilitary settings. The screening tests for HIV antibodies are calibrated to be extremely sensitive, so a significant number of false-positive results occur. All positive tests should be confirmed with a *Western blot analysis*, in which purified, electrophoretically separated HIV antigens incubated with patient serum produce a characteristic pattern. Opportunistic infections such as *Mycobacterium tuberculosis*, *Treponema pallidum*, fungi, *Toxoplasma gondii*, and the herpes viruses define the syndrome and may cause uveitis. CMV retinitis is the most common form of ocular inflammation seen in AIDS and is a poor prognostic sign. A number of immunologic abnormalities have been documented in AIDS, including lymphopenia ($<600/mm^3$), a substantial reduction in the percentage of T cells ($<30\%$), and a reversed helper-to-suppressor T cell ratio (<0.5). T cell subsets can be accurately quantified with immunofluorescent labelling, flow cytometry, and cell-sorting techniques.

10. Chlamydial serology

Chlamydial organisms have been isolated from the joints and the anterior chamber from one patient with Reiter's syndrome. Although chlamydial urethritis and conjunctivitis have been implicated in the pathogenesis of Reiter's syndrome, the presence of antibodies is so common that an elevated titer is of minimal use. A significant convalescent IgG titer rise or high IgM titers might provide a clue to the cause of new-onset Reiter's syndrome in selected patients. The *microimmunofluorescence test*, an indirect antibody test using whole purified chlamydial elementary bodies, provides antibody titers with serotype specificities. Serotype-specific monoclonal reagents are now available for serologic testing in a research setting.

11. Borrelia titers in lyme disease

Either ELISA or indirect IFA tests for IgG and IgM directed against the tick-borne causative agent, *Borrelia burgdorferi*, are available through state laboratories and the CDC in Atlanta. Many patients with the classic cutaneous manifestation of early Lyme disease, erythema chronicum migrans, have ***elevated IgM responses***. Sometimes, however, several weeks of illness are required before the levels of either IgM or IgG antibody become elevated. In these cases, testing of both acute and convalescent sera may increase the chances of obtaining a positive result. Because the antibody response may be aborted altogether by early antibiotic therapy, early Lyme disease cannot be documented in all patients. After the first 5 or 6 weeks of illness, almost all patients have an elevated IgG response, and virtually all patients with arthritis have elevated titers. Titers can be performed on the serum as well as the cerebrospinal fluid. Small amounts of *IgM rheumatoid factor* are produced at certain times in many patients with Lyme disease.

Relapsing fever is due to *Borellia recurrentis* or *Borellia novyi* infection and may be accompanied by uveitis. These Borellia species are transmitted by other members of the Ornithodoros tick family or by the human body louse. All of the Borellia spirochetes can be identified in Giemsa- or Wright-stained blood smears drawn during a febrile episode.

12. Leptospira antibodies

An ***agglutination test*** utilizing commercially available killed organisms is available through most state public health laboratories. A tentative diagnosis of ocular leptospirosis should not be made in the absence of serum antibodies to *Leptospira icterohemorrhagiae*, the major human pathogen. A titer of 1:400 or more is diagnostic. The organisms may be isolated from blood or urine in the early, febrile stages. Many mammals serve as reservoirs, where chronic renal infection leads to passage in the urine. Occasionally, small epidemics of Weil's disease are seen in sewer workers and others exposed to rat urine or contaminated water supplies. Signs and symptoms develop after an incubation period of 10 to 12 days and vary from a mild fever to severe illness, including jaundice, renal failure, and meningitis. Uveitis has not been a frequent component of the disease in the United States,

but mild anterior iritis, membranous vitreous opacities, retinal and papillary haemorrhage, and chorioretinal exudate have been described.

13. Bacterial serology

Serologic testing for antibody responses to gram-negative and gram-positive organisms is not generally believed to be useful in the diagnosis of uveitis syndromes. The rare diagnosis of neisserial endophthalmitis is made by identification of organisms by culture and Gram's stain. Although serum antituberculous antibodies may be useful in identifying pulmonary tuberculous infection, tuberculous serology alone is not useful in isolated ocular tuberculosis. As focal extrapulmonary manifestations assume a greater proportion of tuberculous disease in the United States, ophthalmologists will have to rely more on clinical judgment, diagnostic therapeutic trials with anti-tuberculosis chemotherapy, a precise history, and skin testing rather than serology and the traditional chest roentgenogram in making a diagnosis of tuberculous uveitis.

14. Brucellosis antibody

Brucellosis has been incriminated as a cause of recurrent iritis, nodular choroiditis, and, rarely, a severe endophthalmitic panuveitis. A standard tube agglutination test with acute and convalescent titers should show a fourfold rise in order to establish a presumptive diagnosis of Brucella uveitis. Like leptospirosis, blood cultures may be positive in the early stages of the disease. Brucellosis is usually found in hoofed farm animals: goats, sheep, cattle, and swine. Pregnant animals are particularly susceptible and frequently abort. Human transmission occurs by direct contact with infected animals or consumption of unpasteurized milk. Acute symptoms include fever, chills, and weakness. Chronic infections are characterized by fever, malaise, depression, and abscesses in the bones, spleen, kidneys, or brain.

C. OTHER HAEMATOLOGICAL TESTS

C-reactive protein

Acute phase reactants are proteins that become elevated in response to stressful or inflammatory states such as infection, injury, surgery, trauma, or tissue necrosis. They include globulins, α1-antitrypsin, α1-acid glycoprotein, haptoglobin, ceruloplasmin, fibrinogen, and C-reactive protein (CRP). The CRP is a highly sensitive acute phase indicator and can be measured by ELISA or other immunologic methods. CRP has a molecular weight of 144 kd and reacts with numerous other substances, including DNA, nucleotides, various lipids, and polysaccharides, including the pneumococcal C-polysaccharide. There is still no consensus among physicians for the widespread use of CRP, because other clinical parameters may be just as sensitive, including fever, leucocytosis and the ESR. CRP has been used as a marker for disease activity in the seronegative spondyloarthropathies.

Angiotensin-converting enzyme

Angiotensin-converting enzyme (ACE) is produced by a variety of cells, including capillary endothelial cells, lung tissue, and activated monocytes, macrophages, and epithelioid cells found in noncaseating granulomas. ACE is a dipeptidylcarboxypeptidase, catalyzing the conversion of the decapeptide angiotensin 1 to the pressor angiotensin 2, the cleavage of bradykinin to an inactive metabolite, and a number of other reactions. The serum ACE concentration is probably a reflection of the total amount of granulomatous tissue in the body. The normal level is 55 IU/litre. Serum ACE levels are elevated in about 75% of patients with active, untreated systemic sarcoidosis and about 40% of chronic, untreated patients. However, serum ACE level may be normal in active ocular sarcoidosis as the ocular granuloma load may not be enough to raise the serum concentration.

Lysozyme levels

Lysozyme, or muramidase, is a basic, cationic low-molecular weight enzyme present in tears, saliva, and nasal secretions. It reduces the local concentration of susceptible bacteria by attacking the mucopeptides in bacterial cell walls. Lysozyme originates from phagocytic cells and is normally present in serum at a concentration of 1 to 2 μg/ml. It is actively secreted by monocytes and macrophages. Lysozyme is also secreted by the sarcoid granuloma. In adults, serum lysozyme levels generally parallel elevated serum ACE levels, although lysozyme may be elevated with a normal ACE in occasional patients with sarcoidosis. The lysozyme test is nonspecific and may be elevated in other diseases, including tuberculosis, leprosy, osteoarthritis, and pernicious anaemia. In tuberculosis, lysozyme activity is elevated in over 50% of patients, while the ACE is elevated in only 10%. Serum lysozyme is depressed by systemic corticosteroid administration but, unlike serum ACE, is not normally higher in children when compared with adults. Also in patients on systemic ACE inhibitors, this test is of help. The serum lysozyme value may be elevated, however, in patients older than 60 yrs of age. So age must be taken into consideration when interpreting both ACE and lysozyme levels. Both ACE and lysozyme can be sensitive noninvasive tools in approaching a patient with granulomatous uveitis when the entire clinical presentation is carefully considered.

Lysozyme levels are elevated in tuberculous pleural effusion specimens and may prove to be a useful marker in aqueous paracentesis specimens taken from patients with presumed tuberculous uveitis. Most laboratories quantify lysozyme levels spectrophotometrically, but turbidometric, viscometric, immunologic, and bioassay methods are also available.

D. DETECTION OF MAJOR HISTOCOMPATIBILITY ANTIGENS

The human major histocompatibility complex, containing DNA encoding human leucocyte antigen (HLA) genes, is located on the short arm of chromosome 6. The HLA sites localize to heterodimeric (two different chains) cell surface molecules belonging to the immunoglobulin superfamily. Class I HLA molecules include the A, B, and C loci and are found on the surface of virtually every cell. Class II HLA molecules include the D, DR, DQ, and DP loci and are restricted to lymphocytes, macrophages, and other immunocompetent cells. Humans possess two haplotypes, usually inherited as a unit from each parent. Each haplotype has three class I and four class II alleles. Because HLA expression is codominant, it is theoretically possible to type two antigens at each of these seven loci unless the subject is homozygous for one or more loci or antisera are not yet available for a rare HLA type. There are currently 124 recognized HLA specificities.

The class I molecules provide a recognition target for lymphocytes responsible for cell-mediated immunity. Thus, class I antigens are recognized during graft rejection and they restrict the cytotoxic response against virus-infected cells to lymphocytes expressing the same class I antigens as the infected cells. Class II molecules are essential to antigen presentation and normal interactions between immuno-competent cells.

Genetically predetermined susceptibility to 530 distinct diseases has been linked to certain specific HLA markers in over 4,000 separate clinical studies. None of the HLA markers is, of course, specific for a given disease. The presence of an HLA antigen in a given patient, however, is suggestive of its associated disease and may provide the clinician with an additional clue in establishing a definitive diagnosis. The relative risk of 69.1 for HLA-B27 and ankylosing spondylitis, which was the first such association ever described, indicates that an HLA-B27-positive white person is about 69 times more likely to develop ankylosing spondylitis than someone not carrying this antigen. The HLA-B27 antigen itself characterizes a unique clinical picture in uveitis, making it an important diagnostic tool, unlike the situation in rheumatologic practice in which HLA-B27 typing is less valuable. HLA-B27-positive patients with acute anterior uveitis are more likely to be younger at the age of onset, to be male, to show frequent unilateral alternating eye involvement, to have severe symptoms with each episode (including fibrinoid anterior chamber reactions), to have a higher incidence of ocular complications, to lack mutton-fat keratic precipitates, and to have an associated seronegative spondyloarthropathy.

The HLA type may also help define prognosis. In presumed ocular histoplasmosis syndrome,

HLA-B7 is strongly associated with disciform macular lesions, but not with peripheral atrophic scars. HLA-DR2, however, is associated with both macular and peripheral scarring, suggesting a distinct genetic predisposition to macular neovascularisation in this disease.

Patients with pauciarticular juvenile rheumatoid arthritis are particularly prone to uveitis. HLA-DR5, which is associated with the early-onset form of this disease most frequently seen in girls, characterizes patients more likely to develop a chronic, bilateral disease associated with band keratopathy and the presence of antinuclear antibodies. HLA-B27, on the other hand, is associated with later-onset pauciarticular juvenile rheumatoid arthritis and concomitant uveitis similar to the classic HLA-B27 pattern. Uveitis occurs in 53% of patients with HLA-DR5 related early-onset juvenile rheumatoid arthritis found mostly in females and in 25% of patients with the HLA-B27-related, later-onset form usually found in males.

In general, HLA tests are not ordered on a routine basis and complete histocompatibility typing is never ordered as part of an evaluation for uveitis. Specific HLA types can, however, provide more information to the astute clinician who requires additional data to confirm a suspected diagnosis.

II. URINALYSIS

The urinalysis is also used to assess the general health status of the patient. A urine specimen is a cost-effective, painless liquid tissue biopsy of the urinary tract that rapidly provides a great deal of information. The urinalysis is a useful screening test for renal, genitourinary, meta-bolic, and hepatic diseases. Among the most significant conditions detected by chemical means in a macrourinalysis are proteinuria, glucosuria, ketonuria, and the presence of the pigments haemoglobin and bilirubin. A micro-urinalysis of centrifuged urine sediment should be performed on fresh or refrigerated specimens. White cells, red cells, urinary casts, and crystalluria can all be quantified under the microscope. The presence of a suspected infection can be rapidly confirmed by urine dip-stick nitrite and leucocyte esterase tests

(Chemstrip, Boehringer-Mannheim Diagnostics, Indianapolis). A urine culture should probably be performed in all cases of presumed urinary tract infection including cases of suspected Reiter's syndrome with or without genitourinary symptoms. *Chlamydia trachomatis* may be isolated from the urethra, urine, conjunctiva, or rectum of patients with Reiter's syndrome, although iridocyclitis usually develops after the acute infectious phase. Only a few patients with Reiter's uveitis, however, have responded to tetracycline therapy.

Urine CMV cultures as well as CMV cytology are central to the diagnosis of CMV infection. Hypercalciuria is twice as common as hypercalcaemia in sarcoidosis. Thus, a 24-hour urinary calcium determination may be helpful, however, inconvenient and nonspecific. Twenty-four-hour urine collections for uric acid can be a more sensitive screening test than serum uric acid in establishing a diagnoses of gout. Finally, the ova of *Endolimax nana* have been found in the urine of a patient with exudative chorioretinopathy.

■ III. STOOL EXAMINATION FOR PARASITES

Intestinal parasites are a rare cause of uveitis in the United States: for example, only one case of Ascaris ocular invasion has been proven. *Entamoeba histolytica, Escherichia coli, E. nana,* and *Giardia lamblia* have been described as producing a cystic macular lesion. Although *Toxocara canis* and *T. cati* are recognized causes of uveitis, humans are not natural hosts. Ingested ova from contaminated soil or uncooked vegetables such as lettuce advance to the larval stage in the human intestinal epithelium, penetrate the portal vasculature and lymphatics, and spread to the liver, where eosinophilic granulomas may be produced. Some larvae survive, infect the lungs, enter the heart, and thereafter disseminate throughout the body. The larvae never mature in the human host; thus neither ova nor mature Toxocara parasites are found in human faeces.

■ SKIN TESTS

Intradermal injection of 0.1 ml of soluble antigens prepared from a number of infectious agents can be performed in the office during the initial visit.

MANTOUX TEST

The most useful test antigen is the tuberculin purified protein derivative (PPD). The standard dose is 5 TU (US tuberculin units) or intermediate strength, equivalent to 0.0001 mg (Aplisol, Parke-Davis, Morris Plains, NJ). Current lots of PPD are standardized for biologic activity against PPD-Seibert (PPD-S), a reference bulk lot prepared in 1940. Second strength (250 TU) can be given to patients who do not react to an initial 5-TU injection, whereas first strength (1 TU) should be given to patients who the clinician suspects may have a strong reaction and are therefore at risk for sloughing and ulceration at the injection site (Tubersol, in first and second strength, available through Squibb/Connaught, Princeton, NJ). There is no evidence of booster effects or repeated skin testing leading to conversion from negative to positive. Intracutaneous injection, the Mantoux test, is the most reliable test available. Injection of 0.1 ml of PPD antigen into the volar or dorsal surface of the forearm is made just below the skin surface with a short (½ inch) No. 27 gauge needle, bevel upward, to produce a discrete 6- to 10-mm wheal or bubble. The use of insulin syringes with intrinsic needles will avoid repeated waste of antigen extract in the needle hub of standard tuberculin syringes. If no bubble appears due to a deep injection, the test should be immediately reapplied at a site at least 5 cm away. Skin tests are read 48 to 72 hours following injection. Induration measuring 10 mm or more is considered positive (Fig. 18.1) this indicates a previous infection with *Mycobacterium tuberculosis*, although previous infection with *M. bovis* or photochromogenic mycobacteria may also produce a positive result. Patients may also develop coexistent erythema, a wheal and flare that usually fades after 12 to 18 hours, which is evidence of an immediate hypersensitivity to the same test antigen. Uveitis patients with induration less than 10 mm, or even erythema alone, have had favourable clinical responses to oral antituberculous therapy. On the other hand, patients with proven ocular

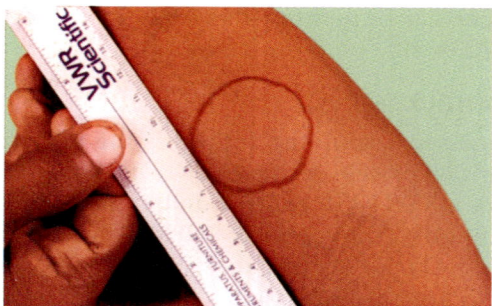

Fig. 18.1: *Mantoux reading.*

tuberculous infection have had insignificant or negative PPD skin tests.

HISTOPLASMIN SKIN TEST

Although the use of histoplasmin skin testing in uveitis is no longer universally recommended, greater than 80% of patients with presumed ocular histoplasmosis syndrome have positive skin tests. Some authors believe that histoplasmin skin testing may increase the danger of activating a macular lesion in susceptible patients.

KVEIM TEST

Approximately 80% of patients with sarcoidosis react positively to skin testing with the Kveim antigen. This antigen is prepared from human sarcoid granulomas, is difficult to obtain, requires several months of incubation followed by a biopsy at the injection site for histologic verification, does not have absolute specificity, and entails a risk of hepatitis or retrovirus transmission. False-positive and false-negative results may occur, limiting its usefulness.

BEHÇET'S SKIN PUNCTURE TEST

Patients with active systemic Behçet's disease show increased dermal sensitivity to needle trauma, owing to their unusual leukotactic tendency. The appearance of a pustule 24 to 36 hours after an intradermal needle puncture, with or without the injection of 0.1 ml of normal saline, is almost diagnostic for Behçet's disease. Erythema and infiltration may appear within a few hours, and occasionally a microabscess can be produced. This test may not be positive in patients with ocular manifestations when the systemic disease is in remission. No universal agreement on the usefulness of this test exists because only 10% of Behçet's patients demonstrate a positive response.

CUTANEOUS ANERGY

This is a phenomenon of reduced or absent cutaneous sensitivity to a given antigen to which the subject was sensitive before. In developing countries where Bacillus-Calmette-Guerin (BCG) vaccination is routinely performed, negative tuberculin test in a BCG-vaccinated patient or in a patient with a previously positive tuberculin skin test is of great value in diagnosis of sarcoidosis. This is the most well-known manifestation of anergy. It has been recommended as one of the diagnostic criteria by the first international workshop on ocular sarcoidosis.

RADIOLOGICAL TESTS

When an ophthalmologist orders a roentgenogram the radiologist should know exactly which diagnoses are being considered.

1. Chest roentgenograms are useful when conditions, such as tuberculosis, sarcoidosis, or histoplasmosis are suspected.

Active pulmonary sarcoidosis characteristically shows bilateral hilar adenopathy (Fig. 18.2) with or without parenchymal disease; hilar adenopathy characteristically precedes the onset of peripheral infiltrates. Chest roentgenographic abnormalities are found in about 80% of patients with ocular sarcoidosis.

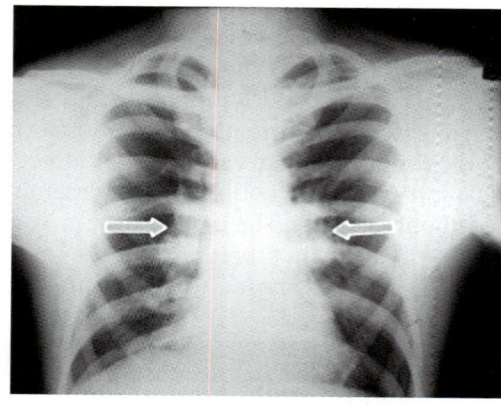

Fig. 18.2: *X-ray chest showing hilar adenopathy suggestive of sarcoidosis.*

Active pulmonary tuberculosis may reveal characteristic wedge-shaped segmental infiltrates, cavitary lesions, calcified granulomas, or diffuse parenchymal nodules accompanied by ipsilateral hilar enlargement. Lordotic views of the relatively oxygen-rich apices may demonstrate old scarring or concentrated active lesions due to the aerobic preferences of mycobacteria.

2. **Ocular and orbital plane films** may show calcification of various parts of the uvea; for example:

- Late degenerative choroidal changes.
- Fine stippling in retinoblastoma, or intraocular calcification seen in retinopathy of prematurity and hyperparathyroidism.
- Intraocular foreign bodies can be identified and localized by plain films as well as ultrasonography and computed tomography.

3. **Sacroiliac joint films** should be ordered when ankylosing spondylitis or other seronegative spondyloarthropathies, such as Reiter's syndrome or psoriatic arthritis, are suspected. It is important to specifically order a sacroiliac series, not a lumbar spine series, since both a straight anteroposterior projection and the more sensitive oblique tunnel view of the joints will be taken.

- *Sacroiliac disease* occurs in 20% of patients with Reiter's syndrome.
- When a patient has psoriasis with sacroiliitis (Fig. 18.3), iridocyclitis is also likely to occur, whether or not the HLA-B27 antigen is positive.

4. **Painful, swollen joints can be X-rayed** if juvenile or adult rheumatoid arthritis, Reiter's syndrome, or sarcoidosis is suspected.

- *In juvenile rheumatoid arthritis*, the knee is most commonly affected. Since children with pauciarticular manifestations develop the worst iridocyclitis, a routine knee roentgenogram is recommended, even though there is no clinically suspected arthritis.
- *In Reiter's syndrome*, the hands, feet, heels, and sacroiliac joints are most commonly affected.
- Weight-bearing joints are also afflicted.
- *In ankylosing spondylitis* and sarcoidosis. Permeating, lytic, and destructive bony changes are also seen occasionally in sarcoidosis.

5. **Radiographic studies for cerebral calcification,** although helpful, are nonspecific and do not differentiate between toxoplasmosis and CMV inclusion disease, as the roentgenographic findings can be the same for both infections. This is not surprising when one realizes that *Toxoplasma gondii* and CMV are both neurotrophic intracellular pathogens and may both be seen together within the same host cell.

6. **Upper gastrointestinal small bowel series and barium enema roentgenograms** may identify anomalies associated with uveitis, including Whipple's disease, Crohn's disease, ulcerative colitis, and abdominal abscess.

7. **Paranasal sinus and dental films** occasionally, may be of value in locating clinically suspected loci of infection in otherwise idiopathic uveitis.

8. **CT scan chest** is very useful in tuberculosis of the lung and also to delineate hilar lymphadenopathy in patients with sarcoidosis (Fig. 18.4).

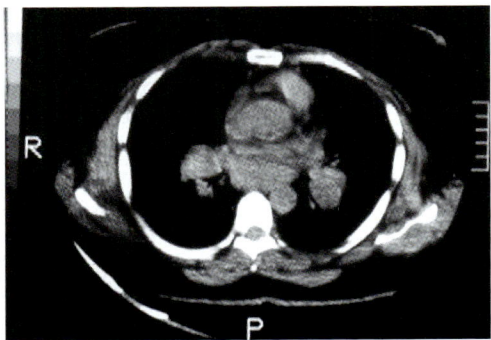

Fig. 18.3: *X-ray sacroiliac joint showing sacroiliitis.*

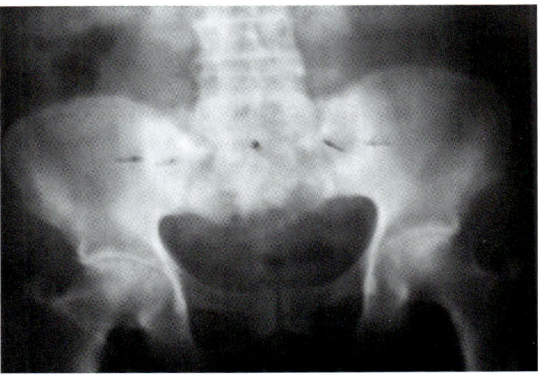

Fig. 18.4: *HRCT showing hilar adenopathy.*

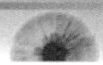

NUCLEAR MEDICINE STUDY

GALLIUM STUDY

Gallium citrate scan can identify inflammatory disease and tumours throughout the body. Gallium is taken up by mitotically active liposomes of granulocytes. The actual scan is performed 48 hours following the intravenous injection of radiolabelled gallium citrate. For the purpose of sarcoid diagnosis, a limited scan of the head, neck, and chest is sufficient and less expensive than a total body scan. Although radiation doses are extremely minute, careful dosimetric consultation with a clinical radiation physicist should be undertaken before performing this test in pregnant women and young children.

- *Gallium scan is more sensitive than routine chest roentgenograms* for showing pulmonary involvement in sarcoidosis. It lacks specificity, however, as numerous other pulmonary diseases show abnormal uptake, including tuberculosis, carcinoma, lymphoma, and silicosis.
- *Increased lacrimal gland uptake of gallium* occurs in over 80% of patients with active sarcoidosis, although this is also nonspecific; as many as 25% of patients with increased lacrimal gland uptake have no other evidence of the disease. Thus, gallium scans may lead to a false-positive diagnosis of sarcoidosis by physicians unfamiliar with these limitations.
- *When combined with determination of serum ACE and lysozyme levels, a skin test panel, chest roentgenogram, and other tests tailored* to a careful history and examination, the gallium scan can be instrumental in establishing a diagnosis of ocular sarcoidosis.

Technetium scans have been used in the diagnosis of Sjögren's syndrome and correspond well to minor salivary gland biopsy findings.

ANCILLARY TESTS IN UVEITIS

Recently, enormous progress has been achieved in investigational procedures for uveitis. A provisional clinical diagnosis can be reached in most cases of uveitis. Ancillary tests help in confirming the clinical diagnosis and are most useful in dilemmatic situations in diagnosis. Increased precision and accuracy in the assessment of the level and degree of inflammation and its monitoring goes parallel with the development of extremely potent and efficacious therapies.

Common ancillary tests used in uveitis include:
- Fundus autofluorescence
- Laser flare photometry and laser flare cell photometry
- Ultrasound biomicroscopy
- Fluorescein angiography
- Indocyanine green angiography
- Optical coherence tomography
- Ultrasonography
- Electrophysiological tests in uveitis.

FUNDUS AUTOFLUORESCENCE

Fluorescence is the capability of absorbing light at a specific wavelength and releasing it at a longer, less energetic wavelength. Autofluorescence is the natural and spontaneous emission of light by a substance.

Excitation wavelength used in fundus autofluorescence (FAF) imaging is generally, but not always, 488 nm (argon laser).

Modalities of FAF imaging could be near-infrared FAF and blue-light FAF imaging.

Source of fundus autofluorescence (FAF) is the lipofuscin of retinal pigment epithelial (RPE) cells. Lipofuscin is the lysosomal metabolic accumulate of non-dividing RPE cells. It accumulates with age and in some retinal disorders as a byproduct of light-related vitamin A cycling. Lipofuscin exhibits a characteristic autofluorescence when excited in ultraviolet (UV) or blue light. The level of autofluorescence represents a balance between accumulation and clearance of lipofuscin.

Normal FAF image of the posterior pole of the retina would show:
- *Optic nerve head or dark* because of the absence of RPE thus lipofuscin.
- *Retinal vessels* are hypoautofluorescent because of absorption of light by the blood.

- *Macular area*, the FAF signal is reduced at the fovea when compared with the surroundings. From the foveola, a distinct increase in the signal can be observed till the margin of the fovea, followed by a further gradual increase of AF toward the outer macula. This is caused by absorption by luteal pigments (i.e. lutein and zeaxanthin) in the neurosensory retina at fovea, especially foveola, and a possible spatial differences in melanin deposition.

Mechanism of autofluorescence

Amount of autofluorescence is dependent on the amount of fluorophores in any given area.

- *Inflammation* can alter the amounts of fluorophores during acute phases.
- *Autofluorescence (FAF) photography complements other methods of imaging, such as colour fundus photography.* Acute inflammatory changes can alter the size and number of fluorophore content of the RPE cells due to a number of factors including RPE cell dysfunction and destruction. Inflammation induces a number of pro-oxidative pathways, which may increase the amount of fluorophores present.
- *Hypertrophy and reactive hyperplasia of the RPE* may increase the thickness of the RPE, contributing to the formation of autofluorescence.
- *Choroidal neovascularization* (CNV) associated with intraocular inflammation produces characteristic autofluorescence findings.
- *Secondary CNV* is often easily recognised by FAF because the surrounding hyperplastic RPE is hyper-autofluorescent and, hence, FAF neatly outlines the neovascularisation.
- *Following treatment, CNV may contract and leave a zone of absent RPE result in hypo-autofluorescent in that particular area.*
- *Areas of RPE with increased pigmentation* also show increased autofluorescence. With time, the areas start to become thinner, and RPE cells are reduced and the area appears darker during autofluorescence photography because of the lack of fluorophores.

Uses of autofluorescence

From autofluorescence imaging, we can estimate the extent of damage due to a particular disease, monitor its progression and can anticipate future complications.

Causes of altered fundus autofluorescence

I. *Causes for an increased FAF signal*

1. *Excessive RPE lipofuscin accumulation*
- *Lipofuscinopathies.* Stargardt disease, Best disease, pattern dystrophy, and adult vitelliform macular dystrophy
- *Age-related macular degeneration*

2. *Occurrence of fluorophores anterior or posterior to the RPE cell monolayer*
- Cystoid macular oedema
- Serous PED
- Druse in the subpigment epithelial space
- Older intraretinal and subretinal haemorrhages
- Choroidal vessel in the presence of RPE and choriocapillaris atrophy
- Choroidal nevi and melanoma

3. *Lack of absorbing material*
- Cystoid macular oedema (displacement of luteal pigment)
- Idiopathic macular telangiectasia type 2 (depletion of luteal pigment)

4. *Optic nerve head druse*
5. *Artefacts.*

II. *Causes for a reduced FAF signal*

1. *Reduction in RPE lipofuscin density*
- RPE atrophy (geographic atrophy)
- Hereditary retinal dystrophies (such as RPE65 mutations).

2. *Increased RPE melanin content*
- For example, RPE hypertrophy.

3. *Absorption from extracellular material/cells/fluid anterior to the RPE*
- Migrated melanin-containing cells
- Crystalline druses or other crystal-like deposits
- Fresh intraretinal and subretinal haemorrhages
- Retinal vessels
- Luteal pigment (lutein and zeaxanthin)
- Media opacities (vitreous, lens, anterior chamber, cornea)
- Fibrosis, scar tissue, borders of laser scars.

Autofluorescence in some posterior uveitic conditions

Choroiditis, multifocal choroiditis, panuveitis syndrome

- *Clinically visible chorioretinal scars* are hypo-autofluorescent due to damage and destruction of the RPE cells. FAF lesions often outnumbers the number of chorioretinal scars seen clinically, correctly delineating the extent of involvement. The hypoautofluorescent spots are very small, and clinically visible scars appear to be composed of multiple smaller hypoautofluorescent spots.
- *Secondary choroidal neovascularisation* is visible as an area of hyperautofluorescence.

Serpiginous choroiditis

- *Active lesions* have been reported to be hypo-autofluorescent. At a very early stage, FAF showed increased autofluorescence and changes from a granular to a speckled pattern within a few weeks, and finally becoming hypoautofluorescent after a few months.
- *In reactivation phase,* the margins of the lesions shows hyperautofluorescence because of the activity of the RPE cells at the margin and deposition of lipofuscin (Fig. 18.5).

VKH

- *In acute VKH disease,* mild and uniform hyper-autofluorescence is seen in the macula and hypoautofluorescence at the area of the serous retinal detachment and fluid pockets.
- *Following treatment,* FAF returns normal. In late presentation, FAF abnormality is scattered and widespread and never returns to normal pattern due to extensive damage to the RPE.

LASER FLARE PHOTOMETRY AND LASER FLARE CELL PHOTOMETRY

Laser flare photometry (LFP) provides a non-invasive, objective and quantitative measure of aqueous humour flare. It is used as a research and an adjunctive clinical tool.

Principle

The LFP is based on the principle that increased protein content of the aqueous humour causes scattering of light. A laser beam of light scans a

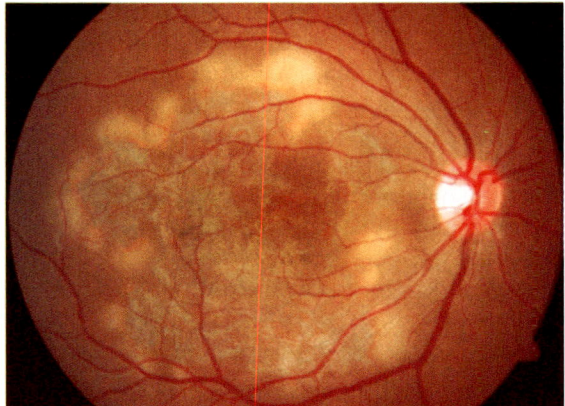

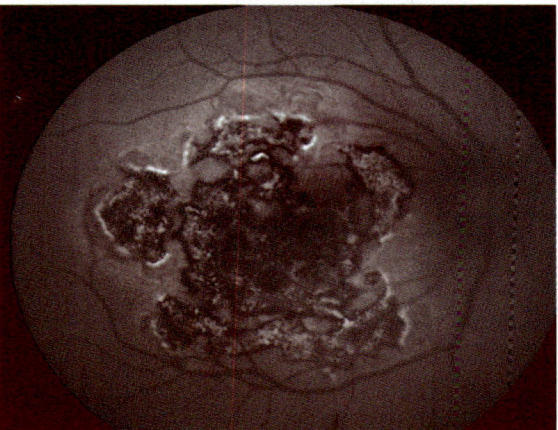

Fig. 18.5: *Fundus autofluorescence in serpiginous choroiditis showing hyperfluorescence of the active edge.*

measurement window projected into the anterior chamber and light scattered by protein particles in the aqueous humour is detected by a photomultiplier. The amount of scattered light in the measurement window is proportional to the concentration and size of the proteins in the aqueous humour.

Method

- *Laser flare-cell photometer* (LFCP) is used for LFP. A fixed volume (0.5 mm) is scanned two dimensionally by the laser beam. The result of aqueous humour flare expressed in photon counts per millisecond (ph/ms).
- *Seven measures are taken.* The highest and lowest values are discarded and the machine automatically calculates the mean and standard deviation of the remaining five readings.

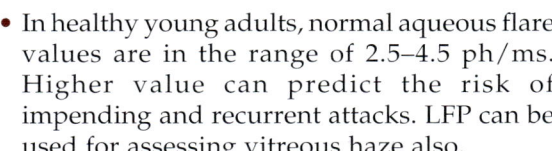

- In healthy young adults, normal aqueous flare values are in the range of 2.5–4.5 ph/ms. Higher value can predict the risk of impending and recurrent attacks. LFP can be used for assessing vitreous haze also.

Uses

- Flare measured by LFP may reflect severity of inflammation during exacerbations and in presence of subclinical inflammation during quiescent periods.
- It may guide both immediate as well as long-term immunomodulatory treatment of panuveitis entities, like Behçet's disease, VKH, etc.
- Laser flare photometry may play an even more important role in monitoring therapy and predicting outcomes in children with uveitis.

Pit falls

- Particles, such as pigment, cannot be differentiated from inflammatory cells and may be counted as cells.
- Differentiation between various cells, such as erythrocytes, ghost cells or leucocytes cannot be done either.

ULTRASOUND BIOMICROSCOPY

- *High frequency ultrasound biomicroscopy* (UBM) enables *in vivo* imaging of the anterior segment structures of the eye, including structures posterior to the iris plane that could not have been previously imaged by conventional ultrasonography.
- *Media opacities* (e.g. corneal opacity, cataract, pupillary membranes, etc.) do not preclude examination.
- *High-magnification and high resolution images* of the iridocorneal angle, posterior chamber, ciliary body, pars plana, vitreous base and peripheral retina and choroid can be obtained using the UBM.

Principle

The UBM uses high frequency transducers (50–100 MHz) incorporated into a B-scan ultrasound. The higher frequency transducers allow better resolution, but lower penetration of ocular tissues, thus are ideal for examination of superficial and anterior ocular structures. A real-time image can be displayed or stored.

Limitations

- Requires an experienced and technically skilled operator (the main disadvantage)
- It is time consuming
- The contact method might be uncomfortable for certain patients.

Method

Conventional UBM transducers are immersed in a cup filled with saline or a coupling media placed on the globe under topical anaesthesia with the patient in a supine position. Imaging with upright position is possible with advanced probes with built-in water bath.

Uses

It is a useful tool for detection of:

- *Ciliary body* inflammation, mass lesions and atrophy
- *Pars plana membranes*
- Exudates, zonular status
- Suspected cases of cyclodialysis cleft
- *Intraocular foreign* body at the angle of anterior chamber or pars plana, in hypotonous eye
- Other inflammatory and non-inflammatory conditions affecting pars plana and peripheral retina.

FLUORESCEIN ANGIOGRAPHY

Fundus fluorescein angiography (FFA) is an indispensable imaging tool for the diagnosis and monitoring of inflammatory diseases affecting the posterior segment of the eye.

Basic principles

The fluorescein dye is a small protein-bound (80%) molecule that absorbs light at 480–490 nm and emits at 530 nm. Remaining unbound dye (almost 20%) produces most of the fluorescence. Neither of the molecules (bound/unbound) can diffuse through the normal retinal vessel wall, the intact retinal pigment epithelium (RPE) or the large choroidal vessels. It diffuses freely through the fenestrated choriocapillaris.

Methodology

- *Fluorescein dye is injected* rapidly through intravenous route, usually through antecubital vein.
- *Blue excitation filter* (wavelength 465–490 nm) is used to project blue light. Blue light is then absorbed by unbound fluorescein molecules, and the molecules fluoresce, emitting light with a longer wavelength in the yellow–green spectrum (520–530 nm).
- *Barrier filter blocks* any reflected blue light so that the images capture only light emitted from the fluorescein molecules.
- *Images are acquired* in the digital media/film immediately after injection and continue for ten minutes depending on the pathology being imaged.

Phases of angiography

Fluorescein angiography has been divided into different phases:

1. *Choroidal flush*. The filling of the choroidal circulation is seen as the choroidal flush 10–12 seconds following injection. A patchy and mottled hyperfluorescence is seen as the choroidal lobules fill. Dye appears in the retinal circulation 1–3 seconds later.

2. *Arteriovenous phase*. The early arteriovenous phase involves the filling of the retinal arteries, arterioles and capillaries. This is followed by the late arteriovenous phase or laminar venous phase as the dye fills the veins in a laminar pattern.

3. *Venous phase*. It is characterised by the laminar flow in the retinal veins followed by venous filling. The peak phase with maximal fluorescence occurs at approximately 30 seconds and is characterised by complete filling of retinal veins.

4. *Recirculation phase*. During the recirculation of the dye, fluorescence gradually decreases with emptying of dye in the retinal vessels. Extravasated dye from the choriocapillaris stains the choroid and scleral rim of the optic disc.

After 10 minutes, the dye is no longer seen in retinal vessels. However, several structures including the optic nerve head, Bruch's membrane, and sclera are stained with the dye and continue to fluoresce.

Pathophysiological interpretations

There is no extravasation from the normal retinal vasculature. Abnormal patterns may be:

1. *Hypofluorescence* may be due to blockage or vascular filling defect in the choroidal or retinal circulation.

Blocked fluorescence may be caused by any opacity (vitreousopacity, blood, inflammatory infiltrate, fluid, pigment, etc.) that obscures the visibility of fluorescein in the choroid and/or in retinal circulation. Colour fundus photograph is sometimes required to differentiate between blockage and non-perfusion.

2. *Hyperfluorescence* may be caused by transmission (window) defects, abnormal retinal or choroidal vessels, leakage, staining or pooling of fluorescein.

- *Retinal pigment epithelial defects* cause transmission of choroidal fluorescence; thus hyperfluorescence (window defect) will have the same size and shape both in early and late phase.
- Pinpoint leaks of RPE are differentiated from window defects by their increasing size and change in shape with pooling of dye in the subretinal space.
- *Inflammation of the optic disc* causes hyperfluorescence due to dilated capillaries on the optic disc in the early phase and staining of the optic disc with leakage in the late phase.
- *Leaky abnormal vessels*, such as retinal neovascularisation (NVE or NVD) cause intense fuzzy hyperfluorescence due to profuse leakage of the dye.
- *Staining of retinal vessel walls* and retinal vascular leakage are the hallmarks of retinal vasculitis in FFA.
- *Leakage of dye* and pooling in the cystoid spaces at the macula give rise to a petalloid pattern of hyperfluorescence.
- *Diffusion of fluorescein into tissue* or material is defined as staining, which is a late phase phenomenon (during recirculation).

Uses of FFA in uveitis

Fluorescein angiography is especially useful in uveitis for the evaluation of:

- Optic disc inflammation.
- Macular oedema.

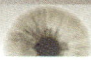

- Occlusive vasculitis.
- Early detection of non-occlusive retinal vasculitis, neovascularisations, retinal pigment epithelial changes, disease activity in choroiditis and the source and pattern of leaks in exudative retinal detachment.
- *Inflammation of the retinal capillaries* can only be detected by angiography, so it has diagnostic importance in Behçet's disease and other vasculitis and intermediate uveitis.
- *In choroiditis, active lesions show early hypo- and late hyperfluorescence* (Fig. 18.6). It is due to oedema which blocks the initial dye but later leakage from the surrounding tissue cause hyperfluorescence.
- *In VKH,* in the acute uveitic stage, bilateral pinpoint RPE leaks and late pooling of dye in the subretinal space are the characteristic angiography findings. Similar findings are also seen in eyes with exudative retinal detachment associated with sympathetic ophthalmia and in posterior scleritis which is unilateral.
- *In active serpiginous choroiditis,* early hypofluorescence and late fuzzy staining are characteristic angiographic signs of an active lesion.

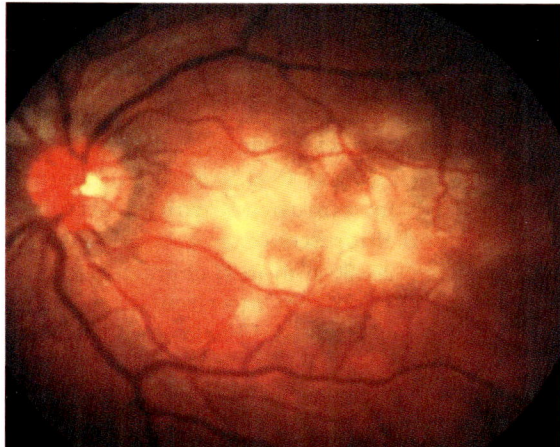

INDOCYANINE GREEN ANGIOGRAPHY (ICGA)

In the diseases which primarily involve the choroid and choriocapillaris, indocyanine green angiography is a better modality of investigation when compared with FFA.

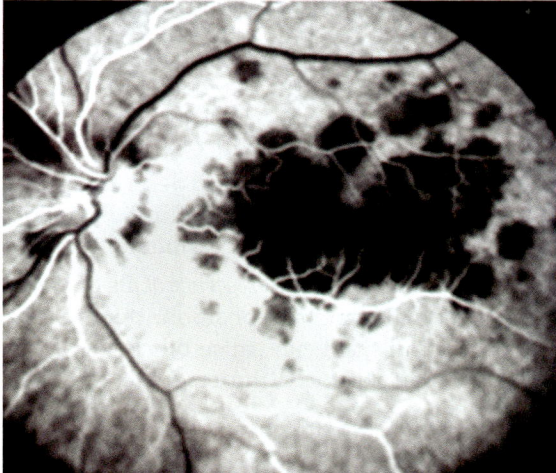

Principle

Indocyanine green is a relatively large molecule than fluorescein with peak absorption of light at 795 nm and emission at 830 nm. Near infrared fluorescence of ICG allows access to the deeper structures. Almost all of the dye binds to serum proteins (80% binding globulins and α-lipoproteins). Therefore, the large ICG-protein complex does not leak from minimally inflamed retinal vessels. It leaks through the fenestrated choriocapillaris at a slower rate than fluorescein and slowly impregnates the choroid and is not readily washed out thus delineating the choroid and choroidal lesions. So the clinical interpretation of ICGA is mainly based on the changes in background choroidal fluorescence in pathologic conditions.

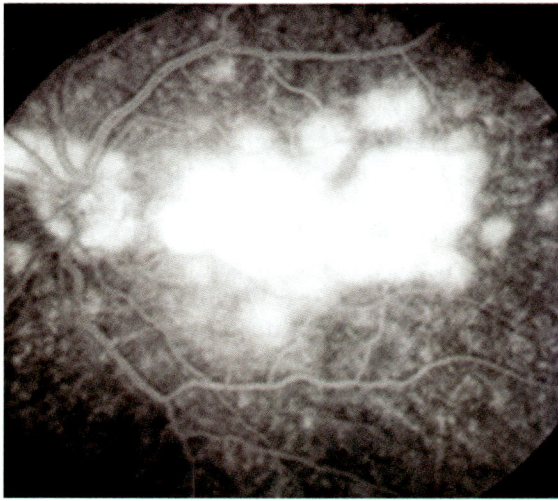

Fig. 18.6: *FFA in APMPPE showing early hypofluorescence and late hyperfluorescence of lesions.*

Phases of ICGA

Three main phases of ICGA have been defined:

1. *Early phase* (up to 3 minutes) characterised by filling of both the choroidal and retinal circulation, seen as superimposed vasculature.
2. *Intermediate phase* (8–12 minutes) characterised by maximum choroidal stromal background fluorescence.
3. *Late phase* (25–30 minutes) characterised by wash-out of dye from the circulation and a relatively dim choroidal background fluorescence.

ICGA in choroidal inflammations

- *Optic disc appears* dark throughout the phases of ICGA.
- *Choroidal vasculitis* may be seen as early stromal vessel hyperfluorescence, but it is best appreciated as fuzziness of choroidal vessels in the intermediate phase ICGA.
- *Hypofluorescent dots* have been described as an ICGA sign of active choroidal inflammation and they disappear after treatment.
- *Because of the infrared fluorescence of the ICG dye,* only heavy pigment deposition, thick blood or subretinal fluid can cause blockage of the background choroidal fluorescence.

Inflammatory choroidal vasculopathy and ICGA

Two types of inflammatory choroidal vasculopathy have been described based on the ICGA patterns.

Type 1 pattern represents *inflammatory choriocapillaropathies* or the white dot syndromes, including APMPPE, serpiginous choroiditis and multifocal choroiditis, where ICGA demonstrates patchy or geographic hypofluorescent areas, which may be associated with choriocapillaris non-perfusion. In multiple evanescent white dot syndrome (MEWDS), ICGA typically shows confluent hypofluorescence around the optic nerve and numerous dark dots throughout the posterior pole, which may not be appreciated on ophthalmoscopy or FA. In MEWDS, it was suggested that early hyperfluorescent lesions on FA associated with intermediate to late hypofluorescence on ICGA could represent RPE damage, while early hypofluorescent lesions on both FA and ICGA could represent perfusion disturbances of choriocapillaris or transient blockage caused by inflammatory lesions at the level of outer retina-RPE (Fig. 18.7).

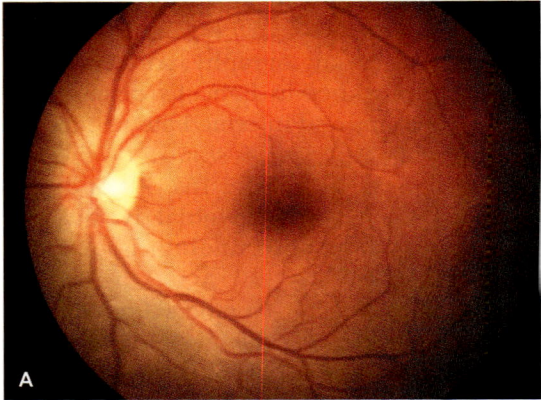

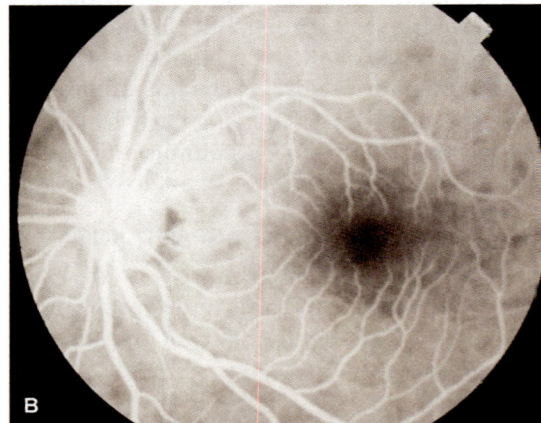

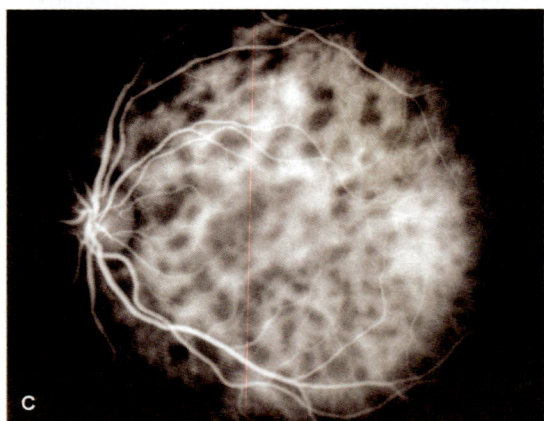

Fig. 18.7: *Fundus photo, (A) FFA; (B) ICG; (C) of a case of MEWDS showing better delineation of choroidal lesions in ICG.*

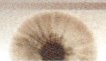

Type 2 pattern represents more diffuse choroiditis with inflamed large vessels appearing fuzzy with the leakage of dye and dark dots associated with inflammatory foci in the choroid. Sympathetic ophthalmia, VKH, birdshot chorioretinopathy, sarcoidosis, tuberculosis and syphilis tend to exhibit the Type 2 pattern. While hypofluorescent dots, best appreciated in the intermediate phase, tend to have a uniform size and distribution in VKH, sympathetic ophthalmia and birdshot chorioretinopathy, a random distribution is usually observed in sarcoidosis and tuberculosis.

Several reports have shown that ICGA revealed choroidal lesions that were not detected by ophthalmoscopy or FA in a variety of chorioretinal inflammatory disorders, including ocular sarcoidosis, ocular tuberculosis, ocular syphilis, ocular toxoplasmosis, sympathetic ophthalmia, VKH disease, multifocal choroiditis, APMPPE, MEWDS, serpiginous choroiditis, the choroidal involvement in birdshot chorioretinopathy, lupus choroidopathy and posterior scleritis. Also, indocyanine green angiography is an adjunct to FFA in the assessment of inflammatory choroidal neovascularisation, especially in eyes with occult membranes.

OPTICAL COHERENCE TOMOGRAPHY

Optical coherence tomography is a non-invasive, non-contact *in vivo* imaging of the retina and the optic nerve head.

Principle

It uses light to acquire high-resolution images of ocular structures. Measurements are obtained by directing a beam of light onto the tissues and measuring the echo time delay and magnitude of reflected or backscattered light using low coherence interferometry. A low-coherence, near-infrared light from a superluminescent diode light source is split into two beams, one goes to a reference mirror and the other to the retina. As the light comes back from the mirror and the eye, it creates an interference pattern, which then is analyzed by a photodetector. Cross-sectional images are generated by scanning the optical beam in the transverse direction, thereby yielding a two-dimensional dataset (B-scan) that can be displayed as a false-colour or grayscale image.

Scan protocol

For an optic nerve head or a macular scan with time domain (TD)-OCT, six radial line scans in a spoke-like pattern are centred on the optic nerve head or the fovea. Higher resolution spectral-domain OCT (SD-OCT) has entered clinical practice with reported resolution of 3–5 µm with improved visualization of retinal morphologic and pathologic features. Spectral-domain OCT technology relies on a spectrometer and high-speed camera and a fixed reference mirror.

Advances in OCT technology have been achieved by exploring ultrahigh-resolution (UHR) OCT, adaptive optics OCT, eye-tracking and Doppler OCT.

OCT interpretation

The currently available SD-OCT allow improved visualization of 4 bright lines in the outer retina, which represent the external limiting membrane (ELM), the photoreceptor inner and outersegment junction (IS/OS), the interdigitation of the photoreceptor outer segments (OS) and the RPE and the RPE-choriocapillary complex. All four layers are diagnostically useful in understanding the pathologies and structural changes of the retina in choroiditis. Integrity of ELM and IS/OS junction are important for vision.

Clinical applications

1. *Macular oedema.* Optical coherence tomography is suitable for detecting and monitoring uveitic macular oedema and provides important information about the type of macular oedema and any abnormality of the vitreoretinal interface. Different types of macular oedema of patients with uveitis are seen, like:

• *Cystoid macular oedema* (CME) with the presence of low reflective intraretinal cystic spaces separated by thin, high-reflective retinal tissue.

• *Diffuse macular oedema (DME)* characterised by increased macular thickness and the presence

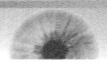

of small low-reflective areas with spongy appearance of the retinal layers.

- *Serous retinal detachment* is seen as a clear separation of the neurosensory retina from the RPE.

Epiretinal membrane (ERM) is an important feature of inflammation, which appears as a hyperreflective line adhering to the retinal layer. OCT also shows concurrent vitreoretinal traction. Higher resolution OCTs can also delineate choroidal layers.

2. Iridocyclitis. A peculiar finding described in eyes with active iridocyclitis using OCT is the occurrence of a ring-like pattern of retinal thickening outside the foveal centre in the inner ring and combined inner and outer rings. The macular thickening has been shown to have a significant correlation with active iridocyclitis.

3. JIA. Macular oedema and/or maculopathy in patients with juvenile idiopathic arthritis associated uveitis has also been observed by OCT.

4. VKH disease. VKH disease is the earliest and most extensively studied by OCT. Early studies involving the use of TD-OCT revealed that serous retinal detachments had two changes in structural patterns, namely, a true serous retinal detachment and an intraretinal fluid accumulation. Based on the observation that the subretinal septa dissolved immediately after pulse corticosteroid therapy, it has been concluded that the subretinal septa were composed of inflammatory products, such as fibrin which acts as a glue between outer segments, forming the membranous structure and the cystoid spaces characteristic of acute VKH disease. The mean choroidal thickness in the acute phase was significantly increased in the acute phase as compared with the convalescent phase of VKH and with normal eye.

5. Sympathetic ophthalmia. In patients with sympathetic ophthalmia (SO), OCT shows serous retinal detachment in the outer segment demarcated by the ELM and RPE, hyperreflective bands indicating fibrous septa within the serous detachment, disruption of the continuity of the RPE and IS/OS junction, and

undulations and bumps on the RPE surface adjacent to the serous retinal detachment. OCT scans of Dalen-Fuchs nodules showed discrete nodules at the level of RPE that were associated with mild shadowing and overlying detachment of the neurosensory retina.

6. Retinochoroidal toxoplasmosis. Vitreoretinal morphology in patients with active ocular toxoplasmosis lesions shows hyperreflectivity of the retina at the site with active lesion and some degree of retinal RPE-choriocapillaris/choroidal optical shadowing. Incongenital toxoplasmosis macular structural changes consist of retinal thinning, RPE hyperreflectivity, excavation, intraretinal cysts and fibrosis.

7. Multifocal choroiditis. OCT shows choroidal and outer retinal involvement and the process extends into the inner retina leading to a circumscribed focal retinal thickening.

8. Serpiginous choroiditis. The acute phase inflammation was limited to the deeper retinal and choroidal structures. There is an increased reflectance of the choroid and deeper retinal layers, along with disruption of the photoreceptor IS/OS junction in both active and inactive lesions.

9. Birdshot chorioretinopathy. OCT (ultra-high resolution) revealed disorganisation of inner retinal layers as well as photoreceptor and RPE atrophy. Decreased visual acuity was shown to be related with abnormal macular thickness and loss of the IS/OS junction, reduction in the total retinal thickness as determined by OCT. Restoration of retinal architecture following therapy has also been described based on OCT.

10. APMPPE. OCT shows hyperreflective area above the RPE in the photoreceptor layer in the early phase of the disease and nodular hyperreflective lesion on the plane of the RPE with mild underlying back scattering in the later phase of the disease.

11. Acute zonal occult outer retinopathy (AZOOR). OCT shows loss or irregularity of the IS/OS junction alone.

12. Multifocal choroiditis and panuveitis (MCP). Patients who had blind spot enlargement

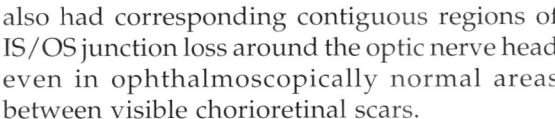

also had corresponding contiguous regions of IS/OS junction loss around the optic nerve head even in ophthalmoscopically normal areas between visible chorioretinal scars.

13. *MEWDS.* OCT described the widespread loss of the IS/OS junction during the acute phases.

14. *Anterior segment OCT (AS-OCT).* An adaptation of OCT technology for better visualisation of the anterior segment has been achieved using longer wavelength light of 1,310 nm as compared with 830 nm used for retinal imaging. Cross-sectional images of the anterior chamber were obtained using anterior segment OCT.

15. *In detecting AC cells in hazy media.* Hyper-reflective spots in the anterior chamber could be quantified. Anterior segment OCT was able to detect anterior chamber cells in eyes with significant corneal oedema.

Limitations

Because the pigmented posterior layer of the iris prevents light transmission beyond this structure, the ciliary body cannot be visualised using anterior segment OCT scans.

ULTRASONOGRAPHY

It is a non-invasive, dynamic imaging modality for rapid evaluation of posterior segment structures in eyes with media opacities that obscures fundal examination. It is a useful adjuvant modality even in eyes with clear media to differentiate between inflammatory and non-inflammatory pathologies of the posterior segment.

Basic principle

The sound wave transmitted from a probe into the eye travels in ocular media of different densities. In ophthalmic ultrasound, both A-scan and B-scan ultrasonography are usually used in combination. A-scan/amplitude scan ultra-sonography is a mono-dimensional scan and shows the distance between surfaces, as well as reflectivity characteristics (high/low reflective). The B-scan/brightness scan ultrasonography gives a two-dimensional cross-section image that shows the location, shape and extension of the lesion. Kinetic B-scan ultrasonography allows real-time assessment of movements of intraocular lesions. A three-dimensional ultrasonography is also possible with newer instruments. The sound reflected back to the probe from the interface of different media is known as an echo. Higher reflectivity produces stronger echo, which is seen as a high spike on the A-scan and brighter dots on the B-scan ultra-sonogram. The sound waves are also absorbed by the media. Dense media absorbs more. Therefore, sound is both reflected and absorbed by dense media resulting in a weaker echo and even shadowing posterior to a dense medium. 10 MHz probe provides useful information on the vitreous cavity, retina, choroid, sclera, optic disc and periocular tissues. 20 MHz probe gives a better resolution and is useful for the evaluation of anterior vitreous cavity and lens.

Clinical applications

- *In the normal eye*, the vitreous is echolucent and the vitreoretinal interface produces a high spike.
- *Vitritis* causes diffusely distributed echoes of low reflectivity, which move freely.
- *Vitreous haemorrhage* produces moderate reflective mobile clump and membrane echoes.
- *Posterior vitreous detachment* is common in eyes with uveitis and appears as a mobile low reflective thin line.
- *Configuration of retinal detachment on ultrasonography* may suggest the underlying pathology. Traction retinal detachment appears as a tented hyperechogenic line (table top configuration) whereas exudative RD shows shifting fluid. Choroidal detachment shows an immobile thick line with higher reflectivity. But they do not appear posterior to equator.
- *Choroiditis.* Peripapillary choroidal thickness is an important measurement in choroiditis/posterior uveitis to understand activity. Choroidal thickening due to diffuse choroiditis has alow to medium reflectivity whereas diffuse posterior scleritis shows high reflective thickening of the posterior wall of the globe.

- There may be widening of the sub-Tenon space due to inflammatory oedema/fluid appearing as an echolucent zone posterior to the thickened wall and the posterior echolucent zone becomes continuous with the optic nerve giving rise to the T sign. It may be evident in diffuse posterior scleritis, sympathetic ophthalmia and VKH.
- *Focal retinochoroidal infiltrates or granulomas* may also be imaged by ultrasonography in the form of localized thickening or focal retinochoroidal elevation.
- *Malignant or benign intraocular tumours* have characteristic ultrasonographic features that differentiate them from inflammatory lesions.
- A high level expertise and quality imaging are essential for the use of ultrasonography as a diagnostic tool.

Limitations

It is an examiner-dependant procedure. Technical skill and experience are important in the performance and interpretation of this imaging modality.

ELECTROPHYSIOLOGICAL TESTS IN UVEITIS

The electrophysiological examination includes the electroretinogram (ERG), visual evoked potentials (VEPs), electrooculogram (EOG), multifocal ERG (mfERG), and multifocal VEPs (mVEPs).

Electroretinogram

- *ERG is an electrophysiological examination* that reflects retinal electrical potential in response to a light stimulus.
- *Wave of ERG.* The a-wave is the first negative wave, and it is followed by the positive b-wave, which is further followed by a second negative wave—the c-wave. d-waves appear, only if the stimulus is applied for sufficient time.
- *Generation of wave.* a-wave is generated by the photoreceptors in the outer retina, b-wave reflects the responses of bipolar and Müller cells in inner retinal layers, c-wave is generated in the retinal pigment epithelium (RPE) and d-wave reflects the activity of 'off' bipolar cells.

- *Evaluation of b:a wave ratio* is used as an index of inner to outer retinal function and the analysis of the waves gives information about the location of a retinal lesion.
- *Amplitudes and implicit times* of the waves are measured in ERG evaluation.
- *Flash ERG* represents the retinal electrical response to photic stimulation.
- *Pattern ERG* (PERG) is generated by a stimulus structure in the form of a black-and-white alternating checkboard or bars on a pattern monitor. The PERG wave consists of three components. The first, a small negative component, is N35, which is followed by a prominent positive component, P50, and finally a large negative component—N95. PERG is used primarily for the evaluation of the function of inner retinal layers and especially the ganglion cell layers of the retina.

Multifocal ERG. mfERG objectively evaluates the macula, allowing functional mapping of the central retina by selecting electrical responses from multiple retinal locations of the macular area, which are tested simultaneously.

Electro-oculography (EOG)

EOG is an electrophysiological test that examines the function of the outer retina and RPE, reflecting metabolic changes in the RPE and giving extra information about retinal function and supporting tissues. It is expressed as a ratio of the peak amplitude in the light to the minimum amplitude in the dark (light/dark or Arden ratio).

Visual evoked potentials

- *VEP is an electrophysiological examination* which objectively reflect the functional integrity of the whole visual pathway, from the photoreceptors in the retina to the visual cortex in the occipital lobe.
- *VEPs are generated* by the electrical activity in the entire visual cortex because of stimulation of the eye.
- *There are three types of stimuli:* The flash, the pattern reversal, and the pattern on/off. VEP examination is useful in the assessment of the visual function in uncooperative patients, in

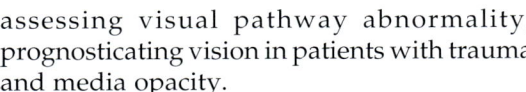

assessing visual pathway abnormality, prognosticating vision in patients with trauma and media opacity.

- *Limitation.* Since VEP reflects the entire visual pathway, an abnormal test does not provide the exact location of the dysfunction and over expression of the macular lesion.

Multifocal VEP. mVEP is an objective electro-physiological examination that evaluates the functional integrity of the visual pathway from the retina to the visual cortex.

Role of electrophysiological examination in posterior uveitis

Electrophysiological examinations have a role in different white dot syndrome entities, VKH, and retinochoroidal toxoplasmosis (Table 18.1).

Table 18.1 *Electrophysiological tests in some posterior uveitis entities*			
Disease	*VEP*	*ERG*	*EOG*
1. MEWDS	In some cases: decrease of P100 amplitude P100 delayed	Acute phase: a- and b-wave amplitude reduced oscillatory potentials abnormal Resolved in recovery. mfERG sensitive indicator for recovery.	Abnormal
2. APMPPE	N/subnormal	Acute phase: Slightly abnormal values of a- and b-wave Recovery: Similar results, contrary to MEWDS	Acute phase: Highly abnormal Scar stage: Significantly improved
3. Birdshot chorio-retinopathy	Selective b-wave amplitude reduction most prominent finding, prolonged implicit times. Late stages: ERGs extinguished. They are useful in monitoring the disease severity and treatment monitoring	Abnormal	
4. Vogt-Koyanagi-Harada	Before treatment: Highly abnormal. During treatment, amplitude and latency initially improve significantly, but amplitude remains significantly decreased compared to normal for at least 1 year	MfERG: Useful test in guiding the therapy and detecting early retinal damage	
5. Behçet's disease	P100 significantly delayed (neuro Behçet, even before clinical signs)	Abnormal	Normal
6. Ocular syphilis	Significantly reduced	Before treatment extinguishing response, after treatment recovery	
7. Fuchs' heterochromic cyclitis		Patterned ERG and flash ERG abnormalities, reduced oscillatory potential amplitude	
8. Toxoplasma retinochoroiditis		Photopic and scotopic ERG abnormal	

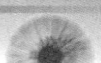

BIBLIOGRAPHY

1. Becker MD, Rosenbaum JT. Essential laboratory tests in uveitis. Dev Ophthalmol 1999;31: 92–108.

2. Centers for Disease Control and Prevention. 2006 sexually transmitted diseases treatment guidelines. MMWR Recomm 2006;55 (RR11):1–85.

3. Chan CC, Shen D, Tuo J. Polymerase chain reaction in the diagnosis of uveitis. Int Ophthalmol Clin 2005;45(2):41–55.

4. Ciardella AP, Borodoker N, Costa DL, et al. Imaging the posterior segment in uveitis. Ophthamol Clin North Am 2002;15:281–96.

5. Kijlstra A. The value of laboratory testing in uveitis. Eye (Lond.) 1990;4(Pt 5):732–6.

6. Mahalakshmi B, Therese KL, Madhavan HN, Biswas J. Diagnostic value of specific local antibody production and nucleic acid amplication technique -Nested polymerase chain reaction (n PCR) in clinically suspected ocular toxo-plasmosis. Ocular Immunology & Inflammation, 1744-5078, Volume 14, Issue 2, 2006, pp. 105–12.

7. Majumder PD, Sudharshan S, Biswas J. Laboratory support in the diagnosis of uveitis. Indian Journal of Ophthalmology 2013;61(6):269–76.

8. Ongkosuwito JV, Bosch-Driessen EH, Kijlstra A, Rothova A. Serologic evaluation of patients with primary and recurrent ocular toxoplasmosis for evidence of recent infection. Am J Ophthalmol 1999;128:407–12.

9. Rosenbaum JT, Wernick R. The utility of routine screening of patients with uveitis for systemic lupus erythematosus or tuberculosis. A Bayesian analysis Arch Ophthalmol 1990;108(9):1291–3.

10. Sandler G. The importance of the history in the medical clinic and the cost of unnecessary tests. Am Heart J 1980;100(6 Pt 1):928–31.

11. Yamamoto S, Pavan-Langston D, Kinoshita S. Detecting herpesvirus DNA in uveitis using the polymerase chain reaction. Br J Ophthalmol 1996; 80:465–8.

Pathological Diagnostic Tests in Uveitis

Chapter Outline

INTRODUCTION
BIOPSY TECHNIQUES USED IN UVEITIS
• Aqueous and vitreous sample

• Iris and ciliary body biopsy
• Chorioretinal biopsy
• Fine needle aspiration biopsy

INTRODUCTION

Examination of a patient with uveitis needs to be very meticulous as the association with systemic autoimmune and infectious diseases is high. Some forms of uveitis, e.g. Fuchs' heterochromic iridocyclitis, serpiginous choroiditis can be diagnosed based on clinical picture alone. Ancilliary tests are also helpful in diagnosing an entity, like HLA-B27 related recurrent anterior uveitis. Importance of biopsy pathology in uveitis lies in certain situations, like Masquerade syndrome:

• Vitreoretinal lymphoma and metastasis
• Intraocular infections
• Undiagnosed, recalcitrant posterior uveitis.

BIOPSY TECHNIQUES USED IN UVEITIS

The following techniques with various modifications have been used in pathological diagnosis of uveitis:[1,2]

• Aqueous and vitreous sample collection
  • Anterior chamber paracentesis (keratocentesis).
  • Diagnostic vitrectomy and vitreous tap.

• Iris and ciliary body biopsy.
• Retinochoroidal biopsy.
• Fine needle aspiration biopsy.

AQUEOUS AND VITREOUS SAMPLE COLLECTION

ANTERIOR CHAMBER PARACENTESIS

Indications

• Masquerade syndrome.
• Hypopyon uveitis.
• Endophthalmitis.
• Lens-induced uveitis.
• Parasitic uveitis.

Technique

Anterior chamber paracentesis is a relatively safe outpatient technique.

Procedure

It should be done under aseptic precautions. Following steps can be followed:

• *Eye is anaesthetised* using topical proparacaine eyedrop for 3 times at 5 minutes interval and an universal eyelid speculum the patient is made to lies supine.

- *Separate the eyelids* and keep the lashes away from the ocular field. An antibiotic drop is instilled just before the procedure.
- *Tuberculin syringe* or 2 cc syringe with a 30 gauge needle is used for the paracentesis. However, if there is a fibrinous reaction in AC, a larger bore needle (25–26 gauge) should be used. In presence of a hypopyon in AC, the needle tip should be kept 1 mm away from the upper margin of the hypopyon.
- *Patient is asked to fixate at the ceiling*. The pupil preferably should be undilated as it reduces the risk of lens touch.
- *Needle is inserted*, bevel down, in an oblique fashion through the onset stroma, near the lower limbus to create a valvular, self-sealing AC entry.
- *One should stay over the peripheral iris tissue* at all times to avoid lenticular or endothelial touch. The plunger is slowly withdrawn to collect 0.1 to 0.3 ml of aqueous.
- *Needle is withdrawn* from the eye, the entry point is massaged with a cotton pledget, a drop of topical povidone iodine is applied
- *Eye* is patched with a sterile dressing, which is removed after 20–30 minutes.
- *Eye* is evaluated for any endothelial or lens touch and AC formation, topical antibiotic eyedrops are prescribed for 3 days and patient is re-evaluated after 1 to 2 weeks.

Complications
- Hyphema
- Endothelial or lens touch
- Wound leak
- Iritis
- Endophthalmitis
- Needle track abscess.

VITREOUS TAP AND DIAGNOSTIC VITREOUS BIOPSY
Indications of vitreous biopsy
Vitreous biopsy is a useful adjunct to the systemic workup of the cases that constitute diagnostic dilemmas and in which intraocular inflammation is mostly confined to the posterior pole.[3] Such cases include:
- Chronic uveitis unresponsive to empirical treatment with systemic anti-inflammatory medications

- Atypical clinical presentation
- Inconclusive non-invasive laboratory workup
- Acute sight-threatening disease
- Endophthalmitis.[4]

Techniques
A vitreous specimen can be obtained by: Vitreous aspiration or pars plana vitrectomy.

Technique of vitreous aspiration
Vitreous aspiration can even be done in an office setting. As perforation of sclera is painful, the procedure is done using subconjunctival anaesthesia, by injecting 0.1 ml of 2% lignocaine over the area of needle insertion. 25 G needle is mostly used in uveitic eyes as the vitreous is liquefied due to the inflammation. In case of organised vitreous, 23 G needle can be used. The needle is attached to a 2 cc syringe along with a stopcock (Fig. 19.1). The needle is inserted 3.5 mm away from the limbus in a phakic eye and 3 mm in a pseudophakic/aphakic eye. 0.1–0.3 ml of vitreous is withdrawn in the

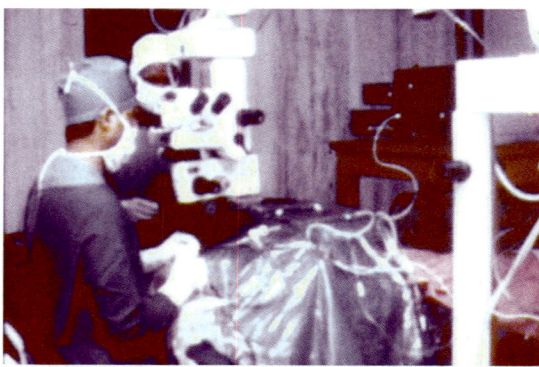

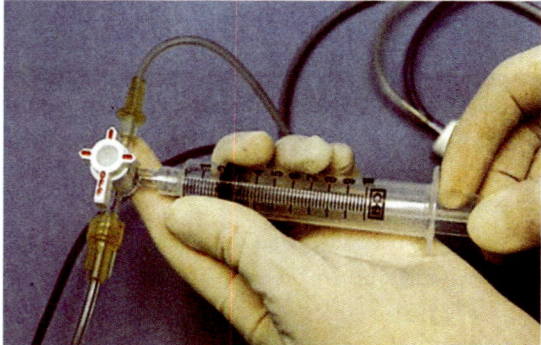

Fig. 19.1: *Vitreous biopsy sample being obtained using three-way stop-cock.*

syringe and manipulating the stopcock, an equal amount of antibiotic is injected.

Complications include:
- Retinal tear
- Refinal detachment
- Vitreous haemorrhage
- Endophthalmitis.

Diagnostic pars plana vitrectomy

The procedure can be done under either general or topical anaesthesia. For vitreous aspiration, the one-port technique can be used. However, in eyes with uveitis, where there can be coexistent media opacities or intraocular inflammation, the three-port technique is preferable. Balanced salt solution (BSS) infusion is used to control the intraocular pressure during the procedure. Control of the pressure can minimise the risk of severe intraoperative hypotony as well as choroidal detachments and expulsive haemorrhage, all of which are more common in eyes with uveitis.[3] However, in diagnostic vitrectomy, the initial vitreous specimen is obtained undiluted (before the infusion port is opened); approximately 1.0 ml of vitreous is obtained directly from the vitrectomy cutter handpiece, with a cutting rate at 1200/minute, through an in-line stopcock and tubing attached to a syringe.[3,5,6] The infusion line is subsequently opened, and a standard, total vitrectomy is performed. Effort is taken to remove as much of the vitreous body as possible by harvesting material from all areas of the fundus including with scleral indentation.[3] Both the undiluted vitreous specimen and the vitreous washings from the subsequent total vitrectomy should be delivered immediately for cytopathological and microbiological analysis.[5,6]

Handling aqueous and vitreous samples

The following tests can be done using an aqueous or vitreous sample.

Microbiological analysis

The aqueous or vitreous specimen can be used for:
- Gram stain
- KOH staining
- Culture.

Smears and stains. The smears and stains are very useful for rapid initial diagnosis of endophthalmitis but their role is limited. Gram stain is positive in 66% of culture proven cases.

However, positive smears can help the clinician choose the appropriate antibiotic for the organism before the results from the cultures are available.

Culture. Routinely, the culture media used for inoculation include blood agar, chocolate agar, thioglycollate broth, brain heart infusion agar, sabouraud dextrose agar, BHIB with gentamicin.

In case of vitreous specimen, cultures can be performed in both diluted and undiluted vitreous. Undiluted samples can be used directly for cultures or smears. Vitreous washings are initially passed through millipore filters. During filtration, microorganisms or any cellular elements concentrate on the filter surface. The filter is then cut under sterile conditions and used for culture.

Bacterial cultures should be kept for 5–14 days, if the presence of a slowly growing anaerobic bacterium (i.e. *Propionibacterium acnes*) is suspected.

Sensitivity of vitreous cultures has been estimated to be 50% and is much higher than that of aqueous.[7] Processing both diluted and undiluted vitreous increases the sensitivity of vitreous cultures to 57.4%.[8]

Molecular biologic study: Polymerase chain reaction

This technique amplifies a specific locus on a DNA sample from a complex mixture of DNA. Approximately 0.05 ml of the sample should be preserved for this test, if viral infection, infectious or *P. acnes* endophthalmitis is suspected.

Nested PCR. In this technique, 2 pairs of primers are used for the same locus. If one locus gets wrongly amplified by a primer, there is very little chance it will get amplified by the second primer, so the proper locus only gets amplified, thus increasing the specificity of the procedure.[2]

Real-time PCR. In this technique, the load of the DNA copies is quantified in real-time by assessing the increasing fluorescence of a detector. So it allows both detection and quantification of a gene locus, thus giving evidence of active multiplication of an organism. Figure 19.2 demonstrates PCR test in a patient with chronic granulomatous uveitis.

Cytological analysis

The entire specimen is spinned down, the supernatant transpipetted, the pellet is resuspended in formalin or glutaraldehyde and then passed through 2 millipore filters. These filters can be used for staining including immunohisto-chemistry. Cytospin method can also be used[15] which involves the use of cytospin slides that are cleaned with alcohol and assembled with a slide filter card and sample delivery chamber, secured by a metal clip. Typically, up to 0.4 ml of fluid sample (3–5 drops) is added to the chamber together with an equal amount of cytospin collection fluid. After spinning at 1800 rpm for 2 minutes, slides are removed from the cytospin chamber, further fixed in cytology fixative (70% alcohol/formalin), and stained with haematoxylin and eosin.

Certain important findings on cytology are given below:

Aqueous aspirate

- *Phacogenic uveitis:* Macrophages engulfing lens particles, chronic inflammatory cells (Fig. 19.3)
- *Parasitic uveitis:* Eosinophils, polymorphs, sometimes parasite (Fig. 19.4)
- *Masquerade syndrome:* Malignant cells.

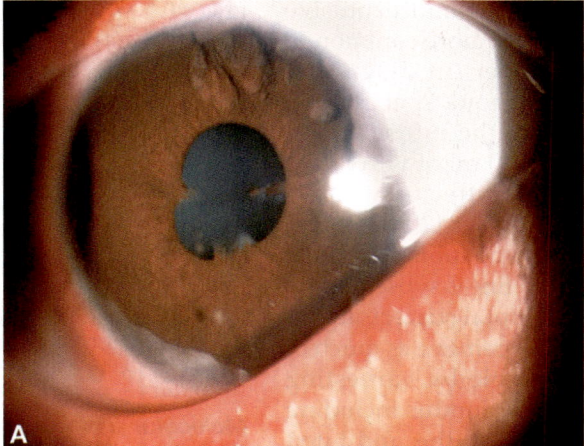

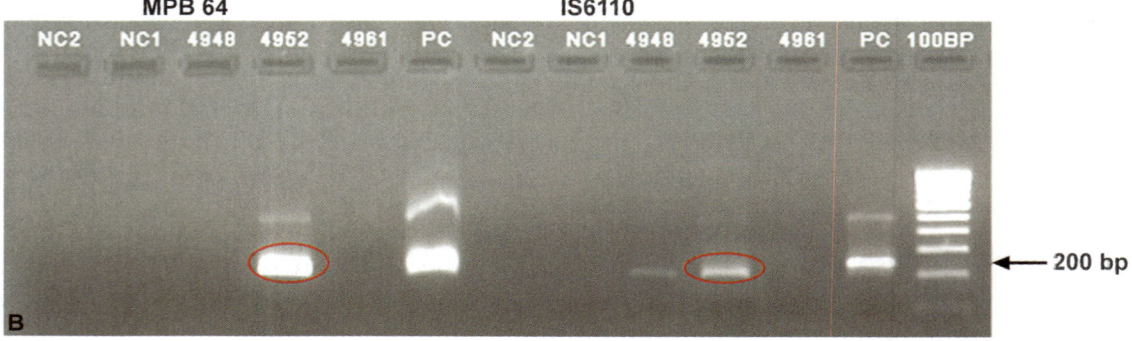

Fig. 19.2: *A, Clinical photograph of a patient with chronic granulomatous anterior uveitis with mutton fat KPs, broad posterior synechiae and peripheral anterior synechiae; B, PCR from aqueous tap positive for MPB64 and IS6110 genome confirming diagnosis of tuberculosis (PC: Positive control, 4962: Specimen well).*

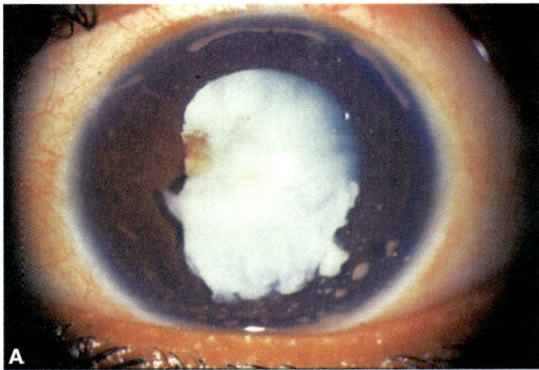

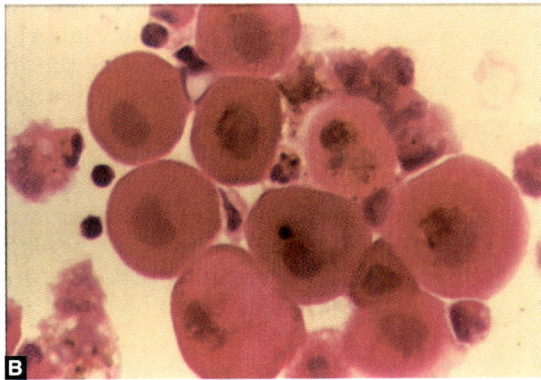

Fig. 19.3: *(A) Granulomatous anterior uveitis in a case of traumatic cataract with ruptured anterior lens capsule; (B) AC tap showing macrophages with engulfed lens matter.*

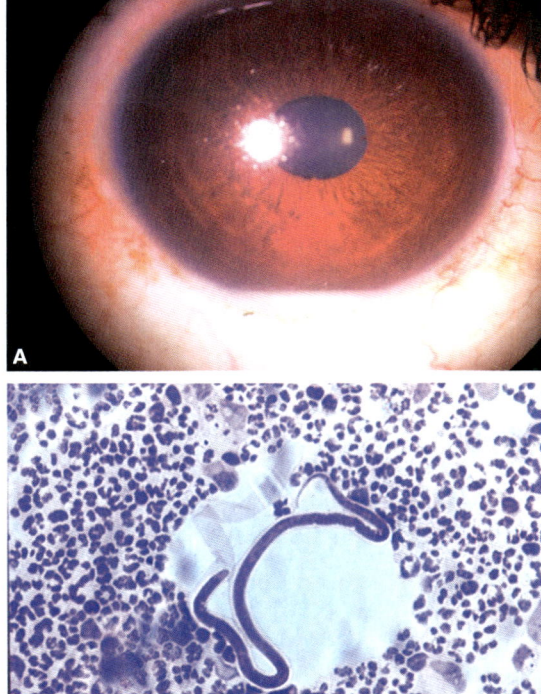

Fig. 19.4: *(A) Hypopyon in anterior uveitis, not responding to topical steroid therapy; (B) AC tap showing microfilaria along with chronic inflammatory cells.*

Vitreous aspirate

- *Large cell lymphoma:* Large pleomorphic cells with round to oval nuclei with scanty cytoplasm, often with micronuclei (Fig. 19.5)
- *Phacoanaphylactic uveitis:* Lens fragments engulfed by macrophages, surrounded by epitheloid cells and giant cells
- *Uveitis:* Heterogenous inflammatory infiltrate.

Antibody detection

The supernatant obtained after centrifugation can be used for antibody detection by ELISA. This is specially useful for conditions, like toxoplasma or toxocara. The ocular antibody production should be analysed using Goldmann-Witmer coefficient.[9]

GW coefficient = Titre of aqueous antibody in serum globulin × Titre of serum antibody in aqueous globulin.

GW coefficient:
- 0.5–2 = No ocular infection
- 2–4 = Probable ocular infection
- > 4 = Diagnostic of ocular infection.

Flow cytometric analysis

This technique analyses the physical and chemical properties of particles or cells moving in a single file in a fluid stream. This technique is specially applicable for analysis of tumours, like retinoblastoma, leukaemia, lymphoma to give an idea about the variation in cell population in the tumuors. This is used as an adjunct to histopathologic examination. Also, at present, ratio between cytotoxic and helper T cells is used to analyse the pathology of ocular inflammation. In a study, CD22+ lymphocyte >20% in the cell population as found by flow cytometric analysis had a positive predictive value of 100% in diagnosis of intraocular lymphoma. A ratio of

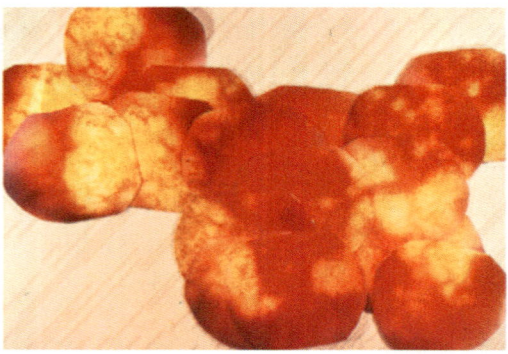

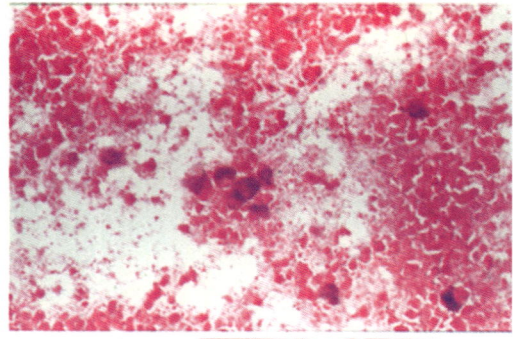

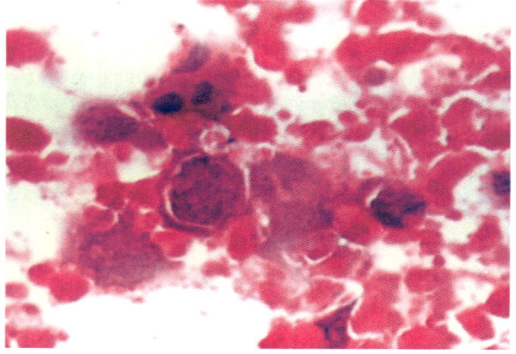

Fig. 19.5: *Colour fundus photograph of a 57-year-old female patient showing subretinal mass (at top). Vitreous biopsy showed large, pleomorphic cells with scanty cytoplasm in a necrotic background suggestive of large cell lymphoma.*

IL10/IL6 of >1 was found to have a sensitivity of 74.3% and specificity of 75% from vitreous biopsy in a study.[10]

IRIS AND CILIARY BODY BIOPSY

Indications

Indications are limited and include the following:
- Metastatic nodules or primary tumours of iris/ciliary body masquerading uveitis.
- Ruptured iris or ciliary body cysts.
- Granulomatous lesions of iris/ciliary body as seen in tuberculosis, sarcoidosis, certain fungal infection, like coccidioidomycosis to confirm the diagnosis.

Technique

A safe procedure has been described.[11] The *punch biopsies* can be performed as an ambulatory procedure under local anaesthesia. A clear corneal incision with a 3.2 mm angled slit knife is made close to the iris lesion. A viscoelastic is injected to fill the anterior chamber. A Kelly Descemet's membrane punch with a 1.0 mm diameter head and a 0.75 mm deep bite is inserted into the anterior chamber to lie over the iris lesion. The Kelly punch is placed with its mouth over the lesion and pressed down firmly before the punch is made. After taking a punch, the Kelly punch is kept closed and removed from the eye to be opened over a dry cellulose sponge. The viscoelastic is left in the anterior chamber. For a ciliary body biopsy, similar procedure can be used with the aid of visualisation by a direct goniolens.

Complications

Bleeding, rise of IOP due to retained viscoelastic, corneal endothelial touch, exacerbation of inflammation.

Advantages

- FNAB, though can be used for solid tumours in this area, it actually yields an aspirate for cytopathology rather than a tissue sample. Punch biopsy yields a tissue sample enabling both histologic and cytopathologic evaluation as well as architecture and level of infiltration.
- The tissue is also sufficient for special stains to aid in diagnosis.
- This technique also does not require much surgical expertise.

CHORIORETINAL BIOPSY

With the advent of new imaging systems, most of the choroidal lesions can be characterized. However, in atypical cases and in suspected intraocular lymphoma where vitreous biopsy comes negative, this technique has a role. Indications include:
- To exclude potential intraocular neoplasms (Masquerade syndrome, e.g. intraocular

lymphoma), which are primarily localised to the retina or choroid.

- To identify infective agents in progressive retinitis/retinal necrosis (e.g. atypical toxoplasmosis).
- To identify a causative organism or neoplasm in immunocompromised patients with uveitis.
- To aid in the diagnosis of uveitis with progressive sight-threatening chorioretinal lesions unresponsive to treatment.

Technique

Choroidal/chorioretinal biopsy can be done through an external or trans-scleral approach or an internal (Fig. 19.6) or transvitreal approach.

External approach

The surgical technique for performing an external chorioretinal biopsy is fairly straight

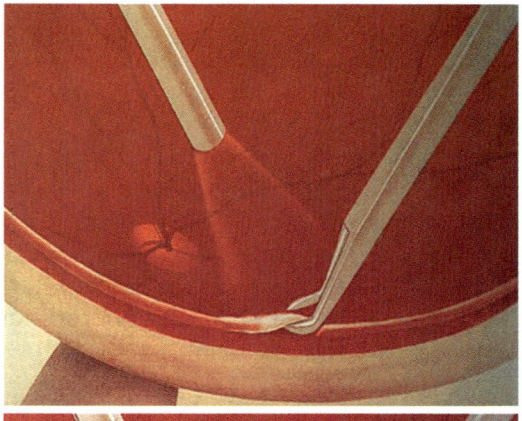
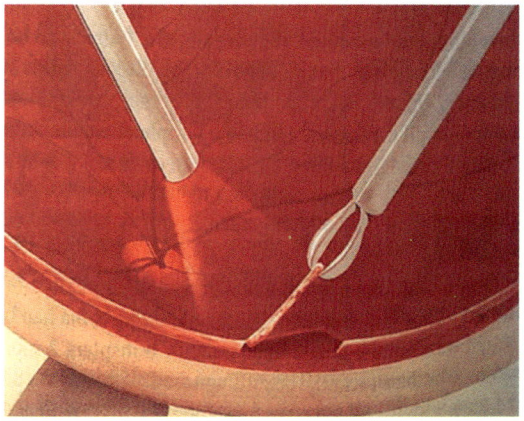

Fig. 19.6: *Technique of chorioretinal biopsy through internal approach.*

forward.[12,13] First, provided that the fundus is clearly visible, laser photocoagulation is applied 1–3 days before surgery in a zone of the area to be biopsied. If the vitreous is too hazy, endolaser is placed immediately following vitrectomy. After a 360° conjunctival incision and isolation and tying of the rectus muscles, a three-port pars plana vitrectomy is performed (in addition to endolaser application in the area to be biopsied, if it was not placed prior to the surgery). The vitreous specimen (dilute and undilute) is sent for cytologic, microbiologic or flow cytometry analysis as required. A nearly full-thickness scleral flap is made, leaving one side attached to act as a hinge. When the flap of sclera is retracted, the surgeon is able to visualize the choroids, which is practically bare. Next, a penetrating diathermy is placed through the choroid and retina along the outer margin of the inner choroidal bed. Two incisions parallel to the limbus are made. Next, by inserting one blade of a 0.12 forceps through the incision, the full thickness of the choroid and retina may be grasped at one edge. Then, two more incisions, perpendicular to the limbus, are made with Vannas scissors, thereby yielding a block of chorioretinal tissue. Extreme care should be taken to grasp the full-thickness tissue only once with the forceps so that the architecture of the tissue remains intact. The scleral flap is then closed over the wound and is sutured closed followed by fluid-gas exchange.

Internal approach

Transvitreal retinochoroidal (endoretinal) biopsy is another approach by which chorioretinal tissue is acquired.[12,13] Briefly, in this technique, a standard three-port vitrectomy is performed (sending undiluted and diluted vitreous sample to the pathology lab for analysis) with endodiathermy used to outline an area of retina that is of interest. Intraocular scissors are introduced into the vitreous space and a small hole is created in the retina such that the area of interest is excised. With intraocular forceps, the retinal tissue is brought to the opening for the vitrector and is gently drained out of the eye using intraocular irrigation. In case of a retinal detachment, the

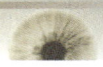

specimen should be taken from the margin of attached and detached retina. Cassoux et al.[14] also devised a technique of subretinal injection of sodium hyaluronate to induce a localized retinal detachment to collect the tissue specimen from the area of interest. The resultant bulging retina was subsequently excised by cutting around the perimeter with scissors and extricating the biopsy with forceps. Endolaser was then applied around the biopsy site.

Handling the specimen

The biopsy tissue is immediately processed by an ophthalmic pathologist in the operating room. It is generally divided into three portions. One-third of the tissue is fixated for routine histopathologic studies, including light and electron microscopic examinations. The second portion is snap frozen in optimal cutting temperature (OCT) embedding compound and is used for immunopathologic and molecular characterization. The third portion is sent for culture with the preference for viral and other microorganisms cultures and/or tissue culture. Sometimes, enough tissue may not be available for dividing in three parts and analysing. In that case, a frozen section analysis should at least be performed.

FINE NEEDLE ASPIRATION BIOPSY (FNAB)

Indications

Indications for FNAB are following:
- Cases of suspected infectious subretinal lesions mimicking as choroidal tumours
- Patients with metastatic disease of choroid where primary is not known
- Cases where patient refuses recommended therapy until histopathological confirmation is obtained.

Technique

Limbal route is used to approach anteriorly located lesions, like iris lesion.

For posterior segment lesions, two routes are available:
- *Pars plana approach.* In this approach, the needle is inserted through pars plana (3.5 mm from limbus) in the quadrant opposite to the lesion and passed through the vitreous to

reach the lesion. For posteriorly located tumours, vitrectomy needs to be performed before aspiration.
- *Corneolimbal approach.* This technique is used in tumours with high-risk of dissemination through needle track, e.g. retinoblastoma. The needle is passed through the limbus, then through the zonules to reach the vitreous. As it passes through multiple planes, the tumour cells are removed as the needle is removed from the eye.

Points to be remembered for biopsy in a case of intraocular lymphoma:[15]

- To stop the steroids before the diagnostic procedure to increase the yield
- If a distinct mass lesion is there, biopsy from it is always preferable than do a vitreous tap
- Vitreous tap may come negative due to apoptosis and degeneration of the lymphoma cells and due to increased inflammatory cell population. Doing a cytokine profile or cell culture can be considered in such cases.

Complications

- Bleeding from the needle track
- Dissemination of tumour cells, though rare, can happen
- Iatrogenic retinal perforation. In fact, when a choroidal lesion is biopsied in this technique, it is unavoidable and theoretically can cause a retinal detachment. But practically, the break is very small and it gets clogged by the blood clot from the underlying choroid.

REFERENCES

1. Van der Lelij A, Rothova A. Diagnostic anterior chamber paracentesis in uveitis: a safe procedure? The British Journal of Ophthalmology 1997; 81(11):976–9.
2. Biswas J, Annamalai R, Krishnaraj V. Biopsy pathology in uveitis. Middle East African Journal of Ophthalmology 2011;18:261–7.
3. Jeroudi A, Yeh S. Diagnostic vitrectomy for infectious uveitis. International Ophthalmology Clinics. 2014;54173–97.
4. Forster R, Abbott R, Gelender H. Management of infectious endophthalmitis. Ophthalmology 1980; 87:313–9.

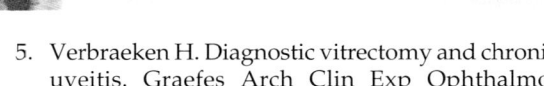

5. Verbraeken H. Diagnostic vitrectomy and chronic uveitis. Graefes Arch Clin Exp Ophthalmol 1996;234:2–7.
6. Bovey EH, Herbort CP. Vitrectomy in the management of uveitis. Ocul Immunol Inflamm 2000;8:285–91.
7. Savitri S, Subhadra J, Muralidhar V, et al. Sensitivity and predictability of vitreous cytology, biopsy and membrane filter culture in endophthalmitis. Retina 1996;16:525–9.
8. Donahue SP, Kowalski RP, Jewart BH, Friberg TR. Vitreous cultures in suspected endophthalmitis. Biopsy or vitrectomy? Ophthalmology. 1993; 100:1597–8.
9. Garweg JG, de Groot-Mijnes JD, Montoya JG. Diagnostic approach to ocular toxoplasmosis. Ocular Immunology and Inflammation. 2011;19255–61.
10. Wolf LA, Reed GF, Buggage RR, et al. Vitreous cytokine levels. Ophthalmology 2003;110(8): 1671–2.
11. Pe'er J, Blumenthal EZ, Frenkel S. Punch biopsy of iris lesions: a novel technique for obtaining histology samples. The British Journal of Ophthalmology 2007;91660–2.
12. Nussenblatt RB, Davis JL, Palestine AG. Chorioretinal biopsy for diagnostic purposes in cases of intraocular inflammatory disease. Dev Ophthalmol 1992;23:133–8.
13. Martin DF, Chan CC, de Smet MD, et al. The role of chorioretinal biopsy in the management of posterior uveitis. Ophthalmology 1993;100:705–14.
14. Cassoux N, Charlotte F, Rao NA, et al. Endoretinal biopsy in establishing the diagnosis of uveitis: a clinicopathologic report of three cases. Ocul Immunol Inflamm 2005;1379–83.
15. Finger PT, Papp C, Latkany P, Kurli M, Iacob CE. Anterior chamber paracentesis cytology (cytospin technique) for the diagnosis of intraocular lymphoma. The British Journal of Ophthalmology 2006;90:690–2.

Section

V

Clinical Evaluation and Investigations for Disorders of Ocular Motility

20. Evaluation of a Case of Strabismus and Orthoptic Instruments
21. Evaluation and Investigations in Paralytic Squint
22. Evaluation and Investigations of a Case of Nystagmus

Evaluation of a Case of Strabismus and Orthoptic Instruments

Chapter Outline

EVALUATION OF A CASE OF STRABISMUS

History, vision evaluation and preliminary examination

History

Vision evaluation

Preliminary examination

- Inspection
- Pupillary reactions
- Media and fundus examination
- Refraction

Motor evaluation

Cover tests

- Direct cover test
- Cover-uncover test
- Alternate cover test

Quantitative measurement of angle of deviation

- Bruckner pupillary red reflex test
- Hirschberg corneal reflex test
- Prism and alternate cover test
- Prism reflex test (Krimsky's test)
- Perimeter method
- Maddox rod test
- Synoptophore method
- Double prism test
- Haploscopic test

Assessment of ocular movements

- Ductions
- Versions
- Vergences

Assessment of accommodation and AC/A ratio

- Heterophoria method
- Gradient method

- Fixation disparity method
- Haploscopic methods

Assessment for extraocular muscle paresis

- Diplopia charting
- Quantitative measurement of action of extraocular muscles
  - Lancaster red-green test
  - Hess screen test
  - Lees screen test
- Field of binocular fixation
- Bielschowsky's phenomenon test
- Bielschowsky's head tilt test

Sensory evaluation: Assessment for binocular cooperation and sensory anomalies

- Tests for fixation behaviour
- Tests for the state of retinal correspondence
- Assessment for grades of binocular single vision
- Tests to assess suppression and amblyopia

ORTHOPTIC INSTRUMENTS

Conventional orthoptic instruments

- Synoptophore
- Livingston binocular gauge
- Visuscope
- Euthyscope

Computer-based orthoptic programs

- Computerised orthoptic diagnostic programs
- Computer-based vision therapy and neurovision therapy programs
- Computer-based combined diagnostic and therapeutic programs

EVALUATION OF A CASE OF STRABISMUS

To avoid repetition, the subject of evaluation is discussed even before the clinical description of different varieties of the squint. Though the list of tests is exhaustive, all of these may not be required in every case. An experienced strabismologist chooses a set of tests to be performed in a particular patient.

Main components of evaluation of a case of strabismus are:

I. *History, vision evaluation and preliminary examination*
- History
- Vision evaluation
- Preliminary examination

II. *Motor evaluation*
- *Head posture evaluation*
- *Evaluation for ocualr deviation*
  - Cover tests
  - Corneal reflex tests
  - Subjective tests for measurement of deviation
  - Measurement for cyclodeviation
- Assessment for ocular movements
  - Evaluation of duction
  - Evaluation of version
  - Evaluation of vergence
- Assessment of accommodation, and AC/A ratio
- Assessment for extraocular muscle paresis

III. *Sensory evaluation*
- Tests for fusion
- Tests for binocularity and diplopia
- Tests for fixation
- Tests for status of retinal correspondence
- Tests for suppression and amblyopia
- Tests for stereopsis.

In general, for a systematic evaluation, following approach may be adopted.

HISTORY, VISION EVALUATION AND PRELIMINARY EXAMINATION

HISTORY

A detailed and meticulous history taking before beginning the examination is very important in the management of a case of squint. A complete history taken should contain the following information:

1. *Age of the patient*

2. *History of present illness.* Information about deviation of eye should include:
- Time when first noticed. It is desirable to document the age of onset of deviation or symptoms. All available old photographs of the child are invaluable for this purpose.
- Onset, sudden or gradual.
- Constant or intermittent deviation.
- Unilateral or alternating deviation.
- If alternating, which eye more frequently fixates (dominating eye).
- Alleged cause, if any, such as trauma, illness, psychologic disturbance, change in occupation, increase in close work, etc.
- Abnormal head posture (ask to demonstrate).
- Associated symptoms such as diplopia, blurred vision, headache, asthenopia.
- Any histroy of closing or covering one eye in bright light indicates intermittent squint.

3. *Birth history.* It is specially important in cases of childhood onset deviations. Enquiry should be made regarding:
- Problems during pregnancy
- Problems during delivery.

4. *Family history.* History regarding any of the following disorders in grandparents, parents, siblings or even in uncles, aunts and cousins is important:
- Strabismus
- Refractive errors
- Lazy eye
- Other ocular defects.

5. *Past history*
- General ill health
- Any systemic disease
- Any ocular defect.

6. *History of previous treatment*
  a. *Optical treatment*
  - *When and how long?*
  - *Were glasses worn constantly?*
  - *Effect of glasses on the deviation.*
  - *Date of last refraction.*

b. *Orthoptic treatment.*
- *Occlusion.* Type, when, how long, effect on vision.
- *Exercises.* When, type, how long, effect on deviation.

c. *Surgical treatment*
- *When performed?*
- *Eye operated: Right, left or both.*
- *Muscle touched: Medial, lateral or both (if known).*
- *Patient's/parents' opinion about the result of surgery.*

VISION EVALUATION

Testing of visual acuity of each eye separately is critical in evaluation of any patient with strabismus. Visual acuity should be tested without glasses and with glasses (if worn); and for near and distance vision.

Methods of testing visual acuity in infants, preschool age children and in schoolage children as well as adults have been described in Chapter 2. However, for a ready reference, these are enumerated below:

Methods of estimating visual acuity in infants
1. Fixation behaviour test
2. Preferential looking test
3. Optokinetic nystagmus
4. Visually evoked response
5. CSM method.

Methods of estimating visual acuity in preschool-age children
1. Marble game test
2. Hand chart
3. Illiterate E-game test
4. Allen's preschool vision test
5. Sheridan-Gardiner test.

Methods of estimating visual acuity in schoolage children and adults
1. Snellen's test types
2. E-chart
3. Landolt's broken-C chart.

Visual acuity in patients with nystagmus. In patients with nystagmus, visual acuity may be better with both eyes open than with one eye occluded. In order to assess this situation, it may be helpful to place a +5.00D sphere lens in front of the eye not being tested, and then reverse this in order to test the other eye.

PRELIMINARY EXAMINATION

Inspection

Large degree squint (convergent or divergent) is obvious on inspection.

Epicanthus, when observed in infants, may be the cause of pseudoesotropia.

Facial asymmetries may also create the impression of pseudostrabismus especially hypertropia.

Abnormal head posture (AHP) when present, becomes obvious during initial inspection of the patient. Infact observation for AHP should always be made without any instructions to the patient, otherwise a lot of information may be lost after the patient becomes concious of being examined. As described in detail in Chapter 2, observation should be made for all the three components of head posture, i.e.
- *Chin* elevation or depression (vertical component)
- *Face turn* to right or left (horizontal component)
- *Head tilt* to right or left shoulder (torsional component).

Interpupillary distance (IPD) should also be inspected and measured. Unusually, narrow IPD may be the cause of pseudoesotropia and an exceptionally wide IPD may be a cause of pseudoexotropia.

Inspection during pen light examination may sometimes erroneously reveal strabismus owing to presence of a large angle kappa. A large positive angle kappa may be a cause of pseudoexotropia and a large negative angle kappa may be a cause of pseudoesotropia.

Pupillary reactions

Light reflexes may be abnormal in patients with sensory deviations due to diseases of retina and optic nerve.

Media and fundus examination

It may reveal associated diseases of the ocular media, retina or optic nerve.

Refraction

It is most important, because a refractive error may be responsible for the symptoms of the patient or for the deviation itself. Though, mentioned in the beginning, in practice, refraction is performed after complete squint check-up. Preferably, refraction should be performed under full cycloplegia especially in children. The commonly used cycloplegics are as follows:

1. *Atropine* is indicated in children below the age of 7 years. It is used as 1% ointment thrice daily for 3 consecutive days before performing retinoscopy. Its effect lasts for 10–20 days.

2. *Homatropine* is used as 2% drops. One drop is often instilled every 10 minutes for 6 times and the retinoscopy is performed after 1 to 2 hours. Its effect lasts for 24–28 hours. It is used for most of the hypermetropic individuals between 7 and 35 years of age.

3. *Cyclopentolate* is a short-acting cycloplegic. Its effects last for 6 to 18 hours. It is used as 1% eyedrops in patients between 7 and 35 years. One drop of cyclopentolate is instilled every 10 minutes for 3 times (Havener's recommended dose) and the retinoscopy is performed 1 to 1½ hours later after estimating the residual accommodation, which should not exceed one dioptre.

MOTOR EVALUATION

EVALUATION FOR OCULAR DEVIATION

COVER TESTS

Prerequisites for cover tests

- Patient should be cooperative enough to fixate a target
- Should have sufficient vision to see the target
- Should have central fixation in both eyes
- Latent nystagmus should not be present.

Methods of cover tests

The cover tests should be performed with and without glasses at distance (6 m) and at near (33 cm). The patient is asked to fixate a 6/12 visual acuity symbol or any object that keeps patient's attention, such as a small picture or a toy (especially in small children), with one eye. This is to prevent the use of accommodation, when torch light is used (which is a common practice). The other eye is then covered with the help of an occluder or palm of the hand. The interpretations are made as described below.

Direct cover test

Aim. *To confirm the presence of a manifest squint.*

Procedure. To perform this test, patient is first asked to fixate (Fig. 20.1) a point with both eyes open. The normal looking eye is covered while observing the movement of the uncovered eye. In the presence of manifest squint, the uncovered eye will move in the opposite direction to take fixation. For example, when an exotropia is present, the eye taking up fixation will move towards nose and in the presence of esotropia, it will move towards the temple.

No movement of the uncovered eye on covering the seemingly fixating eye indicates any of the following:

- No squint (pseudostrabismus)
- Gross eccentric fixation (there may be very small or no movement of redress in the uncovered deviated eye)
- No vision in the deviated uncovered eye.

Cover-uncover test

Aim. *To establish the presence and type of heterophoria (latent deviation).*

Procedure (Fig. 20.2). It is performed, when direct cover test has established that no manifest

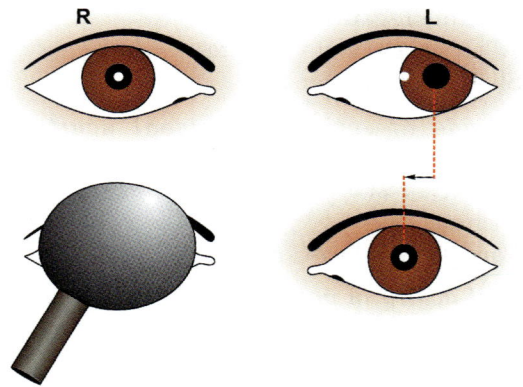

Fig. 20.1: *Direct cover test depicting left exotropia.*

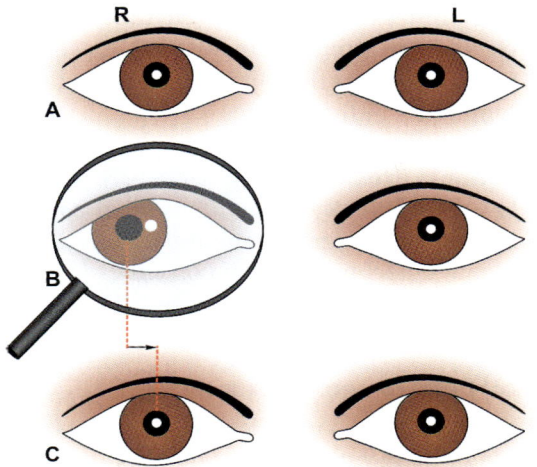

Fig. 20.2: *Cover-uncover test depicting exophoria. Note orthophoria in primary position (A) and immediate inward movement of right eye on removal of the cover (B and C).*

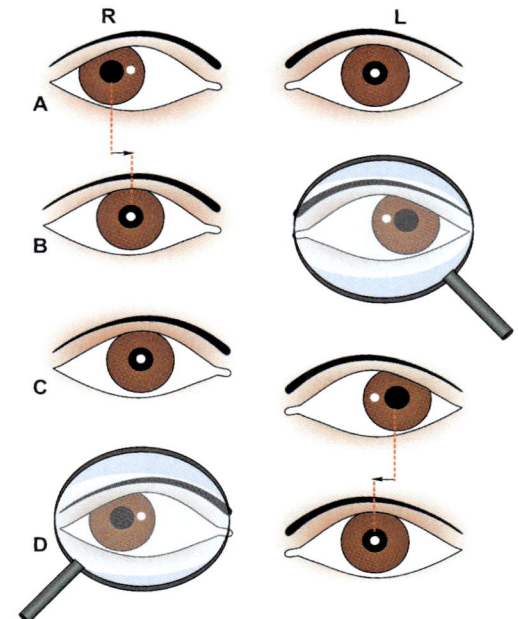

Fig. 20.3: *Alternate cover test depicting alternate exotropia.*

deviation is present. To perform it, one eye is covered with an occluder and the other is made to fixate an object. In the presence of heterophoria, the eye under cover will deviate (since covering one eye of a patient with normal binocular vision interrupts fusion). After a few seconds, the cover is quickly removed and the movement of the eye (which was under cover) is observed. Direction of the movement of the eyeball tells the type of heterophoria (e.g. the eyeball will move towards the nose in the presence of exophoria and towards the temple in the presence of esophoria) and the speed of movement tells whether recovery is slow or rapid.

Alternate cover test

Aim. To *establish whether the squint is unilateral or alternate* and also to *differentiate concomitant squint from paralytic squint* (where secondary deviation is greater than primary deviation).

Procedure (Fig. 20.3). To perform this test, patient is asked to fixate an object alternately with each eye. It is important to place occluder alternately in front of each eye several times to dissociate the eyes and to maximize the deviation. Further, the occluder should be quickly transferred from one eye to other to prevent fusion from occurring. Observations made are as follows: In the presence of an alternate squint, either eye fixates and the opposite eye under cover deviates and maintains the position of deviation on removing the cover; but in the presence of a unilateral squint, after removal of the cover, always the normal looking eye takes up fixation and the squinting eye deviates.

To differentiate concomitant squint from paralytic squint, observation about the degree of deviation in the eye under cover is made while performing the alternate cover test. In concomitant squint, primary deviation is equal to secondary deviation (deviation of the normal eye under cover); while in paralytic squint, secondary deviation is much more than the primary deviation.

Limitations of cover tests

Following deviations may be either overlooked or cannot possibly be diagnosed with cover tests:

- A small heterophoria
- A small angle esotropia (of less than 5$^\Delta$)
- A microtropia
- A monofixation syndrome
- A cyclodeviation.

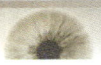

QUANTITATIVE MEASUREMENT OF ANGLE OF DEVIATION

Various methods for quantitative measurement of angle of deviation can be grouped as under:

Objective tests for heterotropia
- Hirschberg corneal reflex test
- Prism and cover test (prism bar cover test)
- Prism reflex test (Krimsky's corneal reflex test)
- Synoptophore test
- Perimeter method.

Subjective tests for heterotropia
- Maddox rod test
- Synoptophore test
- Diplopia test
- Hess/Lees screen test.

Objective tests for heterophoria
- Prism and cover test.

Subjective tests for heterophoria
- Maddox rod test
- Maddox wing test
- Double prism test.

Tests based on corneal reflex
- Hirschberg corneal reflex test
- Prism and cover test (prism bar cover test)
- Prism reflex test (Krimsky's corneal reflex test)
- Perimeter method
- Synoptophore method
- Bruckner test.

Dissimilar image tests
- Maddox rod test for heterophoria or heterotropia
- Double Maddox rod test for cyclodeviations
- Red glass test.

Dissimilar target tests
- Major amblyoscope test
- Lancaster red-green projection test
- Hess screen test.

Bruckner pupillary red reflex test

This is a screening test and does not measure the size of deviation. It is performed with the help of a direct ophthalmoscope. Patient is made to look into the light and examiner compares the brightness of pupillary red reflex of both eyes obtained simultaneously:

- *In orthophoria,* the Bruckner red reflex is symmetric in the two eyes.
- *In strabismus,* the reflex is brighter in the deviated eye.
- *In ocular pathologic conditions* such as large anisometropia, gross retinal pathology, large retinal detachment, media opacities (corneal, lenticular or vitreal), the red reflex is altered in the affected eye.

Hirschberg corneal reflex test

It is a rough but handy method to estimate the angle of manifest squint. In this test, patient is asked to fixate at a point light held at a distance of 33 cm and the deviation of corneal reflex from the centre of pupil is noted in the squinting eye. Hirschberg reported that each 1 mm decentration of corneal reflex corresponds to 7° (14$^\Delta$) of deviation of the visual axis. Thus, roughly the angle of squint is 15° and 45°, when the corneal light reflex falls on the border of pupil and limbus, respectively (Fig. 20.4).

Prism and alternate cover test
(prism bar cover test, i.e. PBCT)

In practice, this test is most popular and a simple method of measuring the angle of deviation objectively in various diagnostic positions of gaze.

Prisms of increasing strength with apex towards the deviation are placed in front of one eye and the patient is asked to fixate a target with the other eye. For large deviations, a loose prism of 30 or 45 prism dioptre is placed in front of one eye and the prism bar is used in front of the other eye.

- *When horizontal and vertical deviations co-exist,* the prisms are placed horizontally in front of one eye and vertically in front of the other eye.
- *Alternate cover test* is then performed till there is no recovery movement of the eye under cover (Fig. 20.5). This will tell the amount of deviation in prism dioptres.

Both heterophoria as well as heterotropia can be measured objectively by this method.

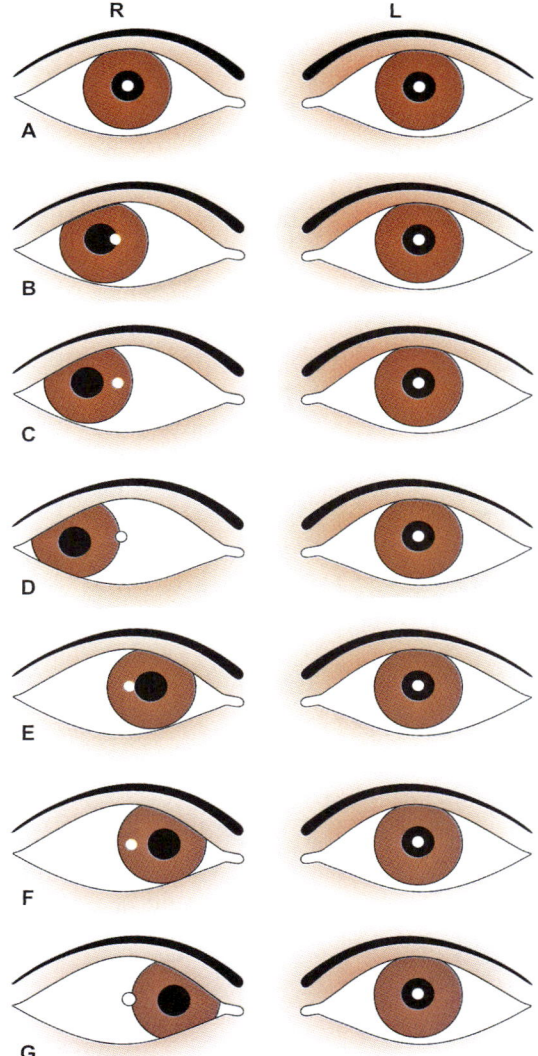

Fig. 20.4: *Hirschberg corneal reflex test depicting ortho-position (A), right exotropia (B:15°, C:30°, D:45°) and right esotropia (E:15°, F:30°, G:45°).*

Test should be performed for distance and near fixation. An accommodative target should be used for near fixation distances.

Test should be performed, preferably in all the nine diagnostic positions of gaze. In Boyce-Smith deviometer (Fig. 20.6), nine prefixed retroilluminated slides (accommodative targets) positioned 35° from the primary position are used to perform cover and prism test in diagnostic positions of gaze.

One great advantage of using a deviometer is that the prism and cover test can be performed in diagnostic positions under exactly the same conditions on different occasions and thus permit meaningful comparison of test results (e.g. preoperative and postoperative).

Comparison of prism and cover test performed in primary position, straight up position and straight down position is very useful in detecting the 'A', 'V' and 'X' pattern heterotropias.

Test should be repeated by holding the prism and occluder before the other eye to detect any difference between right and left fixation, which would indicate incomitance.

Uses of prism and cover test

A carefully performed PBCT can provide following useful information:

1. *Nature of deviation* of esotropia (basic or convergence excess or divergence insufficiency type) and exotropia (basic or convergence insufficiency or divergence excess type) can be known from the results of near and distance measurements.
2. *Accommodative element of deviation* can be known from measuring deviation for far and near with and without glasses (including bifocals, if any).
3. *Incomitance*, if any, can be detected by performing the test in 9 cardinal positions of gaze.
4. *A-V patterns* can be detected by measuring the deviation in upgaze of 25° and downgaze of 35°.
5. *Primary versus secondary deviation* can be detected by measuring the deviation with right and left eye fixating alternately.
6. *Divergence excess versus simulated divergence excess exotropia* can be differentiated by measuring the deviation before and after prolonged occlusion.

Limitations of prism and cover test

- Since, this test requires an accurate fixation, so it cannot be performed, if the deviating eye is blind or has gross eccentric fixation.
- The optical qualities of the prisms also limit the test accuracy. The stronger the prism, the greater the error.

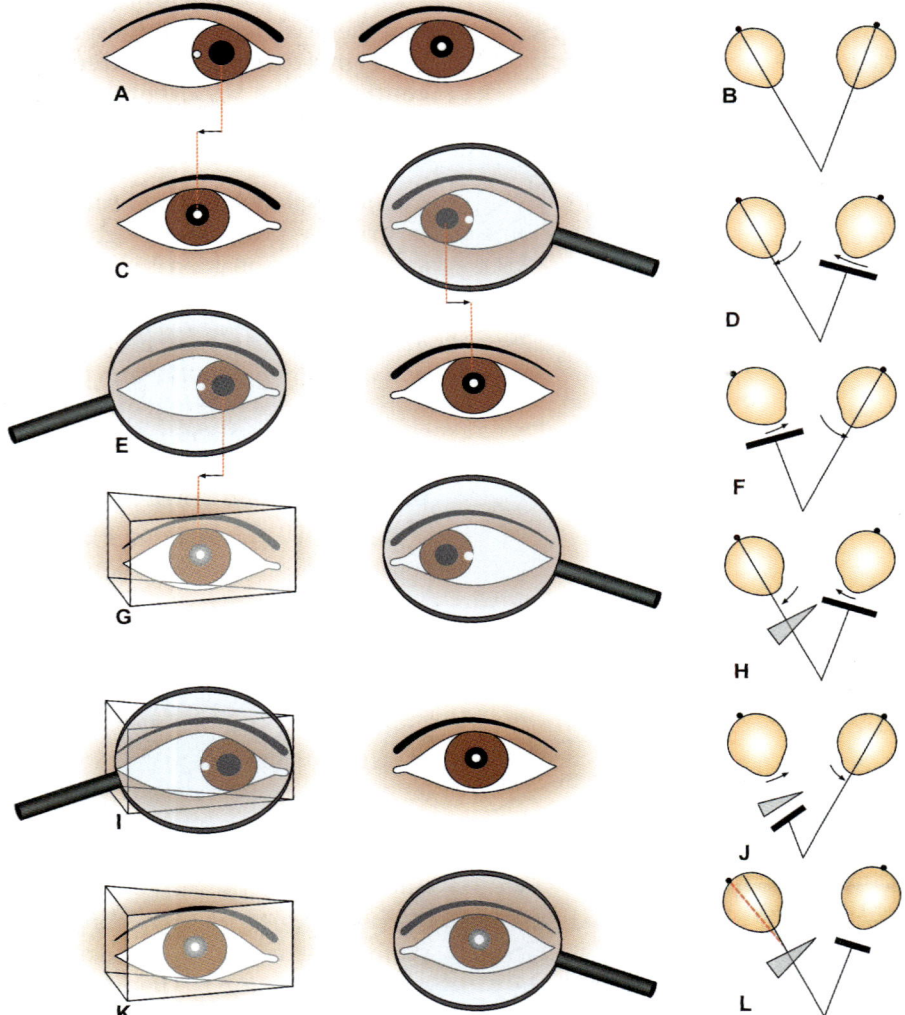

Fig. 20.5: *Prism and cover test with its optical principle. (A) right esotropia; (B) image of the object fixated by left eye is projected on major half of retina of the right eye; (C and D) when left eye is covered, right eye moves outwards to take over fixation and under the cover left eye performs an inward movement of equal amplitude following Hering's law of equal innervation; (E and F) when cover is transferred to right eye, the left eye moves outwards to takeover fixation and under the cover right eye performs an inward movement; (G and H) a prism base-out is held before the right eye and cover is transferred to the left eye. There is still outward movement of the right eye when taking over fixation; (I and J) cover is again transferred and a prism of greater power is held before the right eye; (K and L) transfer of cover to the left eye does not show any outward movement of the right eye indicating that it is the end point of the prism and cover test. At this juncture, prism of sufficient power offsets the nasal displacement and the right eye will no longer change its position when left eye is covered. The power of this prism equals the deviation.*

- The spectacle lenses with power more than ±5D introduce a significant artifact in measurement of deviation. Plus lenses decrease and minus lenses increase the measured deviation.

- The presence of manifest as well as latent nystagmus hinders the accurate measurements by prism and cover test.
- Test accuracy is also limited by the minimum movement of redress that the examiner can detect with naked eye.

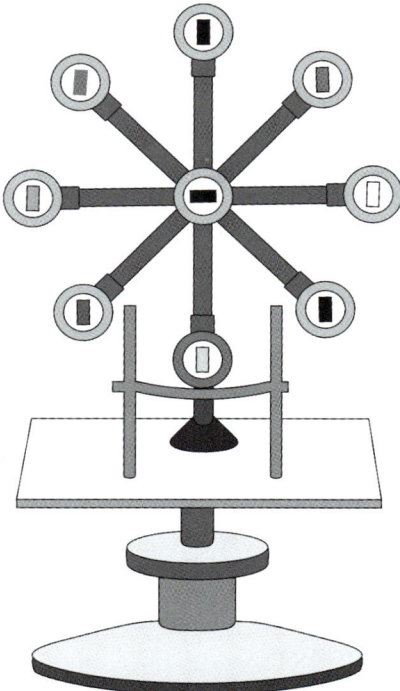

Fig. 20.6: *The Boyce-Smith deviometer.*

Prism reflex test (Krimsky's corneal reflex test)

Prism reflex test first described by *Krimsky* has become universally accepted as a practical method of estimating the size of the angle of squint in patients with a blind or deeply amblyopic eye with or without eccentric fixation.

To perform the test, patient is asked to fixate on a point light and prisms of increasing strength (with apex towards the direction of manifest squint) are placed in front of the normal fixating eye till the corneal reflex is centered in the squinting eye (Fig. 20.7). The power of prism required to centre the light reflex in the squinting eye equals the amount of squint in prism dioptres. To avoid errors from parallax, the examiner must observe the corneal reflex with one eye by sitting directly in front of the deviating eye while keeping his other eye closed.

In an alternative method, prism of increasing power can be placed in front of the deviating eye until the corneal reflexion is centred. However, since the observation of the corneal reflexion through prisms is difficult, therefore, the method described above is preferred.

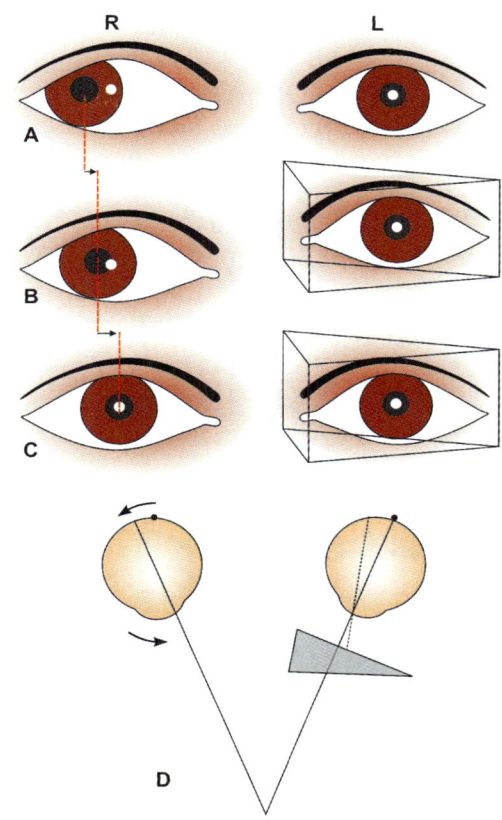

Fig. 20.7: *The Krimsky's corneal reflex test. (A) right ex-otropia; (B and C), prism base-in of increasing powers are placed in front of the fixing left eye till the corneal reflex centres in the right eye (C); (D) optical principle of the prism reflex test.*

Advantages of Krimsky's test
- Since the test requires only that the patient fixate the light, being entirely objective otherwise, it is useful in testing small children
- It is quicker to perform than the prism cover test
- It can be used in patients in whom the deviating eye has a low visual acuity or has lost central fixation.

Limitations of the Krimsky's test
- Since the angle kappa is included in the measurement, the test is inaccurate.
- It is impossible to perform the test for distance fixation, since the position of the examiner's head required to obtain an accurate observation prevents the patient from seeing the fixation light.

Simultaneous prism cover test

Aim. The aim of this test is to measure only the tropia without dissociating the phoria.

This special cover test is used to measure the tropia component of patient with small tropia <10 PD and a larger phoria (i.e. monofixation syndrome). It is not useful for larger tropia (>10 PD), which does not permit fusion and, therefore, does not have an associated phoria.

Procedure. This test is performed as below:

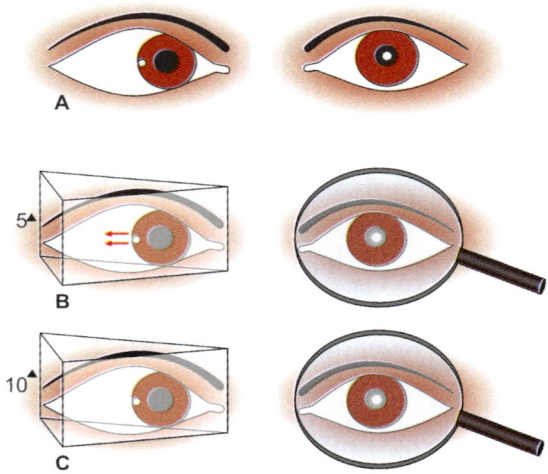

Fig. 20.8: *Simultaneous cover test: Hirschberg test depicting small esotropia (A). Simultaneous placement of prism on the esotropic eye and occluder on the fixing eye will show fixing movement in the esotropic eye when the power of prism is less (B) and no movement when the power of prism is equal to the degree of tropia (C).*

- *Hirschberg corneal reflex test* is performed to estimate the approximate size of tropia (Fig. 20.8A).
- *Simultaneous prism cover test* is then performed by placing the prism of the size of tropia in front of deviating eye and an occluder in front of the fixating eye (Fig. 20.8B). The power of prism with which the deviated eye does not show refixation shift equals the tropia.

Note. For patients with monofixation syndrome, the amount of tropia is measured with simultaneous prism cover test and the total angle (tropia plus phoria) is measured with the alternate prism cover test.

Perimeter method

Patient is asked to fixate at O-mark on the arc perimeter with normal eye and a flash light is moved along its arc till the corneal reflexion is centred in the pupil of the squinting eye. This point on perimeter gives the angle of manifest squint in degrees.

This method, used in the past, is not popular nowadays.

Maddox rod test

It is a subjective test, based on the principle of diplopia, which can be employed to measure both heterophoria as well as heterotropia. The Maddox rod consists of a series of parallel glass cylinders of higher power (usually of red colour) set together in a metallic disc (Fig. 20.9A). The Maddox rod produces a linear

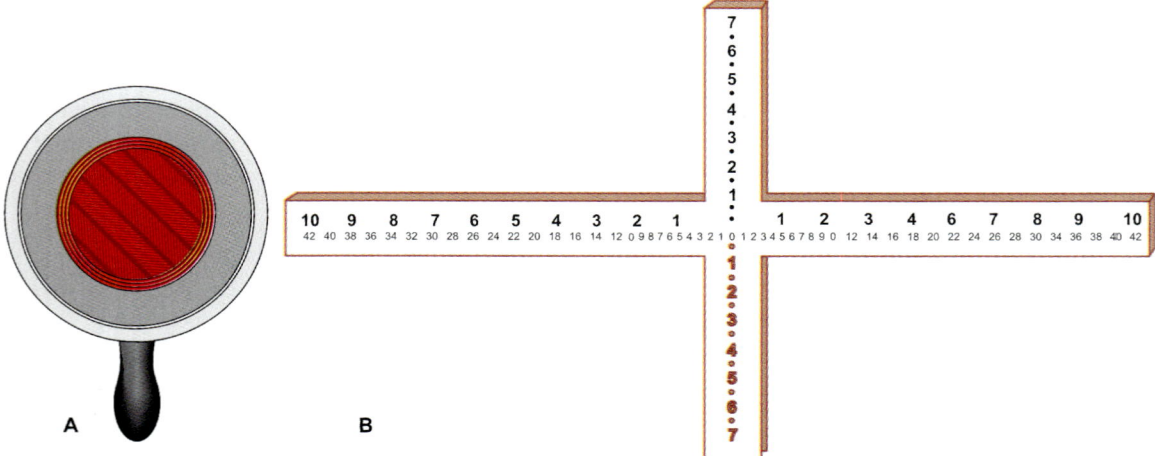

Fig. 20.9: *(A) Maddox rod; (B) Maddox tangent scale.*

image of a point light. When viewed through the rod, the line image is formed perpendicular to the axis of the cylinders.

Measurement of heterotropia

The patient is asked to fix on a point light in the centre of a Maddox tangent scale (Fig. 20.9B) or any point light at a distance of 6 metres. The Maddox rod is placed before one eye with axis of the rod parallel to the axis of deviation (Fig. 20.10). Thus, for measuring a horizontal deviation, the rod is placed in such a way that the patient sees a vertical line of light (Fig. 20.10A). Depending upon the type of deviation, the red vertical line will be seen either to the right or to the left of fixation light. The number on Maddox tangent scale where the red line falls will be the amount of deviation in degrees. Alternatively, prisms of successively increasing power (with apex towards the deviation) are placed in front of the rod until the patient sees the line passing through the fixation light. This gives the amount of heterotropia in prism dioptres. The test should always be repeated with the Maddox rod in front of the other eye, so that deviation during right fixation and left fixation can be compared, and any discrepancy, if there, can be noted. Such an endeavour, specially gives information about:

- Primary and secondary deviations in the presence of paralytic element
- Any change in retinal correspondence with the change in fixation
- Presence of dissociated vertical deviations may be discovered.

Maddox rod test in conjunction with the Maddox tangent scale can be performed successfully in cooperative children as young as 3 to 4 years of age. Such children should be asked to go to the scale and put their finger on the place where they saw the line rather than asked to tell the number from a distance.

In case of vertical deviation, the Maddox rod is rotated so that the line is seen horizontally (Fig. 20.10B) and the deviation is measured directly from the tangent scale or by using prism base-up or base-down depending upon the direction of deviation (apex of prism is kept towards deviation). To measure a cyclotropia, the patient is asked to turn the Maddox rod around the anteroposterior axis, until he/she

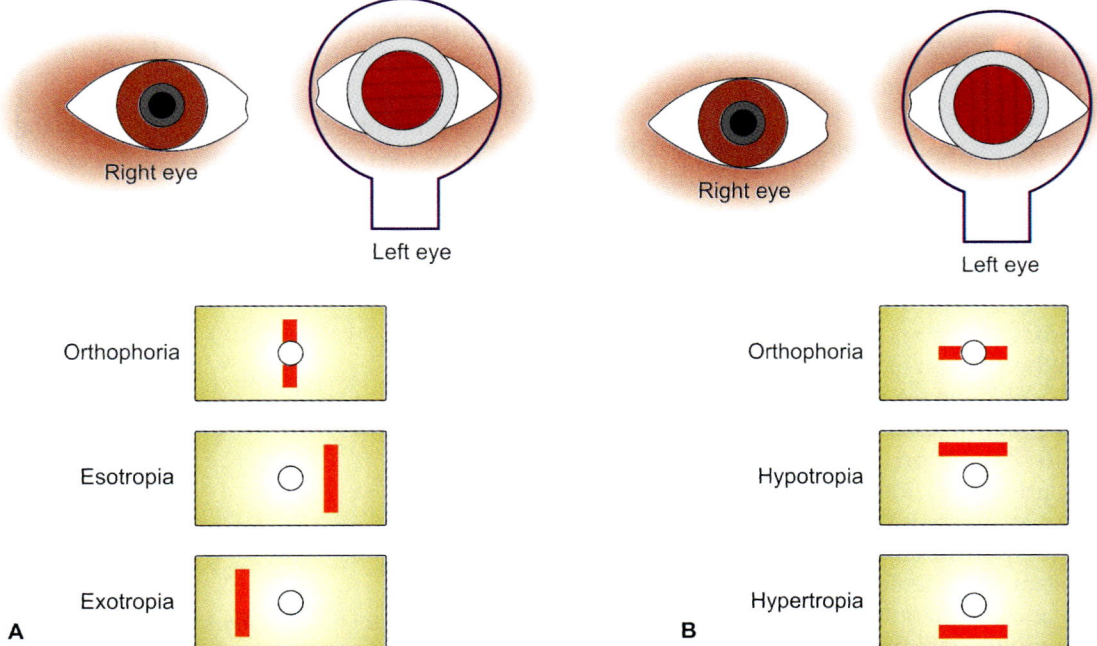

Fig. 20.10: *Maddox rod test for horizontal (A) and vertical (B) heterotropia.*

has the impression that the line is horizontal. The amount of cyclotropia in degrees can be read from the trial frame.

Measurement of heterophoria

To measure heterophoria, the Maddox rod test is performed exactly in a similar manner as performed to measure the heterotropia with the following one exception:

In heterophoria, an occluder is placed before the Maddox rod and while the patient fixates the light source with his/her other eye, the occluder is removed only for a second and the necessary enquiries are made. After making necessary adjustments of the prism, the occluder is again removed for a second. The procedure is repeated till the patient sees red line and point light as superimposed.

The use of a cover is necessary in a phoria, because, if both the fixation light and red line are seen continuously, there will be a constant change in the degree of deviation and the red line will never achieve a steady position relative to the fixation light.

Limitations of the maddox rod test

1. It can be performed, only if there is no suppression under the test conditions.
2. The true angle of deviation is measured, only if the patient has normal retinal correspondence.
3. It is useful only to measure small deviations, since when large prisms are used, it is difficult for the patient to see both the red line and the fixation light, simultaneously.

Maddox wing test

Maddox wing is an instrument (Fig. 20.11) by which the amount of heterophoria for near (at a distance of 33 cm) can be measured subjectively. Like the Maddox rod test, the Maddox wing test is also based on the basic principle of dissociation of fusion by dissimilar objects.

The instrument is designed in such a way that when the patient looks through the eyepiece of the instrument, the right eye sees a vertical white arrow and a horizontal red arrow, while the left eye sees a vertical and horizontal line of numbers. After a few seconds have elapsed to

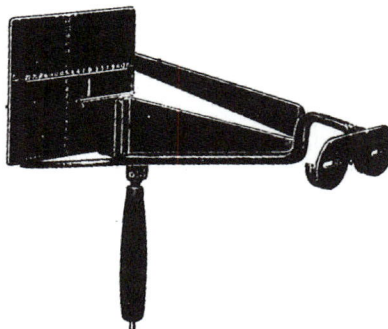

Fig. 20.11: *Maddox wing.*

allow the eyes to assume the fusion free position, the patient is asked to tell the number on the horizontal line to which the vertical white arrow is pointing (this will give the amount of horizontal phoria) and the number on the vertical line at which the red arrow is pointing (this will measure the vertical phoria). The cyclophoria is measured by asking the patient to align the red arrow with the horizontal line of number (Fig. 20.12).

Advantages

1. Since the numbers can be read, only when the patient accommodates sufficiently, this makes the test much more reliable than one in which the patient fixates a light.
2. Horizontal, vertical and cyclophorias can be measured simultaneously.

Disadvantages

1. The interpupillary distance is not adjustable.
2. The test is purely subjective, so the examiner has no objective check.

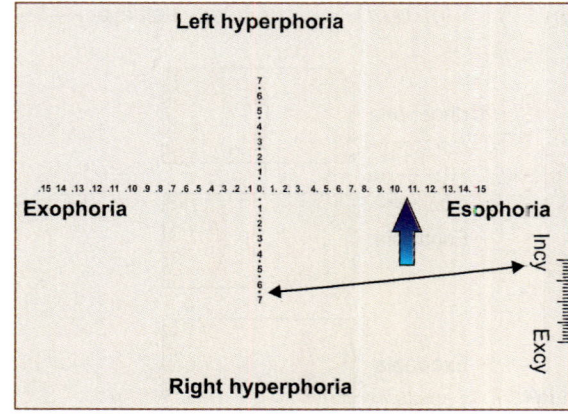

Fig. 20.12: *Maddox wing test.*

Synoptophore method

All types of heterophorias and heterotropias can be measured accurately both objectively and subjectively with the help of synoptophore. Techniques of measuring heterophorias and heterotropias using this instrument are as follows.

Measurement of objective angle of deviation with synoptophore

The synoptophore is set for the patient's height and interpupillary distance. Simultaneous perception slides (e.g. lion and cage) are used. The patient is asked to look at the pictures, and the arm controlling the picture in front of the deviating eye is moved by the examiner until there is no movement of either eye on a cover test performed by alternately turning off the light (Fig. 20.13). The reading on the horizontal scale in front of the deviating eye as well as the one of the vertical scale, represents the objective angle of deviation. For example, if the arm of synoptophore in front of the deviating eye is at 20^Δ base out and has to be raised 2^Δ, the objective angle is recorded as 20^Δ esotropia and 2^Δ hypertropia.

Measurement of the objective angle for near fixation. It can also be made as follows:

To measure the objective angle of deviation for near, a –3.0D lens is inserted in the lens holder situated in front of the eyepiece lenses.

In this way, the patient has to exert 3D accommodation in order to get a clear image of the slides. In doing so, each eye exerts 3^Δ of convergence for each dioptre of accommodation. In other words, 9^Δ of convergence in one eye or

18^Δ of convergence in both eyes—considering the interpupillary distance (IPD) as being 60 mm. For a smaller IPD, the convergence requirement is less and for a bigger IPD, it is more (provided the AC/A ratio is normal). Thus, when recording the angle of deviation, one must keep this in mind and either subtract 18^Δ (for esodeviations) from or add 18^Δ (in case of exodeviations) to the synoptophore readings. In other words, a synoptophore reading of 22^Δ base-out should be recorded as 4^Δ esotropia and a reading of 22^Δ base-in should be recorded as 40^Δ exotropia.

Advantages

Advantages of measuring objective angle of the deviation with synoptophore are as follows:

1. The objective angle can be measured with either eye fixating and in all cardinal directions of gaze.
2. It is possible to measure horizontal, vertical, and torsional deviations fairly accurately.
3. Deviation of any size can be measured since prisms can be used in the lens holder, when necessary.
4. Measurement of objective angle for near fixation can also be made.

Disadvantages

The disadvantages of measuring deviation objectively with synoptophore are as follows:

1. Small children may not cooperate and might be frightened.
2. Though the instrument is optically arranged for distance, there is tendency for the patient to converge as he/she thinks the pictures are close to him/her. Consequently, esotropias usually increase and exotropias decrease in size. Therefore, synoptophore is not being considered a very reliable instrument to measure horizontal deviations.

Measurement of subjective angle of deviation with synoptophore

After measuring the deviation objectively (as above), the patient is asked to comment on the position of the pictures used. If the patient claims superimposition (i.e. the lion seen in the cage) at his objective angle, this angle is also his subjective one. If this is not the case, the arms

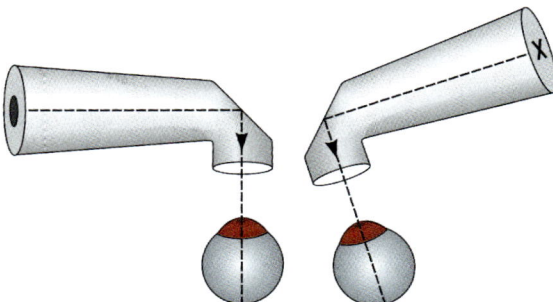

Fig. 20.13: *Measurement of objective angle of deviation with synoptophore.*

are moved back to zero and the patient is asked to move the handle controlling the picture in front of the non-fixating eye until he/she sees the two pictures superimposed (Fig. 20.14). Adjustments can be made for vertical or torsional separation, if necessary. This is the subjective angle. At this point, one should by means of rapid alternate flashing, check whether or not the eyes move, when the patient is asked to fixate on each picture in turn. This is done mainly to make sure that an actual change in the angle between the visual axis has not occurred, as happens frequently through relaxing or increasing the accommodative effort or in cases of a variable angle of deviation.

Problems which may come across while performing this test are as follows:

1. Suppression may prevent the patient from superimposing the pictures. In such cases, simultaneous macular perception or simultaneous paramacular perception slides can be used. The larger the image formed on the retina, the less likely it is to be suppressed.

2. The patient may never succeed in putting the lion in the cage, and it may suddenly be seen on the other side of the cage (in an uncrossed or homonymous position in divergent deviations and in a crossed or heteronymous position in convergent deviations). In such cases, the crossing point is considered to be the subjective angle.

3. It must be realized that the measurement obtained by the subjective method is only the true angle of deviation, if normal retinal correspondence is present.

Measurement of cyclodeviation with synoptophore

There is no way to carry out an objective measurement of a cyclodeviation. The subjective measurement can be performed as follows.

Simultaneous perception slides are used. The slide with lion is kept in front of the right eye and that with cage is kept in front of the left eye. The patient is asked to look at each one in turn and is asked whether the cage appears level. In the presence of cyclodeviation, the cage appears tilted. In incyclotropia, the cage's left-hand side is seen lower than the right-hand side. This is corrected by wheel rotating the slide towards the patient. In the presence of excyclotropia, the cage's right-hand side appears lower than the left-hand side. This can be corrected by wheel-rotating the slide away from the patient (towards the examiner). The amount of deviation is read in degrees from the scale located on the slide-holder of the instrument. It should be remembered that the tilt of the image is in the direction opposite to the tilt of the eye.

Double prism test

Double prism test consists of two prisms which are mounted base to base. It is used to elicit cyclophorias. To perform this test the, double prism is placed before one eye in such a manner that the junction of the two bases intersects the pupil and is horizontal. Then the patient is asked to look at a horizontal line against an empty background which does not offer any fusional stimuli and inferences drawn are as follows:

• Patient will see two parallel lines with the eye having double prism in front of it, i.e. one line displaced above and the other displaced below with respect to the single line seen by the other eye.

• In the absence of any cyclophoria, all three lines will be parallel.

• If a cyclophoria is present, the single line will have an angle relative to the other two lines as follows:

♦ In incyclophoria, the line or lines seen by the right eye will be tilted towards right and those seen by left eye will be tilted towards left.

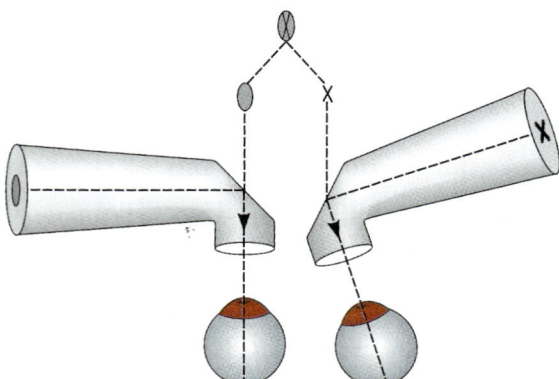

Fig. 20.14: *Measurement of subjective angle of deviation with synoptophore.*

• In excyclophoria, the line or lines seen by the right eye will be tilted towards left and those seen by left eye will be tilted towards right.

Haploscopic tests

Tests based on the haploscopic principle to measure the deviation include Lancaster red-green test, Hess and Lees screen tests. These tests are very useful for measuring incomitant strabismus in patients with diplopia (*see* page 399–404).

ASSESSMENT OF OCULAR MOVEMENTS

ASSESSMENT OF DUCTIONS

1. *Duction test.* Ductions are monocular movements and are measured at near distance. When examining ductions, one eye is covered and the fellow eye fixates a spotlight which is moved to bring the fixating eye to the farthest possible position, in all the cardinal directions of gaze. For interpretation of the observations, following methods are in vogue:

i. In most frequent practice, the examiner observes whether *movement lags or is excessive* in any direction. If no lags are noticed, the ductions are recorded as full; if lags are noticed, the muscle and the eye involved are indicated. Usually, a subjective assessment is made on scale of 7 points (+3 to −3) or 9 points (+4 to −4). Further, a note is also made of the occurrence of any nystagmoid movements in the presence of full ductions.

ii. Judging the *normalcy of adduction and abduction in relation to fixed points.* Following useful guidelines have been suggested:

• In maximal adduction, *an imaginary vertical line through the lower lacrimal punctum should coincide with a boundary line between the inner one-third and the outer two-thirds of the cornea* (Fig. 20.15A).

◆ *In excessive adduction, more cornea is hidden* (Fig. 20.15B).
◆ *In defective adduction, more cornea is visible. Some of the sclera may also be visible* (Fig. 20.15C).

• *In maximal abduction, the lateral limbus touches the outer canthus* (Fig. 20.15D).

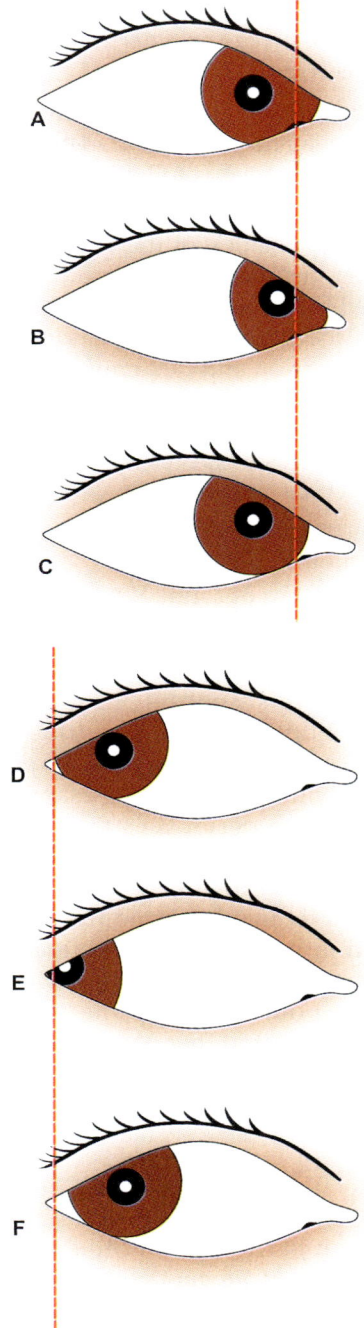

Fig. 20.15: *Judgement of adduction (A, B, C) in relation to lower punctum and abduction (D, E, F) in relation to lateral canthus. For explanation see text.*

• *In excessive abduction, some of the cornea is hidden under the outer canthus* (Fig. 20.15E).

• *In defective abduction, some of the sclera is visible between the outer canthus and the limbus* (Fig. 20.15F).

2. *Kestenbaum's limbus test of motility.* The duction movements are measured with the help of a transparent ruler as follows:

• *Adduction* is measured by noting a difference between the position of the temporal limbus in primary position and maximum adduction.
• *Abduction* is measured by noting a difference between the position of the nasal limbus in primary position and maximum abduction.
• Similarly, *elevation* and *depression* are measured with respect to inferior limbus and superior limbus, respectively.
• Normal values reported are:
  ◆ Adduction : 10 mm
  ◆ Abduction : 10 mm
  ◆ Elevation : 5–7 mm
  ◆ Depression : 10 mm

3. *Subjective perimeter method of measuring ductions.* In this method, to measure the amplitude of duction movements, the patient's head is placed into the chin rest of a perimeter in such a way that the eye to be examined is in the centre of the perimeter arc or perimeter hemisphere. The other eye is occluded and the patient is asked to fixate and follow the perimeter target that is moved from the centre of the field to periphery. He/she is instructed to indicate, when he/she can no longer see the target. This point indicates the limit of the duction movement in that particular direction. Normal values reported by this method are:
  ◆ Adduction : 50°
  ◆ Abduction : 50°
  ◆ Depression : 50°
  ◆ Elevation : 40°

4. *Objective perimeter method or corneal reflex method of measuring ductions.* The amplitude of duction movements can be checked somewhat more objectively by using corneal light reflex. In this method, after closing one eye, patient is asked to turn his/her eye maximally in a given direction. Then the examiner moves a small flash light along the arc of the perimeter until the reflex from the patient's cornea appears to be centred in the pupil. The examiner views it with one eye from the position of flash light. This point gives the limit of the particular duction movement.

Note: It is important to be aware of the fact that, in practice, the measurement of ductions is not of much value in the investigation of strabismus, since only a small fraction of the fibres of a muscle need to function in order to rotate the eye to the limits of its field of duction. A defect in the amplitude of duction occurs, only when almost complete paresis of a muscle occurs. Therefore, a partial paresis usually cannot be diagnosed on testing ductions.

ASSESSMENT OF VERSIONS

In general, study of versions is more important factor than the study of ductions, when deciding on which muscle or muscles to operate.

Further, the investigation of versions is of greatest importance in patients with non-comitant strabismus, because comparison of the extent of movement of the two eyes relative to each other during a version is the most sensitive test to detect underfunction of a muscle.

1. Version test

It is performed at approximately 15 inches. The patient is asked to hold his head straight and still and to make eye movements on command or to follow a fixation light in all the cardinal directions of gaze. The fixation light should be kept at such a distance that one can always observe the corneal reflections in both eyes. The following observations should be made on version test.
• For excessive or defective movements in any direction.
• To detect underaction of one muscle and overaction of its contralateral synergist.
• To detect overaction of one muscle without underaction of its contralateral synergist.
• To note any retraction of the globe and narrowing of palpebral fissure in certain direction of gaze (as seen in Duane's retraction syndrome).
• To detect the overaction of inferior and superior obliques.

Clinically, the overaction of oblique muscles can be graded by following methods:

i. *Depending upon the vertical deviations,* the overactions of obliques is graded as:
   a. *Mild overaction*—when vertical deviation (e.g. hypertropia in inferior oblique overaction) is appreciated only in sursumadduction.
   b. *Moderate overaction*—when vertical deviation is appreciable on adduction itself.
   c. *Severe overaction*—when hypertropia is seen in primary position.

ii. *Depending on the angle, the adducting eye makes with the horizontal line* as it elevates and abducts (if overacting) on lateral version to the opposite side, the overaction of inferior oblique is graded as shown in Fig. 20.16.

Similarly, the overaction of superior oblique also can be graded by observing the angle

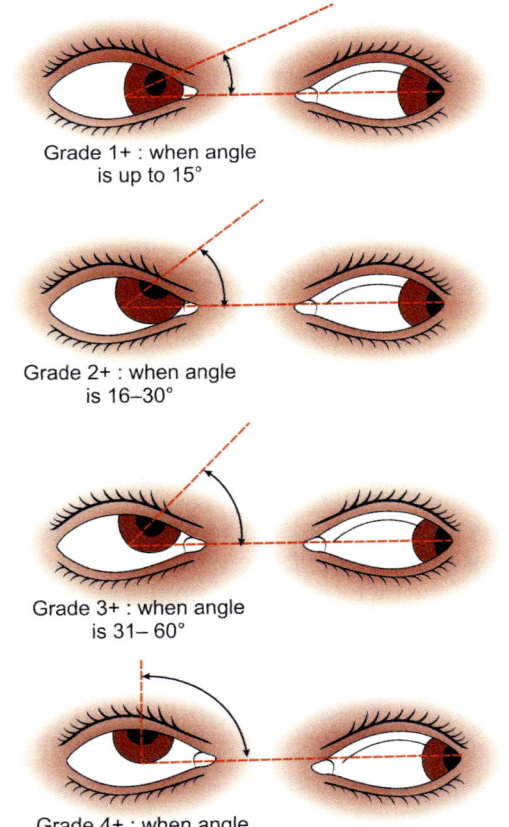

Grade 1+ : when angle
is up to 15°

Grade 2+ : when angle
is 16–30°

Grade 3+ : when angle
is 31– 60°

Grade 4+ : when angle
is 61– 90°

Fig. 20.16: *Grading of inferior oblique overaction depending on the angle adducting eye makes with horizontal line.*

the adducting eye makes with the horizontal line as it depresses and abducts.

2. Perimeteric method of measuring versions

The amplitude of versions can be measured on the perimeter in the same way as ductions except that the patient fixates and follows the test object with both eyes until he/she sees it double or until it moves too far out for him/her to follow.

In general, such a measurement of the absolute amplitude of versions is of little practical value.

MEASUREMENT OF VERGENCES

The status of motor fusion is assessed by measuring the vergences, i.e. the fusional amplitudes. In the presence of heterophoria or an intermittent heterotropia, the fusional amplitudes can be measured both by the prism method or synoptophore method. While, in a patient with heterotropia, only the synoptophore method is useful, since fusion in casual gaze is necessary for testing with prism method. Fusional divergence is measured from the subject's phoria position, whereas relative divergence is measured from the position of fusional demand, i.e. the orthoposition.

Testing of fusional amplitudes with prism method

The test can be performed using a prism bar or a rotatory prism (Risley prism) or single prism. A prism bar consists of a series of prisms of increasing strength (Fig. 20.17). It is held by the examiner in front of one of the patient's eyes and merely needs to be moved higher or lower to bring a stronger or weaker prism into the line of sight.

Amplitudes of divergence are measured first and those of convergence second.

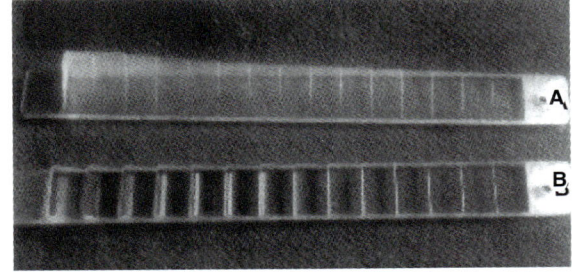

Fig. 20.17: *Prism bars, horizontal (A) and vertical (B).*

Measurement of amplitude of divergence

To perform the test for distance, patient is asked to fixate the 6/12 symbol at 6 metres and the prism bar is used with the prism base directed in BI in front of the one eye (preferably the non-dominant one). By progressively increasing the amount of base in prism power, the eyes are diverged to the limit of bifoveal single vision, i.e. up to the point, when the patient just appreciates diplopia. This point is the end point of the test and is called the *break point*. Its reading is recorded. At this point, the power of the prism is decreased slowly, until he/she again fuses. This point called the *recovery point* is also noted.

To measure the amplitude of divergence for near, the above test is repeated at 33 cm. The end point and the recovery point are recorded. But unlike the test for distance, the end point for the near test is blur point, i.e. the maximum amount of base-in (BI) prism power after which the patient's vision is blurred. The mechanism of blurring of vision is as follows:

The retinal disparity produced by the use of base-in prism evokes fusional divergence that maintains bifoveal single vision until its amplitude is exhausted. At this point, the patient, who is accommodating during near vision, can produce further divergence and maintain single vision longer, if he/she relaxes his/her accommodation, because this simultaneously decreases the amount of accommodative, convergence present. But, due to relaxation of accommodation, the near object becomes blurred.

Measurement of amplitude of convergence

To perform the test for near, patient is asked to fixate 6/12 symbol at 33 cm and the bar is used with prism base directed out (BO). By progressively increasing the amount of BO prism power, the eyes are converged to the limit of bifoveal single vision, i.e. up to the point, when the patient just appreciates diplopia. This point is the end point, of the test and is called the *break point*. Its reading is recorded. At this point, the power of the prism is decreased slowly until he/she again fuses. This point, called the *recovery point*, is also recorded. Theoretically, before the break point, there will be a blur point because after the exhaustion of the fusional convergence patient starts using his/her accommodative convergence to avoid diplopia. This, however, can only be done by accommodating in excess of the requirements for the given distance (pseudomyopia) and consequently the image is blurred. Therefore, it is important to record the *blur point* in order to know what kind of fusional amplitudes are measured.

To perform the test for distance, the same procedure is repeated at 6 m and the blur point, break point and recovery point are recorded.

An example of a recording of fusional amplitudes as tested with the prism bar:

Distance : Diverged to 12^Δ BI/recovered at 9^Δ BI
Converged to 32^Δ BO/recovered at 21^Δ BO
Blurred at 12^Δ BO

Near   : Diverged to 14^Δ BI/recovered at 9^Δ BI
Converged to 36^Δ BO/recovered at 24^Δ BO
Blurred at 18^Δ BO

Synoptophore method of measuring fusional amplitudes

To begin with, the objective angle of deviation is determined using simultaneous macular perception slides. Then, the second-grade fusion slides (similar targets with control marks for each eye) are introduced and if the patient fuses these targets and sees them as one with both control marks, the examiner blocks the arms at the objective angle. Then, first the amplitude of divergence and second the amplitude of convergence are measured as below.

To measure the divergence, the arms of the synoptophore are slowly diverged and the patient is instructed to report occurrence of diplopia or the disappearance of one or the other control mark of the picture (suppression). This point—the *break point*—is recorded and the arms of the synoptophore are slowly converged (i.e. brought to less divergent position) and the *recovery point,* where fusion occurs, is noted.

To measure the convergence, the arms of the synoptophore are further converged slowly till the fusion breaks and the *break point* is noted. Then, the arms are moved back into a less convergent position until fusion is regained and the *recovery point* is noted.

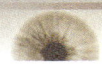

To measure the amplitude of vergences for near with synoptophore, a –3.0 DS lens is placed before each eye. In order to see clearly with –3.0 DS lens, the subject has to overcome these lenses by accommodating as if he/she was fixating an object at a distance of 33 cm. To simulate the orthoposition for near fixation, the synoptophore tubes have to be set according to the convergence requirement for a point 33 cm distant which, in prism dioptres, is three times the patient's interpupillary distance in centimetres.

The procedure of testing for near is the same as for distance.

Normal values of vergences are as follows:

Vergence	Distance (6 m)	Near (33 cm)
Convergence	14–20$^\Delta$	35–40$^\Delta$
Divergence	5–8$^\Delta$	15–20$^\Delta$
Vertical vergence	2–4$^\Delta$	2–4$^\Delta$
Incyclovergence	10–12°	10–12°
Excyclovergence	10–12°	10–12°

An example of recording of fusional amplitudes as tested with the synoptophore:

Distance:
- *30$^\Delta$ ET, objectively and subjectively*
- *First- and second-grade fusion at angle*
- *Convergence to 42$^\Delta$ BO/recovery at 32$^\Delta$ BO*
- *Divergence to 12$^\Delta$ BO/recovery at 20$^\Delta$ BO.*

Near (with –3.0 D):
- *44$^\Delta$ ET objectively and subjectively*
- *First- and second-grade fusion at angle*
- *Convergence to 56$^\Delta$ BO/recovery at 44$^\Delta$ BO*
- *No divergence past angle, suppression OD.*

Measurement of near point of convergence

The near point of convergence (NPC) is the closest point at which an object can be seen single during bifoveal vision. In other words, it is the point at which the two foveal lines of sight intersect, when maximum convergence is exerted.

The NPC practically measures all types of convergence; since an object actually approaches the eyes during testing. That is, the test for NPC simultaneously stimulates fusional, accommodative and proximal convergence and during the last phase, if the patient is cooperative, there will be a strong voluntary effort to converge.

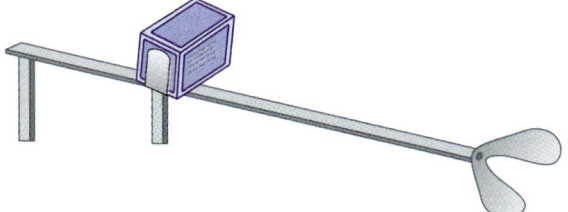

Fig. 20.18: *RAF rule.*

Instruments. Near point of convergence can be measured simply with the help of a graded plastic rule placed at the outer canthus and a fixation target (e.g. tip of a sharp pencil) moved towards the eye; or by use of specially designed rule such as RAF rule (Fig. 20.18), Livingstone binocular gauge (described on page 422) and Prince rule. These specially designed instruments basically consist of a bar or rule made from plastic, metal or wood on which a rider with the test chart can be moved back and forth (fixation target). At one end of the bar is a wing-like support that fits over the nose and rests against the lower orbital margins during the measurement. In Prince rule, the bar is 24 inches long and 1/2 inch square that has different markings on each of its four sides. One side is divided into centimetres (to be used for measurement of NPC and NPA), the second one into inches, and the third one into dioptres (for NPA in dioptres), and the age is indicated in years on the fourth side. The sliding target contains targets for measuring NPA and NPC.

Procedure. For measurement of convergence, a dot or a vertical line may be used as the target. It is advanced towards the patient at, or slightly below the eye level, until the patient has converged maximally and cannot sustain single bifoveal fixation as the target is brought closer. At this break point, the subject's non-dominant eye will diverge *(objective test)* and patient may appreciate diplopia *(subjective test)*. The distance from the canthus to this point is read on the rule and the NPC is recorded in mm or cm. Some of the near point rules have the zero point of their scales at the so-called spectacle point (i.e. 27 mm in front of the baseline). Therefore, with such instruments, 27 mm must be added to the distance that is read off the scale.

Normal values. The normal values of NPC vary considerably among different persons and even in different examinations of the same person. In normal adults, its average value is 70 mm (7 cm) with a range between 50 and 100 mm (5 to 10 cm). A distance closer than 5 cm is excessive, however, in children it may be as close as tip of the nose. NPC further away than 10 cm is defective or remote. In patients with convergence insufficiency (CI), it may be as remote as 25 or 30 cm or more.

Measurement of maintenance of convergence

The ability of the eyes to maintain convergence after the patient has been able to converge his/her eyes to a near vision can be tested by the inappropriately named test—*the drop convergence test*. In this test, after bringing the fixation target into reading distance, patient is asked to maintain convergence at this point and the fixation object is dropped suddenly. Some patients are better able than others to keep their eyes converged in the absence of a fixation object.

ASSESSMENT OF ACCOMMODATION AND AC/A RATIO

ASSESSMENT OF ACCOMMODATION

As we know, accommodation is a unique mechanism, by which our eyes can even focus the diverging rays coming from a near object on the retina in a bid to see clearly (Fig. 20.19). Assessment of accommodation is of great diagnostic value in cases of incomitant strabismus of non-paralytic origin. Assessment of *amplitude of accommodation* (the difference between the dioptric power needed to focus at near point 'P' and far point 'R', i.e. $A = P - R$) in practice can be made either by measurement of near point of accommodation (NPA) or by use of minus lenses as below.

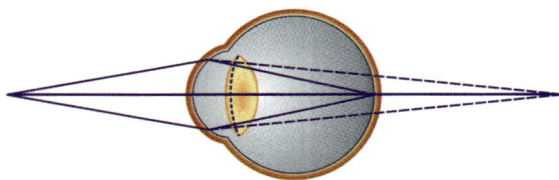

Fig. 20.19: *Effect of accommodation on divergent rays entering the eye.*

Measurement of near point of accommodation

The near point of accommodation (NPA) is the closest point at which small objects can be seen clearly. It is also called 'near point' or 'punctum proximum'.

NPA is measured using a near point rule such as RAF rule (Fig. 20.18) or Prince rule. The description of such a rule has been given in the discussion on the measurement of the near point of convergence.

To determine the NPA, a sliding target with 6/9 letters, numbers or fine lines is moved from or towards the eye until closest point is found at which it still can be seen clearly. During the examination, the patient has to wear his/her full optical refractive correction. The NPA is determined first for each eye separately and then for both eyes together. The NPA is measured in centimetres marked on one side of the instrument bar. The side of bar marked in dioptres will indicate the amplitude of accommodation in dioptres. The third side of the bar shows the age corresponding the accommodation. For example, if the patient reports that the point appears blurred at 25 cm, the dioptric markings will show +4.0 D and the age 40 years.

If, while measuring the NPA, the patient's amplitude of accommodation is found so low that his/her near point is beyond the length of the instrument, plus lenses are added to his/her correction until the near point is brought within range. The dioptric power of these additional lenses is then deducted from the measured values of amplitude of accommodation. Conversely, in young patients with very high accommodative power, minus lenses may be added to his/her distance correction to move his/her near point away from his/her eyes. The dioptric power of those minus lenses is then added to the measured value of amplitude of accommodation.

Measurement of amplitude of accommodation using minus lenses

This test is also performed first for each eye separately and then for both eyes together and during examination patient has to wear his/her full refractive correction. The patient is asked to fixate 6/60 symbol at a distance of 6 metres and

minus lenses of progressively increasing power are added before the eye till he/she can see the target clearly. The power of this minus lens is equivalent to the amplitude of accommodation in dioptres.

ASSESSMENT OF ACCOMMODATIVE CONVERGENCE/ACCOMMODATION (AC/A) RATIO

The AC/A ratio is the relationship between accommodative convergence (AC), expressed in prism dioptres ($^\Delta$) and accommodation (A), expressed in lens dioptres (D). This relationship is linear one and is thought to be relatively stable throughout life. The normal AC/A ratio is about 3 to 5 prism dioptres for one dioptre of accommodation. The concept of AC/A ratio was first clearly defined by Fry who later with Haines introduced the abbreviation AC/A ratio.

Methods of measurement of AC/A ratio

1. *Heterophoria method.* To measure AC/A ratio, in this method, the deviation is measured with full optical correction at 6 metres distance and at 33 cm distance in prism dioptres, and IPD is measured in centimetres. Then the AC/A ratio is calculated from the following formula:

$$AC/A \; = \; IPD + \frac{^\Delta n - ^\Delta d}{d}, \; where;$$

IPD = Interpupillary distance in centimetres

$^\Delta n$ = Deviation at 33 cm or 3 dioptres distance in prism dioptres

$^\Delta d$ = Deviation at 6 metres distance in prism dioptres

d = The fixation distance at near in dioptres

Note: Esodeviations are denoted by positive (+) and exodeviations by negative (–) sign.

For example, if IPD = 6 cm, $^\Delta n = 9^\Delta$ exophoria and $^\Delta d = 3^\Delta$ exophoria, then

$$AC/A = 6 + \frac{-9 - (3)}{3}$$
$$= 4 \, ^\Delta/D$$

2. *Gradient method.* This method is based on the fact that for a given fixation distance, minus lenses placed before the eyes increase the requirement for accommodation and plus lenses relax accommodation. Further, it is assumed that –1.0 D lens produces an equivalent of 1.0 D of accommodation, whereas +1.0 D lens relaxis accommodation by 1.0 D.

In practice, original deviation is found at near while the patient wears his/her optical correction and then with additional +3.0 D lens and the calculations for AC/A ratio are made as follows:

$$AC/A \; = \; \frac{^\Delta L - ^\Delta O}{D}, \; where$$

$^\Delta L$ = Deviation with additional lenses.

$^\Delta O$ = Original deviation without additional lenses.

D = Dioptric power of the additional lenses.

For example, if original deviation ($^\Delta O$) = 2^Δ esophoria, deviation with additional lenses ($^\Delta L$) = 10^Δ exophoria and the power of additional lenses (D) used is +3 D, then:

$$AC/A \; = \; \frac{2 - (-10)}{3} = 4^\Delta/D$$

Alternatively, the patient's original distance phoria ($^\Delta O$) is determined while he/she wears full optical correction. A –3.0 D lens is then placed before his/her eyes and the distance deviation ($^\Delta L$) is measured once more. The AC/A is calculated as above.

The gradient method is inaccurate because it does not take into account the patient's interpupillary distance (IPD).

3. *Clinical distance-near-relationship method.* This is a very simple method in which AC/A ratio is known by substracting distance deviation (D) at 6 metres from the near deviation (N) measured at 33 cm; i.e. AC/A = N – D. For examples:

i. In a patient with esotropia (ET) of 40 PD at near and 20 PD at distance, the AC/A ratio = 40 – 20 = 20 PD.

ii. In a patient with distance orthophoria and near exotropia (XT) 15 PD the AC/A = –15 – 0 = –15 PD

The results are interpreted as below:

• Up to 10 PD of N – D is normal.

- >10 PD of N – D is high AC/A ratio
- <10 PD of N – D difference is less AC/A ratio.

4. *Fixation disparity method.* In this method, AC/A ratio is indirectly derived from the fixation disparity induced either by forced convergence by use of prism or by altering the accommodative stimulus by use of optical lenses. Because of its complexity, this test is not performed in routine clinical practice.

5. *Haploscopic methods.* In haploscopy, the visual fields of the two eyes are differentiated and a separate target is presented to each eye. Hering's original instrument was designed primarily for studying the AC/A ratio. In practice, this method is no more used. However, the haploscopic devices, such as the major amblyoscope, are of fundamental importance for the study of the sensorimotor cooperation of the eyes.

ASSESSMENT FOR EXTRAOCULAR MUSCLE PARESIS

When paresis of one or more extraocular muscles is suspected as cause of squint, in addition to the duction test and version test, following tests should also be performed:

- Abnormal head posture examination
- Diplopia charting
- Quantitative measurement of actions of muscles extraocular
- Field of binocular fixation
- Bielschowsky's, phenomenon test
- Bielschowsky's, three-step test.

I. ABNORMAL HEAD POSTURE EXAMINATION

Note the abnormal head posture, if any, and examine its components in detail *see* Chapter 21.

II. DIPLOPIA CHARTING

Plotting of diplopia fields is indicated in patients complaining of confusion or double vision. The test is easy to perform provided the patient is cooperative. To perform the diplopia charting, patient is asked to wear red-green diplopia charting goggles; red glass being in front of the right eye and green in front of the left eye. The patient is made to sit with his/her head straight in a semidark room and is shown a fine linear light from a distance of 4 feet. The light is moved from primary position into all of the other eight directions of gaze. For each direction, patient is asked to comment on the position, brightness and separation between the red and green images. From the patient's comments, the examiner notes the following points:

- Whether horizontal diplopia is homonymous or heteronymous.
- Whether the image seen by right eye (red image) is higher or lower than the image seen by the left eye (green image) or *vice versa*.
- In which direction of gaze, separation between red and green images is greatest.
- Whether there are any directions in which fusion is present.

In a modified test of Franceschetti, instead of red green goggles, a red Maddox rod is placed in front of right eye and white Maddox rod in front of the left eye and the patient fixates on a spotlight which is seen as vertical red line with right eye and vertical white line with left eye.

Diplopia charts of patients with paresis of different extraocular muscles are shown in Figs 21.5 and 21.6.

Disadvantages of diplopia plotting test

- This test is only qualitative, therefore, it is not possible to comment on the minor changes of the improvement or deterioration from the records of different dates in the same patient.
- The test requires intelligent patient, especially to comment where the separation is maximum.
- It is not possible to perform the test in colour blind patients.
- This test is not of use in congenital palsies and those of long-standing onset, because due to deep suppression diplopia cannot be elicited.

III. QUANTITATIVE MEASUREMENT OF ACTIONS OF EXTRAOCULAR MUSCLES

The quantitative measurement of actions of extraocular muscles is essential to comment about the paretic muscles and the pathological sequelae of the paralysis, *viz.* overaction, contracture and secondary inhibitional palsy.

The tests employed for quantitative measurements of ocular movements are based on haploscopy. The haploscopic tests are based on the principle described by Burian that in the presence of normal retinal correspondence, the two test objects presented to the two eyes will be superimposed, if they stimulate the foveae of the two eyes, irrespective of the position of the two eyes (Fig. 20.20).

Commonly used haploscopic tests to have a graphic record of the relative power of extraocular muscles in all directions of gaze include:

- Lancaster red-green test
- Hess screen test
- Lees screen test.

1. Lancaster red-green test

The Lancaster red-green test is a haploscopic test. It utilizes a Lancaster red-green screen which is window-shade type of screen that can be rolled up when not in use. The screen contains horizontal and vertical lines forming squares of 7 cm (Fig. 20.21). All the squares are of the same size and the tangential error is not taken into account. While performing the test, the patient's

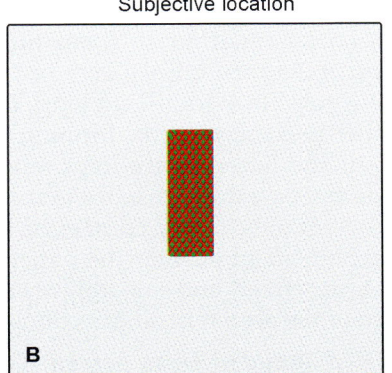

Fig. 20.20: *Burian's principle of haploscopic tests. Note, the right eye is esotropic and two different objects (red and green) presented to the two eyes (A) are stimulating the foveas and are thus subjectively localized as superimposed over each other (B).*

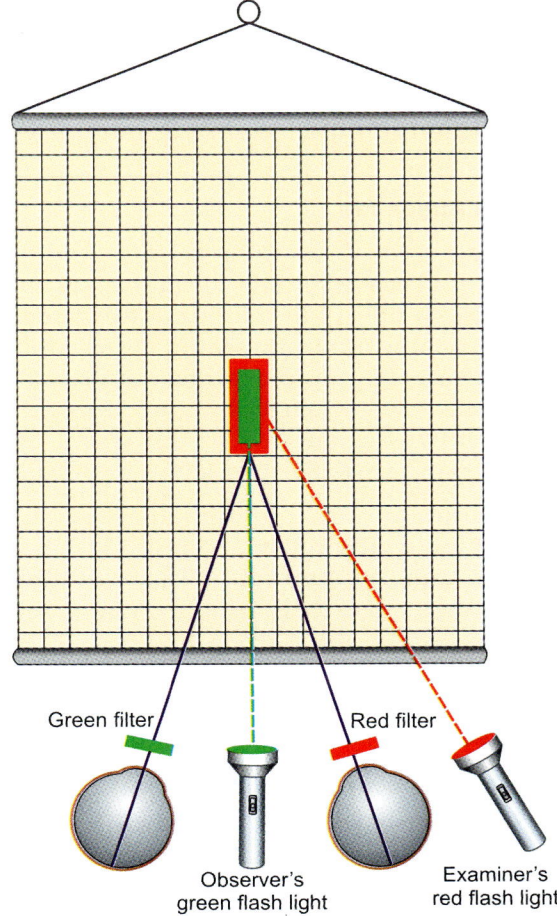

Fig. 20.21: *Lancaster red-green test.*

eyes should be in level with the centre zero mark, and he/she can be seated at either 1 or 2 metres. At 2 metres, each square subtends an angle of $2° = 3.5^\Delta$; at 1 metre it subtends an angle of $4° = 7^\Delta$. The patient is given a red-green reversible goggles (e.g. red glass in front of right eye and green glass in front of left eye) and green flashlight that projects a linear image. The examiner has a similar red flash light and projects the red streak of light on the zero mark on the screen. The patient is asked to superimpose his/her green light on the examiner's red light. This is then repeated in all cardinal directions of gaze. The distance between the streaks of light represents the measurement of the objective deviation provided retinal correspondence is normal. The results are plotted on a chart that is an exact replica of the screen. Since the projected image is a line, the patient's response may indicate the presence of cyclotropia, when his/her streak is tilted. This test is most useful in patients with ocular paralysis and least useful in patients with heterophoria or intermittent heterotropias.

2. Hess screen test

Principle
The Hess screen test is based on the haploscopic principle. It utilizes the Hering's law of equal innervation, which states that in all voluntary movements of the eye, equal and simultaneous innervation flows from the brain to the muscles of both eyes concerned in the respective direction of gaze (yoke muscles).

Prerequisites
Patient should have:
1. Full understanding about what he/she is supposed to do, since the test is purely subjective.
2. Good vision in both eyes.
3. Central fixation.
4. Normal retinal correspondence.

Discription of conventional Hess screen

Original Hess screen consisted of a single tangent screen made up of a black cloth 3 ft wide × 3½ ft long, marked by a series of horizontal and vertical red lines (Fig. 20.22). The distance between each line subtends a visual angle of 5°.

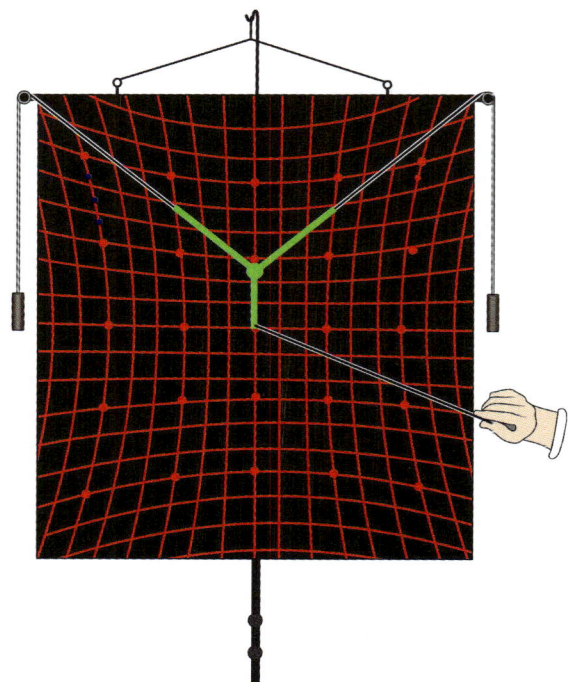

Fig. 20.22: *The Hess screen.*

Fixation points are indicated at the centre of the screen and at the intersections of the 15° and 30° lines by red dots. Thus, the red dots form an inner square of 8 dots along the 15° lines and an outer square of 16 dots along the 30° lines. The inner square represents the 8 cardinal directions of gaze and the outer square the extreme directions of gaze. In the original Hess screen, indicator consists of a knot tying three green cords together to form the letter Y. The end of central vertical green cord is fastened to a movable black rod 50 cm long. The ends of the other two green cords, forming upper two limbs of the letter Y, are kept taut by black threads that pass through loops to small weights at corresponding upper corners of the screen. This arrangement enables the patient to move the indicator freely and smoothly over the whole surface of the screen in all directions.

Modified wooden Hess screen. One of the modifications of the original Hess screen is a wooden screen with small red lights forming the fixation points (Fig. 20.23) and a green dot light projecter as the indicator. Presently, it is more commonly in use.

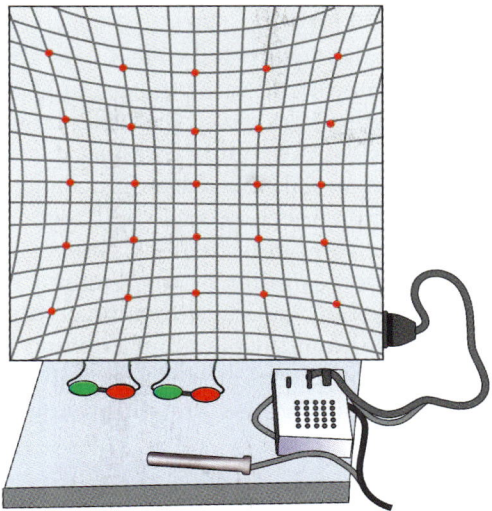

Fig. 20.23: *Modified Hess screen.*

Procedure Hess screen test

The patient wears red-green goggles and sits 50 cm from the commonly used modified wooden Hess screen. The patient now sees the fixation points (red light) with one eye and the indicator (green light of projector) with the other eye. The patient is asked to superimpose the indicator successively on each of the fixation points, and the relative position of the eyes is plotted for each of these directions of gaze on a chart which is replica of the Hess screen.

Digital Hess screen

Digital or the PC Hess screen provides the clinician, a new computer-based tool for assessing patients suffering from paralytic strabismus, using image manipulation technology and software technology. It is designed to run on any computer operating under Windows, with a 19" (or larger) monitor. When the program is run for the first time, the user is required to calibrate the size of the screen (by measuring the dimensions of a box displayed on the screen) and to enter the preferred viewing distance (usually 25–50 cm). It provides integration function of diagnosis of strabismus, data record and analyze.

Key features

- Rapid and accurate assessment of the size and direction of phoria/tropia

- Results plotted in conventional Hess screen format allow the clinician to establish whether a deviation is concomitant or incomitant and which muscle is affected
- A variety of analytical tools to help the clinician form a diagnosis
- Built in database allows results to be archived for future reference
- Results can be printed or pasted into referral letters and reports
- Runs on a standard PC
- Voice instructions, possible.

Operating methods

Digital Hess screen is a computer program which is designed to run on any computer. Steps of use are as below:

- *Patient wears red and green goggles* and is positioned in front of the computer screen at the appropriate distance (Fig. 20.24A).
- *Room lights are extinguished and a red and a blue circle are displayed on the screen* (the right eye sees the red circle and the left the blue). Initially the red circle is placed in the top left of the screen and the patient is instructed to move the blue circle using the mouse until it appears to be centred on the red circle.
- *As the eyes are dissociated*, any deviation in this direction of gaze will result in a misalignment of the circles (Fig. 20.24B). This is repeated for

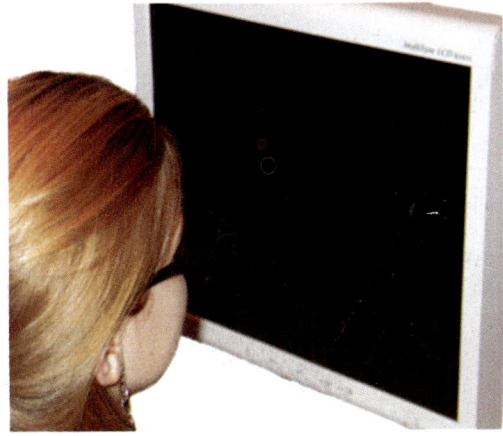

Fig. 20.24A: *Patient is seated in front of a PC Hess screen after wearing red and green goggles.*

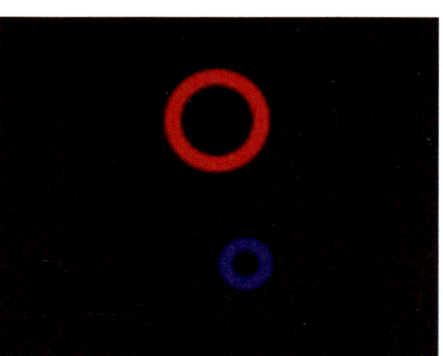

Fig. 20.24B: *Misalignment of the circles seen due to any deviation in the direction of gaze.*

either 9 or 25 directions of gaze (depending on the option selected). The colour of the circles is then reversed and measurements repeated with the left eye fixating. The nine point test takes approximately 4 minutes to complete.

- *Results are then displayed* in the conventional format on the screen.
- *Multiple plots can be superimposed* to assess longitudinal changes and the exact amplitude of any deviation can be displayed at any point on the chart (Fig. 20.25).
- *A number of analytical tools can then be applied* to the data to help the clinician establish a diagnosis. For example, the program will automatically calculate the relative areas of the plots for the left and right eyes, helping the clinician to determine which eye has a palsied muscle and providing an index for monitoring the progression of an incomitant deviation.

3. Lees screen test

Lees screen, also known as the Hess-Lees screen, is another modification of the original Hess screen. The Hess-Lees screen (Fig. 20.26) consists of two tangent screens made of white translucent material placed at a right angle with a plane mirror bisecting this right angle and dissociating the fields of the two eyes. The tangent pattern similar to the original Hess screen printed in black dots (fixation points) on a white background is placed just behind both the translucent screens, and is seen only when the translucent screens are illuminated for performing the test.

Procedure

To perform the test with right eye fixing, the patient sits facing the left tangent screen at 50 cm from it with his/her forehead leaning against the central vertical rim of the mirror. The line bisecting the mirror horizontally lies in the same plane as the centre of the horizontals of the tangent screens. Patient's pupils are levelled with this horizontal line by an adjustable chin rest. The patient is given a pointer with a ring at its tip. The examiner has another pointer with a small disc at its tip, half the diameter of the patient's pointer. The right screen is illuminated and left screen is kept non-illuminated. The patient's right eye vision is intercepted by the mirror, in which he/she sees the right screen projected forward as a virtual image that appears to be superimposed upon the left screen. The patient's left eye sees the left screen directly (he/she is facing that screen) but cannot see the

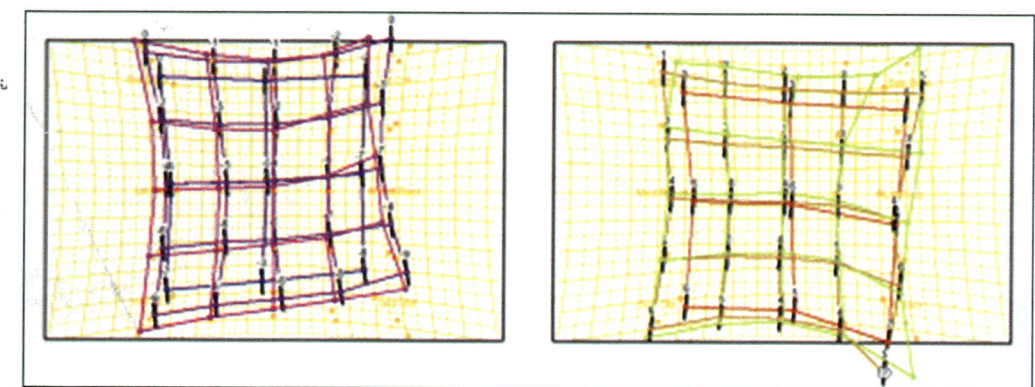

Fig. 20.25: *Hess screen plots superimposed to assess longitudinal changes and the exact amplitude of any deviation.*

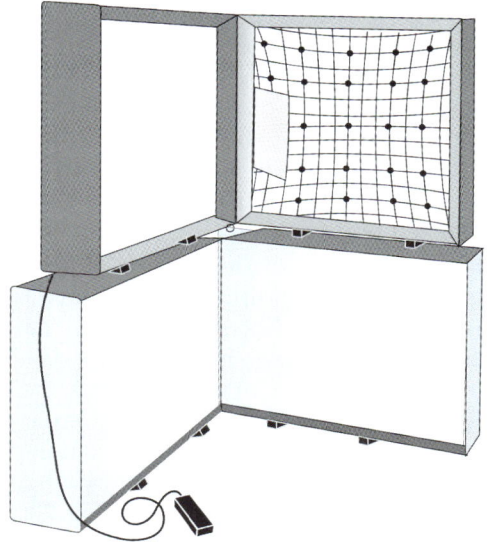

Fig. 20.26: *Lees screen.*

right screen, situated laterally. The examiner now places his pointer on the zero (central) point of the right screen. Its image that appears to be superimposed on the left screen is seen by the patient's right eye. Patient is asked to super-impose his/her pointer on the examiner's pointer with his/her left hand on the left screen. By means of a foot pedal, the left screen is illuminated for 1–2 seconds so that the examiner

can plot on the diagnostic Hess chart the precise location of the patient's pointer on the left screen. The 8 dots of the inner square are then plotted in sequence and, wherever necessary, this is followed by the plotting of the 16 dots of the outer square.

To perform the test with left eye fixing, patient sits facing the right screen which is kept unilluminated while looking with his/her left eye into the mirror, where he/she sees the virtual image of the left (illuminated) screen. The procedure described above is then repeated.

Diagnostic interpretation of the Hess chart

The diagnostic interpretation of the Hess chart is done by comparing the two fields, i.e. one, of the left eye plotted while the right eye fixing and other, of the right eye plotted while the left eye is fixing. The interpretation should be done as follows:

1. *Compression of the space* between the two plotted fixation points indicates underaction of a muscle acting in that direction.

2. *Expansion of the space* between the two plotted fixation points indicates overaction of the muscle acting in that direction.

3. *Smaller field belongs to the eye* with the paretic muscle (Fig. 20.27A).

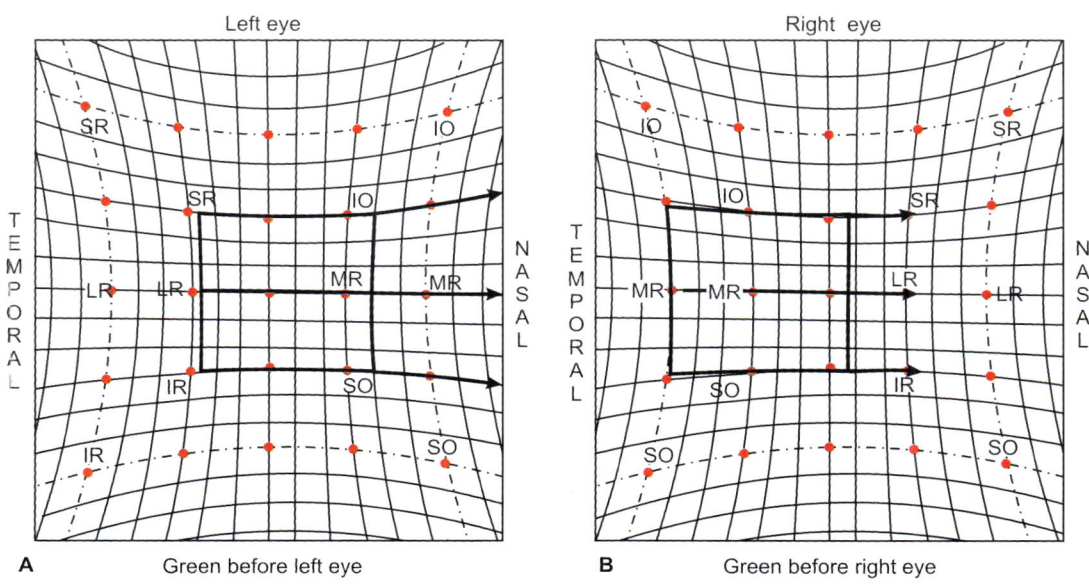

Fig. 20.27: *Hess chart of a patient with right lateral rectus palsy.*

4. *Non-affected eye shows the larger field* expressing the overaction of the contralateral synergist (Fig. 20.27B).

5. *Fields of similar shape and size are suggestive of comitant deviation,* while the fields of dissimilar shape and size indicate incomitance.

6. *In the smaller field, the greatest displacement (compression) away from the normal cardinal direction* will indicate the paretic muscle (underaction). In many cases, displacement in the direction of the field of the antagonist (due to contracture) may also be seen.

7. *In greater field, the greatest displacement (expansion) away from the normal cardinal direction* will indicate the overacting muscle (contralateral synergistic or yoke muscle of the paretic muscle). In many cases (especially in those of long duration), there may also be displacement of the field away from the direction of the antagonist of this muscle (due to inhibitional palsy of the contralateral antagonist).

IV. FIELD OF BINOCULAR FIXATION

It should be tested in patients with incomitant squint, where applicable, i.e. if patient has some field of binocular single vision. The area of binocular single vision is opposite to the direction in which ocular motility is impaired. In general, the field of binocular fixation represents the extreme limits of conjugate movement of the eyes in all directions in the absence of any movement of the head.

Procedure

The test is performed on the perimeter using a central chin rest. The patient fixates a small (3.5 mm) movable white target in the primary position, which is then moved along the arc until diplopia results or it goes out of the fixation limits. This point is recorded. The arc is then moved on successively in 15° steps and the test repeated for each position until the whole field has been examined. Normal field of fixation is shown in Fig. 20.28.

If the patient has diplopia in central position fixation, the target is moved in the periphery till the target becomes single or the target goes out of fixation point. The record of binocular field of fixation is completed as above.

The diplopia as well as binocular fixation is better appreciated, when the test is performed using red and green goggles in front of the eyes and a movable spot of white light as target. In the area of binocular single fixation, the target spotlight will appear as mixture of red and green, and when binocular fixation is lost it will appear red or green.

It is standard to shade the area of binocular single vision after plotting on the chart. In the presence of suppression, the test can be performed with filters, but this may diminish the fusional response. In general terms, the field of binocular fixation is more or less circular with a radius of about 45–50° from the fixation point in the primary position, except below when it is restricted on either side by the nose (Fig. 20.33C).

In a patient with paresis of an extraocular muscle, it may be helpful to record a patient's successive fields of binocular fixation on the same chart, thus making it easy to observe the clinical cause of the condition. As an example, Fig. 20.29 shows field of binocular fixation before and after operation (on the same chart) in a patient having 3rd nerve palsy of 2 years duration.

V. BIELSCHOWSKY'S PHENOMENON TEST

This test is performed for confirming the diagnosis of alternating sursumduction suspected on alternating cover test. The eye under cover deviates upwards and extorts. When the cover is removed, the eye slowly rotates downward to return to its previous position.

To perform the Bielschowsky phenomenon test, patient is asked to fixate a spotlight with one eye and the other eye is covered by an occluder. It is observed that the eye under cover moves up and extorts. Then, a filter is held before the fixating eye, keeping a watch on the eye under cover, which moves downward and intorts. This influence of changing the light stimulus in the fixating eye on the deviation of the covered eye is known as the Bielschowsky phenomenon. Its presence confirms the diagnosis of alternating sursumduction made on alternate cover test.

VI. BIELSCHOWSKY'S HEAD TILT TEST

This test was originally recommended by Bielschowsky to differentiate between superior

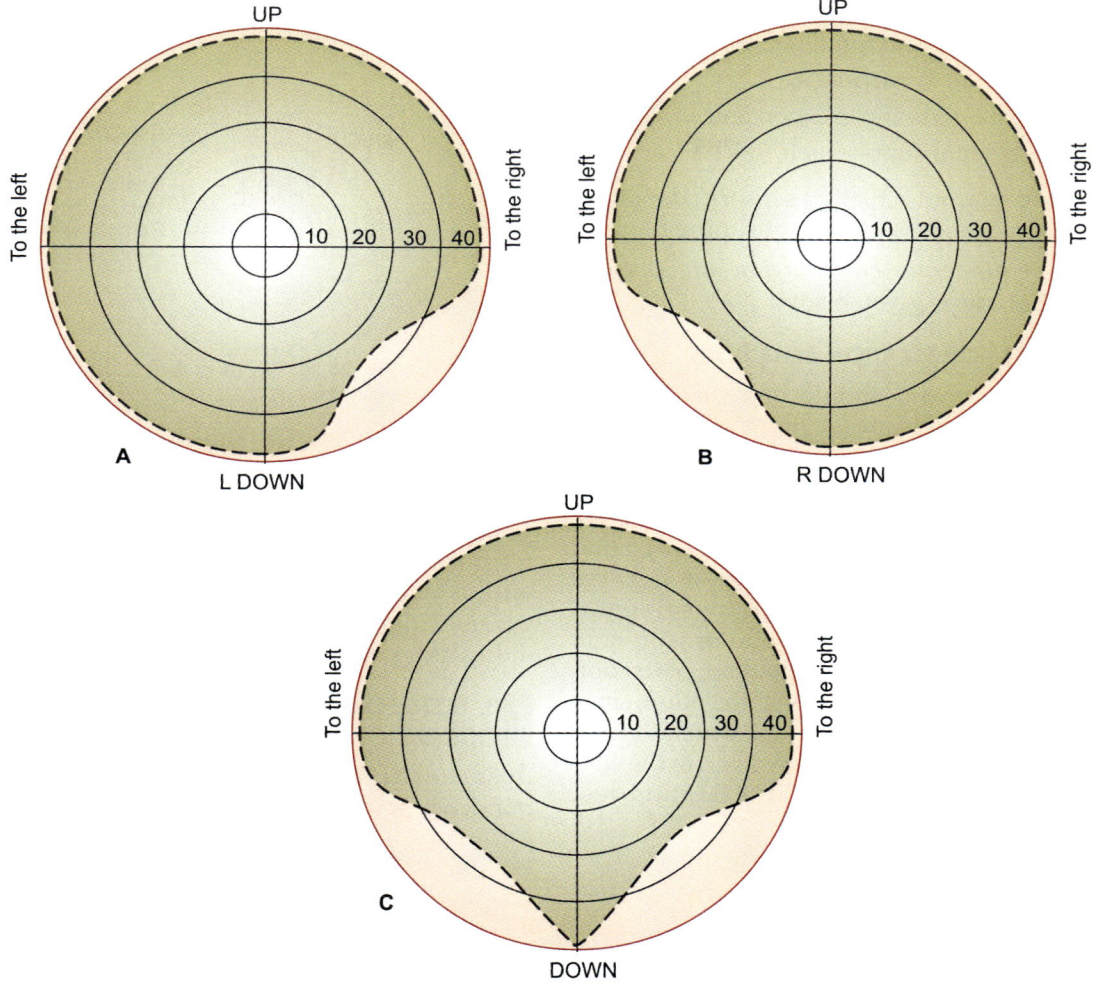

Fig. 20.28: *Field of fixation: (A) left eye, (B) right eye and (C) binocular.*

oblique palsy in one eye and superior rectus palsy in the contralateral side. The modified *three-step technique of Bielschowsky's head tilt test* is used for the diagnosis of paretic vertical recti and oblique muscles. For details, *see* Chapter 21.

SENSORY EVALUATION: ASSESSMENT FOR BINOCULAR COOPERATION AND SENSORY ANOMALIES

Normal binocular single vision consists of three grades: Simultaneous perception, fusion and stereopsis. It is maintained with central fixation and normal retinal correspondence.

There are variety of sensory adoptations that occur in response to clinical situations that disrupt binocular vision. The development of a specific type of sensory adaptation depends on when (age of the patients) the sensory anomaly occurred and the severity and type of binocular disruption.

Visually mature patients may develop following sensory adaptations:

• Diplopia
• Confusion
• Rivalry.

Visually immature patients may develop following sensory adaptations:

- Monofixation syndrome
- Anomalous retinal correspondence (ARC)
- Large regional suppression.

Amblyopia, not actually a sensory adaptation may occur as a consequence of suppression.

Tests for binocular cooperation and sensory anomalies are as given below:

A. TESTS FOR FIXATION BEHAVIOUR

Fixation behaviour should be tested in each patient with strabismus having vision less than 6/6 Snellen's. It can be tested with the help of a visuscope (page 423) or fixation star of the ophthalmoscope. Patient is asked to cover one eye and fix the star with the other eye. Fixation may be *centric (normal on the fovea) or eccentric* (which may be unsteady, parafoveal, paramacular, centrocaecal, paracaecal or temporal; Fig. 20.30). The preliminary checking of fixation should be done without dilating the pupil, since this would be an obstacle to the pursuit of the rest of the diagnostic tests. However, in the end, pupils should be dilated and fixation test

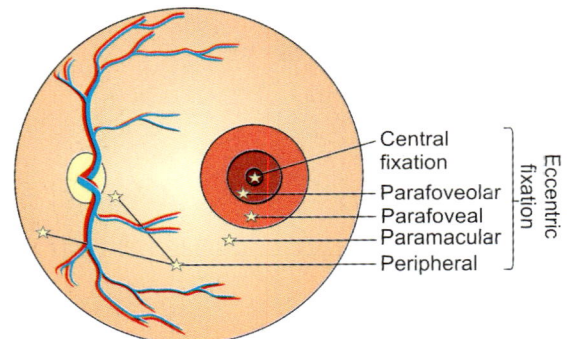

Fig. 20.30: *Types of fixation.*

repeated along with the detailed fundus examination.

A steady central foveal fixation is a good prognostic sign. An unsteady but central foveal fixation indicates a possibility of good vision with conventional occlusion while a steady paramacular or peripheral eccentric fixation indicates a poor prognosis.

B. TESTS FOR THE STATE OF RETINAL CORRESPONDENCE

Assessment for the state of retinal correspondence is neccessary only in the presence of a constant manifest deviation. It is absolutely essential to know the state of monocular fixation, whether it is eccentric or central, so that this can be taken into account, when evaluating the results of the various tests.

In the absence of normal retinal correspondence (NRC), a patient with strabismus may develop anomalous retinal correspondence (ARC). ARC is an unstable secondary adaptation of sensory interaction between the two eyes that has developed under conditions of everyday stimulation and exists under these conditions.

The tests employed to evaluate state of retinal correspondence are described here in decreasing order of their similarity to normal circumstances.

1. Striated glass test *(Bagolini test)*

This test, performed with the Bagolini striated glasses, is closest to everyday visual conditions. The eyes are not dissociated during the test and can be observed by the examiner.

Bagolini's striated glasses (sometimes referred to as lenses) are in fact glass plates without

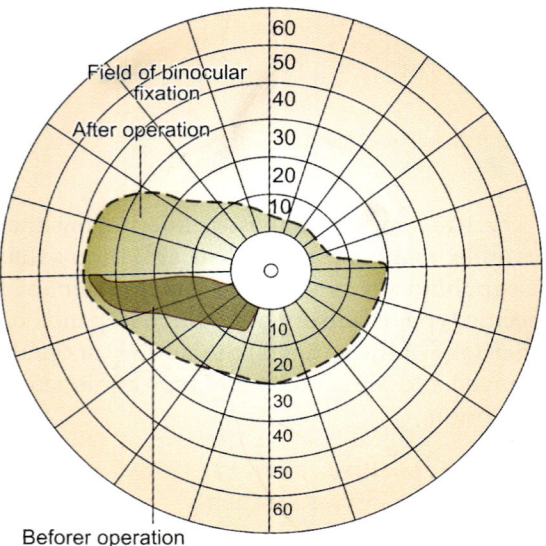

Fig. 20.29: *Field of binocular fixation before and after extraocular muscles surgery in a patient with third nerve palsy.*

refractive power. The glass plates contain extremely fine parallel striations on the surface. When looking through them, a spotlight appears as a fine streak of light perpendicular to the striations. The principle basically is the same as for the Maddox rod except that the patient can actually see through Bagolini's glasses. The glasses are mounted so that they can be inserted into a trial frame. Marks on the glass indicate the direction of the streak seen by the patient.

Procedure to perform the test (Fig. 20.31). Preferably the test should be performed in a room with subdued light. The test is performed for distance (6 metres) as well as near (33 cm). Patient is instructed to fixate on a spotlight. The striated glasses are placed in a trial frame with their axis oriented respectively at 45° and 135°, so that a normal subject would see two streaks of light forming a × intersecting at the spotlight (Fig. 20.31A). In a patient with strabismus, one of the following observations may be made:

1. A patient with a constant tropia having normal retinal correspondence (NRC) with no demonstrable suppression will experience diplopia, i.e. will see two spotlights each one crossed by one streak of light (Fig. 20.31B). According to the deviation, they will be seen either in crossed or in uncrossed diplopia.

2. In the presence of suppression of one eye, the patient will see the spotlight crossed by the line in front of the non-suppressing eye only (Fig. 20.31C).

3. A patient with harmonious anomalous retinal correspondence will see a perfect cross, as seen by a normal person (Fig. 20.31A), but the cover test will show the presence of a tropia.

4. Two streaks, but only one crossing through the centre of the light (the other one being displaced away from the light with a portion of it missing), indicate a suppression area with either normal retinal correspondence or unharmonious ARC (Fig. 20.31D).

5. In the presence of a small angle tropia, if the patient sees a perfect cross as seen by a normal person (Fig. 20.31A), and there is no movement on cover test, NRC is indicated (although there may be lack of bifoveal fixation). Parks records such cases as having 'unknown retinal correspondence'.

Advantages of Bagolini's test
- This test is closest to the everyday visual conditions, i.e. there is minimal interference with normal visual condition since the patient can see with both eyes.
- It is a simple and easy test both for the patient and the examiner. Even a child can describe exactly what he sees.
- The test can be performed for any fixation distance.
- Since the eyes are not dissociated during the test, these can be observed by the examiner.

Disadvantages
- The test is only qualitative since the angle of anomaly cannot be measured.
- Small angles of anomaly may be over-looked.

2. Diplopia test

To perform this test, patient's deviation is first determined objectively and the diplopia test is then performed under the same conditions (i.e. same fixation distance and refractive correction) to permit comparison. In the diplopia test, the patient fixates a spotlight on the centre of a tangent scale through a red filter and the deviating eye is uncovered. To begin with, each eye is covered alternately, so as to show him, that the fixation light and the tangent scale or screen is seen with one eye and red spot of light with the other eye. When both eyes are uncovered, the patient may see one or two lights as follows:
- When the patient sees one red light and one white light, it indicates either normal retinal correspondence or unharmonious ARC (if the separation of the images is not compatible with the angle of deviation).
- When the patient sees only one red light, it indicates suppression of the deviating eye.
- When the patient sees a mixture of red and white or a light red light, it indicates probability of harmonious ARC.

Advantages
The test is very simple and can be performed in children of average intelligence who are as young as 4 years of age.

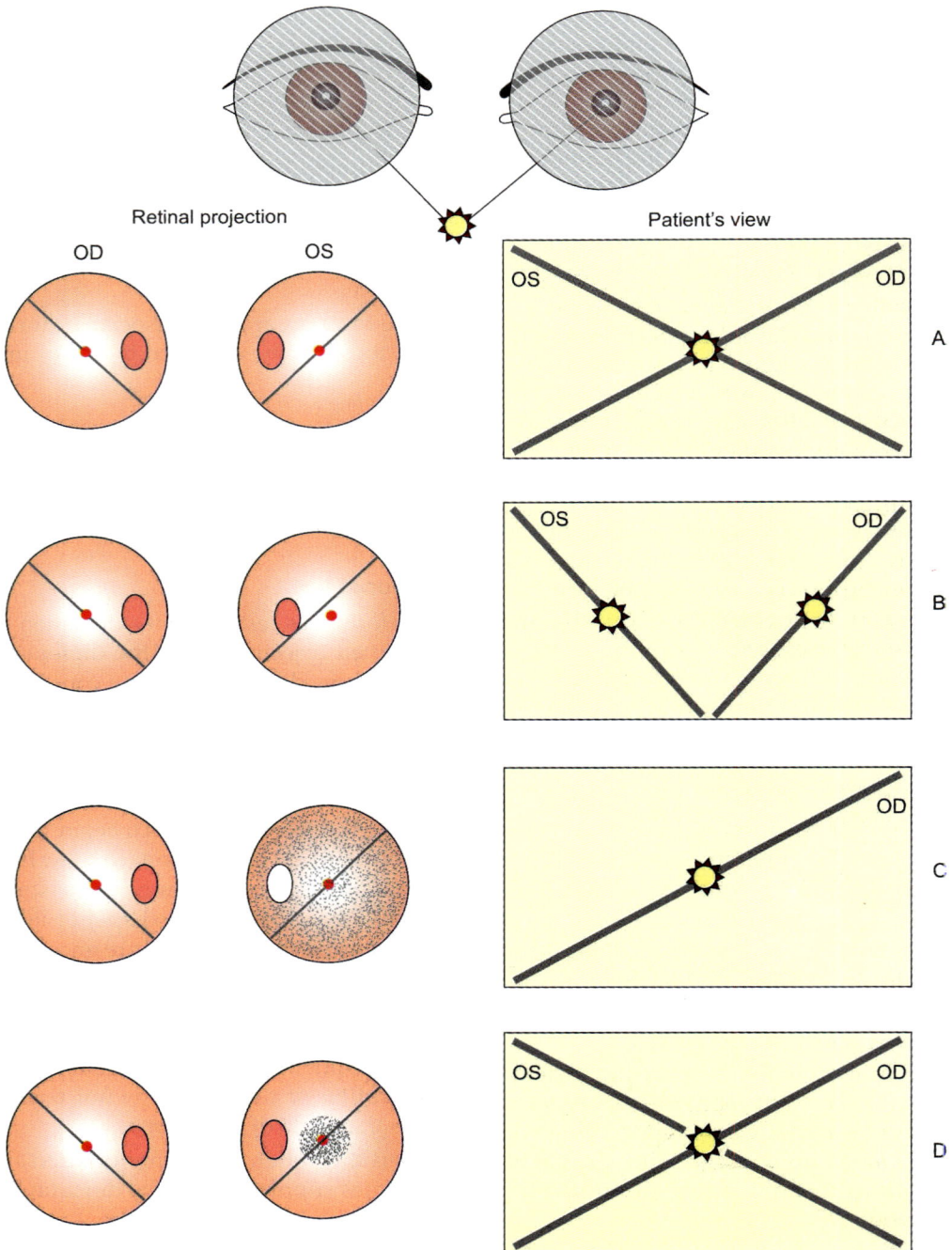

Fig. 20.31: *Bagolini's striated glass test (for explanation see text).*

Disadvantages

It is difficult to differentiate between fusion of the images and suppression of the deviating eye, since even in binocular vision, the fixating eye will be dominant and the image will tend to appear red.

3. Prism bar and red filter test

To perform this test, patient is asked to fixate a spotlight at 6 metres distance and a prism bar cover test is carried out with prism bar in front of the fixating eye, till the deviation is neutralized. The prism bar reading at this point equals the objective angle of squint. A red filter is then placed in front of the deviating eye and the patient is asked to describe what he/she sees. The various possibilities are as below:

1. Patient may suppress one eye, i.e. he/she does not see red light or a mixture of red and white light. This makes the test useless.
2. In the presence of normal retinal correspondence (i.e. when the foveae have a common visual direction), the patient may see the light as a blend of red and white.
3. In the presence of ARC, i.e. when the foveae have different visual directions, the patient will see two lights, a white and a red one. In a patient with esodeviation, the diplopia will be crossed and with exodeviation uncrossed (paradoxical diplopia).
4. To measure the angle of anomaly, in the presence of ARC, the prism bar is now moved slowly (decreasing the base-out strength for esodeviations or the base-in strength in exodeviations) until the diplopia disappears or until the type of diplopia is reversed. The prism bar value at this point equals the subjective angle of squint. The difference between the objective and subjective angles represents the angle of anomaly.

4. Synoptophore test

To detect ARC by synoptophore method, *objective and subjective angles* of the squint are measured using dissimilar slides (e.g. lion and the cage) as discribed on page 389, respectively, and the results are interpreted as below:

1. If the objective and subjective angles of the squint coincide, normal retinal correspondence (NRC) is present.
2. If the objective angle is greater than subjective angle, the anomalous retinal correspondence (ARC) is present; and the difference between these angles is called the angle of anomaly, when the angle of anomaly is equal to the objective angle, i.e. when subjective angle is zero, the ARC is harmonious. In unharmonious

ARC, angle of anomaly is smaller than the objective angle.

5. Worth's four-dot test

For this test, patient wears red-green goggles with red lens in front of the right eye and green lens in front of the left eye and views a box with four lights—one red, two green and one white (Fig. 20.32A). Since the lights are of the colours complementary to those of the filters before the patient's eye, he/she can see the red light only through the red filter and the two green lights only through the green filter. The white light can be seen with both eyes.

Depending upon the patient's observation, the results are interpreted as below:

1. If the patient sees all the four lights (one red, two green and one white or red or green or mixture of red and green) in the absence of manifest squint, he/she has normal binocular single vision (Fig. 20.32A).
2. With abnormal retinal correspondence (ARC), patient sees all the four lights as above even in the presence of a manifest squint (Fig. 20.32B).

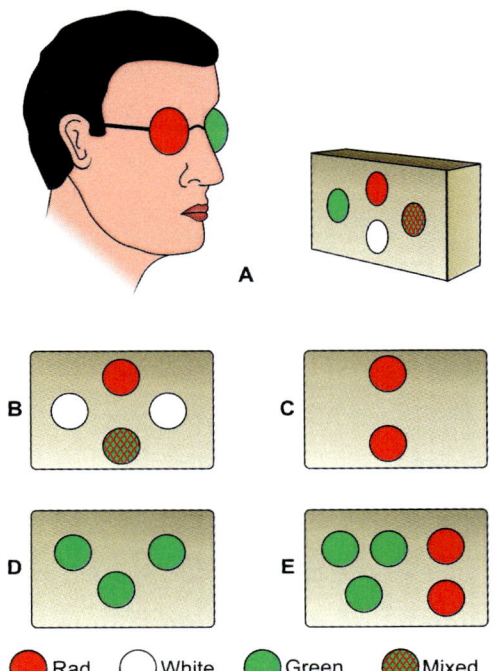

| ● Rad | ○ White | ● Green | ● Mixed |

Fig. 20.32: *Worth's four-dot test.*

3. If the patient sees only two red lights, he/she has left suppression (Fig. 20.32C).

4. If the patient sees only three green lights, he/she has right suppression (Fig. 20.32D).

5. When the patient sees three green lights and two red lights alternately, it indicates presence of alternating suppression.

6. If the patient sees five lights (2 red and 3 green), he has diplopia (Fig. 20.32E).

6. Bielschowsky's after image test

In this test, patient's right fovea is stimulated with a vertical bright light and left fovea with a horizontal bright light (Fig. 20.33A) for 15 seconds each and the patient is asked to draw

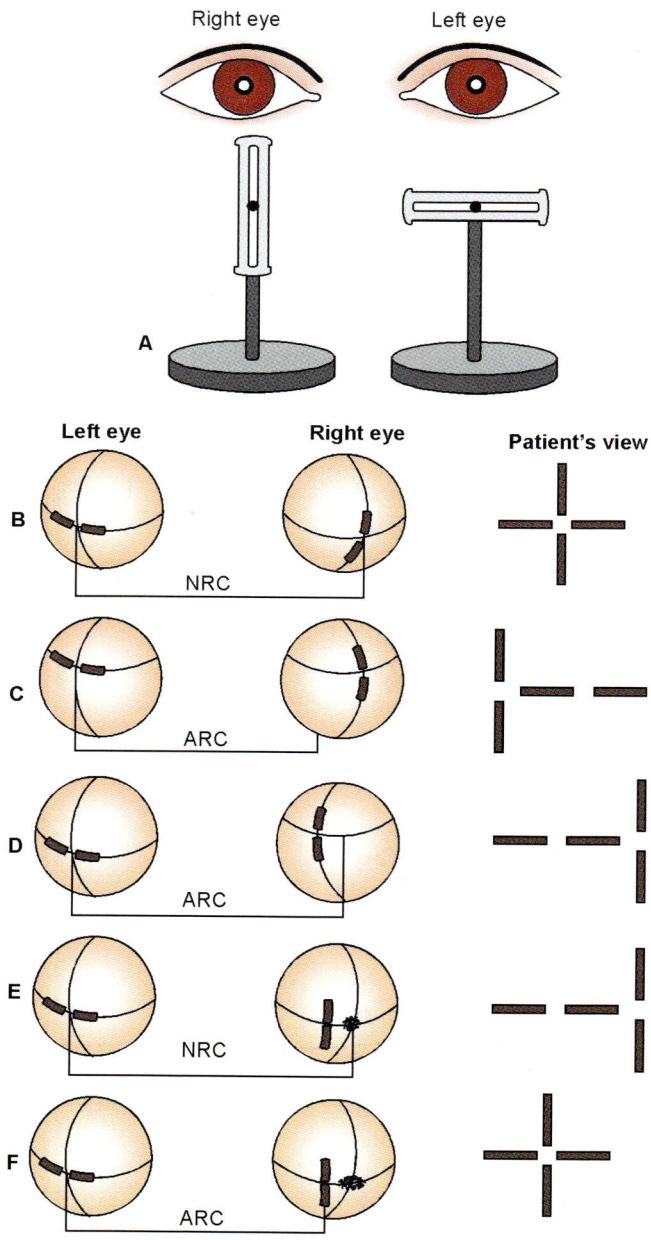

Fig. 20.33: *Bielschowsky's after image test (for explanation, see text).*

the position of after images. Perception of the after images is easiest, when the patient closes his/her eyes or when he/she looks at a blank screen. *The results are interpreted as below*:

1. A patient with normal retinal correspondence will draw a cross (Fig. 20.33B).
2. A right esotropic patient with ARC will draw vertical image to the left of horizontal image (Fig. 20.33C).
3. A right exotropic patient with ARC will draw vertical image to the right of horizontal (Fig. 6.33D).
4. A response showing the images in a crossed position in exotropia (Fig. 20.33E) and in an uncrossed position in esotropia (Fig. 20.33F) indicates the presence of paradoxic diplopia in the presence of ARC with eccentric fixation.
5. The patient may draw only vertical image (in left suppression) or only horizontal image (in right suppression). In alternate suppression, patient sees vertical and horizontal lines alternately.

Disadvantages

1. The after image test is the most unphysiologic of all the tests for ARC, since an after image and a normal visual stimulation are so different that they cannot even be compared.
2. Small children do not understand what they should observe.

7. Cupper's binocular visuscope test

In this test, the patient sits 5 metres away from a Maddox scale and is asked to fixate the light on the centre of scale with fixing eye and the examiner looks the images of the visuscope on the retina of patient's deviated eye. Since it may be difficult for the examiner to look through the visuscope without blocking the patient's view of the fixation object, i.e. the patient is asked to fixate through a plane mirror or prism (which changes the direction of fixation) (Fig. 6.34A).

The examiner projects the star of the visuscope on the patient's fovea and asks the patient to tell its position on the Maddox scale in respect to the central fixation light. The results are interpreted as below:

1. In the presence of normal retinal correspondence, the patient sees star superimposed on the fixation light (Fig. 20.34B).

2. In the presence of ARC, patient sees star to the right or left of the fixation light depending upon the deviation. The number on the Maddox scale coinciding with the star gives the angle of anomaly (Fig. 20.34C).

After the presence of ARC is established, the examiner moves the visuscope until the star and the fixation light coincide, and at this point, the examiner notes the position of the star on the patient's retina. This peripheral point on the retina of the patient's deviated eye has acquired a common visual direction with the fovea of the dominant eye. This point is not always the same as the one used for eccentric fixation. In other words, the angle of anomaly is not always identical with the distance between the fovea and the retinal point used for fixation.

Disadvantages

The binocular visuscope test is difficult to perform with young children.

Evaluation of tests for retinal correspondence

A great disparity between the results of various tests performed for evaluation of state of retinal correspondence is reported in the literature. In general, as stated earlier, the tests that interfere least with the ordinary conditions of seeing (e.g. Bagolini's test) show more ARC response and the tests which cause most dissociating conditions (e.g. after image test) show less ARC response.

C. ASSESSMENT FOR GRADES OF BINOCULAR SINGLE VISION

Assessment for grades of binocular single vision (BSV) is essential, since its achievement is the ultimate goal in the management of a case with strabismus. As stated earlier, the three grades of BSV include simultaneous perception (first grade), fusion (second grade) and stereopsis (third grade). Various tests employed to assess the state of BSV are known.

D. TESTS TO ASSESS SUPPRESSION AND AMBLYOPIA

TESTS FOR DETECTION OF SUPPRESSION

1. Worth's four-dot test. This test can be employed to diagnose the suppression involving the peripheral retina. As described in detail on page 409, the patients having left suppression

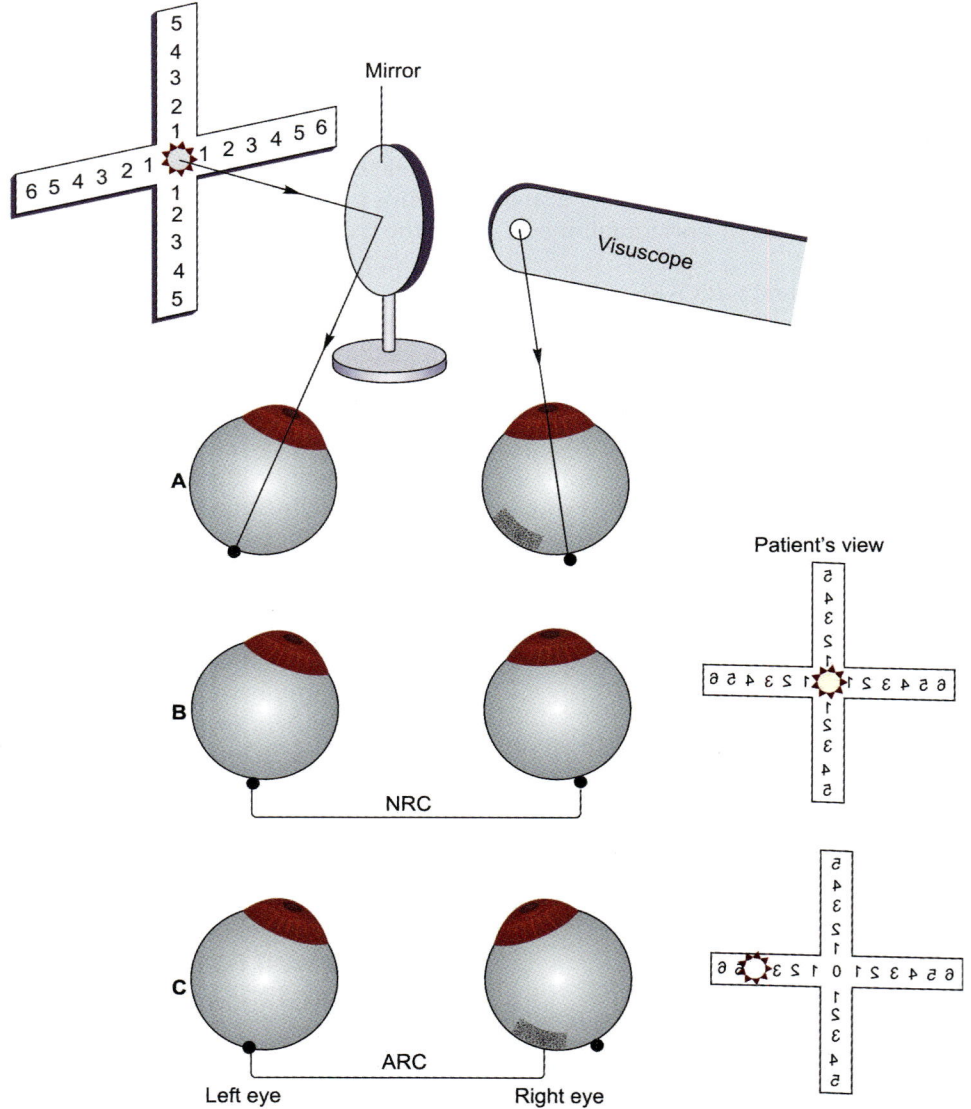

Fig. 20.34: *Cupper's binocular visuscope test (for explanation, see text).*

will see only two red lights and that having right suppression will see only three green lights (Fig. 20.32). In the presence of alternate suppression, patients will see alternately two red lights and three green lights.

Disadvantages. Worth's four-dot test is not a very useful test for suppression because of the following reasons:

• It does not detect foveal suppression.
• Since the eyes are easily dissociated with red-green glasses, a patient with unstable but functionally useful binocular vision may exhibit a suppression response with this test.
• In a patient having ARC, a normal fusion response (the patient sees all four dots in a rectangular arrangement) occurs even in the presence of suppression.

2. The 4D base-out prism test (Fig. 20.35). This test popularized by Jampolsky is performed for detection of small angle heterotropias and the presence of central suppression scotoma.

Technique. To perform this test, patient fixates a penlight (Fig. 20.35A). Then a 4D prism is placed with base-out in front of the right eye and the examiner observes the presence of a biphasic corrective movement of the left eye (Fig. 20.35B and C). This is absent in the presence of a central suppression scotoma (Fig. 20.35D).

Mechanism of biphasic corrective movements can be explained as below:

- The prism displaces the image towards its base, in other words, from the fovea of the right eye towards a point on the temporal half of the retina (4D or 2° away from the fovea). The relaxation movement of the right eye will elicit conjugate movements of both

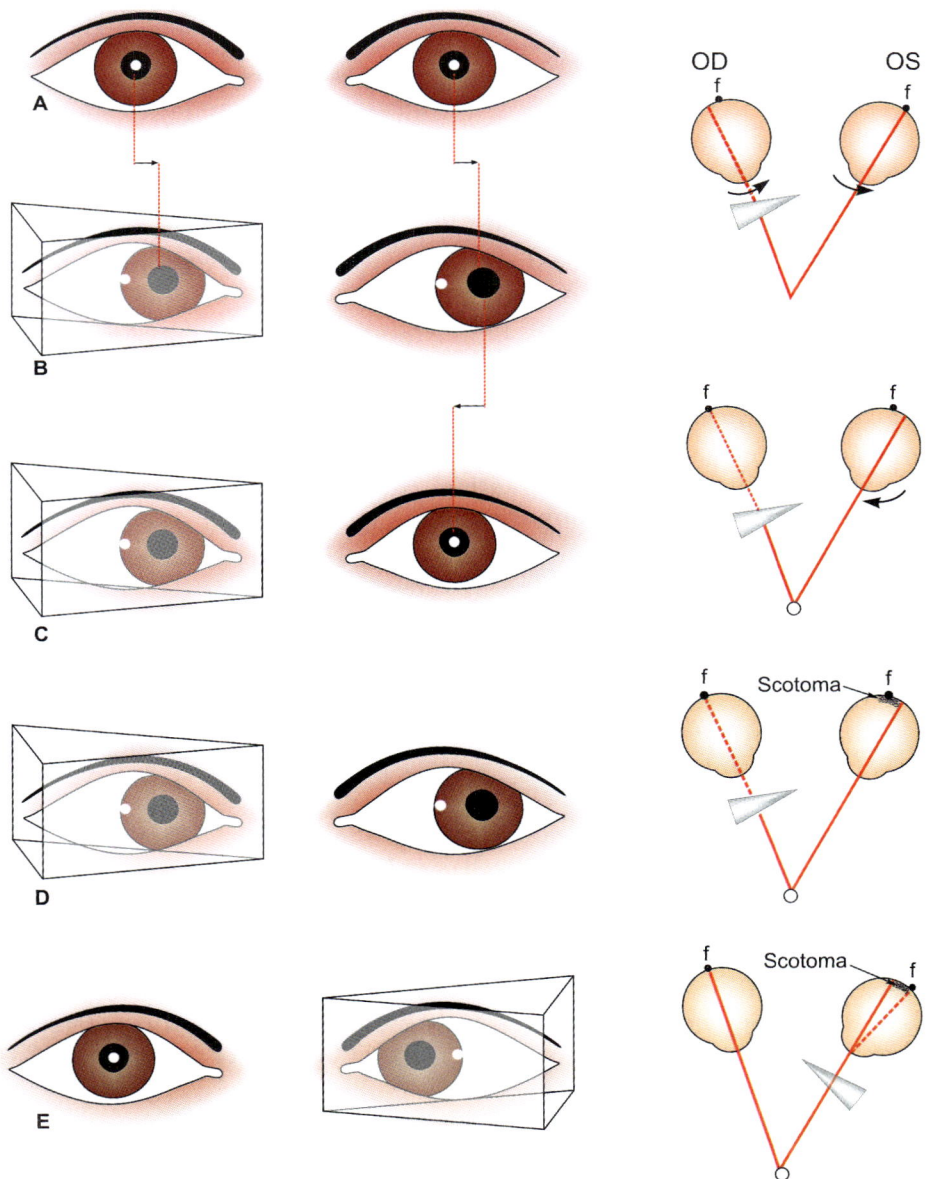

Fig. 20.35: *The 4D base-out prism test with its optical principle (for explanation, see text).*

eyes to the left (levoversion), if the right eye has no foveal suppression (Fig. 20.35B).

- This displaces the image in the left eye from the fovea to the temporal retina and thus, the left eye now makes a fusional movement in the opposite direction, if no foveal suppression is present (Fig. 20.35C). In the presence of central suppression scotomal this will be absent (Fig. 20.35D)

- The test should be repeated with prism over the left eye (Fig. 20.35E) and observation for a biphasic corrective movement in the right eye should be made.

3. Diplopia test or red glass test. *See* page 407.

4. Bagolini's striated glass test. A foveal (central) suppression scotoma in orthotropic patient or a fixation point scotoma in the presence of microtropia can be detected with Bagolini's striated glass test. As described on page 406 and shown in Fig. 20.31, a patient with fixation point suppression will see a central interruption of the light streak.

5. Visual acuity test with Project-O-Chart slide of American optical. It is a very effective test to detect foveal suppression in patients with microtropia or in patients with subnormal binocular vision after surgical correction of essential infantile esotropia. In this test, visual acuity of each eye is measured under binocular conditions with the Project-O-Chart slide of American optical. Presence of decreased visual acuity in one eye that is not present, when the eye is tested under monocular conditions indicates the foveal suppression.

6. Synoptophore test. Suppression can be diagnosed with the use of simultaneous perception slides (e.g. a cage and a lion) as well as fusion slides (e.g. identical pictures of a rabbit, one having a candle and the other having flower). When simultaneous perception slides are used, normally patient should see the lion in the cage. In the presence of suppression, patient sees either lion or cage.

To begin with, simultaneous foveal perception (SFP) slides are used. When foveal suppression is present, the simultaneous macular perception (SMP) slides are used. In the presence of macular suppression, simultaneous paramacular perception (SPP) slides are used and observations are made. While using fusion slides, if the patient sees a rabbit with both the candle and flower, it indicates normal binocular single vision. In the presence of suppression, either the candle or the flower is absent. The fusion pictures are graded according to the size in the same way as the simultaneous perception pictures.

Suppression scotoma can be mapped out, at least in the horizontal meridian with synoptophore. One arm of the instrument is rotated, and the points are noted at which the target carried by the moving arm disappears and reappears.

Test for measurement of depth of suppression

Depth of suppression is not equal in all the patients. The degree to which facultative suppression can produce obligatory suppression probably depends upon the age of the child, when facultative suppression begins. The deeper the suppression, more difficult it is to overcome.

Depth of suppression can be measured with the help of red filter ladder (Fig. 20.36) which contains a series of red filters of increasing density. The red filter ladder usually consists of gelatine fibres, beginning with one layer and increasing to six or eight layers. The more the layers, the darker the filter.

To measure the depth of suppression, the patient is asked to fixate a small light, and the filters in increasing density are placed in front of the fixating eye till the patient sees double lights. Some patients see double with a filter made of single layer; while the others require filters of three or more layers depending upon the depth of suppression. The greater the

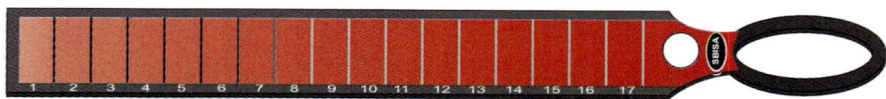

Fig. 20.36: *Red filter ladder used for measuring depth of suppression.*

number of layers needed, the deeper is the suppression.

EVALUATION FOR AMBLYOPIA

Diagnosis of amblyopia is made by a reduced best corrected visual acuity that cannot be entirely explained on the basis of physical ocular abnormalities. Clinical evaluation of a suspected case of amblyopia should include the following:

1. Evaluation of visual acuity.
2. Neutral density filter test.
3. Test for crowding phenomenon.
4. Thorough ocular examination including fundus examination.
5. Refraction.
6. Evaluation for central versus eccentric fixation.
7. Tests for other sensory anomalies.

1. Evaluation for visual acuity. As mentioned above, clinical evaluation of visual acuity is most important for the diagnosis of amblyopia. Generally speaking, a difference of two lines between the best corrected visual acuity of the two eyes (e.g. OD 6/6, OS 6/12 or OD 6/5, OS 6/9) is considered diagnostic for amblyopia. For practical purposes, particularly after amblyopia treatment has started, any acuity difference is considered amblyopia.

Severity of amblyopia. In the Amblyopia treatment study (ATS) group trials, amblyopia has been graded as below:

- *Mild to moderate* amblyopia is defined as visual acuity in the amblyopic eye of 20/80 or betta.
- *Severe amblyopia* is defined as visual acuity in the amblyopic eye of 20/100 to 20/400.

Methods employed to evaluate visual acuity depend upon the age of the patient and have been described in detail on page 48. However, for a ready reference, important points for different age groups are mentioned as follows:

Methods for evaluating visual potential in infants and very young children (up to 2½ years of age). Infancy and early childhood is probably the most important age to be bothered, since it is the most sensitive period to develop amblyopia. At the same time, testing of vision during this period is also not so easy. However, untiring efforts should be made to detect unequality of vision in two eyes. Certain useful methods are as follows:

Fixation behaviour test. Fixation behaviour test is a reliable and useful test in infancy to obtain a rough estimate of visual acuity. Each eye is covered alternately and behaviour of the infant is noticed. If vision is equal or nearly equal in both eyes, an infant or very young child will not object to having either eye covered. However, if the visual acuity is reduced in one eye, the child will show objection (in the form of a cry or pushing the occluder away) when the normal eye is covered. In such cases, one should suspect any ocular disease, high refractive error or amblyopia.

A rough estimate of visual acuity can be made by testing with brightly coloured toys of varying size while occluding one eye. It is noticed whether the child can fix and follow the toy.

Binocular fixation pattern (BFP). The binocular fixation pattern, indicating strength of preference for one eye or the other under binocular viewing conditions, is generally relied upon for estimating the relative level of vision in two eyes for very young children with strabismus. It is important to note that, when the infant's binocular fixation pattern is tested, an accommodative target such as small toy should be used. A child with extremely unequal vision will show great preference for the good eye. A child with nearly equal vision will have only mild preference for one eye. Five grades of binocular fixation pattern described while making the patient fix with the deviated eye (Table 20.1).

Binocular fixation pattern test is quite sensitive for detecting amblyopia but is sometimes false positive (showing a strong preference, when vision is equal or nearly equal in the two eyes), particularly with small-angle strabismic deviations.

Prism-induced tropia test. Prisms can be used in a variety of ways to induce a tropia, thus allowing the binocular fixation pattern to be assessed in children with small angle strabismus:

- *25 dioptre base-in prism test (Cassin, 1982).* A 25 D base-in prism is introduced over one eye

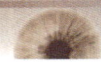

Table 20.1 *Grading of binocular fixation pattern in strabismic patients*

Grade	Description of response
Grade 0	: Spontaneous alternation (no preference for one eye).
Grade 1	: Holds fixation through blink (simply prefers one eye but can use the other eye with nearly equal frequency).
Grade 2	: Holds fixation until blink, i.e. habitually fixing eye resumes fixation with the next blink (moderate fixation preference).
Grade 3	: Holds fixation for 1–2 seconds but switches before blinks (strong fixation preference but the other is used briefly for fixation).
Grade 4	: Immediately switches fixation on removal of cover from non-deviating eye (strong fixation pattern, and patient uses only one eye for fixation).

and the child's eye preference is noticed. The prism is then placed over the other eye and preference is noted. This prism induces a large esotropia that cannot be overcome by most children and results in diplopia. Therefore, a child with equal vision will ordinarily use the eye without the prism to fixate regardless of which eye is viewing through the prism. If a child shows preference for one eye to fixate through the prism, the nonpreferred eye is considered amblyopic.

• *Vertical prism test (induced tropia test).* Ten to fifteen dioptre vertical prism test has also been recommended to assess eye fixation preference by producing tropia with diplopia, similar to 25 D base-inprism test.

Note that the vertical prism test rectifies the high rate of misdiagnosis of amblyopia by standard fixation preference testing in patients with small-angle strabismus and monofixation syndrome. This is because the vertical prism breaks up the peripheral fusion and central scotoma complex, thus allowing the patient to fixate with either eye.

CSM method of rating monocular fixation. CSM method has been used to describe the fixation pattern of a too young patient for visual acuity measurement by some workers after examination with a handlight as follows:

• **C:** Stands for '*central*' which refers to the fact that angle kappa appeared equal in direction and magnitude.
• **S:** Stands for '*steady*' which means that fixation is not aimless or wandering as in amblyopia and also that nystagmus is absent.
• **M:** Stands for '*maintained*', meaning thereby that there is no shift on the cover test, i.e. a manifest squint is not present.

It has been reported that rating of monocular fixation pattern as *central, steady* and *maintained* provides limited information. An eye with extremely poor visual acuity may also have central, steady and maintained fixation. Therefore, use of CSM should be avoided, particularly, if it replaces a visual acuity notation. Similarly the 'maintained' is no alternative to cover and cover-uncover test to detect manifest deviation.

Preferential looking test, optokinetic nystagmus and visually evoked potential. These tests are also used to measure visual acuity in infants and very young children (for details *see* page 35–37).

Methods of estimating visual acuity in preschool children (2½ to 4 years). Commonly employed tests are listed below (for details *see* page 38–41):

• Marble game test
• Hand chart test
• Illiterate E-game test
• Allen's preschool vision test
• Sheridan Gardiner test
• Stycar matching test.

Methods of estimating visual acuity in school children and adults (age 5 and older). Most commonly used tests are as follows (for details *see* page 41–43):

• Snellen's test types
• E-chart for illiterate
• Landolt's broken-C chart.

2. Neutral density filter test. Whenever possible, it is imperative to illucidate this important characteristic of amblyopic eye—that the amblyopic eye sees better under mesopic conditions (between scotopic and photopic condition).

This can be tested with neutral density filter test.

3. Test for crowding phenomenon should be performed to establish the separation difficulties—another important feature—exhibited by amblyopic eyes.

4. Thorough ocular examination including fundus examination. A thorough ocular examination including a detailed fundus examination is very important to rule out any cause, other than amblyopia, of reduced visual acuity.

5. Refraction. The importance of a meticulous refraction cannot be overemphasized in the clinical evaluation of squint and amblyopia (*see* Chapter 36, pages 701–736).

6. Evaluation for central versus eccentric fixation. About one-half of all amblyopic eyes are associated with eccentric fixation. The fixation pattern can be evaluated by following methods:

i. *Angle kappa method.* An idea about eccentric fixation can be made by comparing the angle kappa in each eye. Though it is commonly used but comparatively less accurate method of detecting eccentric fixation. Angle kappa can be estimated by following methods:

• *Hand light method.* After occluding the non-fixing eye, patient is made to fix a hand light held directly below the examiner's eye to avoid an inaccuracy due to parallax. The location of corneal reflex is noted. The same procedure is repeated on the other eye. The angle is positive, when the corneal reflex is displaced nasally and negative, when it is displaced temporally (Fig. 20.37). A positive angle kappa of up to 5° is physiologic in emmetropic eyes.

♦ *In central fixation,* the corneal reflex is located in a similar position in each eye.

♦ *In eccentric fixation,* a significant difference in the location of corneal reflex in fixing and nonfixing eye will be noted.

It is not an accurate method. Small degree of eccentric fixation is often missed. However, it is the only available method of testing eccentricity in infants.

• *Arc perimeter method.* In this technique, after occluding one eye, patient is asked to fix a centre mark on the perimeter, and a very fine

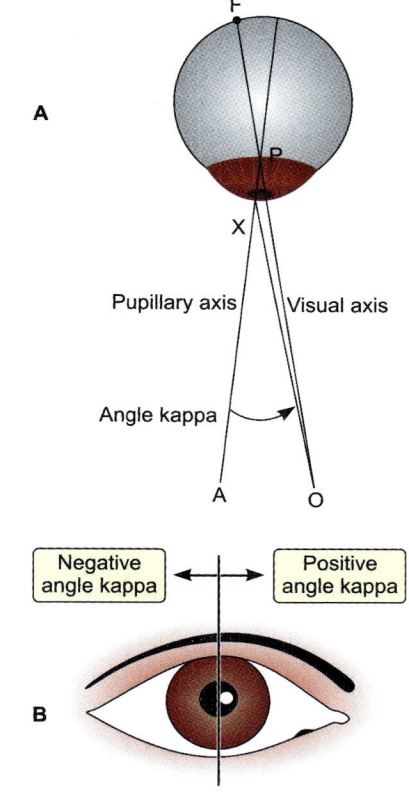

Fig. 20.37: *(A) Angle kappa (OPA) is formed between the visual axis (OF) and central pupillary line (AP). However, clinically angle kappa (OXA) is measured at a point on the cornea (X) that lies in the central pupillary line. (B) Angle kappa is labelled positive when the corneal light is displaced nasally and negative when it is displaced temporally.*

light is moved along the perimeter arc until the light reflex is centred on the cornea. Location of light on the perimeter arc tells the angle kappa in degrees.

• *Major amblyoscope method.* Angle kappa is measured using special slides with synoptophore (*see* page 421).

ii. *Visuscope method.* In most clinical practice, visuscope or its ophthalmoscopic alternative is the most commonly employed method for testing eccentric fixation (*see* page 423). However, this technique requires patient's cooperation and thus can be used in patients above 4–5 years of age.

iii. *Haidinger's brushes method.* Patient is made to perceive the entoptic pattern of the Haidinger brushes and then asked to touch its centre with a pointer. In the presence of central fixation, patient will easily do so. However, if fixation is eccentric, a gross error will be made and patient will be unable, despite repeated attempts to correct the error. Being cumbersome, this method is not used routinely.

iv. *Maxwell's spot method.* Maxwell spot is a round, dark, purplish spot of about 3 arc degrees in diameter. It is perceived entoptically, when the eye is exposed to a homogenous blue or purple field. In central fixation, this spot is centred over the fixation target. In eccentric fixation, the Maxwell spot is displaced to the side of fixation target by an angular amount equivalent to the degree of eccentricity. Like Haidinger's brushes method, this is also sparingly used in common clinical practice.

7. Tests for other sensory anomalies. Amblyopia may be associated with ARC. Therefore, the tests employed for suppression and ARC may also be required for a thorough clinical evaluation of amblyopia.

ORTHOPTIC INSTRUMENTS

GENERAL CONSIDERATIONS

Uses

The orthoptic instruments are required for diagnostic, therapeutic or both purposes.

A. *Diagnostic uses of orthoptic instruments*
1. Measurement of angle of deviation (subjective and objective).
2. Measurement of range of fusion.
3. Measurement of accommodative convergence/accommodation (AC/A) ratio.
4. To know the sensory status of binocular vision and to detect the sensory anomalies such as suppression, amblyopia and ARC.
5. To evaluate for stereoacuity.
6. To evaluate the motor status of binocular vision.

B. *Therapeutic uses of orthoptic instruments*
1. Exercises to improve the fusional range.
2. Exercises to improve the relative convergence or relative accommodation.
3. Anti-suppression exercises.
4. Amblyopia therapy.

Working principle of orthoptic instruments

Working of most orthoptic instruments is based on the fact that they either allow or detect the dissociation of fusion of binocular vision.

The common modes by which an orthoptic instrument can cause dissociation of two eyes are as follows:

1. Use of septum so that each eye sees the different half of the field, as in Maddox wing, diploscope, Remy separator, cheiroscope and Pigeon-Cantonnet stereoscope.
2. Use of two tubes, one in front of each eye as in synoptophore.
3. Use of red and green complimentary glasses one in front of each eye.
4. Use of polaroide glasses.
5. Use of striations as in Bagolini's glasses.
6. Use of cylindrical lenses as in Maddox rod.

Types of orthoptic instruments

- Conventional, i.e. non-computerised orthoptic equipment
- Computerised orthoptic programs *see* page 428–432.

CONVENTIONAL (NON-COMPUTERISED) ORTHOPTIC INSTRUMENTS

Like any other branch of science, the science of orthoptic and strabismus is also advancing and changing fast. With time, certain instruments have become obsolete and some have become less important. For example, even synoptophore is no more considered an essential equipment for orthoptic set-up. However, its persence do adds grace to the orthoptic clinic. Description of certain instruments which are used only for diagnostic purposes has been given along with the diagnostic tests under the evaluation of a case of strabismus.

A few other important orthoptic instruments which have not been described elsewhere will be described in this section. Orthoptic instruments can be grouped as below:

I. Essential orthoptic instruments

The bare minimum equipment required for the clinical work of a patient with strabismus are:

1. A refraction trial set with prism of 1–8 D

2. Snellen's vision chart and single letter E-chart.

3. Prism bars, horizontal and vertical (page 393)

4. Loose prism set

5. Fixation targets, for near and distance

6. Occluders

7. Bagolini's striated lenses (pages 406)

8. Red and green goggles

9. Maddox rods (page 386)

10. Direct ophthalmoscope

11. Transparent foot ruler.

II. Desirable orthoptic instruments

These instruments, when present, add grace and completeness to the orthoptic clinic. These include:

1. Synoptophore

2. Random dot stereo test

3. Hess screen (page 400)

4. RAF rule (page 395)

5. Worth four dot test (page 409)

6. Indirect ophthalmoscope

7. Spielman's occluder.

III. Additional orthoptic instruments

There is no limit to additional orthoptic instruments. Additional orthoptic instruments can be grouped as below.

Priority additional orthoptic instruments

1. Haidinger brushes and after images attachment for synoptophore.

2. Teller acuity cards with screen

3. Optokinetic nystagmus drum

4. VER and electronystagmography

5. System perimeter

6. Camera for documentation

Non-priority additional orthoptic instruments

1. Livingston binocular gauge

2. Remy separator

3. Reading bars

4. Cheiroscope

5. Neutral density filters and graded density bar

6. Maddox wing (page 388)

IV. Orthoptic instruments not used presently

1. Bishop-Harman diaphragm

2. Stereoscope (Holmes, Keystone)

3. Projectoscope

4. Visuscope

5. Euthyscope

6. Coordinator

7. CAM vision stimulator

8. Pigeon-Cantonnet stereoscope

9. Tibbs binocular trainer

10. Diploscope.

SYNOPTOPHORE

Synoptophore (major amblyoscope) is a haploscopic device. Though not an essential instrument but its presence is most desirable in an orthoptic clinic. It essentially consists of two tubes, having a right-angled bend, mounted on a base having a chin rest and a forehead rest (Fig. 20.38). Each tube contains a light source for illumination of slides and a slide carrier at the outer end, a reflecting mirror at the right-angled bend and an eyepiece of +6.5 D at the inner end (Fig. 20.39). The two tubes can be converged, diverged and moved vertically separately or together by means of knobs. The tubes can also be adjusted to the patient's interpupillary distance. Each slide carrier can be rotated to adjust for any torsion. The horizontal, vertical and torsional positions of each tube with regard to normal zero position can be read on scales in either degrees or prism dioptres.

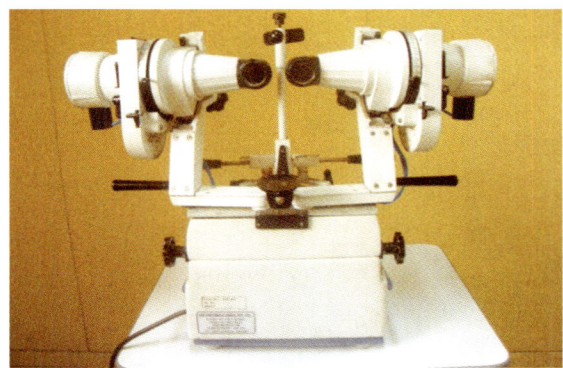

Fig. 20.38: *Synoptophore.*

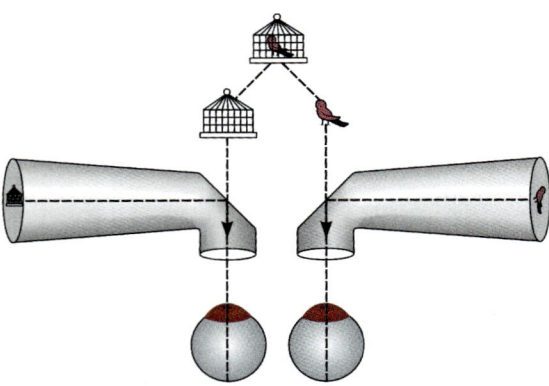

Fig. 20.39: *Optical principle of synoptophore.*

The graduations from the zero mark inward represent base-out prisms or degrees of convergence (+), while those from the zero mark outward represent base-in prisms or degrees of divergence (−).

Light switches permit the simultaneous or alternate illumination of the tubes, useful for performing the cover tests.

Synoptophore slides

The pair of slides used to perform various diagnostic and therapeutic purposes include the following.

1. *Simultaneous perception slides.* Two dissimilar slides, such as one having picture of a bird and the other of the cage, constitute a pair of simultaneous perception slides (Fig. 20.40A). Each slide is presented separately to each eye. Ideally,

the pictures should not have overlapping contour since this will induce suppression. These slides are graded by their size into three groups:

a. *Simultaneous foveal perception (SFP) slides.* This pair consists of small sized pictures, the images of which do not exceed the size of the fovea.

b. *Simultaneous macular perception (SMP) slides.* The pictures in this pair of slides are slightly larger than those on the SFP slides.

c. *Simultaneous paramacular perception (SPP) slides.* These slides have the largest pictures and form images that extend into paramacular areas.

(**Note.** As a routine, if possible, the smallest slides should be used. However, the larger slides may be required in the presence of suppression or amblyopia).

2. *Fusion slides.* Fusion slides consist of two similar pictures, each of which is incomplete in one small detail. For example, there are two rabbits each lacking either a tail or a bunch of flowers. If fusion is present, one complete rabbit with tail and holding a bunch of flowers will be seen (Fig. 20.40B). In the presence of suppression, either tail or bunch of flowers will be missing in the respective eye.

Grading. The fusion slides are also graded according to the size in the same way as the simultaneous perception slides.

3. *Stereoscopic slides.* Stereoscopic slides consist of two pictures of the same object which have been taken from slightly different angles, i.e. the

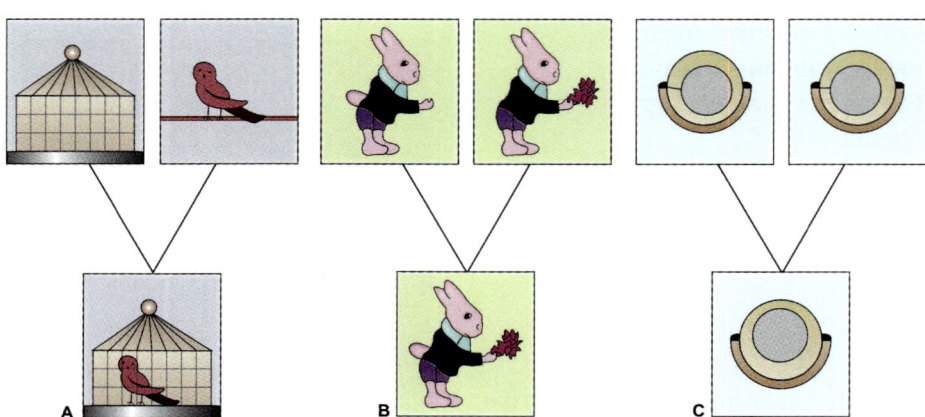

Fig. 20.40: *Synoptophore slides for simultaneous perception (A); fusion (B); and stereopsis (C).*

picture for one eye is in part dissimilar from that for the other eye. These dissimilar parts are imaged on disparate retinal areas in the two eyes and, when the entire picture is fused, the disparity gives rise to the perception of stereopsis of the dissimilar portions (Fig. 20.40C).

Uses of synoptophore

Diagnostic uses

1. Measurement of the objective and subjective angles of deviation (page 389).
2. Measurement of the primary and secondary deviations.
3. Measurement of deviation in cardinal directions of gaze.
4. Measurement of interpupillary distance (IPD).
5. To investigate the state of retinal correspondence (page 406).
6. Estimation of grades of binocular vision.
7. To estimate presence and type of suppression.
8. Measurement of range of fusion or vergence (page 393).
9. Measurement of angle kappa.

Therapeutic uses

It is used in the treatment of:
1. Suppression.
2. Abnormal retinal correspondence.
3. Eccentric fixation.
4. Accommodative esotropia (dissociation training).
5. Heterophorias and intermittent heterotropias (improvement of fusional amplitude).

Measurement of anlge kappa with synoptophore

To measure the angle kappa with synoptophore, a special slide is placed in front of the eye under observation. This slide consists of a row of numbers and letters (4 3 2 1 0 A B C D) and animal pictures (for small children and illiterate patients) placed at 1° intervals (Fig. 20.41). The patient is asked to focus on the '0' mark while the examiner looks for the corneal reflex. If the corneal reflex is on the nasal side of centre of pupil, the angle is positive; if it is on the temporal side, it is negative. The patient is then asked to look in turn either one letter or one number until the reflex is centred. The degree of deviation corresponding to the letter or number is then recorded. For example, if the left eye is being tested and the corneal reflex is centred, when the patient looks at the number 3, the patient has 3° negative angle kappa in the left eye.

Measurement of interpupillary distance with synoptophore

To measure the IPD, arms of the synoptophore are placed at zero and the patient is instructed to look at the centre of the picture in the right hand tube with his/her right eye. The examiner, with his right eye closed, aligns the central white line which is on the mirror unit of the tube, with the reflection of the light on the centre of the patient's pupil. The same procedure is repeated with the patient fixing with the left eye and the examiner closing his right eye. The IPD is then read on the millimetre scale.

Digital synoptophore

Digital synoptophore, introduced recently, is likely to soon replace the currently used electric synoptophore for sensory and motor assessment of strabismus patients as well as measurement of the angle of deviation.

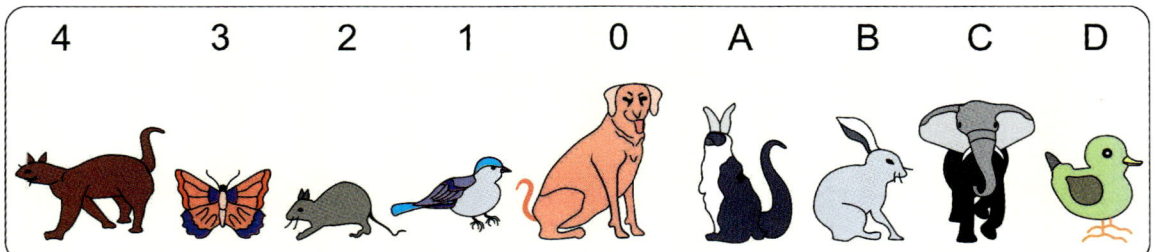

Fig. 20.41: *Synoptophore slide for measurement of angle kappa.*

Features of digital synoptophore

Digital Synoptophore (Fig. 20.42) comprising of a computer controlled display device consists of both hardware and software components:

Hardware component consists of various subunits as described below:

- *Computer system* with colour monitor.
- *Screen divider*. An opaque vertical screen divider, to divide the display screen into 2 equal right and left halves.
- *Input device* to move the generated screen targets, such as mouse, trackball, etc.
- *Two tubes* to carry the images from the display screen to each eye separately which contain a lens system and eyepieces assembly with adjustable interpupillary distance.
- *Adjustable chin-rest and head-rest* for stabilizing the patients head.

Software component consists of various computer programs designed for various orthoptic test.

Procedure

Before examination, the interpupillary distance (IPD) for the patient must be first measured in millimetres. The distance between the eyepieces is then set according to this measurement. The patient places his chin on the chin-rest and his forehead against the headrest. The chin-rest is adjusted in such a way that the eye level is at the centre of screen vertically.

Uses

It is used to perform the following tests on patients with strabismus:

- Simultaneous perception (foveal, macular and paramacular)
- Fusion
- Stereopsis
- Assessing retinal correspondence
- After image testing
- Measure the angle of deviation
- Orthoptic exercises.

LIVINGSTON BINOCULAR GAUGE

Livingston binocular gauge (Fig. 20.43) is an apparatus used for the measurement of convergence and accommodation. Basically, it consists of a 36 cm long wooden ruler marked in centimetres and half-centimetres. In the centre of this ruler, from 6 cm mark to 21 cm mark, there is a slot into which is present a slidable convergence rod (white vertical rod, the centre third of which is painted black). One end of this ruler is so designed that when in position, it

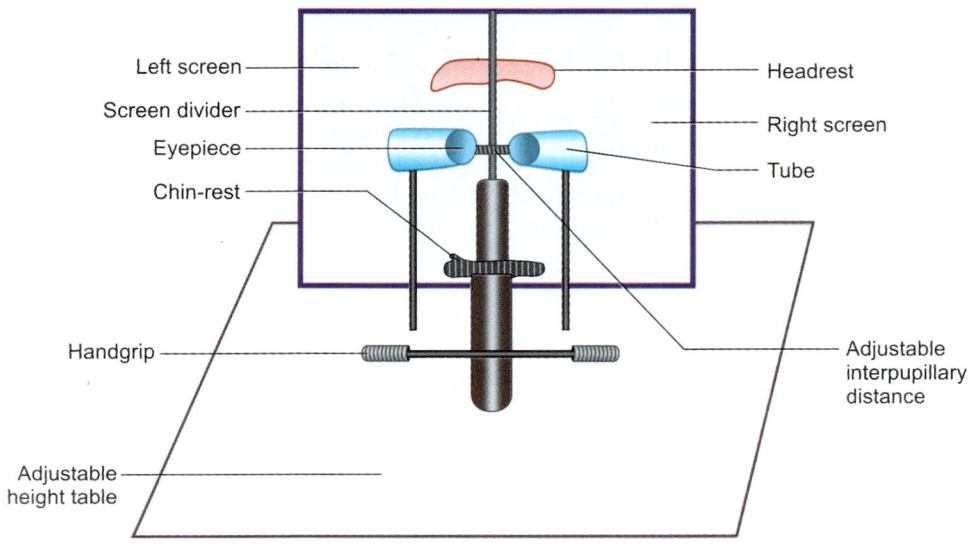

Fig 20.42: *Hardware component of digital synoptophore.*

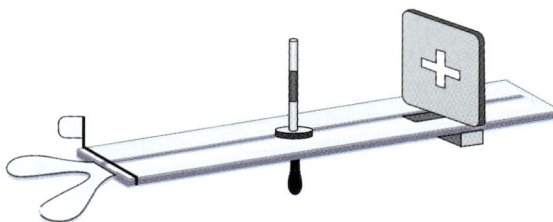

Fig. 20.43: *Livingston binocular gauge.*

straddles the patient's nose and rests upon his/ her cheek bones. At this facial end of the ruler, a detachable occluder is attached which can be used to occlude either eye while measuring uniocular accommodation. In this position, the markings on the ruler indicate distance from the anterior surface of cornea. At the other end of the ruler, there is a box-like attachment which can slide towards the eye. This box-shaped attachment is 6 cm wide and has a cross-like opening (cut in the surface facing the patient) through which the back surface of the box consisting of a white rectangular card with a central black vertical line (opposite the vertical limb of the cross-opening) is seen. The black vertical line is used for measuring the convergence. On either side of the black vertical line, there are three black horizontally placed letters—ALT, opposite the horizontal limb of the cross-opening. These letters are used for measuring accommodation.

Uses of livingston binocular gauge

1. *Measurement of objective convergence.* The ruler is fitted on the patient's cheek bone. The convergence rod is kept farthest from the patient, who is asked to continuously look at the central black section of the rod which is moved steadily towards the patient's eyes. The examiner notes the scale reading, where the patient's one or both eyes diverge on the loss of binocular fixation. Normally, the objective convergence varies between 6 and 10 cm in young adults.

2. *Measurement of subjective convergence.* After fitting the ruler on the patient's face, the central convergence rod is removed and the box-like attachment is kept farthest from the patient. The patient is asked to look at the black vertical line placed in the centre of vertical limb of

cross-opening while the box is slid towards the patient's face. The point where the patient observes that the line has moved slightly to the right or to the left or has become double is noted on the scale. This reading gives the measurement of subjective convergence. The normal value of subjective convergence is less than 20 cm, but is almost invariably greater than that of objective convergence.

3. *Measurement of accommodation.* The instrument is used in the same way as used for measuring subjective convergence; except that now the patient is asked to look at the letters placed corresponding to the horizontal limb of the cross-opening of the box-like attachment. The point where the patient reports blurring of the letters gives the reading of his/her near point (punctum proximum).

VISUSCOPE

It is an instrument similar to ophthalmoscope (Fig. 20.44) which is used to examine the fixation pattern of patients during monocular vision. It was designed by Cupper. With the help of this instrument, examiner projects a disc with a green filter having a star in the centre and surrounded by concentric rings onto the patient's fundus. The distance between the concentric rings is ½°. The patient is asked to look into the star after occluding the eye not being examined. Normally, the foveolar reflex of the patient coincides with the star if the fixation is central. In the presence of eccentric fixation, the star, will not coincide with the foveolar reflex and can be anywhere on either the nasal or temporal retina or above or below the fovea (Fig. 20.30). The degree of eccentricity may be known from the concentric ring with which the star coincides.

EUTHYSCOPE

Euthyscope is a modified form of ophthalmoscope which is used in pleoptics for the re-education of the fovea that has lost its principal visual direction in eccentric fixation.

This instrument projects an approximately 30° wide beam of light in the centre of which an opaque 3° or 5° disc can be moved to cause a black dot. This serves to shield the fovea during the exposure of the surrounding retina. Since the

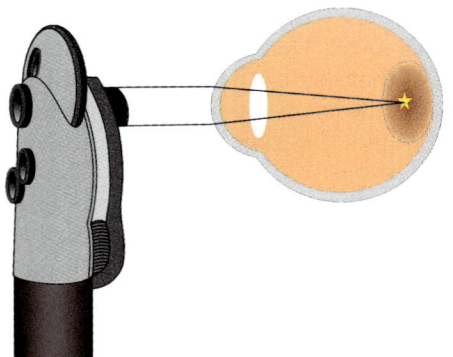

Fig. 20.44: *Examination of fixation pattern with visuscope.*

light intensity used is moderate, the peripheral retina is not dazzled but only stimulated enough to produce an after image. A green filter disc enables the examiner to locate the fovea without dazzling the patient's retina. Since pleoptic treatment is now obsolete, so this instrument is also not used in the modern orthoptic clinics.

DIPLOSCOPE

The diploscope consists of a 25 cm long metal shaft supported by a handle having face-piece at one end and a card holder at the other end. Depending upon the model, the face-piece can rest on the nose (Fig. 20.45), the cheek bones, or the upper lid. The card holder contains a card with white background. On this card are printed letters DOG, with a green sqaure placed centrally above the O and a red square centrally below the O. About 6.5 cm in front and parallel to the card holder is mounted a metal septum

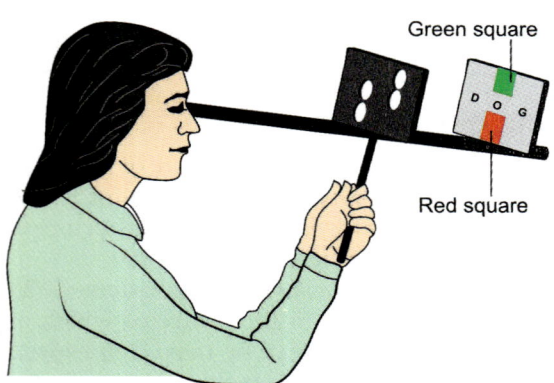

Fig. 20.45: *Diploscope.*

which is perforated by four holes, each 8 mm in diameter. The two holes are situated horizontally 15 mm apart from each other and at an equal distance from the centre of the septum. The other two holes situated vertically, one below the horizontal left-hand hole and other above the horizontal right-hand hole.

When in use, the septum dissociates the two eyes in such a way that each eye can see only two of the three letters on the white card and only one of the two-coloured squares. The left eye sees the letters OG and the lower red square, while the right eye sees the letters DO and upper green square (Fig. 20.46).

Uses

1. Suppression and the presence or lack of binocular vision can be detected. With normal retinal correspondence and bifoveal fixation, when the two images of O are fused, the patient will see three holes with the word DOG in them (Fig. 20.46).

2. The main use of the instrument is to exercise for relative convergence, when binocular single vision is present. To perform exercise, patient is asked to move his/her eyes in relation to septum and card at four different positions (described below). As the patient does so, he/she sees a change in the relative position of the letters and colours as perceived by each eye simultaneously. This movement of letters into a definite pattern is utilized in training the patient to appreciate and control the position to which his/her eyes are directed. Thus, it teaches the patient to switch easily from distant to near fixation and *vice versa* improving the fusional amplitudes which are essential for a comfortable binocular single vision.

Procedure

The four positions of fixation and the various kinds of physiological diplopia, when practising with the diploscope, are as follows (Fig. 20.46).

Position 1. The point of fixation is central letter O on the card. In this position, letter D falls on a point temporal to the fovea in the right eye and is projected to the left of O, while G falls on point

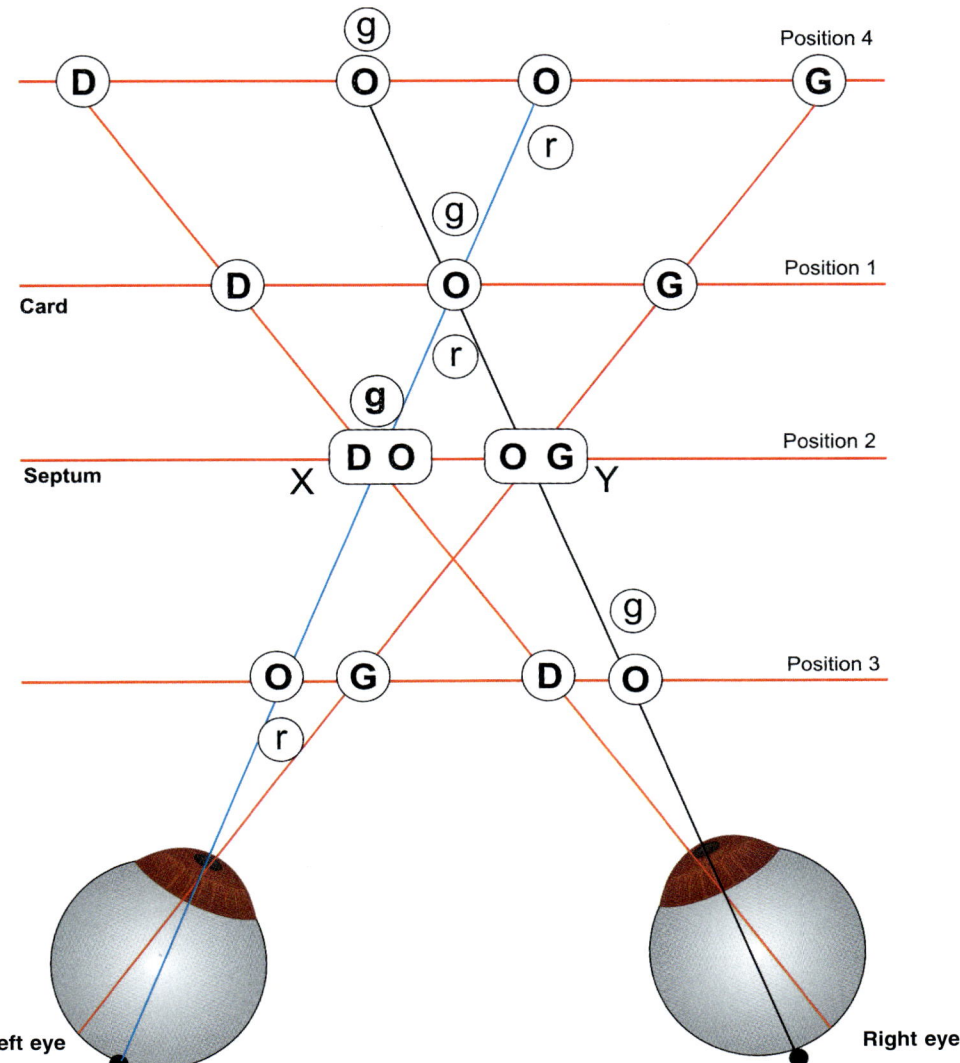

Fig. 20.46: *Principle of diploscope and observations made by the patient while in use at positions 1, 2, 3 and 4 (for explanation, see text).*

temporal to the fovea in the left eye and is projected to the right of O. Thus, the letters DO are seen with the right eye and the letters OG with the left eye and in the presence of binocular single vision patient will perceive three holes with the word DOG in them.

Position 2. The second point of fixation is the centre of metal septum midway between the two horizontally placed holes (Fig. 20.46). When the patient's eyes converge on this point, the images

of O no longer fall on both foveas, but on a retinal element nasal to the fovea in each eye. Consequently, the O will be seen in uncrossed (homonymous) diplopia and the patient sees DO and OG. When the patient will exert a greater amount of convergence, he/she may see only DG, because the D and O and the G and O will overlap.

Position 3. The point of fixation is tip of a pencil or other object held midway between the septum and his/her eyes. When the patient's eyes converge on this point, the images of both D and

O in the right eye and G and O in the left eye fall on a retinal element nasal to fovea in each eye and thus will be projected temporally, and the patient will see OG DO on the card.

Position 4. The point of fixation is an object (such as a picture on the wall) situated beyond the printed card. When the patient fixates at this distant point, the images of D and O and G and O fall on retinal element temporal to fovea in each eye and thus will be projected nasally, and the patient will see DO OG.

Note: The aim of exercise with diploscope is to teach the patient to obtain and maintain all four positions with ease so that effortless convergence and divergence is fully established. It is advisable to practise for 2 to 3 minutes for 2 to 3 times a day. Position four is quite useful in improving the fusional divergence (fusional negative convergence).

REMY SEPARATOR

Remy separator is a simple instrument which consists of a septum with a handle having a transparent slide holder at one end and a nose-piece at other end (Fig. 20.47). The patient resting the septum on his/her nose is instructed to look through the slides at an object beyond them. If his/her eyes are properly focused for the distant object, the picture of the slides (such as a star and a circle) will be imaged one on each fovea and will be seen superimposed by the patient (Fig. 20.48).

Uses. The instrument is designed in such a way that when used properly, it teaches the

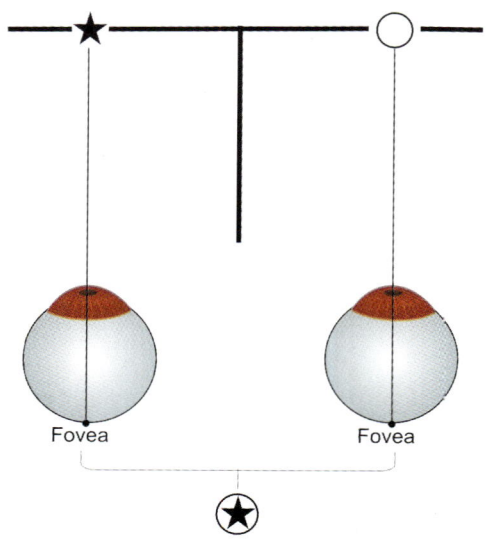

Fig. 20.48: *Optical principle of Remy separator.*

patient to relax his/her convergence and strengthen the fusional divergence.

READING BARS

Reading bars are simple devices used to train the patient for subjectively controlling the maintenance of binocular vision.

Principle. All reading bars are based on the principle of physiologic diplopia.

Common reading bars include thumb bar reader, zig-zag bar reader, the Mayan bar reader, the Jaual grid, Tibb's physiologic diplopia reader.

Method. By introducing a bar between the patient's eyes and the reading material, the patient is made aware of physiologic diplopia (Fig. 20.49). As the patient reads the print binocularly, he/she perceives the bar in crossed diplopia, each image of bar hiding on position of the print from one eye, but not the other, so that the print can be read normally. Maintaining the correct position of his/her eyes despite this obstacle will strengthen the binocular vision of the patient. This is a very useful and simple home exercise.

CHEIROSCOPE

The cheiroscope (Fig. 20.50) is an instrument for anti-suppression exercises. It consists of a

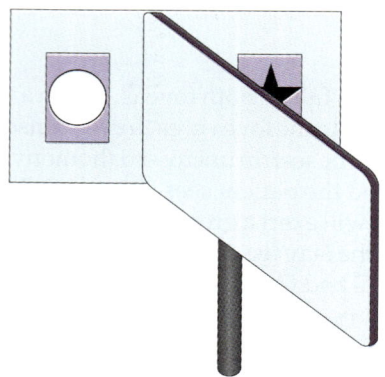

Fig. 20.47: *Remy separator.*

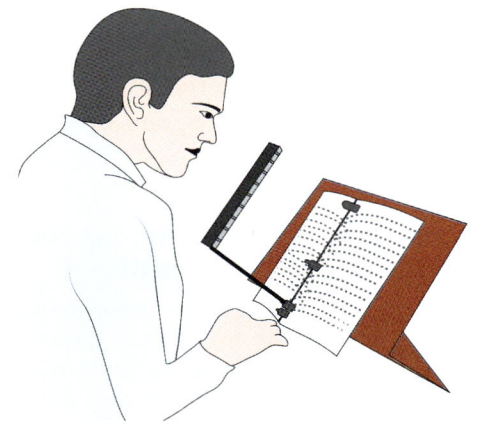

Fig. 20.49: *Zig-zag bar reader in use.*

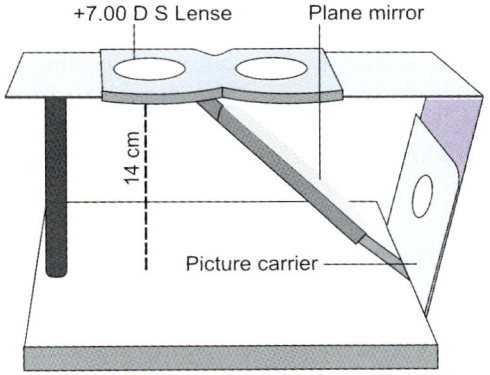

Fig. 20.50: *Cheiroscope.*

working base, a picture carrier to one side, a headrest containing a pair of +7.0 D spherical lenses, and an obliquely placed septum extending from the centre point between the lenses to the base of the picture carrier. A plane mirror is attached to the septum on the side where the picture is located. The distance between lenses and the working base is 14 cm, which is the focal length of each lens and the eyes are consequently focused for distance. Most cheiroscope models may be turned around so that the mirror is in front of the right or left eye, depending upon which eye is required to fixate.

Uses. The instrument can be used in cases of heterophorias, intermittent tropias, or small tropias (in the latter, prisms to neutralize the deviation have to be taped over the eyepiece).

Procedure. The picture to be copied is placed in the picture carrier and a sheet of paper on the base of the instrument. The patient should look with his/her fixating eye into the mirror and with the suppressing one on the paper. He/she is instructed to trace the picture (which has black outlines) on the paper using a pencil (a red-coloured pencil is very helpful, especially in the beginning). Steady fixation of the picture should be stressed to prevent rapid alternation, which can be suspected, if the patient's drawing is either smaller or larger than the picutre or if parts of the picture are missing.

TIBB'S BINOCULAR TRAINER

The Tibb's binocular trainer (Fig. 20.51) is a haploscopic instrument designed for home use. However, in offices where a major amblyoscope is not available, it can also be used as a diagnostic instrument. It consists of three parts: A middle septum and two wingboards that fold together like a book. The middle septum has a mirror on both sides so that it can be used with either eye fixating. Each of the wingboards has a vertical scale of 20^Δ base-up and base-down and a horizontal scale of 40^Δ-base in and base-out. Four cards (target carriers) come with the instrument and consist of peripheral, macular, and foveal superimposition and fusion pictures.

Uses. It can be used for both diagnosis and treatment of suppression and abnormal retinal correspondence and for increasing fusional amplitudes.

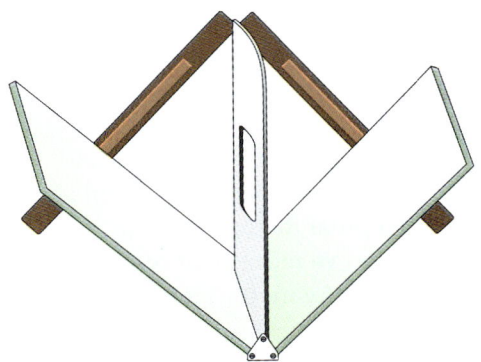

Fig. 20.51: *Tibb's binocular trainer. Direct cover test depicting left exotropia.*

Procedure. One wingboard is placed so that it rests along the table at a slight angle to it. The vertical wingboard is to the right side, when the right eye is the fixating one; it is to the left side, when the left eye is fixating. The patient places the bridge of his/her nose against the curved part of the septum so that his/her visual axis is perpendicular to the table. His/her head should not be tilted.

One target carrier (such as the dog) is taped on the vertical wingboard so the zero mark shows in the window. This target is seen in the mirror. The patient places another target on the horizontal wingboard (such as the cage for superimposition or another dog for fusion) and moves it until the two images are superimposed. This target is not viewed in the mirror.

COMPUTER-BASED ORTHOPTIC PROGRAMS AND INSTRUMENTS

Computer-based orthoptic programs have brought a revolutionary change in the diagnosis and management of orthoptic disorders. Computer-based orthoptic practice includes:

- Computerised orthoptic-diagnostic programs for sensory as well as motor evaluation
- Computer-based orthoptic therapy programs for vision therapy, and neurovision therapy.

Recently many computer-based systems have been developed for orthoptic practice which are either only diagnostic, or therapeutic, or combined diagnostic and therapeutic programs. Some of these are listed below:

I. *Computer-based diagnostic programs*
- Electronic vision testing programs
- Optodrum [Software for optokinetic drum (OKN)]
- Digital Hess chart and diplopia chart
- BVA (Binocular Vision Assessment Program)
- PTS (Perceptual therapy system)
- ReadAlyzer eye movement recording system
- TOVA (Test of variable attention)
- Visagraph.

II. *Computer-based therapeutic programs*
- Vision therapy programs
- Neurovision therapy programs.

III. *Computer-based combined diagnostic and therapeutic systems*
- TRYe vision therapy software
- Computer orthoptics program by HTS INC solutions
- Computer orthoptics.

I. COMPUTERIZED ORTHOPTIC DIAGNOSTIC PROGRAMS AND INSTRUMENTS

Several applications are available for smartphones, tablets, laptop, and PCs that reproduce many eye tests. These can be used by optometrists, ophthalmologists and some programs by the patients also. Computer orthoptics includes complex monocular and binocular stimuli, which allow automatic testing and measurement of the following skills: Oculomotor (pursuits and saccades); fusional ranges; phorias; motor fields; fixation disparities, suppressions; retinal correspondence; accommodative facility; stereopsis, visual memory and aniseikonia.

Some common such programs are described briefly.

Electronic vision testing programs. Electronic charts are available for far as well as near vision testing. Few examples are:
- Chart Pro (*www.eyechartprotoapp.com*)
- Optos' chart remote (*blog.optos.com/index.php/optos.chart.remote.ipad.app*)
- Vision Test (*https://itunes.apple.com/ca/app/vision-test/id380288414?mt=8 or https://play.google.com/store/apps/details? id=com.threesidedcube.visiondroid*)
- With sight Book (*www.digisight.net/patients/vision_testing*)
- AAPOS Vision Screening App.(*www.aapos.org/ahp/aapos_vision_screening_app*) has optotype for both adults and children, and can be used by anyone including healthcare workers.

Optodrum. The Optodrum (www.linsay.com/Linsay_associates_Medical/Optodrum.html) is a good alternative to the expensive and bulky optokinetic drum for adults and children. It even has a version for the iPad that uses its camera to record a video of the patient's eye movement while looking at moving patterns.

BVA is a stand-alone binocular vision screening program. It is capable of automatic testing of

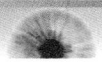

heterophorias, fusional range, saccades, pursuits, accommodation, suppressions, fixation disparities and an asthenopia survey.

PTS test. Computerized perceptual therapy system allows automatic testing for speed of information processing, visual sequential processing, visual simultaneous processing.

ReadAlyzer eye movement recording system. This system allows fixations, regressions, fixation duration, reading speed, cross correlation between right and left eye, play-back of recorded eye movements.

TOVA (test of variables attention). It assesses ADD, ADHD and impulsivity.

Visagraph an eye movement recording system is capable of computerized recordings of reading eye movements, saccades and fixations.

Digital Hess screen See page 401.

Digital syneptophore Described on page 421.

II. COMPUTER-BASED VISION THERAPY AND NEUROVISION THERAPY PROGRAMS

VISION THERAPY PROGRAMS

Vision therapy is effective for:
- Eliminating amblyopia
- Breaking suppressions
- Improving oculomotor skills
- Improving visual memory
- Improving accommodative facility
- Altering retinal correspondence; increasing fusional ranges; and/or treating strabismus.

The gamepad and mouse allow the patient's therapy responses to alter the target demands. The Computer Orthoptics graphics are instantly moved, rotated or changed to create any base-in base-out disparity. A few computer-based orthoptic programs are mentioned below.

Computer vergence system (CVS)

This program uses random dot stereograms to form pictures that require bi-foveal fixation to stimulate the vergence system. The program gradually increases the amount of vergence required to appreciate the stereogram picture and can monitor progression online. This may be used as part of the home therapy program

and the results of the computer program are often followed by an eye care professional with printouts that can be brought into the office visit. A maintenance program consists of activities that preserve the patient's present level of function and/or prevent regression of that function. Maintenance begins when the therapeutic goals of a treatment plan have been achieved, or when no additional functional progress is apparent or expected to occur.

Perceptual visual tracking program (PVT)

This program is designed to improve specific tracking deficits that are often found in persons. Perceptual visual tracking skills are basic to all aspects of reading and other academic areas. Improvement in tracking is often accompanied by improvement in reading, spelling, attention, and speed of working. PVT contains a variety of visual tracking programs that have been clinically proven. They are game-like in nature so that improvement takes place almost effortlessly. Individuals of all ages from five years up can benefit from PVT. It is a sophisticated yet user-friendly computer application that will run on almost any personal computer.

Vision builder: Computer vision training

A home vision training program designed to treat both binocular vision disorders such as convergence problems (i.e. eye-teaming problems), accommodation problems (i.e. non-refractive focusing difficulties), suppression (i.e. 'lazy eye') and eye-tracking difficulties, as well as visual perceptual or visual information processing difficulties that can impact on a student's learning by limiting their ability to understand and remember what they see.

Eyeport @ Vision Training System

Has revolutionized the way people look at their vision. To read more comfortably, learn more easily, work less painfully, and play sports more effortlessly, people everywhere are doing daily eye exercises with the EYEPORT.

Eyelights

Target the weaker functioning side of the brain via the non-dominant eye. Light stimulation

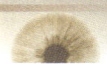

directly to the non-dominant brain causes an excitatory barrage to travel to the mesencephalon, the most metabolic area of the brain, where an increase in cellular activity takes place. The excitatory barrage travels also to the parietal, temporal, and occipital lobes of the brain, while collateral fibers lead to the pineal gland, pituitary gland, and hypothalamus.

AmbP iNet Program

An amblyopia hand-eye coordination program which uses principles of operant conditioning and behaviour modification to appropriately alter stimuli characteristics to improve visual acuity (Fig. 20.52).

- Patients begin therapy with targets that are easily seen and become progressively smaller as therapy progresses. Correct responses are

reinforced with subsequent reduction in the size of the stimuli. Therapy is directed to improve resolving ability with concomitant use of hand-eye coordination tasks. Therapy can be performed monocularly or monocularly in a binocular field (Fig. 20.53A and B).

- The AmbP iNet program provides a cumulative graph depicting each session's performance. The computer denotes date, time, duration and denotes when the patient has performed the assigned tasks as well as if they were performed correctly.

PTS II iNET. It is a home-based computerized perceptual therapy program that has been designed to address a variety of visual perceptual information processing domains, including simultaneous processing, sequential processing, speed-of-information processing, visual

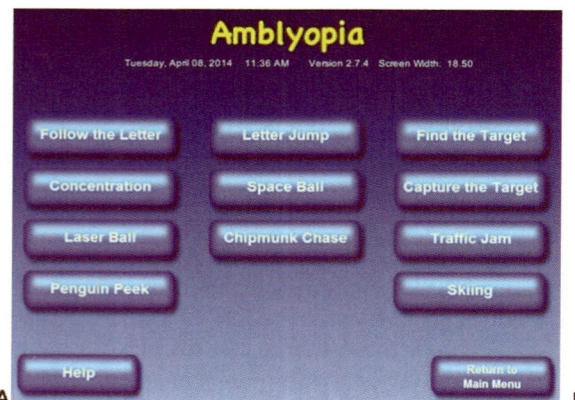
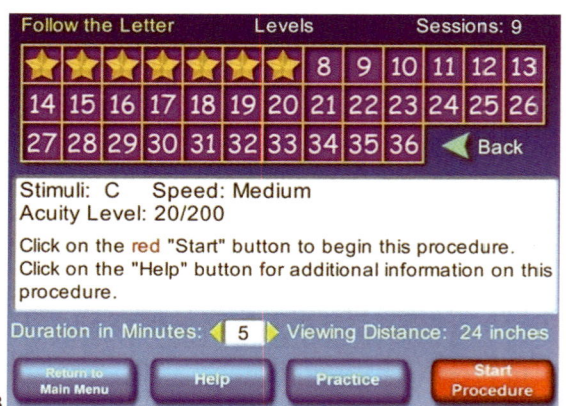

Fig. 20.52: *AmbP iNet program.*

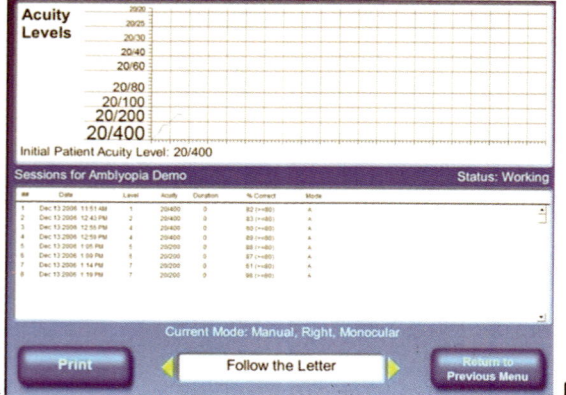
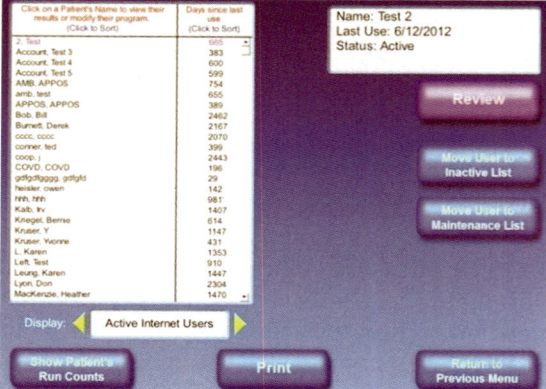

Fig. 20.53: *Protocol of therapy with AmbP iNet program.*

temporal processing, and rapid automatized naming:

- Dyslexia
- Ordinary reading disability
- Word decoding difficulty
- Problems in reading comprehension
- Spelling problems
- Memory disorders
- Laterality-directionality deficits
- Slow speed of information processing
- Non-verbal learning disability
- Mathematics difficulty
- Above average intelligence but not achieving up to potential
- Acquired brain injury with perceptual-cognitive deficits
- Attention disorders
- Diagnosis of perceptual/visual information processing deficits (Fig. 20.54).

Therapy procedure. PTS II iNet presents the patient with a grid that shows the different difficulty levels for each procedure. Each time the patient meets or exceeds a therapy goal they receive a gold star. The program gives the patient verbal reinforcement. It prompts them to 'Get Ready' before a stimulus is presented. PTS II iNet also verbally reinforces correct and incorrect responses. For example, it will encourage them by saying 'Good Job' after they input a correct response.

Dynamic reader. The dynamic reader is a home Vision Training program designed to improve reading eye movements and thus reading fluency and comprehension.

ADR iNet. Moving text, standard, and whole line dynamic reading.

Brainware safari. Therapy for 14 cognitive skills in six areas.

Play attention. Improves attention.

Sanet vision untegrator. Procedures for saccadic trainer, tactile feedback, hand speed function, 'visual search' saccadic, metronome, tachisto-scope functions.

Sub iNet. Addresses subitizing deficits to improve math skills.

Track and read. Twelve therapy procedures for developing saccadic eye movements, span of recognition, and visual sequential memory skills.

NEUROVISION THERAPY PROGRAMS

1. Revital vision. Concept of neurovision therapy is based on the visual plasticity, which is the ability of the visual system to change its responses in order to adapt to the changes in the visual input. Revital vision is a perceptual learning therapy program developed by 'Revital Vision Technology'. Perceptual learning is an alternative treatment option which modifies visual function in adult amblyopia. The perceptual learning therapy program (Revital Vision) is a non-invasive software-based patient-specific, interactive perceptual learning tool based on visual stimulation. It facilitates neural connections at the cortical level through a

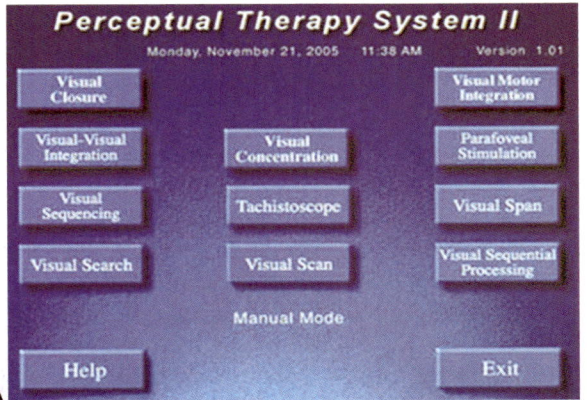
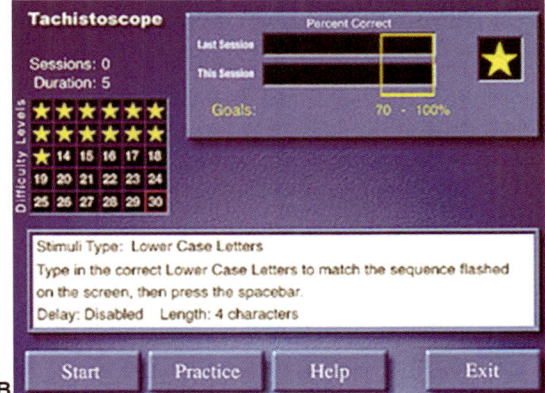

Fig. 20.54: *Diagnosis of perceptual/visual information processing deficit.*

computerized training regimen using Gabor patches to improve contrast sensitivity and visual acuity. The term perceptual learning describes a process whereby practising certain visual tasks leads to an improvement in visual performance. As visual perception depends on both the optical input received from the eye and the neural processing of that input in the visual cortex, Revital vision technology improves quality of vision (visual acuity and contrast sensitivity) by enhancing neural processing in the primary visual cortex.

The typical building blocks of the visual stimulus in the field of visual neuroscience are:

- Gabor patch
- Neuronal lateral interactions
- Brain (neural plasticity)
- Perceptual learning.

Effects of revital vision–perceptual learning. Neurovision technology (Revital) is formed around proprietary algorithms and has proved successful in the following ways:

- Improvement of lateral interactions in amblyopia
- Improvement of CSF in amblyopia
- Improvement of CSF in non-amblyopic groups
- Improvement of VA
- Transfer to improvement of binocular vision.

2. Neurovision rehabilitator used for those with brain injury is useful as ocular vestibular integrator, visual motor enhancer, visuomotor integrator, dynamic ocular motor processing, fixation anomalies.

III. COMPUTER-BASED COMBINED DIAGNOSTIC AND THERAPEUTIC PROGRAMS

1. TrYe (Train your eyes) vision therapy software
TrYe (Train your eyes) vision therapy software has been designed and developed by 'Digital Works Technology Private Ltd', using the domain expertise of 'Sankra Nethralya, Chennai, India'. This program has the ability to run on multiple platforms, such as PC, Laptop, Mobile and Tablet.

Uses of TrYe software include:

- *Binocular vision assessment*, and thus addresses to the binocular vision dysfunctions. Binocular

vision assessment program in TrYe is based on apparent conditioning using random dot stereograms (RDS) as targets. RDS targets are devoid of monocular cues and have been recommended for fusional vergence testing and training.

- *'Office vision therapy'* (TrYe-Doctor's module) program for dysfunctions of binocular vision, accommodation and ocular motor system.
- *Home-based vision therapy program* (TrYe-Patient's module) for vision therapy at home.

2. Computer orthoptics program by HTS INC solutions™. HTS iNet/Computer Vergence System (CVS) is a sophisticated yet easy-to-use vergence exercise computer application that the patients can run on Windows and Mac computers. It encourages and motivates patients by continuously evaluating their progress and making the exercises more challenging whenever the goals are achieved.

To assure compliance, CVS uses random-dot stereograms. Each exercise requires bifovial fixation for correct responses. The responses required are a simple choice of four arrows keys; up, down, left or right. The results of each exercise session are documented as the program notes the date, duration and vergence demand of each exercise. All results are available for your review via the Internet. The HTS iNet program is fully automated and easy to use. *Procedures* include:

- Pursuits
- Saccades
- Base-in/base-out vergence
- Auto slide vergence
- Jump ductions
- Base-up/base-down vergence
- Accommodative rock.

3. Computer orthoptics. It includes both orthoptic therapy and diagnostic procedure:

- *Therapy procedures* include smooth vergence, rotations, jump ductions, multiple choice vergence, accommodative rock, pursuits, saccades, visual memory, cheiroscope and amblyopia therapy procedures.
- *Diagnostic procedures* for heterophobia, fusional ranges, accommodative facility, pursuits, saccades, Worth 4 dot, motor field, fixation disparity, visual memory, aniseikonia.

BIBLIOGRAPHY

1. American Academy of Pediatrics. Learning Disabilities, Dyslexia, and Vision: A Subject Review. Pediatrics 1998; 102(5):1217–9. A statement of reaffirmation for this policy was published on August 1, 2008.

2. Bagolini B. Tecnica per l'esame della visione binoculare sensa introduzione di elementi dissocianti: "test del vetro striato," Boll. Ocul. 37:195, 1958.

3. Bielschowsky A. Application of the afterimage test in the investigation of squint. Am J Ophthalmol 20:408, 1937.

4. Bielschowsky A. Lectures on motro anomalies. Hanover, NH, 1943 (reprinted 1956), Dartmouth College Publications.

5. Birch E, Shimojo S, Held R. Preferential-looking assessment of fusion and stereopsis in infants aged 1–6 months. Invest. Ophthalmol Vis Sci. 26: 366, 1985.

6. Bixenmann WW, Noorden GK von. Apparent foveal displacement in normal subjects and in cyclotropia. Ophthalmologica 89:58, 1982.

7. Brown HW. The cover test. In Allen, JH, editor: Strabismus ophthalmic symposium, II, St Louis, 1958. Mosby–year Book, Inc., p. 225.

8. Capobianco NM. The subjective measurement of the near point of convergence and its significance in the diagnosis of convergence insufficiency. Am Orthopt J 2:40, 1952.

9. Carniglia P, Cooper J. Vergence Adaptation in Esotropia. Opt Vis Sci, 69 (4): 308–13, 1992.

10. Convergence Insufficiency Treatment Trial Study Group. Randomized clinical trial of treatments for symptomatic convergence insufficiency in children. Arch Ophthalmol 2008 Oct;126(10): 1336–49.

11. Cooper J, Burns C, Cotter S, Daum KM, Griffin JR, Scheiman M. Optometric Clinical Guideline: Care of the patient with accommodative or vergence dysfunction. Am. Optom. Ass. 1998.

12. Cooper J, Citron M. Microcomputer Produced Anaglyphs for Evaluation and Therapy of Binocular Anomalies. Journal of the American Optometric Association, 1983;65:185–8.

13. Cooper J, Ciuffreda KJ, Carniglia PE, Zinn KM, Tannen B. Orthoptic Treatment and Eye Movement Recordings in Guillain-Barré Syndrome. A case report. Neuro-ophthalmology 1995;15(5):249–56.

14. Cooper J, Duckman R. Convergence Insufficiency: Diagnosis and Treatment. Journal of the American Optometric Association 49(6):1978.

15. Cooper J, Feldman J, Eichler R. Relative Strength of Central and Peripheral Fusion as a Function of Stimulus Parameters. Opt. Vis Sci, 69:1992.

16. Cooper J, Feldman J, Janus S, Appleman W, Appel S, Horn D. Pupillary Dilation and Funduscopy with 1% Hydroamphetamine Plus 0.25% Tropicamide (Paremyd) Versus Tropicamide (0.5% Or 1%) as a Function of Iris and Skin Pigmentation, and Age. J Am Opt Ass. 1996;67(11):669–75.

17. Cooper J, Feldman J, Pasner K. Intermittent Exotropia: Stimulus Characteristics Affect Tests for Retinal Correspondence and Suppression. Bin Vis & Eye Mus Qtly. 2000;15(2):131–40.

18. Cooper J, Feldman J. Operant Conditioning and the Assessment of Stereopsis in Young Children. American Journal of Optometry & Physiological Optics, 1978;55(8):532–542.

19. Cooper J, Feldman J. Random Dot Stereogram Performance by Strabismic, Amblyopic and Ocular Pathology Patients in an Operant Discrimination Task. American Journal of Optometry & Physiological Optics 1978;55(9):599–609.

20. Cooper J, Feldman J. Operant Conditioning of Fusional Convergence Ranges Using Random Dot Stereograms. American Journal of Optometry & Physiological Optics 1980;57(4):205–13.

21. Cooper J, Feldman JM, Selenow A, Fair R, Bucciero F, MacDonald D, Levy M. Reduction of Asthenopia Following Accommodative Facility Training. Am J Optom Physiol Opt 1987;64: 430–6.

22. Cooper J, Medow N. Correspondence: Sensory Status in Intermittent Exotropia. Bin Vis Eye MusSurg Qtly 1994;9:11–2.

23. Cooper J, Medow N. Intermittent Exotropia of the Divergence Excess Type: Basic and Divergence Excess Type (Major Review). Bin Vis Eye Mus Surg Qtly 1993;8:187–222.

24. Cooper J, Record CD. Suppression and Retinal Correspondence in Intermittent Exotropia. Brit J Ophth 1986;700:673–6.

25. Cooper J, Selenow A, Ciuffreda J, Feldman J, Faverty J, Hokoda S. Reduction of Asthenopia in Patients with Convergence Insufficiency Following Fusional Vergence Training. Am J Opt Physl Opt 1983;60:982–9.

26. Cooper J. 'Diagnosis and Remediation of Accommodative Anomalies', Chapter in Clinical Diagnosis of Optometric Problem, John Amos (Ed). Butterworth Publications, 1987.

27. Cooper J. Review of Computerized Orthoptics with Specific Regard to Convergence Insufficiency. Am. J. of Optom. and Phys. Optics 1998;65(6): 455–63.

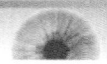

28. Crone RA, Everhard-Halm Y. Cyclofusion. In Moore S, Mein J (eds): Orthoptics: Past, Present, and Future. New York, Stratton Intercontinental, 1976, p 409.

29. Dell Osso LF Daroff RB. Eye movement characteristic and recording techniques. In Glaser JL (ed): Neuro-ophthalmology. Hagerstown MD Harper and Row, 1978, p 187.

30. Duke-Elder S, Wybar K. System of Ophthalmology. In Duke-Elder S (Ed). Ocular Motility and Strabismus, vol 6. St Louis, Mosby, 1973.

31. Eskridge JB, Perrigin DM, Leach NE. The Hirschberg test: correlation with corneal radius and axial length Optom Vis Sci 1990;67:243.

32. Feldman J, Cooper J, Carniglia P, Schiff FM, Sheete TN. Comparison of Fusional Ranges Measured by Risley Prisms, Vectograms, and Computer Orthoptics, Optom and Vis Sci 1989; 66(6):375–82.

33. Feldman J, Cooper J, Reinstein F, Swiatoca J. Asthenopia Induced by Computer-Generated FusionalVergence Targets. Opt Vis Sci 1992;69: 710–6.

34. Fink WH. The vergence test—an evaluation of the various techniques Am J Ophthalmol 1948;31:48.

35. Hardesty HH. Diagnosis of paretic vertical rotators. Am J Ophthalmol 1963;56:818.

36. Jampolsky A. The prism test for strabismus screening J Pediatr Ophthalmol 1964;1:30.

37. Lyle TK, Wybar KC. Lyle and Jackson's practical orthoptics in the treatment of squint (and other anomalies of binocular vision), (Ed). 5, London, 1967, HK Lewis and Company Ltd.; also Springfield, III, 1967, Carles C Thomas, Publisher.

38. Noorden GK von. Atlas of Strabismus. St Louis. Mosby, 1977.

39. Noorden GK von. Infantile esotropia: a continuing riddle (Scobee Lecture). Am Orthopt J 1984;34:52.

40. Pickwell LD. Eye movements during the cover test. Br J Ophthalmol 1973;28:23.

41. Robinson GL, Foreman PJ. Scotopic sensitivity/ Irlen Syndrome and the use of coloured filters: a long-term placebo controlled and masked study of reading achievement and perception of ability. Perceptual and Motor Skills 1999 Augt;89(1): 83–113.

42. Romano PE, Noorden GK von. Limitations of cover test in detecting strabismus. Am J Ophthalmol 1971;77:10.

43. Rubin ML. Optics for Clinicians Gainesville, Fl, Triad, 1974.

44. Ruttum M, Noorden, GK von. The Bagolini striated lens test for cyclotropia Doc Ophthalmol. 1984;58:131.

45. Scheiman M, Mitchell GL, Cotter S, Cooper J, Kulp M, Rouse M, Borsting E, London R, Wensveen J. Convergence Insufficiency Treatment Trial Study Group. A randomized clinical trial of treatments for convergence insufficiency in children. Arch Ophthalmol. 2005 Jan;123(1): 14–24.

46. Schnider C, Ciuffreda K, Cooper J, Kruger P. Accommodation Dynamics in Divergence Excess Exotropia. Investigative Ophthalmology 1984;25: 414–8.

47. Ziring PR, et al. Learning Disabilities, Dyslexia, and Vision: A Subject Review (RE9825). American Academy of Pediatrics Policy Statement Volume 102, No 5 November 1998;1217–9.

Evaluation and Investigations in Paralytic Squint

Chapter Outline

CLASSIFICATION OF INCOMITENT SQUINT

EVALUATION AND INVSTIGATIONS IN PARALYTIC SQUINT

Clinical features

Investigations
- History
- Inspection
- Cover test
- Ocular movements
- Measurement of deviation

- Diplopia test
- Bielschowsky three-step test
- Limitations of Park's three-step test
- Quantitative measurement of extraocular muscle actions
- Field of binocular fixation

Differential diagnosis
- Comitant versus incomitant
- Congenital versus acquired ocular palsy
- Paralytic versus restrictive incomitant squint

CLASSIFICATION OF INCOMITANT SQUINT

Incomitant squint is a type of heterotropia (manifest squint) in which the amount of deviation varies in different directions of gaze. Further, amount of deviation may also vary depending on which eye is fixing. Incomitant deviations include the following conditions:

1. *Vertically incomitant horizontal heterotropias* (A-, V-, X-, Y- and λ-pattern heterotropias)

2. *Paralytic strabismus*
  i. *Paralytic esotropia*
  - Lateral rectus paresis or paralysis
  - Divergence paralysis
  ii. *Paralytic exotropia*
  - Isolated medial rectus paresis
  - Complete third nerve paralysis
  - Paralysis of convergence

  iii. *Paralytic vertical deviation*
  - Single muscle paresis or paralysis
    - Superior oblique paralysis or paresis
    - Inferior oblique paralysis or paresis
    - Superior rectus paralysis or paresis
    - Inferior rectus paralysis or paresis.
  - Part of complete third nerve paralysis
  - Supranuclear lesions
    - Double elevator paralysis
    - Double depressor paralysis.

3. *Restrictive ocular motility defects*
  A. *Restrictive strabismus due to misdirected muscle forces.*
    1. Congenital cranial dysinnervation disorders (CCDDs)
    2. Congenital ectopic extraocular muscle insertion and/or pulley location
    3. Displaced extraocular muscle

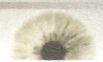

B. *Restrictive strabismus due to mechanical restrictions*

1. *Tight extaocular muscles*
   - Inelastic superior oblique in congenital Brown's syndrome
   - Thyroid ophthalmopathy
   - Entraped inferior rectus muscle in blow-out fracture of orbital floor.
   - Monocular elevation deficiency (MED), caused by fibrotic IR muscle.
   - Strabismus fixus.

2. *Structural adhesions*
   - Fat adherence to extraocular muscles or sclera after strabismus surgery, retinal detachment surgery or periocular trauma
   - Congenital fibrotic bands
   - Acquired Brown's syndrome due to scarring/inflammation around, the trochlea
   - Conjuctival and Tenon's capsule scarring.

3. *Orbital mass lesions*
   - Orbital tumours causing mass effect on the globe movements.
   - Glaucoma explant with large bleb causing mass effect.

EVALUATION AND INVESTIGATIONS IN PARALYTIC SQUINT

Paralytic squint refers to ocular deviation resulting from complete or incomplete paralysis of one or more extraocular muscles. Complete paralysis is also called palsy and incomplete paralysis is called paresis.

CLINICAL FEATURES

For evaluation of a case of paralytic squint, it is imperative to know about its presenting clinical features, which are described here.

1. *Diplopia.* It is the main symptom of paralytic squint. It is more marked towards the action of paralysed muscle. It may be crossed (in divergent squint) or uncrossed (in convergent squint). It may be horizontal, vertical or oblique depending on the muscle paralysed. Diplopia

occurs due to formation of image on dissimilar points of the two retinae (Fig. 21.1).

2. *Confusion.* It occurs due to formation of image of two different objects on the corresponding points of two retinae following misalignment of the visual axes of two eyes (Fig. 21.2).

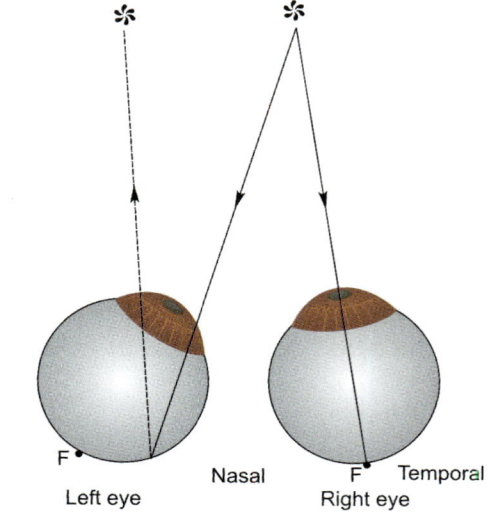

Fig. 21.1: *Uncrossed diplopia in a patient with left convergent squint.*

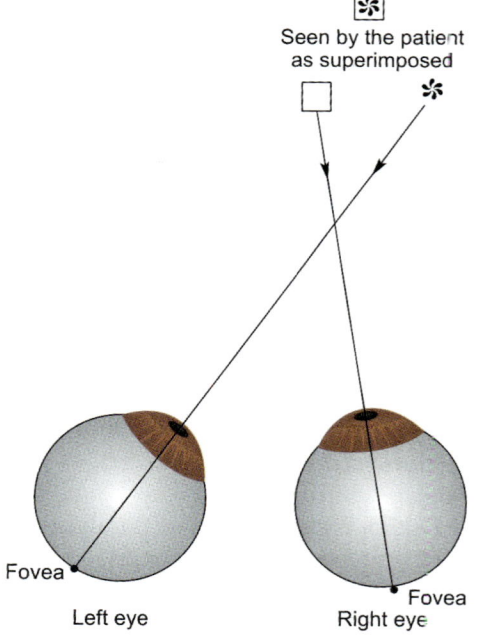

Fig. 21.2: *Confusion due to formation of image of two different objects on the corresponding points of two retinae.*

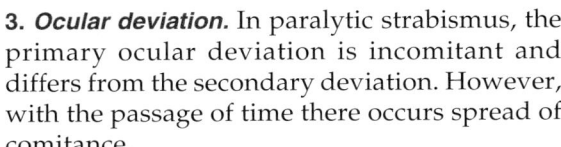

3. *Ocular deviation.* In paralytic strabismus, the primary ocular deviation is incomitant and differs from the secondary deviation. However, with the passage of time there occurs spread of comitance.

Primary deviation. It is deviation of the affected eye, when the unaffected eye is used for fixation and is away from the action of paralysed muscle, e.g. if lateral rectus is paralysed, the eye is convergent.

Onset of paralytic ocular deviation may be of sudden as seen in trauma and vascular occlusions; or gradual as seen in tumours and multiple sclerosis.

Incomitance depending upon gaze. The angle of deviation changes with the direction of gaze. It is greatest in the direction in which maximal activity is required for the involved muscle, i.e. in the diagnostic position of the muscle. For example, in a patient with paresis of right lateral rectus muscle during levoversion, no or little esotropia may be noted in right eye, while in primary position, right esotropia is marked, which will become maximum in dextroversion, i.e. deviation will be maximum in the field of action of right lateral rectus muscle.

Secondary deviation. It refers to deviation of the unaffected eye seen under cover, when the patient is made to fix with the affected eye. In a recently acquired ocular palsy, the secondary deviation is much greater than the primary deviation. This is due to the fact that the strong impulse of innervation required to enable the eye with paralysed muscle to fix is also transmitted to the yoke muscle of the sound eye resulting in a greater amount of deviation. This is based on Hering's law of equal innervation of yoke muscles.

In a long-standing ocular palsy, the secondary deviation is often much the same as the primary deviation because completion of the muscle sequelae leads to comitance.

Spread of comitance. A paralytic deviation undergoes several stages. The first stage is characterized by weakness of the paralyzed muscle during which secondary deviation is much more than the primary deviation as described above. Almost immediately following the paresis of an extraocular muscle, the direct antagonist begins to overact. A contracture of the antagonist muscle will develop within days to weeks, if the patient fixes with the unaffected eye. At this point, the deviation may become greater in the field of action of antagonist than it is in the field of action of weak agonist muscle. During the next stage, the deviation will spread into all fields of gaze and become increasingly comitant, i.e. there occurs a gradual spread of comitance to all fields of gaze. Ultimately, it may then no longer be possible to determine the nature of original deviation since the secondary deviation is often much the same as the primary deviation.

In most cases, spread of comitance occurs within a few weeks, months or even one to two years after the onset of paralysis. However, the spread of comitance is not a rule; in some cases of paralytic squint, it may not occur at all. Spread of comitance is quite common in infants with sixth nerve palsy, and ultimately patient may present with a comitant esodeviation.

4. *Ocular movements.* Restriction of ocular movements occurs towards the direction of action of the paralysed muscle/muscles. When the paralysis is of recent onset, a careful study of duction and version movements will make the diagnosis on the basis of incomplete movements in the field of action of the paralysed muscle. However, in long-standing cases, development of muscle sequelae such as contracture of the direct antagonist muscle and secondary inhibitional palsy of the contralateral antagonist muscle, present difficulties in the identification of the paralysed muscle. Under these circumstances, other tests like head-tilt test and Hess screen charting, etc. may be helpful in diagnosing the paralysed muscle.

5. *Past pointing.* Past pointing also described as *false projection* or *orientation* occurs due to increased innervational impulse conveyed to the paralysed muscle during movement in the direction of action of paralyzed muscle.

It can be demonstrated by asking the patient to close the sound eye and then to fix an object placed on the side of action of paralysed muscle. Patient will locate it further away in the same direction. For example, a patient with paralysis of right lateral rectus will point more towards right than the object actually is.

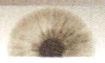

6. *Nausea, vertigo and dizziness.* Nausea, vertigo and dizziness result from diplopia, confusion and false localization. These symptoms are more prevalent in vertical and torsional diplopias than in horizontal diplopia. They do not occur in patients with congenital defects and disappear quickly in children. Adults adapt more slowly.

7. *Muscle sequelae.* Muscle sequelae refer to changes that take place in the extraocular muscles after some time of the paralysis or paresis of one or more of the extraocular muscles. The speed and extent to which they develop in different patients vary markedly. The exact reasons for this are unknown, but the speed and degree of their development depend partly on which eye the patient uses for fixation. Mostly, the patients use sound eye, however, sometimes the paretic eye may be used for fixation if: (1) it has better visual acuity, (2) it is originally dominant eye, or (3) fixation with paretic eye increases the separation of the double picture (due to secondary deviation) which causes less problem.

Muscle sequelae occur to much lesser degrees in patients with congenital paralysis as compared to the acquired paralysis. These occur more in paralysis due to lesions of the nerves than the lesions of muscles and include the following:

i. *Overaction of the contralateral synergistic (yoke) muscle.* Overaction of the yoke muscle develops quickly, when paretic eye is used for fixation and slowly, when the sound eye is used for fixation. This overaction of the yoke muscle is responsible for secondary deviation of the sound eye. With the passage of time, this overaction becomes habitual due to the development of spasm and contracture and remains, even if the original paresis should recover spontaneously.

ii. *Contracture of the direct antagonist.* After paralysis of a particular extraocular muscle, its direct antagonist is more or less unopposed and thus overact and is responsible for the primary deviation. Within a few weeks, the overacting muscle becomes spastic, contracting more and more leading to a greater angle of deviation. Eventually, this leads to a contracture, an organic change in the muscle in which muscle fibres are replaced by fibrous tissue.

iii. *Secondary inhibitional palsy of the contralateral antagonist muscle.* It is a manifestation of Hering's law of equal innervation. Since the direct antagonist of the paretic muscle is more or less unopposed, so it will require less than normal innervation for a particular extent of a movement. According to Hering's law, the same innervation will flow to its yoke muscle (which is contralateral antagonist of the paretic muscle). Consequently, the contralateral antagonist of the paretic muscle will exhibit a weakness; which has been called the secondary inhibitional palsy of the contralateral antagonist muscle. Perhaps the better term will be '*simulated weakness of the yoke's antagonist*' or PAY syndrome: pseudo-weakness of the antagonist of a yoke. This underaction of the yoke muscle of the antagonist occurs earlier and is more pronounced, when the paretic eye is used for fixation than when the sound eye is preferred for fixation.

The muscle sequelae developing following paresis of a particular muscle are shown in Table 21.1.

Table 21.1 *Muscle sequelae following paresis of extraocular muscles*			
Paretic muscle	*Muscle sequelae*		
	Overaction of contra-lateral synergistic (yoke) muscle	*Contracture of directant antagonist muscle*	*Secondary inhibitional palsy of the contralateral antagonist muscle*
Right lateral rectus	Left medial rectus	Right medial rectus	Left lateral rectus
Right medial rectus	Left lateral rectus	Right lateral rectus	Left medial rectus
Right superior oblique	Left inferior rectus	Right inferior oblique	Left superior rectus
Right inferior oblique	Left superior rectus	Right superior oblique	Left inferior rectus
Right superior rectus	Left inferior oblique	Right inferior rectus	Left superior oblique
Right inferior rectus	Left superior oblique	Right superior rectus	Left inferior oblique

Figures 21.3 and 21.4 show the muscle sequelae occurring in a patient with right lateral rectus and left superior oblique muscles, respectively.

8. Abnormal head posture. An abnormal head posture is a common feature of the paralytic strabismus. A compensatory head posture does not necessarily develop in every patient with a paresis or paralysis of extraocular muscles.

However, when present, it can aid in making the diagnosis.

Reasons for abnormal head posture. Abnormal head posture may be adapted for any of the following two reasons:

i. *To achieve binocular single vision.* Most frequently, an abnormal head posture is adapted to achieve binocular single vision, i.e. to avoid

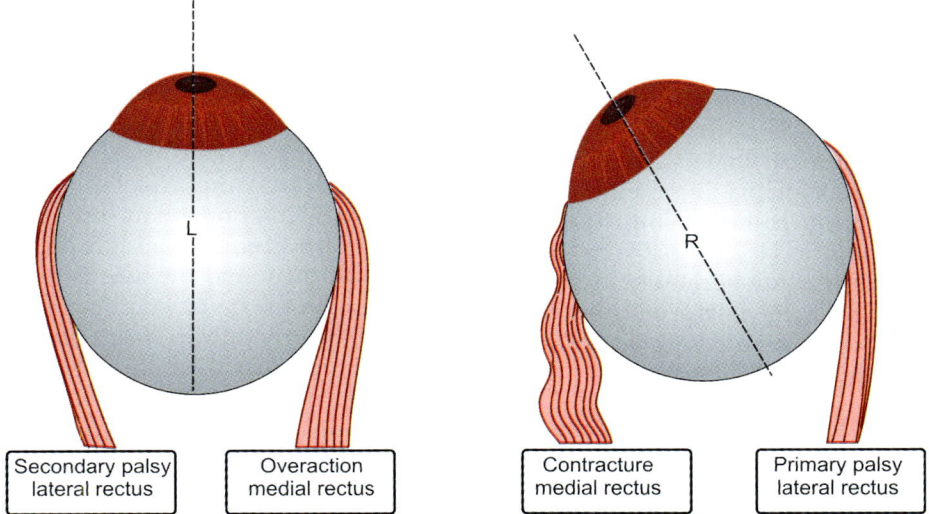

| Secondary palsy lateral rectus | Overaction medial rectus | Contracture medial rectus | Primary palsy lateral rectus |

Fig. 21.3: *Muscle sequelae following paralysis of right lateral rectus muscle.*

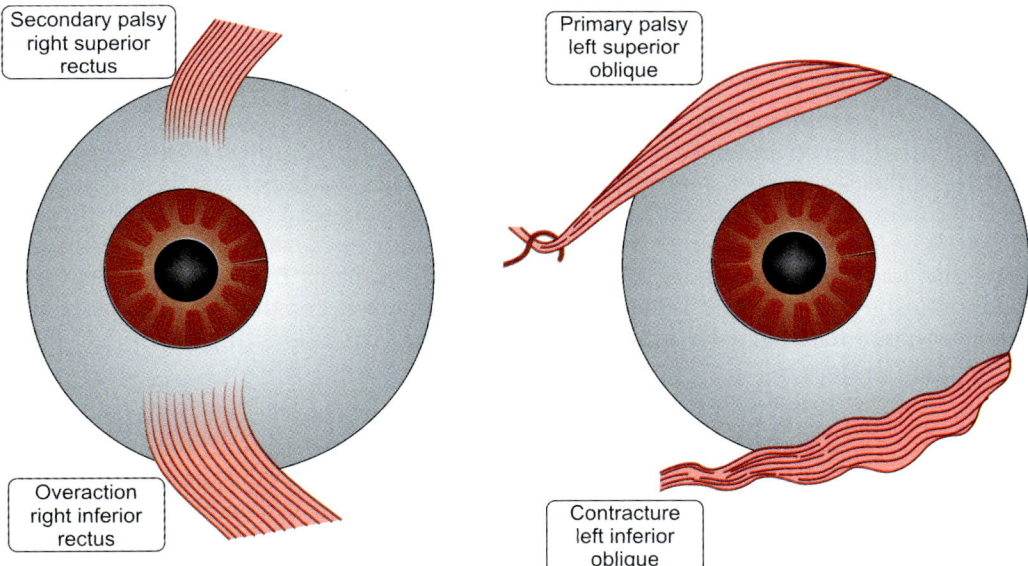

Secondary palsy right superior rectus

Primary palsy left superior oblique

Overaction right inferior rectus

Contracture left inferior oblique

Fig. 21.4: *Muscle sequelae following paralysis of left superior oblique muscle.*

the troubling diplopia and/or confusion. For this purpose, the head is turned into the field of action of the paralysed muscle, and that the eyes are directed by the *doll's head phenomenon*. This process allows the patient to move his/her limited field of single vision so that it coincides with his/her egocentric (straight ahead) position. In other words, the patient can see the things in front of him/her as single.

ii. *To achieve wide separation of the two images.* Less frequently, patients with paralytic strabismus develop abnormal head posture in order to increase the separation between diplopic images. This occurs in patients who have no useful field of bifoveal single vision but suffer from the constant diplopia. Since they have no choice but to live with it, they attempt to separate the double pictures as far as possible by turning the head in the field of paretic muscle. In this field, the deviation of the involved eye will be maximal and, thus, the 'true' and the 'false' image of objects in front will be maximally separated.

Components of abnormal head posture

A. *In horizontal rectus muscle palsy.* If one of the horizontally acting muscles (lateral or medial rectus) is involved, the abnormal head posture will consist of only one component, i.e. *face turn* towards the action of paretic muscle. For example, in a paresis of right lateral rectus muscle, there will be a face turn to the right side, and in a paresis of right medial rectus muscle, there will be a face turn to the left side.

B. *In palsy of cyclovertically acting muscles.* The superior and inferior recti and the superior and inferior oblique muscles are cyclovertically acting muscles and contraction of any one of them alone would produce a combination of vertical, horizontal and torsional movements. If anyone of these muscles is paretic, there will be three components of abnormal head posture as follows:

- Chin elevation or depression
- Face turn
- Head tilt

1. *Chin elevation or depression* occurs in paralysis/paresis of elevators or depressors of the eye, respectively. By doll's head phenomenon, in chin elevation, the eyes move down and in chin depression, the eyes move up. In this way,

the involved eye is brought out of the field of action of paretic elevator or depressor muscle.

2. *Face turn.* As mentioned above, face turn in the paresis of a horizontally acting muscle (medial or lateral rectus) is towards the action of the paretic muscle. However, in the paresis of one of the cyclovertically acting muscles, the face turn is such that the eyes are brought away from the field in which the muscle has its greatest vertical effect. Thus in the case of superior and inferior recti which have their maximal vertical effect in abduction, the face is turned so that the involved eye is adducted, when the patient looks straight ahead, i.e. in paresis of the vertical recti, the face will be turned towards the affected eye. Since the superior and inferior oblique muscles have their greatest vertical effect in adduction, the opposite is true for them and the face is turned so that the eye with the involved oblique is abducted, i.e. face is turned away from the affected eye (towards left in paresis of oblique muscle of right eye).

3. *Head tilt.* The head tilt occurs to compensate for the torsion or to help relieve the vertical separation of the double images as follows:

- In paresis of a oblique muscle, head tilt occurs to compensate the torsion caused by the direct antagonist of the paralysed muscle. For example, in paresis of right superior oblique, the head will tilt towards left to compensate for the extorsion caused by right inferior oblique muscle.

- In paresis of a vertical rectus muscle, the head tilt occurs to compensate the torsion caused by the contralateral antagonist of the paralysed muscle. For example, in paresis of right superior rectus, the head will tilt to the right to compensate for the extorsion of the left eye caused by overacting left inferior oblique muscle.

Diagnostic importance of abnormal head posture. The typical head posture adapted may be a pointer towards the paretic muscle especially in a fresh case of isolated muscle palsy.

Abnormal head postures assumed in paresis of extraocular muscle of right eye are as shown in Table 21.2.

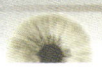

Table 21.2 *Abnormal head posture in extraocular muscle paralysis*

Muscle paralysed	Components of abnormal head posture		
	Chin	*Face turn*	*Head tilt*
Right superior rectus	Elevation	Right	Right
Right inferior rectus	Depression	Right	Left
Right superior oblique	Depression	Left	Left
Right inferior oblique	Elevation	Left	Right
Right lateral rectus	–	Right	–
Right medial rectus	–	Left	–

As discussed above, it is not difficult to understand the different abnormal head postures that would theoretically occur as a result of the deficient eye movements caused by paralysis of individual muscle. However, in practice, conditions are not so clear because of the following factors:

- The paresis may be so slight that a partial compensation is already sufficient and the typical head posture may never develop.
- More than one muscle may be involved leading to a complex picture.
- Muscle sequelae and secondary changes may alter the original condition.

Ocular torticollis. The abnormal head posture adopted by the individuals with congenital and infantile paralytic squint is sometimes referred to as acquired ocular torticollis, because it resembles an orthopaedic deformity called congenital torticollis. In the later condition, the head cannot be straightened due to organic changes in the neck musculature. In contrast, the ocular torticollis is merely a functional position and the head can be straightened passively. In the early stages, if one eye is occluded, the patient with ocular torticollis will straighten the head. However, in late stages, secondary scoliosis may occur as a consequence of ocular torticollis and because of it, patient's head may not straighten with monocular occlusion. Further, if secondary vertebral column changes have been allowed to develop, it may no longer be possible to correct the abnormal head posture even by surgically aligning the eyes.

Facial asymmetry due to atrophy of the lower side of the face is a feature of both long-standing ocular as well as congenital torticollis, so it cannot be considered a differentiating feature.

9. *Sensory adaptations*. Sensory adaptations such as suppression, abnormal retinal correspondence and amblyopia are, in general, less known with paralytic squint vis-á-vis concomitant squint; perhaps, because of the following reasons:

- Patients with paralytic squint can assume abnormal head posture to achieve a single binocular vision which may prevent the occurrence of suppression, ARC and amblyopia.
- Patients with paralytic squint have variable angle of deviation in various positions of gaze; while sensory adaptations usually develop in patients who have stable and constant angle of deviation.

With the passage of time, the deviation becomes increasingly comitant, as discussed under spread of comitance. Under such circumstances, the patient is unable to maintain fusion in any direction of gaze, and as a result, suppression, ARC and amblyopia become established.

Occurrence of comitance in paralytic squint is common but not universal. If the strabismus remains incomitant and onset is during childhood, diplopia in the paretic field of fixation may be prevented by *regional suppression.*

Amblyopia occurs in only those patients of paralytic squint who are unable to maintain

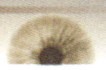

simultaneous binocular vision in any direction of gaze and in whom paralysis occurs in early life. Further, sometimes, presence of amblyopia may cause confusion in the diagnosis of paralytic squint. This is because some patients, who prefer to fixate with the paretic eye because of certain reasons mentioned earlier, develop amblyopia in the non-paretic deviated eye.

◼ INVESTIGATIONS OF INCOMITANT SQUINT

It should include: (1) evaluation from strabismic point of view and (2) investigations to find out the cause of incomitant squint, such as orbital ultrasonography, orbital and skull computerized tomographic scanning and detailed neurological investigations (which are beyond the scope of this chapter).

A detailed work-up of a strabismic patient is described in Chapter 20. However, the salient points relevant to the paralytic strabismus are mentioned herein briefly.

History

A detailed history should be taken with reference to following points:

1. *Subjective symptoms*
- *Diplopia.* Enquiry should be made to ascertain: Onset, constant/intermittent, distance at which diplopia is noticed, relative position of images, field where greatest separation of images occurs, any change since onset, does diplopia disappear, when eye is occluded.
- *Confusion.* It occurs due to formation of images of the different objects on the corresponding points of two retina.
- *Other subjective symptoms* which a patient with paralytic strabismus may experience are: Dificulty in focussing, headache, eye strain, general asthenopic symptoms and discomfort from abnormal head posture.

2. *Objective symptoms*
- Constant/intermittent deviation
- Abnormal head posture
- Ptosis, exophthalmos.

3. *Any attributed cause*
4. *Any previous ocular problems and treatment taken*

5. *General health*
6. *Family history.*

Inspection

1. Ocular posture
2. Abnormal head posture; note its exact components
3. Facial asymmetry
4. Ptosis, exophthalmos.

Cover test

It should be carried out for near and distance; with and without abnormal head posture. The cover test will detect:

1. Presence of any manifest or latent deviation.
2. Type of deviation
3. Incomitance—primary versus secondary deviation
4. Normally fixing eye. Patient usually fixes with the non-affected eye; but this may be influenced by visual acuity or dominant eye.

Ocular movements

Investigation of ocular movements is carried out while the patient watches a fixation target, i.e. moved from the primary position into each of the cardinal positions of gaze.

1. *Version movements.* The examiner compares the movement of the two eyes in all positions of gaze. Symmetric movement indicates that no defect is present. Unequal movements are seen in underactions, overactions and limitations.

2. *Duction movements.* Monocular movements are of value only in differentiating between a paresis and a total paralysis. Testing for ductions also helps to detect mechanical limitation of movements.

3. *Doll's head movements and command movements* testing is of particular use in supranuclear gaze palsies.

Measurement of deviation

1. *Synoptophore method.* Major amblyoscope is the best instrument for measurement of deviation in paralytic squint; since measurements are taken to compare the size of the deviation in each of the cardinal directions of gaze while each eye in turn is used for fixation. To make the comparison valid, it is extremely important that the fixation object be moved an equal distance from the primary position in each direction. For this, synoptophore can be adjusted so that the deviation can be measured while the patient is looking at an equal angle from the primary position in all directions of gaze.

2. Prism and cover test. It is an easy method, while carried out with the help of a prism bar. Measurements should be taken with and without abnormal head posture for near and distance fixation, fixing either eye. Measurements can be made in all the cardinal directions, but for comparison these are not considered very accurate. Since it is not possible to measure at an equal angle from the primary position in all directions; as is possible with the synoptophore.

3. Measurement of torsional deviation can be made with special slides on major amblyoscope, or on adapted Lees screen.

Note. In a paresis or paralysis of an extraocular muscle, the deviation will be greatest in the direction of maximal singular action of the muscle while the affected eye is fixating.

Diplopia test

For details, see Chapter 20. Salient points are as follows:

- Tested with red/green goggles and a linear light, or without dissociation aids.
- Position of maximum vertical and horizontal separation of images and position of maximum torsion is noted.
- Distal image belongs to the affected eye.
- The results are recorded either by written description or as diplopia chart. Diplopia charts of paralysis of extraocular muscles of right eye and left eye are shown in Figs 21.5 and 21.6, respectively.

Bielschowsky three-step test (B3ST)

The classical head tilt test was proposed by Bielschowsky to differentiate between superior oblique palsy in one eye and superior rectus palsy in the contralateral side. However, presently in practice is the three step test as

modified by Parks'. It is useful in diagnosing the paresis of any cyclovertically acting muscle. There are in total 8 cyclovertically acting muscles; 4 work as depressors of the eyes, and 4 work as elevators. The two muscles on each eye that are responsible for depression are the inferior rectus and superior oblique, and the two muscles on each eye that are responsible for elevation are the superior rectus and the inferior oblique.

As expected, at the onset of a cyclovertical muscle palsy, there will be limitation in the field of action of the paralysed muscle. Shortly thereafter, an overaction in the field of the antagonist muscle will be noted. With time, this overaction will produce a contracture of the antagonist. Thereafter, there will be spread of comitance, so that the amount of deviation will gradually increase and become approximately the same in the all fields of gaze. At this point, based on analysis of duction and version movements of the eye, the diagnosis of cyclovertical palsy becomes impossible. At this juncture, the Parks' modification over Bielschowsky's head tilt test can be quite useful. There are three steps of this test, each of which eliminates half of the remaining potential muscles, leaving only one muscle to be blamed after the three steps.

Procedure of three-step test

Step 1
- Perform cover-uncover test in primary position and determine which eye is hypertropic. If the patient's presenting sign is a hypodeviation, consider it hyperdeviation of the opposite eye. Step 1 reduces the number of affected muscles from 8 to 4.
- A right hypertropia (RHT) implies any of the following:
  ♦ Weakness of depressors of right eye (RIR, RSO)
  ♦ Weakness of elevators of left eye (LIO, LSR).
- A left hypertropia (LHT) implies any of the following:
  ♦ Weakness of depressors of left eye (LIR, LSO)
  ♦ Weakness of elevators of right eye (RIO, RSR).

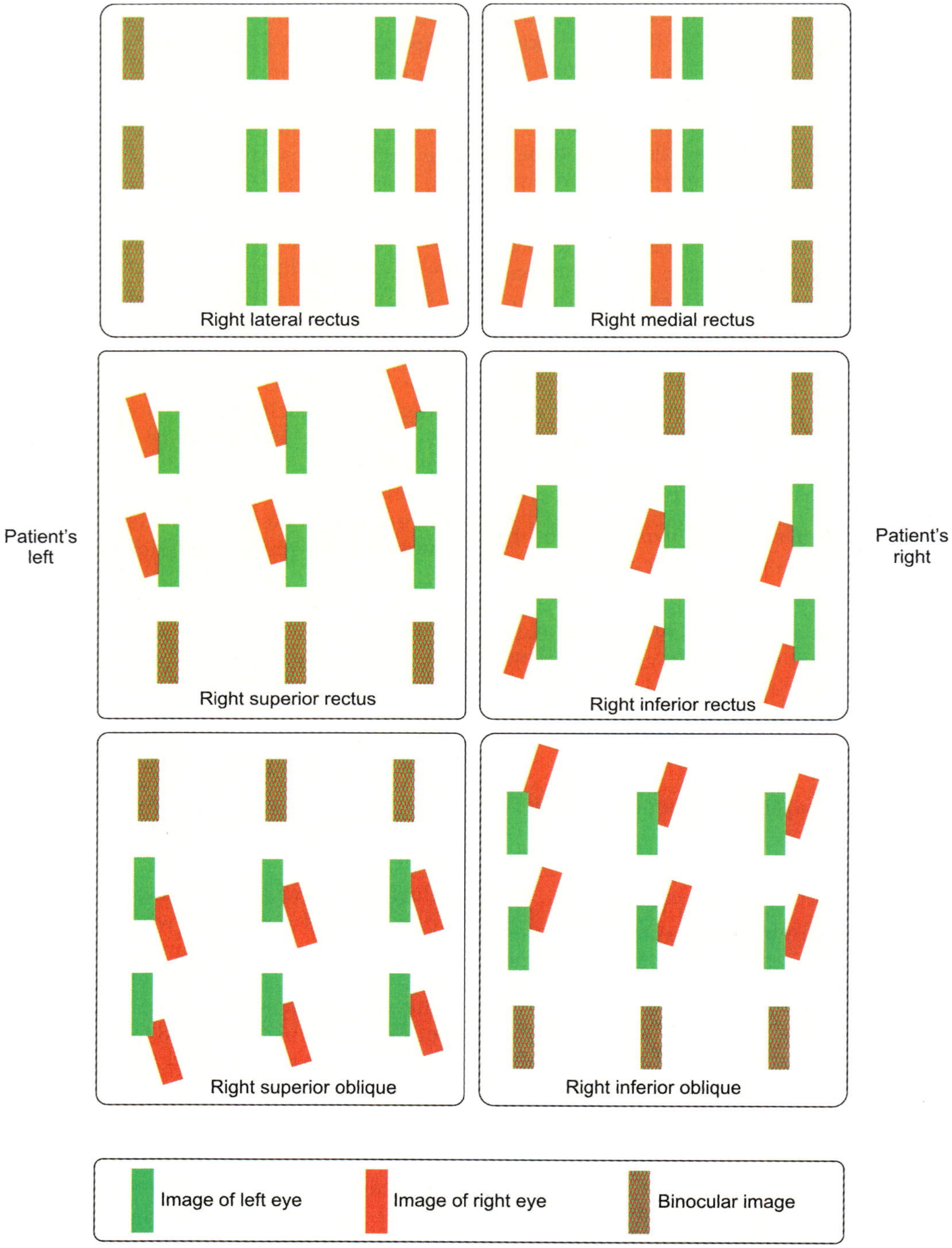

Right lateral rectus

Right medial rectus

Patient's left

Right superior rectus

Right inferior rectus

Patient's right

Right superior oblique

Right inferior oblique

Image of left eye   Image of right eye   Binocular image

Fig. 21.5: *Diplopia charts (patient's view) of paralysis of extraocular muscles of the right eye.*

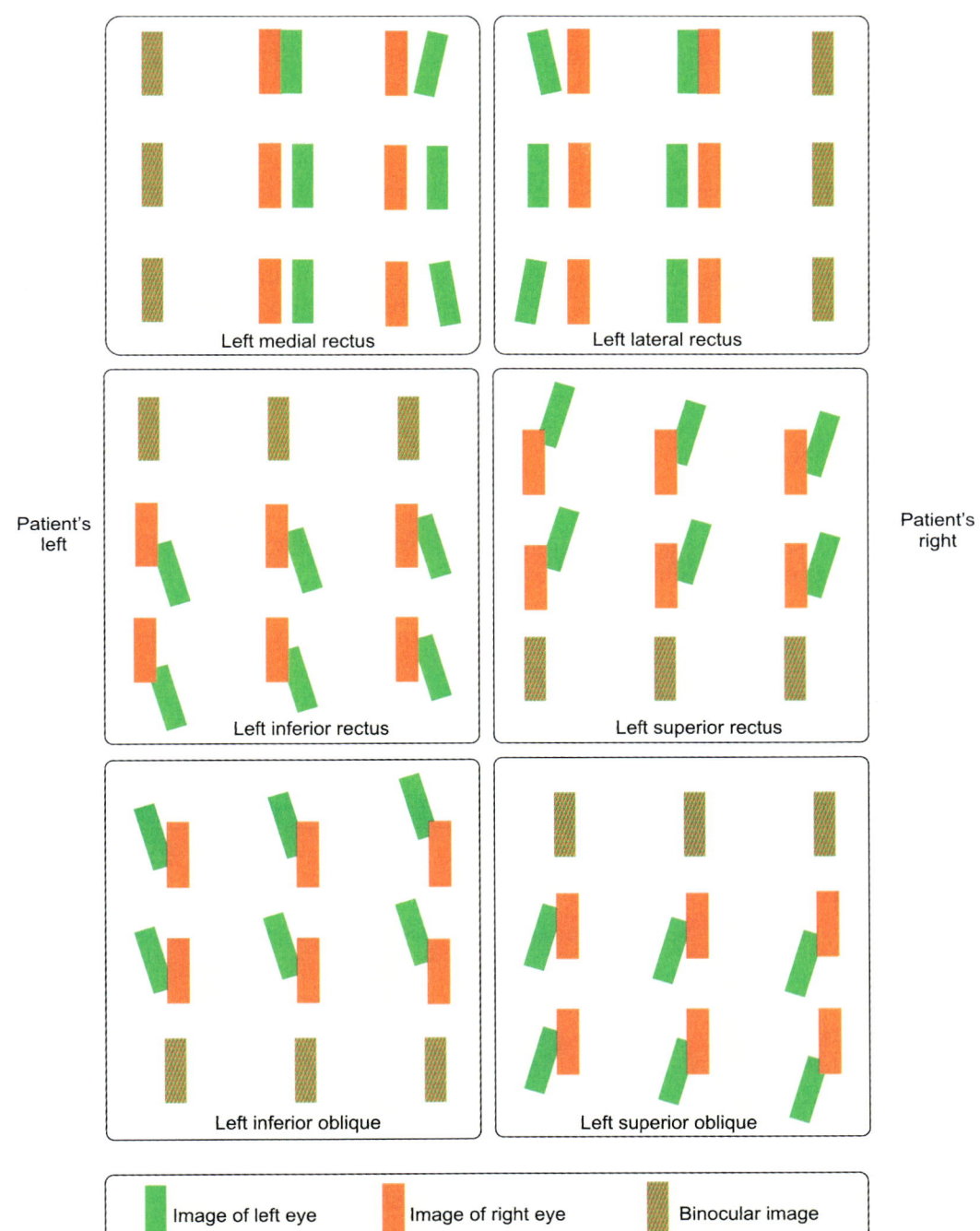

Patient's left

Patient's right

Left medial rectus

Left lateral rectus

Left inferior rectus

Left superior rectus

Left inferior oblique

Left superior oblique

Image of left eye   Image of right eye   Binocular image

Fig. 21.6: *Diplopia charts (patient's view) of paralysis of extraocular muscles of the left eye.*

- Let us assume, e.g. the patient being examined has LHT. Draw an oval (with red lines) around the two possible muscle pairs responsible for LHT (Fig. 21.7A).

Step 2

- Determine whether hypertropia (HT) is larger in right gaze or left gaze.
- If the LHT is larger in right gaze, it implies weakness of any of the 4 vertically acting muscles in right gaze:
  - RSR, RIR
  - LIO, LSO.
- If the LHT is larger in left gaze, it implies weakness of any of the 4 vertically acting muscles in left gaze, i.e.
  - LSR, LIR
  - RIO, RSO.
- Let us say, in the same patient having LHT, the deviation is greater in right gaze. Draw an oval (with green lines) around the two possible muscle pairs (Fig. 21.7B).

- Note that at this point, the paretic muscle must be either the LSO or RSR muscle, since they are the only muscles encircled twice (Fig. 21.7B).

Step 3

- Determine, if the HT is larger, when measured during head tilt to the left or right. For proper measurement, the base of the prism should be held parallel to the floor of the orbit and not parallel to the floor of the room. The Maddox rod and correcting prism should be held so that the line and base are parallel to the floor of orbit (Fig. 21.8).
- If the LHT is larger, when the head is tilted to the right, this implicates any of four muscles that act vertically in right tilt position, i.e. either intorters of right eye (RSR, RSO) or extorters of left eye (LIR, LIO).
- If the LHT is larger, when the head is tilted to the left, this implicates any of the four muscles that act vertically in left tilt position, i.e. either

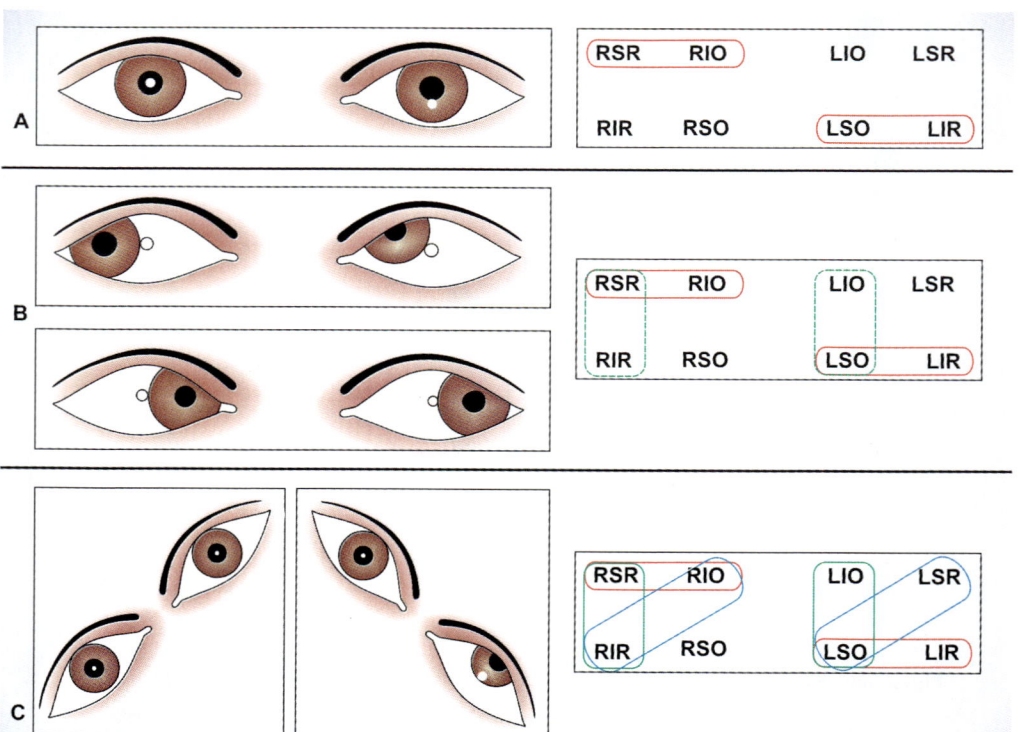

Fig. 21.7: *Bielschowsky's three-step test (B3ST) in a patient with left superior oblique paralysis. (A) step 1; (B) step 2; (C) step 3 (for explanation, see text).*

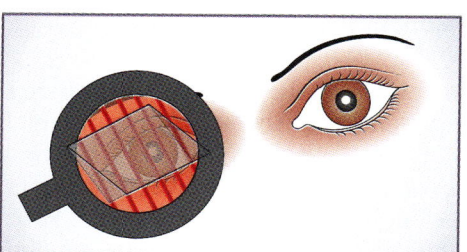

Fig. 21.8: *Measurement of deviation using Maddox rod and prism in a patient with right hypertropia. Note, head is tilted to the right and base of the prism is held parallel to the floor of the orbit. Maddox rod is held in such a way that the red line seen is also parallel to the floor of the orbit.*

intorters of left eye (LSR, LSO) or extorters of right eye (RIR, RIO).

- Now, for the same individual, suppose that the vertical deviation is quite large, when the head is tilted to the left and is almost absent, when the head is tilted to the right. Draw an oval (with blue lines) around the muscle implicated, i.e. (LSR, LSO, RIR, RIO) (Fig. 21.7C).
- Note that at this point, the LSO is the only muscle, i.e. surrounded by three ovals and is connected by the line that represents head tilt to the right (Fig. 21.7C).

Summary of the test shown in Fig. 21.7:
Step 1: LHT (LIR, LSO, RSR or RIO)
Step 2: Worse in right gaze (RSR or LSO)
Step 3: Worse in left tilt (LSO)

Results of B3ST in paralysis of various cyclovertically acting muscles are summarized in Table 21.3.

Limitations of Park's three-step test

This test is quite useful in general, but it is not always diagnostic and can be misleading, especially during following conditions:

- In cases of long-standing paresis
- When more than one muscle are paretic, e.g.
    - Bilateral fourth nerve palsy
    - Multiple other muscle weakness
- In cases with restrictions.
    - Superior rectus overaction
    - Superior rectus contracture
    - Inferior restriction
- Dissociated vertical deviation (DVD)
- Pulley heterotopia
- Superior rectus palsy
- Skew deviation
- Prior extraocular muscle surgery.

Quantitative measurement of extraocular muscle actions

The quantitative measurement of extraocular muscle action is most essential to comment about the paretic muscles and the pathological sequelae of the paralysis, *viz.* overaction, contracture and secondary inhibitional palsy.

Commonly employed tests to have a graphic record of the relative power of extraocular muscles in all directions of gaze are as follows:

- Hess screen test
- Lees screen test
- Lancaster red and green test.

Table 21.3 *Results of Bielschowsky three-step head tilt test in paralysis of cyclovertically acting muscles*

Paralysed muscle	Bielschowsky head tilt test		
	Step 1 (hypertropia in primary gaze)	Step 2 (HT worse in left or right gaze)	Step 3 (HT worse on left or right tilt)
RSO	RHT	Left	Right
RIR	RHT	Right	Left
LIO	RHT	Right	Right
LSR	RHT	Left	Left
LSO	LHT	Right	Left
LIR	LHT	Left	Right
RIO	LHT	Left	Left
RSR	LHT	Right	Right

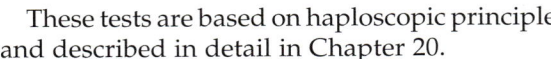

These tests are based on haploscopic principle and described in detail in Chapter 20.

Uses of haploscopic tests

These tests are repeatable and their uses are as follows:

- Diagnose underactions and overactions of extraocular muscles and provide a good pictorial representation of muscle actions
- Diagnose A- and V-phenomena
- Diagnose mechanical/neurological palsy
- Diagnose congenital/acquired palsy
- Aid in plan of surgery—preoperatively
- Show effect of surgery—postoperatively
- Provide an accurate and permanent record of change in state of ocular movements in subsequent visits and thereby form part of serial record of progress of palsy
- Measure torsional movement with linear pointer (Dulley and Harden) or cyclotiltmeter (Brown).

Field of binocular fixation

It must be tested, wherever applicable, i.e. if patient has some field of binocular single vision. It provides, useful and repeatable information. The area of binocular single vision is opposite to the direction in which ocular motility is impaired.

The aim of treatment of muscle paralysis is to provide comfortable field of binocular fixation, i.e. the central field and lower quadrants.

For details of the test, *see* in Chapter 20.

Other tests

Other tests which can be carried out, if necessary, includes forced duction test, EMG, EOG, orbital ultrasonography and computerized tomographic scanning.

▌ DIFFERENTIAL DIAGNOSIS OF INCOMITANT SQUINT

Differential diagnosis to be considered in patients with incomitant squint in general are as follows:

- Comitant (non-paralytic) versus incomitant (paralytic) squint
- Congenital versus acquired palsies
- Paralytic versus restrictive incomitant squint.

Comitant (non-paralytic) versus incomitant (paralytic) squint

As mentioned earlier, by and large, there arises no problem in differentiating comitant (non-paralytic) squint from the paralytic (incomitant) squint of recent onset. However, in patients with long-standing paralysis, there occurs spread of comitance and thus it becomes extremely difficult and at times even impossible to differentiate such a condition from the comitant squint. Anyshow, for a ready reference, the differences between paralytic and non-paralytic squint are depicted in Table 21.4.

Congenital versus acquired ocular palsy

Many a time, patients with congenital paralysis of an extraocular muscle may remain asymptomatic for decades because of either a strong fusion mechanism or by an unnoticed slight abnormal head posture. Such a patient, when reaches adult life, the chances are that, unless the latent deviation is small one, decompensation will begin to occur, especially between the ages of 30 and 40 years. The patient may notice that he/she is beginning to suffer from an intermittent diplopia, especially if he/she is tired, overworked, or suffering from ill health. Some of these patients may develop intermittent squint without diplopia due to suppression of the image of the deviating eye. Such patients may experience difficulty in focussing or have a feeling of using only one eye.

Under these circumstances, one needs to differentiate between cases of congenital paralysis with recent decompensation and those of acquired paralysis of recent onset. It is very essential, since in the former the treatment is invariably operative while the latter requires a diligent search for its cause by a complete medical and neuro-ophthalmologic evaluation and the appropriate treatment. Some of the chief differences between the congenital and acquired ocular palsies are summarized in Table. 21.5.

Paralytic versus restrictive incomitant squint

Incomitant ocular deviations are known both due to palsies as well as restrictions of extraocular muscles and are often confused with one another by even experienced examiners.

Table 21.4 *Differences between paralytic and non-paralytic squint*

S. no.	Feature	Paralytic squint	Non-paralytic squint
1.	Age of onset	Any age	Usually in childhood
2.	Type of onset	Usually sudden, rarely may be slow or since birth	Usually gradual
3.	History of head injury	Common	Uncommon
4.	Diplopia	Usually present	Usually absent
5.	Ocular movements	Limited in the direction of paralysed muscle	Usually full
6.	False projection	It is common in palsy of recent onset, i.e. patient cannot correctly locate the object in space, when asked to do so in direction of paralyzed muscle. There occurs past pointing.	False projection is negative
7.	Head posture	A particular abnormal head posture may be present, depending upon the muscle paralysed.	Normal
8.	Nausea and vertigo	Usually present, due to confusion, diplopia and false projection	Absent
9.	Primary versus secondary deviation	Secondary deviation is more than primary deviation	Secondary deviation is equal to primary deviation
10.	Sensory adaptations (ARC, suppression, amblyopia)	Uncommon	Common
11.	Cyclotropia	Common with cyclovertical paresis	Uncommon, except in A- and V-patterns
12.	Muscle sequelae	Present in old cases	Absent
13.	Neurological findings or systemic diseases	May be present	Usually absent

Though, these are two distinct problems but mere measurement obtained with prism and alternate cover tests with either eye fixing do not differentiate between them, since in both, the secondary deviation is typically greater than the primary deviation. However, a differentiation between the two is most important for the successful treatment of incomitant deviation. It is unequivocal to state that the restrictions must be relieved first, before any other therapy, whether surgical or non-surgical to be effective.

Commonly employed tests to differentiate between palsies and restrictions are as follows:

1. Passive forced duction test (traction test)

As mentioned above, detection of associated restriction is most important for the successful therapy of an incomitant squint. Therefore, it is mandatory to carry out forced duction test (FDT) before any surgical therapy is undertaken.

Steps of the forced duction test (FDT)

i. *Anaesthesia.* In adults and cooperative elder children, FDT can be performed preoperatively under topical anaesthesia with 4% xylocaine instilled every 4 minutes for 4 times. In small and uncooperative children, FDT is done under general anaesthesia during surgery, taking an account of following points:

- To remove the effect of tonic innervational factors, the FDT should be performed, when patient has reached stage 3 of anaesthesia.
- If succinylcholine is to be used, preferably the FDT should be performed while the patient

Table 21.5 *Differences between congenital and acquired ocular palsies*

S.no.	Feature	Congenital ocular palsy	Recent acquired ocular palsy
1.	Onset of symptoms	Usually indefinite and intermittent	Usually definite and sudden
2.	Diplopia	Rare, intermittent diplopia in decompensation	Almost invariably present, but may be limited to paretic field
3.	Primary deviation	May be intermittent or constant angle of deviation may be large; but symptoms may be only slight	Usually constant Angle of deviation may be small and yet the symptoms may be pronounced
4.	Secondary deviation	Only slightly greater than the primary deviation (due to spread of comitance)	Usually much greater than the primary deviation
5.	Past pointing	Usually absent	Present
6.	Abnormal head posture	May persist on covering paretic eye because of secondary scoliosis and contracture of neck muscles	Disappears on covering paretic eye
7.	Facial asymmetry	Common with torticollis of long-standing	Absent
8.	Amblyopia	May be present	Absent
9.	Forced duction test	May be positive due to contracture of antagonist	Negative
10.	Abnormal head posture in old photographs	May be present	Absent

has received an inhalation anaesthetic by mask, but before intubation. Otherwise one will have to wait for at least 20 minutes till the contraction of the extraocular muscles caused by succinylcholine is over.

• Pancuronium, a nondepolarizing muscle relaxant, that does not alter the FDT, should be preferred over succinylcholine.

ii. *Grasping of the globe.* After proper anaesthesia, the globe should be grasped near the limbus with either a forceps without teeth or Pierse forceps to avoid tearing of the conjunctiva. Preferably, the globe should be held with the help of two forceps at right angle to the axis in which restriction is to be tested.

For example, in a patient with divergent squint (Fig. 21.9A), to distinguish between lateral rectus paralysis and mechanical restriction involving the medial aspect of the globe, the forceps should be applied at 6 and 12 o'clock positions (Fig. 21.9B).

iii. *Passive rotation of the globe.* After grasping, the globe should be rotated passively towards the direction of action of suspected weak muscle, e.g. into abduction in patients with lateral rectus weakness versus mechanical restriction involving medial aspect of the globe (Fig. 12.9C), taking following precautions:

• When FDT is being performed under topical anaesthesia, patient should be instructed to look at his/her hand held in the direction in which the eye is to be rotated by the forceps. This will help in avoiding the effect of tonic innervational factor.

• Care should be taken not to push the globe into the orbit posteriorly, since this may conceal a restriction of the movement resulting in a false negative FDT.

• To test the restrictions in the field of action of recti, the globe should be rotated, up, down, medially or laterally.

• To test the restrictions in the field of action of oblique muscles, the globe should be rotated both down and in, and up and in.

Note. FDT should be repeated at the time of surgery and also after completion of the surgery.

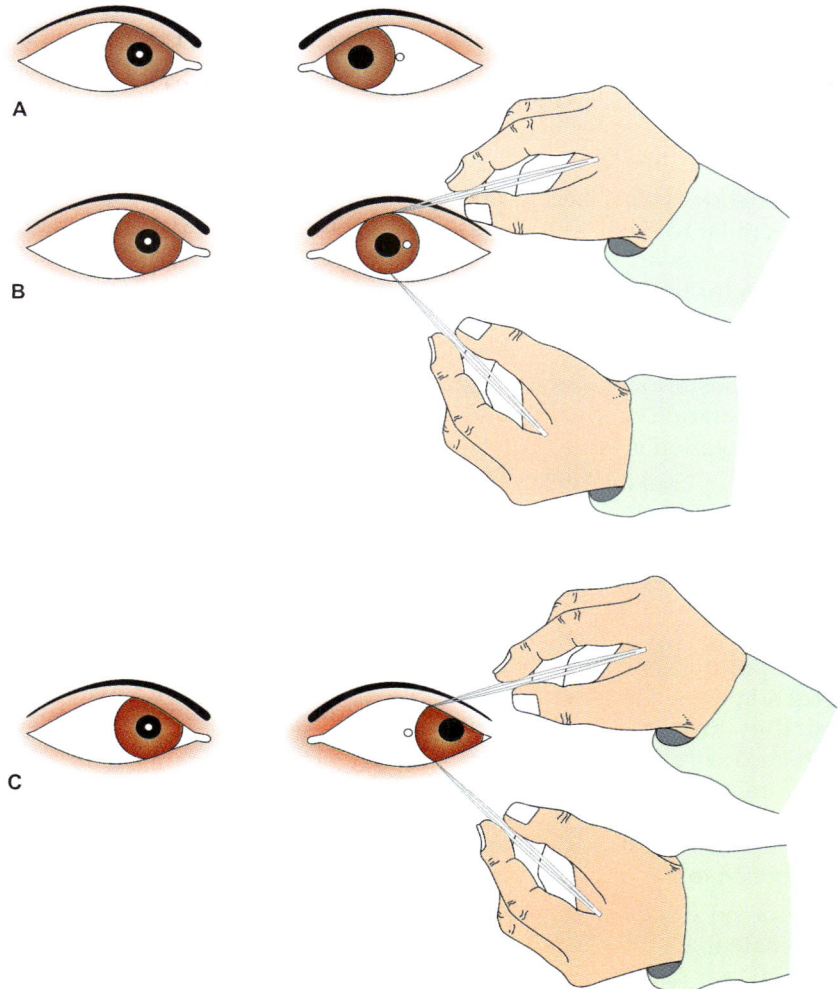

Fig. 21.9: *Technique of forced duction test (for explanation, see text).*

Interpretation of the results of FDT

1. *Forced duction test is labelled negative,* if no resistance is encountered during passive rotation and the examiner can rotate the globe to its full extent. A negative FDT implies that the motility defect is clearly caused by paralysis of the weak muscle.

2. *Positive FDT* is labelled, if a resistance is encountered during passive rotation of the globe. With a feeling of resistance, if the examiner can rotate the globe no further than the patient voluntarily can, the motility defect is purely due to mechanical restriction. However,

with a feeling of resistance, if the examiner can passively rotate the globe beyond where the patient can voluntarily rotate it, but not to its full extent, the motility defect is a combination of mechanical restriction and agonist muscle weakness.

The restriction noted in the positive FDT may be one of the following types:

i. *Leash restriction* is caused by the mechanical factors such as marked scarring of Tenon's capsule and conjunctiva, contracture of an extraocular muscle and/or entrapment of muscle or its facial sheath on the side of globe opposite the limited field of rotation.

The globe can be passively rotated freely up to a point after which tethering effect of restriction does not allow the globe to move further any more. Such a restriction is not only felt but can also be seen as a taut string of conjunctiva (*String sign*).

ii. *Reverse leash restriction*. The tethering effect of restriction is similar to leash restriction as described above. However, the mechanical factors responsible for tethering are marked shortening of conjunctiva and Tenon's capsule, marked posterior scarring of orbital tissues or a tight posterior fixation suture used in Faden's operation on the same side of globe in which rotation is limited.

iii. *Elastic restriction* is caused by an early contracture of a muscle following paresis of its agonist, co-contraction of extraocular muscles due to effect of succinylcholine and orbital cellulitis. In contrast to the leash and reverse leash restriction (in which globe can be rotated to a point after which tethering effect of restriction does not allow the globe to move further any more), in elastic restriction, there occurs a partial resistance over the entire range of ocular movement which can be overcome by an increased force.

2. Exaggerated traction test

It is a modified forced duction test which is performed to estimate the tightness in superior oblique (SO) and inferior oblique (IO) muscles.

Procedure. For checking tightness of RSO, the eyeball is grasped near the limbus at 6 and 9 o'clock positions, as described in FDT. To perform this test, the eyeball is first pushed in the orbit and then elevated, adducted and rolled back and forth by extorting and intorting the globe across the tendon. During this manoeuvre, if the eyeball jumps across the tendon, tightness of the superior oblique is indicated.

Tightness of the inferior oblique is also tested in the similar manner, except that instead of elevating and adducting, the eyeball is pushed down and nasally.

3. Spring-back balance test

It is a continuation of the FDT, when performed under general anaesthesia. It is of specific use in patients who are suspected (after FDT) of having mechanical restriction and not a weak muscle. In this test, after holding near the limbus, eyeball is rotated back and forth vigorously for 2–3 times and then released suddenly. After settling, normally, the globe comes to rest in straight ahead position. However, in the presence of a significant mechanical restriction, the eyeball will be drawn towards the direction of the mechanical pull, e.g. the eyeball will be adducted, if the cause of mechanical restriction is located medially.

4. Active force generation test

In this test, eyeball is stabilized with the forceps applied at the limbus under topical anaesthesia and patient is asked to move his/her both eyes in the direction of the muscle to be tested. For example, if right lateral rectus muscle is to be tested, patient is asked to move his/her eyes in dextroversion. During this movement, the force generated by the contracting muscle of the eye being tested (e.g. Rt LR) is transmitted through the forceps to the examiner's fingers. From the feel of the transmitted force, examiner can judge subjectively whether the contracting muscle is weak or normal (Fig. 21.10). For objectively quantifying this test, calibrated forceps are available which indicate the amount of force generated in grams. A normally acting muscle generates a force of 60–80 g in extreme gaze. This

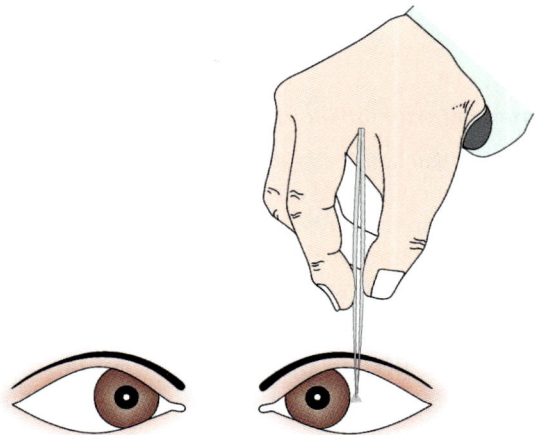

Fig. 21.10: *Technique of judging active force generated during ocular movement (muscle contraction). (For explanation, see text).*

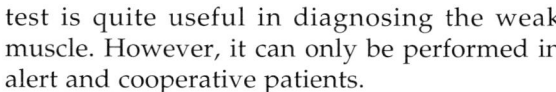

test is quite useful in diagnosing the weak muscle. However, it can only be performed in alert and cooperative patients.

5. *Lid fissure changes on eye movements*

- *Narrowing of lid fissure* along with globe retraction is seen in restrictive squints, as in Duane's retraction syndrome.
- *Lid fissure widening* and a relative proptosis is noted in paralytic squint as the patient looks into the field of action of paretic rectus muscle.

6. *Electro-oculographic measurement of saccadic velocity*

Saccades are sudden, jerky conjugate eye movements, that occur as the gaze shifts from one object to another. These movements bring the object of regard quickly on the fovea with an average velocity of 250°/second in the field of action of the muscle concerned. Measurement of saccadic velocity with the help of specially designed electro-oculographic (EOG) recorder can help in differentiating muscle restrictions from the muscle weakness. The saccadic velocity is decreased in paretic muscle, while it is near normal in mechanical muscle restrictions.

7. *Positional tonometry*

It has been reported that intraocular pressure rises from the compression of a non-relaxing stiff muscle, when attempts are made to move the eye into the field of its antagonist. Perkin's hand-held applanation tonometer or Digilab Pneumotonometer can be used to measure the IOP in different gaze positions. A pressure increase of over 5 mm Hg in a particular field of gaze is indicative of a restriction.

BIBLIOGRAPHY

1. Adler FH. Superior oblique tendon sheath syndrome of Brown. Arch. Ophthalmol 1959;48:264.
2. Aebli R. Retraction syndrome. Arch. Ophthalmol 1933;10:602.
3. Afifi AK, Bell WE, Menezes AH. Etiology of lateral rectus palsy in infancy and childhood J Child. Neurol 1992;7:295.
4. Ahluwalia BK, Gupta NC, Goel SR, Khurana, AK. Study of Duane's retraction syndrome. Acta Ophthalmol 1988;66:728.
5. Albert DG. Personal communication. In Parks, MM. Annual review: strabismus. Arch. Ophthalmol 1957;58:152.
6. Arimoto H. Ocular findings of thalidomide embryopathy. Jpn J Clin Ophthalmol 1979;33: 501.
7. Bahn RS, Heufelder AE. Pathogenesis of Graves ophthalmopathy. N Engl J Med 1993;329:1468.
8. Bell JA, Fielder AR, Viney S. Congenital double elevator palsy in identical twins. J Clin Neuro Ophthalmol 1990;10:32.
9. Berens C, Girard L. Transplantation of the superior and inferior rectus muscles for paralysis of the lateral rectus muscle. Am J Ophthalmol. 1950;33:1041.
10. Berlit P. Isolated and combined pareses of cranial nerves III, IV and VI. A retrospective study of 412 patients. J. Neurol. Sci. 103:10, 1991.
11. Bielschowsky A. 2 Die Motilitatsstorungen der Augen. In Axenfeld T, Elschnig A, (Eds): Graefe Saemisch's Handbuch der gesamten Augenheikunde, ed. 2, vol. 8, Berlin, 1939, Julius Springer.
12. Bielschowsky A. Lectures on motor anomalies, Hanover, NH, 1943 (reprinted 1956). Dartmouth College Publications.
13. Boyd TAS, Leitch GT, Budd GE. A new treatment for "A" and "V" patterns in strabismus by slanting muscle insertions: a preliminary report. Can. J Ophthalmol 1971;6:170.
14. Breinin G. The physiopathology of the A- and V-patterns. In Symposium: the A- and V-patterns in strabismus. Trans Am Acad Ophthalmol. Otolaryngol 1953;57:157.
15. Brosky MC, Pollock SC, Buckley EG. Neural misdirection in congenital ocular fibrosis syndrome: Implications and pathogenesis. J Pediatr. Ophthalmol, Strabismus 1989;26:159.
16. Brown HW. Congenital structural muscle anomalies. In Allen, JH, (Ed). Strabismus ophthalmic symposium I. St. Louis, 1950, Mosby- Year Book. Inc., p. 205.
17. Brown HW. Isolated inferior oblique paralysis. Analysis of 97 cases. Trans. Am. Ophthalmol. Soc, 1957;55:415.
18. Brown HWL. Congenital structural anomalies of the muscles. In Allen, JH editor: Strabismus ophthalmic symposium II, St. Louis, 1958, Mosby-Year Book, Inc., p. 391.

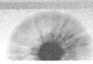

19. Brown HW. True and simulated superior oblique tendon sheath syndromes. Doc. Ophthalmol. 1973;34:123.

20. Brown HW. Vertical deviations. In Symposium, strabismus. Trans. Am. Acad Ophthalmol. Otolaryngol 1953;57:157.

21. Brown WB. Isolated inferior oblique paralysis. Trans Am. Ophthalmol. Soc. 1957;55:415.

22. Burke JP, Ruben JB, Scott WE. Vertical transposition of the horizontal recti (Knapp procedure) for the treatment of double elevator palsy: effectiveness and longterm stability. Br. J Ophthalmol. 1992;76:734.

23. Burian HM, Van Allen MW. Cyclic oculomotor paralysis. Am. J Ophthalmol. 1963;55:529.

24. Costenbader FD. Introduction. In Symposium: the A- and V-patterns in strabismus. Trans. Am. Acad. Ophthalmol. Otolaryngol. 1964;68:354.

25. Dotti MT, Federico A, Palmeri S, Guazzi GC. Congenital oculo-facial paralysis (Moebius syndrome) evidence of dominant inhertance in two families. Acta Neurol 1989;11:434.

26. Duane A. Congenital deficiency of abduction associated with impairment of adduction, retraction movements, contraction of the palpebral fissure and oblique movements of the eye. Arch. Ophthalmol. 1905;34:133.

27. Duane RD, Schatz NJ, Caputo AR. Pseudo Duane's retraction syndrome. Trans. Am. Ophthalmol. Soc. 1976;74:122.

28. Duke-Elder S, Wybar K. System of ophthalmology, vol. 6: Ocular motility and strabismus, St. Louis, 1973, Mosby-year Book, Inc., p. 736 ff.

29. Esswein MB, Noorden GK von. Paresis of a vertical rectus muscle after cataract surgery. Am J Ophthalmol. 1993;116:424.

30. Fells P, Collin JRO. Cyclic oculomotor palsy. Trans. Ophthalmol. Soc. UK 1979;99:192.

31. Fink WH. The A and V syndromes. Am. Orthopt. J. 1959;9:105.

32. Fitzsimmons R, Lee J, Elston J. The role of botulinum in the management of sixth nerve palsy. Eye 1989;3:391.

33. Fitzsimmons R, Lee JP, Elston J. Treatment of sixth nerve palsy in adults with combined botulinum toxin chemodenervation and surgery. Ophthalmology 1988;95:1535.

34. Gobin MH. Sagittalization of the oblique muscles as possible cause for the "A", "V", and "X" phenomena. Br J Ophthalmol. 1968;52:13.

35. Gopal KSS. Acquired double depressor palsy. Indian J. Ophthalmol. 1988;36:35.

36. Gottlob L, Catalano RA, Reinecke RD. Surgical management of oculomotor nerve palsy. Am J Ophthalmol. 1991;111:71.

37. Guyton D. Exaggerated traction test for the oblique muscles. Ophthalmology 1981;88:1035.

38. Hardesty HH. Diagnosis of paretic vertical rotators. Am.JOphthalmol. 1963;56:811.

39. Helveston EM. A new two step method for the diagnosis of isolated cyclovertical muscle palsies. Am. J. Ophthalmol. 1967;64:914.

40. Helveston EM, Krach D, Plager DA, Ellis FD. A new classification of superior oblique palsy based on congenital variations in the tendon. Ophthalmology 1992;99:1609.

41. Huber A. Electrophysiology of the retraction syndrome. Br J Ophthalmol. 1974;58:293.

42. Jampolsky A. Oblique muscle surgery of the A- and V-pattern. J Pediatr. Ophthalmol. 1965;2:31.

43. Jampolsky A. Surgical leashes and reverse leashes in strabismus surgical managemnet. In Symposium on strabismus: transactions of the New Orleans Academy of Ophthalmology, St. Louis, 1978, Mosby-Year Book. Inc., p.244.

44. Khawam E, Scott A, Jampolsky A. Acquired superior oblique palsy. Diagnosis and management. Arch. Ophthalmol, 1967;77:761.

45. Knapp P, Moore S. Diagnosis and surgical options in superior oblique surgery. Int. Ophthalmol. Clin. 1976;16:137.

46. Knapp P. Diagnosis and surgical treatment of hypertropia, Am, Orthopt. J. 1971;21:29.

47. Knapp P. Vertically incomitant horizontal strabismus: the so-called A and V syndrome. Trans. Am. Ophthalmol. Soc, 1959;57:666.

48. Knapp P. A- and V-patterns. In Symposium on strabismus. Transactions of the New Orleans Academy of Ophthalmology, St. Louis, 1971, Mosby-Year Book, Inc., p 242.

49. Kodsi SR, Younge BR. Acquired oculomotor, trochlear, and abducent cranial nerve palsies in pediatric patients. Am. J. Ophthalmol. 1992; 114:568.

50. Manners RM, O'Flynn E, Morris RJ. Superior oblique lengthening for acquired superior oblique overaction. Br J Ophthalmol. 1994;78:280.

51. Metz HS. Saccadic velocity measurements in strabismus. Trans, Am. Ophthalmol. Soc. 1983;81:630.

52. Metz HS, Scott AB, Scott WE. Horizontal saccadic velocities in Duane's syndrome. Am. J. Ophthalmol. 1975;80:901.

53. Noorden GK von, Awaya S, Romano PE. Pastpointing in paralytic strabismus. Am. J Ophthalmol. 1971;71:27.

54. Noorden GK von, Hansell R. Clinical characteristics and treatment of isolated inferior rectus paralysis, Ophthalmology 1991;98:253.

55. Noorden GK von, Murray E, Wong SY. Superior oblique paralysis. A review of 270 cases. Arch. Ophthalmol. 1986;104:1771.

56. Noorden GK von, Ruttum M. Torticollis in paralysis of the trochlear nerve. Am Orthopt. J 1983;33:16.

57. Noorden GK von, Tredici TD, Ruttum M. Pseudo-internuclear ophthalmoplegia after surgical paresis of the medial rectus muscle. Am J Ophthalmol. 1984;98:602.

58. Noorden GK von, Olson CL. Diagnosis and surgical management of vertically incomitant horizontal strabismus. Am J Ophthalmol. 1965; 60:434.

59. Olivier P, Noorden GK. Excyclotropia of the nonparetic eye in unilateral superior oblique muscle paralysis. Am. J. Ophthalmol. 1982;93:30.

60. Olivier P, Noorden GK von. Results of superior oblique tenectomy in inferior oblique paresis. Arch. Ophthalmol. 1982;100–581.

61. Parks MM. Isolated cyclovertical muscle palsy. Arch. Ophthalmol. 1958;60:1027.

62. Parks MM. The weakening surgical procedures for eliminating overaction of the inferior oblique muscle. Am J Ophthalmol, 1972;73:107.

63. Roper-Hall G, Feibel RM. Measurement of the field of binocular single vision in the evaluation of incomitant paralytic strabismus. Am. Orthopt. J 1974;24:77.

64. Rush JA, Younge BR. Paralysis of cranial nerves III, IV, and VI: causes and prognosis in 1,000 cases. Arch. Ophthalmol. 1981;99:76.

65. Ruttam M, Noorden GK von. Orbital and facial anthropometry in A- and V-pattern strabismus. In Reinecke, RD, editor: Strabismus II, New York, 1984, Grune & Stratton, Inc., p. 363.

66. Scott WE, Kraft SP. Classification and surgical treatment of superior oblique palsies: I. Unilateral superior oblique palsies. Tran sactions of the New Orleans Academy of Ophthalmology, New York, 1986, Raven Press, p. 15.

67. Scott WE, Kraft SP. Classification and surgical treatment of superior oblique palsies: II. Bilateral superior oblique palsies. Transactions of the New Orleans Academy of Ophthalmology, New York, 1986, Raven Press, p. 265.

68. Scott AB, Stella SL. Measurement of A- and V-patterns. J. Pediatr. Ophthalmol. 1968;5:181.

69. Stilling J. Untersuchungen iiber die Entstehung der Kurzsichtigkeit, Wiesbaden, 1887, J.F. Bergmann, p. 13.

70. Turk S. Bemerkungen zu einem Falle von Retraction des Auges. Cbl. Pract. Augenheilk. 1899;23:14.

71. Urist MJ. Horizontal squint with secondary vertical deviations. Arch. Ophthalmol. 1951; 46:245.

72. Urist MJ. Recession and upward displacement of the medial rectus muscles in A-pattern esotropia. Am J Ophthalmol. 1968;65:769.

73. Villaseca A. The A and V syndromes. Am. J. Ophthalmol. 1961;52:172.

74. Wilson ME, Hoxie J. Facial asymmetry in superior oblique muscle palsy. J Pediatr. Ophthalmol. Strabismus 1993;30:315.

Evaluation and Investigations of a Case of Nystagmus

Chapter Outline

DEFINITION AND FEATURES OF NYSTAGMUS
- Definition
- Features
- Classification

CLINICAL EVALUATION AND ELECTROPHYSIOLOGICAL RECORDING AND NEUROIMAGING
- Clinical evaluation
- Electrophysiological recording of eye movements
- Neuroimaging
- Other tests

DEFINITION AND FEATURES OF NYSTAGMUS

DEFINITION

Nystagmus comes from the Greek word *nystagmos* (to nod) and may be defined as repetitive, to and fro involuntary movement of one or both eyes that is initiated by a slow phase (drift). The movements which are not regular and rhythmic are called *nystagmoid movements*.

FEATURES OF NYSTAGMUS MOVEMENTS

1. *Type of waveform.* Eye movements that point the retinal fovea at an object of interest are called *foveating* and those that move the fovea away from the object are called *defoveating*. In nystagmus, each cycle of movement is usually initiated by an involuntary, defoveating drift of the eye away from the object of interest, followed by a return movement. Based on the characteristics of defoveating and foveating movements, the nystagmus may be of pendular or jerky type.

- *Pendular nystagmus*, in which both the defoveating and refoveating movements are slow (non-saccadic), and of equal velocity in each direction (Fig. 22.1A). It may be horizontal, vertical, oblique, rotatory or mixed.
- *Jerk nystagmus* is characterized by the slow defoveating movement in one direction and fast refoveating movement (saccadic) component in the other direction; the later being a recovery phenomenon aimed at refixation. The direction of jerk nystagmus is defined by the direction of fast component (phase). For instance, if the fast phase beat to the right, this is called *right beating* nystagmus. Likewise the jerk nystagmus may be left, up, down or rotatory.

Waveform can further be characterized and documented by the nature of the slow phase as shown in Fig. 22.1B to E.

2. *Direction*. Direction or plane of nystagmus can be horizontal, vertical, oblique, torsional or mixed. For a jerk nystagmus, the direction is described according to the fast phase. For

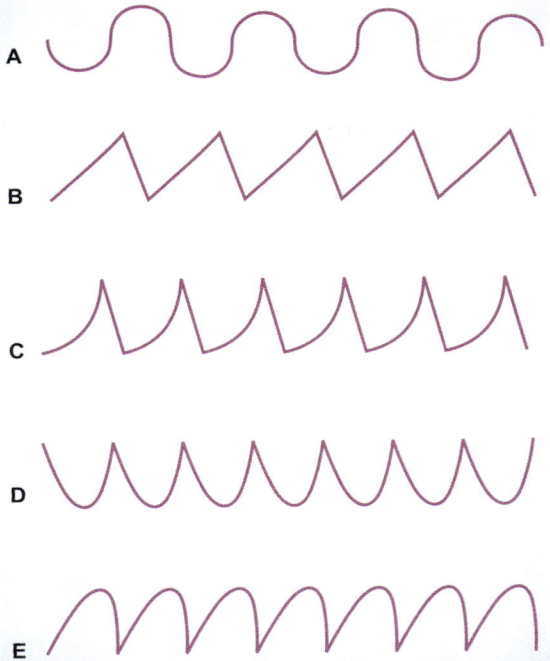

Fig. 22.1: *Waveform characteristics of pendular nystagmus (A) and, jerk nystagmus (B to E). (B) Jerk nystagmus with slow components of constant velocity; (C) Jerk nystagmus with slow components of exponentially increasing velocity; (D) Jerk nystagmus with slow components of exponentially increasing velocity with extended foveation periods that follow slow movements; (E) Jerk nystagmus with slow components of exponentially decreasing velocity.*

simplicity of recording, the direction of nystagmus in case notes the following method may be used:

a. *Pendular nystagmus*

- Horizontal ←→
- Vertical ↕
- Rotatory ↺
- Oblique ↘↗

b. *Jerk nystagmus with quick phase*

- To the right ←
- To the left →
- Up ↑
- Down ↓
- Right rotatory (anti-clockwise) ↶
- Left rotatory (clockwise) ↷

- Oblique up to right ↖ or left ↗
- Oblique down to right ↙ or left ↘

3. *Conjugacy.* Nystagmus may be of conjugate, disconjugate or dissociative type.

- *Conjugate nystagmus.* Binocular nystagmus with symmetric direction, amplitude and rate in both eyes.
- *Disconjugate nystagmus.* Monocular or binocular with different directions and frequencies in two eyes.
- *Dissociative nystagmus refers to* unidirectional but assymetrical nystagmus in two eyes. Such type of nystagmus is seen in internuclear ophthalmoplegia.

4. *Amplitude.* The amplitude is measured in degrees and represents the extent of movement between the start of drift away from fixation and the start of corrective movement in the opposite direction. The amount of movement should be approximately equal. In majority of cases, the amplitude increases, when the patient looks in the direction of the fast phase (*Alexender's law*). When the patient looks in the opposite direction, the amplitude reduces, the oscillation ceasesor the direction of the nystagmus may reverse. There are very few exceptions to this rule, but in some cases of vertical nystagmus, the amplitude increases on looking in the direction of the slow phase.

Grading of amplitude. The amplitude is graded as small, medium or large as below:

- *Fine (small)*—excursions less than 3°
- *Medium*—excursions between 5° and 15°
- *Coarse (large)*—excursions more than 15°

A dissociated nystagmus has different amplitudes in both eyes. Subtle forms of nystagmus, due to low amplitude or inconsistent presence, require prolonged observation over 2–3 minutes. Low amplitude nystagmus may be detected only by viewing the patient's retina with an ophthalmoscope. In case records amplitude is recorded by the thickness of arrows or increasing lines in arrows, e.g.

- Small ➤→ or ——→
- Medium ≫→ or ——→→
- Large ≫→ or ——→→→

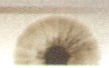

5. *Frequency.* Frequency of nystagmus refers to number of beats, i.e. to and fro movements per second.

Grading and recording of frequency. It is done into low (slow), moderate and high (fast):

- Low (Lo): 1–2 Hz
- Moderate (M): 3–4 Hz
- High (H): > 5 Hz

6. *Intensity.* Intensity of nystagmus is the product of amplitude and frequency.

Grading of intensity. Nystagmus of each type may be seen in the primary position or it may be made apparent, only when the visual axes are deviated. On these grounds, nystagmus may be graded as to its intensity into:

Recording of frequency

- *First degree nystagmus.* In it, the movements occur only in that direction of the gaze in which the quick phase occurs.
- *Second degree nystagmus.* In it, the movements are also present in the primary position.
- *Third degree nystagmus.* In it, movements are also present in the direction of the gaze to the side opposite to that of the quick phase.

7. *Foveation period.* It is the period in the waveform where eye velocity is at minimum and thus visual acuity is maximum (Fig. 22.2). The foveation period is maximum in the null position of gaze and increases with the decrease in intensity of nystagmus.

8. *Null zone and neutral zone*

- *Null zone* refers to the position of eyes where a jerk nystagmus is absent. Some patients may assume a head posture to bring the eyes in the null zone.
- *Neutral zone* is the point from where fast component of nystagmus changes its direction. It may be different than the null zone or may be the same.

9. *Trajectories of nystagmus*

Not infrequently patients with nystagmus show a waveform that has vertical, horizontal and rotary components. When a horizontal and a vertical component coexist and are superimposed on each other, three characteristic nystagmus trajectories can be observed (Fig. 22.3):

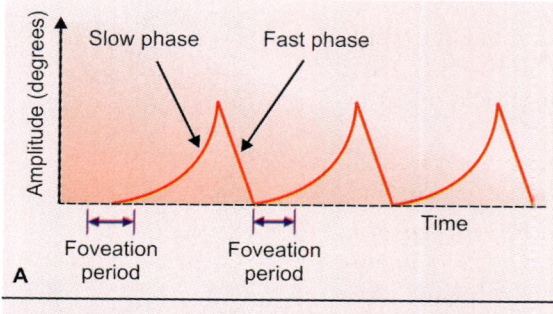

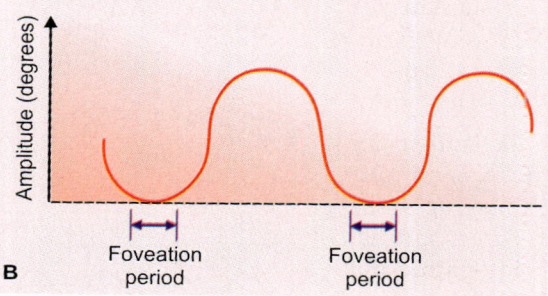

Fig. 22.2: *Foveation period in: (A) Jerk nystagmus; (B) Pendular nystagmus.*

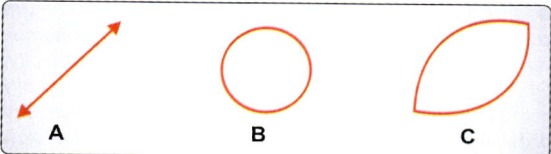

Fig. 22.3: *Trajactories of nystagmus: (A) Oblique; (B) Circular; and (C) Elipticle.*

a. *Oblique trajectory* occurs when vertical and horizontal components are of equal frequency and amplitude and in phase with each other.

b. *Circular trajectory* occurs when vertical and horizontal components are of equal frequency and amplitude and are 90°, out of phase with each other.

c. *Eliptical trajectory* occurs when vertical and horizontal components are of equal frequency but unequal amplitudes and are 90° out of phase with each other.

CLASSIFICATION

Many classifications have been proposed for the nystagmus, and so, the reader will find different classifications in different books. It is important to note here that the terms motor and sensory nystagmus are no longer being considered. National Eye Institute Workshop has developed a new classification in 2001 called the classification of eye movement abnormalities and strabismus (CEMAS). In this volume, a simple classification has been adopted by slightly modifying CEMAS as below:

A. *Physiological nystagmus*
1. Optokinetic nystagmus
2. Endpoint nystagmus (eccentric gaze nystagmus)
3. Physiological vestibular (caloric or rotational) nystagmus
4. Voluntary nystagmus.

B. *Pathological nystagmus*
I. *Early onset (childhood) nystagmus*
1. *Infantile nystagmus syndrome* (includes old names such as 'congenital', 'motor', 'sensory', idiopathic and nystagmus blockage)
2. *Fusion maldevelopment nystagmus* syndrome (old names 'latent, manifest latent,' nystagmus blockage)
3. *Spasmus nutans syndrome*
   • Without optic pathway glioma
   • With optic pathway glioma.

II. *Acquired nystagmus.* This group includes various forms of nystagmus acquired after infancy, which can be further classified as follows:
1. *Nystagmus associated with diseases of visual system*
   • Ocular jerk nystagmus
   • Vertical nystagmus
   • See-saw nystagmus
   • Acquired pendular nystagmus.
2. *Vestibular nystagmus*
   i. Peripheral vestibular nystagmus, e.g. Ménière and drug toxicity nystagmus.
   ii. Central vestibular nystagmus
      • Downbeat
      • Upbeat
      • Torsional
      • Horizontal
   iii. Periodic alternating nystagmus.
3. *Nystagmus due to disorders of gaze holding*
   • Gaze-evoked nystagmus
   • Dissociated nystagmus (ataxic nystagmus)

   • Bruns' nystagmus
   • Convergence-retraction nystagmus
   • Centripetal and rebound nystagmus.

Note. Only a very brief account of the various types of nystagmus is given here just as a passing reference. For detailed accounts, the readers should consult certain standard textbooks on neuro-ophthalmology.

CLINICAL EVALUATION AND ELECTRO-PHYSIOLOGICAL RECORDING AND NEUROIMAGING

A. CLINICAL EVALUATION
It is often possible to diagnose the cause of nystagmus through careful history and systematic examination of the patient.

History
History should include:
• Duration of nystagmus
• Whether it interferes with vision and causes oscillopsia
• Accompanying neurological symptoms
• Whether nystagmus and other visual symptoms are worse with viewing far or near objects, or with patient motion, or with different gaze angles
• If abnormal head posture is present, whether or not these features are evident on old photographs.

Examination of a patient with nystagmus
Comprehensive examination of the visual system
• *Visual acuity* assessment with and without posture, for both near and distance and both binocularly and uniocularly. Binocular acuity should be recorded before occlusion. Methods of measuring monocular vision while avoiding total occlusion include fogging the other eye with plus spheres, polarizing lenses, central field occlusion and the red-green duochrome slide test.
• *Anterior and posture segment examination* to rule out cause of low vision.
• *Measurement of head posture.* In most patients with infantile nystagmus, the head position

corresponds roughly to the null zone. However, an anomalous head posture may be present in patients with INS for reasons other than nystagmus, e.g. uncorrected astigmatism, incomitant squint, muscular torticollis. Nevertheless, presence of AHP in a patient with INS has better visual prognosis than no AHP. All the components of head posture, i.e. face turn, chin elevation or depression and head tilt should be noted. Face turn can be measured using the Goniometer (Fig. 22.4) or by simply using a scale and a protractor.

Systematic examination of each functional class of eye movements (vestibular, optokinetic, smooth-pursuit, saccades, vergence) and their effect on nystagmus.

Examination of nystagmus in a systematic manner. It is essential to have a mental checklist during clinical examination. **ABCDEF** is a suggested pneumonic for systematic examination of nystagmus as below:

Amplitude

Basic shape or waveform

Conjugacy

Direction

Effect of gaze position and fixation, e.g.

- The stability of fixation (with the eyes close to primary position) viewing near and far targets, and at eccentric gaze angles.
- In patients with head turn or tilt, the eye should be observed in various directions of gaze, when the head is in that position as well as when the head is held straight.
- During fixation, occlude each eye in turn to check for latent nystagmus.

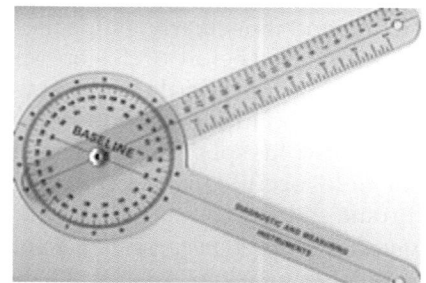

Fig. 22.4: *Goniometer: An orthopaedic instrument which can be used to measure face turn.*

- The effect of removal of fixation (with Frenzelor high-plus spherical lenses).

F is frequency.

B. ELECTROPHYSIOLOGICAL RECORDING OF EYE MOVEMENTS

Electrophysiological recording of ocular motility has provided a new basis for eye movement abnormality classification, etiology and treatment. Only salient features of some of the techniques available for ocular motility recordings are mentioned here.

1. Electro-oculography

Electro-oculography (EOG) is based on the measurement of resting potential of the eye which exists between the cornea (+ve) and back of the retina (−ve).

Technique of recording is shown in Fig. 22.5A and B. Electrodes are placed over the orbital margin near the medial and lateral canthi serve as *active electrodes* (E1–E4 in Fig. 22.5A). A forehead electrode serves as a *ground electrode* or indifferent electrodes (E5 in Fig. 22.5A).

Salient features.
- Horizontal range of measurement of 1 to 40° with a resolution of 1°
- Useful for horizontal and some vertical movements
- A bitnoisy–1°
- Best clinical all rounder with good electrodes.

2. Electronystagmography

Electronystagmography (ENG) is an adaption of electro-oculography (EOG). For ENG like EOG (Fig. 22.5), a ground electrode is attached to the forehead and three recording electrodes are placed one each to the side, above and below each eye which measure the eye movement.

Tests performed with ENG include:
- *Oculomotor tests.* ENG is used to record nystagmus during oculomotor tests such as saccades, pursuit and gaze testing and optokinetics. Abnormal oculomotor test results may indicate either systemic or central pathology as opposed to peripheral (vestibular) pathology.

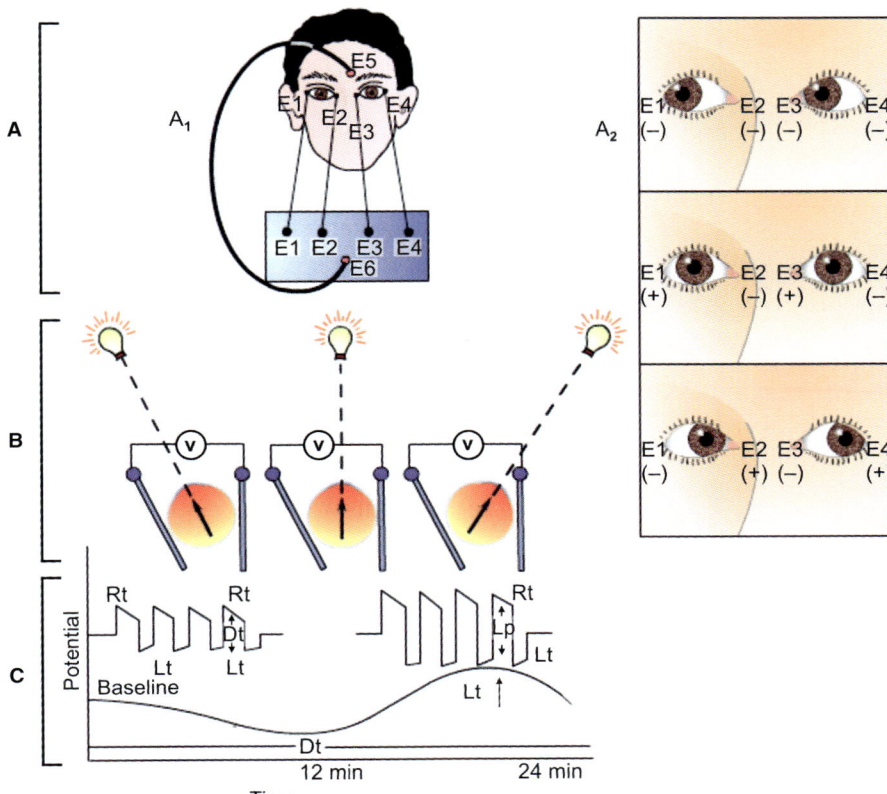

Fig. 22.5: *Technique of recording electro-oculogram: (A) Position of electrodes; (B) Ocular movements during recording; (C) Record of EOG.*

- *Positional testing* is performed to see the effect of head or body movements on the eye movements.
- *Caloric test* is performed to assess the vestibular system.

3. Binocular infrared reflectance oculography (BIRO)

- Useful for horizontal and some vertical movements
- Has a restricted range
- Noise–0.1°.

4. Electromagnetic scleral search coil method

- Useful for horizontal, vertical and torsional movements
- Good resolution and frequency response
- Requires mind bending mathematical analysis

- Eye has to be anaesthetised and a thick silicone lens is needed
- Expensive.

5. Videonystagmography

Videonystagmography (VNG) is a sophisticated technique in which nystagmus is recorded with the help of the infrared video camera which is incorporated in the specially designed infrared camrea goggles worm by the patient during the recording technique (Fig. 22.6). A very sensitive head movement sensors are also incorporated in it.

Tests performed with VNG. Similar to ENG, there are three parts of VNG testing:
a. Ocular and optokinetic testing
b. Positional nystagmus testing
c. Caloric testing.

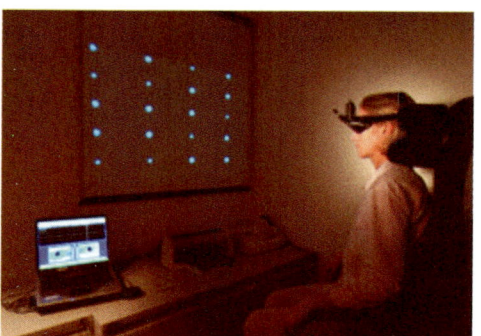

Fig. 22.6: Technique of videonystagmography with infrared goggles worn by the patient.

Advantages of VNG over ENG

- *Less combursome* and less time consuming as electrodes are not required
- *Direct observation* of video images of eye movements available
- *Simultaneous comparison* of waveform can be performed
- *Computerised record* allows storage, processing and analysis
- *Provides more information than ENG.* In addition to information about amplitude, frequency and intensity obtained from ENG; the VNG also provides information about slow phase velocity and foveation window with the help of intrinsic software.

Clinical uses of eye movement recording

Important clinical uses of eye movement recording are as follows:

- *Identifies congenital type of nystagmus* on the basis of waveform. About 40–60% cases of nystagmus have associated squint. About 35% of these patients have FMNS. The best method to differentiate INS form FMNS is eye movement recordings.
- *Allows classification* of acquired nystagmus with greater certainty.
- *VNG helps to evaluate the evolution of nystagmus.* Many INS waveforms begin as pendular nystagmus. Growth and development of the visual sensory system evoke evolution of waveforms during early infancy from pendular to jerk type nystagmus by development of corrective fast phases as well as breaking saccades in slow phases producing the so-called 'mature' waveforms associated with better vision.
- *Measures slowness of saccades* which can be diagnostic, e.g. internuclear ophthalmoplegia.
- *Allows observation of motility* in darkness (vestibular nystagmus).
- *Allows temporal resolution* of very fast eye movements such as flutter, opsoclonus, convergence nystagmus, dysmetria which are difficult to evaluate with the naked eye.
- Trains one to interpret what is 'seen'.
- *Helps in objective assessment of visual functions* of a patient with nystagmus by calculating foveation time, foveation eye position, and eye velocity criteria.
- *Tells about the potential for visual improvement* with treatment.
- *Useful in objective documentation* of response to treatment.
- *Helps in null point evaluation.*

C. NEUROIMAGING

Neuroimaging is indicated to find out associated CNS abnormalities especially in patients with acquired nystagmus, periodic alternating nystagmus, see saw nystagmus, spasmus nutans syndrome and infantile nystagmus syndrome with pallor disc and poor vision.

Hertle's criteria for neurological workup in patients with nystagmus are as follow:

I. *History of*:
- Onset of nystagmus after 6–9 months of age.
- History of prematurity or LBW or developmental delay.
- Abnormal pregnancy/delivery.
- Exposure to toxins/drugs.

II. *Ocular features*:
- Photophobia, delayed visual behaviour.
- Structural abnormalities like foveal or optic nerve dysplasia.
- Nystagmus pattern vertical, asymmetric, dysconjugate or associated with other ocular motor disorders (decrease pursuit, abnormal saccades, paretic gaze).

III. *General features*:
- Patient having manifest hard, soft, focal or diffuse neurologic signs.
- Localising signs of acquired nystagmus.

D. OTHER TESTS

OCT is indicated in retinal dystrophies, degenerations, foveal hypoplasia, schisis cavity, retinal thinning, choroidal thinning.

Autofluorescence can be used for diagnosing accumulation of lipofuschin in macular dystrophies.

ERG is useful in sensory nystagmus associated with conditions like achromatopsia, CSNB, LCA and other atypical retinal dystrophies.

BIBLIOGRAPHY

1. Boyle NJ, Dawson EL, Lee JP. Benefits of Retroequatorial Four Horizontal Muscle Recession Surgery in Congenital Idiopathic Nystagmus in Adults, JAAPOS, 2006;10:404–8.
2. Dell'Osso LF. Tenotomy and congenital nystagmus: a failure to answer the wrong question, Vision Res, 2004;44:3091–4.
3. Erbagci I, Gungor K, Bekir NA. Effectiveness of retroequatorial recession surgery in congenital nystagmus, Strabismus, 2004;12:35–40.
4. Flynn JT, Dell'Osso LF. The effects of congenital nystagmus surgery, Ophthalmology, 1979;86: 1414–27.
5. Hertle RW, Dell'Osso LF. Benefits of retro-equatorial four horizontal muscle recession surgery in congenital idiopathic nystagmus in adults, JPAAOS, 2007;11:313.
6. Schiavi C, Scorolli L, Campos EC. Surgical management of anomalous head posture due to supranuclear gaze palsies and acquired nystagmus. In: Spiritus M (Ed.), Transactions of the 23rd Meeting of the European Strabismological Association, Nancy, 1996;229–32.
7. Sternberg-Raab A. Anderson–Kestenbaum operation for asymmetrical gaze nystagmus, Br J Ophthalmol, 1963;47:339–45.
8. Wang Z, Dell'Osso LF, Jacobs JB, et al. Effects of tenotomy on patients with infantile nystagmus syndrome, JAAPOS, 2006;10:552–60.
9. Wang ZI, Dell'Osso LF, Tomsak RL, Jacobs JB. Combining recessions (nystagmus and strabismus) with tenotomy improved visual function and decreased oscillopsia and diplopia in acquired downbeat nystagmus and in horizontal infantile nystagmus syndrome, JAAPOS, 2007;11:135–41.

Section

VI

Clinical Evaluation and Investigations for Disorders of Ocular Adnexa

23. **Evaluation of a Case of Ptosis**
24. **Evaluation of a Case of Watering Eye**
25. **Evaluation of a Case of Proptosis and Enophthalmos**

Evaluation of a Case of Ptosis

Chapter Outline

INTRODUCTION
- Classification

EVALUATION AND INVESTIGATIONS

Clinical evaluation
- History
- Ocular examination
- Special examination and tests

Neurological examination and investigations
- Neurological examination
- Neuroimaging

CONGENITAL PTOSIS
- Introduction
- Simple congenital ptosis
- Congenital ptosis with superior rectus weakness
- Blepharophimosis syndrome
- Congenital synkinetic ptosis syndrome
- Ptosis with congenital fibrosis of extraocular muscles

ACQUIRED PTOSIS
- Aponeurotic ptosis
- Neurogenic ptosis
- Acquired myogenic ptosis
- Mechanical ptosis

INTRODUCTION

Ptosis or drooping of the upper eyelid is a condition where upper eyelid abnormally covers the cornea. It can be congenital or acquired in nature. It is due to dystrophy of levator muscle in congenital cases. Acquired cases are usually due to dehiscence of levator muscle in elderly patients or can be due to trauma or any disease. If it is severe, it can lead to other problems like amblyopia in children. Management of ptosis requires detailed evaluation and measurement and choosing the most appropriate surgery for a given situation.

CLASSIFICATION
It is broadly classified into:

A. *Congenital ptosis*
I. *Simple congenital ptosis/dystrophic levator muscle*
II. *Complicated congenital ptosis*
- Congenital ptosis with superior rectus weakness
- Synkinetic ptosis
- Blepharophimosis syndrome
- Congenital aponeurotic ptosis
- Congenital third nerve palsy.

B. *Acquired ptosis*
I. *Aponeurotic ptosis (due to levator dehiscence or thinning)*

- Involutional
- Traumatic.

II. *Myogenic ptosis*
- Myasthenia gravis
- Chronic progressive external ophthalmoplegia
- Muscular dystrophy.

III. *Neurogenic ptosis*
- Third nerve palsy
- Horner's syndrome.

IV. *Mechanical ptosis*
- Due to eyelid masses
- Due to scarring.

EVALUATION AND INVESTIGATION

CLINICAL EVALUATION

HISTORY

The history is important in evaluating the patients with ptosis. It should include medical history, family history and history of any drug or allergic reactions.

The following relevant history should be elicited in all patients of ptosis:
- Time of onset
- Diurnal variation
- Whether increasing, decreasing, or constant since the time of manifestation
- Association with:
  - Jaw movements
  - Abnormal ocular movements
  - Abnormal head posture
- History of:
  - Trauma or previous surgery
  - Poisoning
  - Use of steroid drops
  - Any reaction with anaesthesia
  - Bleeding tendency
  - Dysphagia, dysphonia, dysarthria, weakness of any body part
- Photographic documentation is of great help.

OCULAR EXAMINATION

Visual acuity

Best corrected visual acuity should be checked to record any amblyopia, if present in cases of congenital ptosis.

Refraction

Dilated refraction should be done, as astigmatism induced by ptosis is the cause of meridional amblyopia in many cases.

Inspection in diffuse light

1. **Head posture and facial expression** should be noted.

2. **Exclude pseudoptosis** (simulated ptosis) on inspection. Its common causes are:
- *Ipsilateral conditions* such as microphthalmos, phthisis bulbi, enophthalmos, prosthesis, brow ptosis, dermatochalasis, and hypotropia.
- *Contralateral conditions* include: Eyelid retraction, high myopia, and proptosis.

3. **Observe the following features** in each case:
- *Ptosis is unilateral or bilateral.* Causes of bilateral ptosis include congenital ptosis, myasthenia gravis, myotonic dystrophy, Kearns-Sayre syndrome, Lambert-Eaton myasthenic syndrome, and chronic progressive external ophthalmoplegia.
- *Function of orbicularis* oculi muscle.
- *Eyelid crease* is present or absent.
- Height of eyelid crease.
- *Jaw-winking phenomenon* is present or not.
- Amount of lid show.

Palpebral fissure height measurement

Measure the vertical palpebral fissure height (PFH) in the centre in primary gaze, with the help of millimetre scale passing through centre of pupil (Fig. 23.1A) .
- Normal PFH is 9–10 mm in primary gaze
- Decreased in ptosis
- Increased in lid retraction.

Note. PFH should also be measured in downgaze:
- It must be remembered that ptotic lid in unilateral ptosis is usually higher in downgaze due to failure of levator to relax, as dystrophic LPS in congenital cases, neither relaxes nor contracts.
- The ptotic lid in acquired ptosis is invariably lower than normal lid in downgaze.

Measurement of amount (degree and grade) of ptosis

- *In unilateral cases*, difference between the vertical height of the palpebral fissures of the two sides indicates the degree of ptosis (Fig. 23.1B).
- *In bilateral cases,* it can be determined by measuring the amount of cornea covered by the upper lid and then subtracting 2 mm.
- *Severity of ptosis is graded* depending upon its amount as:
  - ◆ Mild ptosis: 2 mm
  - ◆ Moderate ptosis: 3 mm
  - ◆ Severe ptosis: 4 mm

Margin reflex distance

To measure the margin reflex distance (MRD), hold the light source directly in front of the patient looking straight ahead (Fig. 23.1).

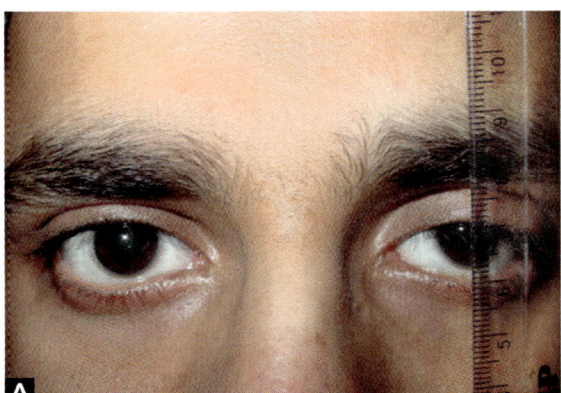

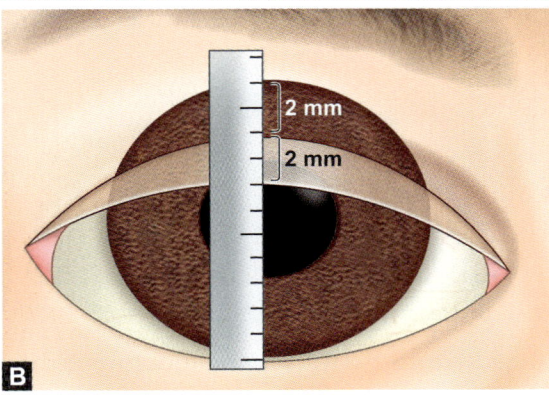

Fig. 23.1: *(A) Measurement of margin reflex distance and palpebral aperture height in primary position; (B) Diagrammatic depiction of mild ptosis.*

MRD-1. The distance between the centre of the lid margin of the upper lid and the light reflex on the cornea would give the MRD-1. If the margin is above the light reflex, the MRD-1 is a +ve value. If the lid margin is below the corneal reflex in cases of very severe ptosis, the MRD-1 would be a –ve value.

- Normal margin reflex distance-1 (MRD-1) is 4–5 mm.
- Measurement of MRD gives more accurate assessment of the amount of ptosis than PFH, as it is independent of the position of lower eyelid.

MRD-2 is the measurement between corneal light reflex and centre of lower lid margin in primary gaze. Sum of MRD-1 and MRD-2 is equal to palpebral fissure height (PFH).

Assessment of levator function

1. *Berke's method (lid excursion method).* Lid excursion is a measure of the levator function.

Patient is asked to look down, and thumb of one hand is placed firmly against the eyebrow of the patient (to block the action of frontalis muscle) by the examiner (Fig. 23.2A and B). Then the patient is asked to look up as far as possible and the amount of upper lid excursion is measured with a ruler (Fig. 23.2C and D) held in the other hand by the examiner.

Levator function is graded as follows:
- Normal: 15 mm or more
- Good: 12–14 mm
- Fair: 5–11 mm
- Poor: 4 mm or less.

2. *Putterman's method.* This is carried out by the measurement of distance between the middle of upper lid margin to the 6'o clock limbus in extreme upgaze. This is also known as the margin limbal distance (MLD).
- Normal MLD is about 9.0 mm
- The difference in MLD of two sides in unilateral cases or the difference with normal in bilateral cases multiplied by three would give the amount of levator resection required.

3. *Illif's test.* It is applicable in early childhood 1 to 2 years of age. In this, upper lid is everted and if LPS function is good, the lid reverts of its own.

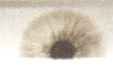

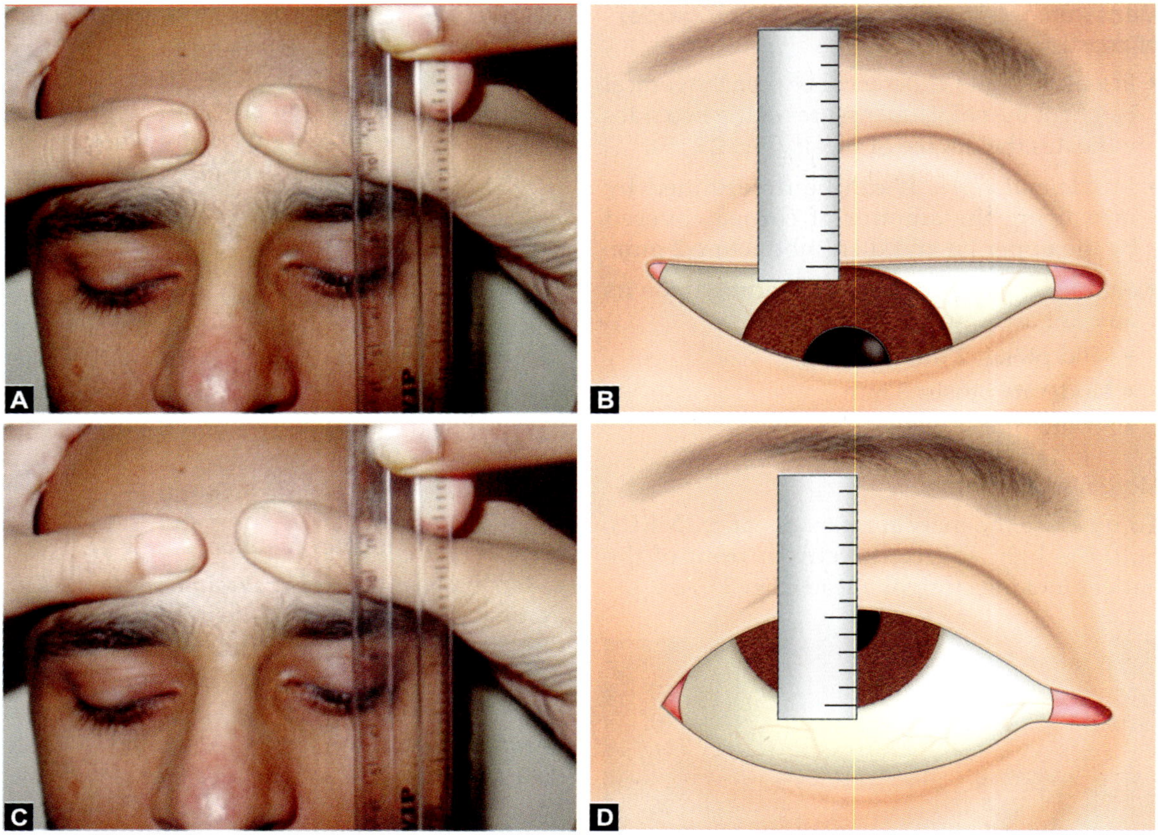

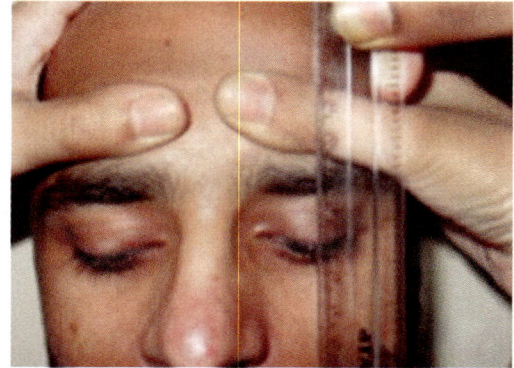

Fig. 23.2: *Measurement of the levator action by Berke's method. Looking down: (A) Clinical photography, (B) Diagrammatic depiction; and looking up; (C) Clinical photography, (D) Diagrammatic depiction.*

4. *MRD-3* refers to the distance from the corneal light reflex to the centre of upper lid margin in extreme upgaze.

- *Amount of LPS resection* in U/L cases = 3 (MRD-3 normal—MRD-3 abnormal) in B/L cases = 3 (7–MRD-3) in mm.

Margin crease distance

Margin crease distance (MCD) is the distance between the centre of upper lid margin to the lid crease. The normal distance is about 10 mm in females and about 8 mm in males and is measured in downgaze (Fig. 23.3). It helps in planning the surgical incision.

Bell's phenomenon

Confirmation of presence of Bell's phenomenon is important before undertaking any surgical

Fig. 23.3: *Measurement of margin crease distance (MCD).*

procedure to avoid risk of postoperative exposure keratopathy. It is the upward and outward rotation of eyeball on closure of the eye. This is referred to as Bell's positive.

It is tested by manually holding the lids open, asking the patient to try to shut the eyes and observing upward rotation of eyeball. Bell's phenomenon is graded as below:

- *Good*: <1/3 of cornea is visible
- *Fair*: 1/3–1/2 of cornea is visible
- *Poor*: >1/2 of cornea is visible.

Associated signs

- *Contralateral lid retraction*. Unilateral ptosis may cause contralateral lid retraction. There may be increased innervation to the ptotic lid as a compensatory mechanism. The increased innervation flows to the contralateral LPS also and leads to lid retraction.
- *Fatiguability test*. Fatiguability is tested by asking the patient to look up for 30–60 seconds. Progressive drooping of the lid or inability to maintain upgaze is suggestive of myasthenia gravis.
- *Marcus Gunn jaw-winking syndrome* may be present in 5% of all cases of congenital ptosis. Stimulation of ipsilateral pterygoid by chewing, sucking or opening the mouth or contralateral jaw movement causes retraction of the ptotic lid.

Examination of eyeball

Examination of eyeball should include:

- *Corneal sensation*. The presence or absence of corneal sensations should be noted.
- *Examination of pupil*. Look for size, shape and pupillary reflexes.
- *Fundus examination* for any disease.
- *Schirmer's test* to assess tear film.
- *Ocular motility*. The extraocular muscle functions, specially of the elevator muscles, should be recorded. Any association of eye movements with change in degree of ptosis should be looked for.

SPECIAL EXAMINATION AND TESTS

Special tests required in acquired ptosis are as below:

1. *Neostigmine/Tensilon test.* This test is done in doubtful cases where an acquired ptosis due to myasthenia gravis is suspected. In adults, 1 mg of neostigmine is injected IM. The ptosis improves in 5 to 15 minutes, if myasthenia gravis

is the cause. Alternately 10 mg of edrophonium (Tensilon) may be injected IV. It is loaded in a tuberculine syringe and 2 mg injected slowly in 15–30 seconds. The needle is left *in situ* and rest injected slowly if no untoward incident is observed. The effect occurs in 1 to 5 minutes, if myasthenia is the cause. If cholinergic reaction occurs, 0.5 mg of atropine is given IV.

2. *Phenylephrine test.* Phenylephrine 10% drops are used to assess mild cases of ptosis. Positive phenylephrine test suggests that patient would respond well to Müller's muscle resection. The test is also useful in Horner's syndrome.

3. *Photographic record* of the patient should be maintained for comparison. Photographs should be taken in primary position as well as in up- and downgazes.

4. *Other special tests* indicated in suspected myasthenic patients include:

- Sleep test
- Ice test
- Morning/evening comparison test.

NEUROLOGICAL EXAMINATION AND INVESTIGATIONS

Neurological examination

Thorough neurological examination should be carried in all acquired cases to rule out neurological diseases.

Neuroimaging

Neuroimaging including CT scan and MRI brain may be required in patients with neurogenic ptosis.

Investigations in acquired ptosis should include:

- Complete haemogram with ESR
- Blood sugar
- Urine examination for albumin and sugar
- Serum T_3, T_4, TSH.

CONGENITAL PTOSIS

INTRODUCTION

Typically, congenital ptosis is associated with congenital weakness (due to developmental

dystrophy) of the levator palpebrae superioris (LPS) muscle. However, some other forms of ptosis may also occur congenitally. So congenital ptosis may include following clinical groups:

- Simple congenital ptosis,
- Congenital ptosis with associated weakness of superior rectus muscle
- Blepharophimosis syndrome
- Congenital synkinetic ptosis syndrome
- Ptosis with congenital fibrosis of extraocular muscles.

SIMPLE CONGENITAL PTOSIS

Simple congenital ptosis is not associated with any other anomaly.

CHARACTERISTIC FEATURES

Characteristic features of simple congenital ptosis are as below (Fig. 23.4):

- *Drooping of one or both upper lids* since birth of variable severity (mild, moderate or severe).
- *Lid crease* is either diminished or absent due to poor levator function.
- *Lid lag on downgaze* (i.e. ptotic lid is higher than the normal) due to tethering effect of abnormal as dystrophic LPS neither relaxes nor contracts. This is in contrast to acquired ptosis in which ptotic lid is lower than the normal in downgaze, whereas it is higher in primary gaze.
- *LPS function* may be poor, fair or good depending upon the degree of weakness.

Levator resection

Levator resection is a very commonly performed operation for moderate and severe grades of

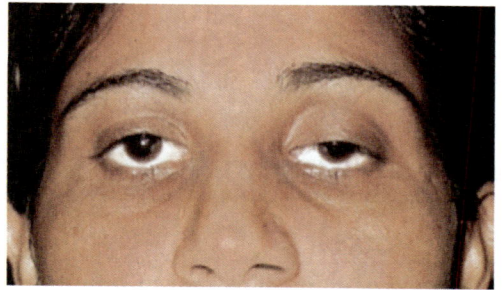

Fig. 23.4: *Simple congenital ptosis.*

ptosis. It is contraindicated in patients having severe ptosis with poor levator function.

Amount of levator resection required: Most of the surgeons find it out by adjusting the lid margin in relation to cornea during operation on the table in individual case. However, a rough estimate in different grades of ptosis can be made:

I. *Moderate ptosis.* Depending on the level of LPS function, the amount of LPS to be resected is as below:

- *Good function*: 16–17 mm (minimal)
- *Fair function*: 18–22 mm (moderate)
- *Poor function*: 23–24 mm (maximum).

II. *Severe ptosis.* Fair levator function: 23–24 mm (maximum LPS resection).

Guidelines for amount of levator resection have been given by Beard (in 1976) and Berke (in 1961). Table 23.1 elaborates Beard's method, which takes into consideration the amount of ptosis and the amount of upper lid excursion and Table 23.2 describes Berke's method for

Table 23.1 *Beard's method for determining amount of LPS resection in congenital ptosis*

Amount of ptosis	Upper eyelid excursion	Amount of resection
2 mm (mild)	0–5 mm (poor)	22–27 mm
	6–11 mm (fair)	16–21 mm
	12 or more (good)	10–15 mm
3 mm (moderate)	0–5 mm (poor)	Maximum (30 mm)
	6–11 mm (fair)	22–27 mm
	12 or more (good)	16–21 mm
4 mm or more (severe)	0–5 mm (poor)	Maximum (30 mm)
	6–11 mm (fair)	25–30 mm
	12 or more (good)	25–30 mm

Table 23.2 *Berke's method for determining amount of LPS resection in congenital ptosis*

Upper eyelid excursion	Superior corneal coverage by upper eyelid
0–5 mm (poor)	0 mm (lid margin at superior limbus)
6–11 (fair)	2 mm
12 or more (good)	4 mm

determining amount of LPS resection. It takes into consideration amount of upper eyelid excursion and intraoperative eyelid placement with respect to the superior limbus.

CLINICAL FEATURES

Blepharophimosis syndrome aptly named blepharophimosis ptosis epicanthus syndrome (BPES) typically comprises four major congenital anomalies—blepharophimosis, ptosis, telecanthus and epicanthus inversus (Fig. 23.5):

1. *Blepharophimosis* is labelled when the horizontal palpebral fissure is narrow (20–22 mm in length) than the normal (25–30 mm).

2. *Ptosis* is usually bilateral symmetrical and often moderate to severe. It is usually associated with bilateral poor levator function.

3. *Telecanthus*, i.e. increased intracanthal distance.

4. *Epicanthus inversus* refers to a skin fold arising from the lower eyelid and growing over the medial canthus.

Other associated features noted not infrequently include:

• *Ectropion of lower eyelid* is also a frequent association.

• *Hypertelorism* refers to widely reported eyeballs resulting from widely reported orbits and broad nasal bridge.

Infrequently associated features include: Strabismus, amblyopia, symblepharon, microphthalmos, lacrimal drainage apparatus anomalies and optic disc coloboma.

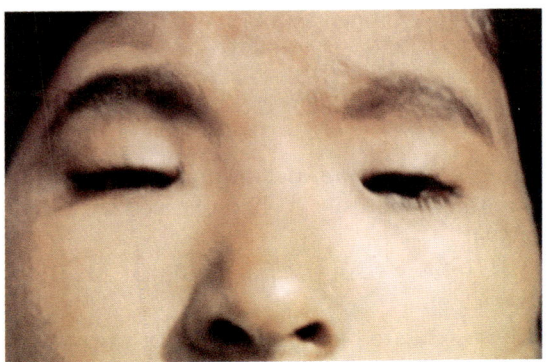

Fig. 23.5: *Blepharophimosis syndrome.*

Types of BPES

Depending upon presence of above features, the BPES has been described into three types:

• *Type I BPES*: Ptosis, telecanthus and epicanthus inversus. Type 1 BPES is associated with premature ovarian failure.

• *Type II BPES*: Ptosis, telecanthus and lower lid ectropion. Type 2 BPES occurs without premature ovarian failure.

• *Type III BPES*: Ptosis, telecanthus, lower lid ectropion and hypertelorism.

◼ CONGENITAL SYNKINETIC PTOSIS SYNDROME

The synkinetic ptosis group includes two conditions:

• Marcus Gunn jaw-winking ptosis
• Misdirected third nerve ptosis.

MARCUS GUNN JAW-WINKING SYNDROME

Clinical features

Marcus Gunn jaw-winking ptosis is characterised by:

• *Occurrence of retraction of the ptotic eyelid with jaw movement*, i.e. with contraction of the muscles of mastication most commonly the ipsilateral external pterygoid muscle (Fig. 23.6).

• *Ptosis is typically unilateral*, and commonly involves the left eye.

• *Eyelid fold is generally better maintained* than in other types of congenital ptosis.

• *Superior rectus muscle weakness* is often associated with this syndrome (75% of cases).

Severity of Marcus Gunn phenomenon has been classified into three grades:

1. *Mild*: Less than 2 mm
2. *Moderate*: 2–5 mm
3. *Severe*: More than 5 mm.

MISDIRECTED THIRD NERVE PTOSIS

Misdirected third nerve ptosis is a rare syndrome in which the ptotic eyelid rises with the ocular movements especially with contraction of medial, inferior and superior rectus muscles supplied by third nerve.

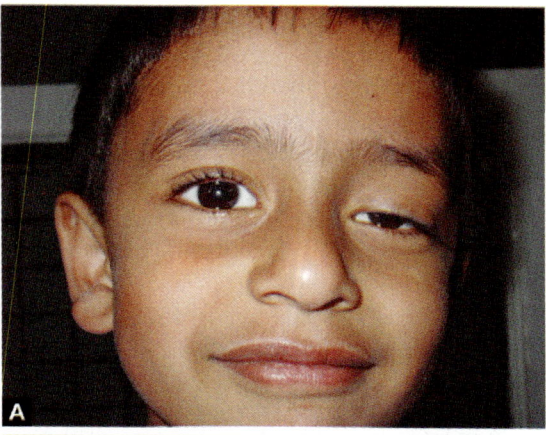

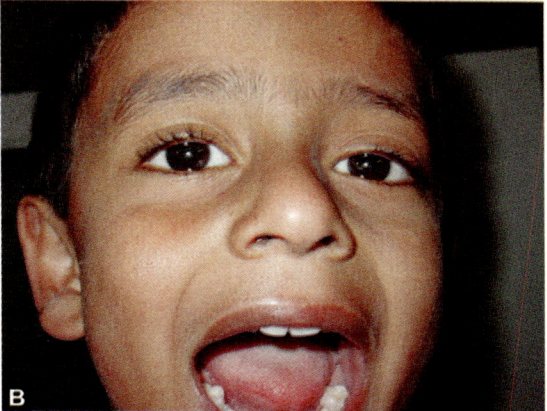

Fig. 23.6: *Marcus Gunn jaw-winking ptosis: (A) Ptosis in primary position; (B) with jaw movement ptosis disappears.*

PTOSIS WITH CONGENITAL FIBROSIS OF EXTRAOCULAR MUSCLES

Congenital fibrosis of extraocular muscles (CFEOMs) may have associated ptosis with following characteristics:

- Eyes are fixed by varying degrees.
- Force duction tests show muscles to be fibrotic.
- Levator function tests show a limited excursion.

ACQUIRED PTOSIS

I. APONEUROTIC PTOSIS

Acquired aponeurotic ptosis is the most common form of ptosis in adults.

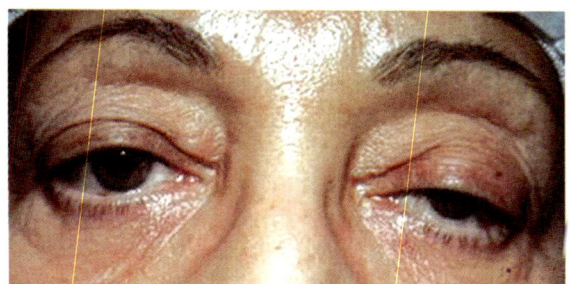

Fig. 23.7: *Aponeurotic ptosis.*

CLINICAL FEATURES

Characteristic features of aponeurotic ptosis are as below (Fig. 23.7):

- *Ptosis* is essentially mild to moderate and increases in downgaze. But the ptosis gets worse at the end of the day simulating myasthenia. This is because the lid is elevated by Müller's muscle, which fatigues by the evening.
- *Eyelid crease* is raised and upper lid sulcus seems deep on the affected side, due to upward drag to the skin associated with dehiscence/disinsertion of aponeurosis.
- *Lid margin* remains lower than the normal side in downgaze in contrast to lid lag seen in congenital ptosis.
- *Lid is thinned*, which can be almost transparent in marked cases.
- *Levator function* is good.

II. NEUROGENIC PTOSIS

Neurogenic ptosis includes cases caused by innervational defects such as:

- Third nerve palsy
- Horner's syndrome
- Ophthalmoplegic migraine
- Multiple sclerosis.

Horner's syndrome, occurring due to oculo-sympathetic paresis, is characterised by classic triad of:

- *Mild ptosis* (due to paralysis of Müller's muscles),
- *Miosis* (due to paralysis of dilator pupillae)
- *Reduced ipsilateral sweating* (anhydrosis)

• *Other features* include mild enophthalmos, loss of ciliospinal reflex, heterochromia, i.e. ipsilateral iris is lighter in colour in case of congenital Horner's syndromes. It occurs due to block of sympathetic stimulation in childhood, which interferes with melanin pigmentation of melanocytes in superior stroma of iris, pupil is slow to dilate, and there occurs slight elevation of the lower eyelid.

III. ACQUIRED MYOGENIC PTOSIS

It occurs due to acquired disorders of the LPS muscle or of the myoneural junction. It may be seen in patients with:

• Myasthenia gravis
• Dystrophia myotonica
• Ocular myopathy
• Oculopharyngeal muscular dystrophy
• Following trauma to the LPS
• Thyrotoxicosis
• Lambert-Eaton myasthenic syndrome.

CLINICAL FEATURES

General considerations

Onset. Ocular MG is characterised by an abrupt or insidious onset of weakness and fatiguability of one or both lids or eye muscles.

Hallmark features of ocular MG are variable and fatiguable ptosis, diplopia, chewing difficulties, dysarthria, dysphagia, dyspnoea, and systemic weakness.

Diurnal variation is exhibited in most patients, as their weakness is better in the morning or after sleep than at the end of the day, when they are weakest.

Variations in clinical presentations are typical in patients with ocular MG, making the diagnosis elusive at times.

Common signs and symptoms of MG can be described under 2 main headings: Lid dysfunction and ocular motility dysfunction.

Lid dysfunctions

1. *Ptosis and fatiguability.* The most common manifestation of ocular MG is unilateral or bilateral ptosis, which can be symmetric or asymmetric. The degree of ptosis is variable and frequently will shift from one eye to the other. It typically becomes worse with fatigue, sustained upgaze and at the end of the day (Fig. 23.8). In cases where the ptosis is subtle, lid fatigue can be enhanced with repeated eyelid closure or sustained upward gaze. Fatiguability test is described on page 477.

• *Levator function in myasthenia is related to the amount of ptosis;* those with marked ptosis will have the most levator weakness.

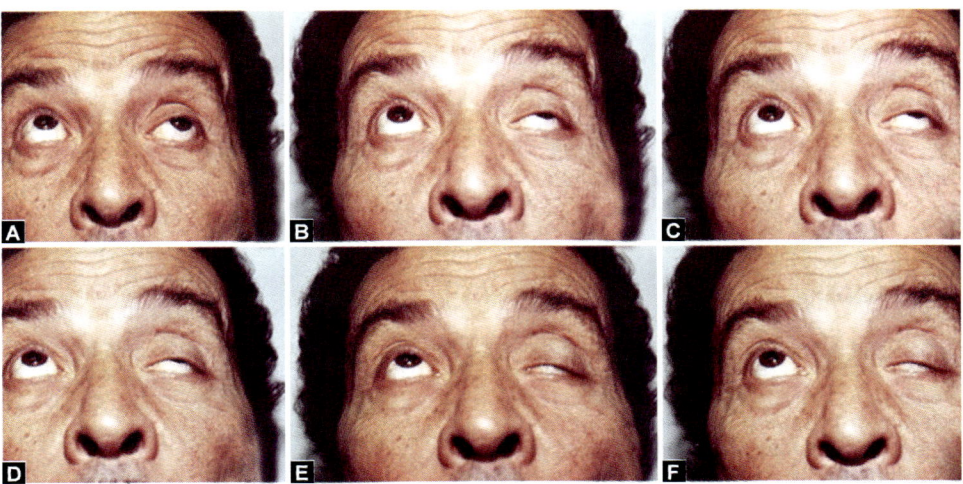

Fig. 23.8: *Fatiguability in a patient with myasthenia gravis (A through F). Note the limited elevation of the left eye denoting superior rectus palsy (A). (A, initially; C, after around 20 seconds; F, after 1 minute).*

- *Normal levator function in the setting of marked ptosis* argues against the diagnosis of myasthenia.

2. **Contralateral lid retraction.** May be present in some patients with unilateral ptosis which will assume its normal position when the ptotic eye is occluded or elevated, a result of Hering's law of equivalent innervations.

3. **Cogan's lid twitch** is characteristic of levator palpebrae superioris muscle involvement. This can be elicited by having the patient rapidly redirect gaze from downward to primary position. If a patient of myasthenic ptosis looks downward for 3–5 seconds, then looks up quickly into primary gaze, the eyelid appears to overshoot upward, then quickly falls (Fig. 23.9). This can be explained by a build-up of acetylcholine in neuromuscular junction of levator muscle fibres while the eyelid is resting in downgaze. Following upward fixation, the levator quickly fatigues and the eyelid droops.

4. **Lid hopping.** During the attempted lateral gaze, the fluttering of ptotic eyelid may be seen, known as lid hopping.

5. **Orbicularis oculi muscle weakness** is seen often in MG. Testing of orbicularis oculi muscle strength is helpful in the diagnosis of patients suspected of having MG. The characteristic 'Peek' sign of orbicularis fatigue is seen in

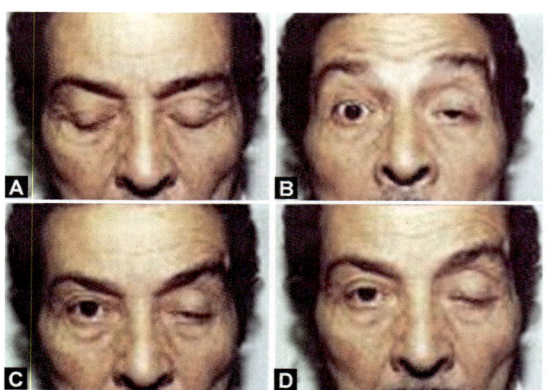

Fig. 23.9: *Cogan sign.* *The patient changes gaze from the downward position (A); to the primary position (B); Both lids are seen to overshoot in a twitch (C); Before gaining their initial ptotic position (D). In this case, the Cogan sign is seen more obviously on the right, whereas the left lid is more ptotic.*

patients with MG. In such patients, upon gentle eyelid closure, the orbicularis oculi muscle will initially contract to achieve eyelid closure. However, orbicularis muscle rapidly fatigues resulting in widening of palpebral aperture.

6. **Curtaining and enhanced ptosis.** In asymmetric ptosis, when the more ptotic eyelid is manually elevated, the fellow eye often droops (curtaining). This sign is nonspecific and can be seen in many other situations like, third nerve palsy. When the ptosis is symmetric, elevation of one eyelid will worsen the other eyelid (enhanced ptosis).

These eyelid signs are consequences of Hering's law, as manual elevation of a ptotic eyelid reduces the patient's required effort to elevate the eyelids and the other eyelid falls.

DIAGNOSIS

The variable course of MG may make the diagnosis difficult and it can mimic a variety of neuro-ophthalmic conditions. In brief, the diagnosis of MG relies mostly on the patients history and physical findings and various tests to elicit the condition.

A. Pharmacological and clinical tests for ocular myasthenia gravis

1. **Tensilon test.** It is a firstline test for diagnosis of MG. It consists of injecting a small amount of tensilon (edrophonium chloride) intravenously. Edrophonium is a rapidly acting and quickly hydrolysed anticholinesterase which temporarily increases the level of acetylcholine at the neuromuscular junction. A 10 mg dose of tensilon is drawn up in a 1cc syringe. Initially, a 0.2 cc test dose is injected intravenously. If the lid or EOM function is not improved within 1 minute, the remaining 0.8 cc is slowly injected over 30 seconds in 2 mg increments, and the lid positions and eye movements are reassessed for improvement (Fig. 23.10). The onset of action begins within 30–60 seconds of intravenous injection and the effect resolves within 5–10 minutes. The advantage of incremental method of administration is that the full 10 mg dose may not be required to produce a positive response. In infants, the dose of edrophorium

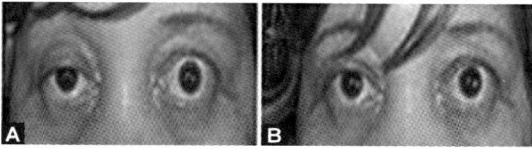

Fig. 23.10: *Ptosis in right eye (A); Which disappears on Tensilon test (B).*

chloride is 0.05 to 1.0 mg subcutaneously and 0.15 mg/kg in children.

Occassionally, patients develop salivation, lacrimation, increased sweating and mild gastrointestinal discomfort. Atropine 0.4 mg should be ready in a separate syringe and administered intravenously, if symptomatic bradycardia occurs.

The Tensilon test is positive in 80–90% of patients with myasthenia gravis. The edrophonium test unfortunately has many false negative and false positive results. It can be false positive in other disorders of neuromuscular transmission, such as Lambert-Eaton myasthenic syndrome, botulism, and organophosphate toxicity, and also in some patients with skull base tumours. Therefore, a positive edrophonium test should not be the sole basis for making a diagnosis of myasthenia gravis.

2. *Neostigmine test.* Intramuscular prostigmin (neostigmine bromide) may be used in children who are uncooperative or too agitated to monitor over a short period of time and also in adults whose signs are subtle and require longer period of observation. Usually 0.6 mg atropine sulphate and 1.5 mg prostigmin are combined in a 3 cc syringe and injected intramuscularly. A change in ocular motility and ptosis is usually evident within 15–30 minutes following the injection.

3. *The 'sleep test'.* It is based on the tendency for MG symptoms to improve following rest; may be used in small children and patients who have allergies or sensitivity to tensilon. The patient is placed in a quiet darkened room and instructed to close their eyes for 30 minutes. The eye movement is measured before and after the rest. The test is considered positive, if there is improvement in ptosis and/or eye movement following the 30 minutes rest period. The

reappearance of the myasthenic signs over the next 30 seconds to 5 minutes adds further confirmation.

4. *The 'ice test'.* It is a simple test for ocular MG in patients who have ptosis. A surgical glove filled with ice is held against the droopy eyelid for 2 minutes. After the ice pack is removed, improvement in ptosis is observed in patients with MG. The test is considered positive when the upper eyelid elevates by at least 2 mm following application of ice pack. The precise mechanism by which cooling improves myasthenic weakness is unclear. Reduced acetylcholinesterase activity and an increased receptor sensitization with lower temperature are the possible mechanisms. This test has a sensitivity and specificity of 76.9% and 98.3%, respectively.

5. *The morning/evening comparison test.* It is similar in concept to the sleep test. The patient is photographed and the ptosis and ocular motility are compared at different times during the day.

6. *The 'fatigue test'.* The patient is asked to look at an object held up by the examiner in front of the patient. After a short period of time, the eyelid(s) will droop in person with ocular MG.

B. Haematological tests

If the diagnosis is suspected, serological tests can be performed such as:

1. *Acetylcholine receptor antibody titre (AChR Ab):* Only about 70% of patients with ocular MG have detectable antibody level while 90% of patients with generalised MG have elevated titre. An elevated titre provides a baseline for future comparisons while monitoring the patient's clinical course and the response to immunosuppressive treatment. Although the blood test when positive is highly specific but not particularly sensitive. The test has a reasonable sensitivity of 80–96%, but in ocular MG, the sensitivity falls to 50%, and they also suggest the presence of thymoma.

2. *Thyroid profile.* Thyroid dysfunction is found in approximate 5–10% of MG patients.

3. *Antibodies against MuSK protein.* A proportion of patients without antibodies against

acetylcholinesterase receptors have antibodies against MuSK protein.

C. Radiological investigations

Chest MRI or CT scan are done to rule out thymic disorders as thymic tumours are present in 10–15% of MG patients, being more common in older individuals and rarely occurring before age of 30 years.

D. Electrodiagnostics

The fatiguability of the muscles in patients with MG can be measured by repetitive nerve stimulation (RNS) test.

A decrement of the compound muscle action potential during electromyographic repetitive nerve stimulation (2 to 5 Hz) of limb or facial muscles is diagnostic in many cases of myasthenia gravis. However, this technique is relatively insensitive in ocular myasthenia. Additional single fibre electromyography (SFEMG) may be helpful in ocular myasthenia, if the repetitive nerve stimulation, edrophonium test, and antibody studies are non-diagnostic or cannot be performed. Normally, two muscle fibres innervated by the same motor axon will exhibit a variation, called jitter, in the time interval between their two action potentials during successive impulses. Jitter can be increased in myasthenia gravis and other disorders of neuromuscular transmission. In patients with mild myasthenia, the combination of single fibre electromyography, antiacetylcholine receptor antibody studies, and the edrophonium test should provide the lab confirmation of myasthenia gravis in at least 95% of patients.

This is considered to be the most sensitive (but not the most specific) test for MG.

CHRONIC PROGRESSIVE EXTERNAL OPHTHALMOPLEGIA

The diagnosis of mitochondrial myopathy depends upon a constellation of findings, family history, type of muscle involvement, specific laboratory abnormalities, and the results of histological, pathobiochemical and genetic analysis. The most common ocular manifestation of mitochondrial myopathy is

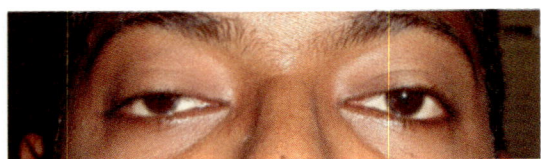

Fig. 23.11: *A patient with CPEO.*

chronic progressive external ophthalmoplegia (CPEO).

The most common form is late-onset bilateral chronic progressive external ophthalmoplegia (CPEO). CPEO is characterised (Fig. 23.11) by ptosis and weakness of extraocular muscles leading to limitation of extraocular movements with relative sparing of downgaze and occasionally dysconjugate ocular movements.

Although, transient diplopia may occur, most patients seldom complain of it and are mostly unaware of their restrictions. The ptosis is often asymmetric. Up to 90% of CPEO patients have additional weakness of the facial, bulbar or limb muscles. Thus, many patients may be classified as "CPEO plus" because they present additional multisystem symptoms such as other neurological symptoms, hearing disturbances, or with diabetes.

OCULOPHARYNGEAL MUSCULAR DYSTROPHY (OPMD)

CLINICAL FEATURES

The combination of ptosis and pharyngeal weakness combined (Fig. 23.12) with

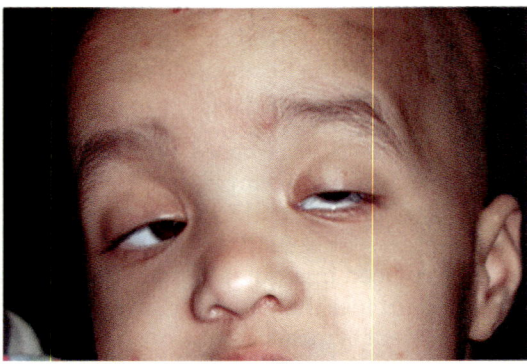

Fig. 23.12: *A patient with oculopharyngeal muscular dystrophy.*

ophthalmoparesis, dysphagia and weakness and wasting of face, neck, and distal limb muscles is quite characteristic for autosomal dominant, late onset OPMD.

MYOTONIC DYSTROPHY TYPE 1 (DM1)

CLINICAL FEATURES

Among the numerous well-known multisystemic features of the classic form of myotonic dystrophy (DM1), e.g. muscle weakness and myotonia, the eye is in any case affected. Not only myotonic cataracts but also retinal abnormalities, ptosis and blepharospasm are common features of the disease.

IV. MECHANICAL PTOSIS

1. Ptosis due to lid masses

Mechanical ptosis may occur due to excessive weight on the upper lid by lid masses, e.g.

- *Multiple chalazia,* if not treated timely, can cause drooping of upper eyelid.

- *Benign tumours* commonly associated with ptosis are neurofibromatosis (Fig. 23.13) and haemangioma.

- *Malignant tumours* involving upper lid such as squamous cell carcinoma, sebaceous gland carcinoma, basal cell carcinoma and even malignant melanoma may cause ptosis.

- *Orbital metastasis* of malignant tumours may produce ptosis as an early sign.

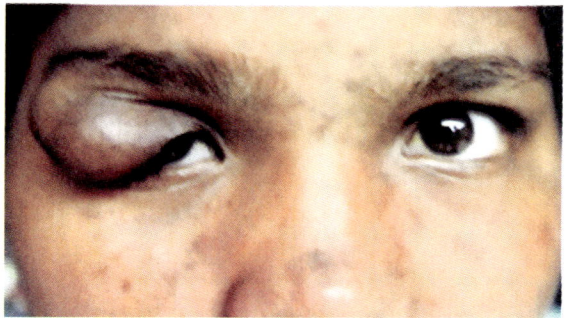

Fig. 23.13: *Mechanical ptosis due to benign tumour upper eyelid.*

2. Ptosis with blepharochalasis

Acquired ptosis may be associated with blepharochalasis.

3. Cicatricial ptosis

It results due to conjunctival scarring in following conditions:

- Ocular pemphigoid
- Erythema multiforme
- Cicatrizing trachoma
- Chemical and thermal burns.

BIBLIOGRAPHY

1. Beard C. Ptosis, 3rd edn. St. Louis: CV Mosby Company 1981.

2. Berke RN. Types of operation for congenital and acquired ptosis – In Trauotman R. Converse J and Smith B (Ed): In Plastic and reconstructive surgery of the eye and adenexa. Washington, DC Butterworths. 1962.

3. Betharia SM, Grover AK, Kalra BR. Br J Ophthalmol 1983;67:58–60.

4. Chan W. Mycophenolate mofetil for ocular myasthenia. J Neurol 2008;255(4):510–3.

5. Crawford JS. Congenital Blepharoptosis in Byron C. Smith Ophthalmic plastic and reconstructive surgery, Vol. 1, CV Mosby Company: 1987;631–53.

6. Gilbert ME, Savino PJ. Ocular myasthenia Gravis. Int Ophthalmol Clin 2007; 47(4):93–103,ix.

7. Grover AK, Mittal Sanjay. A Clinico-pathological study of levator muscle for Congenital Ptosis. Thesis is submitted to Delhi University.

8. Grover AK, Gupta AK. Proceedings of the Golden Jubilee Conference of All India Ophthalmological Society, New Delhi: 1992; 54–6.

9. Grover AK, K Uma Chaturvedi, Sanjal Mittal. Presented at 53 AIOS Annual Conference at Bombay, 1995.

10. Gunn RM. Trans Ophthal Soc UK 1983;3:283.

11. Keesey JC. Clinical evaluation and management of myasthenia gravis. Muscle Nerve 2004;29: 484–505.

12. Mustarde JC. Epicanthus and telecanthus. Int Ophthalmol Cli 4: 1964.

13. Oosterius HJGH. The natural course of myasthenia gravis: a long-term follow-up study. J Neurol Neurosurg Psychiatry 1989;52:1121–7.

14. Pascuzzi RM,Coslett HB, Johns TR. Long-term corticosteroid treatment of myasthenia gravis: Report of 116 patients. Ann Neurol 1984;15:291–8.

15. Putterman: Basis oculoplastic surgery in Peyman GA: Principles and practice of ophthalmology, Vol. 3. Philadiphia: WB Saunders Company, 1980;2246–2333.

16. Seybld ME. Myasthenia gravis: A clinical and basic science review. JAMA 1983;250:2516–21.

17. Smith B, McCord CD, Baylis H. Am J Ophthalmol 1969;68:92.

18. Sommer N, Melms A, Weller M, et al. Ocular myasthenia gravis. A critical review of clinical and pathophysiological aspects. Doc Ophthalmol 1993;84(4):309–33.

Evaluation of a Case of Watering Eye

Chapter Outline

CAUSES OF WATERING EYE

Hyperlacrimation

- Primary hyperlacrimation
- Reflex hyperlacrimation
- Central hyperlacrimation

Epiphora

Lacrimal pump failure

Mechanical obstruction

- Punctal causes
- Canalicular causes
- Lacrimal sac causes
- Nasolacrimal duct causes

CLINICAL EVALUATION OF 'WATERING EYE'

- History taking
- Examination with diffuse illumination using magnification
- Regurgitation on pressure over lacrimal sac

- Fluorescein dye disappearance test (FDDT)
- Lacrimal syringing test
- Diagnostic probing
- Jones dye tests
- Nasal endoscopy
- Lacrimal endoscopy
- Imaging of lacrimal system

MANAGEMENT OF WATERING EYE

Management in adults

- Primary punctal stenosis
- Secondary punctal stenosis
- Canalicular obstruction
- Nasolacrimal duct obstruction

Management in children

- General considerations
- Treatment modalities

CAUSES OF WATERING EYE

It is characterised by overflow of tears from the conjunctival sac. The condition may occur either due to excessive secretion of tears (hyperlacrimation) or may result from obstruction to the outflow of normally secreted tears (epiphora).

HYPERLACRIMATION

1. *Primary hyperlacrimation.* It is a rare condition which occurs due to direct stimulation of the lacrimal gland. It may occur in early stages of lacrimal gland tumours and cysts and due to the effect of strong parasympathomimetic drugs.

2. *Reflex hyperlacrimation.* It results from stimulation of sensory branches of fifth nerve due to irritation of cornea or conjunctiva. It may occur in multitude of conditions which include:

- *Affections of the lids*: Stye, hordeolum internum, acute meibomitis, trichiasis, concretions and entropion.
- *Affections of the conjunctiva*: Conjunctivitis which may be infective, allergic, toxic, irritative or traumatic.

- *Affections of the cornea*: These include corneal abrasions, corneal ulcers and non-ulcerative keratitis.
- *Affections of the sclera*: Episcleritis and scleritis.
- *Affections of uveal tissue*: Iritis, cyclitis, iridocyclitis.
- Acute glaucomas.
- Endophthalmitis and panophthalmitis.
- Orbital cellulitis.

3. *Central hyperlacrimation (psychical lacrimation).* The exact area concerned with central lacrimation is still not known. It is seen in emotional states, voluntary lacrimation and hysterical lacrimation.

EPIPHORA

Inadequate drainage of tears may occur due to physiological or anatomical (mechanical) causes.

Physiological cause is '**lacrimal pump' failure** due to lower lid laxity or weakness of orbicularis muscle.

Mechanical obstruction in lacrimal passages may lie at the level of punctum, canaliculus, lacrimal sac or nasolacrimal duct.

1. *Punctal causes* include:
- *Eversion of lower punctum.* It is commonly seen in old age due to laxity of the lids. It may also occur following chronic conjunctivitis, chronic blepharitis and ectropion.
- *Punctal obstruction.* There may be congenital absence of puncta or cicatricial closure following injuries, burns or infections. Rarely a small foreign body, concretion and cilia may also block the punctum. Prolonged use of drugs like idoxuridine and pilocarpine is also associated with punctal stenosis.

2. *Causes in the canaliculi*: Canalicular obstruction may be congenital or acquired due to foreign body, trauma, strictures and canaliculitis.

3. *Causes in the lacrimal sac*: These include congenital mucous membrane folds, traumatic strictures, dacryocystitis, specific infections like tuberculosis and syphilis, dacryolithiasis, tumours and atony of the sac.

4. *Causes in the nasolacrimal duct*: Congenital lesions include noncanalization, partial canalization or imperforated membranous valves. Acquired causes of obstruction are traumatic/inflammatory strictures, tumours and diseases of the surrounding bones.

CLINICAL EVALUATION OF 'WATERING EYE'

Clinical evaluation of watering eye should include: meticulous history taking, examination, certain diagnostic tests and imaging of the lacrimal system, as descried below.

1. HISTORY TAKING

History taking should include following important points about watering:
- Onset/severity/frequency of watering
- Laterality—unilateral/bilateral
- Continuous or intermittent
- Constant overflowing over cheek or intermittent watering
- Aggravating and relieving factors
- Seasonal variation—worse in winters and windy weather
- History of allergy—medicinal/environmental
- Bloody tears
- Associated history of discharge at medial canthus (mucoid/ropy/stringy), pain, swelling, nasal symptoms, itching, foreign body sensation, redness, and photophobia should be ascertained.

2. EXAMINATION WITH DIFFUSE ILLUMINATION USING MAGNIFICATION

- It should be carried to rule out any cause of reflex hypersecretion located in lids, conjunctiva, cornea, sclera, anterior chamber and uveal tract.
- This examination should also exclude punctal causes of epiphora and any swelling in the sac area.
- Functional epiphora also needs to be ruled out. Important causes of functional epiphora include—lid laxity, lid malposition, facial palsy, incomplete blink and floppy eyelid syndrome.

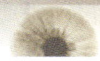

3. REGURGITATION ON PRESSURE OVER LACRIMAL SAC

Regurgitation on pressur over lacrimal sac (ROPLAS); also known as regurgitation test (RT) is a simple, clinical test performed to assess blockage in the lacrimal system. To perform ROPLAS, the anterior lacrimal crest is identified by tracing the inferior orbital margin medially and superiorly. Then, a steady pressure with index finger is applied behind the anterior lacrimal crest, over the lacrimal sac area, above the MPL (Fig. 24.1). The pressure should be applied in upward and medial direction. The observations made on ROPLAS are interpreted as follows:

- Negative ROPLAS, characterised by no regurgitation is seen normally.
- Positive ROPLAS, characterised by regurgitation of clear/mucoid/mucopurulent discharge is suggestive of chronic dacryocystitis.
- Positive ROPLAS with blood tinged fluid warrants ruling out dacryoliths/lacrimal sac tumours.
- False negative ROPLAS may be observed in internal fistula, wrong method of performing the test, if patient has emptied the lacrimal sac before examination, encysted mucocele, atonic lacrimal sac.

4. FLUORESCEIN DYE DISAPPEARANCE TEST (FDDT)

It this test, one drop of fluorescein dye is instilled in both the conjunctival sacs and observations are made after 5 minutes. As per Zappia and Milder classification (1972), the colour intensity remaining after 5 minutes is graded on a scale of 0 to +4. Normally, 0 to +1 dye is seen in the conjunctival sac. Retention of +2 to +4 dye in conjunctival sac indicates inadequate drainage which may be due to atonia of sac or mechanical obstruction.

Advantages of FDDT

- Noninvasive, physiological test
- High specificity and positive predictive value. Hence, a good screening test
- Specially useful in children as OPD procedure as they do not cooperate for syringing.

Pitfalls of FDDT

- Not possible to differentiate between anatomical and functional block
- Not possible to pin point site of block in anatomical obstruction.

5. LACRIMAL SYRINGING TEST

Lacrimal syringing (lacrimal drainage system irrigation) is a simple and most frequently performed test to determine the level of obstruction in patients with epiphora, except in acute dacryocystitis, where it is contraindicated.

It is performed after topical anaesthesia with proparacaine HCl 0.5% or 2 to 4% xylocaine (Fig. 24.2). Normal saline is pushed into the lacrimal sac from lower punctum with the help of a syringe and lacrimal cannula, after dilating the punctum with Nettleship's punctum dilator, a free passage of saline through lacrimal passages into the nose rules out any mechanical obstruction.

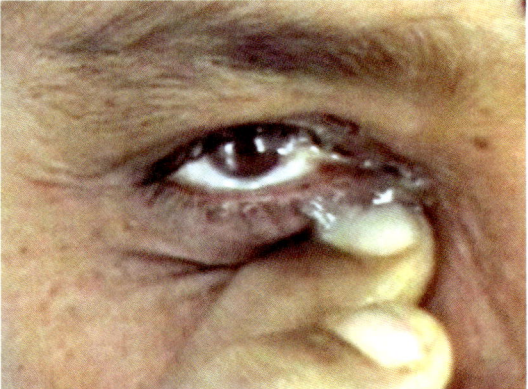

Fig. 24.1: *Regurgitation test.*

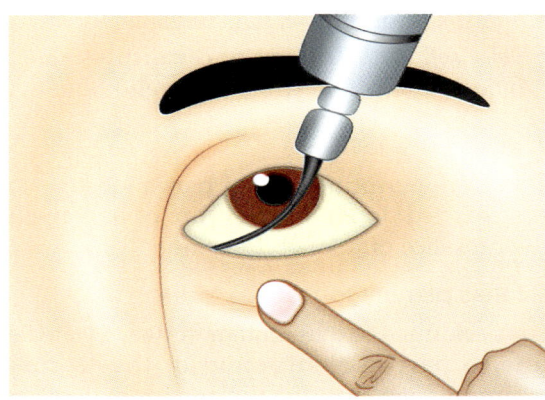

Fig. 24.2: *Technique of lacrimal syringing.*

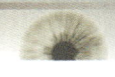

Table 24.1 *Interpretation of results of lacrimal syringing test*

Observation	Interpretation
Immediate regurgitation of clear fluid from same punctum	Same canalicular block
Regurgitation of clear fluid from opposite punctum	Common canalicular block (CCB)/nasolacrimal duct obstruction (NLDO). Probing needed to differentiate (soft stop in CCB, hard stop in NLDO)
Regurgitation of mucoid/mucopurulent fluid after a delay from opposite punctum	NLDO
Patent with considerable pressure on syringe, with regurgitation of some fluid	Partial NLDO
Lacrimal passage patent on syringing (in a patient with positive ROPLAS)	Atonic sac

The interpretation of results of lacrimal syringing test is summarised in Table 24.1.

6. DIAGNOSTIC PROBING

Diagnostic probing of upper lacrimal system is indicated to confirm site of blockage, if syringing reveals non-patent lacrimal system.

Method of diagnostic probing: Punctum is dilated with punctum dilator. Bowman's lacrimal probe is inserted through the punctum, while maintaining lateral stretch on the eyelid, so that the vertical and horizontal part of canaliculus get aligned and iatrogenic damage is prevented.

Interpretation of diagnostic probing is as below:
- *Hard stop*: Nasolacrimal duct obstruction
- *Soft stop*: Common canaliculus block
- *False soft stop*: Kinking of canaliculus due to inadequate lateral stretch of eyelid.

7. JONES DYE TESTS

These are performed when partial obstruction is suspected. Jones dye tests are of no value in the presence of total obstruction.

i. Jones primary test (Jones test I)

It is performed to differentiate between watering due to partial obstruction of the lacrimal passages from that due to primary hypersecretion of tears. One drop of 2% fluorescein dye is instilled in the conjunctival sac and a cotton bud dipped in 2% xylocaine with 1 in 1000 epinephrine is placed in the inferior meatus at the opening of nasolacrimal duct. After 5 minutes, the cotton bud is removed and inspected. A dye-stained cotton bud indicates adequate drainage through the lacrimal passage. Cause of watering is primary hypersecretion. (Further investigations should aim at finding the cause of primary hypersecretion) (Fig. 24.3A). While the unstained cotton bud (negative test) indicates either a partial obstruction or failure of lacrimal pump mechanism. To differentiate between these conditions, Jones dye test II is performed (Fig. 24.3B).

ii. Jones secondary test (Jones test II)

When primary test is negative, the cotton bud is again placed in the inferior meatus. Residual fluorescein is flushed from conjunctional sacs and lacrimal syringing is performed with clear saline. A positive test suggests that dye was present in the sac but could not reach the nose due to partial obstruction. A negative test indicates presence of lacrimal pump failure and is a contraindication for DCR operation.

8. NASAL ENDOSCOPY

Nasal endoscopy is helpful in evaluation of anatomy of the nasal cavity and to diagnose associated diseases.

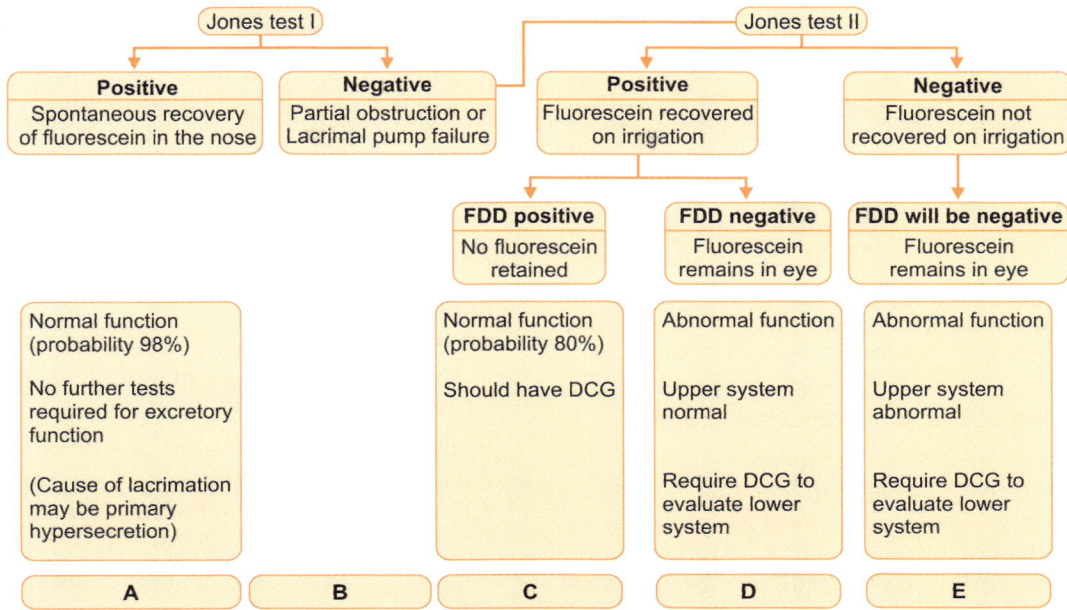

	Jones test I		Jones test II	
Positive Spontaneous recovery of fluorescein in the nose	**Negative** Partial obstruction or Lacrimal pump failure	**Positive** Fluorescein recovered on irrigation		**Negative** Fluorescein not recovered on irrigation

		FDD positive No fluorescein retained	**FDD negative** Fluorescein remains in eye	**FDD will be negative** Fluorescein remains in eye
Normal function (probability 98%) No further tests required for excretory function (Cause of lacrimation may be primary hypersecretion)		Normal function (probability 80%) Should have DCG	Abnormal function Upper system normal Require DCG to evaluate lower system	Abnormal function Upper system abnormal Require DCG to evaluate lower system
A	**B**	**C**	**D**	**E**

Fig. 24.3: *Interpretation of results of Jones dye tests I and II with recommendations for further needful.*

9. LACRIMAL ENDOSCOPY

A rigid endoscope or a fibroptic flexible endoscope of 1.0 mm diameter is inserted through the puncti and canaliculi to inspect the mucosal lining of lacrimal system, and its contents. It is also useful evaluating in DCR fistulae.

10. IMAGING OF LACRIMAL SYSTEM

It is indicated in selective cases where other anatomical and physiological tests do not provide a conclusive diagnosis. The common techniques for imaging of lacrimal system discussed briefly include:

- Dacryocystography (DCG)
- Digital subtraction dacryocystography (DS-DCG)
- Radionucleotide lacrimal scintillography
- CT-DCG
- MR-DCG.

Dacryocystography

It is valuable in patients with epiphora due to mechanical obstruction. It tells the exact site, nature and extent of block (Fig. 24.4). In addition, it also gives information about mucosa of the sac, presence of any fistula, diverticula, stone or tumour in the sac. To perform it, a radio-

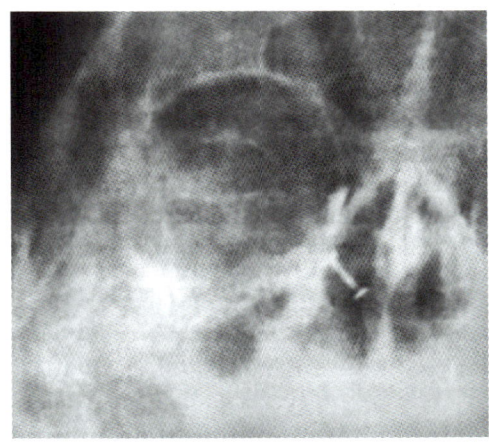

Fig. 24.4: *Dacryocystogram.*

opaque material such as lipiodol, pentopaque, dianosil or conray-280 is pushed into the sac with the help of a lacrimal cannula. X-rays are taken after 5 and 30 minutes to visualise the entire passage.

Digital subtraction-dacryocystography (DS-DCG)

DS-DCG can subtract background images and noises and provide a clear, contrast filled lacrimal image.

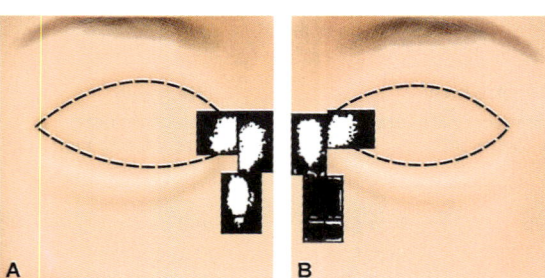

Fig. 24.5: *Lacrimal scintillography showing: (A) Normal lacrimal excretory system on right side; (B) obstruction at the junction of lacrimal sac and nasolacrimal on left side.*

Radionucleotide lacrimal scintillography

It is a noninvasive technique to assess the functional efficiency of lacrimal drainage apparatus. A radioactive tracer (sulphur colloid or technetium 99 m) is instilled into the conjunctival sac with a micropipette and its passage through the lacrimal drainage system is visualised and imaged with a gamma camera (Fig. 24.5).

In contrast to DCG, which is an anatomical test; nuclear scintillography is a physiological test and is useful in determining the site of delay in tear outflow in functional epiphora, partial obstructions and pediatric epiphora.

Computed-dacryocystography (CT-DCG)

Water-soluble iodine-based dye Omnipaque is either instilled into the conjunctival sac or through cannulation of the lacrimal canaliculus. CT scanning of lacrimal sac area with axial and coronal cuts of 2 mm thickness is carried out.

CT-DCG is useful in assessing anatomical variations in lacrimal sac, evaluation of surrounding facial and paranasal structures and traumatic obstructions.

Magnetic resonance-dacryocystography (MR-DCG)

MR-DCG utilizes 0.5% gadolinium meglumine as contrast medium.

Advantages of MR-DCG over CT-DCG include high tissue contrast, better soft tissue delineation, no ionizing radiations.

Disadvantages of MR-DCG over CT-DCG are longer acquisition time, higher cost and lack of bony details.

MANAGEMENT OF WATERING EYE

Management of each cause of epiphora is described in detail in relevant chapters. However, basic principles and brief outline of management in adults and children is outlined below.

MANAGEMENT IN ADULTS

Primary punctal stenosis

1. *Dilatation of punctum* is useful as a short-term measure, but does not give long-term benefits.

2. *Punctoplasty or three snip procedure.* The conjunctival sac is anaesthetised. The punctum is dilated with dilator which is introduced vertically and then pushed inwards along the canaliculus. The posterior wall of canaliculus is incised with the help of a knife. The triangular flap of posterior wall between vertical and horizontal part of canaliculus is cut followed by the insertion of probe to prevent closure of incision.

Secondary punctal stenosis

1. *Ziegler cautery.* Burns applied to palpebral conjunctiva below the puncta resulting in cicatrization of tissue which causes inversion of puncta.

2. *Medial conjunctivoplasty.* A diamond-shaped piece of tarsoconjunctiva is excised 2 mm below the puncta followed by approximation of superior and inferior margins with sutures.

3. *Lower lid tightening.* By lateral canthal sling which may be combined with medial conjunctivoplasty.

Canalicular obstruction

1. *Partial obstruction.* Treated by intubation using silicone stents which is left *in situ* for 6 months.

2. *Total obstruction.* If there is 6–8 mm patent normal canaliculus between puncta and obstruction, the anastomosis of patent part with lacrimal sac with intubation is done (canaliculodacryocystorhinostomy). If there is no patent normal canaliculus between puncta and

obstruction, the conjunctivodacryocystorhinostomy with primary Lester Jones tube insertion is done.

Nasolacrimal duct obstruction

1. *Conventional DCR.* Popular choice for NLDO and dacryocystitis and has a success rate of 80–95%. The operation involves anastomosing the lacrimal sac to nasal mucosa of middle nasal meatus. If there is canalicular damage or a narrow upper nasal cavity, it may be necessary to insert a silicone tube. Results are excellent with success rate of 90%. Causes of failure include inadequate size and position of ostium, unrecognized common canalicular obstruction scarring, too high or small lacrimal opening. Complications include scarring, injury to medial canthal structure, haemorrhage, cellulitis, CSF rhinorrhoea.

2. *Endoscopic DCR.* *Advantages* over conventional include lack of skin incision, less operation time, minimal trauma, blood loss. *Disadvantages* include less success rate, difficulty in examining common canaliculus and difficulty in probing of canaliculus in proximal canalicular obstruction.

3. *Endonasal laser DCR.* It is performed with Holmium: YAG laser under local anaesthesia. It is particularly suited for elderly patients but comparatively has a lower success rate of about 70%.

4. *Balloon dilatation dacryoplasty.* Effective in partial nasolacrimal duct obstruction with a claimed success rate of 60%.

MANAGEMENT IN CHILDREN

General considerations

Symptomatic NLDO occurs in approximately 5–6% of infants. A sticky, watery eye with positive regurgitation on pressure over the lacrimal sac confirms the diagnosis. Treatment depends upon the age of the child.

Treatment modalities

1. *Massage over lacrimal sac area and topical antibiotics* up to the age of 3–4 weeks. It should be carried out at least 3–4 times a day.
2. *Lacrimal syringing* can be performed with normal saline and antibiotic, if the condition does not improve up to the age of 2 months. It should be carried once a week or in two weeks.
3. *Probing of NLD with Bowman's probe* can be considered after up to the age of 6 months. It should be performed under general anaesthesia. Single probing will relieve the obstruction in most of the cases. May be repeated after an interval of 3–4 weeks, if failure occurs.
4. *Balloon catheter dilation* with the help of probe carrying inflatable balloons can be considered in children where repeated probing is a failure.
5. *Intubation with silicone tube* should be considered if repeated probing and balloon catheter dilation are failure. Tube should be kept in place for 5–6 months.
6. *DCR operation* should be considered when the child is brought very late or after repeated failure of probing and balloon catheter dilation. Generally performed after the age of 4 years.

BIBLIOGRAPHY

1. Cahill KV, Burns JA. Management of epiphora in the presence of congenital punctal and canalicular atresia. Ophthal Plast Reconstr Surg. 1991;7:167–72.
2. Esmaeli B, Hidaji L, Adinin RB, et al. Blockage of the lacrimal drainage apparatus as a side effect of docetaxel therapy. Cancer 2003;98:504–7.
3. Fayet B, Koster H, Benabderrazik S, et al. Six canalicular stenoses after 34 punctal plugs. Eur J Ophthalmol 1991;1:154–5.
4. Georgiadis NS, Terzidou CD. Epiphora caused by conjunctivochalasis: Treatment with transplantation of preserved human amniotic membrane. Cornea 2001;20:619–21.
5. Kashkouli MB, Beigi B, Murthy R, et al. Acquired external punctal stenosis: Etiology and associated findings. Am J Ophthalmol 2003; 136:1079–84.
6. Kuchar A, Steinkogler FJ. Antegrade balloon dilatation of nasolacrimal duct obstruction in adults. Br J Ophthalmol 2001;85:200–4.
7. Ko GY, Lee DH, Ahn HS, et al. Balloon catheter dilation in common canalicular obstruction of the lacrimal system: Safety and long-term effectiveness. Radiology 2000;214:781–6.

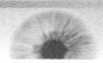

8. Lew H, Lee SY, Kim SJ. The clinical evaluation on the patients complaining of epiphora. J Korean Ophthalmol Soc 2000;41:1112–7.

9. Liu D, Bosley TM. Silicone nasolacrimal intubation with mitomycin-C: A prospective, randomized, doublemasked study. Ophthalmology 2003;110:306–10.

10. Mauffray RO, Hassan AS, Elner VM. Double silicone intubation as treatment for persistent congenital nasolacrimal duct obstruction. Ophthal Plast Reconstr Surg 2004;20:44–9.

11. Meyer DR, Kersten RC, Kulwin DR, et al. Management of canalicular injury associated with eyelid burns. Arch Ophthalmol 1995;113:900–3.

12. Meller D, Tseng SC. Conjunctivochalasis: Literature review and possible pathophysiology. Surv Ophthalmol 1988;43:225–32.

13. Macri A, Rolando M, Pflugfelder S. A standardized visual scale for evaluation of tear fluorescein clearance. Ophthalmology: 2000;107:1338–43.

14. Meller D, Maskin SL, Pires RT, et al. Amniotic membrane transplantation for symptomatic conjunctivochalasis refractory to medical treatments. Cornea 2000;19:796–803.

15. Nerad JA. Diagnosis and management of the patient with tearing, in Nerad JA (ed): Oculoplastic Surgery: The Requisites in Ophthalmology. St Louis, CV Mosby Co 2001;215–53.

16. Otaka I, Kyu N. A new surgical technique for management of conjunctivochalasis. Am J Ophthalmol 2000;385–7.

17. Prasad S, Kamath GG, Phillips RP. Lacrimal canalicular stenosis associated with systemic 5-fluorouacil therapy. Acta Ophthalmol Scand: 2000;78:110–3.

18. Prabhasawat P, Tseng SC. Frequent association of delayed tear clearance in ocular irritation. Br J Ophthalmol 1998;82:666–75.

19. White WL, Bartley GB, Hawes MJ, et al. Iatrogenic complications related the use of Herrick lacrimal plugs. Ophthalmology 2001;108:1085–7.

20. Wormald PJ, Tsirbas A. Investigation and endoscopic treatment for functional and anatomical obstruction of the nasolacrimal duct system. Clin Otolaryngol Allied Sci 2004;29:352–6.

21. Zapala J, Bartkowski AM, Bartkowski SB. Lacrimal drainage system obstruction: Management and Results obtained in 70 patients. J Craniomaxillofac Surg 1992;20:178–83.

Evaluation of a Case of Proptosis and Enophthalmos

Chapter Outline

PROPTOSIS
Definition and classification
- Definition
- Classification

Etiology
- Intraorbital space occupying lesions
- Causes of different clinical types of proptosis

Clinical evaluation
- History
- Clinical examination
- Systemic examination

Investigations
Laboratory investigations
- Thyroid function tests
- Haematological studies
- Urine analysis

Orbital imaging techinques
Noninvasive techniques
- Plain X-rays
- Computed tomography (CT) scanning

- Ultrasonography
- Magnetic resonance imaging (MRI)

Invasive techniques
- Contrast orbitography
- Carotid angiography

Histopathologic studies
- Fine needle aspiration biopsy
- Incisional biopsy
- Core biopsy
- Endoscopic biopsy
- Excisional biopsy

Management of proptosis
- Medical management
- Surgical management

ENOPHTHALMOS
Traumatic enophthalmos
Non-traumatic enophthalmos
- Etiology
- Clinical features
- Clinical work-up and investigations
- Management

PROPTOSIS

DEFINITION AND CLASSIFICATION

DEFINITION

Proptosis is defined as forward displacement of the eyeball beyond the orbital margins. Though the word exophthalmos (out eye) is synonymous with it; but somehow it has become customary to use the term exophthalmos for the displacement associated with thyroid eye disease and the term proptosis for protrusion of the globe secondary to lesions other than thyroid eye disease.

Unilateral proptosis is labelled when one eyeball is protuded by at least 2 mm as compared to the other normal eye.

Bilateral proptosis. Normally, the apex of cornea, in primary position, just touches or lies slightly behind the vertical line joining the superior orbital margin and inferior orbital margin at the level of centre of pupil. In normal individuals, the distance between apex of cornea and lateral orbital margin is about 20 mm (upper limit being 22 mm in Caucasians and 24 mm in African-Americans). In bilateral proptosis, the protrusion of both eyes, symmetrical or asymmetrical, occurs beyond the normal limits.

CLASSIFICATION

Proptosis can be variously classified:

I. *Depending upon laterality*
  1. Unilateral proptosis
  2. Bilateral proptosis

II. *Depending upon axiality*
  1. Axial proptosis
  2. Non-axial proptosis

III. *Depending upon specific clinical presentation*
  1. Acute proptosis
  2. Slowly progressive proptosis
  3. Intermittent proptosis
  4. Pulsating proptosis

ETIOLOGY

INTRAORBITAL SPACE OCCUPYING LESIONS

Orbital lesions cause rise of pressure within the bony orbital cavity and push the eyeball forward (producing proptosis), because this is the only way by which the pressure can be relieved. Intraorbital space occupying lesions may be classified as below:

- *Lesions from the contents of the orbit* like orbital tissue, lacrimal gland, optic nerve, blood vessels, muscles, and nerves.
- *Extension of intraocular malignancy,* e.g. retinoblastoma, malignant melanoma.

- *Invasive lesions from paraorbital regions,* e.g. paranasal sinuses, cranial cavity, nasopharynx, etc.
- *Orbital metastasis* of malignancies from other parts of the body and leukaemias.
- *Inflammations and lymphatic infiltration* of the orbital tissue.

CAUSES OF DIFFERENT CLINICAL TYPES OF PROPTOSIS

A. Causes of unilateral proptosis

1. *Congenital conditions.* These include dermoid cyst, congenital cystic eyeball, and orbital teratoma.
2. *Traumatic lesions.* These include orbital haemorrhage, retained intraorbital foreign body, traumatic aneurysm and emphysema of the orbit.
3. *Inflammatory lesions* can be acute or chronic:
   - *Acute inflammations* are orbital cellulitis, abscess, thrombophlebitis, panophthalmitis, and cavernous sinus thrombosis (proptosis is initially unilateral but ultimately becomes bilateral).
   - *Chronic inflammatory lesions* include pseudotumours, tuberculoma, gumma and sarcoidosis.
4. *Circulatory disturbances and vascular lesions,* such as angioneurotic oedema, orbital varix and aneurysms.
5. *Cysts of orbit.* These include haematic cyst, implantation cyst and parasitic cyst (hydatid cyst and cysticercus cellulosae).
6. *Tumours of the orbit.* These can be primary, secondary or metastatic (*see* page 400).
7. *Mucoceles of paranasal sinuses,* especially frontal (most common), ethmoidal and maxillary sinuses are common causes of unilateral proptosis.

Note. Most common cause of unilateral proptosis in children is orbital cellulitis and in adults is thyroid ophthalmopathy.

B. Causes of bilateral proptosis

1. *Developmental anomalies of the skull:* Craniofacial dysostosis, e.g. oxycephaly (tower skull).
2. *Osteopathies:* Osteitis deformans, rickets and acromegaly.

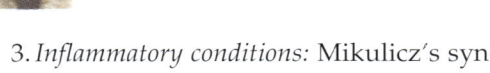

3. *Inflammatory conditions:* Mikulicz's syndrome and late stage of cavernous sinus thrombosis.
4. *Endocrinal exophthalmos:* It may be thyrotoxic or thyrotropic.
5. *Tumours:* These include symmetrical lymphoma or lymphosarcoma, secondaries from neuroblastoma, nephroblastoma, Ewing's sarcoma and leukaemic infiltration.
6. *Systemic diseases:* Histiocytosis, systemic amyloidosis, xanthomatosis and Wegener's granulomatosis.

Note. *Most common cause of bilateral proptosis* in children is neuroblastoma and leukaemia (chloroma) and in adults is thyroid ophthalmopathy.

C. Causes of acute proptosis

It develops with extreme rapidity (sudden onset). Its common causes are—orbital emphysema, fracture of the medial orbital wall, orbital haemorrhage and rupture of ethmoidal mucocele.

D. Causes of intermittent proptosis

This type of proptosis appears and disappears of its own. Its common causes are: Orbital varix, periodic orbital oedema, recurrent orbital haemorrhage and highly vascular tumours. Most important cause of intermittent proptosis is orbital varix, in which proptosis develops intermittently and rapidly in one eye when venous stasis is induced by forward bending or lowering of the head, turning the head forcefully, hyperextension of the neck, coughing, forced expiration with or without compression of the nostrils, or pressure on the jugular veins.

E. Causes of pulsatile proptosis

It is caused by pulsating vascular lesions such as caroticocavernous fistula and saccular aneurysm of ophthalmic artery. Pulsatile proptosis also occurs due to transmitted cerebral pulsations in conditions associated with deficient orbital roof. These include congenital meningocele or meningoencephalocele, neurofibromatosis and traumatic or operative hiatus.

Note. Clinical features of each cause of proptosis and enophthalmos are described in the relevant chapters.

CLINICAL EVALUATION OF PROPTOSIS

HISTORY

As in any other medical problem, the importance of accurate and painstaking history need not be overemphasized. The nature of onset of proptosis and chronology of symptoms and signs may serve as most valuable diagnostic clues to the possible nature of a lesion in the orbit. Meticulous history should provide the following useful information:

Age of onset. It is extremely important to know the age of onset, because the etiology of orbital lesions differs in infants, children, and adults.

  i. *Infants* are more likely to have congenital lesions like craniosynostosis, cephalocele, microophthalmia with cyst, teratoma (Fig. 25.1), retinoblastoma (Fig. 25.2), capillary haemangioma, juvenile xanthogranuloma, and metastatic neuroblastoma.

 ii. *Childhood orbital lesions* include dermoid cyst, lymphangioma, cavernous haemangioma, orbital varices, neurofibroma, rhabdomyosarcoma (Fig. 25.3), glioma of the optic nerve (Fig. 25.4), intraorbital meningioma, orbital cellulitis, leukaemic infiltration, granulocytic sarcoma, Burkitt's lymphoma, eosinophilic granuloma, Hand-Schuller-Christian disease, sinus histiocytosis, hydatid cyst, and fibrous dysplasia.

iii. *Adulthood orbital lesions* are secondary orbital meningioma (Fig. 25.5), thyroid exophthalmos

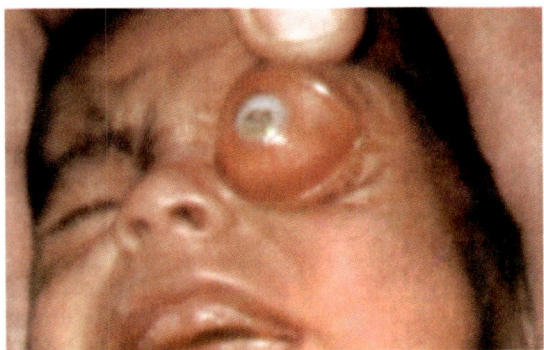

Fig. 25.1: *Congenital cystic teratoma of left orbit in a 5-day-old infant.*

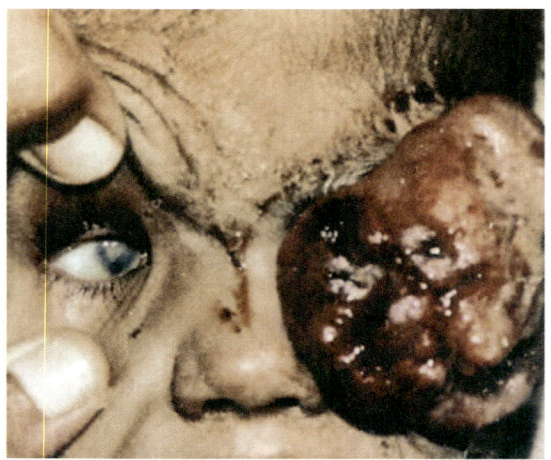

Fig. 25.2: *An extensive growth of retinoblastoma in a 3-year-old child.*

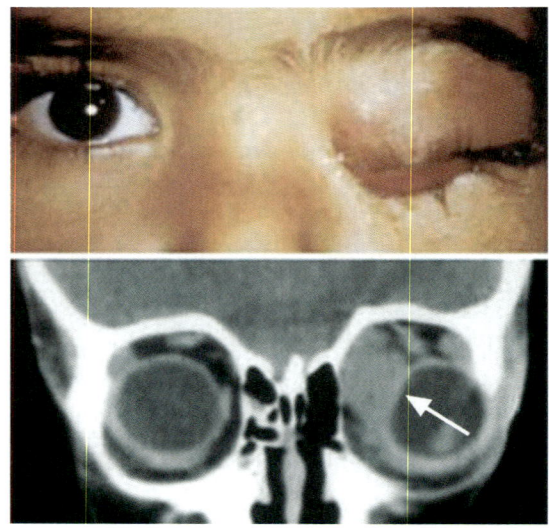

Fig. 25.3: *Proptosis in a child with rhabdomyosarcoma.*

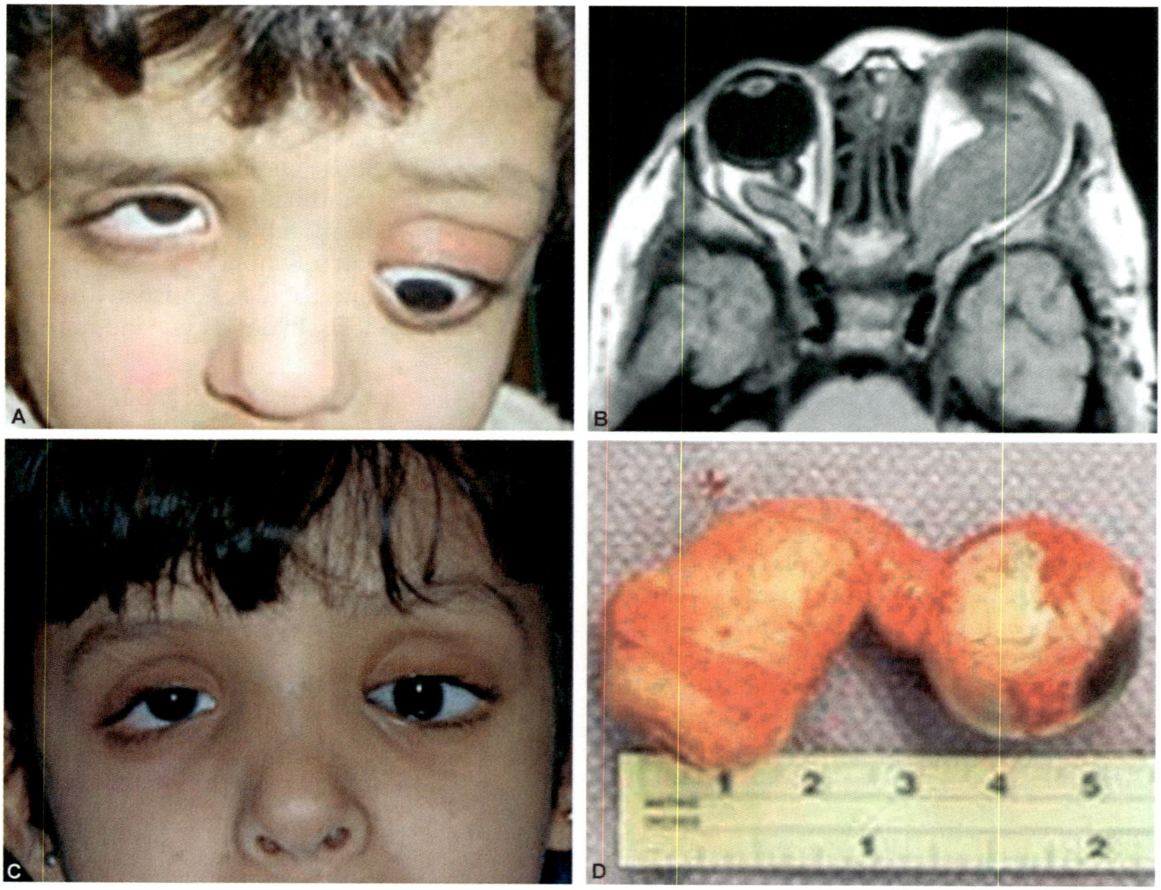

Fig. 25.4A to D: *Axial proptosis in a child with optic nerve glioma.*

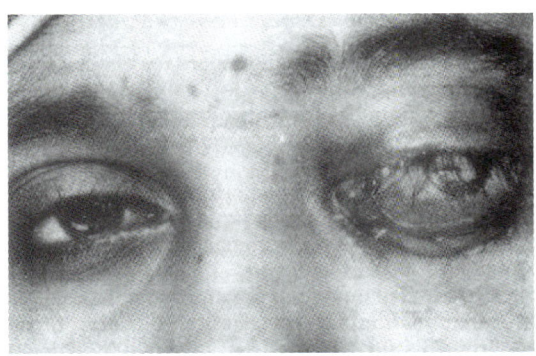

Fig. 25.5: *Secondary orbital meningioma in a 26-year-old female.*

(Fig. 25.6), pseudotumours, lymphoproli-ferative disorders, fibrous histiocytoma, haemangiopericytoma, cavernous haeman-gioma, neurilemmoma, osteoma, mucocele, circulatory disturbances (orbital varices, venous thrombosis, cavernous sinus arteriovenous fistula), orbital involvement secondary to neoplasms arising from adjacent or nearby structures (such as extensions from uveal malignant melanoma), extension from tumours of the lids (such as squamous cell carcinoma, basal cell carcinoma, and sebaceous gland carcinoma), extension from the paranasal sinuses, nasopharynx and cranial cavity, metastatic carcinoma of the orbit, and lesions of lacrimal gland.

Nature of onset. This also provides some important clues for diagnosis, e.g.

• *Proptosis of sudden onset* is seen in orbital emphysema, retrobulbar haemorrhage,

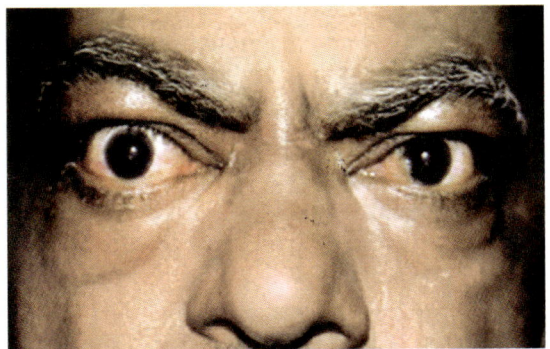

Fig. 25.6: *Bilateral exophthalmos with asymmetric retraction of eyelids.*

rupture and infection of ethmoidal mucocele and acute orbital infections.
• *Proptosis with gradual onset* indicates benign tumours.
• *Rapidly progressive proptosis* is seen in rapidly expanding orbital masses such as rhabdomyo-sarcoma, neuroblastoma, Burkitt's lymphoma, eosinophilic granuloma, capillary haeman-gioma, lymphangioma and traumatic haematoma.

Duration. Long-standing and slowly-progressive lesions are usually benign in nature and malignant lesions are usually of short duration.

Progression pattern of proptosis gives important clues:
• *Continuous progression* is noted in tumours and endocrine exophthalmos.
• *Intermittent postural proptosis* (which dis-appears and reappears) is observed in orbital varices and in 20% cases of angiomas.
• *Variable proptosis* which persists but varies from time-to-time is usually seen in pseudo-tumours and angiomas.
• *Pulsatile proptosis* is a typical feature of arteriovenous aneurysms and cranio-orbital communications.

Chronology of appearance of symptoms. This may also be helpful in localization, e.g. *visual loss followed by proptosis* in a child indicates optic nerve glioma; while reverse chronology, i.e. *proptosis followed by visual loss*, indicates meningioma of optic nerve in adults.

Pain. The painful proptosis occurs in:
• Orbital inflammatory disorders
• Traumatic cases with orbital haematoma
• Later stages of malignancy.

Diplopia. It is a common symptom in orbital disorders related to paralysis of the extraocular muscles or mechanical restriction of ocular movements, as below:
• *Lesions residing in the cavernous sinus or posterior orbit* are responsible for paralytic abnormalities of ocular movements.
• *Anterior orbital lesions* produce diplopia by means of a mechanical restriction caused by lesions that are immediately adjacent to the extraocular muscles.

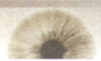

- *Diseases that involve the muscle tissue* include myositis and Graves' disease.

Visual loss. Loss of visual acuity usually implies involvement of optic nerve, either by compression, infiltration, vascular compromise, or inflammation. Relation of visual loss in a patient with proptosis with the nature of lesion may be as below:

- *Marked proptosis with no visual loss* is seen in cavernous haemangioma and neurilemmoma
- *Marked visual loss with mild to moderate proptosis* is observed in optic nerve tumours like optic nerve glioma and optic nerve sheath meningioma.

Lid oedema is a common feature of orbital inflammations and pseudotumours.

History of thyroid disorder may be of particular importance in endocrinal proptosis.

CLINICAL EXAMINATION

Inspection

This is simple but most valuable in eliciting several signs. In many cases, diagnosis may become apparent by careful observation alone. On inspection, following observations should be made:

True proptosis versus pseudoproptosis

Pseudoproptosis is a condition in which the eyeball appears to be proptosed but actually there is no forward displacement.

Causes of pseudoproptosis are:
- Enlargement of the ipsilateral eye as in buphthalmos and high axial myopia
- Enophthalmos of the opposite eye
- Retraction of the upper eyelid on the ipsilateral side
- Shallow orbit (as in craniofacial dysostosis or facial asymmetry).

Unilateral versus bilateral proptosis

Causes of unilateral proptosis
See page 490.

Causes of bilateral proptosis
See page 490.

Axial versus nonaxial proptosis

Axial proptosis usually indicates a mass inside the muscle cone, e.g. optic nerve glioma (Fig. 25.7), haemangioma, meningioma, Schwannoma and metastatic tumours (from carcinoma of breast, lung and prostate).

Non-axial proptosis usually indicates a mass in the peripheral space causing displacement of globe medially, laterally, superiorly or inferiorly, e.g.
- *Proptosis with lateral displacement of globe* is characteristic of ethmoidal sinus mucocele (Fig. 25.8).
- *Proptosis with downward and nasal displacement of globe* suggests a possible mass in the lacrimal fossa.
- *Proptosis with superior displacement of the globe* is a feature of lesion near the orbital floor such as growth in maxillary sinus (Fig. 25.9).

Associated lid signs

Lid signs also provide some diagnostic clues. For example:
- *Swelling of lids associated with ecchymosis of skin* and chemosis of conjunctiva may be seen in orbital cellulitis (Fig. 25.10).

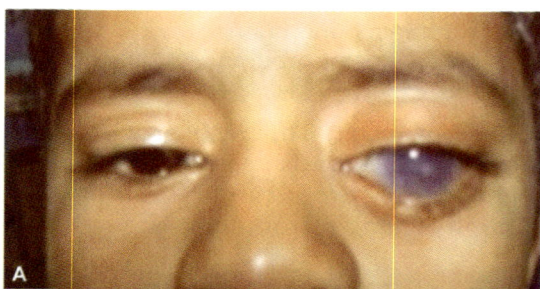
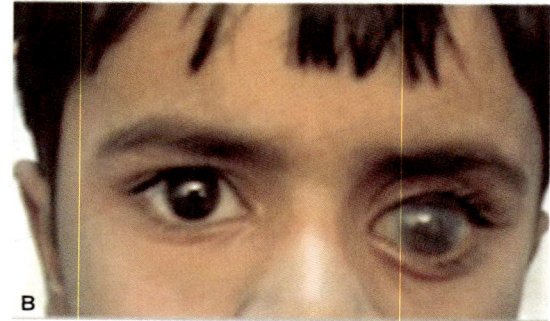

Fig. 25.7: *Appearance of pseudoproptosis due to ipsilateral lid retraction.*

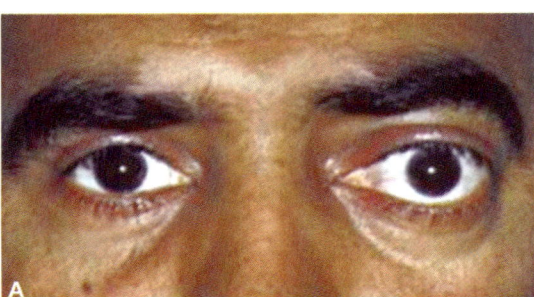

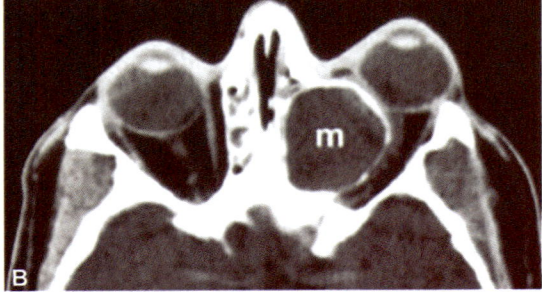

Fig. 25.8A and B: *Mucocele of left ethmoid sinus. Eyeball is displaced laterally.*

position of apex of cornea on each side (Fig. 25.11).
• Patient bends his head forward and cornea should disappear at the same time.

Other observations

Rest of the body surface should be inspected for related skin disturbances, such as haemangioma, melanoma, other metastatic lesions, or the diagnostic cafe-au-lait spots associated with neurofibromatosis.

Palpation

Palpation of the following structures should be done:

I. Retro-displacement/retropulsion of the globe should be estimated by applying equal digital pressure over the two eyes, simultaneously. This is best done with the examiner's thumb over the closed lids.
• *Retro-ocular resistance* is encountered in the presence of solid tumours.

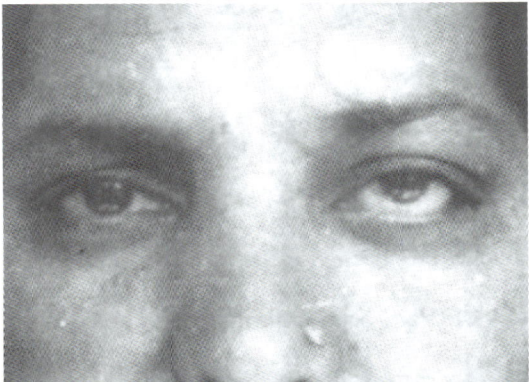

Fig. 25.9: *Proptosis in a 38-year-old female with carcinoma of left maxillary antrum. Eyeball is pushed superiorly.*

• *In the presence of stare and lidlag,* the possibility of proptosis of neoplastic cause can be ruled out.

Inspection for proptosis by Naffziger's method
• Patient sits in front of examiner, head slightly drawn back and looks downwards.
• Examiner stands behind the patient, looks over patient's forehead by bending over the patient's head.
• Examiner raises patient's upper lids with his index fingers from the sides and compares

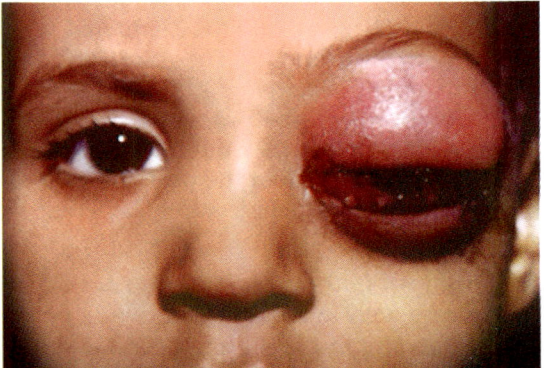

Fig. 25.10: *Orbital cellulitis in a 3-year-old female child.*

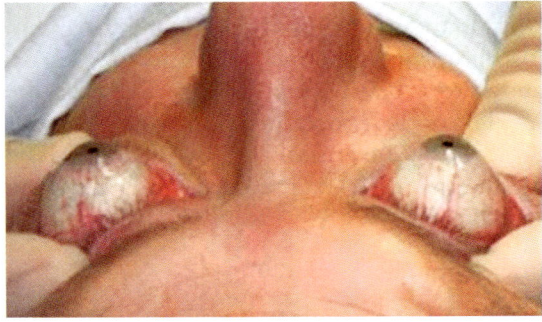

Fig. 25.11: *Naffziger's test for detection of proptosis.*

- *Compressibility* is increased where soft and vascular tumours are present.
- *Any pulsation of the globe* may be confirmed by palpation.
- *Thrill* when present may also be felt in highly vascular tumours.

II. *Palpation of the orbital rims* should be done to note any change in contour or dehiscence of any orbital wall.

III. *Localizing anterior masses.* Palpation of the orbit should be carried out between the globe and the bony orbital rims in all the quadrants. The findings should be compared with the other side in unilateral cases to distinguish between normal and abnormal findings. While palpating a particular quadrant, patient should be instructed to look in the same direction. This gives better access due to relaxation of the orbital septum.

Finger insinuation test can be done by trying to insinuate little finger between the mass and the orbital margin. Patient is asked to look in direction of opposite quadrant, i.e. away from the quadrant being tested.

IV. *Regional lymph nodes to be palpated* are the preauricular lymph nodes. These are the first site of involvement in anterior extension of either infectious or neoplastic processes. In addition, other nearby nodes that might participate in metastatic diseases from the orbits should also be palpated. These include supraclavicular and cervical nodes.

V. *Paranasal (paraorbital) sinuses lend themselves* very well to palpation or gentle percussion, especially in the search for inflammatory disturbances involving both sinuses and orbits.

Auscultation

Auscultation is primarily of value in searching for abnormal vascular communications that generate a bruit, such as carotid cavernous fistula, arteriovenous aneurysm in orbit, etc. The orbit should be auscultated by placing the bell of stethoscope over the closed lids in a quiet room.

Transillumination

Though deep orbital lesions do not lend themselves to transillumination, this modality is often forgotten even in evaluation of anterior orbital or lid lesions. Transillumination of the lids may help to differentiate between solid and cystic lesions and may also reveal certain radiolucent foreign bodies. **Transillumination is useful in unilateral proptosis of elderly persons. A flat sarcoma of the choroid may present as exophthalmos due to early perivascular extraocular extension.**

Ocular examinations

Visual acuity. Any loss of vision preceding exophthalmos suggests tumour of the optic nerve, e.g. glioma in children. Orbital tumours may reduce central acuity of vision by pressing on the back of eyeball producing changes in refraction or Sallman's macular folds. Optic atrophy is responsible for loss of vision in late cases.

Pupillary reactions. Presence of Marcus Gunn pupil is suggestive of optic nerve compression and is an indication for plotting the visual fields in both eyes.

Fundoscopy. Venous engorgement, haemorrhage, papilloedema or optic atrophy may be observed on fundoscopy. These changes are caused by raised intraorbital pressure. Choroidal folds and optociliary shunts may be seen in patients having meningioma.

Ocular motility. Limitation of ocular movements may be caused by restrictive myopathy as in thyroid ophthalmopathy, splinting of the optic nerve as in optic nerve sheath meningioma and neurological deficit resulting from orbital apex lesions.

Forced duction test. This test is done to differentiate defective ocular movements due to neurological lesions from those caused by mechanical restriction. The test is positive when there is mechanical restriction of ocular movements as in fibrotic contracture (thyroid myopathy) and involvement of muscles in malignant growths. It is negative, if the muscle is paretic due to neurological lesions.

Tonometry. Orbital disease may cause raised intraocular pressure. It is usually raised in cases of thyroid exophthalmos especially in upward gaze (positional IOP) changes.

Braley's sign. On upward excursion, tight inferior rectus compresses the globe, causing elevation in intraocular pressure, known as Braley's sign.

Increase in IOP, more than 6 mm Hg, signifies glaucoma.

Increase in IOP, more than 9 mm Hg, signifies optic nerve compression.

Measurement of proptosis

Exophthalmometry (proptometry)

Exophthalmometry measures the protrusion of the apex of cornea from the outer orbital margin (with the eyes looking straight ahead).

- *Absolute exophthalmometry* compares the results of measurement to known normal values which vary between 10 and 20 mm, average range being 16–20 mm (Fig. 25.12), and usually <20 mm is normal. It is not of much clinical significance.

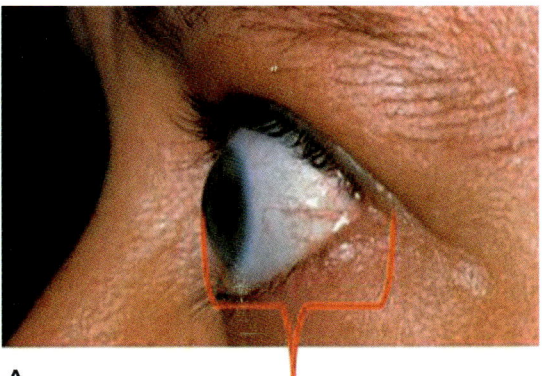

A

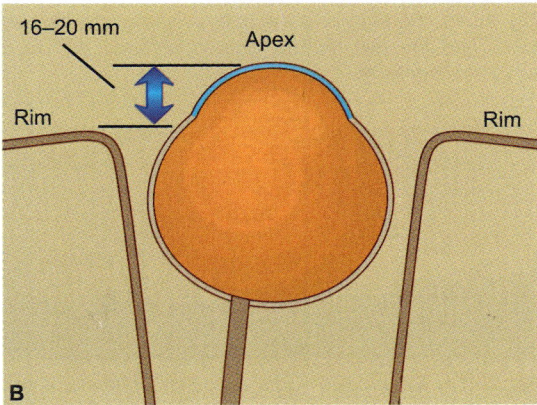

B

Fig. 25.12A and B: *Depicting normal distance from lateral orbital rim to anterior corneal surface or apex (<20 mm).*

- *Relative exophthalmometry* compares results of the two eyes and a difference of more than 2 mm is considered significant. This method is essential to establish the presence of proptosis. Since, the estimation of unilateral proptosis is usually relative to the supposed to be normal other eye, one must not overlook the possibility of natural asymmetry, unequal bilateral proptosis or contralateral enophthalmos.
- *Comparative exophthalmometry* is a follow-up study of proptosis to compare the progress of the disease on subsequent visits.
- *Postural exophthalmometry* changes are diagnostic in Graves' ophthalmopathy.

Common exophthalmometers available include:

1. Luedde's exophthalmometer (Fig. 25.13). It is the simplest form. This is made up of a thick transparent plastic material with a groove which fits into the outer bony margin of the orbit. A scale is engraved on both sides and the observing eye is aligned with them to read off the level of the apex of the cornea.

2. Hertel's exophthalmometer (Fig. 25.14). It is the most commonly used instrument. Its advantage is that it measures the prominence of the two eyes (from the lateral orbit rim), simultaneously.

Technique of Hertel's exophthalmometry is as below:

- Patient is made to sit comfortably with same eye level as that of examiner and asked to close his eyes.

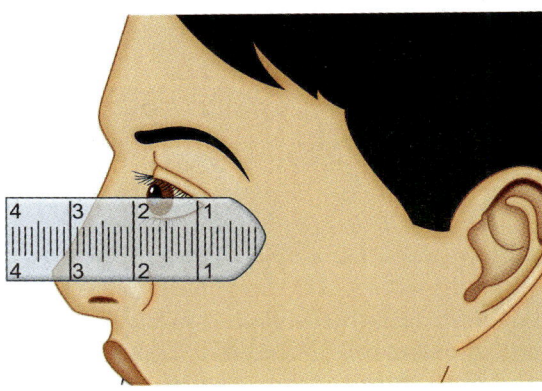

Fig. 25.13: *Luedde's exophthalmometer.*

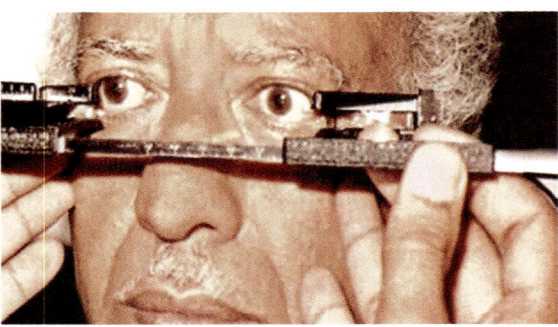

Fig. 25.14: *Simultaneous bilateral exophthalmometry with Hertel's exophthalmometer.*

- The examiner then locates the orbital notch on the temporal side of the orbit with his index finger.
- The exophthalmometer is placed in such a way that its grooved arcs on each end fit into the lateral orbital notches.
- Separation of the exophthalmometer is very important; constant separation reading must be documented as baseline for subsequent measurements (Fig. 25.15).

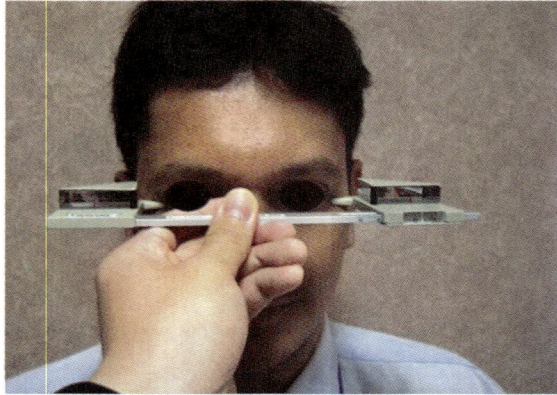

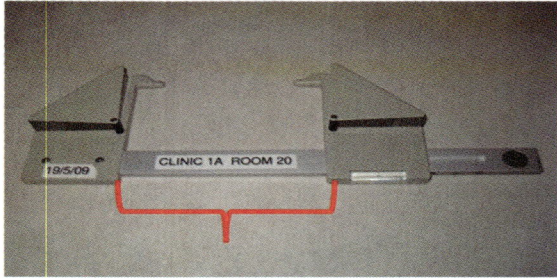

Fig. 25.15: *Constant separation reading in Hertel's exophthalmometer.*

- The patient is then told to open his eyes and look straight towards examiner's closed eye. Poor fixation, convergence, parallax errors, and head movements will affect accuracy of the readings.
- Examiner then looks into the 2 mirrors located at each end of the exophthalmometer (Fig. 25.16). Reading is noted where the apex of cornea in the lower mirror aligns with the measuring scale when the ×2 red lines in the upper mirror are superimposed on each other (Fig. 25.17).

3. Mutch exophthalmometer. It measures each eye separately with the cheek or brow as reference point. It is useful in cases of orbital fractures, etc.

4. Two-scale proptometry. Two-scale proptometry is an easily available and handy method of measuring proptosis. Proptosis can be measured by using 2 scales, one placed at the canthus and the other perpendicular to it, at the level where the apex of cornea coincides.

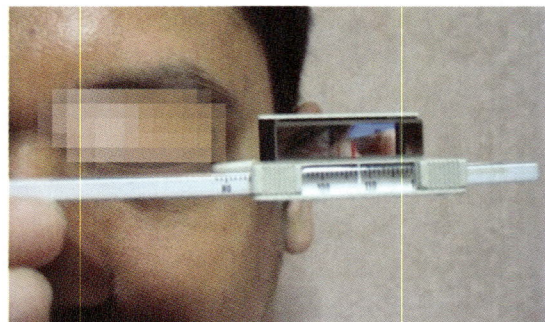

Fig. 25.16: *During Hertel's exophthalometry, the examiner looks into the two mirrors located at each end of the exophthalmometer.*

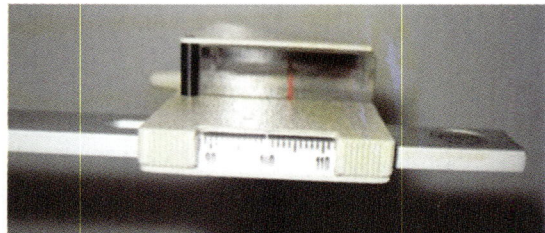

Fig. 25.17: *Reading on Hertel's exophthalmometer is noted where the apex of cornea in the lower mirror align with the measuring scale when the x2 red lines in the upper mirror are superimposed on each other.*

SYSTEMIC EXAMINATION

General systemic examination should be conducted to rule out proptosis (especially when bilateral) associated with systemic diseases such as amyloidosis, histiocytosis or Wegener's granulomatosis.

Thyroid area examination. Since endocrine dysfunction is the most common cause of unilateral as well as bilateral proptosis, *thyroid* evaluation is important in all cases.

Search for primary neoplasm elsewhere in the body whenever metastatic deposits are suspected in the orbit is also essential. The metastatic neoplasms of the orbit are predominantly carcinomas from the breast, lung, stomach, thyroid, kidney, prostate or adrenals. **The second most common metastatic tumour of the orbit is neuroblastoma.** Other metastatic tumours are malignant melanoma, haemangiopericytoma, and Ewing's sarcoma (Fig. 25.18).

Otolaryngological examination is necessary when the paranasal sinus (Fig. 25.19) or a nasopharyngeal mass appears to be a possible etiological factor in producing proptosis.

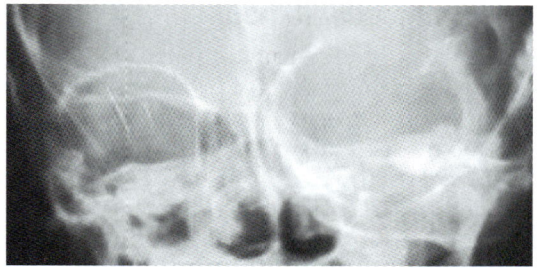

Fig. 25.19: *Enlargement of left orbit in a case of congenital teratoma.*

INVESTIGATIONS FOR PROPTOSIS

LABORATORY INVESTIGATIONS

Thyroid function tests. Extimation of protein bound iodine (PBI), radioactive iodine uptake (RAIU), serum TSH, T3, T4 levels, effective thyroxine ratio (ETR), and thyroid scanning may be necessary when thyroid eye disease (TED) is suspected.

Haematological studies TLC and DLC help in diagnosis of inflammatory lesions or blood dyscrasias, e.g. leukaemias. Relative eosinophilia may indicate hydatid cyst. Casoni's test is done to exclude hydatid disease, but is of value in 50% of cases only.

Urine analysis. Urine analysis for Bence Jones protein may reveal multiple myeloma.

ORBITAL IMAGING TECHNIQUES

Even after a thorough and meticulous clinical examination, the diagnosis of orbital diseases is not clear many a times. Therefore, special investigations are often required in a case of proptosis, which in addition to helping in diagnosis are also useful in planning the management of orbital lesions. Imaging techniques for orbital lesions include noninvasive and invasive techniques.

NONINVASIVE IMAGING TECHNIQUES

- X-rays examination
- Computerized tomography (CT) scanning
- Orbital ultrasonography
- Magnetic resonance imaging (MRI).

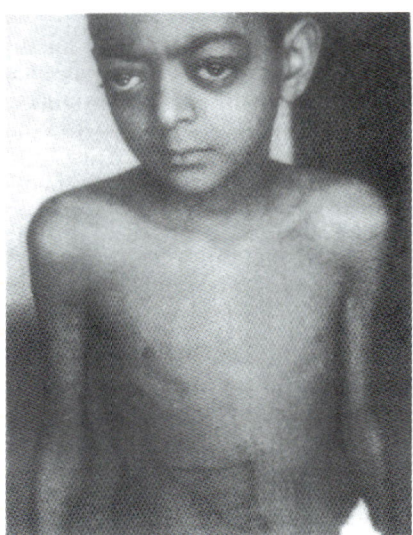

Fig. 25.18: *Bilateral proptosis due to metastatic Ewing's sarcoma in a 12-year-old emaciated child with markings for radiotherapy of primary Ewing's sarcoma of the right iliac crest.*

PLAIN X-RAYS EXAMINATION

Plain X-rays of the orbit are useful to diagnose most extraorbital causes of proptosis. In evaluation of an orbital lesion, a plain skiagram of orbit was the most frequently used investigation till recent past. However, presently CT scan has reduced the role of plain X-ray. The following exposures are frequently required:

I. *Caldwell view* is valuable and frequently employed view for detection of orbital lesions. The skiagram is taken with the patient's nose and forehead touching the film. The beam is angled at about 25° so that the petrous pyramids do not obscure orbital details. This view demonstrates the superior orbital fissure, the greater and lesser wings of the sphenoid bone, the floor of the sella turcica, ethmoid and frontal sinuses, and the innominate or oblique orbital line.

II. *Water view* provides excellent details of the maxillary sinuses, zygomatic arches, and orbits (particularly the orbital rim and roof). This view is obtained with the patient's chin touching the film and nose raised off the film by 2–3 centimetres.

III. *Lateral view* generally shows the anterior clinoid processes, the sella turcica, and the sphenoid sinus clearly.

IV. *Rhese view* is a special projection used to visualize the optic foramina. Views of both optic foramina, preferably on a single film should be obtained for comparison of symmetry and size.

V. *Some other projections* may be helpful but are not usually a part of routine orbital series.

These radiological views provide finite diagnostic information in approximately 50% of orbital cases. The positive yield from such studies is greatly increased by the following dictum: "The roentgenologist should see the patient and the ophthalmologist must see the film."

Commonly observed X-ray signs of orbital diseases

Size of the orbit. Enlargement of the orbit (Fig. 25.19) is not an uncommon finding in orbital space occupying lesions. In infants and children, orbital enlargement occurs within 1 to 3 months while in adults it is a sign of a long-standing benign tumours (1–3 years duration).

   i. *Symmetrical enlargement of the orbit* is observed in mass lesions of the muscle cone (intraconal lesions) like optic nerve glioma, haemangioma, and neurofibroma. Occasionally it may also be seen in pseudotumour and retinoblastoma that extend into the muscle cone.

  ii. *Asymmetrical orbital enlargement* is a sign of extraconal tumours like rhabdomyosarcoma, lacrimal gland tumour, dermoid cyst, haemangioma, etc.

Change in bone density. Increased bone density is observed in sphenoidal ridge meningioma, chronic periosteitis, fibrous dysplasia, Paget's disease, and osteoblastic metastasis.

   i. *Localized decreased density/indentation* of the orbital wall is observed in benign tumours such as dermoid and mixed cell lacrimal gland tumour.

  ii. *Diffuse bony destruction* may signify malignant tumours like lacrimal gland carcinoma and spread of tumours from paranasal sinuses.

Change in orbital shape. This is usually due to fossa formation, as a result of local expansion of the orbital wall. It occurs in orbital dermoids and encapsulated lacrimal gland tumours.

Dehiscence of orbital bones. This may be observed in lesions like mucocele of paranasal sinuses, aneurysm, neurofibroma, lacrimal gland tumours, and fractures.

Intraorbital calcification. This may occur in many lesions such as retinoblastoma (fine-stippled calcification), optic nerve sheath meningioma, lacrimal gland carcinoma, orbital varix (phlebolith), mucocele, parasitic cyst (hydatid cyst), aneurysm, haematoma, and phthisical eyes (Fig. 25.20). Calcified intracranial lesions that may rarely have associated orbital or intraocular lesions are toxoplasmosis, tuberous sclerosis. Sturge-Weber syndrome, and von Hipple-Lindau disease. Actual ossification due to metaplasia of ocular tissue is rarely seen.

Enlargement of superior orbital fissure. This is a classical diagnostic sign of infraclinoid carotid

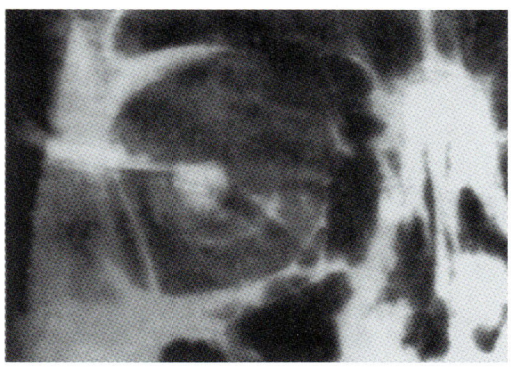

Fig. 25.20: *Calcification in a phthisical eye.*

aneurysms (75% of cases), and therefore, calls for an early carotid angiography. Other causes of widening of superior orbital fissure include intracavenous aneurysm, intracranial extension of orbital tumours, extraseller extension of pituitary tumours, and meningiomas.

Changes in optic canal: Normal adult dimensions of optic canal are reached by the age of 4 to 5 years and its standard size is 4 to 6 mm. Measurements of 7 mm or more are always pathological. However, it is to be stressed that one should always compare the two before giving final verdict on the size of the optic foramina. In normal subjects, the diameter of the two canals should not differ by more than 1 mm.

i. *Uniform regular concentric enlargement* of the optic canal is seen typically in cases of optic nerve glioma (Fig. 25.21).

ii. *Uniform irregular enlargement* may be observed in meningioma of the optic nerve sheath, retinoblastoma, and orbital neurofibromas.

iii. *Erosion of its inferolateral margin* is a sign of infraclinoid lesions such as aneurysms and meningiomas.

iv. *Erosion of its upper margin* is a sign of raised intracranial pressure.

v. *Total destruction of the margins* indicates some malignant neoplasm arising from one of the paranasal sinuses.

vi. *Narrowing and hyperostosis around the optic foramina* may be observed in meningioma en plaque, occasionally.

COMPUTERIZED TOMOGRAPHY SCANNING (CT SCAN)

CT scanning is most valuable, noninvasive method employed in the diagnosis of orbital and related lesions. It uses thin X-ray beams to obtain tissue density values. These values are processed by a computer to provide detailed cross-sectional images. The advent of CT scanning has transformed the investigation of orbital disorders. A combination of axial (CAT) and coronal cuts (CCT) enables a space occupying lesion within the orbit to be visualized in three dimensions. CT scan with contrast medium may further enhance the radiographic shadow of some orbital tumours. CT scanning is, therefore, extremely useful for determining the location and size of a space occupying orbital lesion. Its main disadvantage is its inability to distinguish between pathological soft tissue masses which are radiologically isodense.

Advantage of CT scan is that it is capable of visualizing various structures like globe, extraocular muscles (Fig. 25.22), and the optic nerves (from retroocular space to optic canal). This technique is also useful in examining areas adjacent to the orbit, that is, orbital walls and

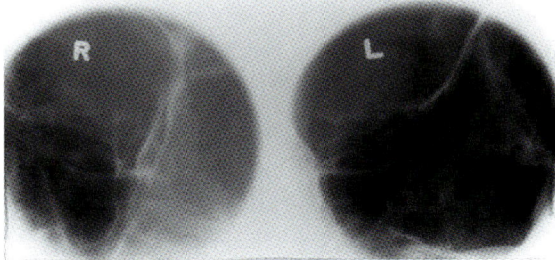

Fig. 25.21: *Enlargement of right optic foramen (R).*

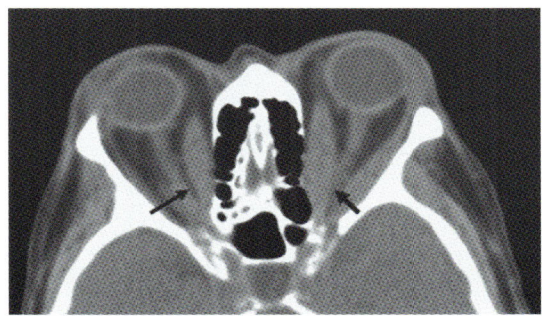

Fig. 25.22: *Thickened extraocular muscles in a case of Graves' ophthalmopathy.*

intracranial structures, if there is a suspicion of diseases such as meningioma (Figs 25.23 to 25.25), optic nerve glioma (Fig. 25.26) or metastasis (Fig. 25.27). Because of these advantages, CT scan has become the single most important investigation for a case of proptosis; and has almost replaced the plain X-rays.

Measurement of proptosis on CT scan

Requirements for reliable assessment of proptosis on CT scan include:

- Plane of the scan must be parallel to the plane passing through the optic nerve head and lens.
- Eyelids must be open, with the patient looking straight ahead.

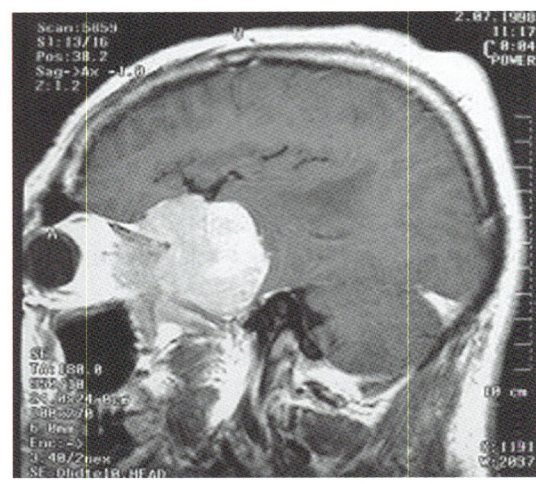

Fig. 25.25: *Extensive bone destruction in a case of sphenoidal ridge meningioma.*

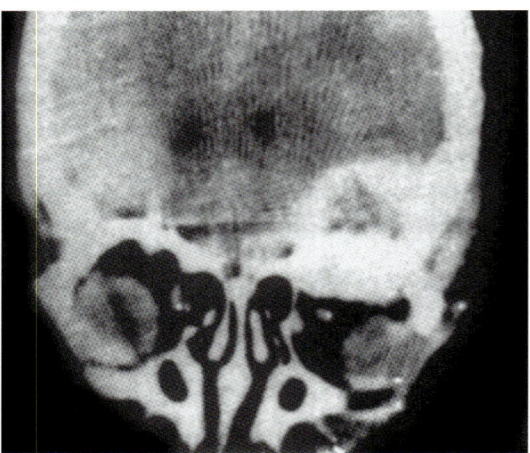

Fig. 25.23: *Sphenoidal ridge meningioma invading left orbit and temporal region; coronal section.*

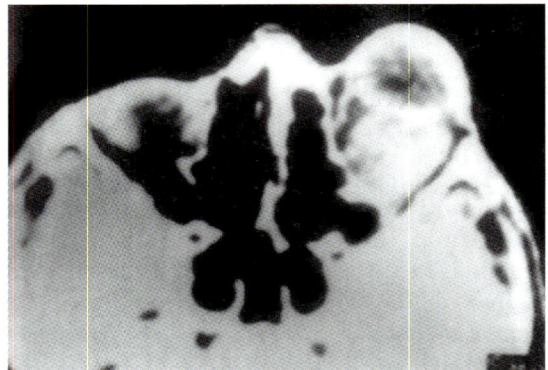

Fig. 25.26: *Very large optic nerve glioma. Note marked proptosis of right eye.*

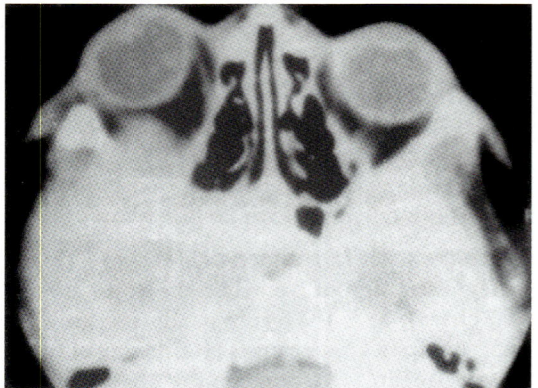

Fig. 25.24: *Sphenoidal ridge meningioma invading left orbit and temporal region; axial section.*

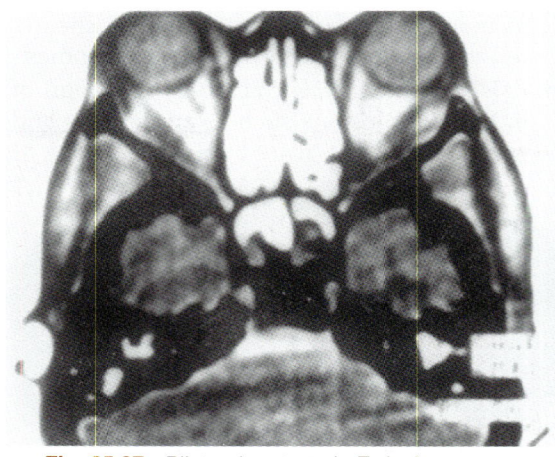

Fig. 25.27: *Bilateral metastatic Ewing's sarcoma.*

Methods of measuring proptosis on CT scan

On CT scan, proptosis can be measured by following methods:

1. *By measuring distance from the anterior corneal surface to interzygomatic line (IZL).* A line between the bony lateral orbital margins drawn on the slice containing the optic nerve head and lens, and the distance of the cornea in front of this line is measured (Fig. 25.28).

2. *Distance from posterior scleral margin (PSM) to interzygomatic line (IZL)* can also be used to measure proptosis. Fig. 21.29A depicts distance between PSM and IZL in a normal patient; which is decreased in a patient with proptosis (Fig. 25.29B).

ULTRASONOGRAPHY

It is a nonradiational, noninvasive, well-tolerated, completely safe technique, and is of particular value as an initial scanning procedure. A-scan produces a unidimensional image and echoes are plotted as spikes. B-scan produces a two-dimensional dotted picture of orbital structures; thus, the latter gives an anatomical display which is much easier for the nonexpert to interpret. C-scan is useful for visualizing soft tissue of the orbit in the coronal plane. In the diagnosis of orbital lesions, ultrasonography is superior to CT scanning in actual tissue diagnosis. It can usually differentiate vascular lesions from metastatic or inflammatory pseudotumour. It is, however, less useful than CT scanning in the evaluation of lesions against bony structures at the apex of the orbit.

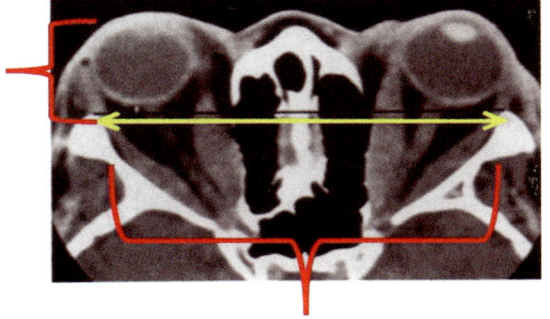

Fig. 25.28: *Measurement of proptosis on CT scan by the distance from the anterior corneal surface to interzygomatic line.*

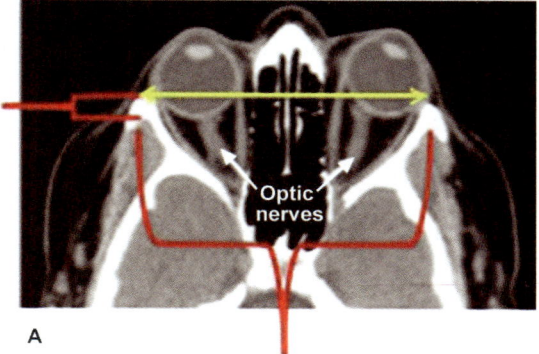

A

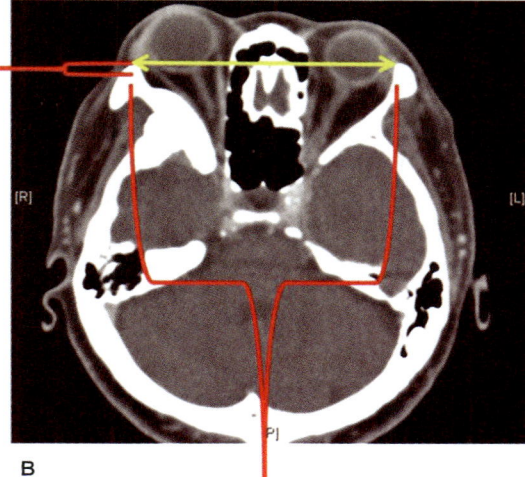

B

Fig. 25.29: *Measuring proptosis from distance between posterior scleral margin and interzygomatic line. (A) Normal person; (B) Patient with proptosis.*

The ultrasonographic patterns of pathological lesions depend mainly on the displacement of the orbital fat. Differential diagnosis is usually based on the patterns of sound reflectivity at the surfaces of the mass and the transmission characteristics of the sound wave as it passes through the lesions. From these, the surface of the mass can be classified as smooth or irregular and, the character of the mass can be sub-classified as solid, cystic, vascular or infiltrative. Commonly observed ultrasonic patterns are discussed below.

Normal echo pattern

When the scan passes through the plane of the optic nerve, the normal echo pattern appears as a W-shaped acoustically opaque area (Fig. 25.30).

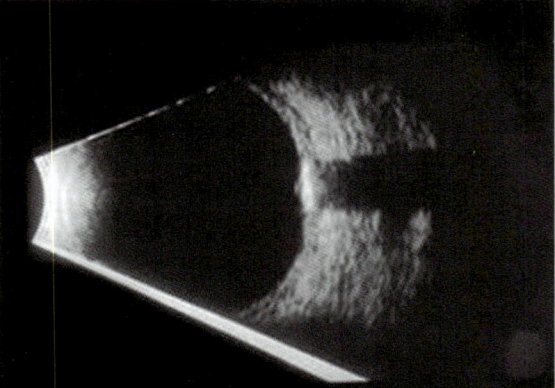

Fig. 25.30: *Ultrasonic pattern (B-scan) of normal orbit at optic nerve plane. Note W-shaped acoustically opaque area.*

Anteriorly, it is separated from the globe by a concavity; and posteriorly it is bounded by an empty notch formed by the optic nerve. The retrobulbar fat pattern is bounded nasally and temporally by the rectus muscles.

Echo pattern in mass lesions

Ultrasonographically, mass lesions of the orbit can be differentiated into the following main groups:

- *Cystic swellings* of the orbit such as mucocele and dermoid cysts are characterized by sharply defined round borders with good sound transmission and no internal reflection, as they are homogenous and fluid filled (Fig. 25.31A).

- *Solid tumours* of the orbit also have round well-outlined borders, but a poor sound transmission and variable encapsulated neurolemmoma, optic nerve glioma, (Fig. 25.31B) and primary orbital meningioma.

- *Spongy lesions* of the orbit, like haemangioma, are diagnosed from irregular shape, good sound transmission, and strong internal echoes from connective tissue septa. Compression of the orbit with the examining probe often demonstrates a spongy consistency (Fig. 25.31C).

- *Infiltrating orbital lesions,* like pseudotumours, lymphangioma, malignant lymphoma and metastatic carcinoma, exhibit irregular variable shape, poor sound transmission, and minimal internal echoes due to homogenous infiltrating tissue (Fig. 25.31D).

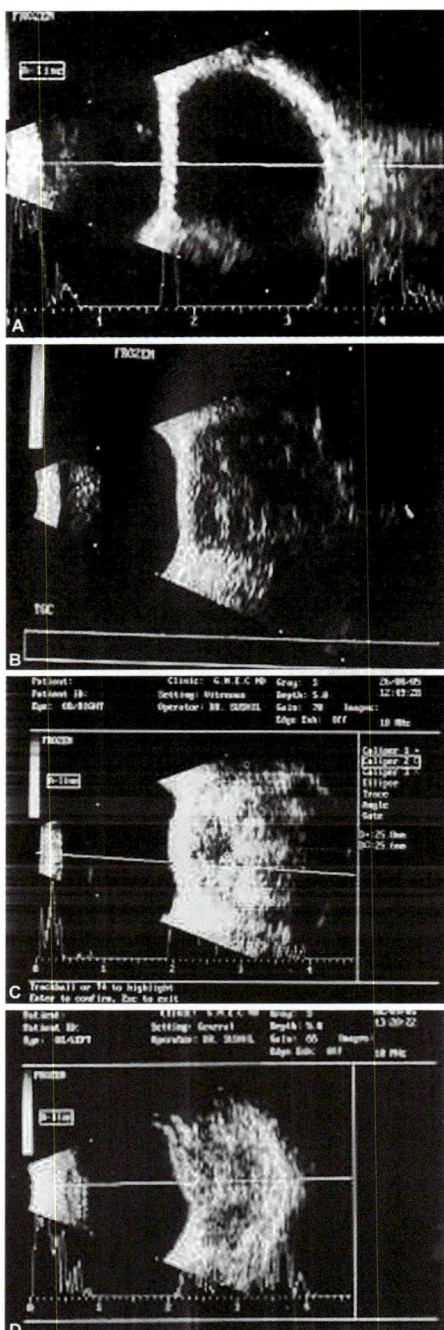

Fig. 25.31: *Ultrasonic pattern (B-scan) of orbital lesion (diagrammatic). (A) Cystic orbital mass having round borders, good transmission and no internal echoes; (B) solid orbital tumour (optic nerve glioma); (C) spongy tumour exhibiting irregular shape, good transmission, and strong internal echoes; and (D) infiltrating lesion, having irregular shape, poor transmission, and minimal internal echoes.*

Ultrasonography in Graves' ophthalmopathy

This is very helpful in diagnosing early cases without manifesting clinical signs of proptosis and in picking up bilateral changes in apparently unilateral cases. The characteristic feature is thickening of extraocular muscles (Fig. 25.32). Usually, the medial rectus is the first muscle to enlarge. **Normal thickness of extraocular muscle in Indians is 3–4 mm.** In Indian population, extraocular muscle thickness is as follows: Inferior rectus> superior rectus>medial rectus>lateral rectus. In addition to enlargement of extraocular muscles, erosion of the temporal wall of the orbit, accentuation of retrobulbar fat, and perineural inflammation of the optic nerve on B-scan, have also been demonstrated in early Graves' ophthalmopathy.

Ultrasonic features of orbital foreign bodies

Localization of orbital foreign bodies by B-scan is difficult, as often these are lost in the highly reflective fatty tissue at high sensitivity settings. The demonstration of a trail of reduplication echoes behind the foreign body is often the first clue of its presence (Fig. 25.33). Reduction of sensitivity is helpful in differentiating stronger foreign body echoes from those of orbital tissue.

Echo pattern in acute inflammation of the orbit. With acute inflammation of the ocular wall or anterior orbit, oedema fluid often collects beneath Tenon's capsule. On ultrasonography, this accumulation of fluid can be easily detected as an echo-free space just outside the strong scleral reflection (Fig. 25.34).

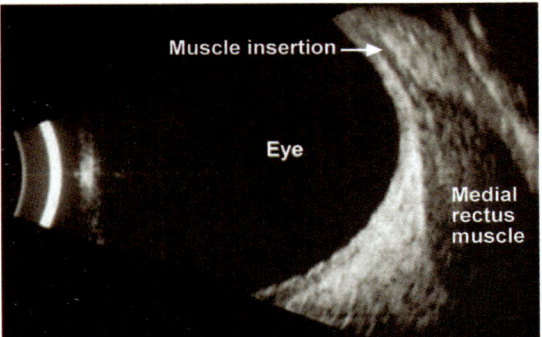

Fig. 25.32: *B-scan ultrasonography in a patient with thyroid eye disease depicting thickening of medial rectus muscle.*

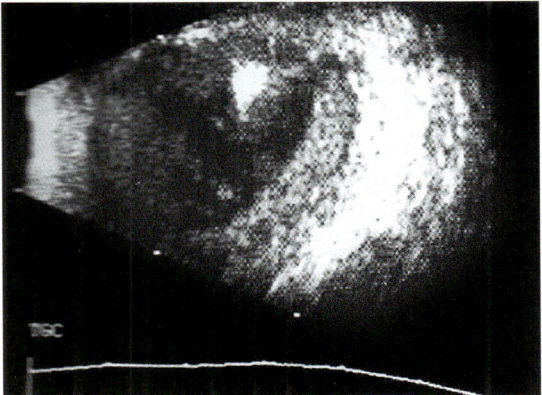

Fig. 25.33: *B-scan ultrasonography in a patient with intraorbital foreign body.*

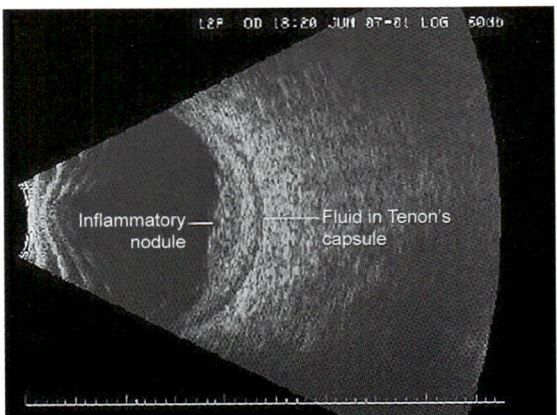

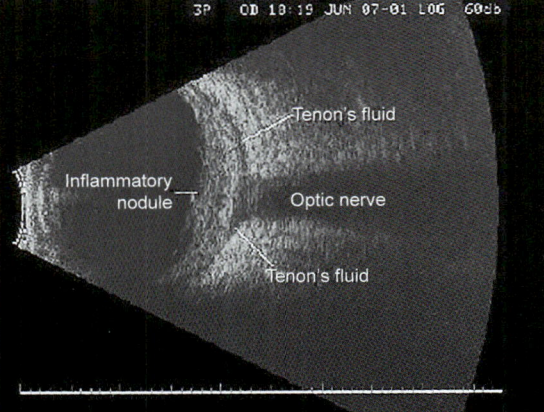

Fig. 25.34: *Ultrasonic pattern (B-scan) (diagrammatic) depicting fluid accumulation within Tenon's capsule and perioptic nerve swelling in a case of acute orbital inflammation.*

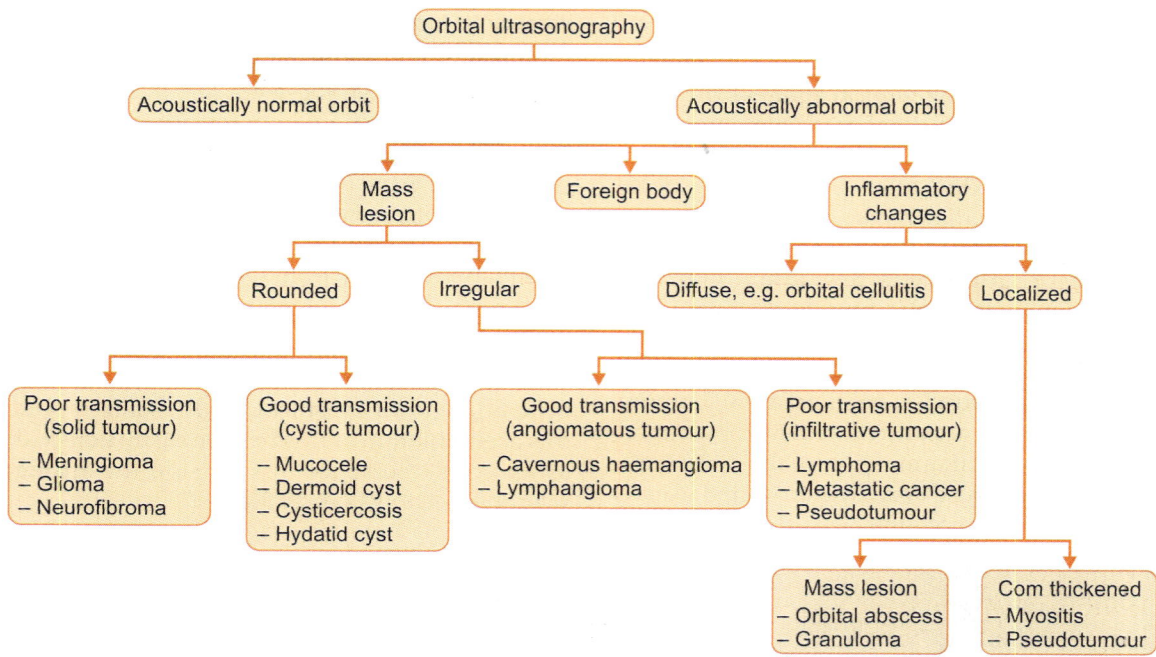

Fig. 25.35: *Ultrasonographic differential diagnosis of orbital lesions.*

Differential diagnosis of orbital lesions based on orbital ultrasonography is summarized in Fig. 25.35.

MAGNETIC RESONANCE IMAGING (MRI)

This technique represents a major advance in imaging methods. It depends on the rearrangement of hydrogen nuclei when tissues are exposed to a short electromagnetic pulse. Sensitive receivers pick up the electromagnetic echoes produced. MRI promises to distinguish between lesions based not only on location and tissue structure, but also on their metabolic profile. It is very sensitive for detecting differences between normal and abnormal tissues and has excellent image resolution. The technique produces tomographic images which are superficially very similar to CT scan but rely on entirely different physical principles for their production. Unlike conventional radiography and CT scanning, MRI does not subject the patient to any ill-effects of ionizing irradiations. So, it is safer for the patient. Further, there is no need for contrast injections.

MRI is superior to CT scan tomography in evaluating intracanalicular (Fig. 25.36), chiasmal, and postchiasmal extension of tumours. It has the added advantage of not being hampered by bone and also proves to be more sensitive in

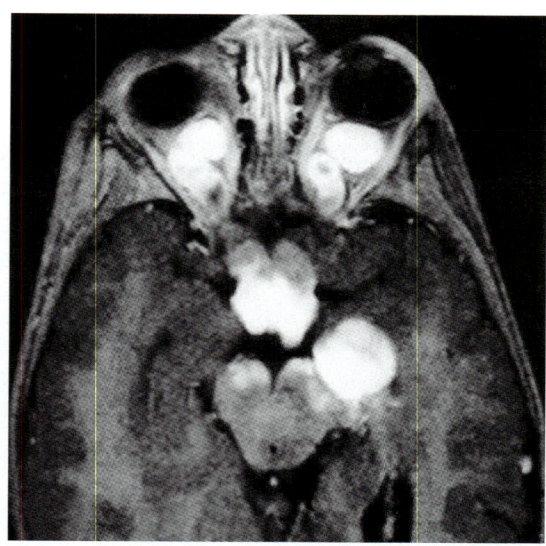

Fig. 25.36: *MRI scan showing extension of intracranial tumour in the optic canal.*

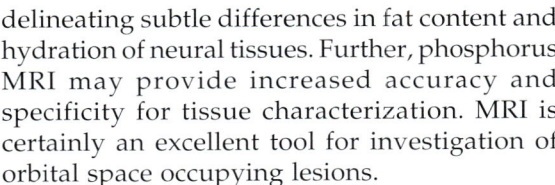

delineating subtle differences in fat content and hydration of neural tissues. Further, phosphorus MRI may provide increased accuracy and specificity for tissue characterization. MRI is certainly an excellent tool for investigation of orbital space occupying lesions.

Contraindications of MRI include pregnancy, epileptic fits, cardiac pacemakers (metallic implants), surgical clips and intraocular foreign body, as the foreign body may move in the magnetic field and cause further damage.

INVASIVE IMAGING TECHNIQUES

The invasive investigations include contrast orbitography, orbital venography and carotid angiography which are sparingly used nowadays.

CONTRAST ORBITOGRAPHY

Orbitopneumography. This old procedure, using retrobulbar injection of air (negative contrast orbitography) is of historical interest only. This invasive technique frequently results in chemical inflammation, allergic reactions, air embolism and even exophthalmos.

Injection of radio-opaque dye in retrobulbar space. This is another abandoned method of contrast orbitography. The dye may cause toxic-optic neuropathy.

Orbital venography. Presently, orbital venography is required in a minority of patients, principally in those who are clinically suspected to have orbital varix. In these cases, venography is indispensable not only to confirm the diagnosis but also, more importantly, to outline the size and extent of the anomaly to facilitate proper surgical planning. Another indication for venography is in the diagnosis of inflammatory processes of orbital veins, e.g. Tolosa-Hunt syndrome, wherein obstruction may be shown in the venous system due to pressure of granulation tissue.

For orbital venography, 10 to 12 ml of suitable contrast medium is injected preferably into the frontal vein on the side of proptosis. Flow of dye into the orbits is facilitated by a tourniquet tied around the forehead, and by digital pressure over the fascial veins. Anteroposterior view (of orbital venogram) provides more information

than lateral view. The venous pattern of the uninvolved orbit may be used as a control for interpretation.

CAROTID ANGIOGRAPHY

The introduction of computerized tomography has made carotid angiography a less frequent investigative procedure for evaluation of cause of proptosis. Arteriography is done in selected cases:

i. *Arteriovenous shunt or other intracranial vascular anomaly*, when suspected.
ii. *Vascular tumour* in the orbit where it is important to identify the feeding vessel prior to surgery.
iii. *Ophthalmic artery aneurysms* to identify the location and extent.
iv. *Arteriovenous communications along the ophthalmic artery–cavernous sinus complex* (that can produce unilateral proptosis), to identify the pathologic circulation.
v. *Pulsating exophthalmos* alone and in cases which are associated with bruit or thrill.

■ HISTOPATHOLOGIC STUDIES

The exact diagnosis of many orbital lesions cannot be made without the help of histopathological studies which can be accomplished by fine needle aspiration biopsy, incisional biopsy, excisional biopsy, core biopsy or endoscopic biopsy.

FINE NEEDLE ASPIRATION BIOPSY (FNAB)

It is a type of non-exfoliative cytodiagnostic technique.

Fine needle aspiration biopsy (FNAB), also known as fine needle aspiration cytology (FNAC), is believed to provide proper identification of most of the lesions. It is performed as outpatient procedure and can be carried out without anaesthesia.

Equipment

Equipment required for FNAB from orbital lesions include:
• Needle, 21–25 gauge, varying in length form 3.0 to 3.75 cm.

- Disposable syringe, 10 ml and 20 ml
- Syringe holder, i.e. pistal
- Glass slides
- Fixative such as 95% ethyl alchol or methanol.

Procedure

I. FNAB for anterior orbital and palpable lesions

Anterior orbital and palpable lesions can be subjected to FNAB directly either trans-cutaneously or transconjunctivally.

Transcutaneously, FNAB is performed as below:
- *Cleaning of skin* of the lids and surrounding area is done with 5% povidone iodine.
- *Fixing of suspected area* is done with the thumb and index finger of left hand.
- *Insertion of needle,* attached to a syringe mounted on a syringe holder, is done through the skin into the suspected lesion (Fig. 25.37A).
- *Vacuum* in the system is created by retracting the plunger to obtain tissue material. In order to aspirate sufficient material, the needle is moved back and forth, and sideways into different areas of the lesion, always maintaining the vacuum (Fig. 25.37B).
- *Pistol is released* at the end of aspiration, pressure is allowed to equalize with the atmosphere, and then needle is withdrawn from the lesion (Fig. 25.37C).

Transconjunctivally, FNAB can be performed for visible lesions. The procedure is same as for transcutaneous approach, except that the conjunctiva is anaesthetized with topical anaes-thetic drops, and antibiotic eye drops are also instilled before and after performing the procedure.

II. FNAB for posterior orbital and non-palpable orbital lesions

In such lesions, the site of FNAB, needs to be localized either with the help of ultrasound, CT scan or MRI.

Ultrasound-guided FNAB is preferred over CT scan and MRI guided, as the former is more economical and requires relatively less set-up and time. However, for deeper orbital lesions, CT scan-guided FNAB is more useful.

Examination of FNAB aspirate

Transfer to glass slide. After completion of FNAB, the needle is lightly touched to a glass slide on which the aspirate is transferred by pushing air through the needle.

Macroscopic examination of the aspirate is then performed, which generally reveals a droplet of fluid with or without blood and/or semisclid material.

Fixation of the aspirate. The aspirate is then spread over the glass slide with the help of an another glass slide and fixation of the smear is then done by two methods:
1. *Dry fixation* is done by using dry air
2. *Wet fixation* is done by using 95% ethyl alcohol.

Staining the slides is then done as below:
- *Air-dried smear* is stained with Poppenheim (May-Grunwald-Giemsa) and Wright stain. The air-dried smears have more differentiated staining of the cytoplasm and extracellular substance such as mucus or colloid.
- *Wet-fixed smear* is stained with Papanicolaou and haematoxylin and eosin stain. This smear gives better presentation of nuclear details.

Microscopic examination of the smears is then performed. Interpretation of the cellular types from FNAB is more difficult as compared to the normal histopathological section and thus needs a more skilled cytopathologist. Nevertheless, the accuracy and reliability of the FNAB in orbital lesions is well-documented and thus is a useful diagnostic tool.

INCISIONAL BIOPSY

Undoubtedly, for accurate tissue diagnosis, a proper biopsy specimen, at least 5 to 10 mm in length, is required and, preferably, it should include material from the periphery as well as interior of the lesion. However, such incisional biopsies, often have a deleterious effect on the course of the tumour, or on symptoms of patients. This embarrassing circumstance may be further compounded, if the results of the incisional biopsy are inconclusive. Therefore, the scope of incisional biopsy in the overall scheme of diagnostic search of orbital tumours is still not clearly defined.

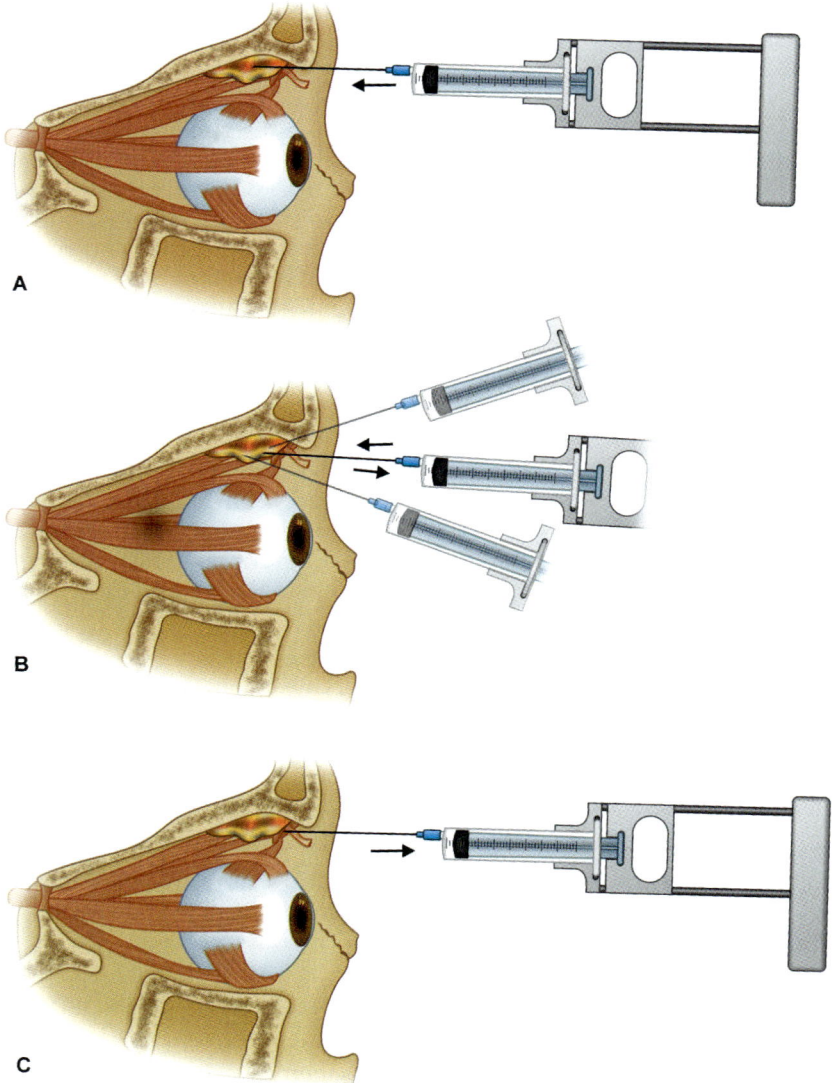

Fig. 25.37: *Technique of fine needle aspiration biopsy from an orbital mass. (A) Insertion of needle in the lesion; (B) Aspiration of material by retracting the plunger and moving the needle side way in the lesion; (C) Release of plunger and withdrawal of needle.*

Incisional biopsy along with frozen tissue study may be undertaken in infiltrative orbital lesions which remain undiagnosed.

CORE BIOPSY

Core biopsy is a new diagnostic technique. The three-part instrument consists of a trephine, an obturator and a tissue fixator. Using local anaesthesia, a 2 mm skin incision is made in the eyelid area nearest the tumour as ascertained by palpation and CT scan. The obturator is then passed through the trephine into the soft tissue tumour. The obturator is then removed and the tissue fixator is passed into the trephine with a clockwise rotating motion, the tissue fixator is bored into the tumour. Once it is fully engaged,

the tissue fixator and the trephine are withdrawn and the cylinder of tissue is removed from the coil of the tissue fixator. The solid tissue obtained by this technique facilitates microscopic diagnosis and has distinct advantage over the cellular specimen obtained by means of a fine needle biopsy.

ENDOSCOPIC BIOPSY

Endoscopic biopsy involves the use of a fiber-optic endoscope to visualize orbital lesion directly and a specially designed instrument to take a biopsy of the lesion. Orbital CT or MRI is used to guide placement of the endoscope for the biopsy. Endoscopic biopsy has an advantage over the fine needle biopsy and core biopsy in that the surgeon can visualize the surface of the lesion directly and select a biopsy site that does not contain large blood vessels and is distant from vital areas. In this technique, sufficient biopsy material is aspirated out endoscopically and is interpreted by a trained cytologist. A distinct disadvantage of the technique is that the orbital fat obscures good visualization.

EXCISIONAL BIOPSY

It should always be preferred to incisional biopsy in orbital masses which are well encapsulated or circumscribed. Further, whatever be the enthusiasm of the ophthalmologist for incisional biopsy, it should be tempered by the understanding that the removal of an orbital tumour, not biopsy, is the main objective. It is the orbital mass which brings the patient to the clinician, and the feature for which he seeks relief.

For excisional biopsy, the following three procedures are available:

i. *Anterior orbitotomy* for a mass in the anterior part of the orbit is readily reached either by transcutaneous or transconjunctival approach (Reese).

ii. *Lateral orbitotomy* for a mass in the posterior part (retrobulbar) or at the apex of the orbit (Kronlein).

iii. *Transcranial approach* is employed when the tumour extends into the cranial cavity (Naffzeiger).

IMMUNOHISTOCHEMISTRY

Immunohistochemistry techniques can be applied to orbital tumours and related lesions to aid differential diagnosis. These highly sensitive tests have contributed greatly to the understanding and classification of orbital tumours. Basically, immunohistochemistry involves the use of antibodies that are specific for certain antigens. The completed antigen–antibody reaction is identified by an enzyme linked to the antibody, that generates a colour reaction when introduced to a certain chemical.

- *Glial fibrillary acidic protein (GFAP)* has been shown to be highly specific for glial cells, thus aiding in the recognition of glial tumours.
- *Factor VIII related* antigen is synthesized by vascular endothelial cells and can be identified in tumours of vascular origin such as capillary haemangioma, cavernous haemangioma and angiosarcoma.
- *S-100 protein* is believed to be a helpful marker for cells of neural crest origin and can, therefore, help to identify tumours of nerve origin and melanomas.
- *Antibodies against surface antigens of B and T lymphocytes* have also been applied recently to the differentiation of orbital tumours.
- *Myoglobin* is the oxygen-binding haem protein found in cardiac and skeletal muscles but not in smooth muscles.

MANAGEMENT OF PROPTOSIS

Depending upon the cause of proptosis, management can be:
- Medical management
- Surgical management

Note. Management of each cause of proptosis is described in relevant chapters.

SUMMARY

- *Thorough evaluation* of a case of proptosis is extremely important before starting any treatment procedures.
- *Systematic approach* with a knowledge of various etiopathogenic mechanisms can help the ophthalmologist to arrive at a relatively short list of differential diagnosis (Fig. 25.38).

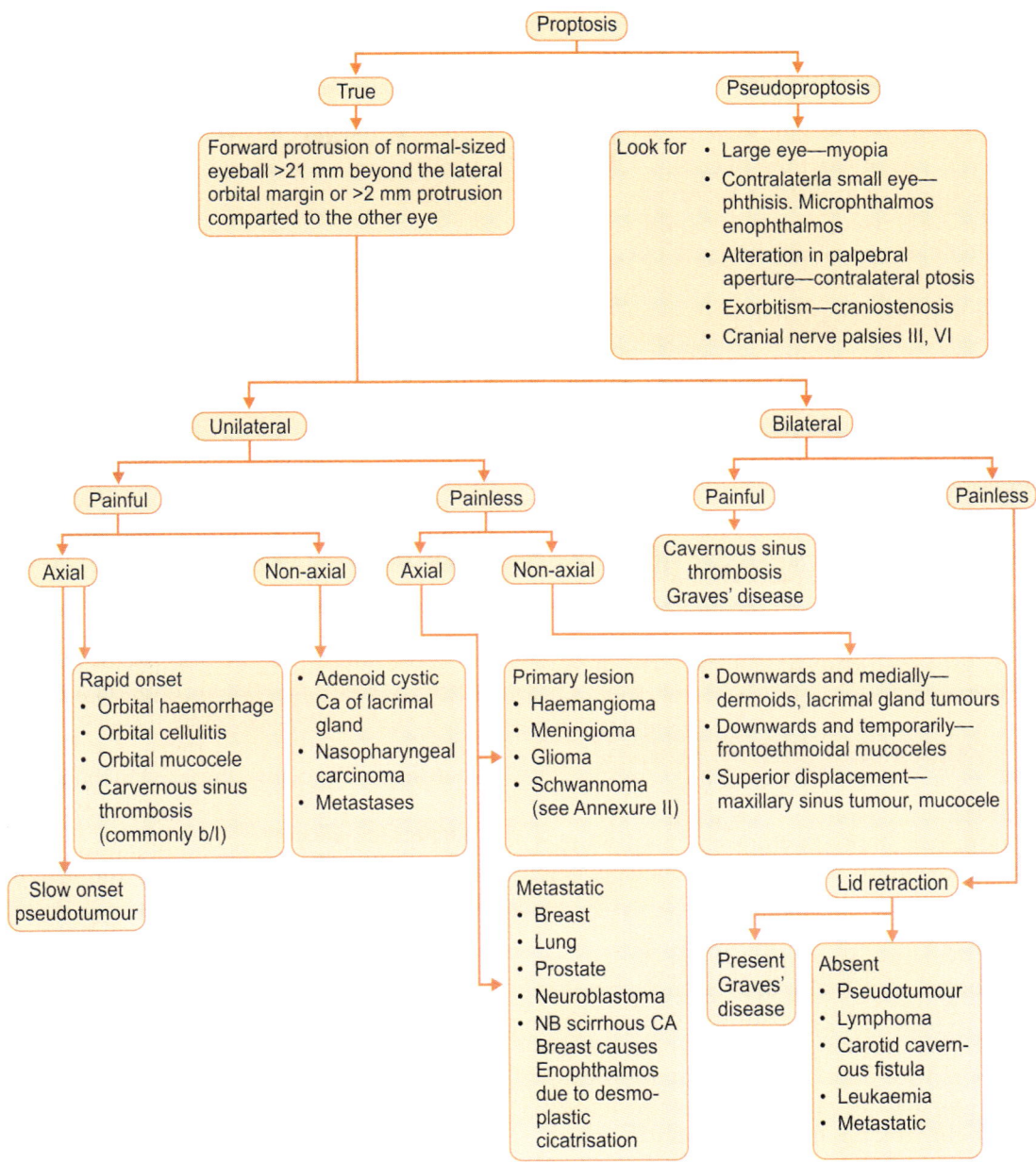

Fig. 25.38: *Scheme to shortlist the differential diagnosis of a case of proptosis.*

- *Orbital imaging techniques* now permit to come to a conclusion rapidly and to precisely plan the approach for prompt and accurate management of a case of proptosis.

ENOPHTHALMOS

Enophthalmos can be defined as a relative posterior displacement of a normal-sized eye in relation to the bony orbital margin. It may be

unilateral or bilateral but comes to the attention of the clinician more often when unilateral. *Unilateral enophthalmos* is said to be present when there is a difference of more than 2 mm on exophthalmometry between the two eyes. However, enophthalmos becomes clinically obvious only when there is a difference of 3–4 mm or more between the two eyes. Etiologically, enophthalmos can be divided into two groups:
1. Traumatic enophthalmos
2. Nontraumatic enophthalmos.

TRAUMATIC ENOPHTHALMOS

Traumatic enophthalmos is associated with blow-out-fracture of the orbital floor (more commonly) and medial wall of the orbit (less commonly).

Factor contributing to development of enophthalmos is mainly herniation of orbital contents in the maxillary sinus. The traumatic enophthalmos increases in degree when there is associated soft tissue prolapse due to medial orbital wall fracture.

NONTRAUMATIC ENOPHTHALMOS

ETIOLOGY

Nontraumatic enophthalmos can be produced by any of the following three main mechanisms:

I. Orbital structural abnormalities

Orbital structural abnormality refers to changes in the bony orbit that result in an increase in orbital volume compared to the volume of its constituents, causing posterior displacement of the globe. Trauma is the most common cause of such structural changes, other structural abnormalities causing nontraumatic enophthalmos include posterior bowing of the floor secondary to chronic sinusitis (silent sinus syndrome); congenital or iatrogenic defects in the greater wing of sphenoid; congenital bony orbital asymmetry; and bone pathology [Paget's disease of the bone (PDB)].

1. *Maxillary sinusitis and silent sinus syndrome.* Chronic maxillary sinusitis with obstruction of the sinus ostium can, in some cases, lead to centripetal collapse of the sinus walls (atelectasis) with subsequent enophthalmos. Often, no prior history of sinusitis is present, and patients present with spontaneous enophthalmos and hypoglobus (silent sinus syndrome). This condition is always unilateral and is seen equally in males and females in their third to fifth decades.

2. *Orbital bony defects.* Defects in the bony orbit may be congenital or iatrogenic (following surgery). Absence of the greater wing of the sphenoid is the most common congenital bony defect and is classically seen in association with neurofibromatosis I. It is hypothesized that the bony changes in neurofibromatosis may be a result of the interaction between the developing orbit and the orbital neurofibromas. Absence of the greater wing of sphenoid can also be an isolated anomaly or associated with orbital varices or (very rarely) with epidermoid cysts.

3. *Paget's disease of the bone.* It is a chronic, progressive disorder in which initial bone destruction is followed by a disorganized reparative process causing distortion. Enophthalmos is a rare manifestation of Paget's disease and is thought to result when there is differential expansion of the orbit compared to the cranium.

II. Orbital fat atrophy

Fat atrophy causes a reduction in the volume of the contents of the orbit, thus allowing the globe to sink backwards within a normal bony orbit. Fat atrophy can be seen in following conditions.

1. *Age-related orbital fat atrophy.* Facial lipoatrophy occurs with aging, starting at the age of 20 and becoming noticeable at the age of 30 in most people. This atrophy may form part of the process responsible for senile enophthalmos, along with redistribution of orbital fat. Descent of the lateral canthus and Lockwood's suspensory ligament occurs with age, and this causes the globe to sink thus pushing the orbital fat pads forward. This is a common cause of bilateral enophthalmos and comparison with old photographs is useful in diagnosis.

2. *Localized scleroderma and Parry-Romberg syndrome.* Scleroderma is a chronic autoimmune disease that can be systemic or localized

to the skin. There are five subsets of localized scleroderma classified by the type and extent of cutaneous involvement: Plaque; generalized; bullous; linear; and deep.

- *En coup de sabre* (ECDS) is a form of linear scleroderma that frequently occurs on the face or scalp, often resembling a stroke from a sword, and may result in orbital tissue atrophy and enophthalmos.
- *Parry-Romberg syndrome (PRS)* is a condition of hemifacial atrophy involving skin and tissues below the forehead that can also cause enophthalmos. Antimalarial medication and methotrexate are the mainstays of treatment.

3. *Lipodystrophy* can be total, partial or localized but enophthalmos is usually seen in association with the partial form. In acquired partial lipodystrophy, women are affected more frequently, and it is usually parts of the upper body and face that are involved. Lupus erythematosus, dermatomyositis and Sjögren's syndrome have all been associated with partial lipodystrophy. The most prevalent acquired form is HIV-associated lipodystrophy, which can result in severe atrophy of facial subcutaneous fat and enophthalmos.

4. *Cockayne's dystrophy.* This rare autosomal recessive disorder was first described by Cockayne as a combination of severe postnatal growth retardation with progressive neurological dysfunction (particularly mental disability and deafness). The average age of death is around 12 years old, with a worse prognosis in those who have structural eye abnormalities. Examination will classically reveal dwarfism and microcephaly as well as a variable number of other problems such as retinal atrophy, cataracts and corneal opacity. Enophthalmos is a well-recognized feature of this syndrome and is believed to be caused by orbital lipodystrophy, but cranial bony orbital malformation may play a role.

5. *Orbital varices* usually present in the third decade of life with exophthalmos, but occasionally may present with enophthalmos. They are vascular hamartomas consisting of a plexus of low-pressure, low-flow, thin-walled and distensible vessels. The varix may eventually cause atrophy of orbital fat, which allows the globe to sink back into the orbit when the vessels are not distended.

6. *Post-irradiation.* Orbital radiation in children, usually for retinoblastoma or rhabdomyosarcoma, is a well-known cause of enophthalmos that develops later in life.

7. *Repeated ocular pressure.* Leber congenital amaurosis is an inherited retinal degenerative disorder that results in blindness at birth. Clinical signs that point to this diagnosis in an infant include pendular nystagmus and a tendency to rub the eyes (oculo-digital sign of Franceschetti). Enophthalmos may be present, which is believed to be related to orbital fat atrophy secondary to constant rubbing of the eye.

III. Posterior traction on eyeball

Enophthalmos can also be caused by posterior traction secondary to fibrosis of the extraocular muscles or connective tissues; this is usually associated with ocular motility problems. This mechanism is responsible for the enophthalmos seen in following conditions.

1. *Orbital metastases.* Orbital metastatic tumours represent 2.5–3.7% of all orbital tumours and usually present with an infiltrative or mass lesion. Enophthalmos is seen in approximately 7–24% of cases. Tumour-induced desmoplasia, fibrosis and muscle invasion are responsible for the enophthalmos; however, fat atrophy could also be a contributory factor.

2. *Restrictive muscle syndromes.* Non-traumatic enophthalmos can be associated with following conditions:

- *Duane retraction syndrome* (DRS) is the most common of the retraction syndromes. Enophthalmos, however, is uncommon and is seen only in the more severe cases.
- *Congenital fibrosis of the extraocular muscles* (CFEOM) is a rare group of disorders characterized by congenital, nonprogressive external ophthalmoplegia. Very rarely, a sporadic form of CFEOM may occur that is characterized by unilateral muscle fibrosis with enophthalmos, ptosis and restricted motility.

- *Acquired retraction syndrome* with enophthalmos has been reported following recurrent pterygium, traumatic enophthalmos repair and decompression.
- *Post-inflammatory restrictive myopathy* with enophthalmos has been reported with orbital involvement in Wegener's granulomatosis, tuberculosis, and sarcoidosis.

CLINICAL FEATURES

Enophthalmos is not always evident clinically and may present with variable signs and symptoms.

Misinterpreted features of approximately 50% of patients with enophthalmos may initially be referred for investigation of:

- Contralateral exophthalmos
- Ptosis
- Diplopia.

Cosmetic concerns include an altered appearance because of:

- Deep-seated globe
- Asymmetric position of the eyes
- Deep superior sulcus
- Pseudoptosis
- Eyelid retraction.

Functional problems include *diplopia, dry eyes* and *corneal desiccation* leading to ulceration.

- *Diplopia.* Although is seen most frequently in traumatic enophthalmos, it also occurs in patients with restricted ocular movements caused by a cicatrizing process.
- *Dry eye disease.* In cases of severe enophthalmos, the globe is drawn away from the eyelids, and this leads to dry eye symptoms and, more seriously, to corneal drying and ulceration.
- *Lagophthalmos* may also be a causative factor for corneal ulceration in some patients.

Pulsating enophthalmos is a very rare condition that is caused by the transmission of intracranial pulsation to the eye via a congenital or iatrogenic bony defect. The pulsation is usually obvious clinically, but is especially noticeable when performing applanation tonometry or Hertel's exophthalmometry.

CLINICAL WORK-UP AND INVESTIGATIONS

Clinical work-up

I. History taking

A thorough history in a patient with enophthalmos includes the time-frame of onset, current and past ocular symptoms, past medical history and a review of systems. For instance, initial proptosis followed by progressive enophthalmos may indicate a fibrosing mass such as scirrhous carcinoma.

II. Local examination

Local examination should include following important features.

1. *Exclusion of pseudoenophthalmos.* Before proceeding to investigations and management, it is very important to rule out a pseudo-enophthalmos. There are a number of conditions that frequently present as enophthalmos such as contralateral exophthalmos, ptosis and microphthalmos. Meticulous clinical examination, exophthalmometry and ocular axial length measurement can usually provide the correct diagnosis.

2. *Measurement of enophthalmos* is an important step in local examination and can be accomplished by following methods:

- *Hertel's exophthalmometer* is the instrument most frequently used to measure the position of the globe in relation to the orbit. It is important to note that any asymmetry between the lateral orbital rims will affect the readings significantly when using this instrument. In such cases, instruments that rest on the superior and inferior rims, such as the Naugle's orbitometer, may be used in all cases of enophthalmos.
- *Measurement of vertical and horizontal displacement of the globe* should also be done. This is performed most simply using a transparent scale to compare the relative pupillary or limbal positions between the two eyes.
- *Radiographic measurements* may be more accurate, but in the absence of any normative data, their validity is doubtful. Traditionally, the *cornea clinoid distance* has been measured on lateral radiographs of the orbit, using a

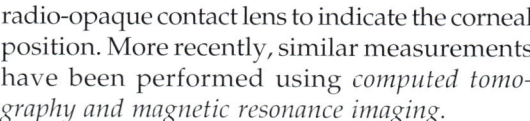

radio-opaque contact lens to indicate the corneal position. More recently, similar measurements have been performed using *computed tomography and magnetic resonance imaging.*

3. *Ophthalmic examination.* A detailed ophthalmic examination should be undertaken, which may reveal clues to the underlying condition (e.g. Lisch nodules).
- Examination for *functional manifestations* of enophthalmos, as discussed above.
- *Testing ocular motility* is important because it is rarely affected by structural changes (except trauma) or fat atrophy, but is frequently affected by *tractional process.*

4. *Examination of old photographs.* Old photographs are a very useful tool for determining the rate of progression of enophthalmos or diagnosing unrecognized congenital asymmetry.

III. Systemic examination

A complete systemic examination should also be performed to get some clue as below.
- *Patient's appearance* may sometimes provide a clue to the diagnosis, as in Cockayne's syndrome.
- Search for *primary carcinomas* (e.g. carcinoma breast).
- *Peripheral stigmata of systemic illness and periorbital signs* of disease (e.g. lid neurofibromatosis) will be pertinent in making an accurate diagnosis.

Investigations

The investigations for a patient with enophthalmos should be tailored according to the history and clinical assessment.

I. *Blood tests* may play a role in narrowing the list of causes, but are rarely diagnostic. Some useful tests may be:
- *Tumour markers, cANCA* (raised in WG)
- *Inflammatory markers* such as *rheumatoid factor* and *anti-nuclear antibodies (ANA)* that are associated with some causes of lipodystrophy.

II. *CT and MRI* are the most useful radiological investigations for enophthalmos.
- These provide a detailed view of the orbital anatomy and delineate any structural abnormalities.

- Imaging also allows an objective assessment of the enophthalmos in comparison to the bony orbit and also in relation to the contralateral eye.
- Soft tissue views can illustrate *fat atrophy, fibrotic changes* and the nature and *extent of any orbital lesions.*

III. *Tissue diagnosis* is useful in a number of settings and is used most frequently in diagnosing orbital lesions such as metastases. Furthermore, *biopsy* can evaluate lipodystrophies or subcutaneous atrophy, as in scleroderma and PRS.

MANAGEMENT
Management includes accurate diagnosis and treatment.

Diagnosis
Nontraumatic enophthalmos is an uncommon condition with a variety of presentations and requires a careful examination for accurate diagnosis. With an understanding of the many possible causes, one can perform an *effective clinical examination* in order to direct further investigations and make the correct diagnosis as described above. This not only directs the management of enophthalmos, but "more importantly" may also reveal a potentially life-threatening systemic illness, which can then be addressed.

Treatment
Treatment of nontraumatic enophthalmos depends upon the causes as below:

I. Enophthalmos due to structural abnormality of orbit

1. *Enophthalmos secondary to maxillary sinusitis and silent sinus syndrome* is usually treated surgically by which involves restoration of normal sinus ventilation with endoscopic/external antrostomy and repair of the orbital floor. Rarely, spontaneous resolution may be seen.

2. *Enophthalmos secondary to orbital bony defects.* Treatment consists of surgical treatment of the cause and orbital implants to cover the defect.

II. *Enophthalmos secondary to orbital fat atrophy*

1. *Treatment of the cause,* e.g.

- *Scleroderma and Parry-Romberg syndrome* are mainly treated by antimalarial medications and methotrexate.
- *Orbital varices.* Trial of radiological embolization followed by elective surgical removal may be performed in selective cases.

2. *Reconstructive surgery* such as lipofilling or silicone orbital implant may be considered.

III. *Enophthalmos due to posterior traction on eyeball*

Enophthalmos secondary *to traction* may require a more complex approach including *removing the cause of the traction* (e.g. releasing tight muscles), *restoration of extraocular motility* and consideration of adjuvant *chemotherapy* or *radiotherapy in cases of metastatic disease.*

Note. It has also been emphasized in a number of scientific papers that clinically evident enophthalmos has a significant psychological effect on patients, and corrective surgery should, therefore, be considered to be *reconstructive* rather than *simply cosmetic.*

BIBLIOGRAPHY

1. Alarcon-Segovia D, Ramos-Niembro F. Association of partial lipodystrophy and Sjögren's syndrome. Ann Intern Med 1976;85:474–5.

2. Aleem MA, Meikandan D, Raveendran S, Ramasubramanian D. Parry Romberg syndrome: newer concepts in pathophysiology. Neurol India 1999;47:342–3.

3. Anderson RL, Dixon RS. The role of Whitnall's ligament in ptosis surgery. Arch Ophthalmol 1979;97:705–7.

4. Ascher B, Coleman S, Alster T, et al. Full scope of effect of facial lipoatrophy: a framework of disease understanding. Dermatol Surg 2006;32:1058–69.

5. Attia S, Zaouali S, Jeguirim H, Njim L, Kriaa S, Yahia SB, Khairallah M. Orbital sarcoidosis manifesting with enophthalmos. Ocul Immunol Inflamm 2006;14:379–81.

6. Aubourg P, Krahn M, Bernard R, et al. Assignment of a new congenital fibrosis of extra-ocular muscles type 3 (CFEOM3) locus, FEOM4, based on a balanced translocation t(2;13) (q37.3;q12.11) and identification of candidate genes. J Med Genet 2008;42:253–59.

7. Babel J, Klein D, Roth A. Leber's congenital amaurosis associated with high hyperopia in four sisters. Ophthalmic Paediatr Genet 1989;10:55–61.

8. Becelli R, Perugini M, Cerulli G, et al. Surgical treatemnt of fibrous dysplasia of the cranio-maxillo-facial area. Review of the literature and personal experience from 1984 to 1999. Minerva Stomatol, Jul-Aug 2002;51(7-8):293–300.

9. Ben Simon GJ, Yoon MK, Atul J, Nakra T, McCann JD, Goldberg RA. Clinical manifestations of orbital mass lesions at the Jules Stein Eye Institute, 1999–2003. Ophthalmic Surg Lasers Imaging 2006;37:25–32.

10. Bikmaz K, Mak R, Al-Mefty O. Management of bone-invasive, hyperostotic sphenoid wing meningiomas. Journal or Neurosurgery Nov 2007;107(5):905–12.

11. Binet EF, Kieffer SA, Martin SH, Peterson HO. Orbital dysplasia in neurofibromatosis. Radiology 1969;93:829–33.

12. Bitar SR, Selhorst JB, Archer CR. Epidermoid-induced pulsating eye. Ann Ophthalmol 1993;25:45–9.

13. Blaszczyk M, Jablonska S. Linear scleroderma en Coup de Sabre. Relationship with progressive facial hemiatrophy (PFH). Adv Exp Med Biol 1999;455:101–4.

14. Buono LM. The silent sinus syndrome: maxillary sinus atelectasis with enophthalmos and hypo-globus. Curr Opin Ophthalmol 2004;15:486–9.

15. Burroughs JR, Hernandez Cospin JR, Soparkar CN, Patrinely JR. Misdiagnosis of silent sinus syndrome. Ophthal Plast Reconstr Surg 2003;19:449–54.

16. Camirand A, Doucet J, Harris J. The aging eye: pathophysiology and management. Surg Technol Int 1996;5:347–51.

17. Chen YR, Wong FH, Hsueh C, et al. Computed tomography characteristics of non-syndromic craniofacial fibrous dysplasia, Chang Gung Med J, Jan 2002;25(1):1–8.

18. Daly BD, Chow CC, Cockram CS, et al. Unusual manifestations of craniofacial fibrous dysplasia: clinical, endocrinological and computed tomographic features. Postgrad Med J. Jan 1994;70(819):10–6.

19. Edgerton TM, Persing AJ, Jane AJ. The surgical treatment of fibrous dysplasia. Ann Surg 1985;202:459–79.

20. Guevara P, Escobar-Arriaga E, Saavedra-Perez D, et al. J Neurooncol. Angiogensis and expression of estrogen and progetstrone receptors as predictive factors for recurrence of meningiomas, (Epubahaed of print), Dec 2009.

21. Lambets SW, Tanghe HL, Avezaat CJ, et al. Mifepristone (RU-486) treatment on meningiomas. J Neurol Neurosurg Psychiatry, Jun 1992; 55(6):486–90.

22. Lisle DA, Monsour PA, Maskiell CD. Imaging of carniofacial fibrous dysplasia. J Med Imaging Radiat Oncol. Aug 2008;52(4):325–32.

23. Minniti G, Amichetti M, Enrici RM, et al. Radiotherapy and radiosurgery for benign skull base meningiomas. Radiat Oncol, Oct 2009;4:42.

24. Mirone G, Chibbaro S, Schiabello L, Tola S, George B. En plaque sphenoid wing meningiomas: recurrence factors and surgical strategy in a series of 71 patients. Neurosurgery, 65(6 Suppl): 100–8; discussion, Dec 2009;108–9.

25. Munro IR, Chir B, Chen YR. Radical treatment for fronto-orbital fibrous dysplasia: the chain link fence. Plast Reconstr Surg, 1981;67:719–29.

26. Park BY, Cheon YW, Kim YO, et al. Prognosis for craniofacial fibrous dysplasia after incomplete resection:age and serum alkaline phosphatise Int J Oral Maxillofac Surg, Mar 2010;39(3):221–6.

27. Paul A. Athanasiov, Venkatesh C. Prabhakaran, Dinesh Selva: Non-traumatic enophthalmos: a review. Acta ophthalmology 2007;1755–3768.

28. Ricciardelli EJ, Borrow JA, Makielski KH. Three-dimensional computed tomography in a case of craniofacial fibrous dysplasia. Ann Otol Rhinol Laryngol 1991;101:275–9.

29. Robert A, Nugent, Rod I, Belkin, Janet M Niegel, Jack Rootman, et al. Correlation of CT and clinical findings. Radiology Dec 1990;177(3): 675–82.

30. Robin D Gibson. Measurement of Proptosis (Exophthalmos) by Computerised Tomography. Australasian Radiology 1979;130:189–94.

31. Schick U, Bleyen J, Bani A, Hassler W. Management ogmeningiomas en plaque of the sphenoid wing. Journal of Neurosurgery, Feb 2006;104(2): 208–14.

32. Schick U. Spheno orbital meningiomas: results in long-term treatment. HNO, Jan 2010;58(1): 37–43.

33. Segni M, GB, Bartley, Garrity IA, et al. Comapribility of proptosis measurements by different techniques. American Journal of Ophthalmology, Jun 2002;133(6):813–8.

34. Shah ZK, Peh WC, Koh WL, et al. Magnetic resonance imaging appearances of fibrous dysplasia Br J Radiol, Dec 2005;78(936):1104–15.

35. Utz JA, Kransdorf MJ, Jelinek JS, et al. MR appearance of fibrous dysplasia. J Comput Assist Tomogr, Sep-Oct 1989;13(5):845–51.

36. Yano M, Tajima S, Tanaka Y, Imai K, Umebayashi M. Magnetic resonance imaging findings of craniofacial fibrous dysplasia. Ann Plast Surg, Apr 1993;30(4):371–4.

Section

VII

Clinical Evaluation and Investigations for Cataract Surgery

26. **Preoperative Evaluation for Cataract Surgery**
27. **Biometry: Calculation of IOL Power**

Preoperative Evaluation for Cataract Surgery

Chapter Outline

PREOPERATIVE EVALUATION AND PREPARATIONS
Review of general medical status of the patient
• Implications and considerations for the associated medical problems
Ocular evaluation
• Present and past ophthalmic history
• Ocular examination

PREOPERATIVE MEDICATION AND PREPARATION
• Consent
• Scrub bath, care of hair and marking of the eye
• Preoperative antibiotics and disinfectants
• IOP lowering
• Mydriasis
Preoperative checklist

PREOPERATIVE EVALUATION AND PREPARATIONS

Once it has been decided to operate for cataract, a thorough preoperative evaluation should be carried out before contemplating surgery. This should include:

A. Review of general medical status of the patient.
B. Ocular evaluation.

A. REVIEW OF GENERAL MEDICAL STATUS OF THE PATIENT

A general medical examination of the patient is recommended to:

• *Exclude the presence of systemic diseases* especially: diabetes mellitus; hypertension and cardiac problems; obstructive lung disorders, history of allergy to drugs, bleeding disorders, use of anticoagulants or immunosuppressants.
• *Presence of any musculoskeletal disorders* like kyphosis, scoliosis or excessive obesity, head tremors or nodding may pose difficulty during sleep.
• *Search for any potential source of infection* in the body such as septic gums, urinary tract infection, etc. should also be made.

Implications and considerations for the associated medical problems

1. Diabetes

It is a commonly found medical problem.

• *Diabetic retinopathy*, if detected, should be treated prior to cataract surgery, since proliferative diabetic retinopathy and macular oedema may develop or worsen following cataract surgery. Sometimes cataract surgery is recommended to improve visualization of the fundus for management of DR. Recommendation for such a situation is to perform a large capsulorhexis.
• *Other anticipated problems* in diabetics include smaller pupil, pigment dispersion, delayed wound healing, fibrinous uveitis and an increased risk of endophthalmitis.

Recommended protocol for a diabetic patient: Blood glucose is checked for everyone who undergoes a cataract surgery and this is re-checked on the day of surgery also for all known diabetics. It is necessary to maintain a special record for the monitoring of blood sugar and medications. The recommended values are: Fasting blood sugar (FBS) <140 mg% and Random blood sugar (RBS) <180 mg% on the day of surgery. Following FBS, patients should be advised to have their normal breakfast. If they are on oral anti-diabetic drugs, they should skip the morning dose of the medications only on the day of surgery. If on insulin, one-third of the dose should be administered in the morning. This is done to avoid hypoglycaemia during the preoperative period. The subsequent doses should be taken as per the routine of the individual patient.

2. Hypertension

Hypertension when associated, may rarely increase the risk of suprachoroidal (expulsive) haemorrhage.

Recommended protocol. Blood pressure (BP) is checked for everyone who undergoes a cataract surgery and this is rechecked on the day of surgery, irrespective of hypertensive status. It is necessary to maintain a special record for the monitoring of BP and the medications. *The recommended maximum blood pressure is 140/90 mmHg or less on the day of surgery. The following recommendations should be followed for all hypertensive patients.*

- The patient should take the prescribed anti-hypertensive medication on the day of surgery.
- Avoid adrenaline in local anaesthesia and phenylephrine eyedrops for dilation.

Use of sedatives a day before starting anti-hypertensive drug may work well in all outreach patients. It is prudent to check BP in the ward before sending them to the OR.

3. Cardiac artery disease

A detailed physician evaluation is required and his recommendations should be followed.
- Sugery may be done a minimum of *3–6 months after myocardial infarction.*

- *Oral antiplatelet need not be stopped for cataract surgery.*

Anticoagulant therapy needs special attention. Warfarin (INR should be less than 2.5) should be stopped at least 3 days prior to surgery in consultation with the haematologist. If required, injectable heparin may be started. If possible, topical anaesthesia should be used to decrease the risk of bleeding.

If on oral anticoagulants, check for prothrombin time (PT). *Surgey can be done, if PT is less than 18 seconds.*
- Continue routine medication on the day of surgery.
- *Phenylephrine should not be used* for pupillary dilation.
- Administer local anaesthesia *without adrenaline* in anaesthetic solution.
- Provide a stretcher or wheelchair to avoid exertions and stress.
- *Cautery should not be used in patients with pacemakers.*

It is preferable to have a *Stand by physician or anaesthetist* during the anaesthetic block and surgery for cardiac monitoring.

4. Asthmatics

Criteria for admission include:
- Asthma under control with drugs.
- Continue the medicines during hospital stay.
- Minimal or no wheeze before surgery and if *present to give IV bronchodilators* or steroids.
- *Avoid plastic drapes* and take *special care for ventilation* while draping for surgery.
- Use oxygen/nebulizer during surgery if the patient is uncomfortable.
- Injection deriphylline/dexamethasone IV, SOS.
- Switch off the air-conditioner (optional).
- *Avoid NSAIDS.* If needed to use tablet nimusulide/paracetamol.

5. Renal failure/renal transplant

- A physician should certify fitness for surgery.
- Avoid tablet acetazolamide and NSAIDS. If painkillers are required, paracetamol is safer.
- Avoid systemic aminoglycosides.

- If already on maintenance dose of oral steroids, double the dosage for a short interval (one to two weeks) following surgery.

6. Septic foci

- Check for dental infection, history of purulent discharge, skin infections, etc.
- Treat adequately before surgery.

Examination and advice of a physician is essential for the following:

- Uncontrolled diabetes mellitus and hypertension
  - If BP > 170/100 mmHg
  - RBS > 200 mg%
- Known cardiac patients
- Recently diagnosed uncontrolled asthmatics
- Renal failure/transplants
- Liver disease
- Known bleeding disorders
- Obese or emaciated patients.

B. OCULAR EVALUATION

Ocular evaluation before cataract surgery should include:

- Present and past ophthalmic history
- Ocular examination.

I. Present and past ophthalmic history

- **Visual complaints.** A cataract patient may be bothered by the glare, diplopia, polyopia or decreased contrast sensitivity apart from decreased visual acuity for near and/or distance.
- **Patient's lifestyle** may be compromised by the cataract. Therefore, cataract surgery should be planned on the basis of need, occupation and lifestyle of the patient.
- **Past ophthalmic history** should include enquiry about previous visual acuity, history of amblyopia, strabismus, previous surgery (especially refractive surgery), trauma and concurrent eye disease.
- **Review the indications for surgery** which include:

1. *Visual improvement.* This is by far the most common indication. When surgery should be advised for visual improvement varies from person to person depending upon the individual visual needs. So, an individual should be operated for cataract, when the visual handicap becomes a significant deterrent to the maintenance of his or her usual lifestyle including the profession.

2. *Medical indications.* Sometimes patients may be comfortable from the visual point (due to useful vision from the other eye or otherwise) but may be advised cataract surgery due to medical grounds such as:

- Lens-induced glaucoma
- Phacoanaphylactic endophthalmitis
- Retinal diseases like diabetic retinopathy or retinal detachment, treatment of which is being hampered by the presence of lens opacities.

3. *Cosmetic indication.* Sometimes patient with mature cataract may insist on cataract extraction (even with no hope of getting useful vision), in order to obtain a black pupil.

II. Ocular examination

A thorough examination of the eyes including slit-lamp biomicroscopy is desirable in all cases. The following useful information is essential before the patient is considered for surgery.

1. Assessment of visual status

Visual status assessment should include:

- *Visual acuity* testing should be done unaided and best corrected and pinhole testing.
- *Perception of light* (PL) must be noted. Absence of PL indicates nil visual prognosis.
- *Projection of rays* (PR). Inaccurate PR may be due to old retinal detachment, visual pathway defects, advanced glaucoma, large area of chorioretinal atrophy and indicates poor visual prognosis. However, at times in dense cataracts, PR may be inaccurate with good visual prognosis.
- *Potential visual acuity tests* which may be required in the presence of opaque media include:
  - Laser interferometry (LI)
  - Potential acuity meter (PAM) test.

2. Examination of pupil

Pupils should be examined to check for:

- Light reactions and RAPD
- Ability of the pupils to dilate adequately before surgery.

Small pupil may result in inadequate capsulorhexis, and uncomplete cortical cleanup. Small nuclear fragments may be left behind the iris because of poor visibility.

Management of small pupil should be planned preoperatively

3. Anterior segment evaluation

Anterior segment evaluation by slit-lamp biomicroscopy is must before cataract surgery.

- *Cornea* should be examined to note any scarring, endothelial status (guttata). In patients with suspicion of endothelial dystrophy, *specular microscopy examination* should be carried out for endothelial cell count and morphology. Normal cell count in elderly patients is 2000–2500 cell/mm^2. Special care is needed in patients with cell counts below 1500 cells/mm^2.
- *Signs of uveitis.* Keratic precipitates (*KPs*) noted at the back of cornea suggest management of subtle uveitis before the cataract surgery. *Other signs of uveitis* which may be noted include pigment dispersal over the anterior lens capsule and presence of posterior synechiae.

Note. Ideally anterior chamber activity should be absent or minimal (+1 cells or less) for three months prior to surgery. In quiet eyes, topical steroids (prednisolone acetate 1% or dexamethasone 0.1%) are used six times a day, starting 1 week before surgery. A course of systemic steroids should also be considered.

- *Cataractous lens* should be evaluated for morphology and maturity of cataract and for grade of nuclear sclerosis (especially important for planning phacoemulsification surgery.
- *Anterior chamber depth* assessment and detection of associated iridodonesis and pseudoexfoliation are very important.
  - *Shallow anterior chamber* is associated with reduction in safe zone for phacoemulsification. Therefore, protection of endothelium with OVD to create space is essential.
  - *Very deep anterior chamber* predisposes to difficulty in manipulation of nucleus.
  - *Pseudoexfoliation* is associated with poor pupillary dilation and weak zonules. Use

of capsular tension ring (CTR) may minimize the risk of dropping the lens into the vitreous.

4. Intraocular pressure

Intraocular pressure (IOP) should be measured in each case, preferably by applanation tonometry. Presence of a raised IOP needs a priority management. The risk of postoperative steroid-induced rise in IOP especially in patients with POAG should also be kept in mind.

5. Examination of lids, conjunctiva and lacrimal apparatus

- *Search for local source of infection* should be made by ruling out conjunctival infections, meibomitis, blepharitis and lacrimal sac infection.
- *Conjunctival swab culture and sensitivity* should be carried out in following cases:
  - One-eyed patients
  - Prior dacryocystectomy (DCT)
  - History of chronic infection, e.g. blepharitis
  - Recently healed corneal ulcer.
- *Lacrimal sac* should receive special attention. Lacrimal syringing should be carried out in a patient with history of watering from the eyes. In cases where chronic dacryocystitis is discovered, either DCR (dacryocystorhinostomy) or DCT (dacryocystectomy) operation should be performed, before the cataract surgery.
- *Trichiasis and entropion* should be looked for and corrected prior to cataract surgery.

6. Posterior segment evaluation

i. *Fundus examination,* wherever possible, should be carried out using direct ophthalmoscope and/or +90 D/+78 D lens, with special attention on the macula, to rule out other causes of decreased vision, especially age-related macular degeneration. Indirect ophthalmoscopy may be useful in hazy media.

ii. *Macular function tests* are important to predict the visual potential in patients with very dense cataracts where fundus examination is not possible. A few simple macular functions tests are as below:

- *Projection of rays (PR).* It is a crude but an important and easy test for function of the peripheral retina. It is tested in a semi-dark room with the opposite eye covered. A thin beam of light is thrown in the patient's eye from four directions (up, down, medial and lateral) and the patient is asked to look straight ahead and point out the direction from which the light seems to come.

- *Two-light discrimination test.* The patient is asked to look through an opaque disc perforated with two pinholes behind which a light is held. The holes are 2 inches apart and kept about 2 feet away from the eye. If the patient can perceive two lights, it indicates normal macular function.
- *Maddox rod test.* The patient is asked to look at a distant bright light through a Maddox rod. An accurate perception of red line indicates normal function.
- *Colour perception.* It indicates that some macular function is present and optic nerve is relatively normal.
- *Entoptic visualization.* It is evaluated by rubbing a point source of light (such as bare-lighted bulb of torch) against the closed eyelids. If the patient perceives the retinal vascular pattern in black outline, it is favourable indication of retinal function. Being subjective in nature, the importance of negative test can be considered if the patient can perceive the pattern with the opposite eye.
- *Potential acuity meter (PAM) test.* It is a subjective method to determine the potential of vision in patients with hazy media. This test is performed with dilated pupil, with the help of PAM devise attached to the slit-lamp. This device projects the image of Snellen's acuity chart to the macula of the patient, who is asked to read the chart. A reasonably accurate assessment of potential visual acuity may be made with this test.
- *Laser interferometry (LI).* Like PAM test, LI is also a subjective test for estimating visual acuity in patients with mild to moderate hazy media. It utilizes the principle of light interference. The interference fringes generated by a Helium-Neon laser are focused on the eye from two sources, which overlap behind the lens. By changing size of the fringes, visual acuity can be ascertained. This test is not possible in patients with very dense cataracts.

iii. *Objective tests for evaluating retina* are required, if some retinal pathology is suspected. These tests include ultrasonic evaluation of posterior segment of the eye; electrophysiological studies such as ERG (electroretinogram), EOG (electro-oculogram) and VER (visually-evoked response).

7. Keratometry and biometry

Keratometry and biometry to calculate power of the intraocular lens (IOL) to be implanted are performed in each case to be taken up for cataract surgery (For details *see*, Chapter 9 pages 179–187).

PREOPERATIVE MEDICATION AND PREPARATION

1. Consent

Consent with detailed information about the procedure, risks involved and outcome expected, should be obtained from each patient. (Annexure I).

2. Hygiene (scrub bath, care of hair and marking of the eye)

- Each patient should be instructed to have a scrub bath including face and hair wash with soap and water.
- Male patients must get their beard cleaned and hair trimmed.
- Female patients should comb their hair properly.
- Eye to be operated should be marked.
- Change of street clothes to operating room clothes is mandatory on the day of surgery.

3. Preoperative antibiotics and disinfectants

These are required to prevent postoperative endophthalmitis:

- *Topical antibiotics* such as fourth-generation fluoroquinolone (0.3% moxifloxacin or 0.3% gatifloxacin) may be used QID for 3 days before surgery and every 15 minutes 4–6 times just before surgery to eradicate conjunctival bacterial flora.
- *Povidone-iodine (10%) solution* should be used to paint the lids, brow region, and facial skin 3 hours before surgery.

- *Povidone-iodine (5%) solution* should be used to irrigate the conjunctival sac 5 minutes before surgery. It is the most important preoperative measure.

4. IOP lowering

IOP lowering is must for conventional extracapsular cataract extraction (ECCE). A few surgeons also prefer to lower IOP in manual small incision cataract surgery (SICS) and phacoemulsification. It can be accomplished by mechanical pressure (digital massage or Honan balloon) and/or by IOP lowering drugs (IV mannitol or acetazolamide).

5. Mydriasis

Mydriasis, sustained throughout the procedure is essentially required. It can be obtained by:
- *Topical tropicamide* 1% (or cyclopentolate) + phenylephrine 2.5% instilled every 15 minutes 4 times before surgery.
- *Topical cyclo-oxygenase inhibitor,* e.g. flurbiprofen 0.3% or, ketorolac 0.5%, or diclofenac 0.1% instilled 3 times, a day before the surgery and every 15 minutes, 4 times immediately before the surgery helps in maintaining mydriasis during the procedure.

PREOPERATIVE CHECKLIST

It is always advisable for the ward nurse to prepare a preoperative checklist to varify whether the preoperative preparation has been done properly (Annexure II).

ANNEXURE I

Sample of consent form for cataract surgery

Name of the patient ....
Father's name ....
Address ....
Date of birth ....
Sex: M ( )   F ( )   I ( )

A. Interpreter needs

An interpreter service is required?   Yes ( )   No ( )

B. Condition and treatment

The doctor has explained that you have the following condition: (Doctor to document in patient's own words) ....

....
This condition requires the following procedure. (Doctor to document include site and/or side where relevant to the procedure)

....
....
Left eye ( )   Right eye ( )

The following will be performed:

The cataract is surgically removed. The lens in the eye is replaced by an artificial lens or what is commonly known as an implant.

C. Risks of this procedure

There are risks and complications with this procedure. They include but are not limited to the following:

General risks
- Infection can occur, requiring antibiotics and further treatment.
- Bleeding could occur and may require a return to the operating room. Bleeding is more common, if you have been taking blood thinning drugs such as warfarin, asprin, clopidogrel or dipyridamole.
- Small areas of the lung can collapse, increasing the risk of chest infection. This may need antibiotics and physiotherapy.
- Increased risk in obese people of wound infection, chest infection, heart and lung complications, and thrombosis.
- Heart attack or stroke could occur due to the strain on the heart.
- Blood clot in the leg (DVT) causing pain and swelling. In rare cases, part of the clot may break off and go to the lungs.
- Death as a result of this procedure is possible.

Specific risks
- A cloudy cornea which may or may not settle. This may require further surgery.
- An acute inflammatory reaction causing pain. This may need further treatment.
- A fragment of the cataract may fall into the back of the eye. This may require further surgery.
- Infection of the eye which could cause loss of vision or loss of the eye.
- Glaucoma (eye disease). This may need further treatment.
- Macular oedema (collection of fluid); and retinal haemorrhage (bleed). This usually settles with time.
- Retinal detachment may occur. This will require further treatment.

- Any of these complications may occur but these complications are now rare.
- Any of these complications may permanently damage sight.
- Any of these complications may involve a second operation being necessary.

D. Significant risks and procedure options

(Doctor to document in space provided. Continue in medical record, if necessary)

....
....
....

E. Risks of not having this procedure

(Doctor to document in space provided. Continue in medical record, if necessary)

....
....
....

F. Anaesthetic

This procedure may require an anaesthetic. (doctor to document type of anaesthetic discussed)

....
....

G. Patient consent

I acknowledge that the doctor has explained;

- My medical condition and the proposed procedure, including additional treatment, if the doctor finds something unexpected. I understand the risks, including the risks that are specific to me.
- The anaesthetic required for this procedure. I understand the risks, including the risks that are specific to me.
- Other relevant procedure/treatment options and their associated risks.
- My prognosis and the risks of not having the procedure.
- That no guarantee has been made that the procedure will improve my condition even though it has been carried out with due professional care.
- The procedure may include a blood transfusion.
- Tissues and blood may be removed and could be used for diagnosis or management of my condition, stored and disposed of sensitively by the hospital.
- If immediate life-threatening events happen during the procedure, they will be treated based on my discussions with the doctor or my Acute Resuscitation Plan.
- A doctor other than the consultant may conduct

the procedure. I understand this could be a doctor undergoing further training.

I have been given the following Patient Information Sheet/s:

( ) Anaesthetic eye operation

( ) Cataract surgery

- I was able to ask questions and raise concerns with the doctor about my condition, the proposed procedure and its risks, and my treatment options. My questions and concerns have been discussed and answered to my satisfaction.
- I understand I have the right to change my mind at any time, including after I have signed this form but, preferably following a discussion with my doctor.
- I understand that image/s or video footage may be recorded as part of and during my procedure and that these image/s or video/s will assist the doctor to provide appropriate treatment.

On the basis of the above statements.

I request to have the procedure

Name of patient ....

Signature ....

Date ....

Patients who lack capacity to provide consent

Consent must be obtained from a substitute decision maker/s.

Name of substitute decision maker/s ....

Signature ....

Relationship to patient ....

Date ....

      Ph No ....

H. Doctor's statement

I have explained to the patient all the above points under the patient consent section (G) and I am of the opinion that the patient/substitute decision-maker has understood the information.

Name of Doctor: ....

Designation:..

Signature: ....

Date:...............................

I. Interpreter's statement

I have given a sight translation in ....
(state the patient's language here) of the consent form
and assisted in the provision of any verbal and written
information given to the patient/parent or guardian/
substitute decision-maker by the doctor.

Name of interpreter ....

Signature ....

Date ....

ANNEXURE II

Preoperative checklist

Name of patient..
Medical record no..

1. Investigation
Hb (if under GA)......... Blood sugar.......... BP ......
Weight .... Others ....

2. Eye examination: Eye ....
Vision .... Sac ....
Xylocaine sensitivity ....
IOP .... IOL power ....

3. Obtained written consent? Y......... , N ....
Attached GVP consent form?

4. Does the patient have DM? Y......... , N ....

5. Does the patient have hypertension?
   Y......... , N ....

6. Eye prepared for operation? Y......... , N ....

7. Eyebrows and eyelashes painted with povidone
   iodine.   Y......... , N ....

8. Eye dilated for operation? Y......... , N ....
   Dilated adequately?

9. Is it cataract (IOL) surgery? Y......... , N ....
   IOL brought as per No.?

10. Did medical officer examine?
    Y......... , N ....

11. Examination by anaesthetist ....

12. Did patient have a bath/wash face? (comment
    on patient hygiene)

....
....

Suggestion of doctor

....
....
....

Date ....
Signature of ward nurse ....

BIBLIOGRAPHY

1. American Academy of Ophthalmology (2008–2009). Basic and clinical science course: Lens and cataract, San Francisco.

2. Becker D. Preoperative medical evaluation: Part 1: General Principles and cardiovascular considerations. Anesthesia progress 2009;56(3):92–103.

3. Fischer S, Bader A, Sweitzer B. Preoperative evaluation. In: anesthesia, Miller R (Ed). 2010;1001–66. Churchill Livingstone, ISBN 978-0-443-06959-8, Philadelphia.

4. Fleisher L. Routine Laboratory Testing in the Elderly: Is it indicated? Anesthesia and Analgesia, 93:249–50;2001.

5. Fong K, Malhotra R. Assessment of the patient with cataract. In: cataract (eye essentials), Malhotra R (Ed). 2008;18–32, Elsevier, ISBN 978-0-08-044977-7, USA. Gwinnut, C. Clinical Anaesthesia (2nd edn), Blackwell, 2004 ISBN 978-1-4051-1552-0, Massachusetts.

6. Hata T, Moyers J. Preoperative patient assessment and management, In: clinical anesthesia, Barash PP (Ed). 2009;569–97. Lippincott Williams & Wilkins, ISBN 978-0-7817-8763-5, Philadelphia.

7. Hepner D. The role of testing in the preoperative evaluation. Clevel and clinic journal of medicine, 2009;76(4):S22–27.

8. Ismael S, Mowafi H. Melatonin provides anxiolysis, enhances analgesia, decreases intraocular pressure, and promotes better operating conditions during cataract surgery under topical anaesthesia. Anaesthesia and snalgesia 2009;108(4):1058–61.

9. Kubitz J, Motsch J. Eye surgery in the elderly. Best practice and research clinical anaesthesiology 2003;17(2):245–57.

10. Lichtor, J. Ambulatory Anesthesia, In: clinical anaesthesia, Barash PP (Ed). 2009;833–46, Lippincott Williams & Wilkins, ISBN 978-0-7817-8763-5, Philadelphia.

Biometry: Calculation of IOL Power

Chapter Outline

INTRODUCTION

CRUDE METHODS OF IOL POWER CALCULATION IN THE PAST
• IDEM lenses
• Standard lens
• Emmetropia lens

IOL POWER CALCULATION WITH BIOMETRY
Biometry
• Measurement of AL and essentials of biometers
• Measurement of refracting power of cornea

Effective IOL Position Optical Biometers
• IOL master
• Lens star
• IOL master vs lens star

Formulae for Calculating IOL Power
• First generation formulae

• Second generation formulae
• Third generation formulae
• Fourth generation formulae
• Fifth generation formulae
• Errors in IOL power calculation

Biometry in Special Conditions
• Biometry for toric IOLs
• Biometry in aphakic eyes
• Biometry in pseudophakic eyes
• Biometry in vitrectomized eyes
• Paediatric biometry and IOL power calculation
• Biometry and Calculation of IOL power after keratorefractive surgery

OPTIMIZATION OF IOL POWER

IMPORTANT CONSIDERATIONS AND FINAL SELECTIONS OF IMPLANT POWER

INTRODUCTION

Calculation of accurate IOL power is an important step in modern cataract surgery. It is an important step in successful IOL implantation. The refractive power of the pseudophakes is final, and the patient must live with any mistake committed or be subjected to repeat operation, i.e. the removal/replacement of the IOL with all the potential risks. Later correction, in other words, can only be achieved with lens exchange or extraocular aids like glasses or contact lenses, or corneal refractive surgery.

To ensure that our patients will have the optimal correction, the power of the lens to be implanted must be determined individually in every case. The development of modern ultrasonography units has made it possible to conveniently and accurately measure the AL of the eye. In the absence of ultrasonography in the past, IOL power was determined using asn intelligent guess-work approach. However, now various formulae have been developed to calculate the IOL power on the basis of various measurements (biometry).

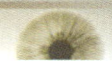

CRUDE METHODS OF IOL POWER CALCULATION USED IN THE PAST

In the 1980s, IOL power was a guess work based on the patient's previous refractive status. However, ethically as well as legally 'guess-work' approach for calculating IOL power should not be employed presently since it is a far less accurate method and its widespread use rapidly revealed that there were occasional unexpected and unsatisfactory results, deviating very widely from the targeted final refraction.

The use of 'guess-work' approach for determining IOL power in the past led to the development of following concepts:

• IDEM lenses
• Standard lens
• Emmetropia lens

Note. These concepts have no place in the present day practice. However, they are described here as historical events.

IDEM LENSES

These lenses are so named since the pre- and post-operative refraction with them is the same. Therefore, IDEM lenses were recommended for the patients who were emmetropic before the onset of cataract. Gernet and Zorkendorfer (1982) have shown that the refractive power of the natural lens is 23.70 D. The cardinal plane of this lens is approximately 6 mm behind the corneal apex. The distance for the cardinal plane of the posterior chamber lens is less; that is, it is further removed from the retina. In order to focus parallel rays of light on the retina, it must be weaker than the natural lens. Therefore, a 20 D artificial lens in the posterior chamber will restore the preoperative refractive error. Similarly IDEM lenses can be calculated for other sites of implantation as shown in Table 27.1.

Here, it is must to mention an important limitation. An IDEM artificial lens will restore the preoperative refractive error, only if the natural lens indeed had about 23.70 D refractive power. This, however, is not always the case. The refractive power of an eye is the result of the combination of different factors, such as the corneal curvature, the distance of lens from the cornea (the depth of anterior chamber), the dioptric power of the lens and the length of the eye. Each of these values can deviate and still an eye can be emmetropic as the different components compensate for each other. Therefore, deviations of 2 D are common and of more than 3 D are rare with the concept of IDEM lens.

STANDARD LENS

The standard lens is one that is approximately 2 D stronger than the IDEM lens, thereby rendering the pseudophakic eye about 1.5 D myopic as compared to preoperative emmetropic refraction. Since 80% of eyes are less than 1D nearsighted or farsighted, this will be a correct, or at least not an incorrect, result for the majority of patients. Further, in emmetropic patients, these were useful in keeping a balance between the distance and near vision. Because these lenses were the most commonly used implants, they were called standard lenses.

• The standard PCIOL had a refractive power of +22.0 D.

• The standard ACIOL had a refractive power of +20 D.

Table 27.1 *Power of different IDEM lenses*

Description of lens	Description of lens in short	Power (D)
Angle-supported lenses	AACL	+17.0
Iris clip lenses	ACL	+18.0
Iris plane lenses		+19.0
Posterior chamber lens (convexity of optic: anterior)	PCL	+20.0
Posterior chamber lens (nodal point closer to retina than with PCL)	PPCL	+21.0
Posterior chamber lens (convexity of optic: posterior)	PPPCL	+22.0

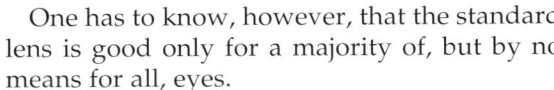
One has to know, however, that the standard lens is good only for a majority of, but by no means for all, eyes.

EMMETROPIA LENS

The emmetropia lens was used with the intention of restoring emmetropic status in previous ammetropic patients. The power of an 'emmetropia lens' was calculated by multiplying primary refractive error by 1.25 and then adding (for hypermetropia) or subtracting (for myopia) this number from the IDEM lens power. Thus,

- *Power of emmetropia lens in hypermetropic patients* = Power of IDEM lens + (Preoperative refractive error ×1.25).
- *Power of emmetropia lens in myopic patients =* Power of IDEM lens – (Preoperative refractive error ×1.25).

For this, a careful history has to be taken, including the kind of glasses the patient wore comfortably in the past. Old refractive values should be accepted, only if they come from reliable records or unequivocal history, or if they match our clinical findings. However, as mentioned in 'IDEM lens' description, deviation of 2–3 D is not rare; therefore, using primary refraction as the basis to determine the power of IOL to be implanted also entails the possibility of significant errors.

IOL POWER CALCULATION WITH BIOMETRY

With the advent of mini-science of biometry, now it is possible to calculate the power of IOL fairly accurately.

Major aspects of IOL power calculation are:

- Biometry
- Formulae for calculating IOL power
- Clinical variables, i.e. IOL power calculation in special situations
- Optimization of IOL power.

BIOMETRY

Biometry essentially includes:

- Measurement of axial length (AL)
- Keratometry (K-reading), i.e. measurement of corneal power
- Effective IOL position.

I. MEASUREMENT OF AXIAL LENGTH AND ESSENTIALS OF BIOMETERS

Axial length is the most important factor in biometric calculations. A 1 mm error in AL measurement results in a refractive error of approximately 2.35 D in a 23.5 mm eye, the error with wrong AL assessment being less in case of longer eyes as compared to shorter eyes.

Methods of measurement of axial length

1. Ultrasonic measurement of axial length can be made by applanation method or immersion technique, the latter being more accurate. A-scans measure the time required for a sound pulse to travel from the cornea to retina. In eyes more than 25 mm, staphyloma should be suspected especially when multiple disparate readings are obtained. To measure these eyes and to obtain the true measurement to the fovea, a B-scan technique must be used.

2. Optical measurement of axial length uses partial coherence laser. The IOL master measures time required for infrared light to travel to the retina. This technique does not require contact with the globe, so corneal compression artifacts are eliminated.

Essentials of A scan biometry

Settings of the biometer

Calibration check. The calibration of the biometer using the model eye provided with it should be checked from time-to-time to ensure accuracy. Instructions for the calibration check are specific and are provided with each instrument by the manufacturer.

Gain or sensitivity setting. Gain refers to the electronic amplification of the sound waves received by the transducer. The amplification factor is called a decibel (dB).

- Normal setting of gain is 70% in most of the biometers.
- Increase in gain may be required when the height of echoes achieved is inadequate as in very dense cataracts, other ocular opacities and high myopia. Increase in the gain produces taller echoes.

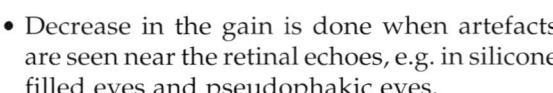

• Decrease in the gain is done when artefacts are seen near the retinal echoes, e.g. in silicone filled eyes and pseudophakic eyes.

Sound velocity setting should be done appropriately according to the type of eye, i.e.
• Normal
• Cataractous (mild, moderate or dense),
• Aphakic
• Pseudophakic (silicone or acrylic).

Note. Change in the sound velocity due to materials like silicone oil in the eye can produce an error of 3–4 D.

Operative instructions

Operative instructions to be kept in mind while performing the A-scan for measuring AL are as follows: *Placing of probe on the anaesthetized cornea should be such that:*
• It points towards macula, this is specially important in myopes, who may have a staphyloma.
• There is no fluid bridge between the probe and cornea.
• Cornea should not be depressed, otherwise it will result in inadvertent shortening of AL.

Mode settings may be manual or automatic, depending on the operator's preference:
• Manual mode setting allows the examiner to choose the best echo pattern produced by the eye. However, there may be delay in pressing the foot pedal, and one may miss the right reading.
• Automatic mode is operated by a software algorithm inside the instrument which controls the interpretation of echo pattern. Most of the surgeons use this mode. It is particularly useful in uncooperative patients.

Note. (1) It is always better to have an observer who should decide whether the best echo pattern has been selected by the automatic mode or not. In this way, one can have advantage of manual dynamic biometry as well as that of static graph of automatic biometry. (2) AL of both eyes should be measured for comparison.

Characteristics of a good scan

A-scan produces one-dimensional images in which echo strengths are displayed as vertical deflections or spikes of varying heights, on a display screen. Characteristics of a good scan are:
• Corneal echo is seen as a tall single peak
• Aqueous chamber does not produce any echo
• Anterior and posterior lens capsules produce tall echoes
• Vitreous cavity produces a few to no echoes
• Retina produces tall, sharply rising echoes with no staircase at the origin
• Orbital fat produces medium to low echoes.

Selection of the scan

The scan with the maximum AL, within the range obtained, should be selected.

II. MEASUREMENT OF REFRACTING POWER OF CORNEA

The central corneal power is the second most important factor in the calculation formulae, with a 1.0 D error in corneal power resulting in 1.0 D postoperative refractive error. Central corneal power can be measured by:
• *Keratometry or corneal topography,* neither of which measures the corneal power directly.
• *Pentacam* is relatively new imaging system that uses a single Scheimpflug camera to measure the radius of curvature of the anterior and posterior corneal surfaces, as well as corneal thickness, for the calculation of corneal power.
• *Galilei,* an another device, which measures corneal power in a similar fashion similar to pentacam.

Keratometry

It is the most frequently used method to measure the refractive power of cornea. *Important points to be considered for keratometry* are summarized here:
• While performing keratometry, the patient should be instructed to look into the keratometer. Majority of the patients with immature cataracts can fixate the reflection of their own eye, so they should be instructed to fixate into the centre of this reflection. Patients with mature cataract can be instructed to fixate the pin with the other eye.
• Mires should be focused in the centre of the eye to take care of the refractive error of the observer.

- Both the minus signs and the vertical component of the plus signs should be superimposed completely. If there is any angle between them, rotate the keratometer till they can be completely superimposed.
- Keratometry may be difficult or impossible in conditions with irregular or distorted corneal surface. In such cases, keratometric readings of opposite eye may be used or K-reading may be calculated from the corneal topography map.

III. EFFECTIVE IOL POSITION

Effective IOL position is influenced by several factors:

1. Anatomical factors include axial length, the steepness of cornea, limbal white to white measurement, preoperative anterior chamber depth and lens thickness. Holladay showed in a study that the depth of anterior chamber had a positive and partial relationship to the limbal white-to-white measurement.

2. IOL-related factors include shape, length, flexibility, anterior angulation (if any) and the material of the haptic of IOL.

3. Surgeon-related factors. Surgeon's individual surgical technique can also influence the ELPo.

4. Bag to sulcus shift. In situations like posterior capsule rent or loss of anterior capsule integrity, the IOL needs to be placed in ciliary sulcus instead of the normal 'in the bag' position. This requires deduction from the calculated IOL power in order to compensate for increase in effective IOL power, depending upon the base power of IOL, empirically taken 0.50–0.75 D less by most surgeons.

OPTICAL BIOMETERS

The introduction of optical biometry has significantly improved the accuracy of axial length measurement from 0.12 mm in immersion ultrasound to 0.02 mm in optical methods. The fact that the retinal pigment epithelium is the end-point of an optical measurement (refractive axial length), whereas the interface between the vitreous and the neuroretina is the end-point of an ultrasonic measurement (anatomical axial length), makes measurements by optical methods longer than those taken with ultrasound. In general optical biometers are reported to give accurate measurement of IOL power as compared to conventional A scan biometry. However, in eye with dense cataract and posterior staphyloma the axial length measurement is more accurate with immersion A/B scan (Holladay or Shamma's method) than with optical biometer. Commercially available optical biometer include:

- IOL master
- LenStar.

IOL MASTER

IOL Master™ (Zeiss Humphrey System) is a combined biometric instrument that measures quickly and precisely parameters of human eye needed for IOL power calculation by a non-contact technique. It also incorporates the software to calculate IOL power from various formulae.

Working principle

It is a non-contact optical device that measures the various parameters based on the following principles:

1. AL measurement is based on a patented interference optical method known as 'Partial Coherence Interferometry (PCI)'. This technique relies on a laser Doppler technique to measure the echo delay and intensity of infrared light reflected back from the tissue interfaces—cornea and retinal pigment epithelium. The instrument is calibrated against the ultrahigh resolution 40 MHz Grieshaber Biometric System. An internal algorithm approximates the distance to the vitreoretinal interphase for the equipment of an immersion A-scan ultrasonic AL.

2. Corneal curvature (K) is determined by measuring the distance between reflected light images as in conventional keratometry (principle of reflection).

3. Anterior chamber depth (ACD) is determined as the distance between the optical sections of the crystalline lens and the cornea produced by lateral slit-illumination.

4. White-to-white is determined from the image of the iris.

5. Calculation of IOL power by the software incorporating internationally accepted calculation formulae.

Advantages of the IOL Master

Operative advantages

1. *Patient comfort*, as the technique involves noncontact measurements.
2. *User-friendly*, as the operator can learn the technique very quickly.
3. *Single instrument* for measuring AL, corneal curvature (K) and ACD.
4. *Cross-infection* risk is not there, as the technique is non-contact.

Technical advantages

1. *LC Display* functions both for monitoring patient's eye alignment and displaying the results of calculation of IOL power.
2. *Safety features* are extensively integrated.
3. *More accurate AL measurement* as compared to A-scan (five times) of the eyes, with AL ranging between 14.0 and 40.0 mm.
4. *Specially useful in certain ocular conditions* where conventional methods are not so accurate, which include:
   - Small corneal scars
   - Anterior cortical spokes
   - Posterior subcapsular plaques
   - Other localized media capacities
   - High to extreme myopia with a type 1, peripapillary posterior staphyloma (ability to measure to the fovea in such a condition is an enormous advantage over conventional A-scan ultrasonography).
5. *Incorporates five IOL power calculating formulae* in an integrated manner. These include Haigis, Hoffer f, Holladay, SRK-II and SRK/T formulae.
6. *Individual optimization of formulae* is possible for every user. Data of the desired lenses need to be entered in the database. On the basis of postoperative refraction results, the lens constants that are entered in the calculation formulae may be personalized (i.e. individually optimized).
7. *Biometry in patients undergone corneal refractive surgery* is possible by use of:
   - Refractive history or contact lens method
   - Haigis-L formula for calculation of IOL power following myopic laser-assisted

in situ keratomileusis (LASIK) or photo-refractive keratometry (PRK).

Procedure

The procedure and operational details of the instrument are beyond the scope. The interested readers may consult the company's manual.

LenSTar

LenStar LS900 (Haag-Streit diagnostics) provides highly accurate laser optic measurements for every section of the eye and is the first optical biometer that can measure the thickness of the crystalline lens. With its integrated Olsen formula and the optional Toric Planner featuring the Barrett Toric Calculator, the LenStar provides the user with latest technology in IOL prediction for any patient.

Working Principle

It is a non contact optical device which measures multiple parameters based on following characteristics:

1. Central corneal thickness. As for every other LenStar axial measurement, optical coherence biometry is used to measure CCT with stunning reproducibility of ±2 μm. CCT is a key parameter in glaucoma diagnosis, and is also used for laser refractive surgery and/or to differentiate prior myopic or hyperopic LASIK procedures when there is no patient history.

2. Keratometry/Topography. LenStar's unique dual zone keratometry, featuring 32 marker points, provides perfect spherical equivalent, magnitude of astigmatism and axis position, making it the biometer of choice for toric IOL's. With the optional T-Cone topography add-on, LenStar provides full topography maps of the central 6 mm optical zone that are crucial for cataract planning.

3. White-to-white. Based on high-resolution colour photography of the eye, every white-to-white measurement can be reviewed and adjusted by the user if necessary. As such, it is fully reliable for use with anterior chamber and sulcus-fixated phakic IOLs. It can also be used to determine advanced IOL calculation formulae.

4. Pupillometry. Measurement of the pupil diameter in ambient light conditions can be used as an indicator for the patient's suitability for apodized premium IOLs, as well as for laser refractive procedures.

5. Lens thickness. Accurate measurement of the lens thickness is key to optimal IOL prediction accuracy when using the latest IOL calculation formulae, Olsen or Holladay 2. Measuring the lens thickness with LenStar significantly improves the IOL prediction accuracy of Holladay 2 and leads to a different IOL power selection in 30% of cases.

6. Anterior chamber depth. Like all axial dimensions captured by the LenStar, ACD is measured by optical coherence biometry, providing more precision and reproducibility. This allows ACD to be measured on phakic as well as on pseudophakic eyes. Additionally, the LenStar is able to display the anatomical anterior chamber depth (endothelium to anterior lens surface).

7. Axial length. It uses a superluminescent diode as the laser source which enables measurement of the axial length of the patient's eye, precisely on the patient's visual axis and in the presence of dense media. The user can review and move all of the measuring gate positions on the A-scan if necessary.

8. Special eye conditions. All of the described measurements are available for use on the regular eye, as well as for aphakic, pseudo-aphakic and silicone oil-filled eyes. In case of error, users may even change the selected eye condition after completion of the measurement procedure.

Advantages

In addition to all the advantages provided by IOL master, LenStar also allow the user to calculate power for Toric IOL implantation using Barrett toric calculator which is incorporated in its software.

IOL MASTER VS LenStar

The LenStar LS 900 device enables to perform accurate and repetitive biometric measurements and implant power calculations. Implant calculation results obtained using the LenStar LS 900 device are comparable to those achieved using the IOL master V.5 device, which has been commonly accepted as standard for over a decade.

- IOL master is based on the principle of partial coherence interferometry (PCI) with 780 nm infrared diode as the source, which emits a dual beam and a short coherence length of 160 microns. LenStar is based on the principle of low coherence reflectometry with 820 nm super luminescent diode as the light source and a 3 db fibre coupler.

- The use of both devices is limited by significant lens opacification, posterior capsule calcification and in presence of posterior staphyloma. In such cases, additional ultrasound biometry should be performed.

- Keratometry results obtained using both devices should not be used alternatively because of the different measurement methods and different refraction indexes.

- The LenStar takes two sets of keratometric readings: one at 1.65 mm and one at 2.3 mm, with 16 points each which is more accurate than IOL master which takes a single set at 2.5 mm with 6 points each.

- The LenStar LS 900 device comparing to the IOL master additionally enables pachymetry, macular retinal thickness, lens thickens and pupil diameter measurement.

- Newer IOL power calculation formulae like the Barrett universal II formula, Oslen formula and Hill-RBF are availabile in LenStar LS 900 but not in IOL master V.5.

- LenStar can also calculate power for Toric IOL implantation using Barrett toric calculator which is not possible in the case of IOL master.

- LenStar software runs on an external PC, which allows direct communication with electronic medical record programs; the software can automatically fill in data fields in a chosen formula.

■ FORMULAE FOR CALCULATING IOL POWER

Depending upon the basis of their deviation, the various formulae for calculating IOL power have been grouped into theoretical formulae and regression formulae.

- *Theoretical formulae.* These are based on mathematical principles revolving around the 'schematic eye'.
- *Regression formulae.* These were arrived at by looking at postoperative outcomes retrospectively.

Taking into consideration the time when they were evolved and the corrections incorporated into them with newer developments, the IOL power calculating formulae have been grouped into various generations, i.e.

- First-generation formulae
- Second-generation formulae
- Third-generation formulae
- Fourth-generation formulae.

A. FIRST-GENERATION FORMULAE

The earliest formulae used for IOL power calculation were the first-generation theoretical and regression formulae.

I. Theoretical formulae

Various theoretical formulae derived from the geometric optics as applied to the schematic eyes, using theoretical constants, had been developed to calculate the power of IOL required for postoperative emmetropia. These formulae were based on three variables:

- The AL of eyeball
- K-reading
- The estimated postoperative ACD.

A few of the first-generation theoretical formulae include the following:

1. Binkhorst formula

$$P = \frac{1336\,(4r - a)}{(a - d)\,(4r - d)}$$

where,

P is the IOL power in diopters.

r is the corneal radius in millimetres (average).

a is AL in millimetres.

d is assumed postoperative ACD plus corneal thickness.

2. Colenbrander–Hoffer formula

$$P = \frac{1336}{a - d - 0.05} - \frac{1336}{\dfrac{1336}{K} - d - 0.05}$$

where, K is average keratometry in dioptres.

3. Gill's formula

$$P = 129.40 + (-108 \times K)$$
$$= + (-2.79 \times L\ eye)$$
$$+ (0.26 \times LCL)$$
$$+ (-0.38 \times Ref)$$

where,

P is the desired IOL power.

K is the refractive power of cornea in dioptres.

L eye is the AL in millimetres.

LCL is the distance of apex of anterior corneal surface to apex of IOL in millimetres.

Ref is the desired postoperative refraction.

4. Clayman's formula

Assume:

Emmetropizing IOL = 18 D

Emmetropic AL = 24 mm

Emmetropic average keratometer reading = 42.0 D

1 mm in AL = 3 D of IOL power

1 D in keratometry = 1D of IOL power

If IOL power >21 D, deduct 0.25 for every dioptre >18.0 D

For example, AL = 22 mm; K = 43.0 D.

It leads to 6 D hyperopia in length; 1.0 D myopia in keratometry

Hence, IOL power = 18 + 6 − 1 = 23.0 D − (23 − 18) × 0.25 D = 21.75 D

5. Fyodorov formula

$$P = \frac{1336 - LK}{(L - C) - CK}$$

where,

P is the implant power for emmetropia.

L is the AL in millimetres.

K is the corneal curvature in diopters.

C is the estimated postoperative ACD.

Algebraic transformation of theoretical formulae

These apparently different formulae are in fact identical except for the correction factors.

They can all be algebraically transformed into

$$P = \frac{N}{L-C} - \frac{NK}{N-KC}$$

where,

P is the implant power for emmetropia.

N is the aqueous and vitreous refractive index.

C is the estimated postoperative ACD in millimetres.

L is the AL in millimetres.

K is the corneal curvature in diopters.

Drawbacks of theoretical formulae

Although the theoretical formulae in practice generally are reliable for eyes with AL between 22 and 24.5 mm, they have following drawbacks:

1. They tend to predict too large an emmetropic value in short-eyes (<22 mm) and too small a value in long-eyes (>24.5 mm).
2. They are too cumbersome to apply without the assistance of a calculator or a computer.
3. They still require a guess about the ACD, and the ultimate result depends on the accuracy of that guess.
4. Most of these formulae were developed and iris-supported lenses were commonly used. So the estimate for the distance between the cornea and implant (postoperative ACD) are different for the presently used PCIOLs.
5. These formulae are based on theoretical simplistic assumption about the optics of the eye.

II. Regression formulae

In view of the drawbacks of theoretical formulae, there had been a tendency to use the simpler empirical formulae in clinical practice. The empirical formulae are based on regression analysis of the actual postoperative results of implant power as a function of the variables of corneal power and AL. In other words, a 'best-fit' line or curve is plotted from the known ALs and K-readings and is subsequently used to predict the implant power needed for future patients.

A number of regression formulae are available. The commonly used are the SRK formula and its modifications.

SRK-I formula

It was introduced by Sanders, Retzlaff and Kraff, based on the regression analysis, taking into account the retrospective computer analysis of a large number of postoperative refractions. The postoperative ACD was not included but was replaced with A-constant which is unique to each different type of IOL and is determined by the manufacture depending upon its material, position of the eye and optic and haptic design angulation, etc. The SRK formula is:

$$P = A - 2.5\,L - 0.9\,K$$

where,

P is IOL power.

A is constant specific for each lens.

L is AL in millimetres.

K is average keratometry in dioptres.

This formula has become the most widely used formula for IOL power calculation. However, like theoretical formulae, it also performs well for eyes with AL between 22.0 and 24.5 mm. In converse to theoretical formulae, the regression formula tends to predict too small a value in short-eyes and too large a value in long-eyes. To address this problem, SRK-I formula has been modified twice.

B. SECOND-GENERATION FORMULAE

I. Theoretical formulae

Modified Binkhorst formulae

Binkhorst in 1981 improved the prediction of effective lens position by using a single variable predictor, the AL, as a scaling factor for effective lens position and presented a formula to better predict ACD.

II. Regression formulae

SRK II formula

The basic equation of the formula is same; i.e. $P = A - 2.5\,L - 0.9\,K$, but the A-constant is modified on the basis of the AL as follows:

- If L is <20 mm: A+3.0
- If L is 20.00–20.99:   A+2.0
- If L is 21.00–21.99:   A+1.0
- If L is 22.0–24.5:   A
- If L is >24.5:   A–0.5

Modified SRK II formula

In this formula, based on the AL, A-constant is modified as given:

- If L is <20 mm: A+1.5
- If L is 20–21 mm: A+1.0
- If L is 21–22 mm: A+0.5
- If L is 22.0–24.5 mm: A
- If L is 24.5–26.0 mm: A–1.0
- If L is >26 mm: A–1.5

C. THIRD-GENERATION FORMULAE

Most of the third-generation formulae are a hybrid of both theoretical and regression (empirical) formulae.

Holladay I formula

In 1988, Holladay proved that the use of a two-variable predictor (AL and keratometry) could significantly improve the predictor of effective lens position, particularly in unusual eyes. He proposed the formulae based on geometric relationship of the anterior segment (third-generation theoretical formula). However, soon this formula was modified and now the Holladay I formula, though theoretical, also uses an empirically derived constant which is then added to the ACD estimate.

Hoffer's Q formula

Hoffer's Q formula is a third-generation theoretical formula, optimized with regression techniques for ACD. This formula performs best for short-eyes.

SRK/T formula

It is a non-linear theoretical optical formula, empirically optimized for postoperative ACD, retinal thickness and corneal refractive index. It thus combines the advantages of both the theoretical and empirical analysis. This formula seems to be significantly more accurate for extremely long eyes (>28 mm).

D. FOURTH-GENERATION FORMULAE

Holladay II formula

It is being considered more accurate because of its enhanced ability to predict the position of the implants. Software programmes are available in the modern biometers to use the Holladay formulae. Otherwise the Holladay formulae are very exhaustive. The various constants and equations used in this formula are as below:

Measured values

K = average K-reading (dioptres)

R = average corneal radius (millimetres) = 337.5/K

AL = measured ultrasonic axial length (millimetres)

Recommended constants

C = refractive index of cornea = 4/3

A = refractive index of aqueous = 1.336

RT = retinal thickness factor = 0.200 mm

Chosen values

V = vertex distance of pseudophakic spectacles (millimetres); default=12 mm

Ref = desired postoperative spheroequivalent refraction (SER) (dioptres)

SF = 'surgeon factor' = distance (millimetres) from aphakic anterior iris plane to optical plane of IOL. It is analogous to A-constant of SRK formula.

Definitions of other variables

AG = anterior chamber diameter from angle to angle (millimetres)

ACD = anatomic ACD (millimetres), distance from corneal vertex to anterior iris plane

Alm = modified AL (millimetres) = AL + retinal thickness factor (RT)

I = power of IOL (dioptres)

A Ref = actual postoperative SER (dioptres).

Holladay consultant IOL programme

It uses Holladay II formula with seven variables.

Refractive formula

It is a theoretical formula described by Holladay to calculate IOL power for aphakic, ametropic, pseudophakic and PRLs. According to this formula, AL measurement is not required. This formula calculates IOL power from the following parameters:

- Preoperative refractive power
- Corneal power
- Desired postoperative refraction
- Vertex distance.

However, this formula was not found to be very good for aphakic eyes as it is difficult to measure the vertex distance accurately, and this may result in high errors.

Haigis formula

Haigis introduced his formula in 1999. The formula is built on the same theoretical base as all others, and differs only in the way the ELP is calculated. Haigis proposed using three different constants to better define the ELP. These constants are called the a0, the a1 and the a2 constants. The three constants can be used as standard, optimized, or triple optimized. In the standard form, none of the constants is optimized. The first constant, a0, is derived from the A-constant using a standard equation (a0 = 0.62467 × A-constant-72.434). The a1 and a2 constants are set at default values, a1 = 0.4 and a2 = 0.1. Single or triple optimization of the Haigis constants can improve prediction accuracy, but requires a large number of cases.

E. FIFTH GENERATION FORMULAE

Hoffer H-5 Formula

The Hoffer H-5 formula is the first fifth generation IOL power formula introduced in 2013, which uses the structure of the Holladay 2 formula and takes into account the demographic specifics of the individual patient based on race and gender. Fourth generation formulas use arbitrary average biometric values. These values are completely different in males and females and in different races. The gender/race specific average is used for a specific patient rather than the overall human average.

NEWER IOL POWER CALCULATION FORMULAE

1. Barrett universal II formula

Barrett universal II formula determines lens position via anatomical depth, utilizes a lens factor related to the physical position of the principal planes of the IOL, and calculates the change in principal planes for positive and negative IOLs. It is termed 'universal formula' because it is designed for use with multiple lens styles and with short, medium, and long axial lengths. It is available in LenStar optical biometer.

2. Olsen formula

The Olsen formula uses exact ray tracing which allows better prediction effective lens position (ELP) as a function of lens thickness (LT) and anterior chamber depth (ACD) to account for the true physical dimensions of an eye's optical system. It uses the same technology employed by physicists to design telescopes and camera lenses.

A key feature of the Olsen formula is accurate estimation of the IOL's physical position using a newly developed concept, the C-constant (Fig. 27.1). The C-constant can be thought of as a ratio by which the empty capsular bag will encapsulate and fixate an IOL following in-the-bag implantation. This approach predicts the IOL position as a function of preoperative anterior chamber depth and lens thickness. It is also available in LenStar optical biometer.

3. Hill–RBF formula

The new Hill-RBF method is a pure data driven IOL calculation approach and, therefore, it is free of the limitation of lens-position estimation. RBF stands for *Radial Basis activation Function*. It is driven by an advanced, self-validating method using pattern recognition based on artificial intelligence and sophisticated data interpolation. Starting with a large number of cases where the biometry and the outcomes are known, RBF is capable to find distinct patterns in the apparently random cloud of data-points.

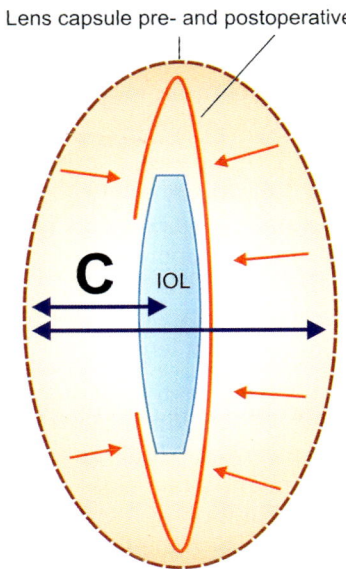

Fig. 27.1: *Concept of C-constant in Olsen formula.*

The current algorithm is based on outcome data of more than 3400 eyes, with LenStar biometry data and the Alcon SN60WL IOL implanted. It works best with this combination of biometry device and IOL but works also very good with biometry data from other optical biometry devices and with other biconvex IOL's from +6 to +30 D.

Reliable calculation results are labeled with 'In Bounds', results that deserve more attention of the surgeon, since the prediction algorithm was not able to determine the desired level of reliability, are labelled 'Out of bounds'. An out of bounds labelled result does not need to be inaccurate but the Hill-RBF method informs the surgeon that the respective pattern of biometric measurements is not well-studied by the algorithm and it is recommended to use the Olsen and the Barrett formula to confirm the proposed IOL.

Limitations of newer IOL power calculation formulae

These newer formulae have recently become available for use on the Haag-StreitLenStar. However, they are not currently available on the Zeiss IOLMaster and other biometers.

USES OF DIFFERENT FORMULAE

Most of the IOL calculation formulae work well for eyes with axial lengths between 22.0 and 24.5 mm. However, in case of longer and shorter axial lengths, their inaccuracy needs to be compensated by optimization.

Optimization is the process of increasing the accuracy of a formula by altering and refining the manufacturer's lens constant. It is worked out by analysing postoperative outcomes with respect to targeted refraction for a particular surgical technique, in a specified IOL design and for given range of axial lengths (*see* page 546).

Albeit controversial, some guidelines have been developed for which formulae to use under specific circumstances. Although earlier widely used, the SRK 2 and older ones now obsolete. Appropriate calibration of settings and adjustments of constants is a must before IOL power prediction. No single formulae has been found to be useful in all circumstances. So depending

upon the circumstances, possible recommendation is as below:

Circumstance	Choice of formulae
AL - <20 mm	Holladay II/Hoffer Q
- 20–22 mm	Hoffer Q
- 22–24 mm	SRK/T; Hoffer Q; Holladay
- 24.5–26 mm	Holladay I
- >26 mm	SRK/T
Myopic LASIK	Haigis L
Piggy Back	Holladay's refractive formulae

The newer formulae Barrett universal II formula; Oslen's formula, Hill-RBF formula and Hoffer H-5 formula are still not widely available in the biometry software. Due to the absence of compelling comparative evidence of the superiority of these formulas over each other, it is justifiable to continue using an appropriate combination (according to axial length) of the two variable - single constant formulae.

Note. Ultimately, the choice of formula is up to the surgeon, but whatever the method, every effort should be made to ensure the highest possible accuracy.

ERRORS IN IOL POWER CALCULATION

Even with the recent advances like IOL master and Orbscan, which have greatly improved the accuracy of ocular biometry, errors in the prediction of IOL power still exist in almost all the methods. These could be subjective or intrinsic in nature.

Most of the existing methods of IOL power calculation are based on the *mean zero error (MZE)* concept, where the empirically fit parameters (such as ELPo) are defined by regression formulae with one-constant optimization. The current MZE methods have personalised the following factors for improved accuracy:

1. *Axial length.* The factor with maximum contribution to error. Sources of error in AL include:
• Corneal indentation
• Improper calibration
• Anatomical thickness of retina
• Failure to recognise appropriate echo patterns on A-scan ultrasound.

2. *Corneal power errors.* These can arise due to inaccuracies in keratometric evaluation.

3. *Estimated lens position,* also known as effective anterior chamber depth (ACD), this can result in an error of 0.5–2.5 D for every 1.0 mm error in calculating ELPo. This parameter takes into account both placement of the IOL during surgery and thickness of the lens to be implanted.

4. *Errors from formula used.* As discussed above, certain formulae have more accuracy in the setting of long and short ALs. Selecting inappropriate formula can produce an error of 0.50–2.5 D in the final IOL power.

5. *Manufacturer labelling error.* The higher the IOL power, the higher will be the error.

■ BIOMETRY IN SPECIAL CONDITIONS

1. BIOMETRY FOR TORIC IOLS

For Toric IOL power calculation, commonly used calculators are (Fig. 27.2):

- ASSORT calculator
- Holladay IOL consultant toric planner
- Barrett Toric calculator.

The ASSORT calculator has a unique feature of calculating the most effective implant available and to compare IOLs based on the target postoperative refraction. The software also includes optimized lens constants for commonly used formulae, such as Hoffer, Haigis, Holladay, and SRK/T, to obtain the effective lens position (ELP). The astigmatic effect of the phaco incision can be dynamically adjusted based on incision placement. The new parameter of corneal topographic astigmatism (CorT Total) can be employed to include an accurate measure of corneal astigmatism with inclusion of the posterior cornea. So, it displays all pre and postoperative toric implant requirements.

The Holladay IOL consultant software features both a ToricPreOp Planner for forward calculation and a ToricPostOp Back Calculator for back calculation. The ToricPreOp Planner allows the user to determine the ideal toricity and axis of placement for a toric IOL using K readings and the expected SIA from the cataract incision. It does not use a constant ratio of 1.46 to

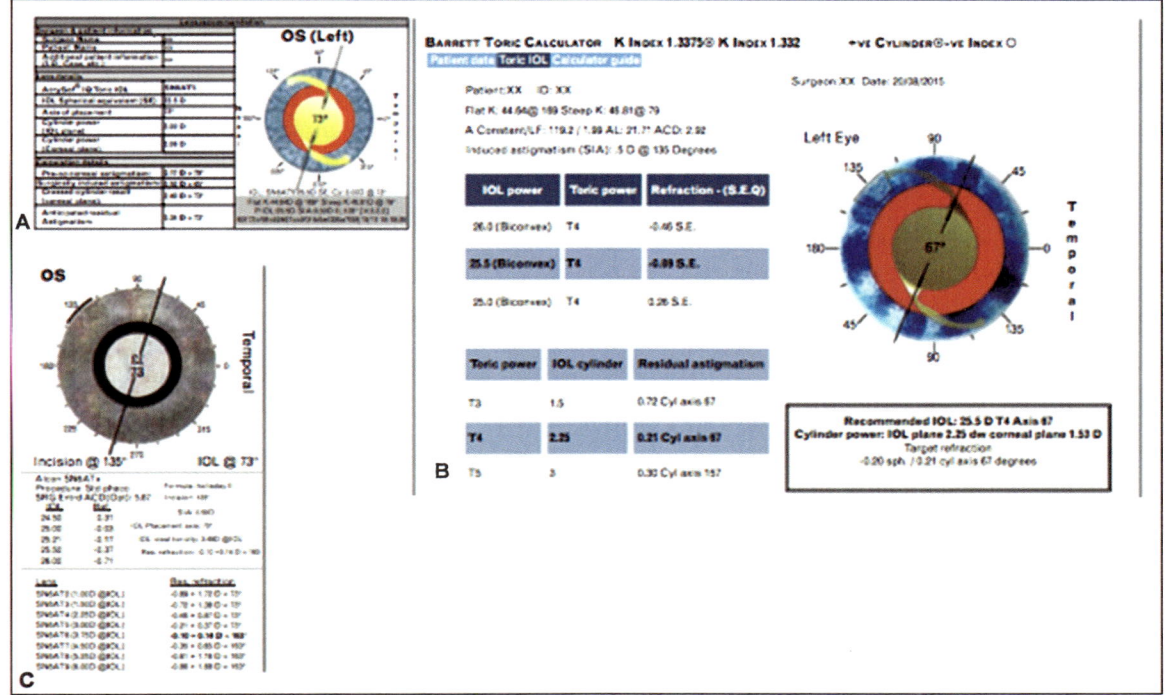

Fig. 27.2: *(A) The Alcon Toric IOL calculator; (B) The Barrett Toric calculator; (C) The Holladay IOL consultant Toric IOL calculator.*

determine the ideal toricity of the IOL from the corneal astigmatism, which is used by some other calculators that can result in errors with low- and high-powered IOLs. Before using the planner, the surgeon should confirm that the K readings and the axes for the flat and steep Ks are correct. The ToricPostOp Back Calculator allows the surgeon to determine the exact amount that the toric IOL should be rotated to produce the smallest residual astigmatism.

2. BIOMETRY IN APHAKIC EYES

It is required for secondary IOL implantation. In an aphakic eye, sound travels at the speed of 1532 m/s. The two lens spikes are absent in these cases or may be replaced by a single spike obtained by the anterior vitreous face and posterior lens capsule. Therefore, if available, immersion technique of biometry is the method of choice for aphakes rather than the contact technique. In modern biometers, options are available for aphakic mode as well.

3. BIOMETRY IN PSEUDOPHAKIC EYES

It is required in those cases, needing an IOL exchange. Such eyes have an extremely high spike at the lens followed by artificial chain of reduplication of echoes which can be misinterpreted as spikes from the retina. This can be avoided by lowering the gain, which eliminates the artificial spikes and increases the retinal spikes. In cataractous eye, the velocity of sound speed is about 1550 m/s but this is not so in pseudophakic eye. In such an eye, sound speed depends on the sound transmission characteristics and the centre thickness of the IOL in that particular eye. In modern biometers, options are available for phakic, pseudophakic or aphakic mode. This should be rechecked while measuring routine cataract cases to avoid miscalculation of IOL power.

Apparent axial length (AAL) and true axial length (TAL). When AL is measured in apseudophakic eye with an ultrasonic probe with a velocity setting of 1550 m/s, which is the standard setting for the normal cataractous eye, the result obtained is labelled as AAL. This is not TAL because unlike the cataractous eye the average sound speed in the pseudophakic eye is not 1550 m/s. Sound speed in pseudophakic

eye depends both on the 'sound transmission characteristic' and the 'centre thickness' of the IOL in that particular eye.

Holladay formula for pseudophakic biometry

$$TAL = (0.988 \ AAL) + T \ [1-(1532/V)]$$

where,

TAL is true axial length, AAL is apparent axial length measured at 1550 m/s, T is the thickness of IOL and V is the velocity of sound in the IOL.

Secondary piggyback IOL for pseudophakia

It has been suggested that in patients who have a significant residual refractive error following the primary IOL implantation, it is often easier surgically and more predictable optically to leave the primary implant in place and calculate the secondary piggyback IOL power to achieve the desired refraction; rather than doing the IOL exchange. The formulae to calculate IOL power in such cases include:

- *Holladay's refractive formula.* This method does not require knowledge of the primary implant or the AL. This formula works for plus as well as minus lenses.
- Gill's nomogram for secondary piggyback IOL.

Apart from Holladay's refractive formula, Gill's nomogram can also be used to calculate power for secondary piggyback IOL. It requires axial length (AL) and spectacle spherical equivalent (SE) to calculate the required power. Gill's nomogram for residual hypermetropia and residual myopia is as below:

For residual hyperopia

Axial length (mm)	IOL power (P)
≤22	1.5 × S.E. + 1
22–25	1.4 × S.E. + 1
≥25	1.3 × S.E. + 1

For residual myopia

Axial length (mm)	IOL power (P)
≤22	1.5 × S.E. − 1
22–25	1.4 × S.E. − 1
≥25	1.3 × S.E. − 1

4. BIOMETRY IN VITRECTOMIZED EYES

Measuring the AL of eyes in which the vitreous has been replaced with silicone oil is difficult

because sound attenuation within the liquid silicone causes the retinal spike to be small and confusing to identify. The difficulty can be overcome simply by increasing the 'system gain'. The result obtained is the AAL, which must be converted to TAL.

Formula suggested by Professor John Shammus:
Velocity of sound wave in silicone oil medium is 990 m/s in an average eye.
TAL = 1133/1550 AAL
For example, a cataractous eye containing silicone oil
AAL = 30.00 mm
TAL = 1133/1550 AAL
= 1133/1550 × 30
= 21.93 mm.

As the silicone oil alters the optics of the eye due to its index of refraction, further adjustment is required after calculation of IOL power using the TAL. Usually these eyes require an IOL which is 2–3 D stronger than indicated by standard power calculation.

5. PAEDIATRIC BIOMETRY AND IOL POWER

Power of IOL. Most surgeons follow the following protocol:
- In older children (> 8 years), emmetropia is the target.
- In children between 2–8 years of age, 10% undercorrection from the calculated biometric power is recommended to counter the myopic shift.
- Below 2 years, an undercorrection by 20% is recommended from the biometric readings.

Note. *Most surgeons follow Dahan et al's simplified approach* based on the axial length only, which is as below:

Axial length	IOL power
17 mm	28 D
18 mm	27 D
19 mm	26 D
20 mm	24 D
21 mm	24 D
22 mm	23 D
23 mm	23 D
>24 mm	Axial length –1 D

Similarly, Vasa vada et al have suggested the following approach.

Age	Under correction
0–3 months	35%
3–6 months	30%
6–12 months	25%
1–2 years	20%
2–4 years	15%
4–6 years	10%
>6 years	5%

6. BIOMETRY AND CALCULATION OF IOL POWER AFTER KERATOREFRACTIVE SURGERY

Routine IOL power calculation based on the AL and the keratometry is often inaccurate in eyes that have undergone previous keratorefractive surgery and often leads to an unacceptable hyperopic error, which inconveniences the patient for both near and distance visions. Infact, the corneal refractive surgeries alter the basic assumptions on which the biometry for IOL calculations is based—namely the perfectly spherical nature of cornea. The refractive surgeries mainly affect the central cornea, as well as alter the posterior corneal curvature, which is not routinely measured. The errors occur due to instruments, index of refraction and formulas used. This incorrect IOL power alteration occur due to three errors: instrument error, index of refraction error and formulae error.

1. Instrument error. Keratometers and corneal topographers used to calculate corneal power cannot obtain accurate measurements in eyes that have undergone corneal refractive surgery. The major cause of error is that the most keratometers measure at the 3.2 mm zone of central cornea, which often misses the central flatter zone of effective corneal power; the flatter the cornea, the larger the zone of measurement.

2. Index of refraction error. The assumed index of refraction (IR) of normal cornea is based on the relationship between the anterior and posterior corneal curvature. This relationship is changed in PRK, LASIK and LASEK eyes but not in RK eyes where alteration in curvature occurs but relation between anterior and posterior corneal curvature is maintained. The manual keratometers measure only the front

surface curvature leading to error in calculation. This overestimates the corneal power by 1D for every 7D of correction of refractive error.

3. Formula errors. All modern formulae except the Haigis formula use AL and K reading to predict position of IOL postoperatively (ELP). In postcorneal refractive surgery, eyes flatter K causes error in calculation.

Note. Because of above errors special methods need to be adopted to measure the actual corneal power after any keratorefractive procedure.

Special methods to calculate IOL power after keratorefractive surgery

There are more than 20 methods proposed over the years to calculate true corneal power or adjust the calculated IOL power to account for the errors caused. Methods to measure IOL power postrefractive surgery can be divided as 'Indirect' or 'Direct' based on the measurement of the corneal power after surgery. Direct involves actual measurement, while indirect makes assumptions based on historical data or theoretical analysis (Table 27.2).

INDIRECT METHODS

1. Clinical history/calculation method. This is the most accurate method, but requires that the keratometry and refraction prior to the kerato-refractive procedure be known, in addition to the stabilized postoperative refraction. In this method, the change in refraction at the corneal plane is subtracted from the original K-reading prior to the procedure, to obtain a calculated postoperative K-reading. Although this is the most accurate method, the preoperative

parameters may not be available since there is usually a long-time interval between the refractive surgery and the cataract extraction. In addition, one must be careful to measure the postoperative refraction before any myopic shift occurs due to nuclear sclerosis.

$K\,postReSx = K\,preReSx - \text{difference in Spherical Equivalent}$
{ReSx = Refractive surgery}

- Convert the pre- and post-operative refraction into spheral equivalent refraction (SER) [sphere 0.5 (cylinder)].
- Now convert these SERs at the spectacle plane (SEQS) with a given vertex distance (V) (in millimetres) into SER at the corneal plane (SEQC)

$SEQC = 1000 / [(1000 / SEQS) - V]$

  Therefore the change in refraction at the corneal plane = Preoperative SEQC–Post-operative SEQC.

- Now subtract this from the mean preoperative K-reading to get the mean postoperative K-value. This is to be used for IOL power calculation.

It is most accurate as the pre-op values are precise up to +/−0.25 mm (30).

2. Contact lens over refraction method. In this method, the SER is determined by normal refraction and then repeated with a hard contact lens in place. If the SER does not change with the contact lens, then the K-reading of the cornea must be equal to the base curve of the plano contact lens. If the patient has a myopic shift in refraction with the contact lens, then the base curve of the contact lens is greater than that of the cornea by a magnitude equal to the amount

Table 27.2 *Direct and indirect methods to measure IOL power in patients with status postrefractive surgery*

Indirect	Direct
Clinical history method or calculation method	Modern theoretical formulae with modifications (Haigis, Holladay), Gaussian optics and regression formulae
Contract lens (CL) over-refraction	Aramberri "double K"
Vertexed IOL power	Topographical methods
Intraoperative autorefraction measurement	Camellin and Calossi method
DBR method	Rosa method
	Direct measurements

of the shift. If there is a hyperopic shift in refraction with the contact lens, then the base curve of the contact lens is less than that for the cornea by the amount of the shift.

Formulae for corrected k value needs 4 parameters:
Base curve of contact lens in Diopters (BC),
Power of contact lens (P),
Refraction without contact lens (R_{base}), and
Refraction with contact lens (R_{CL})

The formula is:
$$K\ postReSx = BC + P + (R_{CL} - R_{base})$$

Limitation is the reliability of refraction in the patient with cataract.

For example a patient with current base SER(R_{base}) = +0.5 sphere.
SER with plano contact lens (R_{CL})= –2.0D (myopic shift)
Suppose base curve (BC) of contact lens used is 35 D. Then,
$$K\ postReSx = 35 + 0 + [-2.0\ D - (+0.5\ D)]$$
$$= 35 + (-2.5)$$
$$= 32.5\ D$$

Use this K for IOL power calculation.

This is also an accurate method for determining the K-value, but the main limitation is that the cataract itself may prevent an accurate refraction.

3. Vertexed IOL method. Based on theoretical studies by Feiz, Latkany and their colleagues, various nomograms were developed after calculating IOL power post LASIK with SRK/T and three other formulas. The change in the spherical equivalent after LASIK was used to modify the IOL power. Its main limitation is the theoretical nature of the study and the lack of large published data with regards to its accuracy.

4. Intraoperative retinoscopy/autorefraction method. In this technique, retinoscopy or autorefraction by hand-held autorefractometer is performed intraoperatively in the aphakic eye after completion of the cataract extraction. The IOL power is then calculated from the aphakic refraction.

Advantage. Theoretically, it seems to be a simple method.

Disadvantages. Asepsis during surgery may be jeopardized and inaccuracy is possible in retinoscopy specially in the eyes which had refractive surgery for hyperopia.

5. DBR method. In this method, like calculation method, preoperative patient data is essential. For it, the refractive surgeons need to measure AL along with refraction and keratometry during refractive surgery and keep a record of the IOL power calculated for emmetropia. The record of residual refractive error after stabilization of the postsurgery refraction is also needed. The calculation is explained with an imaginary example:

Prerefractive surgery data
- Refraction: –5.25 D
- Keratometry: 46.20 D
- Axial length: 25.00 mm
- IOL power for emmetropia (A-constant 118.0): 16.80 D

Postrefractive surgery data
- Refraction: Plane

Calculation
- 0.7 D change at spectacle plane (known fact) = 1.0 D change at IOL plane
  Therefore, 5.25 D change at spectacle plane = 5.25/0.7 = 7.5 D change at IOL plane
  Thus, IOL power for emmetropia = 16.8 + 7.5 = 24.3 D

DIRECT METHODS

So named as one actually measure the corneal power postoperatively to calculate the effective keratometricdioptres. Although most modern devices do not directly measure the posterior corneal curvature, they use alternative algorithms to approximately assume the RI change induced or simply use different variables to predict ELP.

1. Gaussian optics and linear regression. The Gaussian formula uses: Anterior and Posterior radius of curvature - RI of air (1.0); of Anterior K (1.376) and of Aqueous humour (1.336) - Corneal thickness To calculate the Effective Refractive Power (EffRP), the posterior corneal curvature is not directly measured but predicted from the data of Oslen et al. EffRP was then used to predict ELP, along with the application of linear regression analysis. Errors of nearly 0.5 D are still noted.

2. Corneal topography/ keratometry method. These systems are based on the assumption that the posterior radius of curvature of the cornea averages 1.2 mm less than the anterior surface and use an index of refraction of 1.33. This assumption is no longer true in corneas subjected to keratorefractive surgery and it leads to an overestimation of the keratometry by 14% of the change induced by the refractive surgery, i.e. after LASIK, if there is a 7 D change in the refraction at the corneal plane with a preoperative K = 44 D, the actual power of the cornea is 37 D, but the topography/keratometric system reads 38 D. Hence, there is a 1 D overestimation for a change of 7 D, and a 2 D overestimation for a change of 14 D. Therefore, whatever the change in postoperative K-reading, undercorrect it by 14% to get an accurate postoperative K-reading. If this correction is not made, then the end result will be a hyperopic refractive error due to an underestimation of the IOL power.

3. Aramberri double K method. It is one of the most important methods. It uses pre-LASIK corneal power (or 43.5 if unknown) for calculation of ELP and post-LASIK corneal power for the calculation of the IOL power. This can be done automatically in the Hoffer programmes (for the Hoffer f, Holladay I, SRK/T formulas) and in the Holladay IOL consultant programme (for the Holladay II).

4. Camellin and Calossi method. They reported a formula which uses induced refractive change as well as anterior and posterior curvature of cornea to predict IOL power.

5. Rosa method. This uses a correction factor (R factor) for corneal radius which was derived from a regression formula and then compared with the calculation method and double K method. In their study of 19 eyes R factor was found to be superior when applied to the SRK/T and Holladay I. The actual formula for IOL power is derived from manual measurements of corneal power (K) and axial length (AL).

$$K = (0.0276 \times AL + 0.3635) \text{ manual K}$$

6. Direct measurements of anterior and posterior corneal power. With the invention of these newer instruments direct measurement of the posterior corneal power is also possible, which then gives more accurate results for IOL calculation after refractive surgery. The Orbscan and the Pentacam both have been used to measure posterior corneal power, with the Pentacam having slight advantage. But these need more study and data.

7. IOL power calculation in patients with corneal transplants. It is extremely difficult to accurately predict corneal power in transplant patients. If a triple procedure is planned it is suggested that K readings of other eye be used. An alternative option is to use the average k readings from a series of previous transplants. If there is a corneal scar, but no graft is planned, other eye readings can be used or even the power calculated using AL and refractive error of affected eye.

Conclusion

For accurate calculation of IOL power in patients who have undergone keratorefractive surgery, an access to pre- and post-operative patient data is essential. Therefore, it becomes mandatory for the refractive surgeons to maintain detailed records. It may also be prudent to provide all the patients undergoing refractive surgery with a copy of the relevant data, in case they approach another ophthalmologist for cataract surgery. This endeavour will definitely result in more accurate refractive outcomes following cataract surgery and IOL implantation, in patients who had undergone keratorefractive surgery.

Note. Always use more than one modern third-generation and fourth-generation formula (SRK/T, Hoffer f, Holladay II, Haigis) to calculate IOL power in such patients and choose the highest value. Never use a regression formula (SRK I or SRK II).

OPTIMIZATION OF IOL POWER

Optimization of IOL constants is the process by which a constant is refined for a particular surgical technique, lens, formula, surgeon, or measurement device based on previous

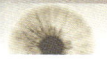
outcomes. This has been shown to improve outcomes significantly and can be done with any formula, lens, or specific situation.

The need for optimization of IOL power is felt due to the fact that with the exception of the Haigis formula, all other currently popular IOL formulae utilize a single 'lens-constant' for completion of the calculation, the rest of the terms of the formula being derived from measurable data. These constants are named differently for different formulae. For example:

- *SRK group* of formulae uses the term A-constant, while
- *Holladay employs* a different constant called the Surgeon's Factor (SF)
- *Hoffer-Q formula* is characterized by the pACD, or the personalized anterior chamber depth.

Since each of these formulae is constructed differently, the constants are also different and cannot be used interchangeably between formulae.

Optimization is the process of finding the specific value of a lens constant, which when used for that particular IOL type, will result in the most accurate IOL power calculations. For a group of patients for whom a particular type of IOL has been implanted, optimization is performed by calculating the lens constant in such a manner that the formula produces the exact refractive error that was actually encountered in that eye. Such a value of the lens constant would make that formula 'perfect' for that specific case.

SOME OBSERVATIONS ABOUT IOL POWER OPTIMIZATION

- *Surgeons optimize their IOL constant* using data from a sample of operated eyes.
- *The IOL master manual* recommends the use of 200 eyes with deviations in postoperative refractions within 2 standard deviations (SD) of the mean.
- *Aristodemou et al evaluated optimization of IOL constant.* They assessed the benefits of intraocular lens (IOL)-constant optimization for IOL Master biometry on refractive outcomes after cataract surgery for all surgeons and individual surgeons. Optimization of IOL

constants reduced the mean absolute errors from 0.66 diopters (D) and 0.52 to 0.40 D and 0.42 D for the Sofport AO IOL and Akreos Fit IOL, respectively. The percentage of eyes within G0.25 D, G0.50 D, and G1.00 D of target refraction improved from for both IOL models.

- *Bonfadini et al have also described optimization of IOL constant for DSAEK triple cases.* In this study, prediction errors were calculated retrospectively for consecutive DSAEK triple procedures. These prediction errors then were used to determine an IOL constant for this cohort of patients. The new optimized IOL constant subsequently was compared with the manufacturer's IOL constant, allowing evaluation and quantification of refractive benefits of optimization. This showed significantly improved accuracy of predicted postoperative refraction compared with the manufacturer's IOL constant, which may help to improve the postoperative refractive outcomes in patients undergoing the DSAEK triple procedure.

OPTIMIZATION VERSUS PERSONALIZATION

The process of optimization can be taken further, by only considering data from a specific pool. For instance, one such pool might consists of eyes that have been operated upon by surgeon Dr X, using biometry device B, keratometry device C, and the measurements having been performed by Mr D. Such narrow focussing is called personalization, and it refines optimization. Personalization allows the incorporation of systematic errors of the measurement devices, as well as individual bias of the surgeon or technician. This further improves IOL power prediction accuracy to an extent.

DYNAMIC IOL OPTIMIZATION

One of the more recent strategies for IOL power optimization is called Dynamic IOL Optimization.[*] This is a powerful personalized analysis system that bypasses the conventional optimization of the lens constants, and instead

---

[*]From: Saurabh Sawhney, Ashima Aggarwal, DOS times, Sept-Oct, 2016

focuses on the relative performance of the formulae as a whole. Conceptually, it can compare an infinite number of IOL power calculation algorithms.

The software has a user-friendly interface that runs on the MS Excel (TM) platform. The user is required to fill in the IOL model names, the surgeons' names, etc. as a one-time exercise, with an option for later additions. Following this, the database is created, wherein the user enters case details including biometry, IOL details, and postoperative refraction. A minimum of eleven complete entries are required before the program can generate optimized IOL powers. This is a safeguard to ensure statistical robustness.

When IOL power calculation is required, the user enters the case-specific biometry details and chosen IOL model. The program then automatically scans the database and chooses a niche cohort.

This cohort comprises of eyes that have a structural configuration that is similar to the test eye. The parameters for this selection are axial length and keratometry. This ensures that when optimizing the IOL power for an unusual eye, for example, a myope, only the matching portion of the database that contains similarly myopic eyes will be evaluated.

Once the niche cohort is chosen, the program then automatically evaluates the relative performance of different IOL formulae in that cohort. Out liers are automatically excluded. This information is then prospectively applied to the test case, yielding a single, usable IOL power.

Advantage of Dynamic IOL optimization:
- First and foremost, it is easy to use.
- There is no need for additional equipment purchase, as it works to make the most of the existing data. The user need not choose a formula as per the ocular configuration. Instead, there is a smooth surface of prediction based on the surgeon's own clinical outcomes.
- Since lens constants are bypassed, there is no need to consider separate values for the contact, immersion or optical methods of measuring axial length.
- The program works continuously. As new data is added, the optimization protocol

recalculates everything. New information is thus constantly incorporated into the system. This is better than optimizing the lens constants every now and then, doing it for different formulae, and for different axial length ranges.
- Since cohort selection is continuous rather than discrete, there is zero data wastage. The entire process.
- Of DIO is facilitated by a very simple user interface.

IMPORTANT CONSIDERATIONS AND FINAL SELECTIONS OF IOL POWER

BIOMETRY: IMPORTANT CONSIDERATIONS

- The surgeon should prefer to do biometry himself or herself, or should have a reliable technician.
- Take care to select the correct mode/velocity.
- Data input should be done very carefully.
- Selection of the appropriate formula is very important.
- Always check and compare the ALs of both eyes.
- To minimize errors in IOL power calculation, recheck the preoperative measurement under following circumstances:
  - AL <22 mm or >25 mm.
  - Average corneal power <40 D or >47 D.
  - Calculated emmetropic implant power is >3 D from the average for the specific style used.
  - The difference in corneal power >1 D, AL >0.5 mm and emmetropic implant power >1 D is found between two eyes.
- IOL power choosen should be compatible with history.
- Always choose a power that is suitable for patient (age, profession and needs).
- Surgeon factor should always be estimated.
- Optimization of IOL power should also be done.

FINAL SELECTIONS OF IMPLANT POWER

After the measurements have been obtained, and the implant power formula chosen has been applied, the surgeon armed with the calculated

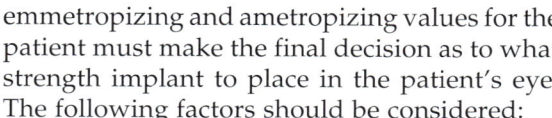

emmetropizing and ametropizing values for the patient must make the final decision as to what strength implant to place in the patient's eye. The following factors should be considered:

1. Fellow-eye refraction and cataract, if any. If the refractive error of opposite eye lies between −2.0 and +2.0 D, then emmetropia should be aimed for. These patients can usually tolerate an anisometropia of 2.0 D. If the refractive error is more than ±2.0 D and both eyes have got cataract, then stepwise reduction can be done by choosing suitable implant powers; e.g. −4.0 D preoperative refraction can be reduced by aiming for 2.0 D undercorrection in one eye and then emmetropia in the other.

2. Lifestyle of patient. Active patients are best served by near emmetropia; sedentary patients may prefer myopia.

3. Hedging. It has been found that the actual postoperative refraction varies by more than 1D from the calculated refraction in over 10% of the cases, and so it is preferable to hedge towards myopia.

RECOMMENDATIONS FOR SELECTION OF IOL IN THE OPERATING ROOM

- The surgeon and a responsible assistant should personally select the primary and backup implants from stock.
- IOL power and style to be used should be mentioned in the OT list against each patient's name and fixed on the operating room wall.
- OT staff should be made aware of the importance of proper IOL power.
- Avoid using varieties of IOL styles.
- Corresponding ACIOL power should also be calculated preoperatively for use in case of need.

- Before IOL implantation, the assistant and the operating surgeon must recheck the IOL power.

BIBLIOGRAPHY

1. Khurana AK. Intraocular Lenses: Optical aspects and Power calculation: Chapter 9, Theory and Practice of Optics and Refraction, 4th ed. 2018.
2. Fedorov SN, Kolinko AI, Kolinko AI. Estimation of optical power of the intraocular lens. Vestn Oftalmol 1967;80:27–31.
3. Hoffer KJ. The Hoffer Q formula: a comparison of theoretic and regression formulas. J Cataract Refract Surg 1993;19:700–12.
4. Sahin A, Hamrah P. Clinically relevant biometry. Curr Opin Ophthalmol. 2012;23:47–53. doi:10.1097/ICU.0b013e32834cd63e.
5. Holladay JT. Standardizing constants for ultrasonic biometry, keratometry, and intraocular lens power calculations. J Cataract Refract Surg 1997;23(9):1356–70.
6. Hoffer KJ. The Hoffer Q formula: a comparison of theoretic and regression formulas. J Cataract Refract Surg 1993;19:700–12.
7. Binkhorst RD. Intraocular lens power calculation manual. A guide to the author's TI 58/59 IOL power module. 2nd ed. New York: Richard D Binkhorst; 1981.
8. Olsen T, Corydon L, Gimbel H. Intraocular lens power calculation with an improved anterior chamber depth prediction algorithm. J Cataract Refract Surg 1995;21:313–9.
9. Hoffer KJ. Modern TOL power calculations: Avoiding error and planning for special circumstances. Focal Points: Clinical Modules for Ophthalmologists. San Francisco: American Academy of Ophthalmology; 1999, module 12.
10. Haigis VV. The Haigis formula. Intraocular Lens Power Calculations. Shammas HJ, ed. Thorofare, NJ: Slack Inc; 2003:chap 5, pp 41-57.
11. Fedorov SN, Galin MA, Linksz A. A calculation of the optical power of intraocular lenses. Invest Ophthalmol 1975;14:625–8.

Section

VIII

Special Investigations for Retina, Vitreous and Optic Nerve

28. Fundus Angiography and Autofluorescence
29. Macular Optical Coherence Tomography
30. Electrophysiological Tests in Ophthalmology

Fundus Angiography and Autofluorescence

Chapter Outline

FUNDUS FLUORESCEIN ANGIOGRAPHY

Basic principle, equipment and technique
- Basic principle
- Equipment
- Procedure
- Contraindications

Normal and abnormal fundus fluorescein angiogram
- Normal fundus fluorescein angiogram
- Abnormalities in fundus fluorescein angiogram
  - Hyperfluorescence
  - Hypofluorescence

Complications and their Management

INDOCYANINE GREEN ANGIOGRAPHY
- Introduction
- Properties of ICG molecule
- Procedure
- Adverse effects
- Phases of ICGA
- Interpretation of ICGA
- Indications
- Contraindications

FUNDUS AUTOFLUORESCENCE
- Introduction
- Principle
- Clinical applications
- Summary

FUNDUS FLUORESCEIN ANGIOGRAPHY

BASIC PRINCIPLE, EQUIPMENT AND TECHNIQUE

Fundus fluorescein angiography (FFA) is the backbone of the retina services of any institute. It was first used in eye in 1961. A careful evaluation and interpretation of FFA are essential to diagnose, treat and follow-up the disease. The most important is its role in guiding laser treatment of the retinal vascular and choroidal diseases.

BASIC PRINCIPLE

Sodium fluorescein is used for fluorescence. It absorbs light energy which is blue (465–490 nm)

and fluoresces at green yellow (520–530 nm) (Fig. 28.1A). In addition to green yellow light reflected back by sodium fluorescein, there is blue light reflected back from structures that do not contain sodium fluorescein. This blue reflected light and green yellow light falls on the filter (barrier filter) which allows green yellow light to pass and keeps away blue reflected light. Failure of this filter leads to pseudofluorescence which may cause difficulty in interpretation and decreased resolution of FFA pictures (Fig. 28.1A).

EQUIPMENT

Both digital and film angiography can be used. Trends are shifting towards use of digital angiography in view of low incurring expenditure and

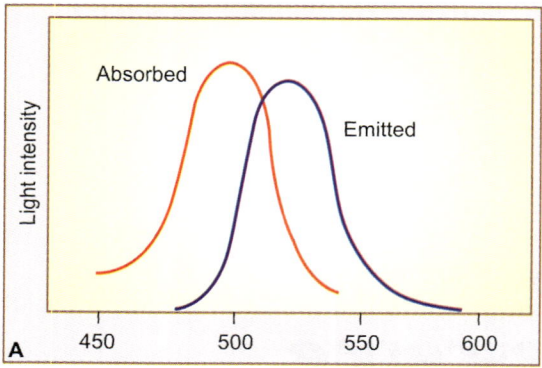

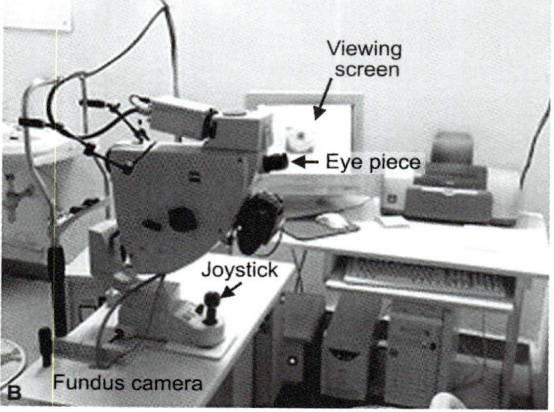

Fig. 28.1: *(A) Graph depicting fluorescein absorption and emission spectra; and (B) Fundus digital imaging system showing screen for simultaneous view of the acquired data and various parts.*

immediate results. Camera with flash unit, timer and matched fluorescein filter form an important part of equipment (Fig. 28.1B). Timer is most important for arm to retina circulation time in diseases with decreased arterial perfusion. Fluorescein dye reaches the eye through systemic circulation after injecting in brachial vein. The exciter filter of the equipment transmits blue light from 465–490 nm which excites the sodium fluorescein dye and barrier filter transmits light from 525–530 nm which is reflected back by sodium fluorescein dye. The transmission of both filters should have minimum overlap. If there is overlap, pseudo-fluorescence will result. After the machine becomes old, the filters become thin, and transmission of more light is there leading to pseudofluorescence compromising the quality of FFA.

Sodium fluorescence is a low molecular weight dye (376.27 daltons) $C_{20}H_{12}O_5Na$ used for fundus fluorescein angiography. It diffuses through most of the body fluids and chorio-capillaris. When injected, 80% of sodium fluorescein is protein bound and only 20% is available for fluorescence. Inner and outer blood retinal barrier are impermeable to it in healthy state. It is eliminated through liver and kidney in less than 24 hours. Urine and skin may develop yellowish tinge.

PROCEDURE

Before proceeding with the test, photographer must settle the field that is to be centered, whether he wants 30° or 60°. Detailed macular evaluation is done by 30° FFA and wider patho-logies need 60°. The camera must be adjusted for vertical adjustment and the eyepiece for accommodation keeping cross hair in sharp focus. The photographer ascertains pupillary diameter also by moving camera from side to side. This also helps him to ascertain focusing peculiarities of particular cornea and lens. By doing this he finds out the best position for a clear fundus photograph.

Before starting the procedure one must ensure availability of emergency tray including hydro-cortisone vial, injection adrenaline 1:1000, injec-tion phenergan, injection atropine, venous cannula, at least three 5 cc and 10 cc syringes with needles intravenous fluid bottles of normal saline as well as dextrose, guide airways of pediatric and adult sizes, laryngoscope with both small and large blade, working battery cells, endotracheal tubes, oxygen cylinder with flow meter and transparent face mask (Fig. 28.2A to D). There should always be supply of light sources. Fluorescein dye used could be in 10 ml (5%), or 5 ml (10%) or 3 ml (25%) vials.

Informed consent has to be taken before the procedure and the procedure and adverse reac-tions must be told. Apart from discolouration of skin and urine, anaphylactic reaction and vasovagal shock are the other rare complications (Fig. 28.2D).

Position the patient with chin at chin rest and forehead touching the head bar. Inject dye slowly with syringe and 23 gauze scalp vein set

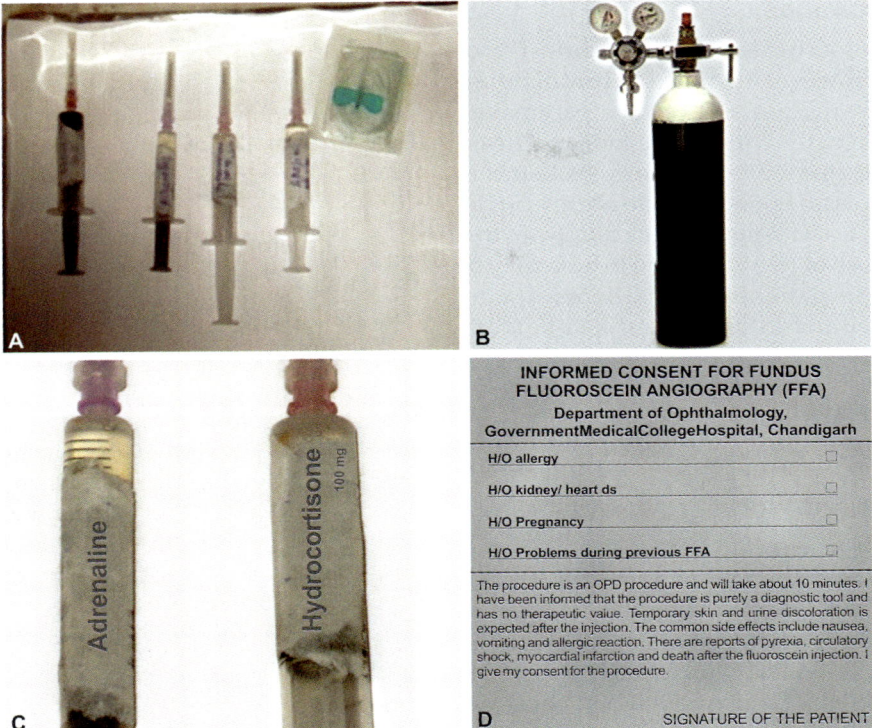

Fig. 28.2: *Emergency equipment tray including oxygen cylinder before start of FFA.*

and start timer. The most frequently accessed vein is antecubital vein and we expect to see the dye in the eye in 9 seconds after injection. The injection must be given in 4–6 seconds and too fast an injection may lead to nausea though it gives better picture.

Fluorescein injection has to be coordinated with fundus photograph. This must be injected after identification and control picture. The first frames should be area of interest which we call primary eye/macula. Initially, capture primary macula every 2 seconds after the dye is visible in choroidal circulation for 30 seconds. The secondary macula is clicked after primary macula followed by disc. The time interval between frames is increased. The periphery should be recorded by tilting the camera. Pictures of other important areas can be taken as evident from clinical examination. We must cover all fields in both eyes in diabetic retinopathy according to airlie house classification as shown in Fig. 28.3. The eye is

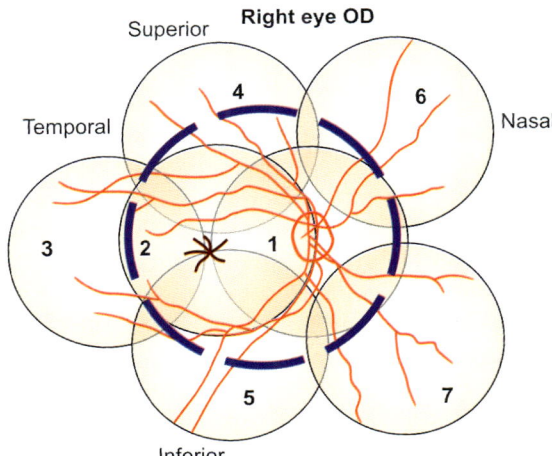

Fig. 28.3: *The 7 airlie house fundus fields to ensure proper clicking of all fields to include relevant data especially in diabetes mellitus.*

moved with the help of fixation light. FFA takes 4–10 minutes. Late pictures after 10 minutes are rarely required except CSCR, CME, etc. to note dye pooling.

CONTRAINDICATIONS

It should be avoided in first trimester of pregnancy. However, there are no contraindications in heart disease and cardiac pacemaker. Avoid FFA in cases with severe kidney disease as dye is excreted by the kidneys. Its better to avoid FFA in cases known to have allergy to dye. A sensitivity test is done to check allergy to dye before full dose of dye is injected in vein may be done in these patients. For patients having cardiac, respiratory disease, test can be done under anaesthetist doctor's supervision.

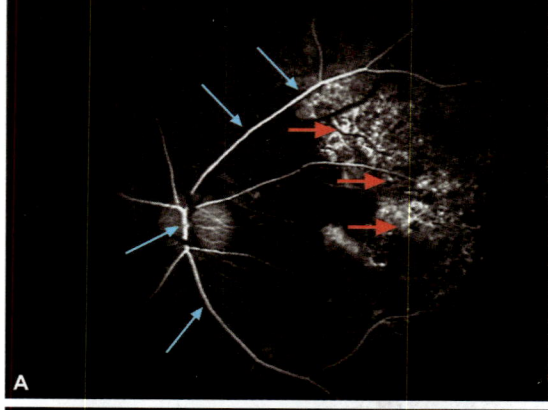

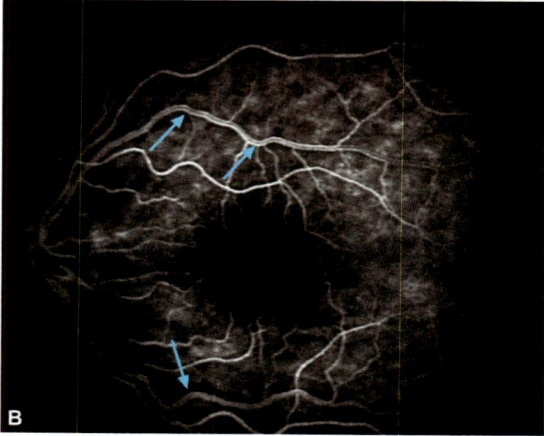

Fig. 28.4: *(A) Choroidal flush appears as irregular patchy hyperfluorescence at posterior pole seen very early and increases over subsequent frames; and (B) Early venous phase shows lamellar flow due to differential blood flow velocity in vessel and increase in choroidal hyperfluorescence.*

NORMAL AND ABNORMAL FUNDUS FLUORESCEIN ANGIOGRAM

NORMAL FUNDUS FLUORESCEIN ANGIOGRAM

In normal FFA, **choroidal flush** (Fig. 28.4A) appears first and arm to retina time for the dye is 10–12 seconds in normal adult . It could be faster in young and delayed in elderly. It is faint, patchy and irregularly scattered throughout posterior fundus. This also fills cilioretinal artery simultaneously, if present. Central retinal artery begins to fill with fluorescein dye 1–3 seconds later. After the arteries are filled, **early venous phase** is seen as lamellar flow phase (Fig. 28.4B) as fluorescein dye enters the veins along the walls. The flow of fluorescein is lamellar and it flows faster in the center of the vessel than on the sides (trilaminar flow). The dark central lamella is nonfluorescent blood that comes from periphery and which takes longer to fluorescene because of its more distant location. The laminae become thicker in next 5–10 seconds and finally merge to give complete fluorescence to the veins. **Arteriovenous phase** starts after this and fluorescene reaches peak in 20–25 seconds (Fig. 28.5A and B). The dye starts to empty from eye circulation after 30 seconds of dye injection. After this **recirculation phase** starts in which lower dye concentration continues to flow in eye circulation. The retinal circulation is completely free of dye in ten minutes. The dye might be retained in some eye tissues leading to pooling of dye (Fig. 28.6A and B) or staining like Bruch's membrane, choroid, sclera, disc and adjacent visible sclera. We see a dark foveal avascular zone because of high columnar retinal pigment epithelial cells and more xanthophylls here than rest of fundus. There is also absence of vessels in center 400–500 microns. Anatomically we know that there are only 4 rows of retinal cells here (ILM, OPL, ONL, rods and cones). This helps us to understand stellate pattern of edema in macula and honey comb appearance +90 D slit-lamp biomicroscopy.

Optic disc FFA needs to be understood clearly. It has a dual blood supply from the retinal vascular system and posterior ciliary vascular system. We see extensive vascular anastomotic channels between these two circulations in case of disease. There are many layers of nerve fibers and glial tissue. The lamina cribrosa portion of nerve is supplied by short posterior ciliary

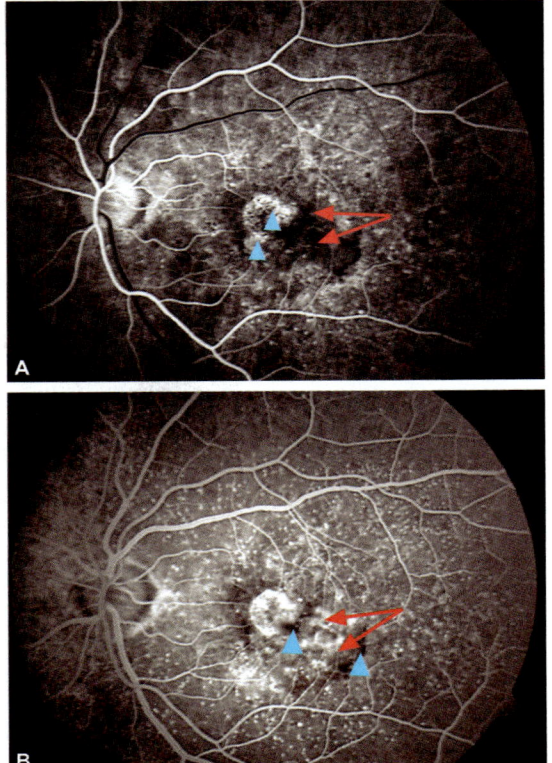

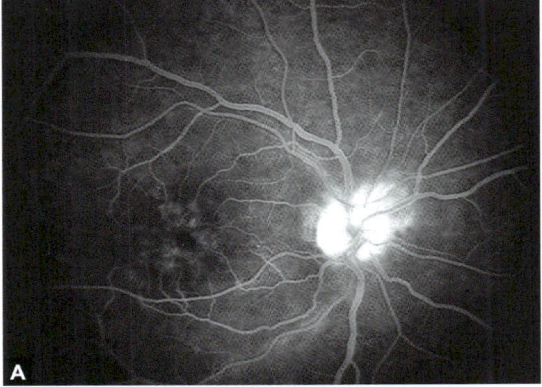

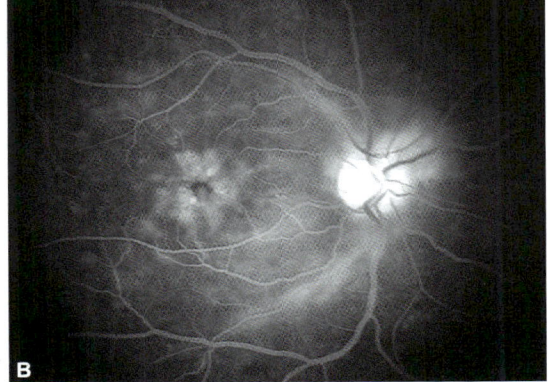

Fig. 28.5: *(A) Early venous phase shows trilaminar flow and abnormal finding of hyperfluorescence (arrow heads) in foveal area with adjacent area of hypofluorescence (arrows); and (B) Arteriovenous phase shows increase in fluorescence which peaks in 20–25 seconds (arrows). There is increase in hyperfluorescence in macular area along with block fluorescence (arrow heads) corresponding to CNVM with retinal hemorrhages.*

Fig. 28.6: *(A) Arteriovenous phase shows decrease in fluorescence and abnormal finding of macular hyperfluorescence; and (B) Which increases in late phase suggestive of dye pooling in patelloid pattern in a case of cystoid macular edema.*

arteries (SPCA) and prelaminar portion is supplied by centripetal branches from peripapillary choroid. There are small branches of retinal arterioles at peripapillary region. As most of the disc is supplied by ciliary system fluorescein dye at disc is seen much before retinal vessels fill up. Main venous drainage is into central retinal vein and peripapillary choroid.

ABNORMALITIES IN FUNDUS FLUORESCEIN ANGIOGRAM

These appear as hypo- and hyper-fluorescent areas which may be traced over subsequent angiogram frames to give proper diagnosis.

HYPERFLUORESCENCE

To interpret abnormal hyperfluorescence check the phase of angiogram in which it first appears and then look at it in subsequent phases. Hyperfluorescence could due to:

- Autofluorescence/pseudofluorescence, i.e. abnormal preinjection fluorescence
- Leakage of dye
- Transmission defect
- Staining.

Abnormal preinjection fluorescence

- *Pseudofluorescence* will be visible at beginning of FFA in red free pictures or due to defect in filter matching which is unusual in modern machines and with frequent change in filters.

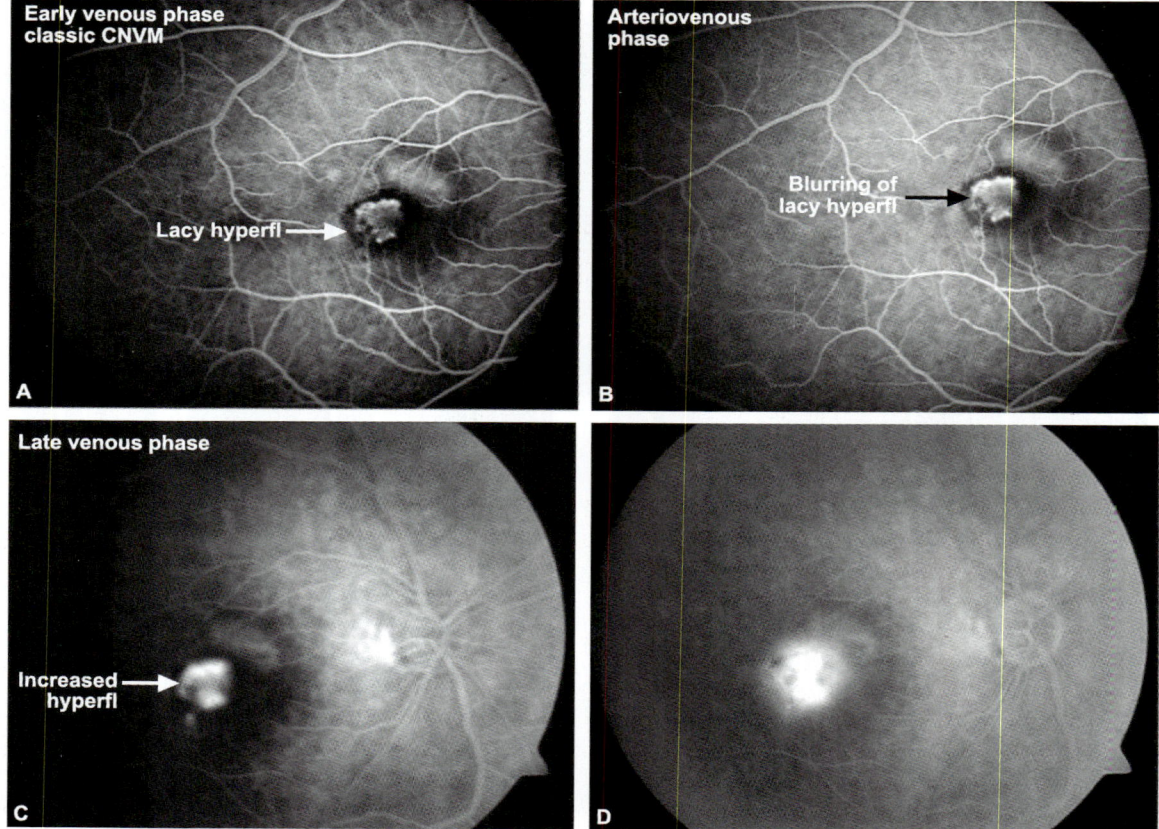

Fig. 28.7: *(A) Early venous phase showing juxtafoveal lacy heperfluorescence; (B) Arteriovenous phase showing blurring of lacy hyperfluorescence; (C) Late venous phase showing increase in hyperfluorescence; and (D) Late phase of FFA showing increase in hyperfluorescence suggestive of classic CNVM.*

- *Autofluorescence* is seen in optic nerve head drusens and astrocytic hamartoma.

Leakage of dye

Hyperfluorescence which appears early in FFA and then increases in subsequent phases both in size and intensity due to leakage from abnormal vessels in retina or choroid as in CNVM.

Thus leakage is any hyperfluorescence that persists 15 minutes after injection after retinal or choroidal vessels are emptied of fluorescence (Figs 28.7 and 28.8). Leakage could be into vitreous as diffuse white haze in inflamed eye. It could also be in case of intraocular tumours or flat/raised neovascularisation.

Transmission hyperfluorescence (Fig. 28.9)

Hyperfluorescence which matches the background choroidal fluorescence, i.e first increases in AV phases and then decreases in recirculation phase, e.g. RPE atrophy in dry AMD.

Thus, transmission hyperfluorescence occur due to RPE atrophy leading to window defect which increases visibility of choroidal fluorescence. Normally pigment epithelium forms a barrier for choroidal fluorescence to be visible. Transmission hyperfluorescence starts in early frames along with choroidal flush and then increases as choroidal fluorescence increases in arteriovenous phase and decreases in late phases as choroidal flush decreases with washing away of dye. It neither increases in size nor changes in shape.

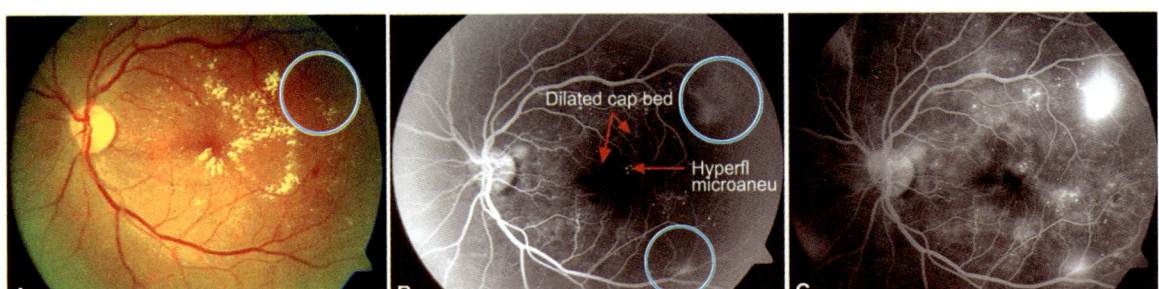

Fig. 28.8: *(A) Fundus picture showing clinically significant macular edema (CSME) encroaching the foveal centre; (B) Arteriovenous phase shows hyperfluorescent dots corresponding to microaneurysms and dilated capillary bed and also hyperfluorescence corresponding to neovessels. There is increase in hyperfluorescence in late phases; and (C) The patient has proliferative diabetic retinopathy and CSME involving the foveal centre.*

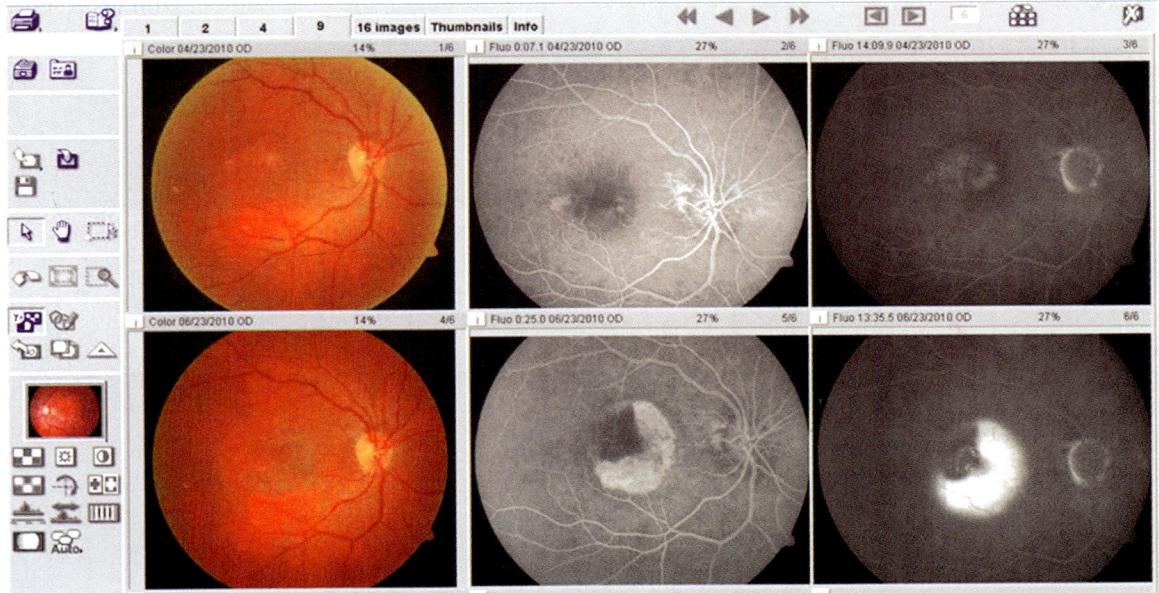

Fig. 28.9: *Case of occult CNVM: The top row showing patchy macular hyperfluorescence increasing in late phase. The bottom row is after injection bevacizumab leading to RPE rip. Hypofluorescence corresponds to RPE folded on itself. Hyperfluorescence is transmission defect due to absent RPE.*

Staining

Some tissues take-up the dye and this hyperfluorescence does not increase over time but persists in late phases which is called staining (Fig. 28.10). Hyperfluorescence which increases in subsequent phases in intensity but not size, e.g. staining of scar tissue.

Disc leakage should be differentiated from normal disc hyperfluorescence due to late staining of lamina cribrosa and leakage from peripapillary choroid.

Pooling of dye

Pooling of dye under sensory retina after breakdown the outer blood-retinal barrier. The pattern of hyperfluorescence in some diseases could be diagnostic like central serous chorioretinopathy (CSCR) (Fig. 28.11).

HYPOFLUORESCENCE

Hypofluorescence refer to decrease or absence of fluorescence during the course of FFA. Depending upon whether it is due to barrier

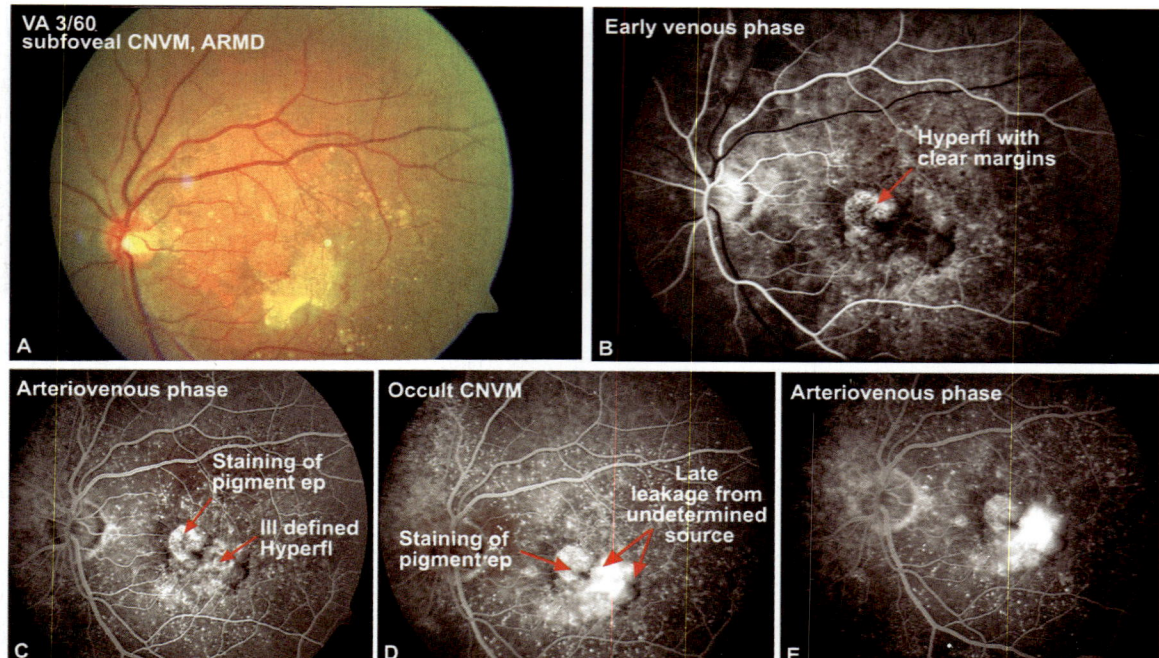

Fig. 28.10: *Scar of old CNVM with fresh recurrence at temporal edge seen as grayish membrane. Early hyperfluorescence with well-defined borders which increases in intensity on late phases with adjacent late leakage from undetermined source (Fig. A to E) suggestive of occult CNVM.*

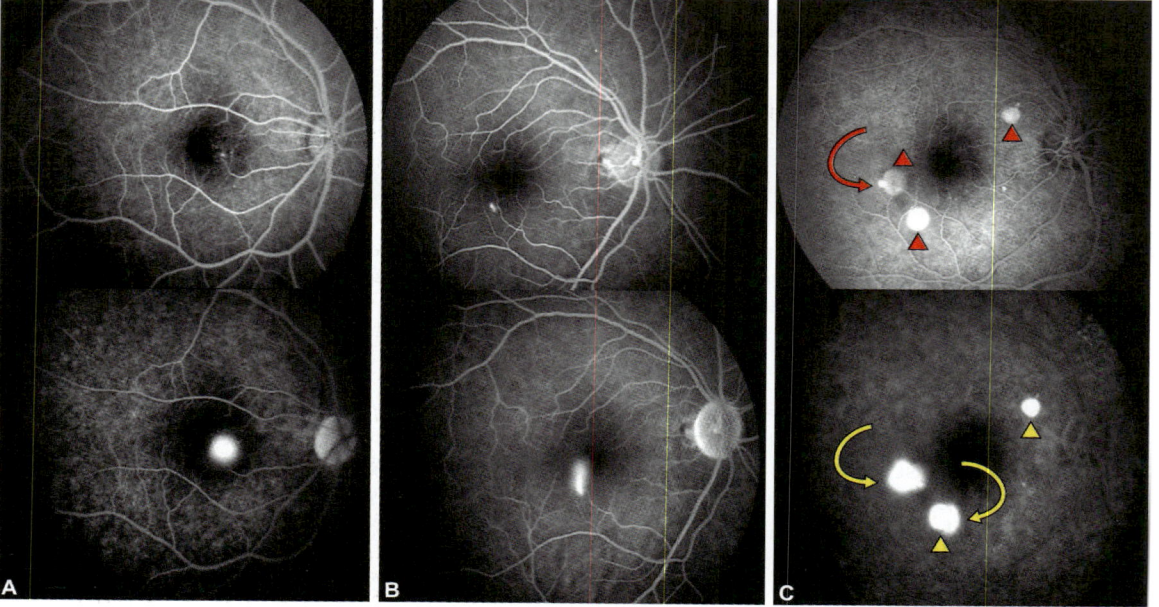

Fig. 28.11: *Top row shows early phase of FFA and bottom row shows corresponding late phases showing various patterns of leakage in CSCR: (A) Expanding dot sign; (B) Smoke stack sign; and (C) Multiple leaks with fuzzy borders (curved arrow) and PED with well-defined borders (arrow heads).*

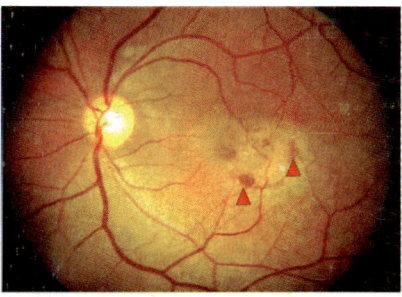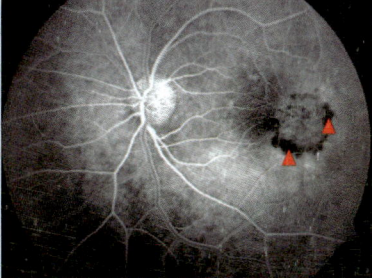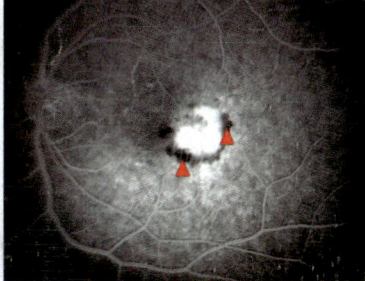

Fig. 28.12: *A case of CNVM showing increasing hyperfluorescence suggestive of active disease surrounded by hypofluorescent area persistent throughout the FFA sugestive of blocked fluorescence due to haemorrhage.*

effect or due to nonperfusion it can be classified as blocked fluorescence or vascular filling defect.

Blocked fluorescence

The transmission of fluorescence could be decreased in choroid or retina. In choroid it can be decreased by retinal haemorrhages and vitreous opacities. In retina the fluorescence can be decreased by preretinal bleed or vitreous haemorrhage (Fig. 28.12) or preretinal pigment clump. This can be differentiated from vascular filling defect by sequential study of FFA. There will be no change in fluorescence of an area with blocked fluorescence. The depth of lesion can be seen by vessels it blocks. If it is in nerve fiber layer it will block all vessels and if it is in inner nuclear layer, only retinal capillaries are blocked. In blocked fluorescence, hypofluorescence persists in all phases of angiogram.

Nonperfusion or vascular filling defect

Hypofluorescence due to nonperfusion, atrophy, absence of circulation or vascular insufficiency is present in early phases of angiogram but it may not persist after some time. If the vessel obstruction is complete or there is total tissue atrophy, it may persist through all phases of angiogram (Figs 28.13 and 28.14). In partial obstruction the filling is delayed or reduced compared to other areas with normal fluorescence. The level could be retinal or choroidal. Choroidal vascular filling defects are most difficult to pick. Early FFA frame should be seen. Normally in choroidal diseases due to nonperfusion, RPE is depigmented or atrophied and it becomes easier to discern choroidal

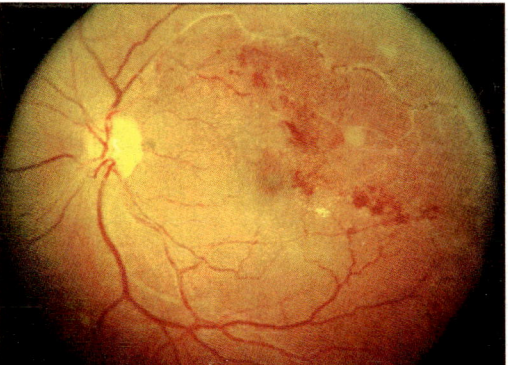

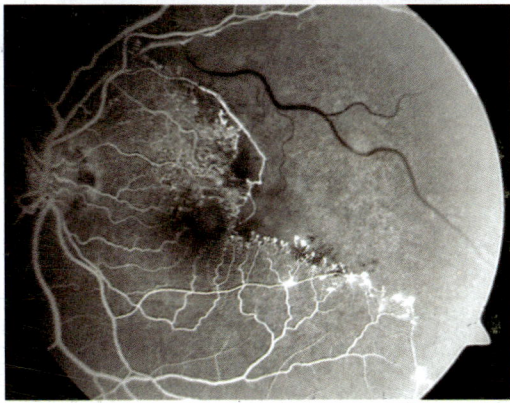

Fig. 28.13: *In a case of branch retinal vein occlusion, hypofluorescence in quadrant of retina corresponding to venous distribution of superotemporal BRV which appears in early frames persists throughout suggestive of both arterial and venous block.*

filling defect. Normally RPE forms a barrier for choroidal fluorescence to be visible. Hypofluorescence in choroidal circulation appears in early phase and disappears in late phases due to pooling of dye from surrounding lobules 2–5 seconds later (Fig. 28.15). In some

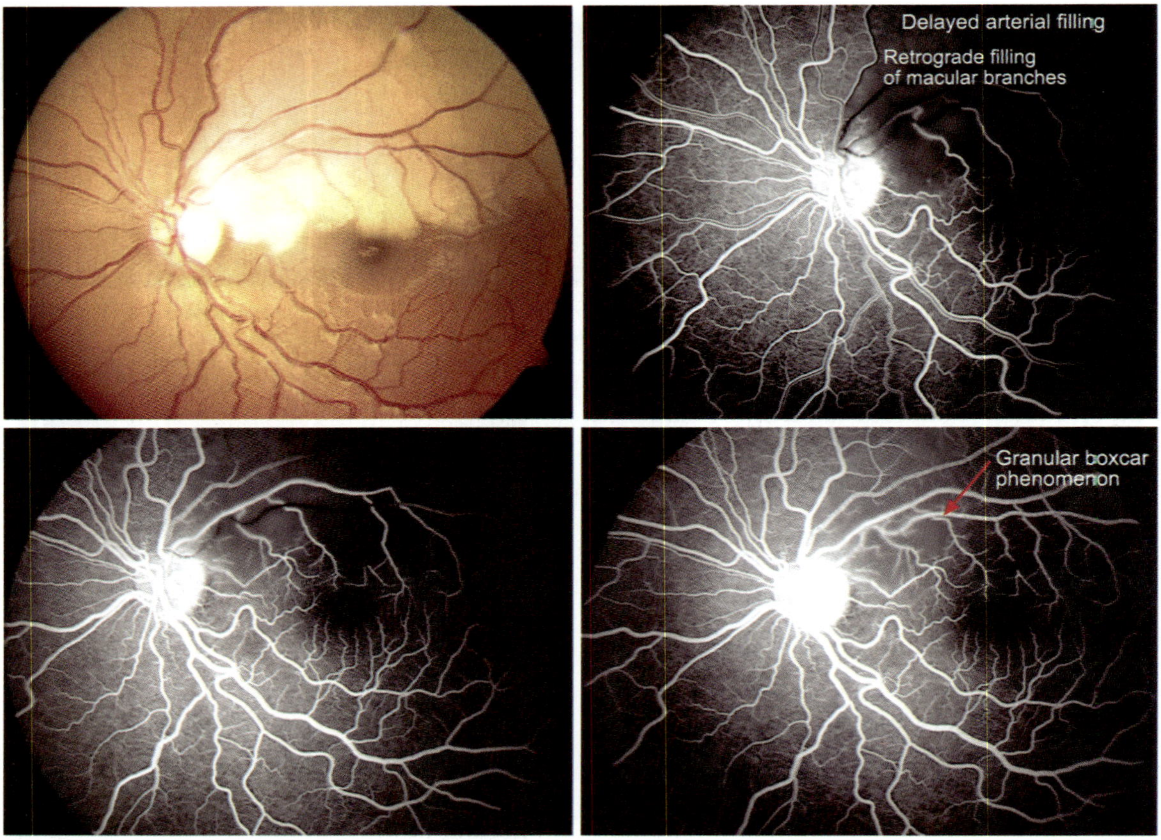

Delayed arterial filling

Retrograde filling
of macular branches

Granular boxcar
phenomenon

Fig. 28.14: *In a case of branch retinal artery occlusion there is delayed arterial filling and retrograde filling of macular branches. We can appreciate the granular boxcar phenomenon in late phases (arrow).*

cases even large choroidal vessels are non-perfused and there is total choroidal hypo-fluorescence staining at edge later from surrounding choriocapillaris. The blocked fluorescent areas continues to be hypofluorescent throughout the angiogram (Fig. 28.16).

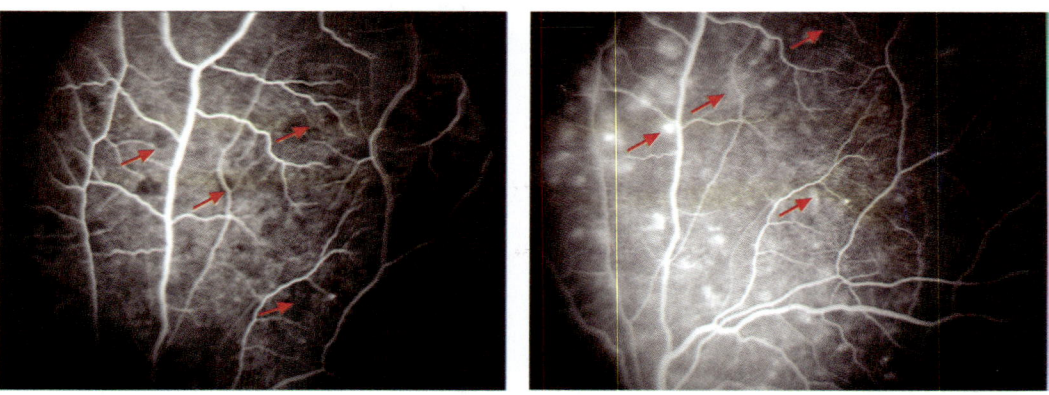

Fig. 28.15: *A case of active multifocal choroiditis showing well-defined hypofluorescence seen in early phases and pooling of dye from adjacent lobules in late phases leading to hyperfluorescence of the same area.*

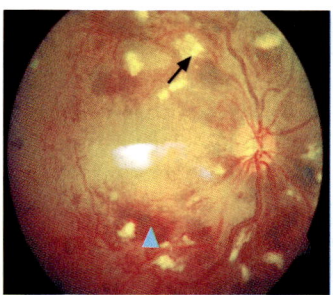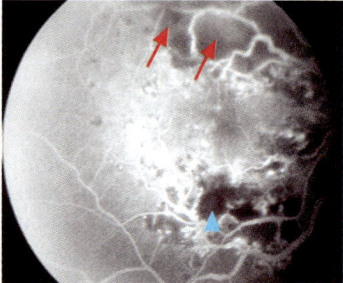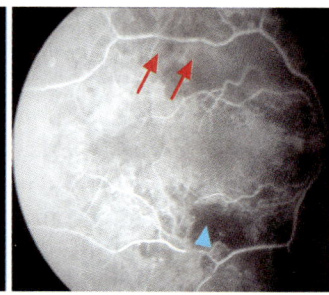

Fig. 28.16: *A case of severe non-proliferative diabetic retinopathy showing retinal hemorrhages leading to blocked fluorescence (arrowheads) and areas of capillary nonperfusion (arrows).*

COMPLICATIONS AND THEIR MANAGEMENT

Complications

In case of problem during FFA, it can be repeated at 30–60 minutes after first injection.

1. *Extravasation of fluorescein dye* can occur rarely. It is extremely painful and may lead to problem like superficial phlebitis, painful granuloma, toxic neuritis, sloughing of skin and necrosis. Local anaesthetic and ice packs at the site of extravasation might help. If the whole dye extravasates choose another vein and reinject full dose and if the extravasation is at end then there is no need to reinject.

2. *Nausea* (5%) which occurs for 30–120 seconds and disappears slowly. Nausea usually occurs after initial pictures are already taken.

3. *Vomiting* is seen in 0.3–0.4% patients and usually 4 hours fasting is recommended before FFA to decrease nausea. In case of history of vomiting in a patient during previous FFA procedure, 25–50 mg of promethazine can be administered prior to procedure.

4. *Vasovagal attacks* can be therein anxious patients. A more severe form of vasovagal attack is syncopal attack (sweating, fainting, hypotension, bradycardia, decreased cardiovascular perfusion).

5. *Anaphylactic reaction* which is characterized by hypotension, tachycardia, bronchospasm, hives and itching) need to be differentiated from syncopal attack. The treatment for both vasovagal and anaphylactic shock lies in treating hypotension as a priority as prolonged hypotension will affect the perfusion of vital organs.

It might be difficult to find intravenous access later thus maintain intravenous line till the end of the procedure.

6. *Allergic reaction* usually appears 2–15 minutes after injection of the dye in form of hives and itching. FFA sometimes gives rise to diffuse hypersensitivity reaction which occurs 48 hours later with diffuse rash and fever.

7. *Death and acute pulmonary edema after FFA* have also been reported.

Treatment of anaphylactic shock/vasovgal reaction/allergic reaction

- Attach oxygen with face mask immediately.
- Start a normal saline infusion through the prior established intravenous access.
- If no IV access, then dilute the 1 cc injection adrenaline to 10 cc so that the effective concentration is 1:10000. Ideally the injection should be ready before the start of procedure. Take 1 cc from this and inject subcutaneously or intravenous to the patient. It should bring the blood pressure (BP) to higher side in no time. Once the BP is achieved, have a IV access immediately, now start fluid through this.
- *Give injection hydrocortisone* 100 mg immediately.
- Monitor blood pressure regularly at one minute interval.

Treatment of vasovagal reaction

- *Supine position.* Make sure the patient is lying the supine position
- *Attach* oxygen with face mask immediately
- *Start a normal saline infusion* through the prior established intravenous access
- *Monitor blood pressure* regularly at one minute interval.

INDOCYANINE GREEN ANGIOGRAPHY (ICGA)

INTRODUCTION

Indocyanine green is a water-soluble tricarbo-cyanine dye, which was used to measure hepatic blood flow and cardiac output. Developed for use in photography during the Second World War, it got FDA approval in 1959 for human use. Its use in ophthalmology is mainly to image the posterior segment, especially the layers deeper to the retina. Due to its fluorescence spectrum in the infrared region, it is ideally suited to image the choroid.

PROPERTIES OF ICG MOLECULE

1. Molecular weight of 775 Daltons.
2. Fluorescent molecule with peak absorption at 790–805 nm and peak emission at 830 nm.
3. 98% protein bound (mainly to alpha-1 lipoprotein)-does not leak under normal conditions and stays in the intravascular compartment.
4. Eliminated exclusively in bile by the liver.
5. Half-life of 3–4 minutes.
6. Has 5% sodium iodide to enhance solubility.
7. Infrared spectrum of fluorescence enables it to image the choroid through blood, lipid and melanin.

PROCEDURE

Indocyanine green dye is injected in the antecubital vein and flushed. This is followed with a 5 ml bolus of saline. 25 mg of dye as lyophilized powder is available for dilution with 5 ml of aqueous solvent, giving a concentration of 5 mg/ml. Extravasation of dye does not lead to pain and burning.

Two types of imaging systems are used to do ICGA:

1. *Conventional high resolution digital imaging systems*
2. *Scanning laser ophthalmoscope (SLO) based systems* — Provide better quality images as compared to conventional imaging systems. Simultaneous FFA and ICGA are also possible. Same syringe can be used to inject both fluorescein and indocyanine green.

Colour, red free, green free and control photographs are taken before dye is injected. ICG is then injected and images are clicked after 8–10 seconds. As ICG fluoresces beyond the visible spectrum, images are difficult to focus. It is difficult to visualise vasculature and hence, visible pathology should be focused. Images are clicked every 8–10 seconds till blooming occurs. Blooming occurs when retinal and choroidal vessels have same concentration of dye and image quality deteriorates. Following this, images are taken at 3, 5, 7, 10 and 25–30 minutes.

ADVERSE EFFECTS

Adverse effects occur in only 0.15% patients and are both mild and transient. ICG has a better safety profile than fluorescein. Hot flushes, urticaria, hypotension, tachycardia, nausea and vomiting seldom occur. Death is reported to occur in 1 in 333333 patients.

PHASES OF ICGA

1. *Early phase*—Occurs at 2–3 minutes and shows superimposed retinal and large choroidal vessels (Fig. 28.17).
2. *Intermediate phase*—Occurs at about 10 minutes and shows maximal choroidal stromal fluorescence due to impregnation with indocyanine green dye (Fig. 28.18).
3. *Late phase*—Occurs at 28–30 minutes and shows dark choroidal vessels against background stromal fluorescence (Fig. 28.19).

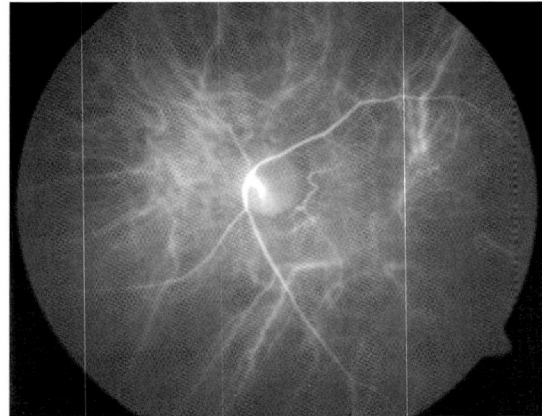

Fig. 28.17: *Early phase—Filling of both retinal and large choroidal vessels.*

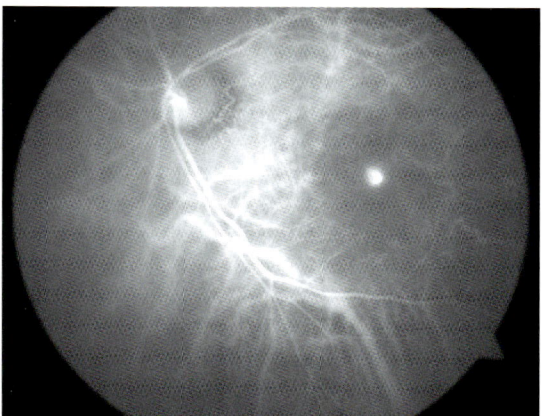

Fig. 28.18: *Intermediate phase—Choroidal vessels with stromal background fluorescence.*

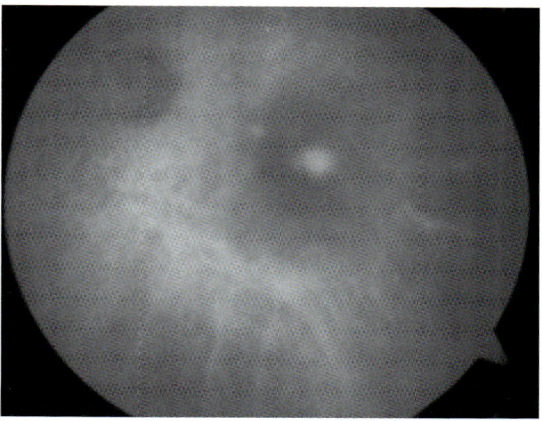

Fig. 28.19: *Late phase—Washout of dye from the circulation, showing dark optic disk and vessels on the background of stromal fluorescence.*

INTERPRETATION OF ICGA

Interpretation of ICGA is more difficult as compared to FFA as both retinal and choroidal circulations are superimposed on each other. Transmission fluorescence is not applicable to ICGA, as retinal pigment epithelium does not act as a barrier to ICG imaging. Standard angiograms for ICGA do not exist. The resolution of ICGA is 11 microns. Two patterns of fluorescence are noted—hypofluorescence (Fig. 28.20) and hyperfluorescence (Fig. 28.21).

INDICATIONS

1. *Choroidal neovascular membrane (CNVM)—* Occult CNVM, pigment epithelial detachment (PED), ICGA is used in suspected cases of occult CNVM. Subtle membranes, which are undetectable on FFA, can be easily picked up. Imaging of PEDs on FFA shows increasing fluorescence in late phases and hence obscures the detection of underlying pathology. ICGA is able to image the choroid below the PED and aids in arriving at a morphological diagnosis. Serous, fibrovascular or haemorrhagic PEDs can be equally well-imaged using this modality. ICGA mediated photodynamic therapy (PDT) is used to reduce the need for recurrent injections of Anti-VEGFs in nonresponsive patients (Fig. 28.22).

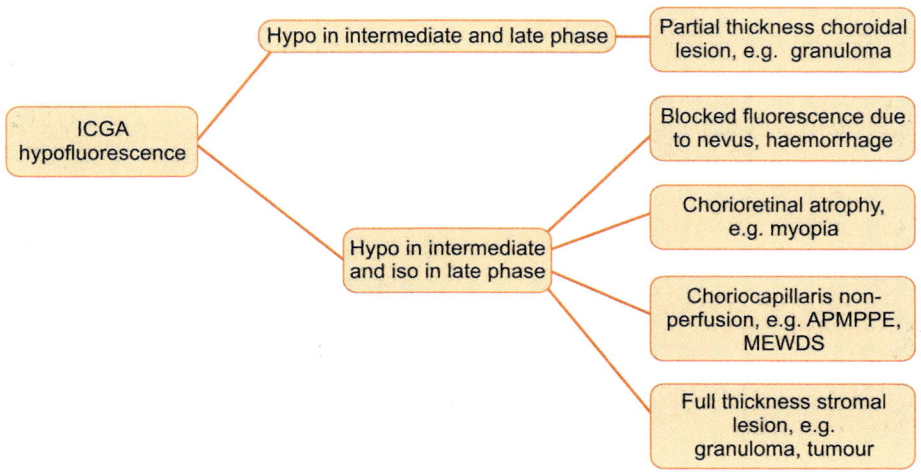

Fig. 28.20: *Causes of hypofluorescence of IGCA.*

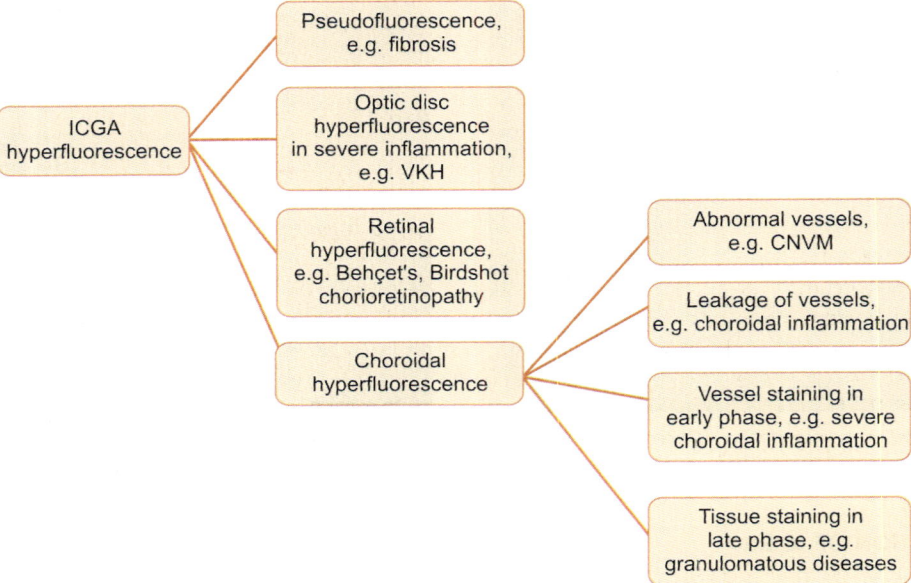

Fig. 28.21: *Causes of hyperfluorescence of IGCA.*

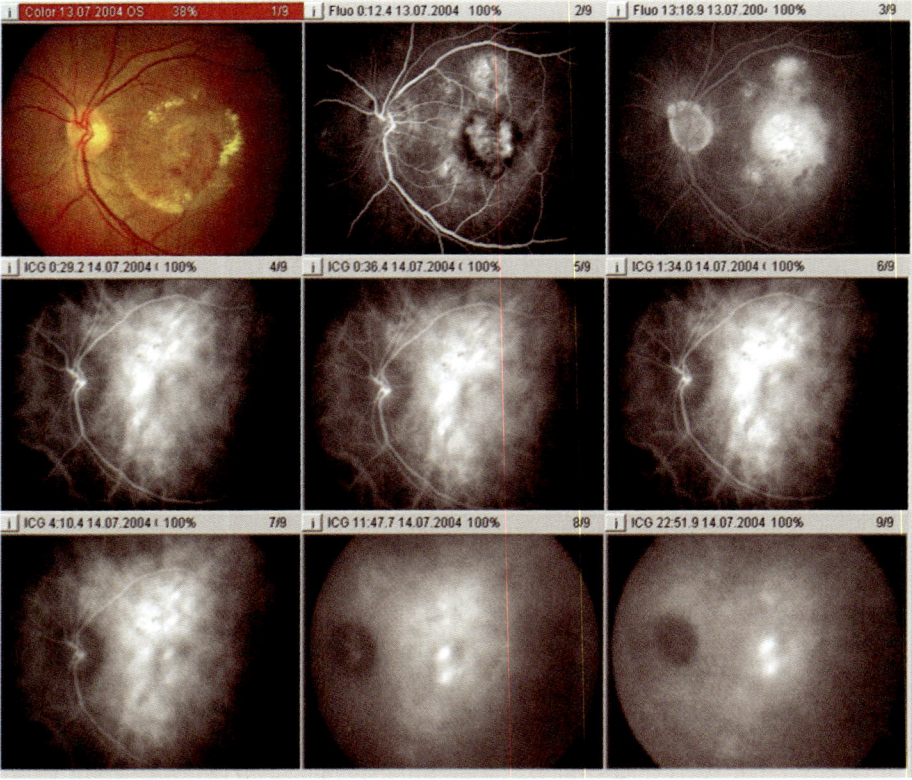

Fig. 28.22: *Top row shows a CNVM with lacy hyperfluorescence in early phase and late leakage on FFA. Middle and bottom row show ICGA images of hyperfluorescence from abnormal vessels which persists in the late phase.*

2. *Retinal angiomatous proliferation (RAP)*—It is a relatively recently recognized entity and classified as type 3 CNVM. Retinal circulation is said to be the site of origin of blood vessels, instead of the choroidal circulation in types 1 and 2 CNVM. ICGA has helped stage this entity into 3 stages: stage 1–Intraretinal neovascularisation (IRN), stage 2–Subretinal neovascularisation (SRN) and stage 3–retinochoroidal anastomosis (RCA). Laser photocoagulation of retinal vessel is recommended for stages 1 and 2. ICGA mediated PDT and anti-VEGF agents are recommended for stage 3 RAP.

3. *Polypoidal choroidal vasculopathy (PCV)*—PCV is increasingly being considered as a type of CNVM. Up to 50% cases of CNVM are said to be due to PCV in Asian patients. Presentation is generally with subretinal haemorrhage or PED (haemorrhagic or fibrovascular). FFA is unable to pick up the lesion. ICGA outlines the areas of polyp like outgrowths of the choroidal vessels responsible for the symptoms. ICGA mediated PDT + anti-VEGF is recommended as the treatment of choice for this condition (Fig. 28.23).

4. *Central serous chorioretinopathy (CSC)*—It is generally a self-resolving disease, with spontaneous recovery in 60–70% cases. However, recurrent and non-resolving cases cause permanent vision loss and metamorphopsia. ICGA has a role in demarcating the points of choroidal hyperpermeability, which are more in number than points of leakage on FFA. These points of choroidal leakage, are subjected to low-fluence or half dose PDT and lead to decrease of leakage on ICGA. Hence, ICGA is used to demarcate areas for application of PDT and prognosticate patients of chronic CSC. Those patients showing clear areas of choroidal leakage respond better to therapy as compared to those showing diffuse choroidal leakage (Fig. 28.24).

5. *Choroidal tumours*—Longer wavelength of ICGA makes it ideally suited to image mass lesions of the choroid. Choroidal melanoma, choroidal metastasis and choroidal hemangioma are common tumours. ICGA aids in diagnosis of all of the aforementioned. In cases

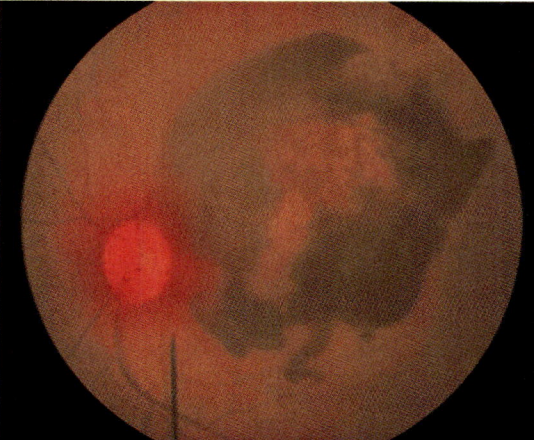
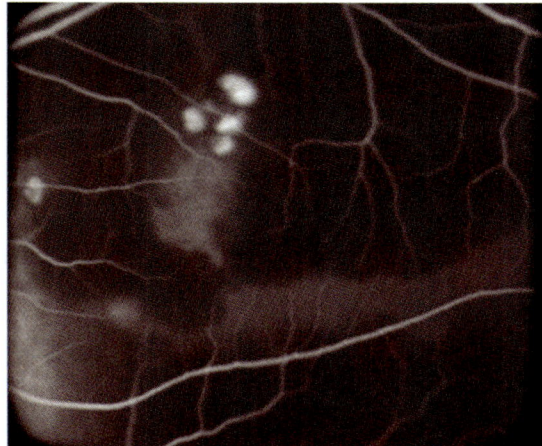

Fig. 28.23: *Fundus photo showing subretinal bleed in macular area with corresponding ICGA showing 4 grape like hyperfluorescent structures, suggestive of polypoidal choroidal vasculopathy.*

of circumscribed choroidal hemangioma, ICGA shows early filling of the vessels in the tumour with late washout of dye surrounded by a hyperfluorescent rim. ICGA mediated PDT has now become the treatment of choice for circumscribed hemangiomas, and leads to regression of the tumour and resolution of surrounding subretinal fluid.

6. *Choroidal inflammation*—Choriocapillaropathies, stromal choroiditis. Pattern of early and late phases of ICGA are the cornerstone for diagnosis of inflammations of the choroid. Inflammation of the choriocapillaris is characterized by hypofluorescence in the early phase, which persists in the late phase.

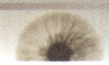

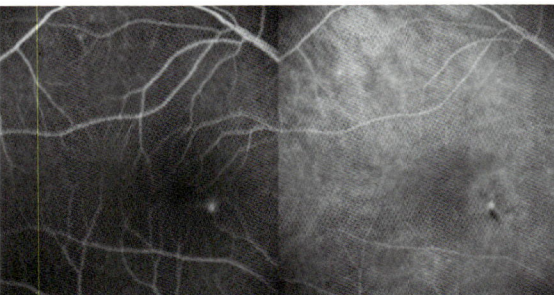

Fig. 28.24: *FFA, on the left, showing point of RPE leakage nasal to the optic disc. ICGA image, on the right, shows a greater area of hyperfluorescent choroid surrounding the point of retinal leakage. Widespread areas of choroidal hyperpermeability are characteristic of central serous chorioretinopathy.*

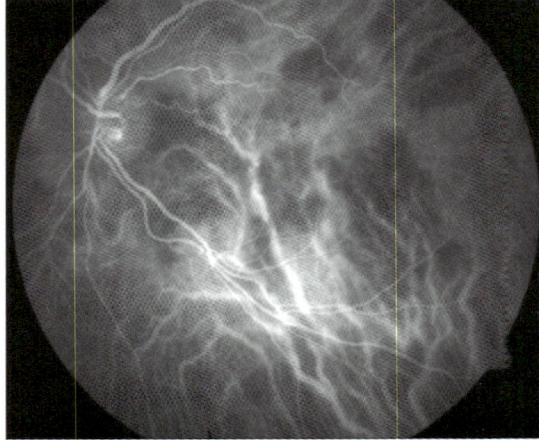

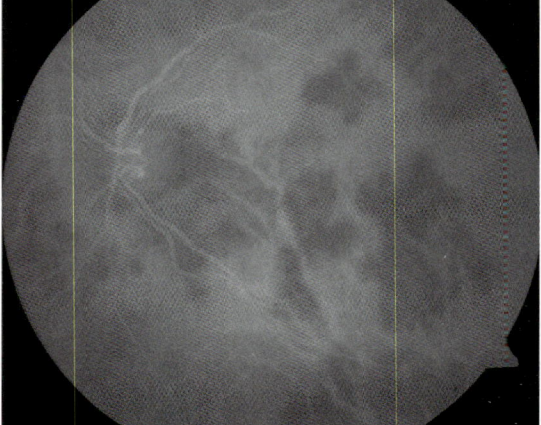

Fig. 28.26: *ICGA showing hypofluorescence in the intermediate and late phases, due to choriocapillaris non-perfusion.*

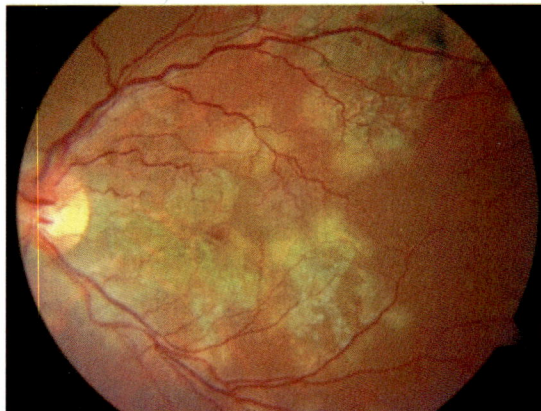

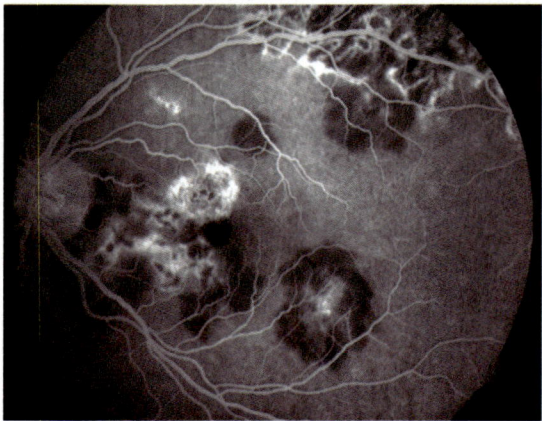

Fig. 28.25: *Fundus photo showing active and healed serpiginous choroiditis lesions with corresponding FFA showing hypo- and hyper-lesions.*

Choroidal stromal inflammations are characterized by leakage from choriocapillaris in the early phase, with hypofluorescence in the intermediate phase, which may (full thickness granulomas) or may not (partial thickness granulomas) persist in the late phase (Figs 28.25 and 28.26).

CONTRAINDICATIONS

1. Documented allergy to iodine
2. Liver disease
3. Pregnancy (Group C drug)
4. Previous allergy to ICG.

FUNDUS AUTOFLUORESCENCE

INTRODUCTION

Fundus photography, fundus fluorescein angiography (FFA), indocyanine green angiography (ICG) and optical coherence tomography (OCT) have been conventionally used as end-points for diagnosing and monitoring retinal diseases in routine clinical practice for several years. Fundus autofluorescence (FAF) is a newer imaging modality for assessing retinal health by allowing metabolic mapping of the fluorophores present in the fundus. It is a non-invasive, and an *in vivo* imaging method that is now being increasingly used for diagnosing retinal diseases.

The dominant fluorophores are lipofuscin (LF) granules that accumulate in the postmitotic retinal pigment epithelium (RPE) cells as a by-product of the incomplete degradation of photoreceptor (PR) outer segments during a normal visual cycle. Lipofuscin consists of a mixture of pigments, including A2E, isomers of A2E and all-transretinal dimer. According to Eldred and Katz, the RPE LF contains at least 10 different fluorophores with discrete emission spectra in the green, golden yellow, yellow-green, and orangered emitting range. Lipofuscin accumulates naturally in the RPE cells and its pattern of distribution in the retina decides its normal FAF pattern. It is the stimulated emission of light chiefly from the LF in the RPE from which the autofluorescence images of the fundus arise. The metabolic activity within the RPE-PR complex can be indirectly judged by the LF content in the RPE. The RPE cells have no means to degrade or transport LF material and these granules are trapped in the cytoplasmic space. Minor fluorophores such as collagen and elastin in choroidal blood vessel walls may become visible in the absence or atrophy of RPE cells.

PRINCIPLE

The FAF signals are emitted across a broad-spectrum ranging from 500 to 800 nm. Ultraviolet light is routinely used to visualize LF with fluorescence microscopy *ex vivo* or *in vitro*. However, its transmission to the retina is limited in the living eye due to the absorption charac-teristics of the ocular media. The LF molecules exhibit a broad range of excitation (300–600 nm). Hence, visible light can be used to elicit its fluorescence *in vivo*. The emission spectrum is broad (480–800 nm) and maximal in the 600–640 nm region of the spectrum. The crystalline lens contributes to normal autofluorescence signal. Hence, modifications are made in the flashlight and detector to minimize the contribution of autofluorescence from the lens, and to allow absolute measurements of FAF. Excitation when using the fundus camera is usually done in the green spectrum (535 to 580 nm) and emission is recorded in the yellow-orange spectrum (615 to 715 nm) (Fig. 28.27A). With the confocal scanning laser ophthalmoscope (cSLO), excitation is usually induced in the blue range (488 nm), and an emission filter between 500 and 700 nm is used to detect emission of the FAF signal (Fig. 28.27B). Because of the difference in excitation and emission spectra, in addition to technical differences between the cSLO and the fundus camera, the types of detected FAF signal may vary between the systems, and it may be possible to visualize different fluorophores. In a normal subject, the fundus shows a diffuse normal FAF signal. Typically, marked hypo-autofluorescence of the optic nerve head (absence of autofluorescent material) and of retinal blood vessels (absorption phenomena by blood contents) are observed. Decreased autofluorescence is also seen in the foveal secondary to absorption from luteal (lutein and zeaxanthin) pigments. The parafoveal area shows mildly decreased intensity compared with the normal background signal at the outer macula (Fig. 28.27A and B).

CLINICAL APPLICATIONS

Abnormal accumulation of LF produces abnormally increased FAF (hyperauto-fluorescence). Accumulation of A2E is toxic and interferes with normal cell functioning. Diseases of the retinochoroid that cause an increased shedding of PR outer segments, disrupted RPE phagocytic function or an inability of the RPE to recycle metabolites produce hyperfluorescence due to LF accumulation as seen in age-related macular degeneration (ARMD) and inherited retinal

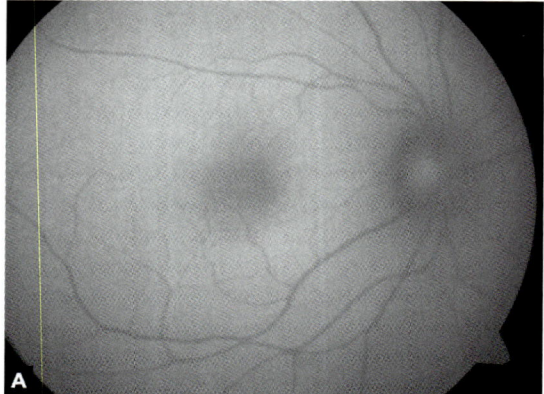

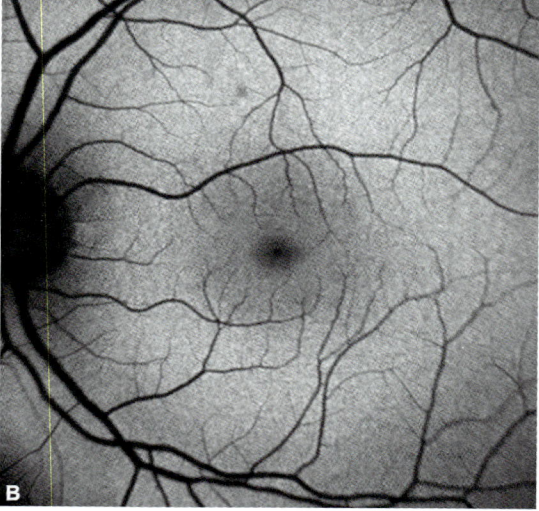

Fig. 28.27: *Fundus autofluorescence photograph of a normal right eye using fundus camera. (A) Where excitation is usually done in the green spectrum (535 to 580 nm) and emission is recorded in the yellow-orange spectrum (615 to 715 nm). Fundus photograph of a normal left eye using the confocal scanning laser ophthalmoscope; and (B) Where excitation is usually induced in the blue range (488 nm), and an emission filter between 500 and 700 nm is used to detect emission of the fundus autofluorescence signal.*

diseases. With the death of PR cells causing disruption of the visual cycle, there is atrophy of the RPE cells and a reduced metabolic turnover leading to decreased FAF (hypoautofluorescence). Deep hypoautofluorescence is observed over areas with advanced atrophic AMD, melanin pigment migration, or fibrotic scar tissue, suggesting RPE atrophy. This finding on FAF denotes extensive damage to the RPE, leading to compromised PR function.

1. Age-related macular degeneration (AMD)

Early AMD

A key role has been attributed to RPE in the disease process. Early manifestations include focal hypopigmentation and hyperpigmentation at the RPE level and drusen with extracellular material accumulating in the inner aspects of Bruch membrane. An international workshop on FAF phenotyping in early AMD reported an analysis of the variability of FAF findings in early AMD. Eight different FAF patterns were classified, including normal, minimal change, focal increased, patchy, linear, lacelike, reticular, and speckled patterns. A relatively poor correlation exists between visible alterations on fundus photographs and notable FAF changes. In early AMD, FAF findings may indicate more widespread abnormalities and diseased areas than clinically seen (Fig. 28.28A and B). The changes seen by FAF imaging may precede the occurrence of visible lesions as the disease progresses and may help to identify specific high-risk characteristics for disease progression as well as to design and monitor future interventional trials.

Geographic atrophy

It represents the atrophic late-stage manifestation of 'dry' AMD. Due to loss of LF, outer retinal atrophy is characterized by severe hypoautofluorescence. Areas of increased intensity signals are observed in the junctional zone surrounding the atrophic patches by FAF imaging, which do not correlate well with funduscopically visible pigmentary changes (Fig. 28.29A and B). The identification of elevated levels of FAF intensities in the junctional zone of atrophy is of particular interest because these changes precede cell death and, therefore, absolute scotoma.

Pigment epithelial detachment (PED)

Most PEDs demonstrate a marked, evenly distributed hyperautofluorescence corresponding to the lesion surrounded by a well-defined, less autofluorescent halo delineating the entire border of the lesion. Some PEDs may also show an intermediate or decreased FAF signal over the lesion that may or may not correspond to areas of RPE atrophy or fibrovascular scaring.

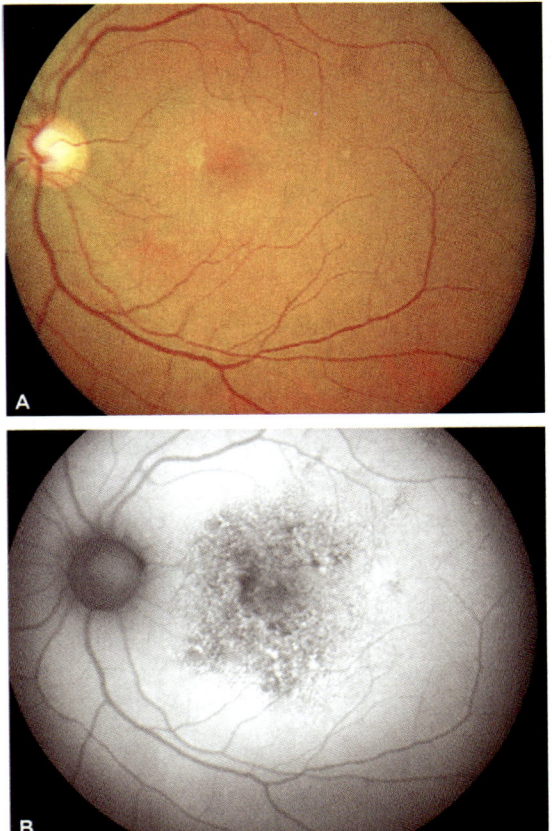

Fig. 28.28: *Fundus photograph. (A) Showing early age-related macular degeneration which are seen as more widespread abnormalities and diseased areas on fundus autofluorescence and (B) Than clinically seen.*

Choroidal neovascular membrane (CNV)

Patches of 'continuous' or 'normal' autofluorescence corresponding to areas of hyperfluorescence on FFA are seen in early CNV secondary to AMD. This indicates that RPE viability is preserved at least initially in CNV development. By contrast, eyes with long-standing CNV typically have increasing hypoautofluorescence, suggesting PR loss, RPE atrophy, development of scar, and increased melanin deposition (Fig. 28.30A and B). Abnormal FAF signals typically extend beyond the edge of the angiographically defined lesion, indicating a more widespread involvement than seen in other imaging studies. Increased FAF signal around the edge of lesions may reflect the proliferation of RPE cells around the CNV.

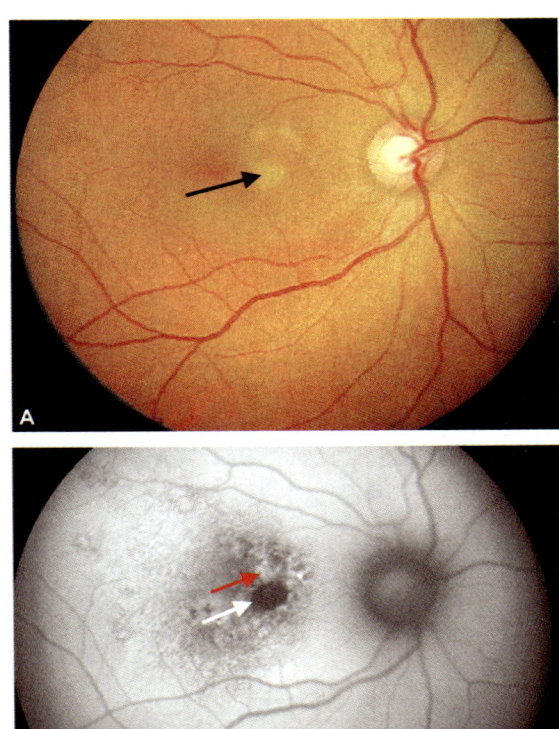

Fig. 28.29: *(A) Fundus photograph. Showing geographic atrophy. Fundus autofluorescence (B) Showing severe hypoautofluorescence corresponding to outer retinal atrophy (white arrows). Areas of increased intensity signals (red arrow) are observed in the junctional zone surrounding the atrophic patches by FAF imaging, which do not correlate well with funduscopically visible pigmentary changes.*

2. Central serous chorioretinopathy (CSR)

It is characterized by idiopathic leaks at the level of the RPE leading to serous retinal detachment. The FAF findings correspond well with the disease stage and are in accord with RPE involvement. Patients with acute leaks show minimal abnormalities with a mild hyperautofluorescence of the serous detachment. Over time, irregular hyperautofluorescnce increases in the area of detachment, corresponding to pinpoint subretinal precipitates seen clinically. Mixed pattern of autofluorescence appears in eyes with chronic disease with atrophic areas showing marked hypoautofluorescence

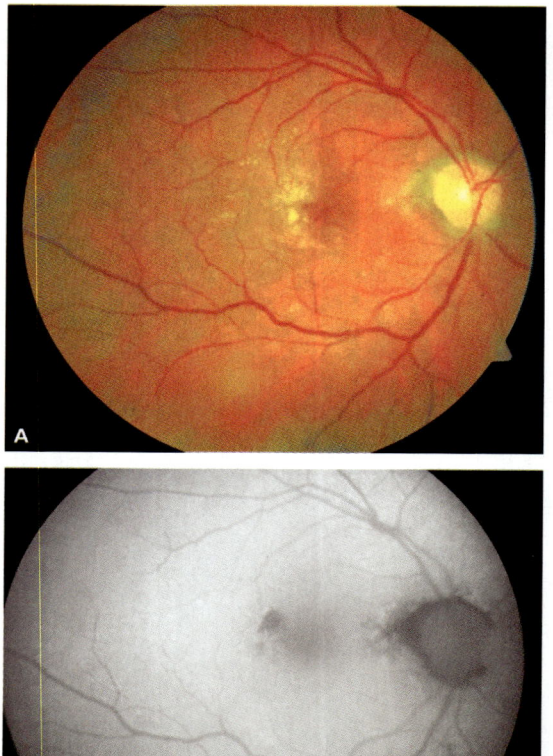

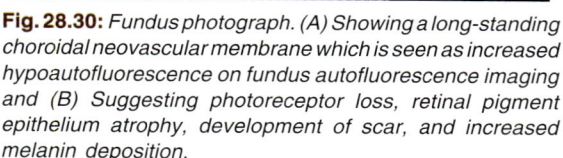

Fig. 28.30: *Fundus photograph. (A) Showing a long-standing choroidal neovascular membrane which is seen as increased hypoautofluorescence on fundus autofluorescence imaging and (B) Suggesting photoreceptor loss, retinal pigment epithelium atrophy, development of scar, and increased melanin deposition.*

(Fig. 28.31A and B). Visualization of fluid tracks in the inferior retina is a typical finding.

3. Macular hole

In early stages (1 and 2) of macular hole, mild to moderate hyperautofluorescence is noted centrally in the area of the hole. In stage 3 full thickness macular hole, a central hyperauto-fluorescence is noted. In stage 4 full thickness macular holes, an increased autofluorescence is noted corresponding to the hole with a surrounding ring of hypoautofluorescence corresponding to the cuff of subretinal fluid (Fig. 28.32A and B). This hyperautofluorescence

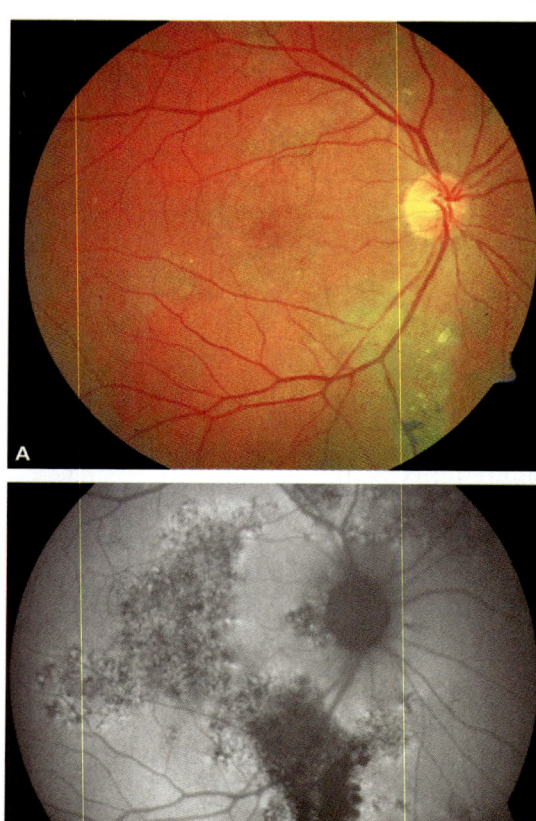

Fig. 28.31: *Fundus photograph. (A) Chronic central serous retinopathy and fundus autofluorescence and (B) Mixed pattern of autofluorescence, with atrophic areas showing marked hypoautofluorescence.*

of the macular hole is no longer visible following a successful surgery (Fig. 28.32C).

4. Retinal dystrophies

Localized abnormalities of FAF intensities are observed in many dystrophies. In patients with retinitis pigmentosa (RP) and cone dystrophies, parafoveal rings of hyperautofluorescence have been identified in absence of funduscopically visible correlates. As the disease progresses, these tend to shrink in RP or enlarge in cone dystrophies. These rings demarcate areas of preserved PR function. In patients with RP, these hyperautofluorescent rings correlate with results from visual function testing. Larger rings tend to correlate with a smaller peripheral visual

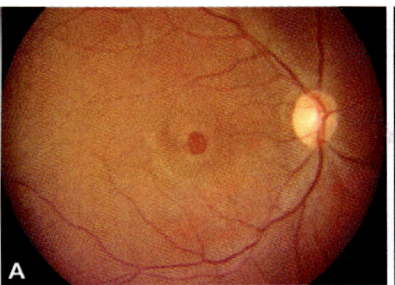
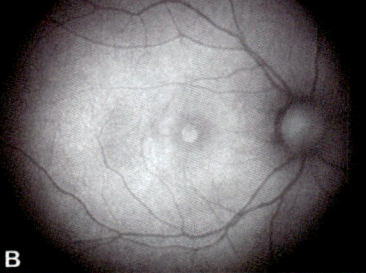
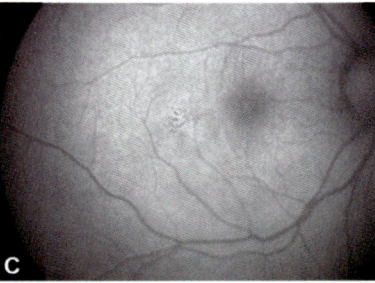

Fig. 28.32: *Stage-4 full thickness macular hole (A and B) showing an increased autofluorescence corresponding to the hole with a surrounding ring of hypoautofluorescence corresponding to the cuff of subretinal fluid; and this hyperautofluorescence of the macular hole is no longer visible following a successful surgery (C).*

field defect. In Stargardt disease, focal hyper-autofluorescent areas correspond to flecks seen on FP suggesting excessive localized LF accumulation. The FAF imaging also allows detection of the abnormal phenotype in some disorders when it is not otherwise clinically evident.

5. Chloroquine/Hydroxychloroquine toxicity

Early RPE alterations can be detected by FAF imaging or multifocal electroretinography when ophthalmoscopy and FFA are less sensitive. A pericentral ring of hyperautofluorescence is seen on FAF imaging in mild toxicity. As it advances, a pericentral mottled hypoautofluorescence is seen. In more advanced cases, a complete pericentral hypoautofluorescence develops (Fig. 28.33A to D).

7. Optic nerve head drusen

Optic nerve head drusens are sometimes not visible on clinical examination because they are subpapillary in nature. They get partially calcified from accumulation of axoplasmic derivatives of degenerating retinal nerve fiber and become increasingly visible with age. They must be differentiated from acquired disc edema, which warrants immediate neurological evaluation and treatment. These bodies are highly auto-fluorescent that can be detected on FAF imaging, besides B-scan ultrasonography (Fig. 28.34A to D).

8. Chorioretinal inflammatory disorders

In multifocal choroiditis, macular hyperauto-fluorescence is seen in areas of active chorio-retinitis that completely disappears and becomes hypoautofluorescent with resolution

of the disease activity after therapy. In APMPPE, placoid areas of hypoautofluorescent corresponding to areas of RPE scarring have been shown in the quiescent phase of the disease. Fundus AF changes have been described in other chorioretinal disorders, including acute syphilitic posterior placoid chorioretinitis which is a rare entity that may mimic APMPPE. Increased FAF corresponds to active geographic lesions at the posterior pole. In multifocal choroiditis and panuveitis (MCP), Haen and Spaide found that all chorioretinal scars visible by autofluorescence imaging were not visible by colour fundus photography. The FAF revealed that patients with MCP have much more widespread involvement of the RPE than would be suspected by any other means of imaging. During an exacerbation of disease activity in a previously quiescent eye with serpiginous choroiditis, a hyperautofluorescent signal on FAF imaging may highlight the active lesion which may be very subtle on FFA. We have described four stages of changing patterns of autofluorescence in tubercular serpiginous like choroiditis as the lesions evolve from an acute stage to the stage of complete healing.

SUMMARY

FAF is a novel imaging modality that provides critical information in various retinal diseases. It is easy, simple, quick, efficient, and non-invasive, and is promising in improving the quality of care for patients with retinal disorders. It provides information over and beyond conventional imaging techniques, and is a reliable tool for disease monitoring.

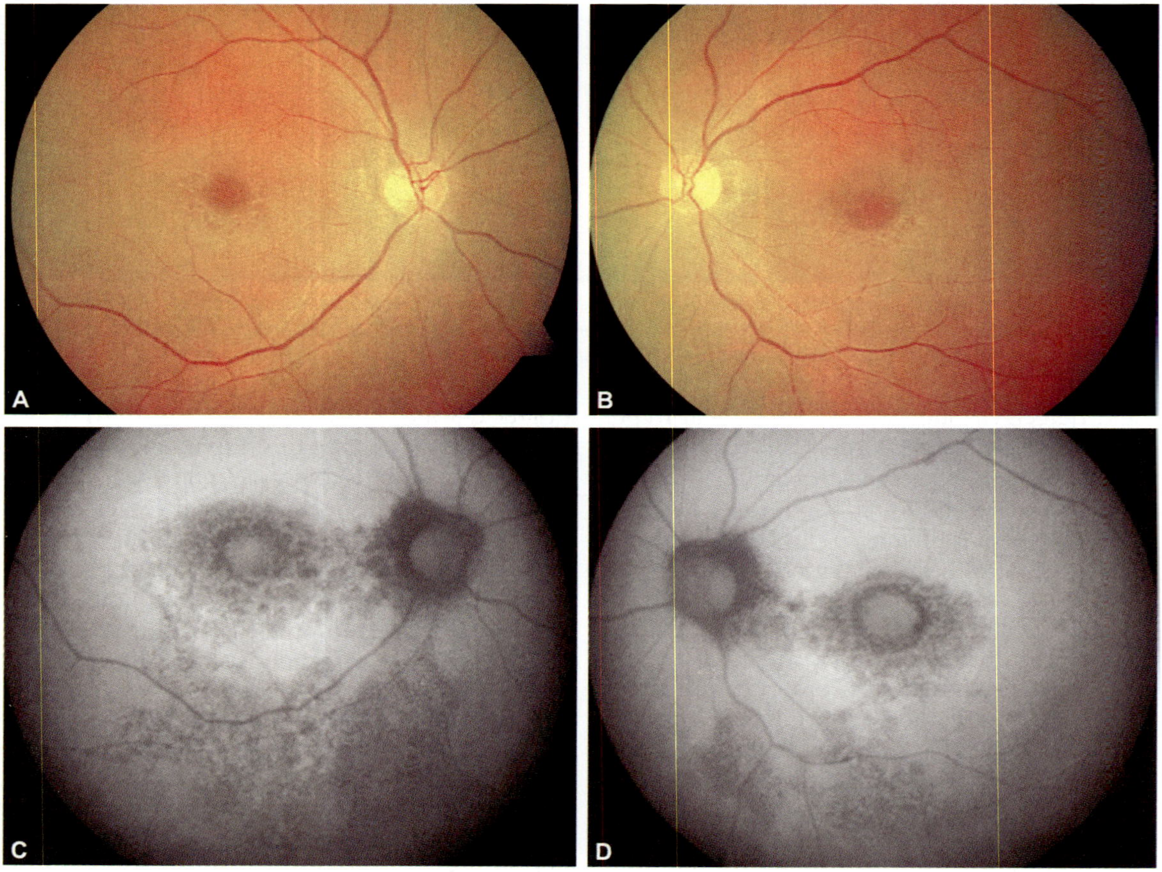

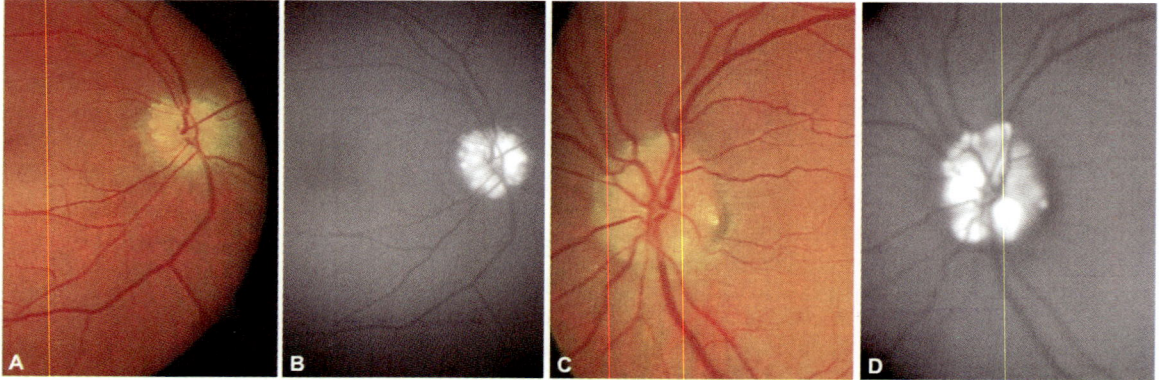

Fig. 28.33: *In advanced stages of chloroquine/hydroxychloroquine toxicity (A and B) and a complete pericentral hypoautofluorescence develops with surrounding mottled hypoautofluorescence (C and D).*

Fig. 28.34: *Optic nerve head drusens may not be clinically apparent (A and C), but can be easily detected on fundus autofluorescence imaging as highly autofluorescent lesions on the optic nerve head (B and D).*

BIBLIOGRAPHY

Fundus Fluorescein Angiography

1. Early Treatment Diabetic Retinopathy Study Research Group. Classification of Diabetic Retinopathy from Fluorescein Angiograms: ETDRS Report Number 11. Ophthalmology 1991;98(5):807–22.
2. Kunimoto, Derek; Kunal Kanitkar, Mary Makar. The Wills eye manual: office and emergency room diagnosis and treatment of eye disease (4th ed.). Philadelphia, PA: Lippincott Williams & Wilkins. 2004;p. 365.
3. Schatz Howard. Fluorescein angiography: basic principles and interpretation. In Retina Volume 2 (Eds) Ryan SJ. St Louis CV Mosby Company, 2006 p. 3.

Indocyanine Green Angiography

1. Carl P Herbort. Fluorescein and Indocyanine Green Angiography in Uveitis. Middle East Afr J Ophthalmol 2009 Oct-Dec;16(4):168–187.
2. Herbort CP, Guex-Crosier Y, LeHoang P. Schematic interpretation of indocyanine green angiography. Ophthalmology 1994;2:169–76.
3. Lim JI, Flower RW. Indocyanine green angiography. Int Ophthalmol Clin 1995;35:59–67.
4. Stanga Paulo E, Lim Jennifer I, Hamilton Peter. 'Indocyanine green angiography in chorioretinal diseases: Indications and interpretation: An evidence-based update'. Ophthalmology, 2003;110(1):15–21.

Fundus Autofluorescence

1. Bellmann C, Holz FG, Breitbart A, Völcker HE. Bilateral acute syphilitic posterior placoid chorioretinopathy-angiographic and autofluorescence characteristics. Ophthalmologe 1999; 96(8):522–8.
2. Bindewald A, Bird AC, Dandekar SS, et al. Classification of fundus autofluorescence patterns in early age-related macular disease. Invest Ophthalmol Vis Sci 2005;46:3309–14.
3. Bird A. Age-related macular disease. Br J Ophthalmol 1996;80:2–3.
4. Delori FC, Dorey CK, Staurenghi G, et al. *In vivo* fluorescence of the ocular fundus exhibits retinal pigment epithelium lipofuscin characteristics. Invest Ophthalmol Vis Sci 1995;36:718–29.
5. Delori FC. Spectrophotometer for non-invasive measurement of intrinsic fluorescence and reflectance of the ocularfundus. Appl Optics 1994;33:7429–52.

6. Eandi CM, Ober M, Iranmanesh R, et al. Acute central serous chorioretinopathy and fundus autofluorescence. Retina 2005;25:989–93.
7. Eldred GE, Katz ML. Fluorophores of the human retinal pigment epithelium: separation and spectral characterization. Exp Eye Res 1988;47: 71–86.
8. Feeney L. Lipofuscin and melanin of human retinal pigment epithelium. Invest Ophthalmol Vis Sci 1978;17(7):583–600.
9. Fishkin NE, Sparrow JR, Allikmets R, Nakanishi K. Isolation and characterization of a retinal pigment epithelial cell fluorophore: an all-trans-retinal dimer conjugate. Proc Natl Acad Sci USA. 2005;102:7091–6.
10. Framme C, Walter A, Gabler B, et al. Fundus autofluorescence in acute and chronic-recurrent central serous chorioretinopathy. Acta Ophthalmol Scand 2005; 83:161–7.
11. Gupta A, Bansal R, Gupta V, Sharma A. Fundus autofluorescence in serpiginous like choroiditis. Retina 2012;32:814–25.
12. Haen SP, Spaide RF. Fundus autofluorescence in multifocal choroiditis and panuveitis. Am J Ophthalmol 2008;145:847–53.
13. Holz FG, Bellman C, Staudt S, et al. Fundus autofluorescence and development of geographic atrophy in age-related macular degeneration. Invest Ophthalmol Vis Sci 2001;42:1051–6.
14. Kellner U, Renner AB, Tillack H. Fundus autofluorescence and mfERG for early detection of retinal alterations in patients using chloroquine/hydroxychloroquine. Invest Ophthalmol Vis Sci 2006;47:3531–8.
15. Kurz-Levin MM, Landau K. A comparison of imaging techniques for diagnosing drusen of the optic nerve head. Arch Ophthalmol 1999; 117(8):1045–9.
16. McBain VA, Townend J, Lois N. Fundus autofluorescence in exudative age-related macular degeneration. Br J Ophthalmol 2007;91:491–6.
17. Robson AG, Michaelides M, Saihan Z, et al. Functional characteristics of patients with retinal dystrophy that manifest abnormal parafoveal annuli of high density fundus autofluorescence; a review and update. Doc Ophthalmol 2008 Mar;116(2):79–89.
18. Robson AG, Saihan Z, Jenkins SA, et al. Functional characterisation and serial imaging of abnormal fundus autofluorescence in patients with retinitis pigmentosa and normal visual acuity. Br J Ophthalmol 2006;90:472–9.

19. Schmitz-Valckenberg S, Holz FG, Bird AC, Spaide RF. Fundus autofluorescence Imaging. Review and perspectives. Retina 2008;28:385–409.

20. Spaide RF, Klancnik JM Jr. Fundus autofluorescence and central serous chorioretinopathy. Ophthalmology 2005;112:825–33.

21. Sparrow JR, Boulton M. RPE lipofuscin and its role in retinal pathobiology. Exp Eye Res 2005; 80:595–606.

22. Vaclavik V, Vujosevic S, Dandekar SS, et al. Autofluorescence imaging in age-related macular degeneration complicated by choroidal neovascularization. A prospective study. Ophthalmology 2008;115:342–6.

23. Von Rückmann A, Fitzke FW, Gregor ZJ. Fundus autofluorescence in patients with macular holes imaged with a laser scanning ophthalmoscope. Br J Ophthalmol 1998;82:346–51.

24. Weiter JJ, Delori FC, Wing GL, Fitch KA. Retinal pigment epithelial lipofuscin and melanin and choroidal melanin in human eyes. Invest Ophthalmol Vis Sci 1986;27(2):145–52.

25. Wing GL, Blanchard GC, Weiter JJ. The topography and age relationship of lipofuscin concentration in the retinal pigment epithelium. Invest Ophthalmol Vis Sci 1978;17(7):601–7.

26. Yeh S, Forooghian F, Wong WT, et al. Fundus auto fluorescence imaging of the White Dot syndromes. Arch Ophthalmol 2010;128(1):46–56.

Macular Optical Coherence Tomography

Chapter Outline

INTRODUCTION AND PRINCIPLE OF OCT

- Introduction
- Principle

COMPARISON OF CURRENTLY AVAILABLE OCT MACHINES

- Stratus OCT
- Cirrus OCT
- Spectralis OCT

INTERPRETATION OF OCT IMAGING

Layer wise interpretation of OCT

OCT findings in common macular lesions

- Central serous retinopathy
- Cystoid macular edema
- Age related macular degeneration
- Macular hole

Conclusion

INTRODUCTION AND PRINCIPLE OF OCT

INTRODUCTION

There are changing trends in imaging of retina. Earlier fluorescein angiography was regarded as gold standard and then the trends shifted to doing optical coherence tomography (OCT) in conjunction. As the understanding of OCT increased trends shifted to preference of OCT due to non-invasive nature of procedure. But the recent trends are for multi-modality imaging (OCT, FFA, ICG, autofluorescence) to achieve a comprehensive description of retinal morphology and function. Diverse retinal images acquired by different modalities at the same time and different time instants must be mutually registered. Retinal autofluorescence provides information about retinal pigment epithelium. Indocyanine green angiography tells about choroidal vasculature and OCT provides overview of neurosensory retina, retinal pigment epithelium (RPE) and choriocapillaris. OCT has become the most important adjunct tool for diagnosis, assessment and management of macular diseases. Leakage is quantified and this is important for monitoring disease progression and seeing response to treatment. Increased resolution of OCT with newer machines gives us insight into well-being of photoreceptors and functional outcome also.

PRINCIPLE OF OCT

The basic principle of OCT is low coherence interferometry (Fig. 29.1).

Time domain (TD) OCT

In time domain OCT the light beam is split into reference beam and measurement beam and both travel different path but with same length before these are picked up by a detector to produce interference signal. In the reference beam a single echo is generated after reflection

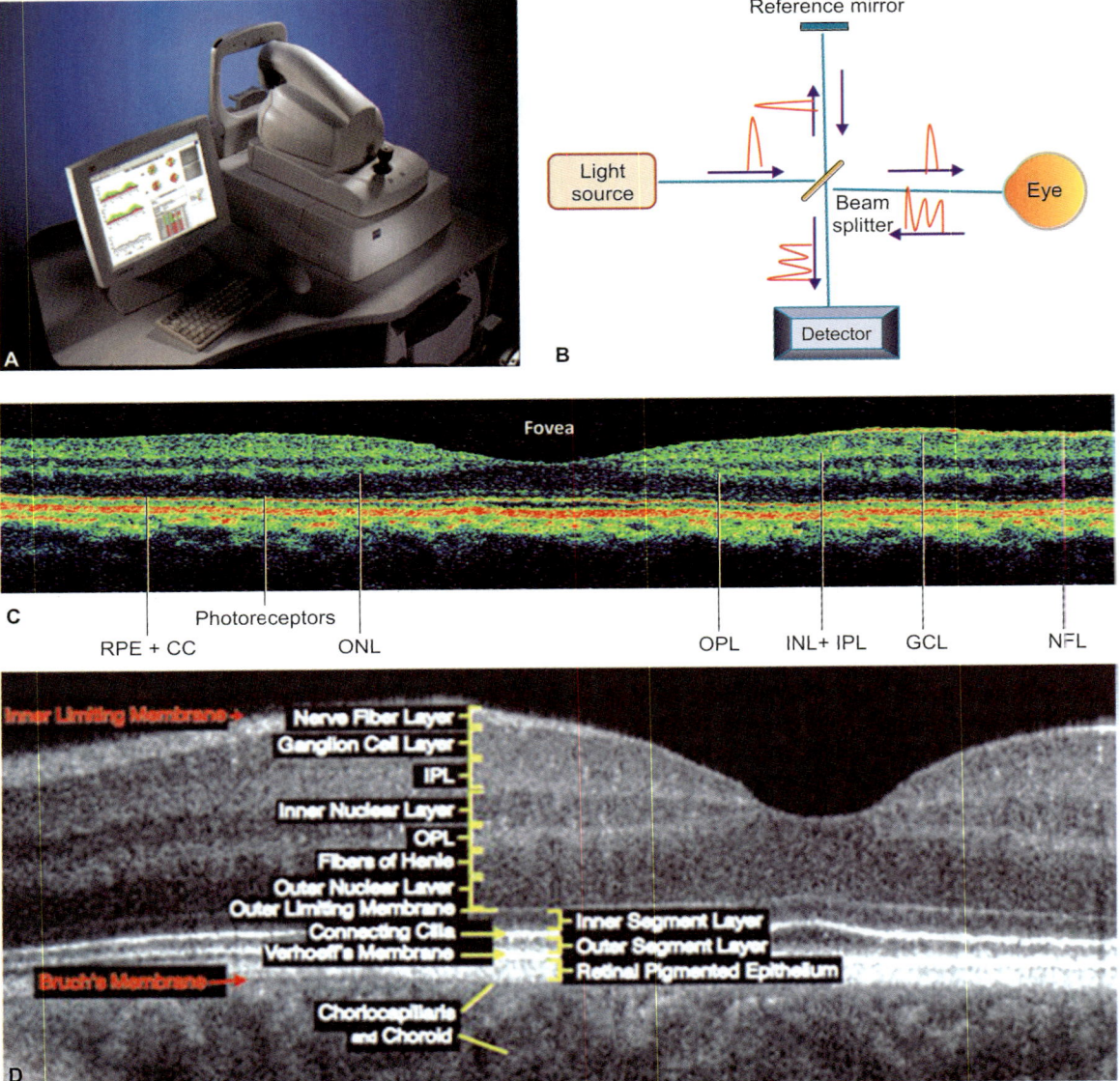

Fig. 29.1: *(A) Photograph of stratus OCT machine (Carl Zeiss meditech) showing simultaneous viewing screen; (B) Line diagram showing principle of the OCT machine; (C) OCT scan of normal macula on stratus OCT showing correlation with various histological layers; and (D) OCT scan on spectral domain OCT showing correlation with different layers on histological examination.*

from the mirror and in the measurement beam various micro structures reflect these at variable intervals giving rise to multiple echoes. The intensity of echoes and time interval between these generate 2-D anteroposterior view of different layers of retina which is comparable to *in vivo* histology of retina. This was first demonstrated by Huang in 1991. With the advent of new machines the resolution has improved and the time required has also decreased. In time domain OCT (TD OCT-stratus by Zeiss) the mirror of reference beam moves back and forth so the image acquisition time is more. Various retinal layers appear as hypo- and hyper-reflective layers on OCT as shown in Fig. 29.1C.

Images are now obtained by newer machines in 2–3 dimensions.

Spectral domain OCT

Spectral domain OCT (SD OCT) is based on the principle of Fourier transform mathematical equation (1807), where movement of mirror in the path of reference beam is not required and interference signal is a function of wavelength and all echoes of light from various tissue interfaces are analysed simultaneously. SD OCT is 50 times faster than TD OCT. SD OCT gives us best visualisation of various layers of retina:

- Examination can be simultaneously performed in different planes and 3 D reconstruction and more precise quantitative measurement is possible.
- SD OCT gives clearer visualization and differentiation of each layer as compared to TD OCT.
- **Nerve fiber layer** is inner most layer and borders are sharper than on TD OCT.
- **Ganglion cell layer** can identify single hyperfluorescent spots as corresponding cells.
- **Nuclear layers** are hyporeflective. Intraretinal vessels are hyperreflective with posterior shadowing in TD OCT but vessel wall and lumen clarity is seen on SD OCT.
- **Outer layers of retina** can be analysed more clearly on SD OCT due to high speed and volume and appear as three bands. This helps in functional information on these tissues especially photoreceptors.
  - ♦ **External limiting membrane** is a moderately reflective membrane under ONL. It is almost always seen with SD OCT while it is seen with difficulty on TD OCT.
  - ♦ The first hyperreflective band under ONL is inner segment/outer segment junction (IS/OS junction) of photoreceptors.
  - ♦ **The outer layer is RPE,** composed of two distinct hyperreflective bands separated by thin hyporeflective strip. The outer band is composed of RPE but the inner band origin is unclear, which sometimes is thought to be Verhoef's membrane (constituted by tight junctions of RPE cells) (Fig. 29.1C and D).
- Due to longer wavelength with spectral domain OCT even choroid can be visualized.

In SD OCT the moderately hyperreflective outermost structure corresponds to sclera.

- **Newer OCT machines acquire retinal cube sections** (512 vertical, 528 horrizontal in cirrus OCT in approximately 11 seconds) which can simultaneously show tomography in 3 sections. The acquisition time with newer software is so short that even motion artifact can also be removed. RPE and ILM can further be isolated from other retinal layers. Retinal thickness can further be evaluated in 3 D maps. White and red are the colours for thicker area and green and blue represent thinner areas.

COMPARISON OF CURRENTLY AVAILABLE OCT MACHINES

Currently available OCT machines include:
- Stratus OCT
- Cirrus OCT
- Spectralis OCT.

Comparison of some commercially available OCT machines is summarized in Table 29.1.

Different scan protocols with stratus OCT

1. *Line.* This protocol allows one to take a scan through a specified area of retina. The angle and length of the line can be altered. The longer the length of the lesser is the resolution.

2. *Radial lines.* This protocol contains 6 to 24 line scans which pass through a common axis. It is useful to measure the retinal thickness in a given area.

3. *Raster lines.* Multiple parallel line scans are taken to cover a larger rectangular area. The default setting is 6 lines with 3 mm rectangle.

4. *Macular thickness and fast macular thickness.* They are the same as radial line scans, but the aiming circle has a fixed diameter of 6 mm. The fast macular scan reduces the time taken to acquire scans.

Different scans protocols with cirrus and spectralis OCT

1. *Raster lines.* Similar to the protocol in time domain OCT.

2. *Raster lines HD.* Higher density images are acquired for better tissue detail.

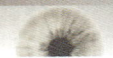

Table 29.1 *Comparison of different OCT machines available*			
	Stratus (time domain)	*Cirrus (spectral domain)*	*Spectralis (spectral domain)*
Axial resolution	10 μ	5 μ	3.9 μ axial resolution 14 μ transverse resolution
Scan velocity	400 axial scan/sec	27,000 axial scan/sec	40,000 axial scan/sec
Enhanced depth imaging	Not possible	Not possible	Possible
Scanning time	Slower scanning time	0.017–0.25 sec	0.005–0.01 sec
Tracking eye movement	Absent	Absent	Present
Simultaneous ICG, FFA, red free picture and auto-fluorescence	Not possible	Not possible	Possible
Central macular thickness measurement	Measures between RNFL and inner boundary of RPE	Measures between RNFL and outer boundary of RPE	Measures between RNFL and outer boundary of RPE
Central macular thickness	230 ± 33.2 microns	270 ± 43.7 microns	

3. *Macular cube (512×256).* Multiple scans are taken in a rectangle of set dimensions and retinal thickness can be calculated at any point within the rectangle. 3-dimensional reconstruction can also be done to look for anteroposterior traction in addition to transverse changes.

4. *Macular cube HD.* Similar to the macular cube protocol, but high density images are taken to improve tissue detail.

INTERPRETATION OF OCT IMAGING

LAYER WISE INTERPRETATION OF OCT

We must look at OCT layer wise, in addition to determining the central macular thickness, maximum retinal thickness and looking at the foveal contour, as below.

1. Retinal pigment epithelium (RPE)

For proper OCT interpretation we must try to trace RPE and its separation from Bruch's membrane. Normally these two are in close association with each other and RPE has very high reflectivity. In diseased state we can see RPE as separate from Bruch's membrane. In serous pigment epithelial detachment (PED) we can see RPE lifted up and Bruch's membrane appears as moderately reflective band under RPE (Fig. 29.2A and B). If posterior reflectivity is blocked then it is haemorrhagic PED (Fig. 29.3). It is also blocked in deposits of Best's

disease. Drusens appear as PED filled with moderately reflective homogenous material. There is no serous detachment or cystic spaces associated with it (Fig. 29.4A and B).

Follow RPE band and look for any irregularity, thickening in contour, or fragmentation all of which are suggestive of occult CNVM (Fig. 29.5A to C). Associated neurosensory

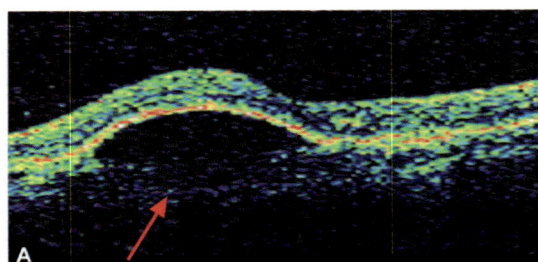

Serous PED

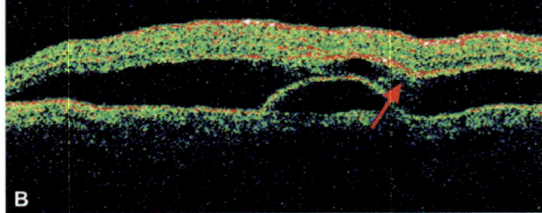

Fig. 29.2: *(A) Retinal pigment epithelial detachment showing optically clear center and Bruch's membrane (arrow) is visible suggestive of serous pigment epithelial detachment (PED) and (B) Serous PED with nerosensory detachment in a case of CSCR, subretinal space shows moderate reflectivity suggestive of fibrin (arrow).*

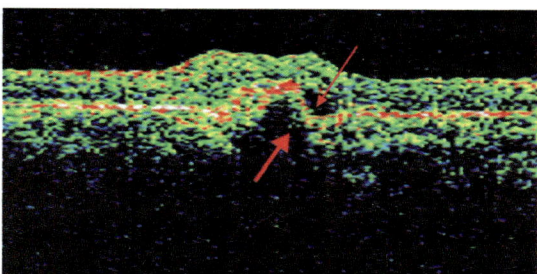

Fig. 29.3: *Retinal pigment epithelial detachment with fibrovascular proliferation in the PED (thick arrow) and block reflectivity posteriorly (thin arrow) and the Bruch's membrane is not seen.*

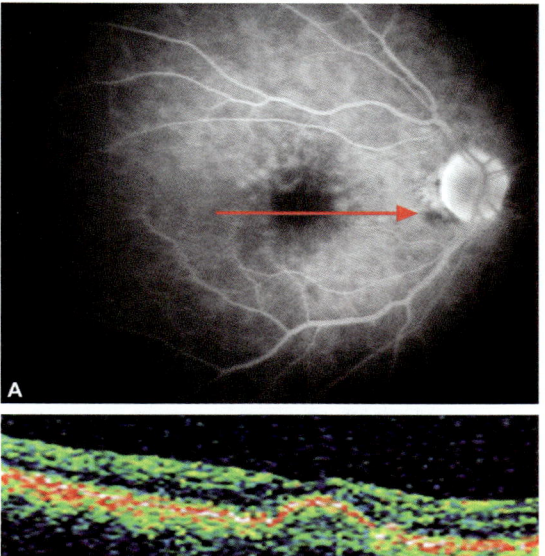

Fig. 29.4: *(A) FFA arteriovenous phase shows point like hyperfluorescence not increasing in late phases consistent with drusens and (B) OCT horizontal scan shows RPE detachment with moderately reflective homogenous material in the PED, suggestive of drusen.*

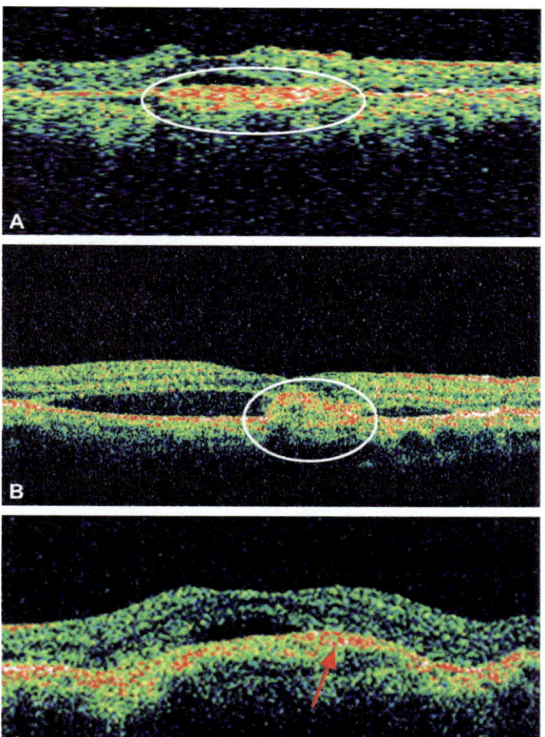

Fig. 29.5: *(A) RPE is irregular and thickened with overlying serous detachment suggestive of CNVM; (B) Type 1 (classic) CNVM, hyperreflective membrane anterior to RPE with serous detachment; and (C) Fibrovascular PED with serous detachment anterior to it suggestive of Type 2 (occult) CNVM.*

detachment/sensory macular detachment (SMD) and cystic spaces can be seen (Fig. 29.6A and B). Hyperreflective dots represent inflammatory reaction and are present in active CNVM (Fig. 29.7). Sometimes effraction of RPE is seen and retinochoroid anastomosis is seen clearly suggestive of retinal angiomatosis proliferans (Fig. 29.8). Numerous PEDs are seen in idiopathic polypoidal choroidovasculopathy (IPCV) and some choroidal polyps are seen reaching till inner retinal layers also. PEDs in IPCV are more steep and abrupt.

Three main landmarks for outer retinal layers (outer nuclear layers ONL external limiting membrane ELM, inner segment outer segment junction IS/OS junctions) help us to prognosticate the patient. The integrity of photoreceptors is important for good functional outcome. Ischaemic damage may lead to disruption of these layers. Branch retinal vein occlusion is a good example of disruption of these layers in the region of ischaemia (Figs 29.9 to 29.11).

2. Evaluate structures anterior to RPE

The neurosensory retina anterior to RPE is evaluated for vitreous and vitreoretinal adhesions, foveal depression/contour, various retinal layers, presence of cavities and deposits, serous

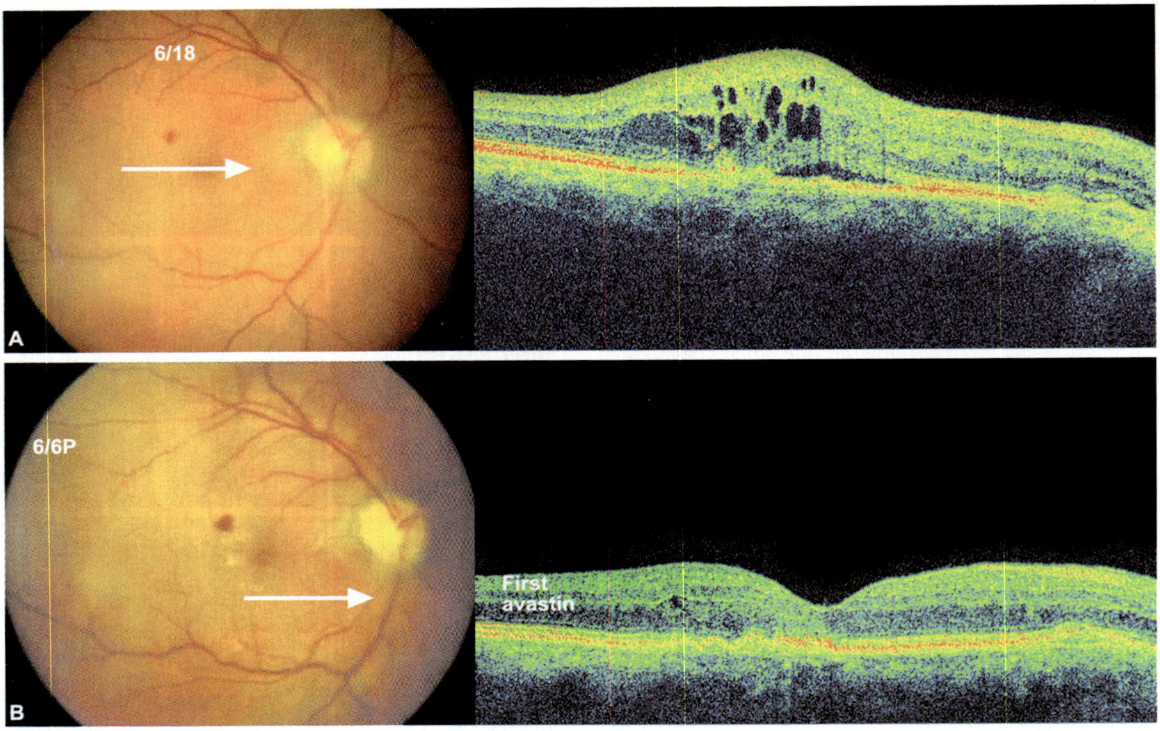

6/18

6/6P

First avastin

Fig. 29.6: *(A) Horizontal OCT scan shows fragmented and disrupted RPE without any thickening with overlying cysts in occult CNVM; and (B) Horizontal OCT scan after intravitreal bevacizumab showing resolution of serous detachment and cysts. (Courtesy: Professor MR Dogra).*

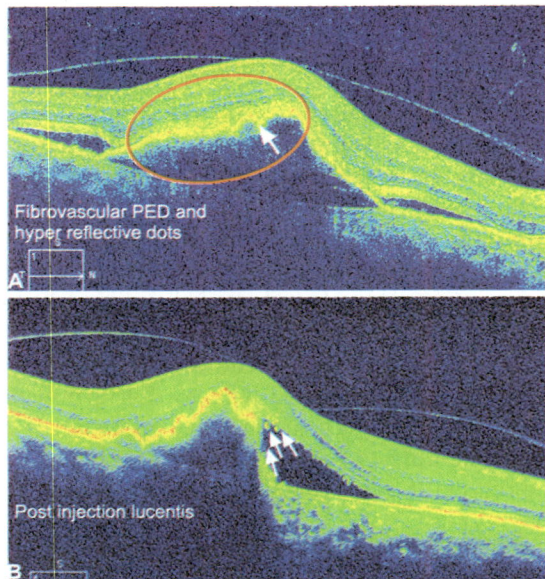

Fibrovascular PED and hyper reflective dots

A

Post injection lucentis

B

Fig. 29.7: *(A) RPE detachment with fibrovascular proliferation with hyperreflective dots suggestive of inflammation seen in active membrane and (B) Same pattern RPE rip after injection lucentes. (Courtesy: Professor MR Dogra).*

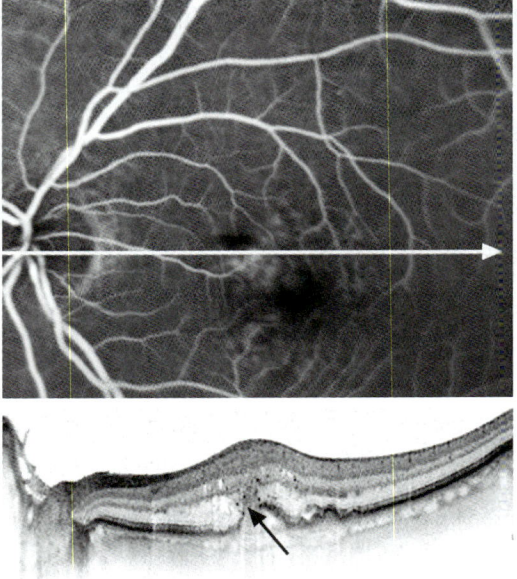

Fig. 29.8: *Effraction of RPE and retinochoroid anastomosis seen in retinal angiomatosis proliferans (Courtesy: Dr. Etnan Priel).*

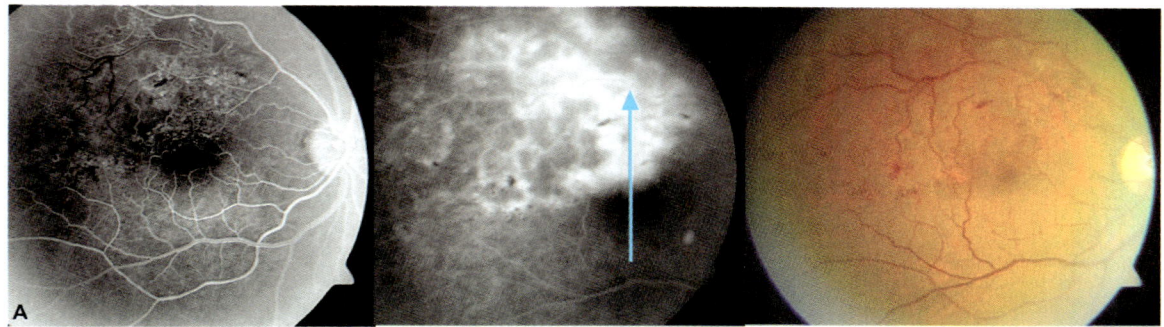

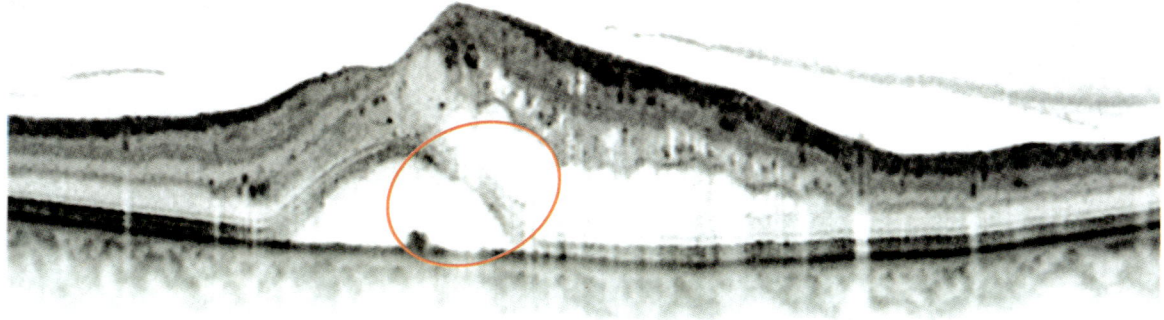

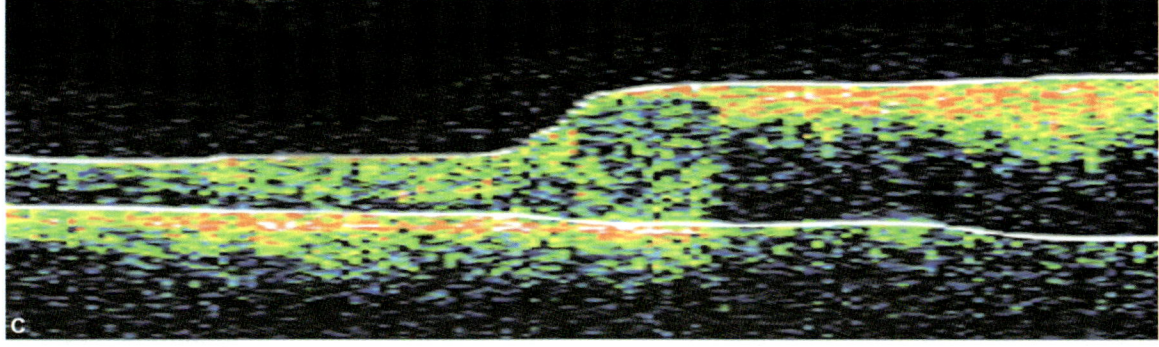

Fig. 29.9: *Case of BRVO. (A) Showing leakage on FFA; (B) Spectralist OCT scan showing increase in thickness with disruption of ELM, IS/OS junction; and (C) Stratus OCT scan of the same patient showing differential increase in thickness and loss of foveal dip.*

macular detachment (SMD) (Figs 29.12 to 29.15). Any hyporeflective structures or hyperreflective structures are looked for. Hyper- reflective lesions could be linear beneath neurosensory retina or within retinal layers (pigment, haemorrhage, fibrous scar) or dots hyperreflective dots (HRD) suggestive of active inflammation especially in active CNVM.

3. Evaluate structures posterior to RPE band

Hyperreflectivity is suggestive of atrophy and hyporeflective is shadowing due to structures in anterior layers (Figs 29.16 and 29.17).

4. Thickness measurement

It is done by an inbuilt software. For reliable thickness measurement, we must evaluate the

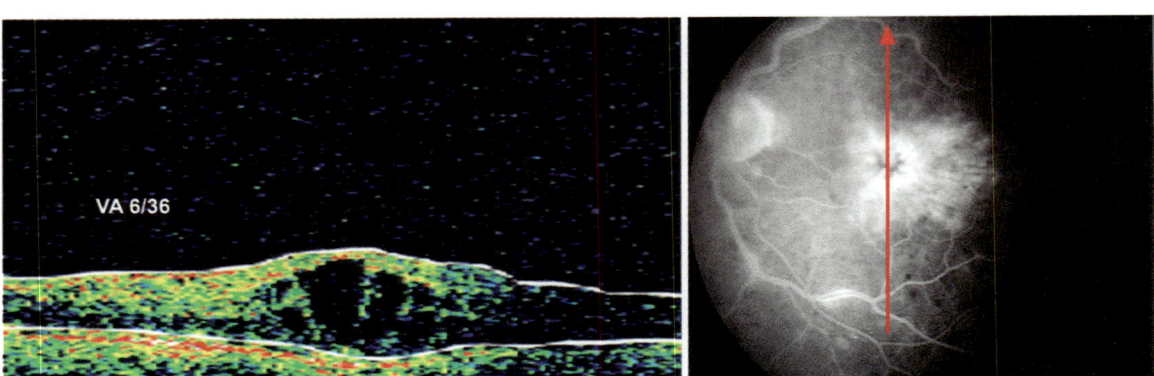

Fig. 29.10: *Vertical OCT scan in a case of CRVO showing cystoid macular edema separated by hyperreflective septa.*

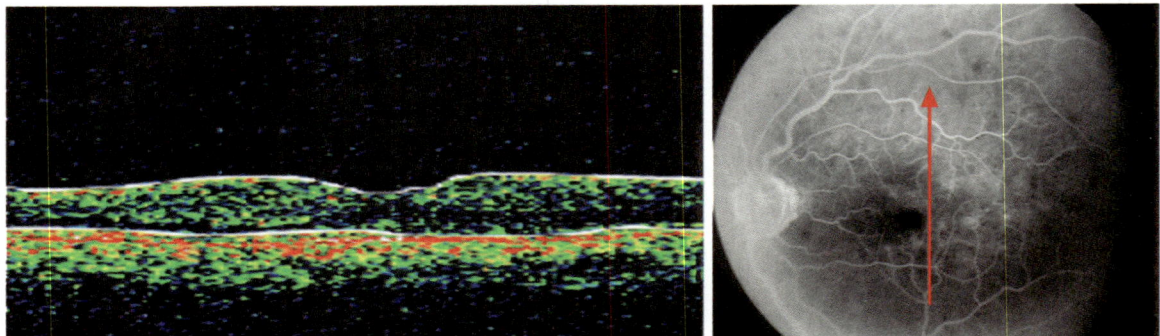

Fig. 29.11: *Resolution of macular edema and restoration of foveal contour after injection bevacizumab in the same patient as seen in Fig. 29.12.*

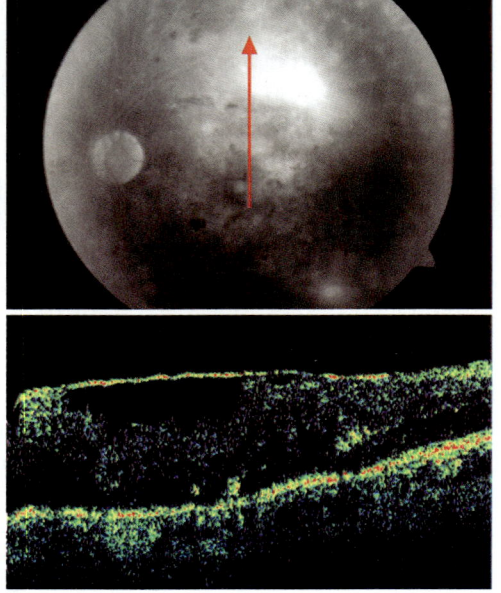

Fig. 29.12: *Vertical macular scan showing vitreomacular adhesions in a case of refractory CSME.*

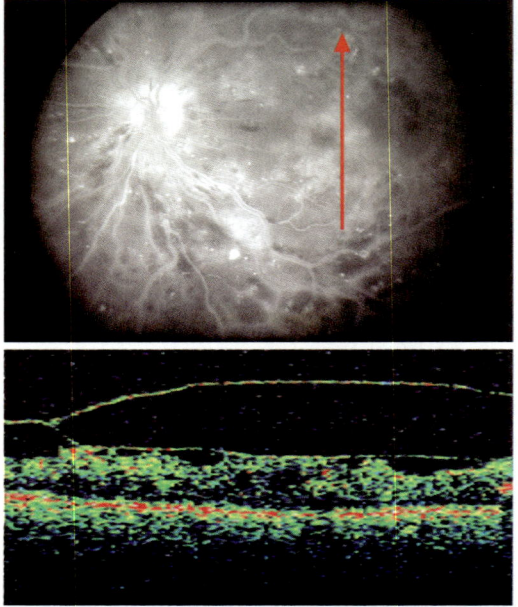

Fig. 29.13: *Vertical scan showing taut posterior hyaloid and vitreoschisis in a case of refractory CSME.*

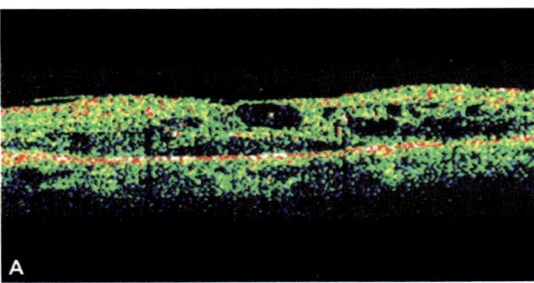

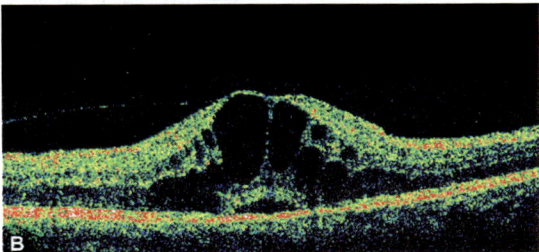

Fig. 29.14: *(A) Horizontal OCT scan of CSME patient showing increased foveal thickness, loss of foveal contour, spongiform pattern of retinal thickening with submacular detachment; and (B) Horizontal OCT scan of CSME patient showing increased foveal thickness, loss of foveal contour, cystoids pattern of macular edema with hyperreflective septa separating cysts.*

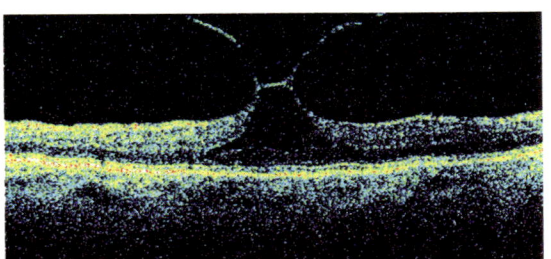

Fig. 29.15: *OCT scan showing clinically significant macular edema with vitreomacular traction.*

scan quality and center the measurement at the fovea (Fig. 29.18). Automated segmentation in high resolution OCTs gives more accurate retinal thickness measurements.

SD OCT measures thickness by incorporating RPE. The posterior line selected is line representing Bruch's membrane. The Cirrus HD-OCT segmentation algorithm identifies the thickness of the retina from the retinal pigment epithelium (RPE) to the internal limiting membrane (ILM). Stratus OCT segmentation algorithm identifies the thickness of the retina

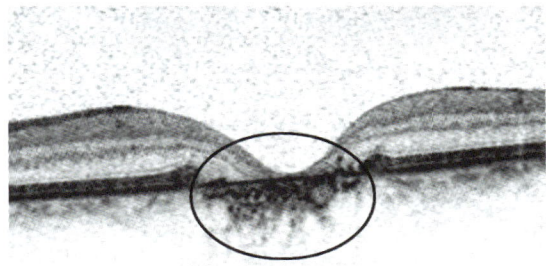

Macular dystrophy

Fig. 29.16: *OCT scan showing marked decrease in foveal thickness and hyperreflectivity under fovea suggestive of foveal atrophy.*

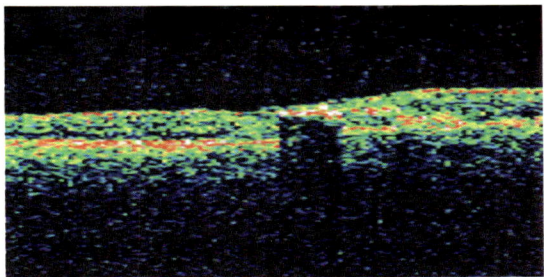

Fig. 29.17: *OCT scan showing hyperreflectivity from pigmented scar and blocked reflectivity posterior to it.*

based on the distance between the ILM and junction of the outer segments (OS) and inner segments (IS) of the photoreceptors. SD OCT thickness measurement are 40–80 µ higher than TD OCT.

OCT FINDINGS IN COMMON MACULAR LESIONS

Central serous retinopathy

Optical coherence tomography is an excellent, non-invasive imaging modality for the diagnosis and for following the resolution of subretinal fluid in CSC. It can pick up subtle fluid accumulation beneath the sensory retina and the RPE not detectable clinically or on FFA. Recently, spectral domain OCT has been used to study ultrastructural abnormalities including external limiting membrane (ELM) and photoreceptor inner segment outer segment junction (IS-OS junction) discontinuities in patients with active and inactive CSC. These studies may provide further insight into the microstructural abnormalities in patients with

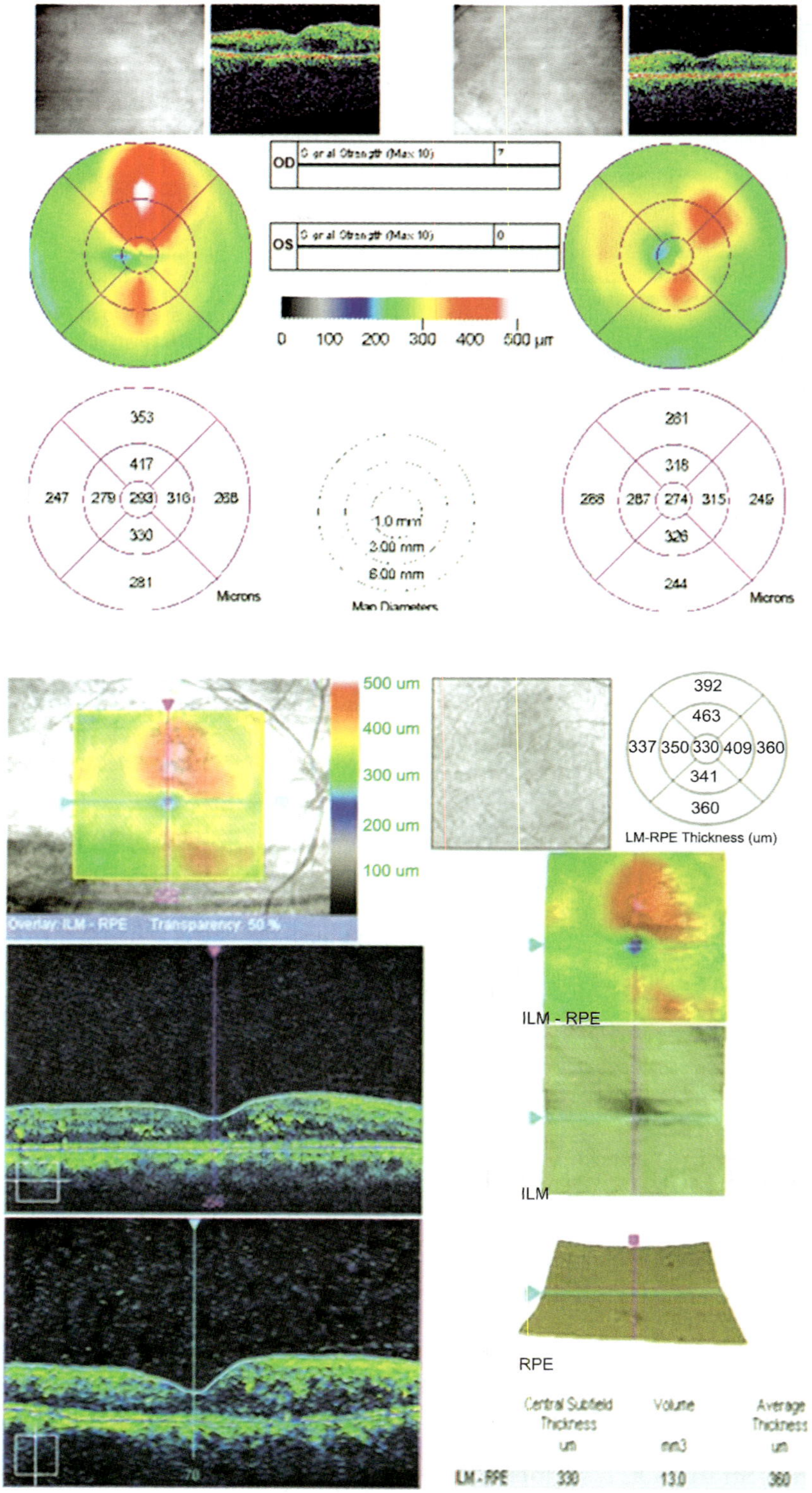

CSC and correlation with visual acuity outcomes following resolution.

Cystoid macular oedema

Optical coherence tomography is a non-invasive device that obtains cross-sectional, high-resolution images of the retina and thus may detect retinal thickening (Huang et al. 1991). Microstructural features are determined by measuring the 'echo' time it takes for the light to reflect from the different structures at varying distances, analogous to A-scan ultrasonography. As the OCT operates with a near-infrared wavelength (about 840 nm), the examination is of minimal discomfort for the patient (Ripandelli et al. 1998). Optical coherence tomography examination is possibly indicated in the early detection and follow-up of patients with macular oedema (Hee et al. 1998). It has been shown to produce highly reproducible measurements and it is as effective at detecting macular edema as fluorescein angiography, but is superior at demonstrating axial distribution of the fluid. The typical OCT picture shows large cystic spaces in the macula having CME (Fig. 29.19).

The RTA (retinal thickness analyser) is a rapid screening instrument that generates a detailed map of retinal thickness.

Age-related macular degeneration

1. OCT can help characterize retinal pathology, even when this information is difficult to discern on clinical examination or

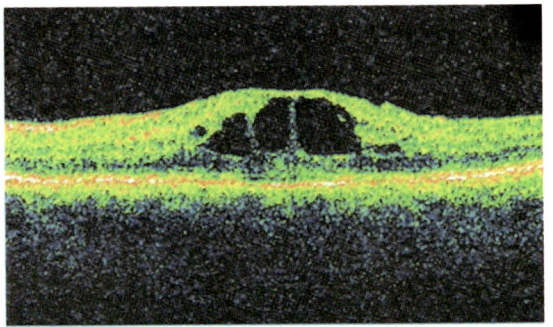

Fig. 29.19: *OCT shows large cystic spaces in the retina having CME.*

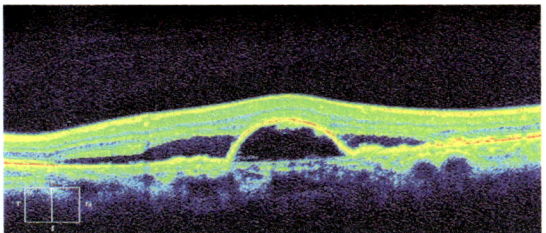

Fig. 29.20: *OCT image of an occult CNV.*

angiography. It is possible to define the location of choroidal neovascular membranes above or below the RPE (Fig. 29.20).

2. Solid fibrous tissue can be differentiated from subretinal fluid when these findings may be angiographically equivocal.

3. Other features of AMD, including cystoid macular oedema (CME), drusenoid RPE detachments and RPE tears can be imaged by OCT.

4. Optical coherence is useful for quantitative assessment of retinal thickness and subretinal fluid when associated with choroidal neovascularization (CNV).

A characteristic appearance of CNV has also been described, consisting of thickening and fragmentation of the reflective layer corresponding to the RPE and choriocapillaris. The extent and location of subretinal fluid associated with CNV can be used to assess whether the pathology is subfoveal, as long as there is preservation of some foveal architecture. As noted on clinical examination and FA, CME is frequently associated with CNV in wet AMD. However, the presence of CME may be difficult to definitively diagnose through those modalities alone.

In addition to imaging subretinal fluid, OCT is effective in identifying intraretinal edema, compared to both clinical stereoscopic images and FA. The appearance of CME on OCT images is seen as hyporeflective, dark spaces within retinal tissue. Its presence is important clinically, since CME as seen on OCT scan in wet AMD correlates with decreased visual acuity. RPE detachments and sub-RPE neovascularization has been associated with occult CNV in AMD as defined histopathologically.

Macular hole

Optical coherence tomography (OCT) is novel non-invasive, non-contact imaging technique capable of producing cross-sectional images of ocular tissue *in vivo* of high resolution (10 μm) which has now become a mandatory and investigation of choice because it not only establishes the diagnosis but also provides important prognostic clue with reference to surgical outcomes.

OCT is useful in the diagnosis of full-thickness macular holes, especially where there is uncertainty on biomicroscopy, and is able to distinguish full-thickness macular holes from partial thickness holes, macular pseudoholes, and cysts.

OCT is also useful for defining the stage of macular hole development and providing a quantitative measure of hole size [which can be used to calculate the hole form factor (a+b/c >0.8 and macular hole index: height/base >0.5 has good closure rate (Fig. 29.21)].

Diameter Hole Index (DHI): Ratio of minimum diameter of MH to base diameter, it is an Indicator of extent of tangential traction.

Tractional Hole Index (THI): Ratio of maximal height of MH to minimum diameter. It is a indicator of antero-posterior traction and retinal hydration. Patients with higher THI values (1.41) and low DHI values (<0.50) had best post-op VA recovery.

OCT has been used to evaluate the vitreo-retinal interface in the fellow eyes of individuals with macular holes and enables the detection of subtle separations of the posterior hyaloid from the retina that are not evident clinically.

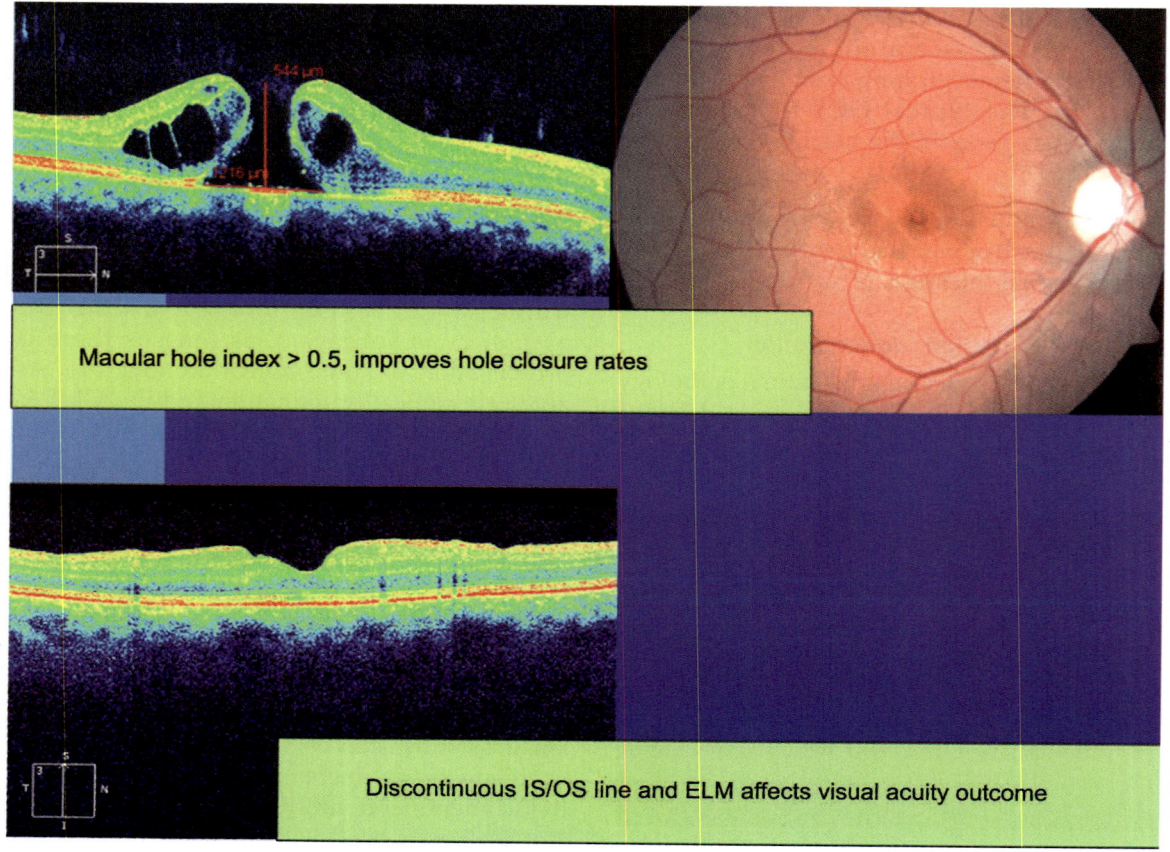

Fig. 29.21: *Fundus photograph and OCT picture of stage IV MH depicting macular hole index.*

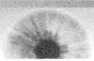

CONCLUSION

OCT is easy to perform and can give a lot of information besides the retinal thickness if read carefully layer wise. With OCT the disease is diagnosed and activity assessed by numerous direct and indirect signs. OCT cannot actually demonstrate vascular component, neovascular network or analyse whether it is an active CNVM or prefibrotic CNVM. Interpretation of OCT should be after correlation with other imaging modalities.

BIBLIOGRAPHY

1. Fercher AF, Hitzenberger CK, Drexler W, Kamp G, Sattmann H. *In vivo* Optical Coherence Tomography. Am J Ophthalmol 1993;116:113–4.
2. Interpretation of OCT scans. In: Gupta V, Gupta A, Dogra MR (Eds). Atlas Optical Coherence tomography of macular diseases and Glaucoma. Jaypee Brothers Medical Publishers 2006;17.
3. Keane PA, Patel PJ, Liakopoulos S, Heussen FM, et al. Evaluation of age-related macular degeneration with optical coherence tomography. Survey of Ophthalmology 2012; 57(5):389–414.

Electrophysiological Tests in Ophthalmology

Chapter Outline

GENERAL CONSIDERATIONS
- Which electrophysiological test tells what?
- When do we order electrophysiological tests?
- Standards of electrophysiological tests

ELECTRORETINOGRAM
- Principle
- Types
- Technique
- Indications
- Interpretation
- Limitation

ELECTRO-OCULOGRAM
- Principle
- Technique

- Indications
- Clinical interpretation
- Limitations

VISUAL EVOKED POTENTIAL
- Types
- Technique
- Indications
- Interpretation
- Limitations

ELECTROPHYSIOLOGICAL TEST: TIME TAKEN, POTENTIAL INDICATIONS AND PRACTICAL STATUS
- Time taken
- Potential indications
- Practical status

GENERAL CONSIDERATIONS

Visual electrophysiology is an indispensable diagnostic support service to clinical ophthalmology as it helps to ascertain the functional integrity.

We have come a long-way since 1849 when DuBois-Reymond first time described how to measure the electrical activity in the visual system. He discovered that excised fish eyes had a potential difference of about 6 mV between the cornea and posterior scleral surface. Einthoven and Jolly, and later, Granit, described the electroretinogram (ERG) in considerable detail in animal eyes using galvanometers (Einthoven, 1908; Granit, 1947) in the early years of the twentieth century. With the advancement in technology for recording, in early 1940s the human ERG was carried out in the clinical setting.

Marked improvements in equipment for generating and recording electrophysiological responses such as solid-state electronics, microprocessors and light emitting diodes (LEDs) have led to a greatly increased understanding of the workings of the visual system in health and disease.

Which electrophysiological test tells what?

The visual electrophysiology tests follow a hierarchal pathway along the various cell layers of the visual system.

Full field electroretinogram (ERG). It measures the mass response generated from the cells of entire retina.

Flash electroretinogram (fERG). Electrical responses from retinal photoreceptors and the inner retinal cells are ascertained by the a- and b-wave components of the flash ERG.

Pattern electroretinogram (pERG). Pattern ERG tells about the macular photoreceptor function and the ganglion cells function is revealed and separated by the technique of recording.

Electro-oculogram (EOG). Examines the function of the retinal pigment epithelium (RPE).

Visual evoked potential (VEP). Tells the integrity of the visual pathway from optic nerve via optic chiasma to the occipital cortex.

A clear understanding of the nature of each of these tests is essential to derive a valid interpretation. This chapter gives an overview of various tests available and some idea of basic interpretation.

When do we order electrophysiological tests?

In some cases, even the detailed clinical examination of the eye cannot explain the exact cause of vision loss. These tests help to provide a piece of *'diagnostic jigsaw'* to detect and categorize the site of lesion in the visual pathway.

Common uses of visual electrophysiology in the clinical setting include the following:
- To provide evidence to confirm or exclude a specific diagnosis
- To indicate the level in the visual system at which a problem lies
- To monitor the progress of a known condition
- To provide an approximate objective measurement of visual acuity
- To provide an indication of the maturity of the visual system in infants
- To detect early disease or carrier status in relatives of an affected individual
- To provide an indication of visual potential in an injured or diseased eye
- To detect a drug or metal toxicity
- To assess the extent of ischaemia of the inner retinal layers in a vascular pathology.

Standards for electrophysiological tests

For each of these recordings in the clinic, certain minimum standards have been laid down by the International Society for Clinical Electrophysiology of Vision (ISCEV). In 1989, they published the first internationally agreed standard for ERG. Standards for other electrophysiological tests and for calibration of recording equipment have been published more recently. These are available on the website www.iscev.org.

The adage *'Man before the machine'* holds very true for visual electrophysiology as the visual electrophysiologist is the key component of the system. The process of recording electrophysiological responses requires special training and meticulous attention to detail. Factors which can influence responses include:
- Placement of recording electrodes
- Ambient lighting levels
- Pupil size
- Extraneous electrical interference
- Calibration errors of the recording equipment.

Each laboratory should maintain their own database of normal values for each test, which must be updated if the equipment is changed or testing protocols revised.

ELECTRORETINOGRAM

Electroretinogram (ERG) is a measurement of retinal electrical response to a light stimulus. It measures the generalized loss of rods or cones or both.

PRINCIPLE

Due to selective transport of ions, the inside of the photoreceptor cells is more negative than the outside resulting in a standing membrane potential in the dark. Once light falls on the retina, it induces a change in the transmembrane movement of especially sodium and potassium ions, making the cells hyperpolarized, that is, they become more negative to the extracellular space than in the dark. These voltage changes are reflected in various ERG components.

TYPES OF ERG

The electrical response of retinal cells to light can be ascertained by the following forms of ERG:

- Full-field flash ERG
- Pattern ERG (pERG)
- Macular or Focal ERG
- Multifocal ERG (mfERG)
- Direct-current ERG
- Long-duration flash ERG (on-off responses)
- Bright-flash ERG
- Double-flash ERG.

Flash ERG generates data appropriate for whole-eye disorders. The basic mfERG result is based on the calculated mathematical average of an approximation of the positive deflection component of traditional ERG response, the b-wave. Multifocal ERG programs measure electrical activity from more than a hundred retinal areas per eye, in a few minutes. The enhanced spatial resolution enables scotomas and retinal dysfunction to be mapped and quantified.

TECHNIQUE OF ERG

- Recordings can be made from both eyes simultaneously and a common earth electrode is usually placed in the middle of the forehead. The corneal electrode may consist of a conducting foil or fiber placed at the lid margin in contact with the cornea or may be mounted in a special contact lens.
- The pupils are dilated and the subject's head is positioned within a bowl with a white, reflective inner surface and a radius that allows the whole retina to be evenly illuminated by light reflected from the surface. This is known as a Ganzfeld stimulus. The light source for the ISCEV standard ERG is a xenon discharge tube, but arrays of bright LEDs may also be used.
- The subject is dark-adapted for 20 minutes.
- *Scotopic threshold response (STR).* Initially recordings are made of the response to very

dim flashes of white light. STR is a negative deflection of a few microvolts in amplitude. The response from many flashes must be averaged in order to detect the response above background noise.

- *Scotopic b-wave.* Flashes of progressively higher intensity are shown. As the flash intensity increases in intensity the implicit time decreases.
- *Scotopic a-wave.* At higher intensities, the a-wave appears and also increases in amplitude with increasing flash intensity. The earliest part of the a-wave originates from the photoreceptors, but the later part reflects the activity of Müller cells.
- *Oscillatory potential.* Next, a bright white flash (the 'standard flash') is used, which produces a mixed rod and cone response with a large a-wave and b-wave, and wavelets or oscillatory potentials superimposed on the ascending limb of the b-wave. The oscillatory potentials can be recorded separately by repeating the recording with a filter to remove the lower-frequency components of the response.
- *Single flash cone response; Cone a-wave and b-waves.* The subject is now light-adapted for 20 minutes to suppress rod activity, and a response is recorded to a bright light flickering at 30 Hz. This is a pure cone response. A recording is made of responses to single flash of bright light. The cone a-wave and b-wave so generated are of smaller amplitude and are faster than their rod counterparts. There is often a distinct peak (I-wave) on the descending limb of the cone b-wave.
- *30 Hz Flicker Cone Response.* Under the photopic condition repetitive standard flashes are presented at a frequency of 30 stimuli per second.

NEWER NOMENCLATURE FOR BASIC ERG RESPONSES

As per the revisions made in 2008 an ISCEV Standard ERG includes the following responses, named according to conditions of adaptation and the stimulus (flash luminosity) (Fig. 30.1):

- Scotopic 0.01 ERG (formerly 'rod response') (Fig. 30.1A)

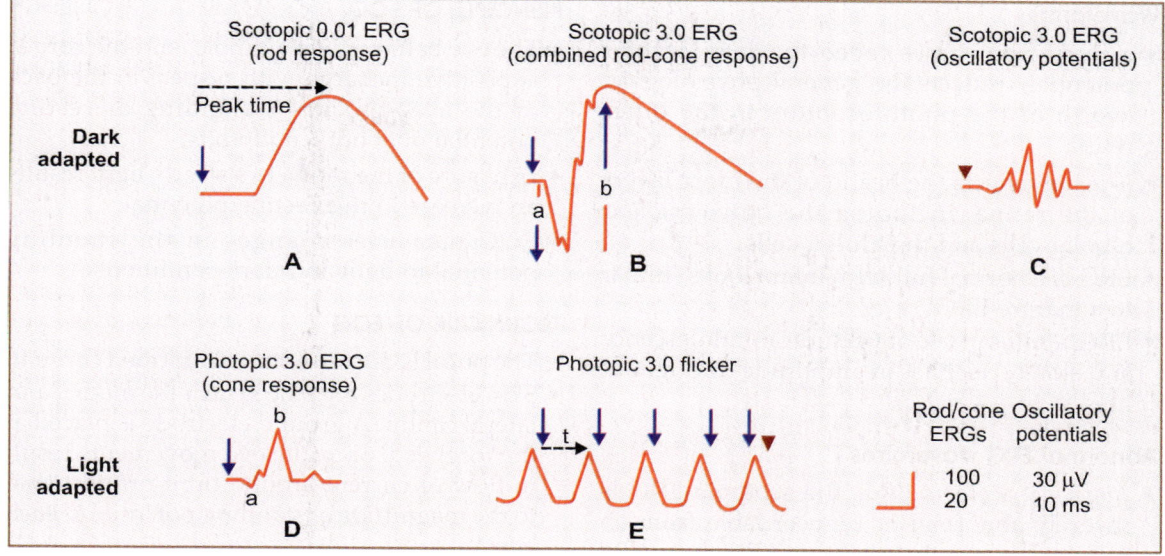

Fig. 30.1: *Exemplary waveforms of the six basic ERG responses.*

- Scotopic 3.0 ERG (formerly 'maximal or standard combined rod-cone response') (Fig. 30.1B)
- Scotopic 3.0 oscillatory potentials (Fig. 30.1C)
- Photopic 3.0 ERG (formerly 'cone response') (Fig. 30.1D)
- Photopic 3.0 flicker (Fig. 30.1E).

INDICATIONS

Inherited retinal degenerations in which the ERG can be useful include:
- Retinitis pigmentosa and related hereditary degenerations
- Retinitis punctata albescens
- Leber's congenital amaurosis
- Choroideremia
- Goldman-Favre syndrome
- Gyrate atrophy of the retina and choroid
- Congenital stationary night blindness
- X-linked juvenile retinoschisis
- Achromatopsia
- Cone dystrophy
- Disorders mimicking retinitis pigmentosa
- Usher syndrome.

Other ocular disorders in which the standard ERG provides useful information include:
- Diabetic retinopathy

- Other ischaemic retinopathies including central retinal vein occlusion (CRVO), branch vein occlusion (BVO), and sickle cell retinopathy
- Toxic retinopathies, including those caused by plaquenil and vigabatrin
- To monitor retinal toxicity in many drug trials
- Autoimmune retinopathies such as cancer associated retinopathy (CAR), melanoma associated retinopathy (MAR), and acute zonal occult outer retinopathy (AZOOR)

Note. Other ERG tests, such as the photopic negative response (PhNR) and pattern ERG (PERG) may be useful in assessing retinal ganglion cell function in diseases like glaucoma.

INTERPRETATION OF ERG

Principal measures of the ERG waveform

Two measures are taken:
(1) The amplitude (a) from the baseline to the negative trough of the a-wave, and the amplitude of the b-wave measured from the trough of the a-wave to the following peak of the b-wave; and (2) the time (t) from flash onset to the trough of the a-wave and the time (t) from flash onset to the peak of the b-wave.

Waveforms

- *a-wave*, sometimes called the 'late receptor potential,' reflects the general physiological health of the photoreceptors in the outer retina.
- *b-wave* reflects the health of the inner layers of the retina, including the outer nuclear bipolar cells and the Müller cells.
- ERG of a normal full-term infant looks similar to a mature ERG.
- ERG attains peak amplitude in adolescence and slowly declines in amplitude throughout life.

Abnormal ERG waveforms

- *Abnormal scotopic ERG*, the scotopic ERG is severely abnormal or unrecordable from an early stage and the photopic ERG is usually better preserved, but deteriorates as the disease progresses.
- *Negative ERG.* Preserved a-wave, but reduced b-wave. This is found in conditions such as central retinal artery occlusion and congenital stationary night blindness.
- *No ERG response* is seen in Batten's disease, Leber's congenital amaurosis.
- *Increased a wave* is seen in albinism.

Note. If the full field ERG is normal and the patient has an unexplained visual loss then a focal or multifocal ERG should be done.

LIMITATIONS OF ERG

A limitation of traditional full-field ERG for the diagnosis of retinopathy is its lack of sensitivity. ERG results are normal unless more than approximately 20% of the retina is affected. So, a patient might be legally blind as a result of macular degeneration and still appear normal.

ELECTRO-OCULOGRAM

The electro-oculogram (EOG), assesses the function of the outer retina; retinal pigment epithelium (RPE) and the interaction between the RPE and the rod photoreceptors. Since the test is carried under photopic-conditions, it cannot distinguish between photoreceptor and RPE dysfunction.

PRINCIPLE OF EOG

- The eye behaves like a dipole, and the cornea is positive incharge with respect to the back of the eye, and has a standing or resting potential of about 6 millivolts.
- Exposure of the retina to a steady light results an increase in this resting potential.
- EOG measures changes in the standing potential to light and dark conditions.

TECHNIQUE OF EOG

- The pupil is dilated after an informed consent.
- Skin electrodes are placed near the medial and lateral canthi. A ground electrode is placed at the forehead. Saccadic eye movements result in flow of current around orbit proportional to the magnitude of standing potential of each eye.
- A Ganzfield is used to illuminate the retina uniformly. The test recordings are initiated after allowing the patient about six minutes for light adaptation.
- The patient is then asked to move his eye first in one direction, and then the other for a fixed 30 degrees, using diode fixation lights (green fixation light in the center and red on the sides).
- The voltage changes so generated are recorded by the skin electrodes during 20 minutes of dark adaptation, and then during a 12–15 minute period of light adaptation.
- The voltage changes are amplified and displayed by the acquisition system of the machine.
- The interpretation of these voltage changes includes the calculation of the amplitude of the light peak in relation to the dark trough as a percentage, the Arden index (Fig. 30.2).

An Arden index >185% or an Arden quotient of >2, is considered as normal. An Arden quotient of <1.65 is significantly abnormal.

INDICATIONS OF EOG

Light response is affected in diffuse disorders of RPE and the photoreceptor layer of retina including some characterized by rod dysfunction, chorioretinal atrophy and by inflammation. In most of these disorders, there is correlation between effects on the EOG and on the ERG,

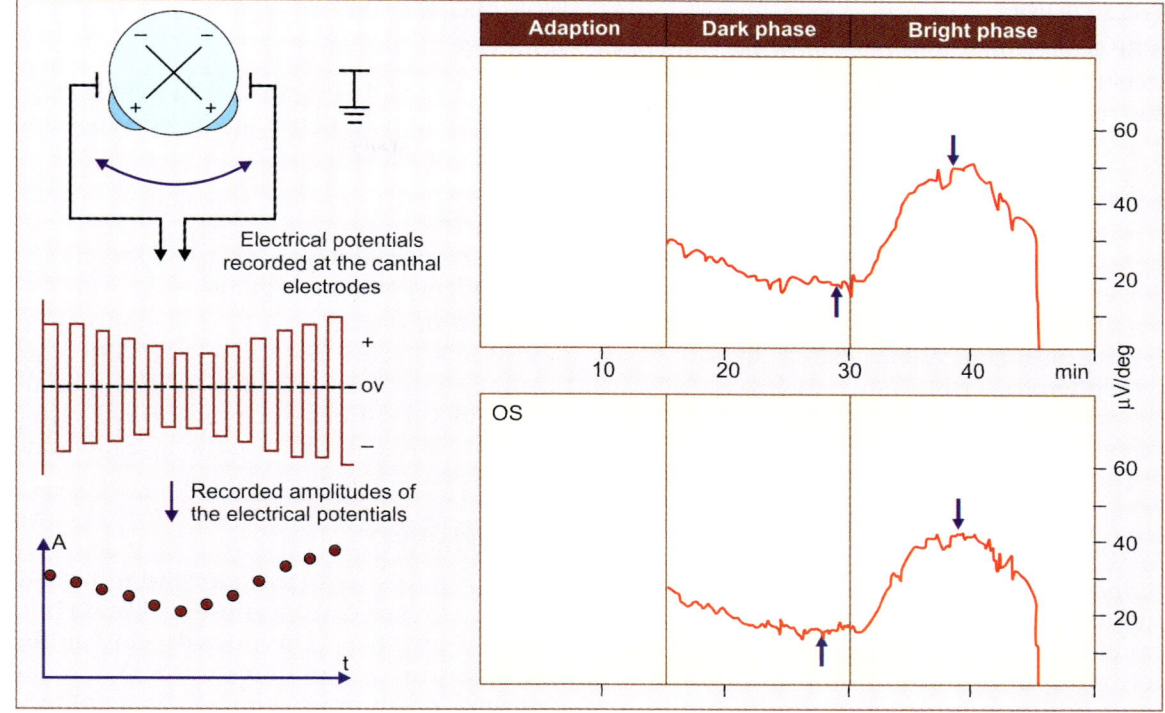

Fig. 30.2: *Light peak and dark troughs recorded during EOG.*

with exception of disorders of bestrophin gene, including Best vitelliform maculopathy, autosomal recessive bestrophinopathy and autosomal dominant vitreoretinochoroidopathy (AD-VIRC) in which the clinical EOG can be highly abnormal even with normal ERG.

CLINICAL INTERPRETATION OF EOG

- *Arden index* (light peak/dark trough × 100) of greater than 185 is considered as normal.
- *A normal ERG and abnormal EOG* are classically seen in patients, as well as asymptomatic carriers of Best's vitelliform macular dystrophy.
- *EOG abnormality is seen in RPE and rod-photoreceptor disorders* including retinitis pigmentosa, choroideremia and age-related macular degeneration.
- *EOG can be used to distinguish* between choroidal melanomas and nevi, since it is abnormal in the former.
- EOG abnormalities are also detected in drug and heavy metal toxicities.

- Oscillatory potentials are decreased when retinal ischaemia is present.

LIMITATIONS OF EOG

- The test cannot be performed in patients with poor fixation, children, infants and unco-operative adults.
- Media opacities and illumination levels can influence the voltage amplitude and therefore, EOG abnormalities must be interpreted with caution.

VISUAL EVOKED POTENTIAL

Visual evoked potential (VEP) is an evoked electrophysiological signal that can be extracted, using signal averaging, from the electro-encephalographic activity recorded at the scalp. It is a sensitive indicator of visual function, with the typical response measuring only 5–10 microvolts in amplitude, which are masked by the electroencephalographic (EEG) noise of 50 microvolts or greater.

TYPES OF VEP

VEP is classified into the following subtypes, depending on the visual stimuli used to elicit the response:

1. *Flash VEP.* Where standard ERG flash is used.

2. *Pattern VEP*

- *Pattern reversal.* Where the pattern of an isoluminant checkerboard or grating of various spatial frequencies is reversed to elicit the VEP. This is the preferred technique for most clinical purposes as the results of pattern reversal stimuli are less variable in waveform and timing than the results elicited by other stimuli.

- *Pattern onset/offset.* Where the VEP is recorded as the patterned stimulus of the pattern reversal is presented.

3. *Special VEPs.* Steady state VEP, sweep VEP, motion VEP, chromatic VEP, binocular VEP, multichannel VEP, LED google VEP, are other forms of VEP.

TECHNIQUE OF VEP

- Each eye is tested separately after an informed consent.

- Silver-silver chloride or gold disk electrode are placed using conducting paste on the scalp relative to bony landmarks in relation to the head size as per the international 10/20 system.

- The active electrode is placed on the midline over the visual occipital cortex (OZ), reference electrode is placed at the frontal pole (FZ) while the ground electrode is at the forehead or earlobe.

- Recordings are done with refractive correction without mydriasis using monocular stimulation.

  Extreme pupil sizes and any anisocoria should be noted.

- For pattern stimulation, the visual acuity of the patient should be recorded and the patient should be optimally refracted for the viewing distance of the screen.

INDICATIONS OF VEP

Flash VEP

- In difficult and uncooperative patients
- In patients with dense media opacities and very poor vision.

Pattern VEP

- Pattern-reversal for pre-chiasmal lesions and for patients with nystagmus
- Pattern-onset/offset VEP for malingerers VEP is a useful tool along with ERG and other clinical assessments to differentiate various conditions such as cortical visual impairment, delayed visual maturation and amblyopia.

INTERPRETATION

The VEP traces (two reproducible records of each) can be presented as positive upwards or negative upwards. The polarity convention and stimulus parameters used should be indicated in the report besides the amplitude and latency. Latency is measured from the stimulus onset to peak of the component measured. It must be remembered that interocular difference in the pattern-reversal VEP indicates dysfunction of the entire pre-chiasmal pathway and includes ocular, retinal and optic nerve causes (Fig. 30.3).

Normal waveforms

1. *Flash VEP.* It consists of a series of positive and negative peaks that are designated in numerical sequence. Commonest components recorded are N2 and P2 at 90 and 120 msec, respectively.

2. *Pattern-reversal VEP.* The peaks are named as negative or positive followed by the latency. Commonest wave used for clinical cases is the P100 component (positive peak at 100 msec) since it is a very robust measure with minimal interocular and inter-subject measurement variation.

3. *Pattern-onset/offset VEP.* Three components described are C1 (positive at 75 msec),

C2 (negative at 125 msec) and C3 (positive at 150 msec). With a stimulated hemifield, the response will appear contralateral to the hemifield stimulated (Fig. 30.3).

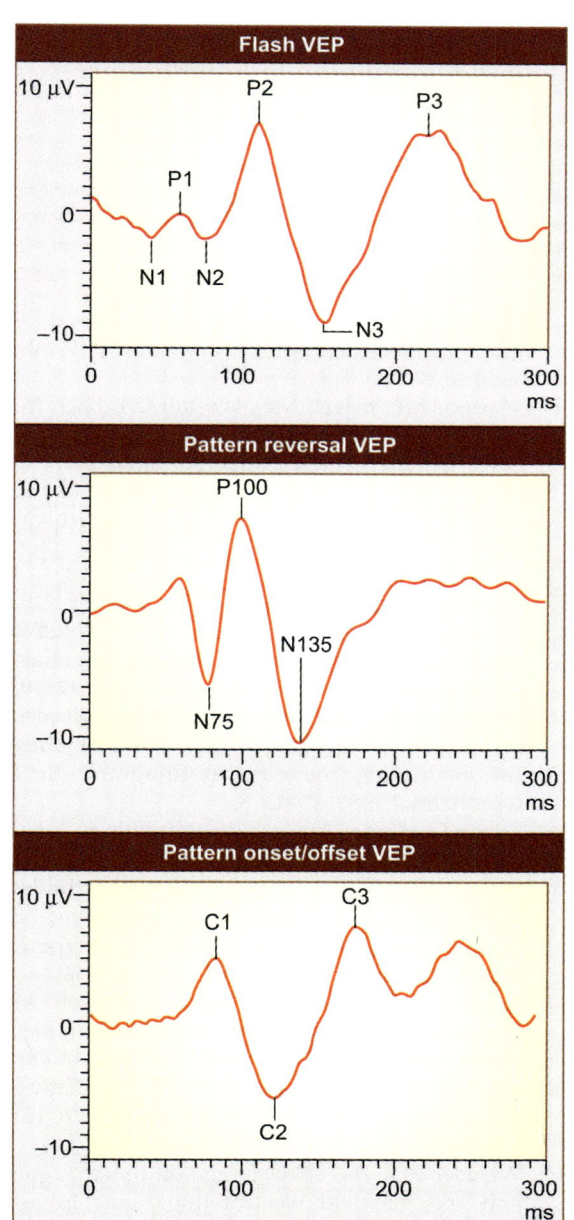

Fig. 30.3: *Normal waveforms for flash VEP, pattern VEP and pattern onset/offset VEP.*

LIMITATIONS OF VEP

VEP has following limitations:

• Age, refractive error, inattention and conscious defocusing of the pattern affect the VEP latency.

• Stimulus parameters such as contrast, luminance, check size and field size are important determinants of the waveform and it is essential for each laboratory to establish their own normal controls.

• Since the amplitudes of VEP are very small, surrounding noise can easily contaminate them and, therefore, strict vigil has to be kept on the recording equipment, recording technique and the stimulus parameters used.

• Numerous specialized types of VEP are being assessed and these are still used as investigational tools. Knowledge in these areas is still evolving.

ELECTROPHYSIOLOGICAL TESTS: TIME TAKEN, POTENTIAL INDICATIONS AND PRACTICAL STATUS

TIME TAKEN FOR VARIOUS ELECTROPHYSIOLOGICAL TESTS

Time taken for various electrophysiological tests is as follows.

• ERG: 60 minutes (40 min DA + drops)
• EOG: 45 minutes
• Pattern ERG: 30 minutes
• Flash or pattern VEP: 30–45 minutes
• Special VEPs: 30–60 minutes

In case of pediatric assessment (under 7 years), multiply time by 1.5.

POTENTIAL INDICATIONS OF VARIOUS ELECTROPHYSIOLOGICAL TESTS

Outline of potential indications of specific electrophysiological tests as summarized in Table 30.1.

Table 30.1 *Outline of potential indications for specific electrophysiological tests*

Provisional diagnosis	EOG	ERG	Bright flash ERG	Pattern ERG	Flash VEP	Pattern VEP	Special VEP
Inherited retinal dystrophies	+	+					
Vascular diseases including diabetes		+		+		+	
Opaque media or trauma		+	+		+		
Retrobulbar neuritis				+		+	
Unexplained visual loss		+		+		+	
Infant with questionable vision		+			+		+
Albinism		+					+
Toxic and nutritional eye disease	+	+		+	+		
Glaucoma				+			
Suspected intracranial lesion				+		+	+

PRACTICAL STATUS OF ELECTROPHYSIOLOGY

- *ERG* is an extremely helpful tool in detecting or confirming retinitis pigmentosa, even in the absence of typical bony corpuscles.
- *EOG* is useful in differential diagnosis of abnormalities of the retinal pigment epithelium such as Best's disease.
- *VEP* is a useful tool along with ERG and other clinical assessments to differentiate various conditions such as cortical visual impairment and delayed visual maturation.

BIBLIOGRAPHY

1. Brigell M, Bach M, Barber C, Moskowitz A, Robson J. Guidelines for calibration of stimulus and recording parameters used in clinical electrophysiology of vision. Doc Ophthalmol 2003;107:185–93.

2. Holder GE, Brigell MG, Hawlina M, Meigen T, Vaegan, Bach M. ISCEV standard for clinical pattern electroretinography-2007 update. Doc Ophthalmol 2007;114:111–6.

3. Hood DC, Bach M, Brigell M, Keating D, Kondo M, Lyons JS, Marmor MF, McCulloch DL, Palmowski-Wolfe AM. ISCEV Standard for clinical multifocal electroretinography (2011 ed).

4. Jasper HH. Report of Committee on Methods of Clinical Examination in Electroencephalography. Electroenceph. Clin. Neurophysiol., 1958;10:370–5.

5. Marmor MF, Brigell MG, Westall CA, Bach M. ISCEV Standard for Clinical Electrooculography (2010 Update), Doc Ophthalmol 2011; 122:1–7.

6. Marmor MF, Fulton AB, Holder GE, Miyake Y, Brigell M, Bach M. Standard for clinical electro-retinography (2008 update). Doc Ophthalmol 2009;118:69–77.

7. Odom JV, Bach M, Brigell M, Holder GE, McCulloch DL, Tormene AP, Vaegan. ISCEV standard for clinical visual evoked potentials (2009 update). Doc Ophthalmol 2010;120:111–9.

8. Perlman I. Relationship between the amplitudes of the b wave and the a wave as a useful index for evaluating the electroretinogram. Br J Ophthalmol.1983;67:443–8.

9. Regan D. Human brain electrophysiology. New York: Elsevier, 1989.

10. Sutter EE. Noninvasive Testing Methods: Multifocal Electrophysiology. In: Darlene A. Dartt, editor. Encyclopedia of the Eye, Vol 3. Oxford: Academic Press; 2010. pp. 142–60.

11. Towle VL, Cakmur R, Cao, Y Brigell M Parmeggiani L. Locating vep equivalent dipoles in magnetic resonance images. 1995;80:105–16.

12. Wachtmeister L, Dowling JE. The oscillatory potentials of the mudpuppy retina. Invest Ophthalmol Vis Sci. 1978;17:1176–88.

13. Weleber RG. The effect of age on human cone and rod ganzfeld electroretinograms. Invest Ophthalmol Vis Sci. 1981;20:392–9.

Section

IX

Imaging Techniques in Ophthalmology

31. Plain X-rays in Ophthalmology
32. Ultrasonography in Ophthalmology
33. Ultrasound Biomicroscopy (UBM) in Ophthalmology
34. Computed Tomography Scanning in Ophthalmology
35. Magnetic Resonance Imaging in Ophthalmology

CHAPTER
31

Plain X-rays in Ophthalmology

Chapter Outline

X-RAYS ORBIT: GENERAL CONSIDERATIONS

Common views of exposure for orbit roentgen

- Water's view
- Lateral view
- Caldwell view
- Rhese view
- Base view

Role of X-rays orbit

- Indications

- Advantages
- Disadvantages

Protocol to describe an X-rays orbit

X-RAYS ORBIT: CLINICAL OBSERVATIONS

- Commonly observed X-ray signs of orbital diseases
- Findings in some common ophthalmic diseases on X-ray
- Methods of localizing ocular foreign body on an X-rays

X-RAYS ORBIT: GENERAL CONSIDERATIONS

X-rays were discovered by William Roentgen in 1895 for which he was awarded the Nobel Prize in 1901. X-rays are a form of electromagnetic radiations which are produced when an electron beam generated at the cathode (by a heated tungsten filament) strikes the anode (also made of tungsten most commonly). The wavelength of these radiations varies from 0.01 to 0.10 nanometres and they have a photographic effect. Film focus distance for all types of X-rays is 100 cm. The X-rays can pass through most soft tissues of the body but leave the bones and most metals visible as they absorb most of the rays. Soft tissues which allow the rays to pass through them appear black on the film while bones which absorb the rays appear white on X-ray film.

COMMON VIEWS OF EXPOSURE FOR ORBIT ROENTGEN

Plain X-rays of the orbit are useful to diagnose most extraorbital causes of proptosis. In evaluation of an orbital lesion, a plain skiagram of orbit was the most frequently used investigation till recent past. However, presently CT scan has reduced the role of plain X-ray. The advantages of plain X-ray skull when compared to other investigations like CT scan are:

- Low cost
- Easy availability and usage
- Preliminary test to detect gross abnormality

Human eye is a soft tissue structure which appears black normally. X-ray helps in determining the presence of metallic foreign body and calcification in the eye. Various views used in the field of ophthalmology include:

- Water's view

- Lateral view
- Caldwell view
- Rhese view
- Submentovertex (base) view.

Water's view

Water's view (occipitomental view) is used to best view the maxillary sinus and orbital floor. It is created by placing the chin of the patient against an X-ray cassette with cantho-meatal line forming an angle of 45° with the cassette. The maxillary region is seen clearly in this view because bony shadow of the petrous temporal bone is excluded. Structures clearly seen in this view are frontal sinus, maxillary sinus, inferior orbital floor, ethmoidal air cells, superior and inferior orbital margin.

Lateral view

This is the most commonly done X-ray of the orbit for foreign body localization. The X-ray is performed with patients head against the X-ray cassette with infraorbital line at a right angle to the cassette. The side to be visualized is kept towards the cassette while performing the X-ray. *Structures seen in this view* are frontal sinus, orbital cavity with orbital roof, ethmoid sinus, anterior clinoid process, sella turcica, pterygo-palatine fossa and hard palate.

Caldwell view

Caldwell view, also known as occipitofrontal or posteroanterior view is performed by positioning both the forehead and the nose against the X-ray cassette. The X-ray beam is directed at an angle of 23° to the canthomeatal line in this view. *Structures visualized* in this view include frontal sinus, ethmoid sinus, posterior part of orbital floor, greater wing of sphenoid, foramen rotundum, floor of sella, lamina papyracea, shape and size of orbits and superior orbital fissure.

Rhese view

Rhese view is also called optic foramena view. With the advent of CT scans, this view has lost its importance but can be handy in low resource settings because of the vital structures visualized in this view. It is performed by placing patient's zygoma, nose and chin against the cassette with

X-ray beam directed posteroanteriorly at an angle of 40° to the mid-sagittal plane. Important structures visualized in this view include optic canal, optic strut, ethmoidal sinus, superior orbital fissure, and lacrimal fossa.

Base view

Base view, also known as submentovertex view, is taken with the patient erect or supine, the head is hyperextended touching the vertex to the couch and shoulders rasied. The film is placed lengthwise with its lower border just below the occipital protuberance. The baseline and the film are parallel. The central ray passes submentally and perpendicular to the X-ray plate and the tragocanthal line.

Structures seen on it are:
- Anterior wall of middle cranial fossa
- Posterior wall of maxillary antrum
- Basal foramina
- Petrous temporal bones
- Posterior wall of orbit
- Foramen ovale and spinosum.

Townes projection

In the supine position the canthomeatal line and the median sagittal line is perpendicular to the film (fronto-occipital/half axial). With the patient erect or supine, and the chin well down on the chest, the head is adjusted so that the radiographic baseline is at right angles to the film. The film is placed length wise with its upper border 5 cm above the vertex. This view is not used commonly because of increased X-ray radiation to the eyes.

Structures seen are:
- Infraorbital fissure
- Superior orbital fissure.

ROLE OF X-RAYS ORBIT

Indications of X-ray

- Open globe injury
- Proptosis
- To rule out multiple foreign bodies
- Foreign body localization
- Blow out fracture
- Screening modality before MRI
- To identify tumours causing calcification.

Advantages of X-ray

- Cheap
- Easily available
- Less radiation exposure
- Good screening tool.

Disadvantages of X-ray

- Gives only two-dimensional image of a three-dimensional body part
- Poor contrast resolution
- Less sensitivity to small changes in attenuation.

PROTOCOL TO DESCRIBE AN X-RAY ORBIT

One should always start by mentioning, if it is a plain X-ray or a digital X-ray followed by patient data (if available). Radio-opaque markers are used to mark the side being viewed. The part of body imaged should be mentioned along with a mention of the view in which the X-ray was taken. This should be followed by a comment on the quality of the X-ray film, whether it is properly exposed or not.

It is a good practice to begin by describing the normal areas of film followed by an elaborate description of the abnormal areas. It is important to describe the appearance in simple words and give a comparative overview with regards to the normal structures in the film. One should always try to avoid jumping to a diagnosis immediately. For example, if one is describing an X-ray with foreign body, one should describe the appearance of foreign body in terms of its approximate size, its shape and radio-opacity of the substance with reference to a normal structure (like whether it is more radio-opaque or less radio-opaque than the bone). Certain cues to a lesion are like benign lesions usually cause localized changes while malignant lesions are associated with diffuse changes.

Most important structure to be looked for in X-ray skull is the base of the skull. In this the pituitary fossa is the most important structure. Other landmarks are:

- Anterior clinoid process
- Planum sphenoidale
- Charismatic sulcus
- Tuberculum sellae
- Floor of the pituitary fossa
- Dorsum sellae
- Posterior clinoids.

X-RAYS ORBIT: CLINICAL OBSERVATIONS

COMMONLY OBSERVED X-RAY SIGNS OF ORBITAL DISEASES

Size of the orbit. Enlargement of the orbit (Fig. 31.1) is not an uncommon finding in orbital space occupying lesions. In infants and children, orbital enlargement occurs within 1 to 3 months while in adults it is a sign of a long-standing benign tumours (1–3 years duration).

I. Symmetrical enlargement of the orbit is observed in mass lesions of the muscle cone (intraconal lesions) like optic nerve glioma, haemangioma, and neurofibroma. Occasionally it may also be seen in pseudotumour and retinoblastoma that extend into the muscle cone.

II. Asymmetrical orbital enlargement is a sign of extraconal tumours like rhabdomyosarcoma, lacrimal gland tumour, dermoid cyst, haemangioma, etc.

III. Causes of small orbit include: anophthalmos, post-enucleation, microphthalmos, mucocele.

Change in bone density. Increased bone density (hyperostosis) is observed in sphenoidal ridge meningioma, chronic periosteitis, fibrous dysplasia, Paget's disease, osteoblastic metastasis, acromegaly, osteopetrosis, craniostenosis and anaemia in childhood.

I. Localized decreased density/indentation of the orbital wall is observed in benign tumours such

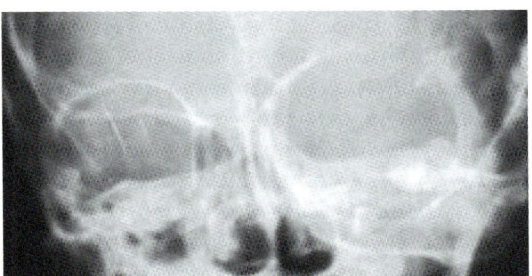

Fig. 31.1: *Enlargement of left orbit in a case of congenital teratoma.*

as dermoid and mixed cell lacrimal gland tumour.

II. Diffuse bony destruction may signify malignant tumours like lacrimal gland carcinoma and spread of tumours from paranasal sinuses.

Change in orbital shape. This is usually due to fossa formation, as a result of local expansion of the orbital wall. It occurs in orbital dermoids and encapsulated lacrimal gland tumours.

Dehiscence of orbital bones. This may be observed in lesions like mucocele of paranasal sinuses, aneurysm, neurofibroma, lacrimal gland tumours, and fractures.

Bare orbits. This is seen in X-ray orbit PA view:
- Due to hypoplasia of the lesser wing of sphenoid
- Seen in neurofibroma.

Intraorbital calcification. This may occur normally and in many lesions. **Causes of normal calcification** of X-ray skull. *Structures in the midline that produce calcification are:*
- Pineal body
- Falx cerebri
- The pacchonian granules
- The labenular commissure.

Normal structures away from midline that produce calcification are:
- Choroid plexus
- Petroclinoid ligament
- The lateral edge of diaphragm sellae
- The carotid artery.

Causes of abnormal calcification seen in X-ray skull include retinoblastoma (fine-stippled calcification), optic nerve sheath meningioma, lacrimal gland carcinoma, orbital varix (phlebolith), mucocele, parasitic cyst (hydatid cyst), aneurysm, haematoma, and phthisical eyes (Fig. 31.2). Calcified intracranial lesions that may rarely have associated orbital or intraocular lesions are toxoplasmosis, tuberous sclerosis. Sturge-Weber syndrome, and von Hipple-Lindau disease. Actual ossification due to metaplasia of ocular tissue is rarely seen.

Enlargement of superior orbital fissure. This is a classical diagnostic sign of infraclinoid carotid

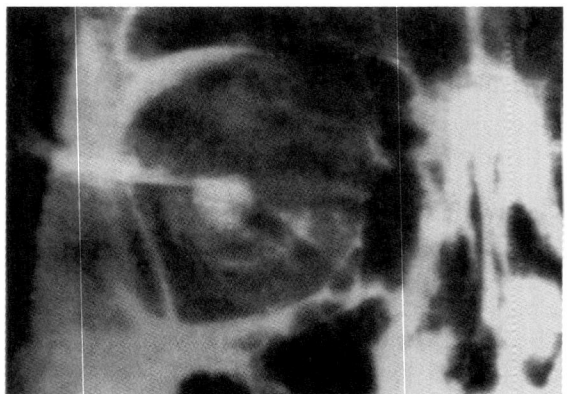
Fig. 31.2: *Calcification in a phthisical eye.*

aneurysms (75% of cases), and therefore, calls for an early carotid angiography. Other causes of widening of superior orbital fissure include intracavenous aneurysm, intracranial extension of orbital tumours, extrasellar extension of pituitary tumours, and meningiomas.

Narrowing of superior orbital fissure: Diseases causing increased density and thickness of bone like:
- Fibrous dysplasia
- Paget's disease.

Changes in optic canal: Normal adult dimensions of optic canal are reached by the age of 4 to 5 years and its standard size is 4 to 6 mm. Measurements of 7 mm or more are always pathological. However, it is to be stressed that one should always compare the two before giving final verdict on the size of the optic foramina. In normal subjects, the diameter of the two canals should not differ by more than 1 mm.

I. Uniform regular concentric enlargement of the optic canal is seen typically in cases of optic nerve glioma (Fig. 31.3).

II. Uniform irregular enlargement may be observed in meningioma of the optic nerve sheath, retinoblastoma, and orbital neurofibromas.

III. Erosion of its inferolateral margin is a sign of infraclinoid lesions such as aneurysms and meningiomas.

IV. Erosion of its upper margin is a sign of raised intracranial pressure.

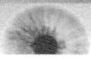
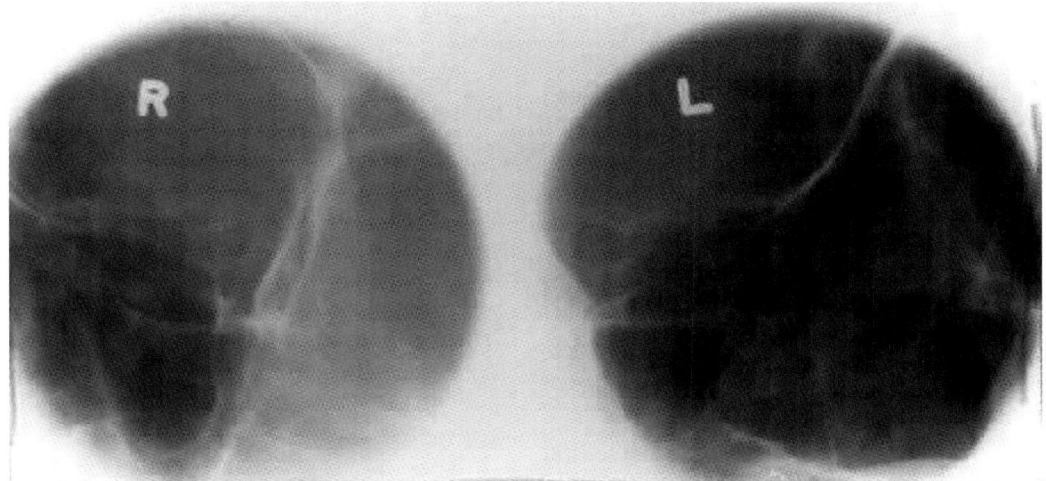

Fig. 31.3: *Enlargement of right optic foramen (R).*

V. Total destruction of the margins indicates some malignant neoplasm arising from one of the paranasal sinuses.

VI. Narrowing and hyperostosis around the optic foramina may be observed in meningioma en plaque, occasionally.

VII. Optic canal compression is seen in:
- Fibrous dysplasia
- Paget's disease
- Microphthalmos.

Changes in orbital fractures. Radiographs no longer have a real role to play in the assessment of facial trauma. However, if they are obtained, the diagnosis of fractures involving the inferior or medial wall may be suspected by visualisation of fluid with the maxillary sinus and ethmoidal air cells respectively. Orbital emphysema may also be visible. Under certain circumstances this may give a black eyebrow sign. Herniation of orbital fat inferiorly may give a 'tear drop' sign.

Sella turcica.
Normal dimensions of the sella turcica:
- Anteroposterior diameter: 4–16 mm (average – 10.5 mm)
- Depth: 4–12 mm (average 8.1 mm)

Most common lesion causing enlargement of the sella: pituitary adenoma X-ray finding in chromophilic adenoma include:
- Enlargement of the sella
- Erosion of the floor of sella
- Erosion of the undermargins of the anterior clinoid process.

Double flooring of the sella—irregular and symmetrical enlargement of the fossa mainly in posterior sellar lesions giving the appearance of double flooring on X-ray skull lateral view.

Causes of calcification in and around sella:
- Atheroma
- Meningioma
- Arterial aneurysm
- TB meningitis
- Optic disc glioma.

Empty sella syndrome—asymmetrical enlargement of the sella due to downward herniation of the subarachnoid space into sella due to raised intracranial tension.

Causes of enlarged sella include:
- Chromophobe adenoma
- Gliomas
- Teratomas
- Craniopharyngiomas
- Empty sella syndrome

- Arachnoid cyst
- Ectopic pinealomas.

Most common cause of suprasellar classification: craniopharyngioma.

FINDINGS IN SOME COMMON OPHTHALMIC DISEASES ON X-RAY

- *Orbital floor fracture*: Tear drop sign is seen
- *Orbital hemangioma*: Calcification with a soft tissue shadow is seen
- *Rhabdomysarcoma*: Erosion of bones of the orbit, appearing as disruption of continuity of bony margins
- *Meningioma* appears as a soft tissue swelling with significant amount of calcification. Other causes of intracranial calcifications include orbital varix, retinoblastoma and phthisical eye
- *Neurofibromatosis* causes enlargement of the superior orbital fissure, best seen in Caldwell view. Causes of superior orbital fissure enlargement include infraclinoid carotid aneurysm, extrasellar extension of pituitary tumours, etc.
- *Foreign body localization* with limbal ring (obsolete nowadays)
- *Congenital toxoplasmosis*: Intracranial calcification might be seen
- *Signs of raised intracranial tension (ICT) in children:* Increased separation of the sutures, increased convolutional markings, thinning of bone and silver beaten appearance—due to pressure of sulci and gyri
- *Signs of raised intracranial tension in adults:* The changes that occur in sella turcica, constitute the most important signs in raised ICT
- *In the earliest phase* there is demineralisation of the cortical bone leading to loss of the normal 'lamina dura' (white line of the sellar floor)
- This is followed by thinning of the dorsum sellae and the posterior clinoid processes. The dorsum sellae becomes shortened and pointed resulting in a shallow turcica
- In extreme cases, the sella becomes very shallow and flattened anterior wall gets demineralised and the floor and dorsum sellae are destroyed.

METHODS OF LOCALIZING OCULAR FOREIGN BODY ON AN X-RAYS

Although CT scans have replaced X-rays almost completely, we considered describing these methods in historical interest. They can come handy in peripheral centers where CT scan are not available yet. These methods can be divided into 3 broad categories:

1. Methods based on rotation movements of the eyeball
2. Methods based on different angles of X-ray exposure
3. Methods using various markers to localize the foreign body

1. Methods based on rotation movements of the eyeball: In this method, lateral view orbit is done on the same film three times with eyes looking straight, up and down. Movement of foreign body with the eye signifies that foreign body lies within the eyeball. An important prerequisite for this method is steady head placement, which can be a problem in children and adults with altered consciousness.

2. Methods based on different angles of X-ray exposure: Various methods have been described like Sweet's method, Mac Kenzie's method, Mc Rigor's method and Dixons' methods, etc. Different markers are placed at different positions and then multiple exposures are given from different angles on the same X-ray film. The location is determined by superimposition of the images. Disadvantage of this method is the cumbersome calculations involved in determination of location of the foreign body.

3. Methods using various markers to localize the foreign body: Radio-opaque markers like suturing a limbal ring to the cornea or placing a contact lens with 4 radio-opaque dots for 3, 6, 9 and 12 o'clock positions have been used. Another method described is injection of radio-opaque dye in the sub-tenon space. All these methods are used to delineate the anatomy of globe and then localize the foreign body. PA view is taken to determine the meridional

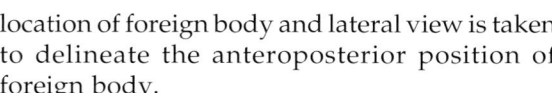

location of foreign body and lateral view is taken to delineate the anteroposterior position of foreign body.

BIBLIOGRAPHY

1. Curtin HD, Wolfe P, Schramm V. Orbital roof blow-out fractures. AJR Am J Roentgenol (citation) [pubmed citation] 1982;139(5):969–72.
2. Fueger Gerhard, Albert Milauskas, William Britton. 'The Roentgenologic evaluation of orbital blow-out injuries.' Am. J. Roentgenol. 1966, July 1;97(3):614–7. [Link].
3. Hammerschlag SB, Hughes S, O'Reilly GV, et al. Another look at blow-out fractures of the orbit. AJR Am J Roentgenol (abstract) [pubmed citation] 1982;139(1):133–7.
4. Harris GJ, Garcia GH, Logani SC, et al. 'Orbital blow-out fractures: correlation of preoperative computed tomography and postoperative ocular motility.' Transactions of the American Ophthalmological Society 1998;96:329–53. [Link].
5. Rothman MI, Simon EM, Zoarski GH, et al. Superior blowout fracture of the orbit: the blowup fracture. AJNR Am J Neuroradiol (abstract) [pubmed citation] 1998;19(8):1448–9.
6. Zilkha A. Computed tomography of blow-out fracture of the medial orbital wall. AJR Am J Roentgenol (citation) [pubmed citation] 1981; 137(5):963–5.

Ultrasonography in Ophthalmology

Chapter Outline

GENERAL CONSIDERATIONS
- Introduction
- Principle
- Ultrasonography machine
- Basic steps of ultrasonography

Ocular and Orbital Scans
- Ocular scan
- Orbital scan
- Immersion B scan
- Ultrasonographic appearance of the structures of the normal eye
- Indications for ophthalmic ultrasound

ULTRASONOGRAPHY FINDINGS IN COMMON INTRAOCULAR LESIONS

Congenital Anomalies
- Retinochoroidal coloboma
- Nanophthalmos
- Persistent hyperplastic primary vitreous

Vitreoretinal Diseases
- Retinopathy of prematurity
- Vitreous hemorrhage
- Posterior vitreous detachment
- Retinal breaks and retinal detachment
- Choroidal detachment
- Asteroid hyalosis
- Coat's disease

Ocular Trauma
- Intraocular foreign body
- Lens trauma
- Scleral rupture

Ocular Infections and Inflammations
- Endophthalmitis
- VKH syndrome
- Scleritis
- Toxocariasis

Ocular Tumours
- Choroidal melanoma
- Choroidal hemangioma
- Choroidal metastases
- Retinoblastoma
- Choroidal osteoma

Miscellaneous Ocular Conditions
- Phthisis bulbi
- Dislocated intraocular lens
- Dropped nucleus
- Silicone oil filled eyeball
- Scleral buckle

ULTRASONOGRAPHY FINDINGS IN ORBITAL LESIONS

Orbital Tumours
- Orbital cavernous hemangioma
- Orbital lymphangioma
- Orbital lymphomas
- Orbital Schwannoma
- Rhabdomyosarcoma
- Orbital varix

Orbital Infections and Inflammation
- Orbital cysticercosis
- Orbital echinococcosis
- Idiopathic orbital inflammatory disease
- Orbital abscess

Optic Nerve Lesions
- Optic disc drusen
- Optic nerve glioma
- Optic nerve sheath meningioma

Disorders of Extraocular Muscles
- Grave's orbitopathy
- Idiopathic orbital myositis

Lacrimal Gland Tumours
- Pleomorphic adenoma
- Adenoid cystic carcinoma
- Lymphomas

Colour Doppler Imaging
- Procedure
- Indications and advantages
- CDI in ocular and orbital disorders

ULTRASOUND BASED SPECIAL INVESTIGATIONS
Ultrasound Biomicroscopy

High-intensity Focused Ultrasound Circular Cyclo-coagulation in Glaucoma Patients

Ultrasound-Guided Fine Needle Aspiration Biopsy

Ocular Ultrasound-Guided Anaesthesia

RECENT ADVANCES IN ULTRASONOGRAPHY
- Contrast enhanced ultrasonography
- Compound imaging
- Three and 4-dimensional ultrasound
- C-scan ultrasound
- Ultrasound elastography
- Fusion imaging
- Remote and robotic ultrasound
- Photoacoustic imaging

GENERAL CONSIDERATIONS

INTRODUCTION

Ophthalmic ultrasonography is an essential diagnostic ocular imaging modality. Modern ultrasound systems provide detailed images of the ocular structures in a rapid, noninvasive manner, thus causing no significant tissue damage. It is a safe diagnostic tool for the evaluation of many ophthalmic and ocular disorders. Ultrasonic imaging of orbital disease and blood-flow pattern complements data obtained by CT scan and other imaging modalities. Diagnostic ophthalmic ultrasonography is most useful in the presence of opaque ocular media due to corneal opacities, anterior chamber opacities, cataract, vitreous haemorrhage or inflammatory opacities. Ophthalmic ultrasonography is also valuable in the presence of clear media, for evaluation of the iris, lens, ciliary body and orbital structures. It is also used for diagnosis and follow-up of ocular diseases, measurement of ocular dimensions and providing information regarding orbital diseases.

PRINCIPLE

Acoustic wave

Sound is the energy that produces alternating compression and rarefaction of the conducting medium as it travels as a wave. Humans can hear sound from 20 Hz to 20 kHz. Ultrasound is an acoustic wave with a frequency above 20 kHz. Echoes are produced when ultrasound waves encounter an interface where two different materials have different acoustic impedances. A short acoustic pulse is generated mechanically by a piezoelectric crystal, which acts as a transducer to convert electrical energy into ultrasound. At every acoustic interface, some of the echoes are reflected back to the transducer, indicating a change in tissue density. The echoes returned to the probe are converted back into an electrical signal and processed. Based on the parameters and design of the specific ultrasound receiver, processing can include amplification, compensation, compression, demodulation, and rejection. A-mode, or A scan, systems graphically display these echoes as a function of time on a video monitor. B-mode systems generate cross-sectional grey scale images by scanning the transducer to address a series of lines through the eye; the amplitudes of received echoes control the brightness (or gray scale) along corresponding lines of a video image (B scan).

• *A scan:* One dimensional time—Amplitude display in which the echoes, represented by spikes from the baseline, are spaced depending on their distance from each other and the probe. The amplification is linear in A scan used for axial biometry, logarithmic when combined with the B scan and S shaped in the standardized A scan for tissue differentiation.

• *B scan:* Two-dimensional—**B**rightness display where the strength of the returning echo is displayed as a dot on the screen, the brightness being directly proportional to the echo strength.

Laws of acoustic energy

Ultrasound is dependent on the laws of acoustic energy: reflection, refraction, and absorption. To accurately access structures based on the intensity of the returning echoes, the sound beam needs to be directed perpendicular to the desired structure. Sound beams directed at an oblique angle towards an interface result in the reflection of some of the sound beams away from the probe causing a weaker signal. Ultrasound directed at a coarse, irregular surface results in significant loss of echo strength due to diversion of reflected echoes.

Frequency and resolution

Frequencies used in ophthalmic ultrasound machines range from 8–80 MHz while in other fields of diagnostic ultrasound, 2–6 MHz is used. The use of higher frequencies allows for increased resolution, which is essential in the evaluation of small ophthalmic structures. The high frequencies are achieved by transducers. The high frequencies (typically 10 MHz) and small wavelengths (e.g. 150 µm) available with ultrasound can provide the detailed resolution required for ocular examinations. Frequencies of 8–12 MHz comprise conventional ophthalmic ultrasound, while high frequency systems utilize a 20 MHz probe. Probe frequencies of 40–100 MHz comprise ultrasound biomicroscopy.

Gain

Ultrasonography machines allow the user to manually adjust the amplification of echo signals displayed on the screen by adjusting the gain. Gain is a measurement of intensity labelled in decibels (dB). Adjusting the gain only changes the intensity of the echo pattern and does not affect the frequency or pulse length of the emitted ultrasound waves. Gain settings range from 30 to 100 dB. At low gain, only strong echo sources are visible. Lowering the gain has the effect of decreasing the depth of sound penetration and narrowing the sound beam resulting

in increased resolution. The choroid, sclera and orbital structures are usually best examined at a low gain. At a high gain, weaker echo sources are detected, but resolution is effectively lost. Vitreous opacities and thin vitreous membranes are best examined at high gain.

Basic physics of ultrasound

Ultrasonic waves transmitted from the probe into the eye

⬇

Waves strike intraocular structures and reflected back to the probe

⬇

Converted into an electric signal

⬇

Signal reconstructed as an image on a monitor

ULTRASONOGRAPHY MACHINE

Ultrasound system (Fig 32.1) consists of the following components:

• Transducer/probe
• Servo (for B mode systems)
• Pulser
• Receiver
• Scan converter and display.

1. Transducer/probe is enclosed within a sealed, fluid-filled housing with an acoustically transparent cap at one end. It is pivoted at an angle of 45 to 60°. It sweeps the ultrasound beam across a scan plane.

2. Servo is a device that controls the motion of the transducer within the probe and registers the orientation of the transducer. As the transducer

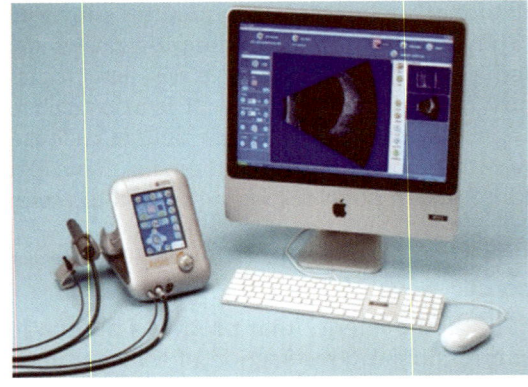

Fig. 32.1: *B scan ultrasonogram machine.*

moves, the servo continously monitors its position and issues signals to the pulser and other components such that pulse/echo vectors are acquired at appropriate positions.

3. Pulser repeatedly 'shock excites' the transducer with short voltage pulses applied across the electrodes of its piezoelectric element. Each excitation results in the generation of an ultrasonic pulse. The nature of the ultrasonic pulse is an important factor in determining the characteristics of the emitted acoustic pulse, and hence, of the attainable resolution of the ultrasound system.

4. Receiver amplifies the minute voltages generated by the transducer excitation.

5. Scan converter and display. An analog-to-digital converter (ADC) is needed to use digital display devices. Analog-to-digital conversion involves transformation of a continuous signal into a discrete binary representation. The ADC samples the output of the amplifier at a specific rate, which is normally at least twice the highest frequency component present in the signal.

BASIC STEPS OF OCULAR ULTRASONOGRAPHY

- *Position.* Ultrasound examination of the eye and orbit is performed in the supine or sitting position.
- *Placing of probe.* The probe is placed directly over the conjunctiva or cornea or placed over closed lids. The former has the advantage of reducing the sound attenuation caused by the lids.
- *Coupling solution* is used to provide standoff and avoid attenuation caused by the air.
- *Once a pathology* is detected, clock hour noted on the transverse scan. Patient asked to look in the direction of the pathology with the probe perpendicular to the lesion of interest.
- *More information* is then obtained by longitudinal scan, A scan and change of gain.

OCULAR AND ORBITAL SCANS

OCULAR SCAN: PROBE POSITIONS

- **Axial:** Demonstrates the lesion in relation to the lens and the optic nerve. The patient fixates in the primary gaze and the probe is placed

on the globe and directed axially. Depending on the clock hour location of the marker, axial-horizontal, axial-vertical and axial-oblique pictures are obtained. These sections demonstrate lesions at the posterior pole and the optic nerve head.

- **Transverse:** Gives the lateral extent of lesion. The mark is kept parallel to the limbus and probe is shifted from limbus to the fornix and also sideways. This scan gives the lateral extent of the lesion.
- **Longitudinal:** Gives the anteroposterior extent of the lesion The mark is kept at right angle to the limbus to determine the anteroposterior limit of the lesion.

During the procedure, the probe is moved from limbus to fornix in different clock hour meridians and the picture seen is of diagonally opposite meridian as follows:

Position of probe (in clock hours)	Area screened (in clock hours)
• 3-Limbus	9-Posterior
• 3-Equator	9-Equator
• 3-Fornix	9-Anterior
• 6-Limbus	12-Posterior
• 6-Equator	12-Equator
• 6-Fornix	12-Anterior

ORBITAL SCANS: PROBE PLACEMENT

- **Transocular:** Best for demonstrating lesions of the mid and posterior orbit
- **Paraocular:** Demonstration of lesions of the lids and anterior orbit.

IMMERSION B SCAN

- Immersion B scan refers to the use of balanced salt solution between the probe and the surface of the eye.
- The vessel holding the balanced salt solution, usually a bottomless cup is placed in a fixed position.
- The mobility of the probe is significantly limited, which prohibits the sound beams from reaching posterior structures in the desired perpendicular manner. For this reason, immersion B scan is not routinely used for the evaluation of posterior segment structures.

- Immersion B scan is valuable in the evaluation of pathology located near the ora serrata (anterior limit of the retina), an area that is too anterior to image with contact B scan and too posterior to image with ultrasound biomicroscopy.
- It is a two-dimensional modality with brightness modulation, and allows the intuitive visualization of various biometric reference interfaces, especially the morphology of the macula and the posterior scleral staphyloma.
- In addition, patients can be guided in the adjustment of eye positions at any time on the basis of the visual content of the images.

ULTRASONOGRAPHIC APPEARANCE OF THE STRUCTURES OF THE NORMAL EYE

On ultrasonography examination: Ocular structures are seen as (Fig. 32.2):

- *Cornea* is visualized as the most superficial echogenic curved line.
- *Iris* appears as a thin echogenic line.
- *Anterior chamber* is an anechoic area that lies between the cornea and the iris.
- *Lens* is seen as an anechoic structure with thin anterior and posterior echogenic capsules.
- *Ciliary body* is seen as a hypoechoic line on either side of the lens.
- *Vitreous* is an anechoic area posterior to the lens.
- *Posterior wall*, comprising the retina, choroid, and sclera (RCS complex), appears as a concave echogenic line extending from the iris plane to the optic nerve and forms the wall of the posterior ocular segment.
- *Optic nerve* sheath is seen as a hypoechoic tubular structure extending away from the globe posteriorly. This is seen as a wedge-shaped acoustic void in the retrobulbar region on an axial scan. The circular area where the ON connects to the retina is the optic disc or papilla. The vertical transverse approach at low gain settings is the ideal view for imaging the optic nerve.
- *Extraocular muscles* are seen as echolucent to low reflective fusiform structures within the orbit, extending posteriorly from their tendinous insertions towards the orbital apex.

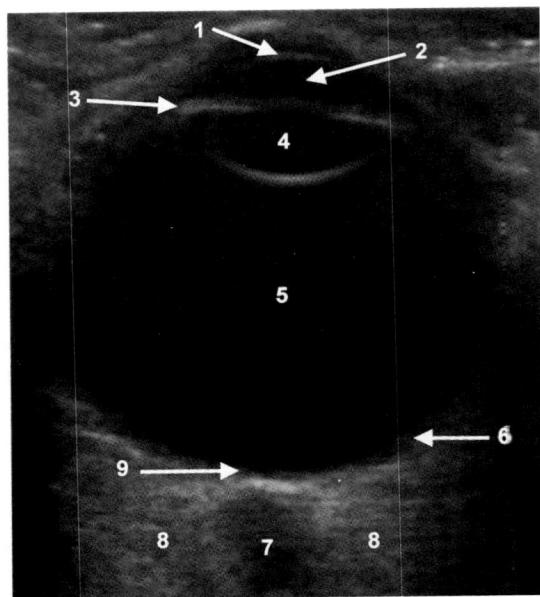

Fig. 32.2: *Sonographic appearance of the structures of the normal eye. The cornea (1) is visualized as the most superficial echogenic curved line; the anterior chamber (2) is anechoic. The iris (3) appears as a thin echogenic line. The lens (4) is defined by anterior and posterior boundary echoes, but the lens itself is echo-free. The vitreous chamber (5) is filled with a clear gel-like substance that is normally echo-free, although the formation of spots and linear echoes with aging is considered normal. The RCS complex (6) forms the wall of the posterior ocular segment; it is seen as an echogenic concave line extending from the iris plane to the optic nerve (ON; 7). The ON is seen as a hypoechoic band surrounded by echogenic retrobulbar fat (8). The circular area where the ON connects to the retina is the optic disc or papilla (9).*

The superior rectus: LPS complex is the thickest and the inferior rectus is the thinnest of the muscles. The inferior oblique is usually not imaged except in pathological conditions.

- *Central retinal artery and vein*, which supplies the inner two-thirds of the retina, and short posterior ciliary arteries are seen on colour Doppler US. The ophthalmic artery and superior ophthalmic vein can also be seen at the retrobulbar orbital fat.

DESCRIPTION OF A LESION

- **Location** in relation to the easily demonstrable landmarks, e.g. optic disc or lens in an intraocular lesion; optic nerve, globe and extraocular muscles in an orbital lesion.

- **Extent**—both anteroposterior and lateral.
- **Dimensions**—in case of tumours and other solid lesions.
- **Shape and configuration**—whether point like, membrane like or mass.
- **Internal reflectivity**—whether echolucent, low, moderate or highly reflective. The sclera is considered as 100% reflective and the reflectivity of other structures is compared with that of the sclera.
- **Structure**—whether solid or cystic, regular or irregular.
- **Degree of sound attenuation**, if any.
- **Mobility**—includes active movements, such as internal vascularity within a mass, movement of a live intravitreal cysticercus; and after-movements such as that seen with a complete posterior vitreous detachment.

INDICATIONS FOR OPHTHALMIC ULTRASOUND

Ocular

Evaluation of ocular structures in following circumstance:

- Opaque media
- Occluded or markedly miotic pupil
- Ophthalmoscopically visible mass lesion
- Suspicion of tumour underlying retinal detachment
- Ocular trauma
- Ocular foreign body.

Orbital

- Unilateral or bilateral exophthalmos
- Unexplained optic atrophy
- Papilledema without evident cause
- Retinal striae
- Suspected intraorbital foreign body.

ULTRASONOGRAPHIC FINDINGS IN COMMON INTRAOCULAR LESIONS

CONGENITAL ANOMALIES

Retinochoroidal Coloboma

- Coloboma is visible as an excavation of the ocular wall.
- B scan in a patient with retinochoroidal coloboma shows a well-defined excavated

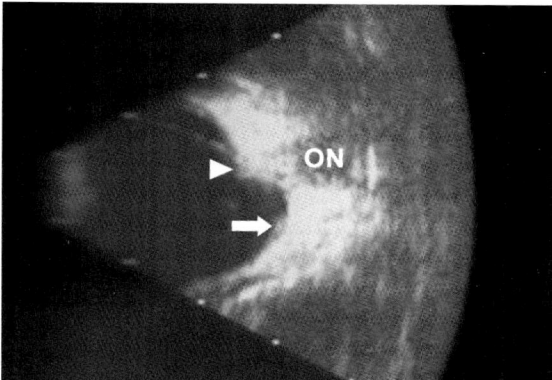

Fig. 32.3: *B scan image in a patient with retinochoroidal coloboma.*

area with the absence of retinochoroidal layer (Fig. 32.3).
- The contour may be smooth or have an outpouching with overhanging edges.

Nanophthalmos

Nanophthalmos is characterized by bilateral and symmetrical small eyes, associated with **shortened axial length (20 mm or less**; at least two standard deviations below age-matched controls), high corneal curvature, high lens/eye volume ratio with narrow iridocorneal angle, high hyperopia (ranging from +8.00 to +25.00) and scleral thickening.

Common B scan findings in nanophthalmos (Fig. 32.4) include:
- Reduced axial length with normal sized lens.

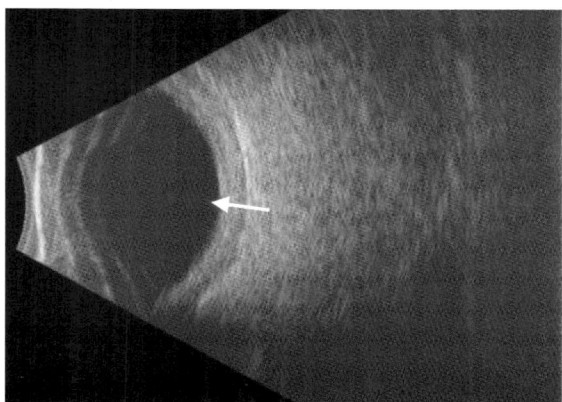

Fig. 32.4: *B scan findings in a patient with nanophthalmos.*

- Increased retinochoroidal scleral thickness (1.37 to 4.00 mm).
- Presence of exudative retinal detachment and choroidal detachment.

Persistent hyperplastic primary vitreous

Common B scan findings in a patient with persistent hyperplastic primary vitreous include (Fig. 32.5):

- Decrease in axial length.
- Thin lens with irregular posterior capsule.
- Retrolental high reflective membrane.
- Vitreous band of variable reflectivity extending from the lens to the optic disc.
- Peripapillary tractional retinal detachment (TRD).
- B scan ultrasonography can also be used to rule out introcular masses, fibrovascular stalk, microphthalmia and to look for calcification.

VITREORETINAL DISEASES

Retinopathy of prematurity

Retinopathy of prematurity is characterised by multiple vitreous membranes and retinal detachment in the periphery. Common B scan findings in retinopathy of prematurity include:

- *Stage 1 ROP* shows shallow retinal thickening.
- *Stage 2 ROP* shows retinal thickening with ridge.
- *Stage 3 ROP* shows a giant ridge with vitreous fibrous band traction.
- *Stage 4a* shows a partial retinal detachment as the retina is drawn anteriorly towards the lens margin by vitreous condensation (Fig. 32.6).

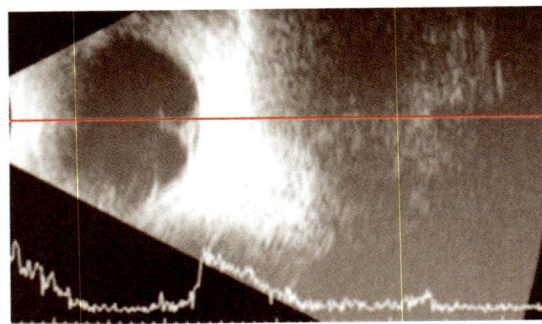

Fig. 32.6: *B scan image in a patient stage 4 ROP showing partial retinal detachment as the retina is drawn anteriorly toward lens margin by vitreous condensation.*

- *Stage 4b* displays a more severe form of partial retinal detachment with doughnut appearance.
- *Stage 5 ROP* reveals a folded and scrolled retina into funnel shape. Funnel-shaped high reflective membrane attached to the optic disc suggestive of a total retinal detachment (Fig. 32.7).

Vitreous haemorrhage

Common B scan findings in a patient with vitreous haemorrhage include (Fig 32.8):

- *Fresh vitreous haemorrhage* is echolucent or very low reflective. These dot-like echoes on B scan may need higher gain settings for detection. On dynamic B scan, fresh vitreous haemorrhagic echoes show distinct after movements
- *Resolving vitreous haemorrhage* is seen as homogenous hypo- to isoechoic vitreous echoes clumped together with distinct after movements.

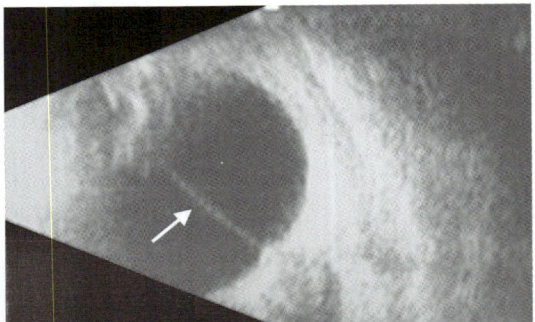

Fig. 32.5: *B scan image in a patient with persistent hyperplastic primary vitreous.*

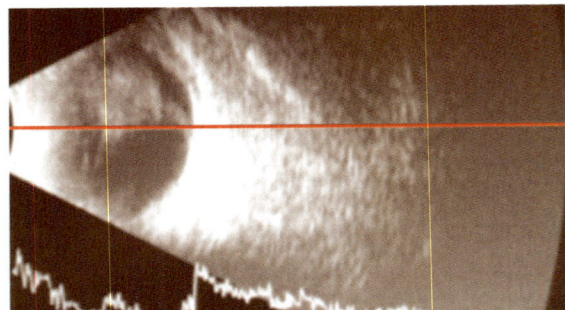

Fig. 32.7: *B scan image in a patient stage 5 ROP showing folded and scrolled retina in funnel shape.*

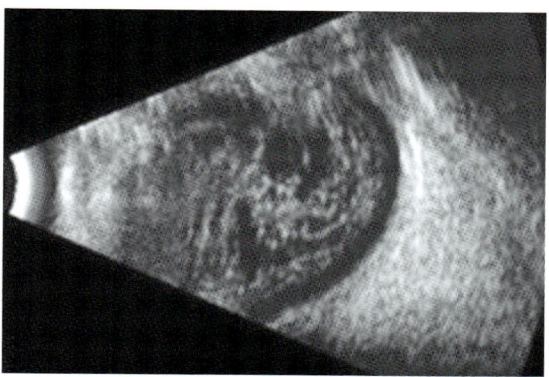

Fig. 32.8: *B scan image in a patient with vitreous haemorrhage.*

- *In old or long-standing vitreous haemorrhage,* the dot like echoes organize to form multiple dense vitreous membranes and bands of varying reflectivity across their extent. These are most dense inferiorly as a result of gravity. These bands have no movements due to the presence of fibrin within them. The sites of attachment of the vitreous membranes to the retina are potential sites for tractional retinal detachment.

Posterior vitreous detachment

- On B scan, posterior vitreous detachment seen as a freely mobile membranous echo with variable attachments to the optic nerve head or retina (Fig. 32.9).
- These could be focal or broad, single or multiple. This is in contrast to a rhegmatogenous retinal detachment where the attachment is to the optic disc, unless it is a peripheral or localised detachment.
- The mobility of the PVD is more than that of a retinal detachment; this helps in differentiation between the two. USG also shows marked mobility and elasticity of the detached vitreous, with a mirror image configuration

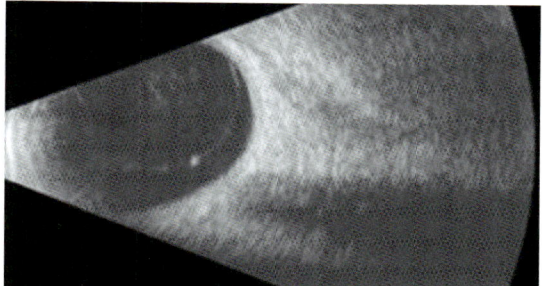

Fig. 32.9: *B scan through macula showing total PVD with Weiss ring.*

when the eye is deviated to one side and then to the other.

Retinal breaks and retinal detachment
Retinal breaks

- Retinal break appears as a breach of tissue on B scan (Fig. 32.10) and on A scan it appears as a highly reflective tissue separate from the other fundus spikes.
- Giant retinal tears are seen as convoluted membranes often with unusual configuration. There is often a free end which is very mobile. Giant retinal break with detachment appears as a rolled out tissue on B scan with clear breach of tissue.

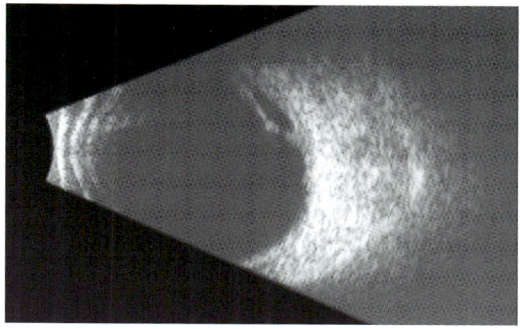

Fig. 32.10: *B scan image in a patient with retinal break.*

Ultrasonographic differentiating features between PVD and retinal detachment

Feature	Posterior vitreous detachment	Retinal detachment
Echogenicity	Low–medium	High
Mobility	High mobility	Low mobility
Change with gain (Db)	Disappears with low gain	Visible with low gain
Optic disc attachment	Present or absent	Always present

Rhegmatogenous retinal detachment

B scan findings in a patient with rhegmatogenous retinal detachment include (Fig. 32.11):

- Tall 100% amplitude spike separated from the choroid and attached at the disc and ora with little after movements.
- After movements become further reduced with PVR changes.
- Finally funnel-shaped membrane is formed which can be closed or open.
- Long standing cases may show retinal cysts and cholesterol debris in subretinal space.

Tractional retinal detachment

On B scan findings tractional retinal detachment is typically seen as a concave membrane with a varying extent of vitreous adhesion, may be either focal or broad depending upon the extent of vitreoretinal adhesion.

- Broad causing table top traction of the retina (Fig. 32.12A)

- Focal vitreoretinal adhesion causing tent like lesion (Fig. 32.12B).

Exudative retinal detachment

- Typical features on B scan in a patient with exudative retinal detachment include the presence of smooth bullae and shifting fluid (Figs 32.13A and B).

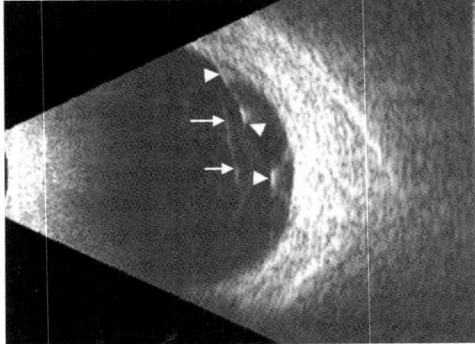

Fig. 32.12B: B scan findings in a patient with tractional retinal detachment showing tent like appearance.

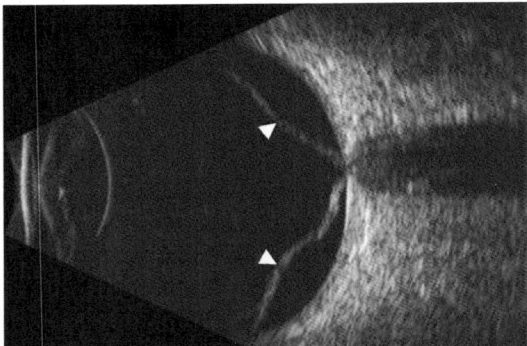

Fig. 32.11: B scan findings in a patient with rhegmatogenous retinal detachment.

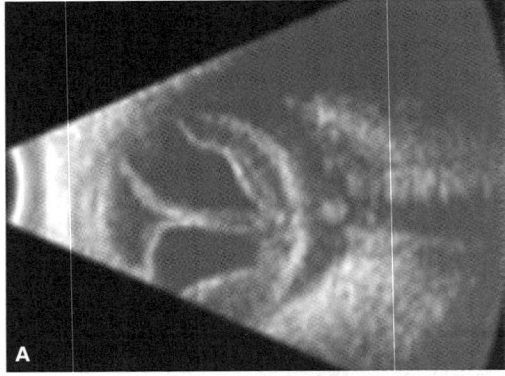

A

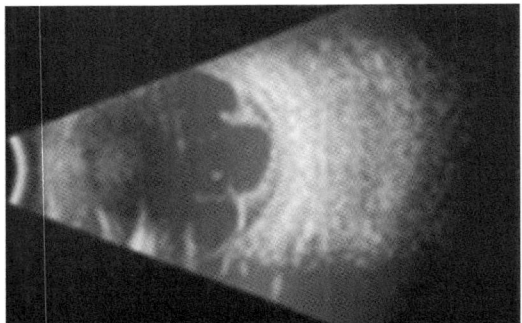

Fig. 32.12A: B scan findings in a patient with tractional retinal fetachment showing table top traction of the retina.

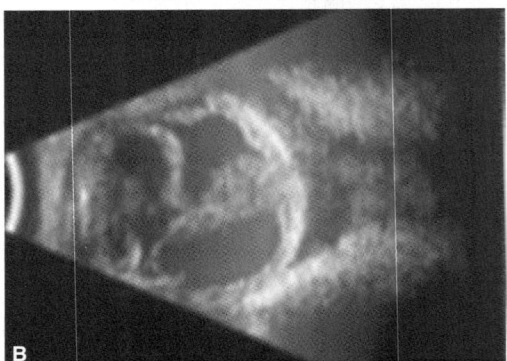

B

Fig. 32.13: B scan image showing shifting fluid in exudative retinal detachment.

- The configuration of the detachment is convex and bullous.
- It can be diagnosed by having the patient sit up or change head position which changes the configuration of the RD.
- Presence of retinochoroidal thickening would indicate an inflammatory etiology such as scleritis, VKH or sympathetic ophthalmia.
- It is necessary to look for a tumour mass or granuloma, if no break or inflammatory signs are noted.

Choroidal detachment

- B scan in a patient with choroidal detachment reveals smooth, thick, dome-shaped membrane in the periphery with little or no after movements, which usually does not extend beyond the equator as it is limited by the exit of vortex veins (Fig. 32.14).
- The A scan shows a typical double peak or M-shaped spike signifying echoes from the choroid and the retina.
- In haemorrhagic choroidal detachment, supra-choroidal space shows multiple dot like moderate to high reflective echoes.
- Shallow peripheral detachments may be flat or concave instead of dome-shaped.

Asteroid hyalosis

- The vitreous cavity shows a varying number of discrete mobile point like bright echoes on the B scan with a high spike on the A scan (Fig. 32.15).

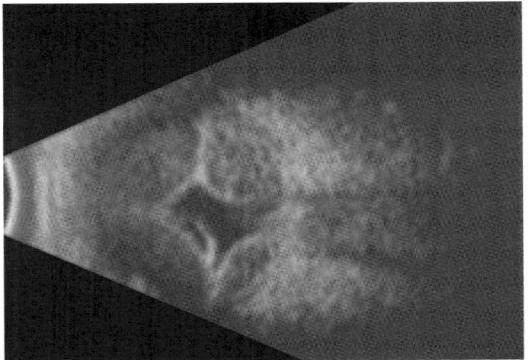

Fig. 32.14: *B scan in a patient with choroidal detachment showing classical kissing choroidal detachment with scalloped appearance. Pinpoint echoes inside the dome-shaped choroidal detachment is suggestive of haemorrhagic type.*

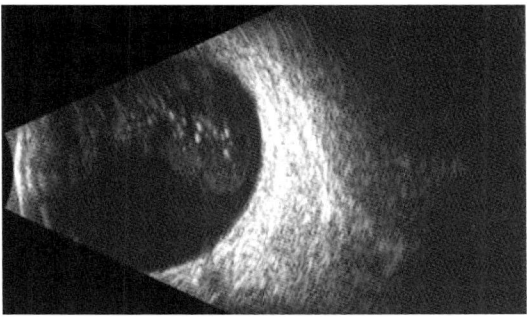

Fig. 32.15: *B scan in a patient with asteroid hyalosis.*

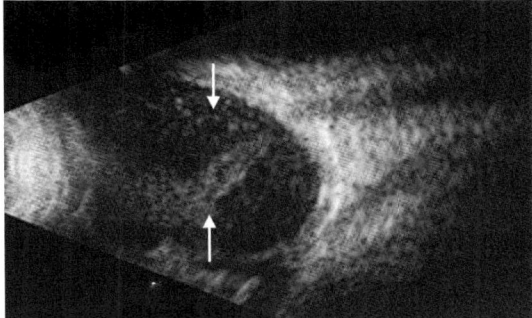

Fig. 32.16: *B scan image in a patient with Coats' disease.*

- There is classically a clear space between the particles and the posterior globe wall, and this can mimic a posterior vitreous detachment.

Coats' disease

- In early Coats' disease on B scan, there is localized, dome-shaped exudative retinal detachment in the posterior pole (Fig. 32.16)
- In severe Coats' disease on B scan, there is a funnel-shaped retinal detachment and opacities from subretinal cholesterol
- B scan through temporal globe shows marked retinal thickening
- Total retinal detachment which can touch the lens
- Absence of mass
- Absence of calcifications.

OCULAR TRAUMA

Intraocular foreign body

- B scan in a patient with intraocular foreign body shows echodense signal with shadowing (Fig. 32.17).

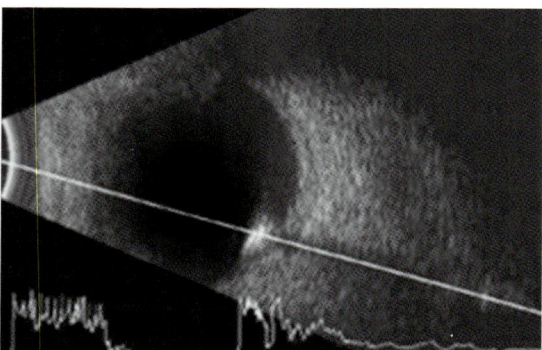

Fig. 32.17: *B scan image in a patient with intraocular foreign body.*

- Reduction of gain is helpful in differentiating stronger foreign body echoes from those of orbital tissues.
- The foreign body may be quite small and linear, and may be missed if the probe is not perpendicular to the flat side of the foreign body.
- Metal and stone being prominent reflectors of ultrasound, produce higher amplitude echoes than any normal structure except bone.
- Stone foreign bodies are usually larger and more irregular in shape.
- Glass has specific echographic characteristics. It is only when the sound beam strikes the long, smooth surface of a glass sliver with perpendicular incidence, that it is likely to be picked up by ultrasound.
- Spherical IOFBs produce very strong reverberations due to their regular structure.

Lens trauma

- The normal clear lens is low reflective. This feature is lost when the lens is damaged either by blunt or penetrating injury.
- The lens may be subluxated or dislocated, either anteriorly or posteriorly, or even expelled out of the globe.
- In case of penetrating, or sometimes even after blunt trauma, a posterior capsule rupture may be seen. The lenticular contents may be disturbed within the capsule, in which case the lens appears very high reflective due to hydration of the cortex. In other situations, the lens matter may prolapse into the vitreous where it can get admixed with vitreous and blood.

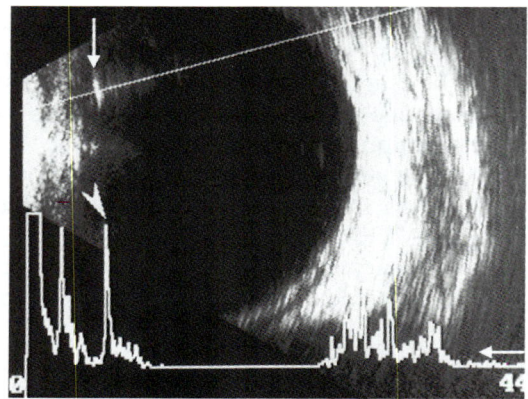

Fig. 32.18: *B scan image in a patient with intralenticular foreign body.*

- In penetrating injuries, one may even see an intralenticular foreign body on B scan (Fig. 32.18).

Scleral rupture

- Can occur either in penetrating or severe blunt trauma.
- Presents as chemosis, subconjunctival and/or vitreous haemorrhage and hypotony.
- B scan at the site of rupture include an area of irregular scleral echolucency often with incarceration of vitreous and retina (Fig. 32.19).
- Other features include choroidal detachments and scleral folds due to hypotony.

OCULAR INFECTIONS AND INFLAMMATIONS

Endophthalmitis

- B scan in endophthalmitis include low reflective vitreous echoes—dot-like or cobweb-shaped membranes suggesting of vitreous inflammation (Fig 32.20).

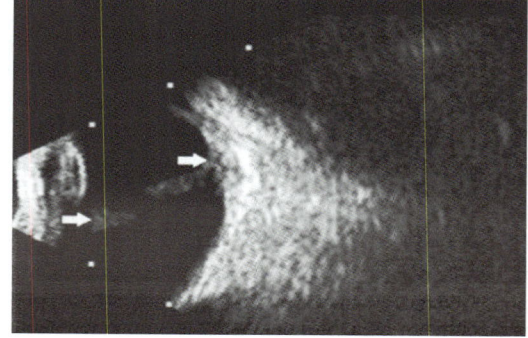

Fig. 32.19: *B scan image in a patient with scleral rupture.*

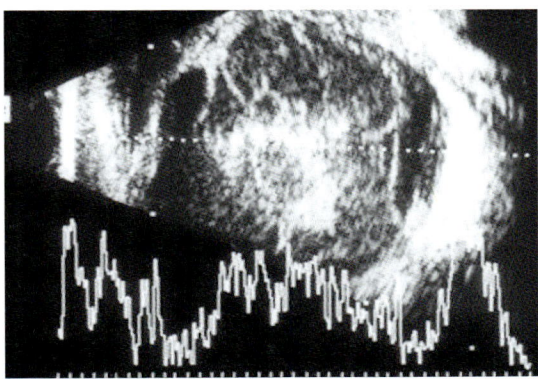

Fig. 32.20: *B scan image in a patient with endophthalmitis.*

- In more severe cases, thick high reflective membrane like echoes may be seen.
- Dispersed vitreous opacities with vitritis.
- Chorioretinal thickening.
- It can also pick-up associated features like retinal detachment, choroidal detachment, or retained intraocular foreign body.
- In cases with opaque cornea or significant cataract, serial B scan ultrasound examination is helpful in documenting improvement or worsening by assessing the intensity of the echoes.

VKH syndrome

- B scan in VKH syndrome shows diffuse low to medium reflective thickening of the choroid at the posterior pole (Fig. 32.21)

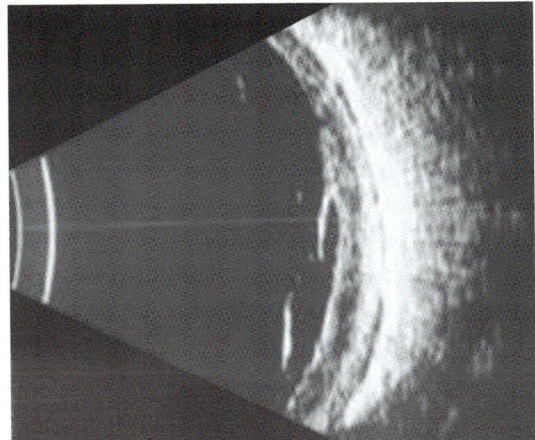

Fig. 32.21: *B scan image in a patient with VKH showing posterior choroidal thickening with overlying retinal detachment.*

- Serous retinal detachment, located inferiorly or at the posterior pole.
- Mild vitreous opacities with no posterior vitreous detachment.
- Thickening of the sclera and/or episclera posteriorly.
- Optic disc elevation.

Scleritis

- B scan ultrasonography shows diffuse or localized highly reflective scleral thickening (Fig. 32.22).
- Associated with swelling of the underlying Tenon's and episclera causing an echolucent area. When peripapillary in location this causes a 'T' sign.
- Exudative retinal and choroidal detachment, optic nerve edema and nerve sheath edema may be seen.

Toxocariasis

- B scan in a patient with toxocariasis shows a granuloma which appears as a mass lesion, commonly peripheral, but can also occur near the disc (Fig. 32.23).

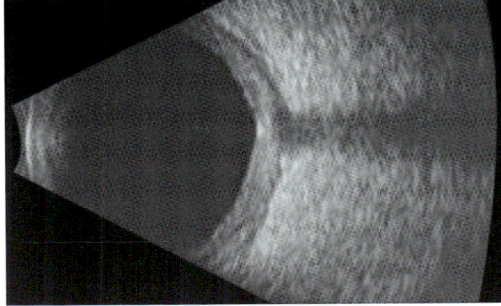

Fig. 32.22: *B scan image in a patient with scleritis.*

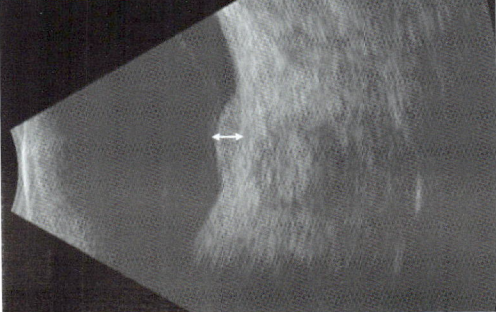

Fig. 32.23: *B scan image in a patient with toxocariasis.*

- This can be highly reflective, with a surrounding tractional retinal detachment.
- Tractional retinal folds extend from the mass to the disc. Multiple vitreous membranes can be seen, some of which can be high reflective. Characteristic pseudocystic degeneration of the peripheral vitreous has been described in patients with ocular toxocariasis.

OCULAR TUMOURS

Choroidal melanoma

- B scan in choroidal melanoma shows a solid dome-shaped or mushroom collar button configuration due to tumour growth through a ruptured Bruch's membrane (Fig. 32.24).
- Regular internal structure on B scan.
- Low to medium internal reflectivity on A scan. Demonstrable internal blood flow seen as flickering spikes on the A scan.

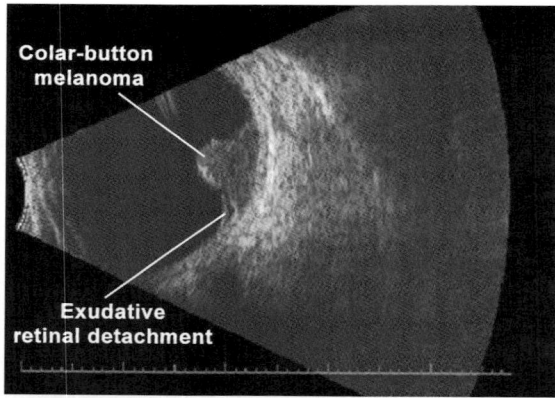

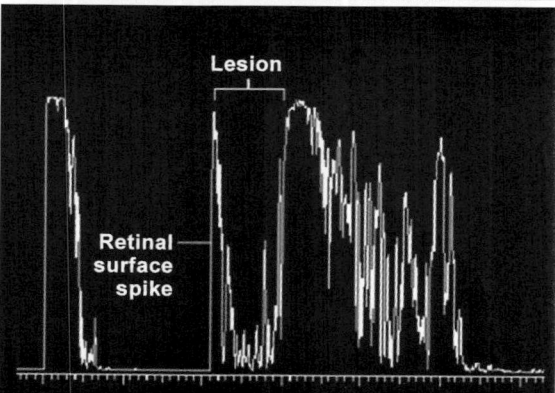

Fig. 32.24: *Orbital B scan image in a patient of choroidal melanoma.*

- USG is used to assess scleral erosions and extraocular extension into orbital fat.
- B scan three classic features of choroidal melanoma are: An acoustically silent zone within the melanoma, choroidal excavation and shadowing in the orbit.
- Vascular pulsations can be seen as fine oscillations of the internal spiking pattern within the tumour.
- Color Doppler reveals tumour vessels as pulsating channels or lakes of colour entering the base of the lesion. Not all tumours are vascular.

Choroidal haemangioma

- Ultrasonographic findings of circumscribed choroidal haemangioma reveals a smooth-contoured, dome-shaped choroidal mass with characteristic high internal reflectivity due to dense fibrous or osseous metaplasia of the overlying RPE (Fig. 32.25).
- Intrinsic vascular pulsations are generally not present.
- A scan echography revealed high internal reflectivity, which is typical for these lesions.
- Diffuse haemangioma shows diffuse marked thickening of choroid.

Choroidal metastases

- B scan in choroidal metastasis shows a solid mass at the posterior pole with irregular or bumpy contour (Fig. 32.26).
- Variable internal structure which can be regular, irregular or have a central excavation.
- Moderate to high internal reflectivity on A scan.

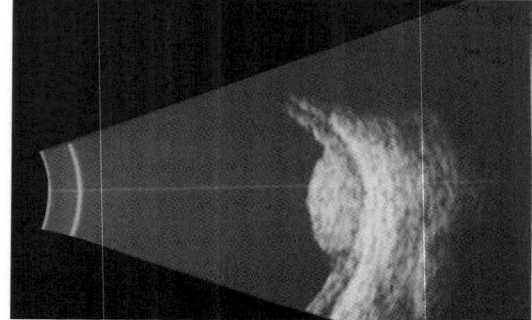

Fig. 32.25: *Orbital B scan image in a patient of choroidal haemangioma.*

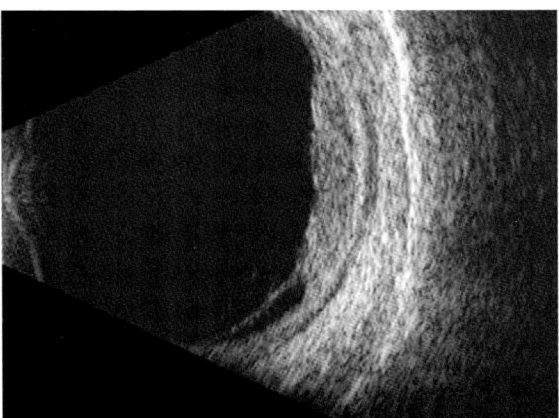

Fig. 32.26: *Orbital B scan image in a patient of choroidal metastasis.*

- Extensive exudative retinal detachment usually over the tumour surface as well.
- Bullous choroidal detachment.

Retinoblastoma

- B scan in retinoblastoma shows single or multiple mass lesions in the vitreous cavity arising from the retina (Fig. 32.27).
- Presence of calcium seen as high reflective specks or clumps within the lesion, causing orbital shadowing are pathognomonic.
- The vitreous cavity can show echoes due to vitreous seeds in an endophytic lesion.
- In an exophytic lesion, an exudative retinal detachment may be seen overlying the mass, with subretinal echoes, suggestive of subretinal seeds.

- A funnel-shaped total retinal detachment with a thick solid mass with similar shape just behind it may be seen.
- B scan helps to detect extrascleral spread as well as to detect optic nerve invasion.

Choroidal osteoma

- On ultrasound, the A scan shows a high intensity echo spike (Fig. 32.28).
- B scan shows slightly elevated, highly reflective choroidal mass with acoustic shadowing that gives an appearance of 'pseudo-optic nerve'. The mass persists at lower scanning sensitivity after the other soft tissue echoes have disappear
- If the intensity (gain) of the ultrasound machine is decreased, there is persistent reflectivity or 'brightness' from the tumour. Ultrasound can also be used to measure the thickness of a choroidal osteoma.

MISCELLANEOUS OCULAR CONDITIONS

Phthisis bulbi

Phthisis bulbi refers to the end stage of many ocular disorders, commonly seen after trauma, failed surgery, and congenital ocular abnormalities

- On B scan, the eye looks shrunken, usually with calcified walls and hyperechoic fibrous tracts from the retina to the posterior lens that can result in retinal detachment (Fig. 32.29).

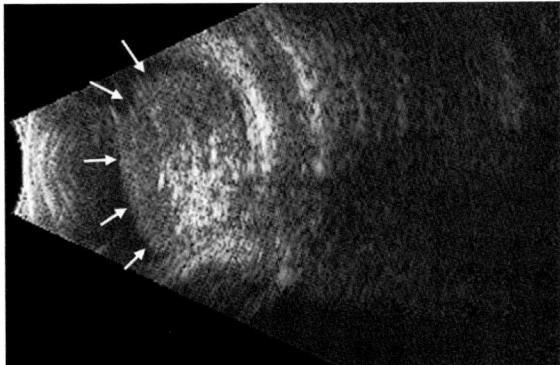

Fig. 32.27: *Orbital B scan image in a patient of retinoblastoma.*

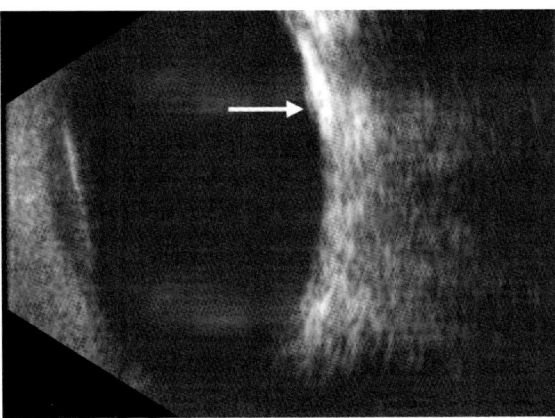

Fig. 32.28: *Orbital B scan image in a patient of choroidal osteoma.*

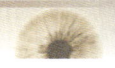

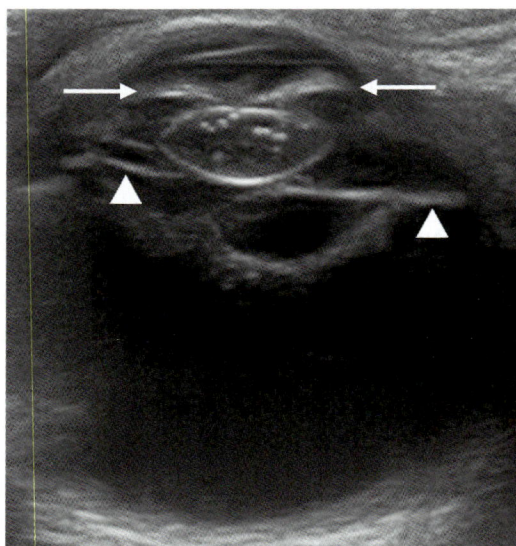

Fig. 32.29: *Axial orbital B scan image in a patient of phthisis bulbi showing increased echogenicity of both walls of the lens, with intraocular echoes. There is also a synechia between the iris and the lens, causing the iris to curve forward (arrows)—the so-called iris bombé. This condition prevents the flow of aqueous humour from the posterior to the anterior chamber. Also note the thick posterior membranes between the lens and the vitreous.*

Dislocated intraocular lens

- Intraocular lens behaves as an IOFB with multiple reflecting surfaces (Fig. 32.30)
- It may be subluxated, freely mobile in the vitreous or lying on the retinal surface
- Depending on the probe direction, the optic, optic-haptic junction and haptics can be made out.

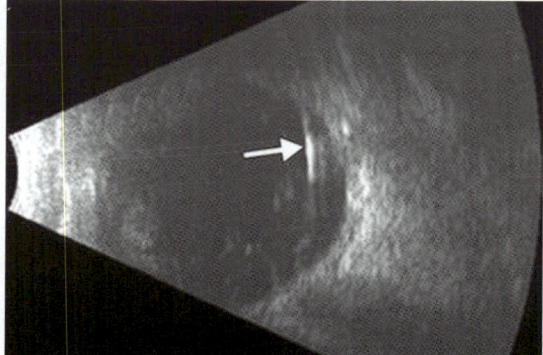

Fig. 32.30: *Orbital B scan image in a patient with intraocular lens in vitreous cavity.*

Dropped nucleus

- The features depend on the clarity of the lens
- The clear lens appears as globular structure, which is echolucent
- The cataractous lens appears highly reflective and the internal echoes vary depending on the amount of cortical hydration (Fig. 32.31)
- A brunescent nucleus causes very high reflectivity with shadowing
- In cases with a long-standing dislocated lens, it may become calcified and cause dense shadowing.

Silicone oil-filled eyeball

- B scan shows apparent lengthening of the globe (Fig. 32.32)
- Silicone oil which is not emulsified produces pronounced sound attenuation and difficulty in imaging the retina
- Emulsified oil presents as high reflective dot-like echoes similar to asteroid hyalosis

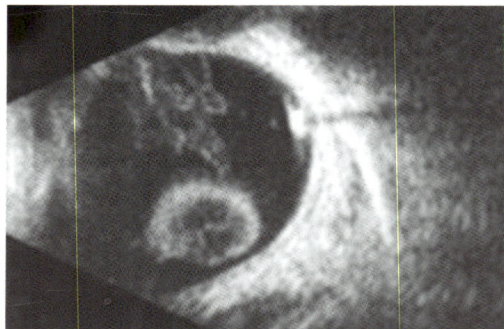

Fig. 32.31: *Orbital B scan image in a patient with dropped nucleus in the vitreous cavity.*

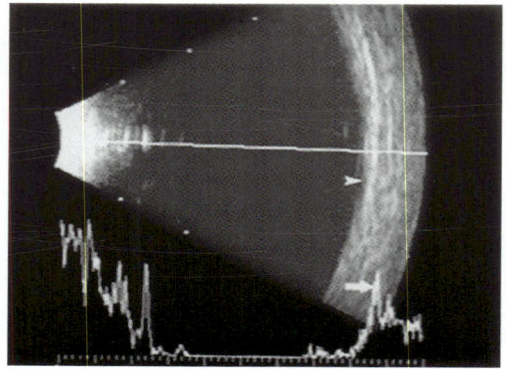

Fig. 32.32: *Orbital B scan image in a patient with silicon oil.*

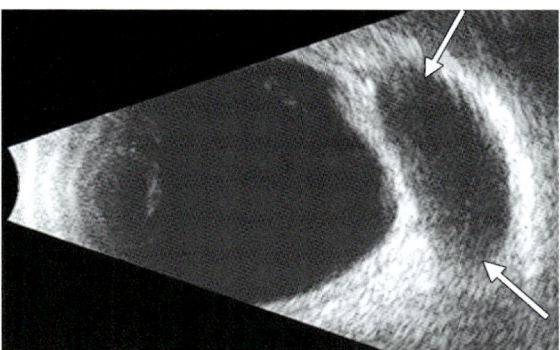

Fig. 32.33: *Orbital B scan image in a patient with scleral buckle.*

- In the presence of an incomplete fill, the posterior surface of the oil bubble may be mistaken for the retinal surface.

Scleral buckle

- On B scan, they appear as echogenic spots with the globe indentation towards the vitreous body and echolucent spot (shadowing) behind the scleral explants (Fig. 32.33).
- The explant shows high reflectivity on A scan.
- Silicone sponge has different echographic features. The air filled cavities in buckling material give a characteristic hyperechoic shadow.
- It may be possible to distinguish an area of echolucency around the buckle if there is associated scleritis and buckle infection.
- The extent of a buckle can be made out if removal is planned, especially if the primary surgery has been done elsewhere or partial removal has been done and no details are available. This is important as the buckle effect seen internally persists for months to years after removal.

ULTRASONOGRAPHY FINDINGS IN ORBITAL LESIONS

ORBITAL TUMOURS

Orbital cavernous haemangioma

- B scan in orbital cavernous haemangioma shows a smooth well-defined round to oval mass (Fig. 32.34A)

- Commonly intraconal, causing globe indentation
- Moderate to strong sound attenuation
- Moderate to high internal reflectivity with regular acoustic structure (Fig. 32.34B).

Orbital lymphangioma

- B scan in orbital lymphangioma shows irregular infiltrative mass lesion with evidence of echolucent spaces separated by highly reflective septae (Fig. 32.35).
- The compressible nature of the lesion is lost when haemorrhage occurs and may return at a later date.

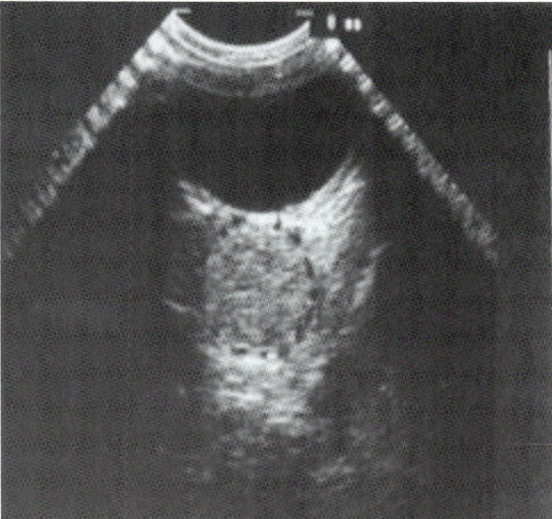

Fig. 32.34A: *B scan ultrasonogram in a patient with cavernous haemangioma.*

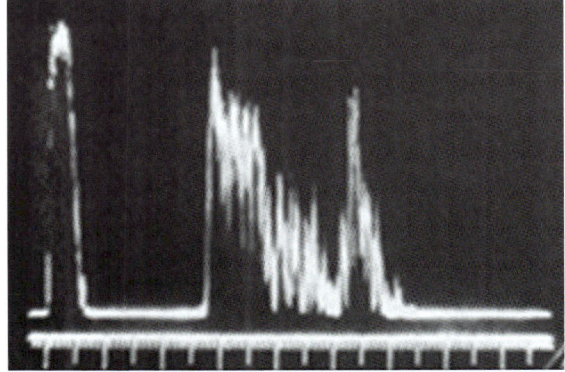

Fig. 32.34B: *A scan USG of cavernous haemangioma demonstrating moderate internal reflectivity.*

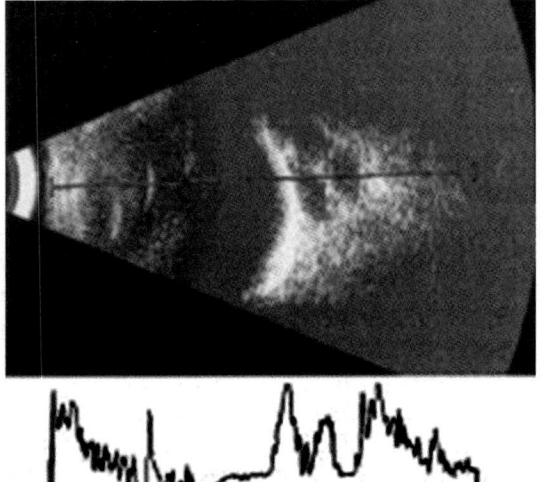

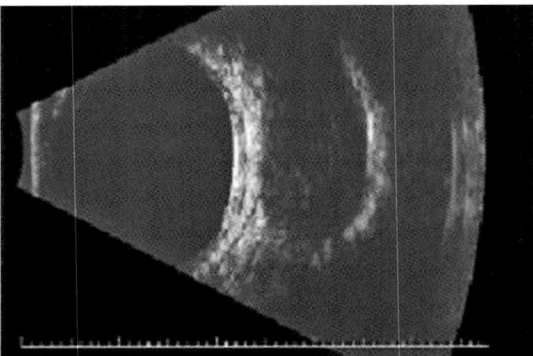

Fig. 32.37: *B scan ultrasonogram in a patient with orbital schwannoma.*

Orbital Schwannoma

- B scan can be used for rapid evaluation, follow up, or progression of schwannomas.
- B scan in orbital schwannoma reveals round, well-defined, solid lesions.
- Regular structure with low internal reflectivity (Fig. 32.37).
- May have septae or cystic spaces with different tissue interfaces that affect the signal intensity.
- Acoustic hollows on ultrasound are suggestive of intratumour haemorrhage.

Fig. 32.35: *Ultrasonography in orbital lymphangioma showing low reflective multicystic lesion within orbit.*

- Occasional lesions may show specks of high reflectivity suggestive of calcium and may even show phleboliths.

Orbital lymphomas

- B scan in orbital lymphoma reveals homogenous, well-defined, ovoid or elongated low reflective lesion, mostly in the superior orbit (Fig. 32.36).
- Essentially extraconal.
- Tendency to mould to either the globe or orbital structures.
- Can be bilateral.

Rhabdomyosarcoma

- B scan in orbital rhabdomyosarcoma shows a well-circumscribed lesion (Fig. 32.38).
- Tend to be unilateral and extraconal.
- Low to medium internal echoes.

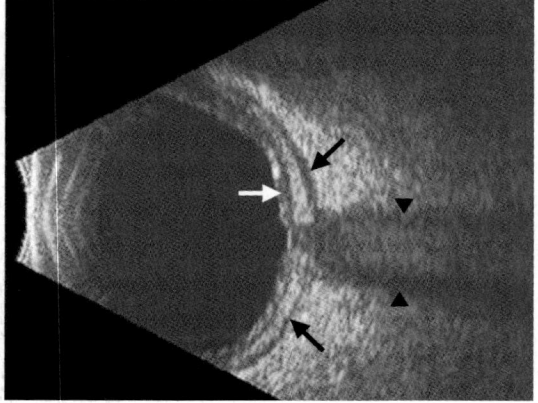

Fig. 32.36: *B scan ultrasonogram in a patient with orbital lymphoma.*

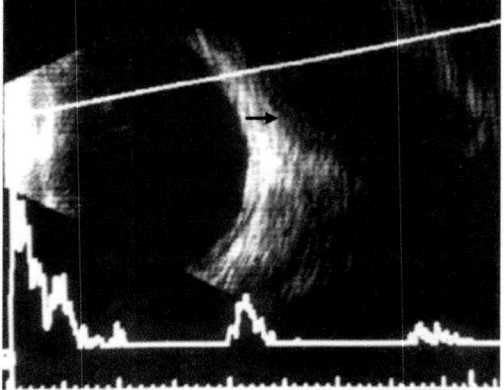

Fig. 32.38: *B scan ultrasonogram in a patient with orbital rhabdomyosarcoma.*

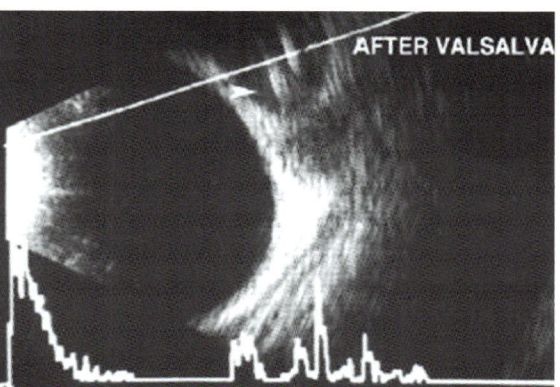

Fig. 32.39: *B scan images showing an irregular echolucent tubular lesion (arrowhead) in the orbit that has increased in size after Valsalva manoeuvre.*

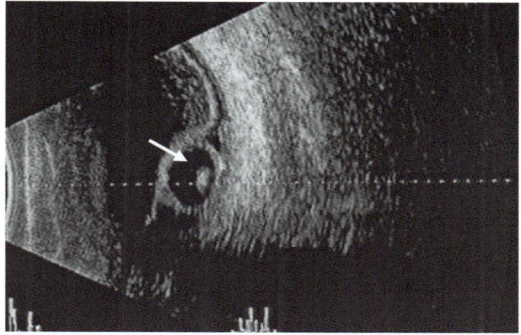

Fig. 32.40: *Orbital B scan ultrasonogram in a patient with orbital cysticercosis showing a well-defined cyst lined by a cyst wall and a hyperreflective scolex.*

- Adjacent bone may be intact or eroded.
- Internal vascularity may be demonstrated on the A scan.
- A 'pseudocystic' appearance has been reported as characteristic, and that is thought to be due to spindle cells in embryonal RMS which have abundant cytoplasm and are separated loosely by edematous fluid.

Orbital varix

- B scan in a patient with orbital varix demonstrates the venous channel (Fig. 32.39).
- Echolucent or very low reflective lesion.
- In case of a phlebolith, the reflectivity may be irregular with some areas that are highly reflective. In such cases the lesion may not change in size with the Valsalva manoeuvre.
- A thrombosed varix may also appear as a large low reflective mass lesion.
- Other orbital contents like EOMs and optic nerve appear normal.
- They typically appear like dilated blood vessels with well-differentiated borders. They have a soft consistency, collapsing on compression and increasing with Valsalva manoeuvre.

ORBITAL INFECTIONS AND INFLAMMATION

Orbital Cysticercosis

- B scan in a patient with orbital cysticercosis reveals a well-outlined round to oval echolucent cyst (Fig. 32.40).

- Echodense nodule adjacent to the inner wall of the cyst represent the scolex.
- Preferentially involves the muscle belly, but can involve the orbital soft tissues as well. The shape of the cyst wall is irregular and may mould to the globe contour in case of soft tissue involvement.
- The scolex is the first to disappear with adequate medical therapy with albendazole, followed by the cyst itself.
- Serial ultrasounds can be performed to note the response to treatment.

Orbital echinococcosis

- B scan in a patient with orbital echinococcosis reveal a single/multilobulated cysts with echolucent centres (Fig. 32.41).

Idiopathic orbital inflammatory disease

- B scan in a patient with idiopathic orbital inflammatory disease reveals ill-defined

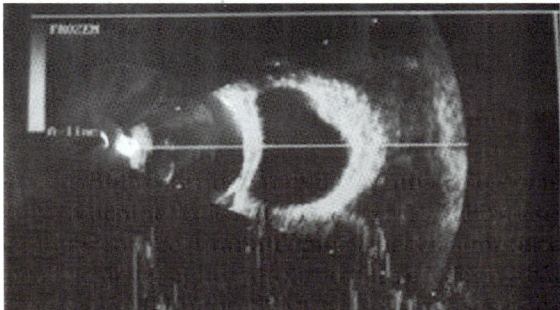

Fig. 32.41: *Orbital B scan ultrasonography showing a large orbital hydatid cyst.*

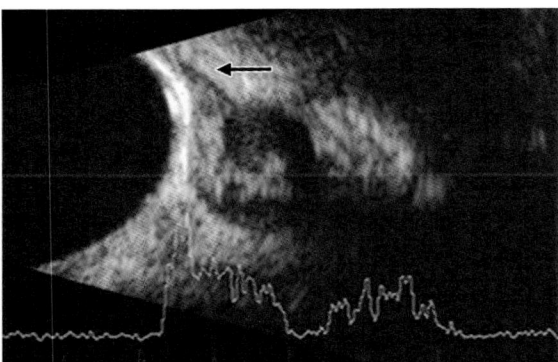

Fig. 32.42: *Orbital B scan ultrasonogram in a patient with idiopathic orbital inflammatory disease.*

orbital mass lesion which may be diffuse and involve adjacent structures (Fig. 32.42).

- Low reflective enlargement of a single or multiple extraocular muscles, which may appear irregular in shape. The low reflectivity is due to diffuse infiltration of the muscle fibres with inflammatory cells.
- Associated scleritis or Tenon's widening adjacent to the involved muscle tendon.
- Widening of the perineural space may be seen.
- Absence of orbital bone contour alteration.
- Lacrimal gland enlargement may be seen.
- In chronic cases, the reflectivity may be high due to fibrotic and sclerotic changes.

Orbital abscess

- B scan in a patient with orbital abscess reveals a well-circumscribed lesion with low internal reflectivity (Fig. 32.43).

- May be multiloculated or solitary.
- If sub periosteal in nature, the lesion may be well-separated from the orbital soft tissues and communication with the adjacent paranasal sinuses may be demonstrable.
- In the case of an abscess, adjacent Tenon's widening or muscle thickening may be present. The T sign may be visible.

OPTIC NERVE LESIONS

Optic disc drusen (ODD)

- On B scan, optic nerve head with ODD is elevated and highly reflective (Fig. 32.44); even on decreasing the sensitivity of the display, calcified drusen maintains high signal intensity, whereas with papilloedema, the signal intensity decreases along with the remainder of the ocular signal.

Optic nerve glioma

- On B scan, optic nerve gliomas present as a smooth fusiform thickening of the optic nerve shadow (Fig. 32.45).
- The reflectivity is homogenous and low. In long-standing cases, cystic areas may be seen.

Optic nerve sheath meningioma

- On B scan, optic nerve sheath meningiomas shows thickening of the optic nerve shadow, but have an irregular structure, and may show areas of calcification (Fig. 32.46).

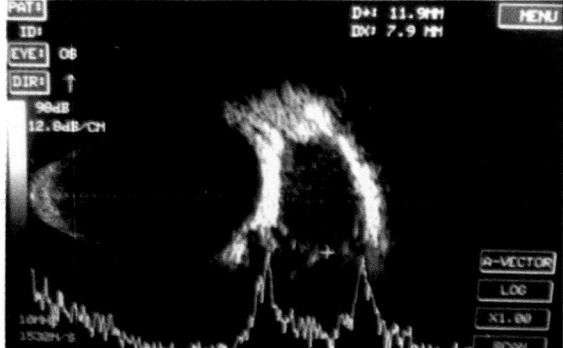

Fig. 32.43: *Orbital B scan ultrasonogram in a patient with orbital abscess.*

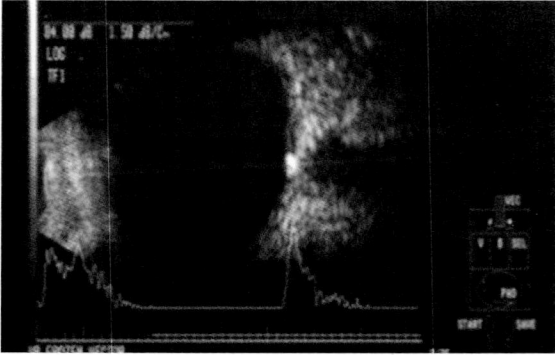

Fig. 32.44: *Orbital B scan ultrasonogram in a patient with optic disc drusen.*

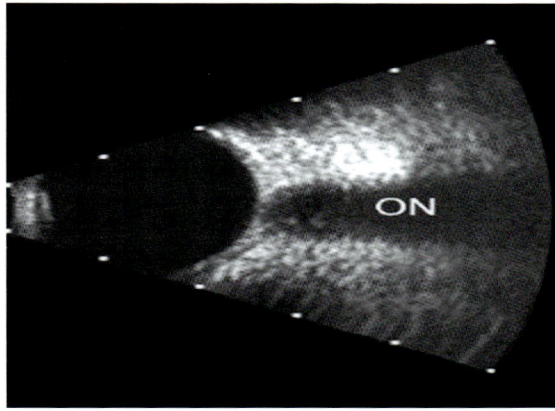

Fig. 32.45: *B scan images of the patient with disc oedema and optic nerve glioma.*

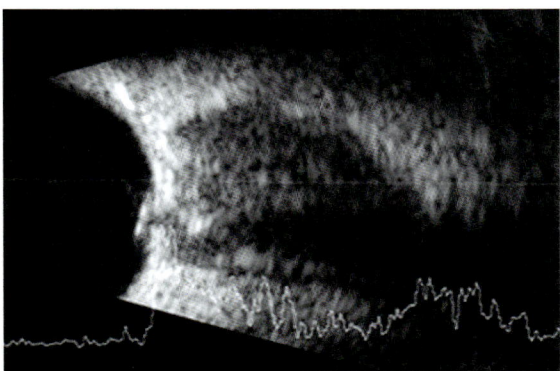

Fig. 32.46: *B scan image of the patient with optic nerve sheath meningioma.*

DISORDERS OF EXTRAOCULAR MUSCLES

Graves' orbitopathy

- Ultrasonography confirms the diagnosis and is useful in following the response to therapy.
- B scan shows characteristic fusiform thickening of the muscle belly which typically spares the tendon (Fig. 32.47).
- The most commonly affected muscle is inferior rectus followed by medial, superior and lateral rectus.
- The thickened muscle is highly reflective due to deposition of hydrophilic mucopolysaccharides. This, along with inflammatory edema creates interfaces within the bundles of muscle fibers which themselves are infiltrated by inflammatory cells.

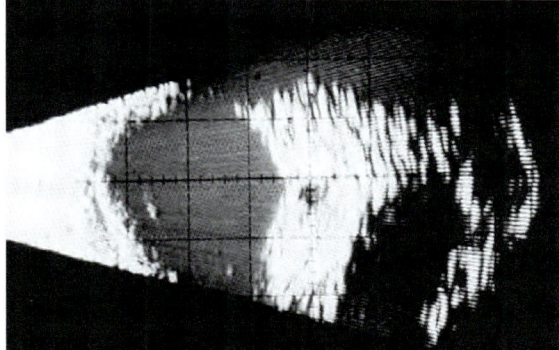

Fig. 32.47: *B scan ultrasonography image of the patient with Graves' orbitopathy.*

- Increase in the amount of orbital fat, enlargement of the lacrimal gland and dilatation of the superior ophthalmic vein due to apical crowding are other features.

Idiopathic orbital myositis

- B scan in a patient with idiopathic orbital myositis shows diffuse thickening of one or more extraocular muscles (Fig. 32.48).
- Involvement of the tendon and belly is characteristic.
- Internal reflectivity is homogenous and low due to diffuse infiltration of the muscle fibres by inflammatory cells.
- Adjacent involvement of the episclera in the form of Tenon's widening may be seen.
- In addition, lacrimal gland enlargement and optic nerve thickening may occur.

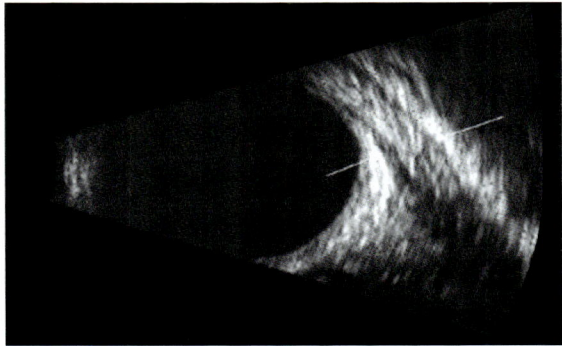

Fig. 32.48: *B scan of the orbit in a patient with nonspecific myositis.*

LACRIMAL GLAND TUMOURS

Pleomorphic adenoma

- B scan in a patient with pleomorphic adenoma shows a well-defined round to oval encapsulated lesion (Fig. 32.49A)
- Medium to highly reflective regular internal structure (Fig. 32.49B)
- Moderate sound attenuation
- May contain cystic cavities
- Bony excavation of the adjacent orbital wall may be seen but there is no bone destruction.

Adenoid cystic carcinoma

- B scan in a patient with adenoid cystic carcinoma reveals a well-circumscribed infiltrative lesion (Fig. 32.50)
- Medium to highly reflective irregular internal structure

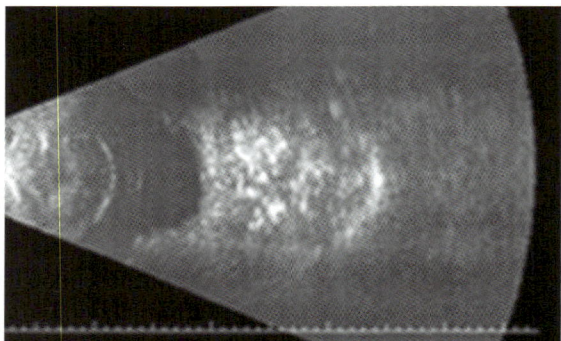

Fig. 32.49A: *B scan ultrasonography orbit showing lacrimal gland tumour with well-defined borders and multiple foci of calcium.*

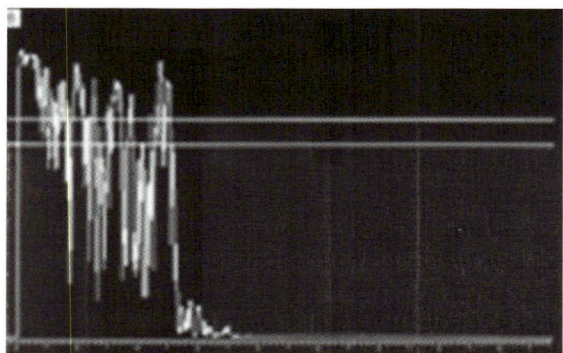

Fig. 32.49B: *A scan ultrasonography showing internal structure and high reflectivity produced by calcium.*

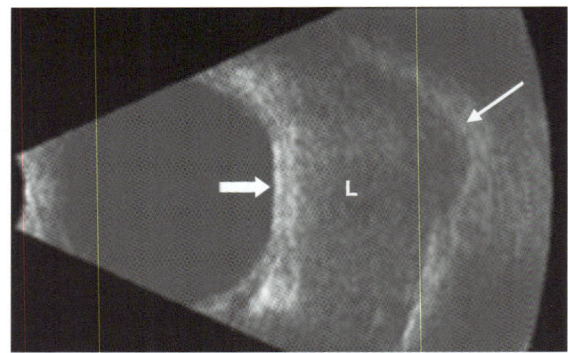

Fig. 32.50: *B scan of the orbit in a patient with adenoid cystic carcinoma lacrimal gland.*

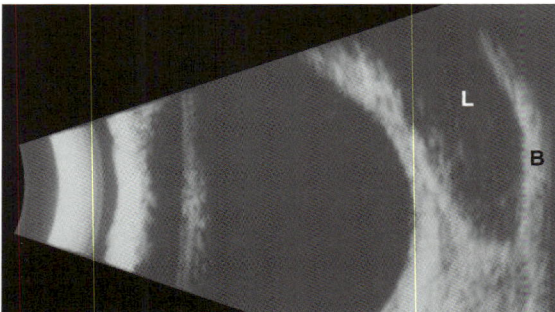

Fig. 32.51: *B scan of the orbit in a patient lymphoma lacrimal gland.*

- Moderate to strong sound attenuation
- Often contain cystic cavities
- Calcification may be seen
- Bony destruction of adjacent orbital wall.

Lymphomas

- B scan in a patient with lymphoma shows an irregular mass due to lack of a capsule (Fig. 32.51)
- Low reflective
- Low sound attenuation
- Do not indent the globe but tend to mould around it
- Do not cause changes in the adjacent bony wall.

COLOUR DOPPLER IMAGING

Colour Doppler ultrasonography (CDI) is a useful diagnostic tool for assessment of orbital, ocular and optic nerve blood flow. It allows the display of blood flow characteristics on a real-time grey-scale B-mode background. Role of CDI in investigation of orbital disorders was first reported in 1989. This noninvasive method is suitable to study vascular abnormalities involving central retinal artery, central retinal vein, posterior ciliary artery, ophthalmic artery and superior ophthalmic vein. It is also applied to assess hemodynamic changes in the orbital vasculature. Doppler imaging is based on the Doppler principle that frequency of sound waves emanating from a source depends on the relative movement between the source and the receiver. Conventional B-mode (brightness modulated) ultrasound imaging requires the use of a transducer to provide information about an acoustical cross-section of a tissue which is eventually displayed in a two-dimensional grey-scale. Duplex scanning is a technology combining B scan with Doppler analysis that enables the gathering of Doppler information from known locations as represented in the B scan image.

PROCEDURE

CDI examination of the globe and orbit is performed with the patient in the supine position, through closed eyelids. The transducer is applied to the closed eyelids using an ultrasonic contact gel (sterile methylcellulose). Doppler imaging is ideally performed parallel to the direction of movement, i.e. at an angle of 0°. Scans can be performed in vertical and horizontal planes. Pressure on the globe should be avoided as it can lead to artifactual decrease in blood flow velocity. For ophthalmic applications, linear transducers with sound frequencies ranging from 7.5 to 15 MHz are preferred. Colour flow information is used to depict the major vascular structures in the orbit, which can be displayed in either blue or red. Colour parameters can be subjectively assigned regarding the direction of the blood flow with respect to the transducer. In general, the flow moving towards the transducer is displayed in red and away from it, is showed in blue. Orbital vessels are frequently parallel to the sound beam, thus, for the majority of the time arteries are displayed

in red and veins in blue. A pulsed Doppler spectral analysis is also obtained to distinguish between arterial and venous flow.

INDICATIONS AND ADVANTAGES OF COLOUR DOPPLER IMAGING

Indictions

- Differentiation of neoplasms from subretinal and choroidal haemorrhages.
- Characterisation of vascularity of intraocular and orbital tumours.
- Follow up of orbital tumours treated with radiotherapy.
- Study of vascular disorders of the orbit such as central artery or vein occlusions, orbital arteriovenous malformations, superior ophthalmic vein thrombosis and orbital varix.
- Optic nerve head pathologies or miscellaneous disorders such as severe myopia, glaucoma or diabetes.
- Diagnosis of caroticocavernous fistula and their follow-up after embolisation.
- Transient ischaemic attack.
- Significant arteriosclerosis on ophthalmoscopy.

Advantages of CDI

- Not using radiation
- Ease of use
- Portability of equipment.

COLOUR DOPPLER IMAGING (CDI) IN OCULAR AND ORBITAL DISORDERS

Carotid Disease

- Reduced blood flow velocities in the ophthalmic artery (OA) or reversal of flow, indicated by blue encoding of OA blood flow on the colour image and negative blood flow measurements with temporal spectral analysis (Fig. 32.52).
- If reversal of flow is present, this may also be detected in the supraorbital and supratrochlear arteries.

Central retinal artery occlusion

- The most important signal demonstrated in CRA occlusion is lack or minimum blood flow in the CRA, with both decreased maximum systolic amplitude and diastolic flow (Fig. 32.53).

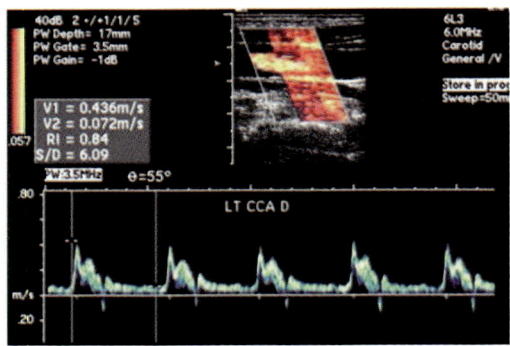

Fig. 32.52: *Colour Doppler imaging in a patient with carotid disease.*

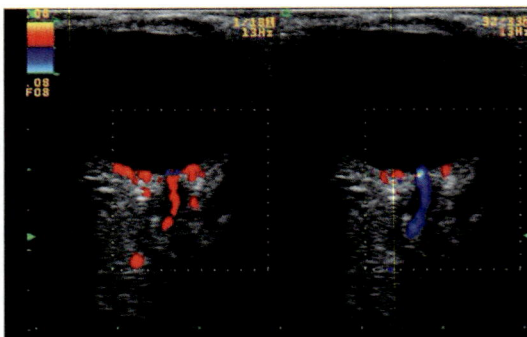

Fig. 32.54: *Colour Doppler imaging in a patient with central retinal vein occlusion.*

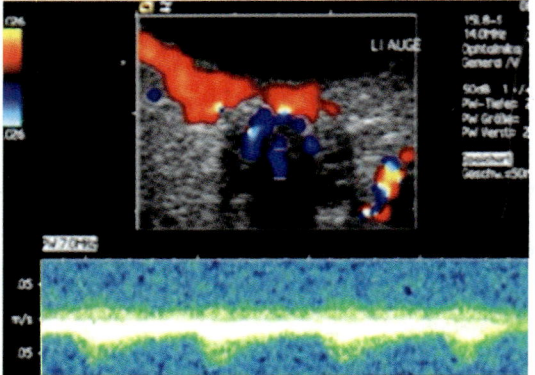

Fig. 32.53: *Colour Doppler imaging in a patient with central retinal artery occlusion.*

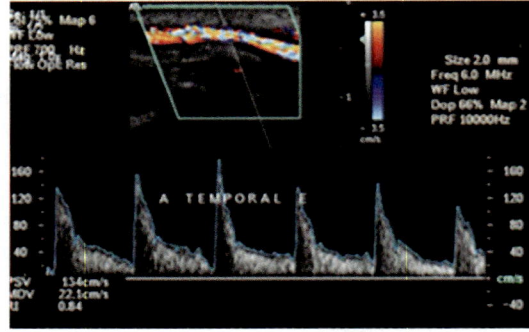

Fig. 32.55: *Longitudinal colour Doppler image of temporal artery showing a zone of stenosis.*

- Reduced blood flow velocities and increased pulsatility of flow on spectral analysis.

Central retinal vein (CRV) occlusion

- In CRV occlusion, the blockage of venous outflow generates a condition of high resistance microvasculature.
- This is demonstrated by CDI as an absence or decrease in magnitude of both maximum and minimum venous velocity in the CRV, as well as decreasing in peak systolic velocity and decreasing in end-diastolic velocity (Fig. 32.54).

Giant cell arteritis

- Markedly reduced blood flow velocities
- Highly elevated pulsatilities in posterior ciliary arteries and central retinal artery (Fig. 32.55)

- In temporal arteritis a hypoechoic, dark area may be found around the perfused lumen of the temporal arteries.

Ocular ischaemic syndrome

- Markedly reduced peak systolic velocity and increased vascular resistance in ocular end arteries such as the central retinal and posterior ciliary arteries (Fig. 32.56).
- Ophthalmic artery reversal of flow seems to represent collateral blood flow to lower resistance vascular beds.

Carotid-cavernous fistula

- CDI studies show increased blood flow velocity with arterialisation of flow, i.e. development of a pulsatile arterial-type flow pattern in superior ophthalmic vein (Fig. 32.57).
- Reduced OA flow is also sometimes detected.

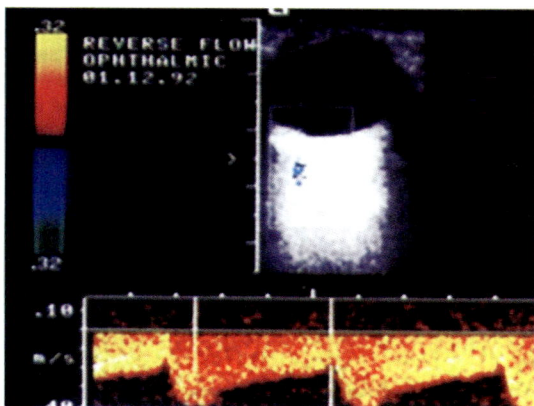

Fig. 32.56: *Colour Doppler image showing reversal of flow in ophthalmic artery.*

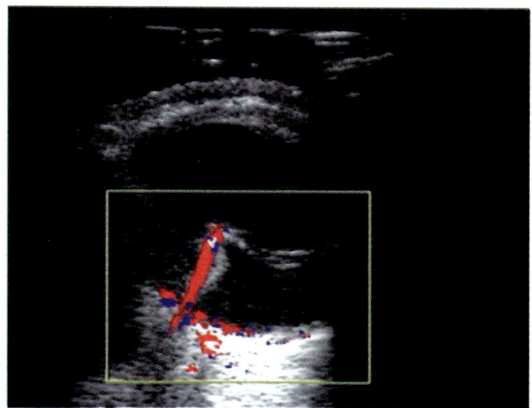

Fig. 32.58: *Colour Doppler image in a patient with retinal detachment.*

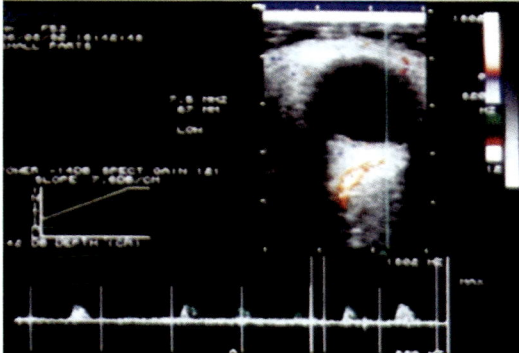

Fig. 32.57: *Colour Doppler image showing reversed pulsatile waveform and reversal of flow in superior ophthalmic vein.*

- CDI may also show normalisation of blood flow parameters following active treatment of CCF.

Retinal detachment

- CDI is helpful in differentiating a detached retina from a dense vitreous band through retinal vasculature in cases where ophthalmoscopy is not feasible.
- The blood flow velocity in the retrobulbar central retinal, short posterior and ophthalmic arteries was decreased in eyes with retinal detachment compared to those of control subjects (Fig. 32.58).
- Eyes with proliferative vitreoretinopathy had lower blood flow velocity and higher RI in the ophthalmic artery than eyes without proliferative vitreoretinopathy, indicating a possible

role of altered circulation in the development of this condition.

Persistent hyperplastic primary vitreous

- Persistent hyperplastic primary vitreous demonstrates the patency of the persistent hyaloid artery.
- Using CDI, blood flow is demonstrable in the persistent hyaloid artery (Fig. 32.59).

Orbital varix

- Orbital varix demonstrate dilated superior ophthalmic vein with low blood flow velocities (Fig. 32.60).
- Hemodynamic changes induced by position or by Valsalva manoeuvre can be recorded by CDI.

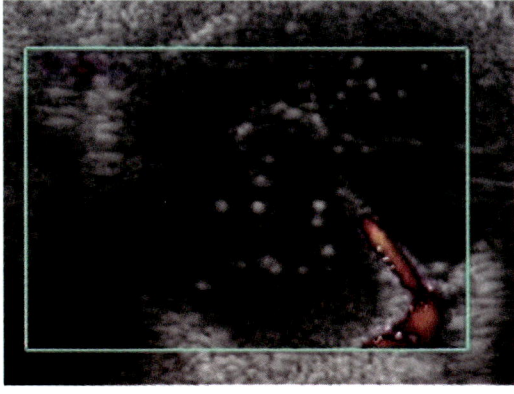

Fig. 32.59: *Colour Doppler image in a patient with persistent hyperplastic primary vitreous.*

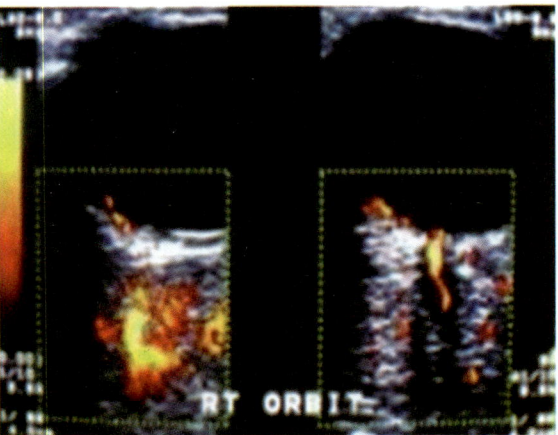

Fig. 32.60: *Colour Doppler image in a patient with orbital varix.*

Anterior ischaemic optic neuropathy (AION)

* CDI of AION demonstrates decreased flow velocities of the posterior ciliary arteries (PCAs) with preserved flow of the CRA and CRV (Fig. 32.61).

Orbital tumours

* Assessment of the vascularity of the tumours.
* Differentiation of vascular from nonvascular tumours and malignant from benign lesions.

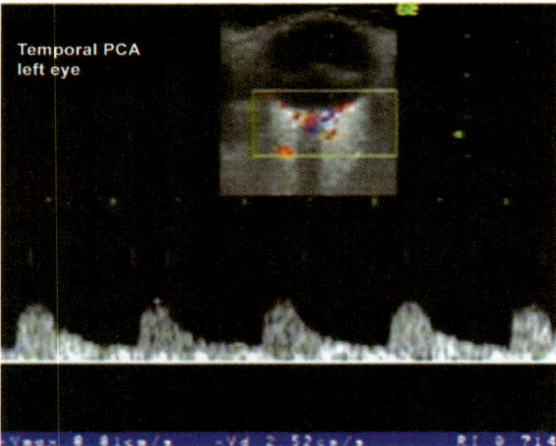

Fig. 32.61: *Colour Doppler image in a patient with anterior ischaemic optic neuropathy diminution of blood flow velocities (especially end-diastolic velocities) in the temporal PCA of the affected left.*

Ocular tumours

* Malignant intraocular lesions have easily demonstrable pulsatile and nonpulsatile blood flow as compared with benign lesions.
* Effective treatment of intraocular tumours results in a reduction of Doppler frequency shift signals recorded from such lesions, indicating reduced vascularity with therapy.
* CDI has come to play an important role in tumour blood flow assessment, not only in displaying tumour microvasculature (Colour Doppler signals) but also in allowing functional analysis (spectral analysis).

Diabetic retinopathy

* The blood flow velocity in the central retinal artery in diabetic patients without diabetic retinopathy was significantly decreased than in control subjects (Fig. 32.62).
* In nonproliferative and in proliferative diabetic retinopathy the reduction of blood flow velocity and the increase of the indices of resistivity was most evident in the central retinal, but also in the short posterior ciliary artery and in the ophthalmic arteries.
* The blood flow velocities in the central retinal, short posterior, ophthalmic arteries and in the central retinal vein decreased after panretinal photocoagulation of diabetic retinopathy.

Retinopathy of prematurity

* The blood flow velocity in the central retinal and ophthalmic artery of premature infants

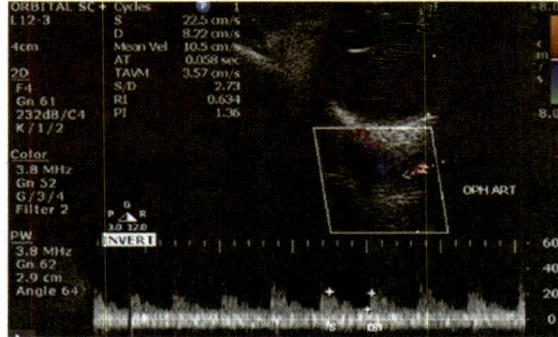

Fig. 32.62: *Colour Doppler image in a patient with diabetic retinopathy.*

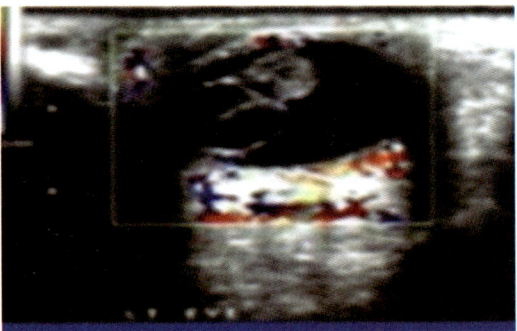

Fig. 32.63: *Colour Doppler image in a patient with retinopathy of prematurity.*

with retinopathy of prematurity (ROP) was significantly increased than in control subjects (Fig. 32.63).

Age-related macular degeneration

- In non-exudative ARMD (including early, intermediate and advanced stages of ARMD) the blood velocity in the central retinal artery and short posterior ciliary arteries decreased and the RI in those arteries increased (Fig. 32.64).
- In exudative ARMD, the blood flow parameters were altered in the short posterior ciliary artery that suggests a compromised choroidal circulation.
- The alteration typically consisted of increased RI in the short posterior ciliary artery.
- After treatment with intravitreal anti-VEGF (bevacizumab), an initial decrease of the blood flow velocity in the central retinal and short

posterior ciliary arteries had been detected in the early postoperative period, but returned to preoperative values after one month.

Myopia

- Colour Doppler imaging in myopia shows decreased blood velocity in the central retinal artery and vein and in the short posterior ciliary artery in affected eyes versus control eyes (Fig. 32.65).
- The pathoanatomic aspects of degenerative myopia include thinning and atrophy of the choroid and retina, decrease of the caliber and straightening of the retinal blood vessels, scarce choroidal arteries and thinning and loss of choriocapillaris.
- All of these characteristics are consistent with the CDI findings that suggest a decreased blood flow in the retina and choroid in degenerative myopia.
- In patients with myopic choroidal neovascularisation, the RI in the short posterior ciliary arteries was increased, suggesting that compromised choroidal circulation may be involved in the pathogenesis of choroidal neovascularisation.

Retinitis pigmentosa

- The blood flow velocity and the RI in the central retinal artery was decreased in patients compared with those of control subjects (Fig. 32.66).
- Peak systolic blood velocity was also decreased in the short posterior and ophthalmic arteries of patients as compared to normal subjects.

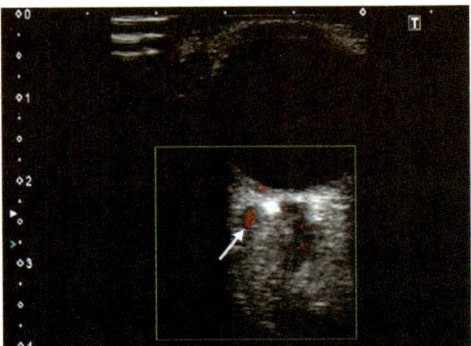

Fig. 32.64: *Colour Doppler echography of the posterior temporal ciliary artery in patient with age-related macular degeneration.*

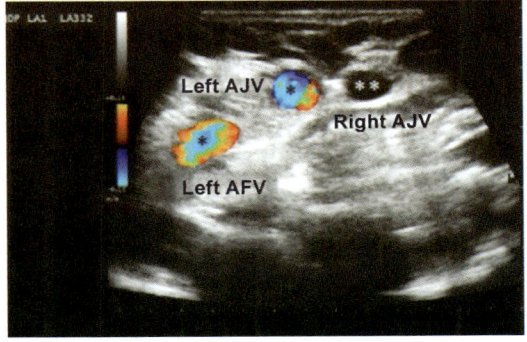

Fig. 32.65: *Colour Doppler image in a patient with myopia.*

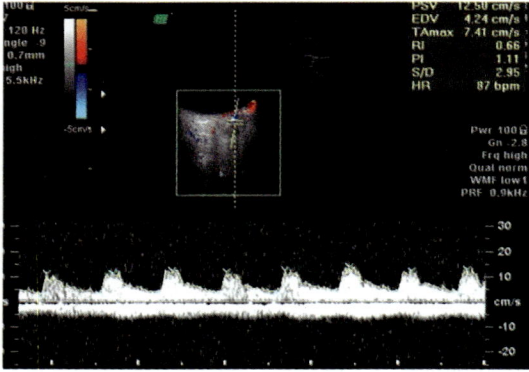

Fig. 32.66: *Colour Doppler image in a patient with retinitis pigmentosa.*

ULTRASOUND BASED SPECIAL INVESTIGATIONS

ULTRASOUND BIOMICROSCOPY

Ultrasound biomicroscopy is a method of imaging the eye at microscopic resolution. It can be used to image any ocular disorder that falls within the penetration limits of sound at high frequencies.

Comparison of B scan and UBM

Characteristic	B scan	UBM
Probe frequency	10 MHz	50 MHz
Depth	4 cm	4 mm
Resolution	940 μ	30–40 μ
Use	To evaluate posterior segment disorders	To evaluate anterior segment disorders

Note: For details on UBM *see* Chapter 33.

HIGH-INTENSITY FOCUSED ULTRASOUND CIRCULAR CYCLOCOAGULATION IN GLAUCOMA PATIENTS

High-intensity focused ultrasound (HIFU) is a technique that uses high-powered transducers to noninvasively treat lesions with volumes as small as 20 mm^3 without affecting intervening tissues (Fig. 32.67). HIFU induces hyperthermia and cavitation, resulting in coagulative necrosis. HIFU systems consist of a power amplifier, pulse generator, therapeutic transducer and a 3D positioning system. HIFU systems generally emit ultrasound frequencies in the range of 1 to 5 MHz and generate focal intensities on the order of 1000 to 10000 W cm^2 in less than 3 seconds. Consequently, temperatures greater than 80°C are routinely attained within lesions during HIFU therapy. Coupling cone made of polymer is placed in direct contact with the eye, which allows good placement of the transducers in terms of centration and distance. At the base of the coupling cone, a suction ring allows the application of a low-level vacuum and enables the cone to maintain contact with the eye. A 30 mm diameter, 15 mm-high ring containing six active piezoelectric elements is inserted in the upper part of the coupling cone. The cavity created between the eye, the cone and the probe (4 ml) is filled with saline solution at room temperature. It aims to achieve a selective and precise cyclocoagulation of the ciliary body while sparing the adjacent ocular structures. The most common complications of ocular HIFU

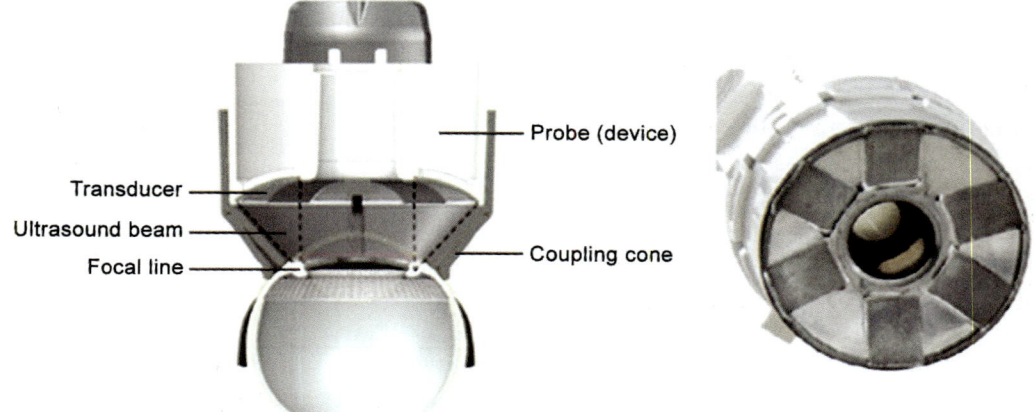

Probe (device)

Transducer

Ultrasound beam

Focal line

Coupling cone

Fig. 32.67: *High-intensity focused ultrasound circular cyclocoagulation machine placed over eye.*

procedures include an immediate rise in intra-ocular pressure and mild iritis. The development of cataracts, phthisis bulbi, and thinning of the sclera are less common complications, with incidences of about 2.5% or less.

ULTRASOUND-GUIDED FINE NEEDLE ASPIRATION BIOPSY

Indications

- Suspected orbital metastasis
- Orbital abscess
- Orbital mass
- Orbital haematoma.

Procedure

- The lesion is first evaluated on ultrasound
- 22 gauge needle mounted on a 5 cc syringe is used
- Infiltration of a local anaesthetic is performed around the proposed site of needle puncture. In children it is performed under general anaesthesia
- The area of the biopsy site is cleaned
- As the needle is introduced, the probe is used to scan longitudinally along the path to visualize the needle along its length
- Once the needle is inside the lesion, the required quantity of material is aspirated
- The needle is withdrawn along the same path, visualizing its exit on ultrasound.

Complications

- Globe perforation with the needle
- Orbital haemorrhage
- Damage to the optic nerve
- Seeding of the tumour along the needle path
- Ocular motility disturbances
- Ptosis.

OCULAR ULTRASOUND-GUIDED ANAESTHESIA

Ophthalmic regional anaesthesia can be achieved through retrobulbar block, peribulbar block, sub-Tenon's block and topical anaesthesia with or without intracameral injection. The choice of specific anaesthesia delivery technique is influenced by patient desires, the extent, type and duration of surgery, and the preferences and experience of the ophthalmologist.

Rationale for USG-guided anaesthesia

Needle misadventure and penetration or perforation of the globe, leading to the potential long-term visual compromise are the most feared complications of ophthalmic anaesthesia. Needle-based eye blocks are 'blind' techniques that are dependent upon surface anatomy landmarks in order to position the needle correctly. Ultrasound A or B scan may provide information as to the globe's axial length and morphology of the eye in order to detect an atypically long or asymmetric, possibly staphylomatous eye. Fundamentally, an RBB is conducted by intentionally angling the needle steeply and deeply within the orbit behind the globe. If the globe is longer than anticipated, or a staphyloma is prominent, greater risk of needle injury to the eye's posterior portion exists. Using ultrasound to visualize important anatomy during the procedure may be of utility.

Purportedly, there is less likelihood to puncture or perforate the globe when one is using a PBB, which entails shallower needle placement with less angulation towards the orbital apex. However, longer globes have greater volume and increased superior/inferior girth, thus exposing the inferior aspect to needle trauma. A transducer frequency of 6 to 13 MHz can readily distinguish between orbital contents and needle and may be an optimal compromise between penetration and resolution frequency priorities.

A regional ophthalmic block is performed only after confirming the correct patient, procedure, and side of surgery. In order to maintain the optic nerve in a slack state, such that it does not impinge upon the needle's path, the patient is instructed to remain in neutral gaze. The proper orientation between the operator and the ultrasound monitor is obtained by standing nearest to the side to be blocked and positioning the monitor in line of sight on the opposite side of the patient's head, such that one may visualize the surgical field and the monitor simultaneously. Water-soluble ultrasound transmission gel is liberally applied to the eyelid. The transducer is positioned just below the supraorbital rim over the upper eyelid and a transocular image of the globe wall and surrounding orbital space are obtained. Incremental angulation of the transducer can bring the needle into clearer view. Altering the depth and sound wave frequency, using medium gain, is also useful.

RECENT ADVANCES IN ULTRASONOGRAPHY

CONTRAST ENHANCED ULTRASONOGRAPHY

Contrast agents used in ultrasonography consist of air- or gas-filled micronized bubbles surrounded by a lipid shell. These agents may be easily introduced intravascularly without generating a host response. Contrast imaging can be performed in either linear or nonlinear fashion.

- The linear mode of acquisition involves B mode imaging of tissue perfused with contrast agents followed by application of a reference subtraction algorithm to enable segmentation of contrast from tissue.

- Nonlinear acquisition and analysis provides a more sensitive method for delineation of contrast and tissue.

Microbubble contrast agents can be non-targeted for general imaging and analysis of tumour volume or organ perfusion, or tagged with specific ligands (streptavidin–biotin system) to quantify expression of endothelial cell surface receptors. Currently available targeted contrast agents include microbubbles conjugated to ligands that target receptors involved in tumour angiogenesis and inflammation such as vascular endothelial growth factor receptor 2 (VEGFR2), p-selectin, integrins, vascular cell adhesion molecule, and platelet cellular adhesion molecule. It improves the contrast differences between tissues through enhancing the strength of reflection signals, and in particular, it can improve the detectable rate of the microvascular, low-velocity and low-flow blood signals, and can display the blood perfusion features in tissues. Use of contrast agent enhances the backscatter echo, so as to signifi-

cantly improve the resolution, sensitivity and specificity of the ultrasonic diagnosis.

Procedure of CEUS

A 22-gauge needle is inserted into the antecubital vein of the left arm and a 4.8 ml contrast agent is injected as a rapid bolus. The line is then flushed with 10 ml saline to accelerate entry of the contrast medium into the bloodstream. The vasculature can then be observed for about 180s, the duration of the perfusion time prior to complete washout.

As compared to CT and MRI, CEUS is cost-effective, portable, produces no ionizing radiation, has no nephrotoxicity, and, most importantly, can provide comparable diagnostic information. Current applications of CEUS are for imaging visceral organs, abdominal aorta. Genitourinary system, and breasts when standard ultrasound is inconclusive. In the realm of ophthalmic ultrasonography, UCA has been reported to slightly improve the detection of small vessels in uveal melanoma and helps differentiate a solid tumour from subretinal haemorrhage or effusion. However, CEUS does not distinguish normal vessels from tumoural vessels. CEUS has been combined with Doppler ultrasound to improve differentiation of retinal detachment from vitreous membrane. Microbubble contrast agents may also be used to deliver drugs or genes to cells.

COMPOUND IMAGING

Spatial compound ultrasound imaging is a technique that uses electronic beam steering to acquire several overlapping scans of an object from different view angles. Each single angle scan is then averaged to create a multi angle image. This can be performed in real-time. The advantage of compound imaging over conventional ultrasound is reduction of speckle and clutter, resulting in better defined tissue boundaries. This technique is particularly well-suited for imaging rounded structures such as the globe.

THREE- AND FOUR-DIMENSIONAL ULTRASOUND

Three-dimensional ultrasonography is a system developed in Toronto, Canada that reconstructs multiple consecutive two-dimensional B scan images to create a three-dimensional block. The probe is held in fixed, transscleral orientation and serial images are rapidly obtained as the transducer rotates. Software transforms the data into a three-dimensional image that is able to be sectioned in longitudinal, transverse, oblique, and coronal views. Three-dimensional ultrasound has been shown to be useful in clinical settings, including estimating the volume of intraocular lesion and evaluating the retrobulbar optic nerve.

Three-dimensional (3D) ultrasound is a technique in which an image of a volume is acquired in real time, whereas 4D ultrasound consists of acquiring a set of 3D images over time. Image acquisition can be accomplished using 2D arrays or 1D probes with attached or integrated position sensors. 3D/4D ultrasound allows for evaluation of the foetal face using surface rendering, multiplanar, and multislice displays for interactive section. 3D and 4D ultrasound provide additional diagnostic information for evaluating the orbit. For example, these modalities enable prenatal diagnosis of anophthalmia when the fetal head position is unfavourable on 2D ultrasound. The reverse face view function is particularly helpful. 3D ultrasound also has applications beyond the prenatal period. This technology can readily depict retinoblastoma and associated features, such as retinal detachment, intratumoural calcifications, and orbital shadowing. Oblique and coronal views of the tumour and optic nerve can be retrospectively derived from 3D ultrasound data and are useful for analyzing intraneural spread of tumour. 3D ultrasound can also be used for ocular and tumour-volume analysis.

C SCAN ULTRASOUND

C scan images are produced by sampling the ultrasound signal amplitude at fixed time intervals while the interrogating sensor is scanned over a surface. C scan ultrasound is particularly useful for measuring the optic nerve diameter and evaluating optic nerve sheath meningiomas and retinoblastoma invasion of the optic nerve. The C scan facility permits imaging of the orbital contents in the coronal plane. It has high resolution and sensitivity, thus it is a useful technique for demonstrating orbital lesions and helps in the accurate measurement of the diameters of the optic nerve along its length. The C scan technique used in conjunction with the B scan also permits three mutually perpendicular planes within the orbit to be visualised, such that the full extent and shape of a lesion can often be determined.

ULTRASOUND ELASTOGRAPHY

Elastography or elasticity imaging is a technique used to map tissue stiffness. Three main types of ultrasound elastography can be implemented: Compression strain imaging; external vibrations; acoustic radiation force or shear wave propagation through tissue using the ultrasound waves to determine the elastic modulus. Indeed, the greater stiffness of malignant tissues with respect to benign or normal tissues can be differentiated with this modality. Furthermore, ultrasound elastography can be used to monitor the effects of high intensity focused ultrasound during treatment. Treated lesions become stiffer, which manifests as decreased strain on elastograms. Orbital ultrasound elastography also appears to be feasible. The anterior vitreous has intermediate elasticity, while the posterior vitreous has low elasticity. The elasticity of the rectus muscles varies with position, being higher in neutral position than in adduction or abduction. In the case of the eyeball, the vitreous cavity displayed a heterogeneous appearance in both gray scale and colour-coded elastographic images. The signal from the anterior vitreous cavity corresponded to intermediate or high elasticity, whereas the signal from the posterior vitreous cavity corresponded to low elasticity.

FUSION IMAGING

Fusion imaging technique accurately assess the mechanical properties of tissues, differentiate normal from abnormal tissues and provide indications for the nature of tumours. The eye differs from other organs in which elastography has been applied so far because it is not solid and has a heterogeneous internal structure. The calculation of the elastic modulus of a tissue depends on assumptions on its properties (ideally the tissue should be incompressible, isotropic, and solid). Nevertheless, the fact that images obtained from all subjects were reproducible and compatible with the histologic characteristics of tissues examined imply that ultrasound electrography may be applied for the study of ocular and periocular structures. The possibility of evaluating the elastic properties of extraocular muscles by ultrasound elastography may be applied in conditions in which muscle rigidity is altered, such as Graves' orbitopathy, in which restrictive fibrotic changes render the affected tissues inelastic.

Fusion imaging is a process in which previously obtained corresponding MRI, CT, or positron emission tomography/CT images are overlaid upon or displayed adjacent to an ultrasound image during real-time scanning. This method is based on global positioning system technology and requires sensors situated next to the patient for coregistration. This technology allows ultrasound-guided procedures to be carried out for lesions that are otherwise inconspicuous on ultrasound. This modality can depict the position of various anatomical structures with respect to the surgical approach. Fusion of intraoperative ultrasound with preoperative CT or MRI has proven useful for guiding resections of complex frontobasal tumours affecting the orbits.

REMOTE AND ROBOTIC ULTRASOUND

There is a trend for compact, portable ultrasound units that can produce images of diagnostic quality for immediate expert interpretation over long distances. Lightweight six degrees-of-freedom robots have been developed. The robot holds and scans an ultrasound probe on a distant patient according to the expert hand movement. The acquired images can be transmitted via satellite or integrated digital network lines. These systems are feasible and effective, but are currently under testing.

PHOTOACOUSTIC IMAGING

Photoacoustic (PA) imaging is a noninvasive modality that combines optical and ultrasound imaging technology. The photoacoustic effect is a phenomenon in which ultrasound waves are generated by light absorbers in soft tissues exposed to a very short duration (~nanoseconds) pulsed laser beam in the near-infrared (NIR) region (wavelengths 700 to 1000 nm). These photoacoustic (PA) waves can be detected by one or more ultrasound sensors located on the surface of the structure being imaged. PA imaging has potential applications in early detection of cancer, guiding biopsy, imaging with targeted nanoparticles, and blood oxygen level determination. In addition, the differential tissue absorption spectra in the NIR can enable PA spectroscopy and functional imaging. Photoacoustic imaging is particularly useful for imaging optically deep structures without compromising the spatial resolution. The photoacoustic images show clear signals from the deep layers in the eye, including the choroid, sclera, and optic nerve. Such blood distribution information may be important for the diagnosis of wet age-related macular degeneration, as well as prove useful as a preclinical imaging tool for ophthalmic drug development. Photoacoustic imaging has been widely reported to be capable of visualizing various biological tissues. Compared to other ocular imaging modalities, photoacoustic imaging can achieve relatively deep penetration depth and more functional and cellular information based on photoacoustic signal generation from endogenous contrast agents such as hemoglobin and melanin. Moreover, a photoacoustic imaging system, such as a transducer and a data acquisition unit, is similar to a conventional ophthalmic ultrasound imaging system and effectively combined with it so that it is feasible to offer mechanical and morphological information in addition to functional and cellular data.

BIBLIOGRAPHY

1. Byrne SF, Green RL. Ultrasound of the eye and orbit. 2nd ed. St. Louis: Mosby Year Book; 2002.

2. Chaudhari HD, Thakkar GN, Gandhi VS, Darji PJ, Banker HK, Rajwadi H. Role of Ultrasonography in evaluation of orbital lesions. Gujarat Medical Journal 2013;68(2):73.

3. Coleman DJ. Reliability of ocular and orbital diagnosis with B scan ultrasound. Ocular diagnosis. Am J Ophthalmol. 1972 Apr;73(4):501–16.

4. Harrie RP. The ongoing role of ophthalmic ultrasound. Review of ophthalmology online 2011.

5. Sobottka B, Schlote T, Krumpaszky HG, Kreissig I. Choroidal metastases and choroidal melanomas: Comparison of ultrasonographic findings. Brit Journ Ophthal 1997;82:159–61.

6. Teismann N, Shah S, Nagdev A. Focus on: Ultrasound for acute retinal detachment. American College of Emergency Physicians 2009.

7. Waldron RG. Contact B scan Ultrasonography. Emory Eye Center. 2003:1–9.

Ultrasound Biomicroscopy (UBM) in Ophthalmology

Chapter Outline

UBM MACHINE
- Feachers
- Technique
- Advantages
- Indications

UBM APPEARANCE IN NORMAL AND DISEASED EYE
- UBM appearance of normal eye
- UBM appearance in eye diseases
  - UBM in patients with low vision after cataract surgery with IOL implantation

- UBM in glaucoma
- UBM in uveitis
- UBM before penetrating keratoplasty
- UBM for evaluation of ocular trauma
- UBM for mass lesions
- UBM in paediatric patient
- Measurements with UBM
- UBM after sugeries

UBM MACHINE

Ultrasound biomicroscopy (UBM) is the high frequency ultrasound imaging of the eye at microscopic resolution. The technique was originally developed by Charles J Pavlin, Francis Stuart Foster and Michael Sherar around 1990 at Toronto, Canada. Very high frequency (VHF) of ultrasound in the range of 40 to 100 MHz is utilized to provide subsurface details with resolution of optical microscopy without violating the integrity of the globe.[1]

Features

UBM is carried out with ophthalmic ultrasound machine. B scan transducer (10 MHz) uses lead zirconate titanate piezoelectric material. To achieve higher resolution at very high frequency (>35 MHz) for UBM transducer uses polymeric material known as polyvinylidene fluoride. Increased acoustic attenuation at VHF limits the penetration of sound waves in the tissues making only superficial structures accessible to UBM (Fig. 33.1).

Technique of Examination

The technique of examination using UBM is similar to conventional B scan examination. Patient lies down in supine position. Topical anaesthetic drops are instilled. Eye cup is placed to hold the eyelids open and filled with 1% methyl cellulose or sterile saline. Moving transducer is placed perpendicular to the structure of interest (Fig. 33.2).

The transducer moves linearly about 4 mm over the imaging field collecting back scatter data at each of 512 equally spaced lines. At higher frequencies penetration of sound waves is less. The resolution ranges from 20 to 60 micrometers with depth of penetration of

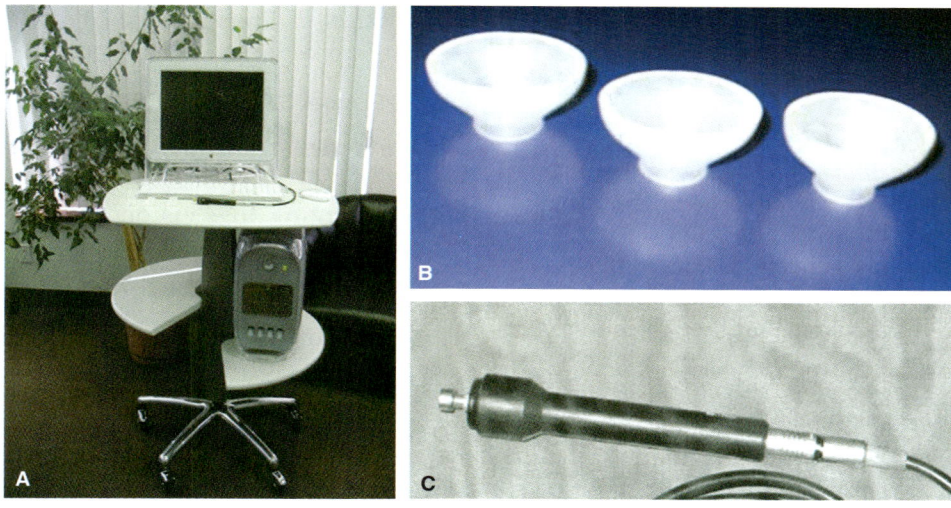

Fig. 33.1: (A) UBM machine; (B) Silicon cups; (C) Transducer.

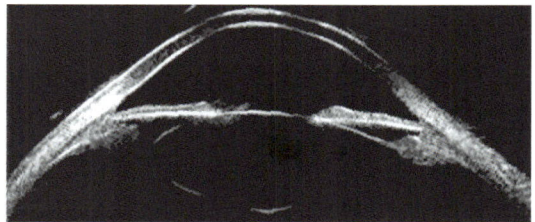

Fig. 33.2: Ultrasound biomicroscopic appearance of a normal eye.

approximately 4 mm². Practically this technique can be used to image any ocular structure that can be approached directly over the surface and falls within the penetration limits of sound waves. Cornea and anterior segment can be examined in any meridian. Conjunctiva, sclera and peripheral retina are examined by rotating the eye away. Adnexal structures having surface exposed can be examined. Penetration through skin and keratinized epithelium is poor due to sound attenuation. As shorter wavelength of high frequency sound allows finer positioning of end points, measurements of various ocular structures are more accurate.

Advantages of UBM

Initially it appears to be time consuming and inconvenient but once mastered, this technique gives excellent information. Its advantages are:

• This technique is very useful in presence of opaque media like corneal oedema, opacity, hyphaema and with non-dilating pupil as in uveitis with posterior synechiae.

• Deep angle structures, ciliary body and sulcus can be explored only by this technique.

• *Images derived by UBM are reproducible* and there is no inter observer variation. While inter observer variations are therein gonioscopy.

• *Anterior segment OCT is difficult in children*, in presence of corneal opacities and posterior boundary of pigmented lesion is inaccessible while UBM gives clear images in these situations.

Indications

UBM is very useful to study patients having low vision due to anterior segment complications after cataract surgery with IOL implantation, glaucoma diagnosis, glaucoma measurements, trauma, paediatric ocular problems, corneal edema due to various causes, ocular mass lesion, uveitis, congenital anterior segment anomalies, for identification and localization of anterior segment foreign bodies and pre/post kerato-plasty.

• *Adnexal and anteriorly placed ocular structures* must be subjected to UBM examination when-ever clinical examination falls short to arrive at the diagnosis.

• *Open globe injuries*, recent surgeries and gross ocular infection are the contraindications for the fear of contamination.

UBM APPEARANCE OF NORMAL AND DISEASED EYE

UBM APPEARANCE OF NORMAL EYE

- *Corneal epithelium and Bowman's* membrane appear asa high reflective layer. Features of normal eye UBM are (Fig. 33.2).
- *Stroma* is a homogeneous low reflective layer.
- *Endothelium and Descemet's membrane* cannot be differentiated; together they form a single, highly reflective line at the posterior corneal surface.
- *Aqueous human* appears echo free.
- *Iris* shows hypoechoic stroma and a high reflective posterior pigment epithelium.
- *Anterior and posterior lens capsule* appears as a bright line.
- *Lens cortex* is echo free.

- *Pars plicata and pars plana* of ciliary body and sulcus are very well-delineated.

UBM APPEARANCE IN EYE DISEASES

I. UBM in patients with low vision after cataract surgery with IOL implantation

Patients having low vision (<6/60) due to anterior segment complications after cataract surgery with IOL implantation can be studied. IOL malposition,[3] pseudophakic papillary block glaucoma with extensive iris bombé, pseudophakic corneal edema[4] and uveitis[5] are the commonest findings. In patients with pupillary block glaucoma with iris bombé, post LASER flattening of iris can be demonstrated by UBM.

1. IOL malpositions. When cornea is hazy UBM unravels different positions of IOL (Fig. 33.3A to F).

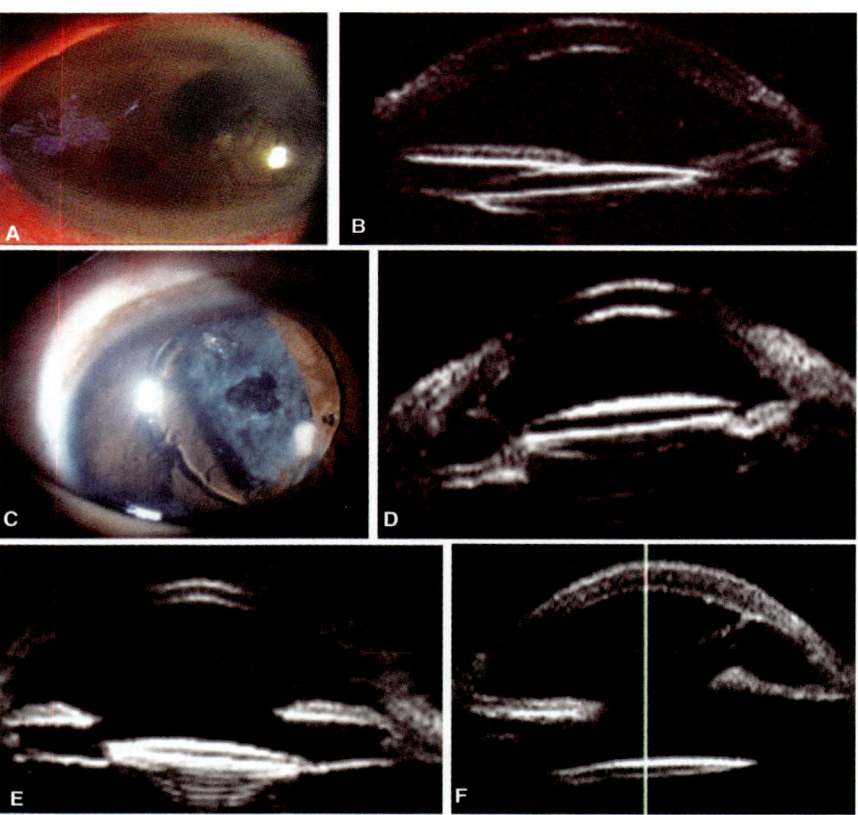

Fig. 33.3: *UBM findings in a patient with postsurgical corneal oedema: (A) Corneal oedema; (B) Tilted IOL, thick cornea echogenic stroma, inferior haptic in sulcus elevating the iris; (C) Thick capsule; (D) AC IOL vitreous in wound; (E) Scleral fixation IOL, away from iris, haptics approaching ciliary body; (F) IOL in vitreous, vitreous toughing endothelium.*

2. Pseudophakic glaucoma. Mechanism of raised intraocular pressure in a pseudophakic eye can be easily understood from its UBM appearance. (Fig. 33.4A to G).

3. Chronic postoperative uveitis. Uveal tissue irritation by optic or haptic touch or sighns of inflammations are well-delineated on UBM (Fig. 33.5A to D).

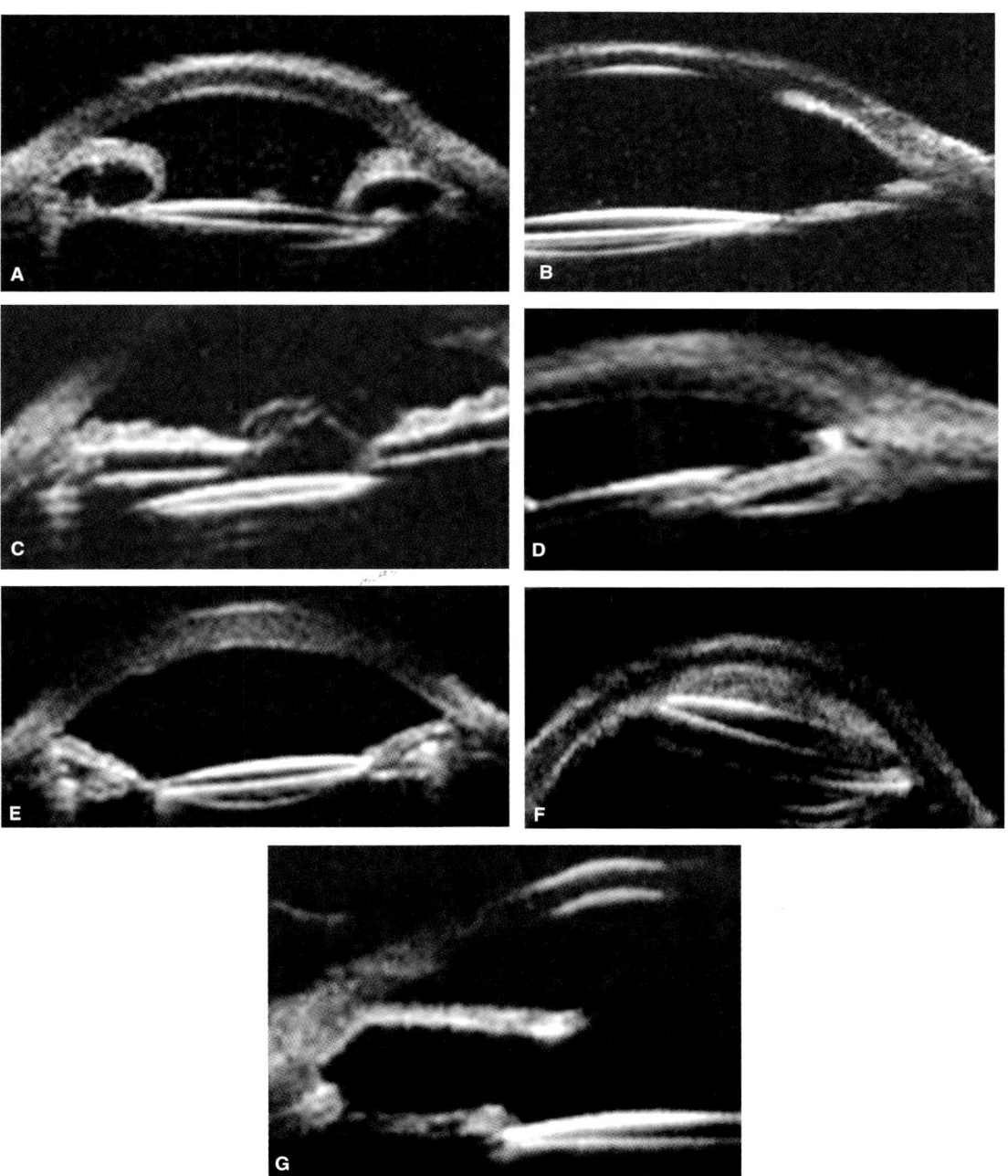

Fig. 33.4: *Common UBM finding in patients with pseudophakic glaucoma: (A) Posterior synechiae, iris bombé, PAS; (B) Anterior synechiae iris totally adherent to cornea; (C) Vitreous in pupil; (D) PC IOL in AC; (E) Optic capture thick haptic in angle; (F) Malignant glaucoma anterior chamber absent; (G) Neovascular glaucoma (angle zipped).*

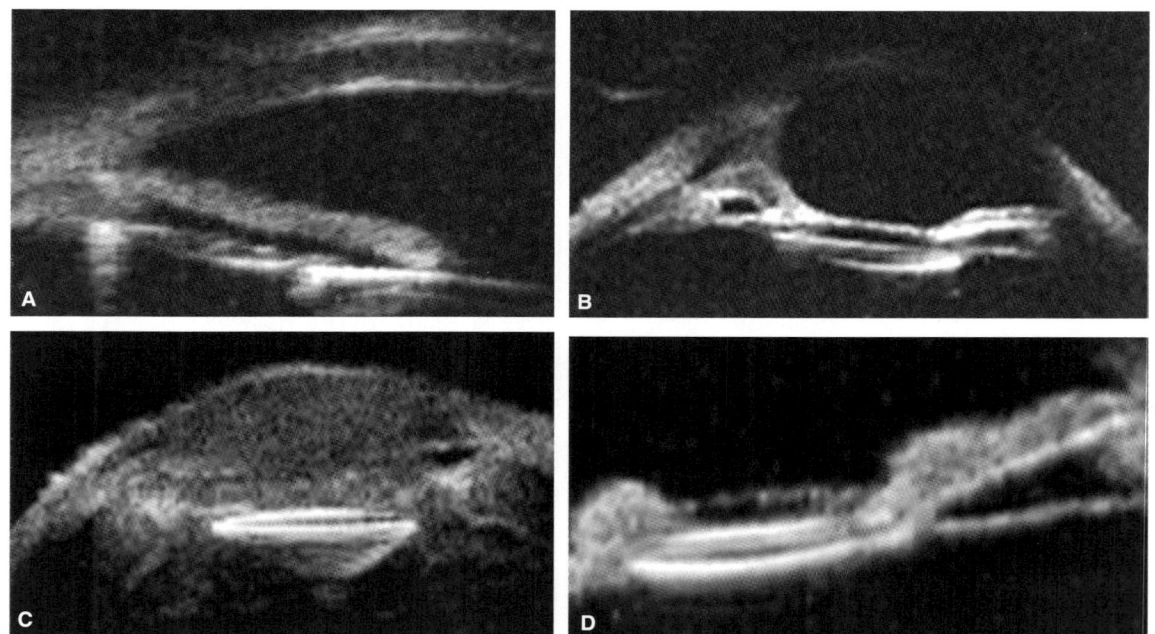

Fig. 33.5: *Common UBM finding in patients with chronic postoperative uveitis: (A) Haptic irritating CB; (B) Anterior and posterior synechiae;(C) Exudates in AC, corneal oedema; (D) Exudative membrane over IOL.*

4. Pseudophakic corneal oedema. Anterior chamber details that are hazy on slit-lamp can be well-visualized by UBM through corneal oedema. (Fig. 33.6A to C).

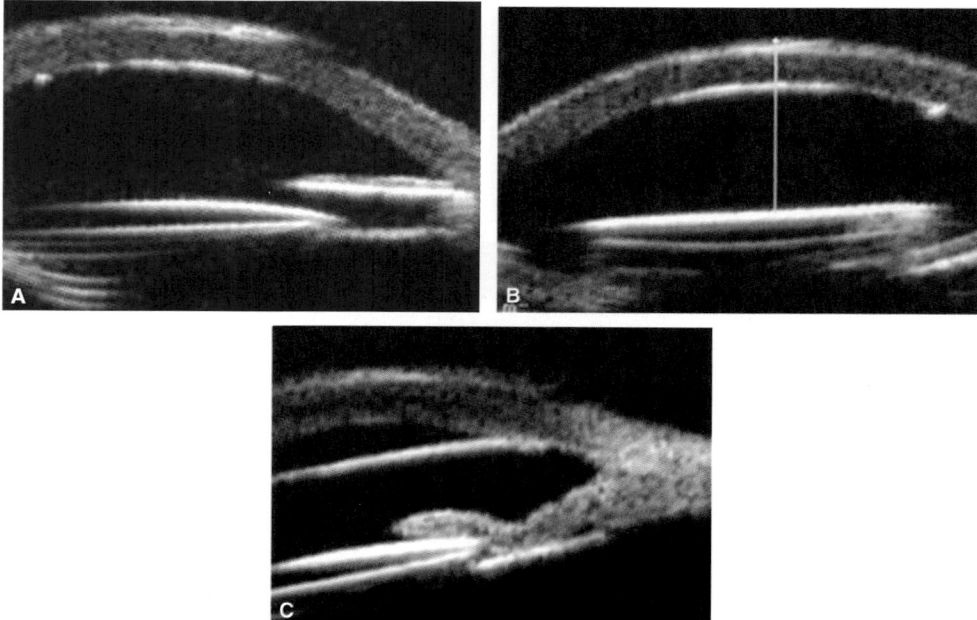

Fig. 33.6: *Some UBM finding in patients with pseudophakic coneal oedema: (A) Endothelial damage with PC IOL; (B) Endothelial damage with AC IOL; (C) Descemet's tear, optic capture, iris adherent to low.*

5. **Miscellaneous postoperative conditions** seen are depicted in Fig. 33.7A to F.

II. UBM in Glaucoma

Various types of glaucomas can be diagnosed with UBM (Fig. 33.8A to N). Apart from primary open angle and angle closure glaucoma and accurate measurements of various angle structures UBM helps to document Plateau iris very well. Flattening of iris following LASER iridotomy and effect of medicines and light on angle configuration can be demonstrated. Glaucoma due to iris and ciliary body mass is well-documented.

Post-traumatic glaucoma. Lesions due to injury to angle structures causing changes in intraocular pressure can be observed (Fig. 33.9A to C).

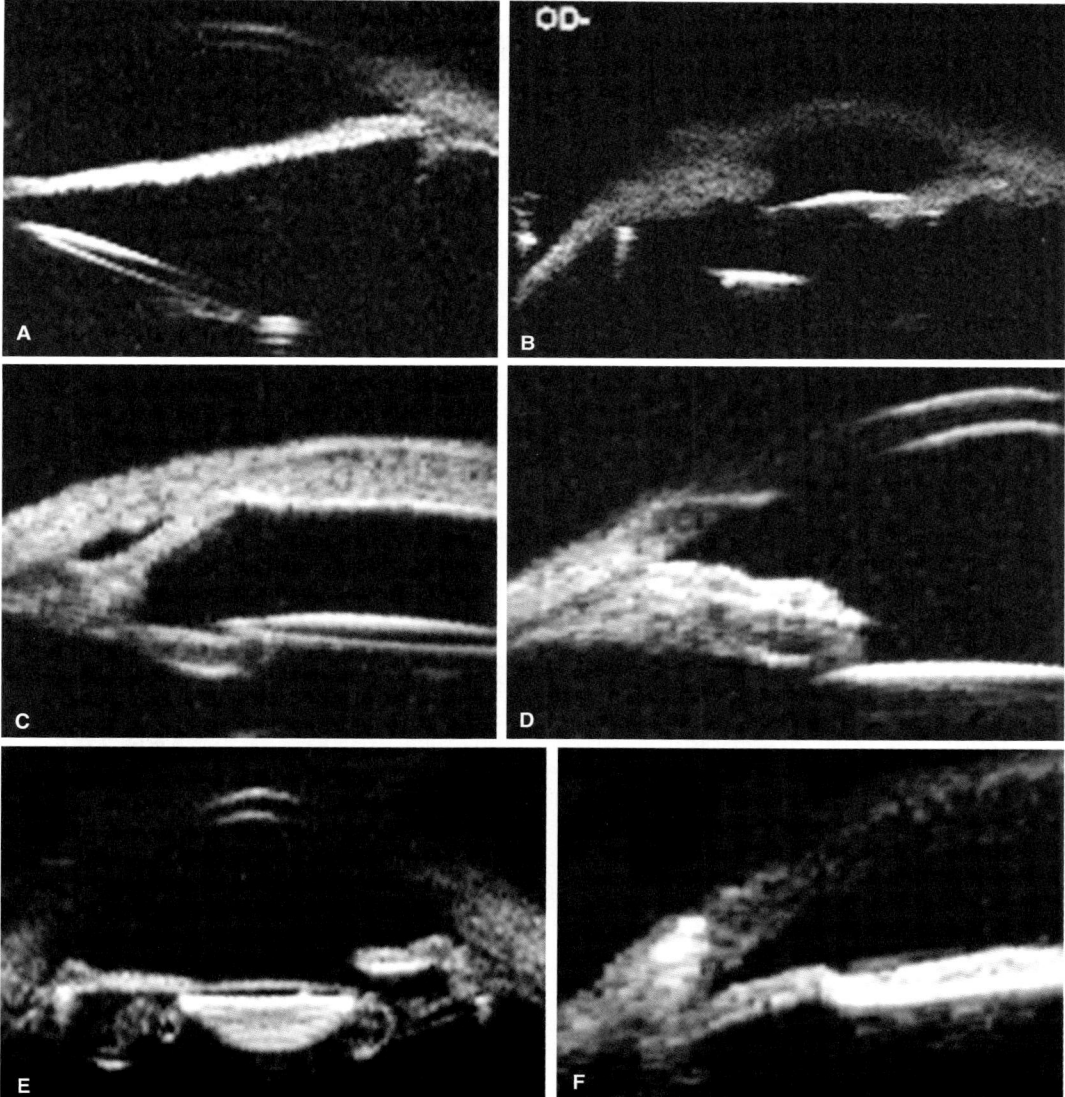

Fig. 33.7: *Some miscellaneous finding seen on UBM in patients with postoperative low vision: (A) Missing on slit-lamp examination seen floating in vitreous; (B) Two IOLs in the eye; (C) Corneal graft with pupil and vitreous synechiae at graft margin; (D) Surgical wound well-apposed; (E) Lens matter behind IOL after cataract; (F) Steel wire sutures optic capture.*

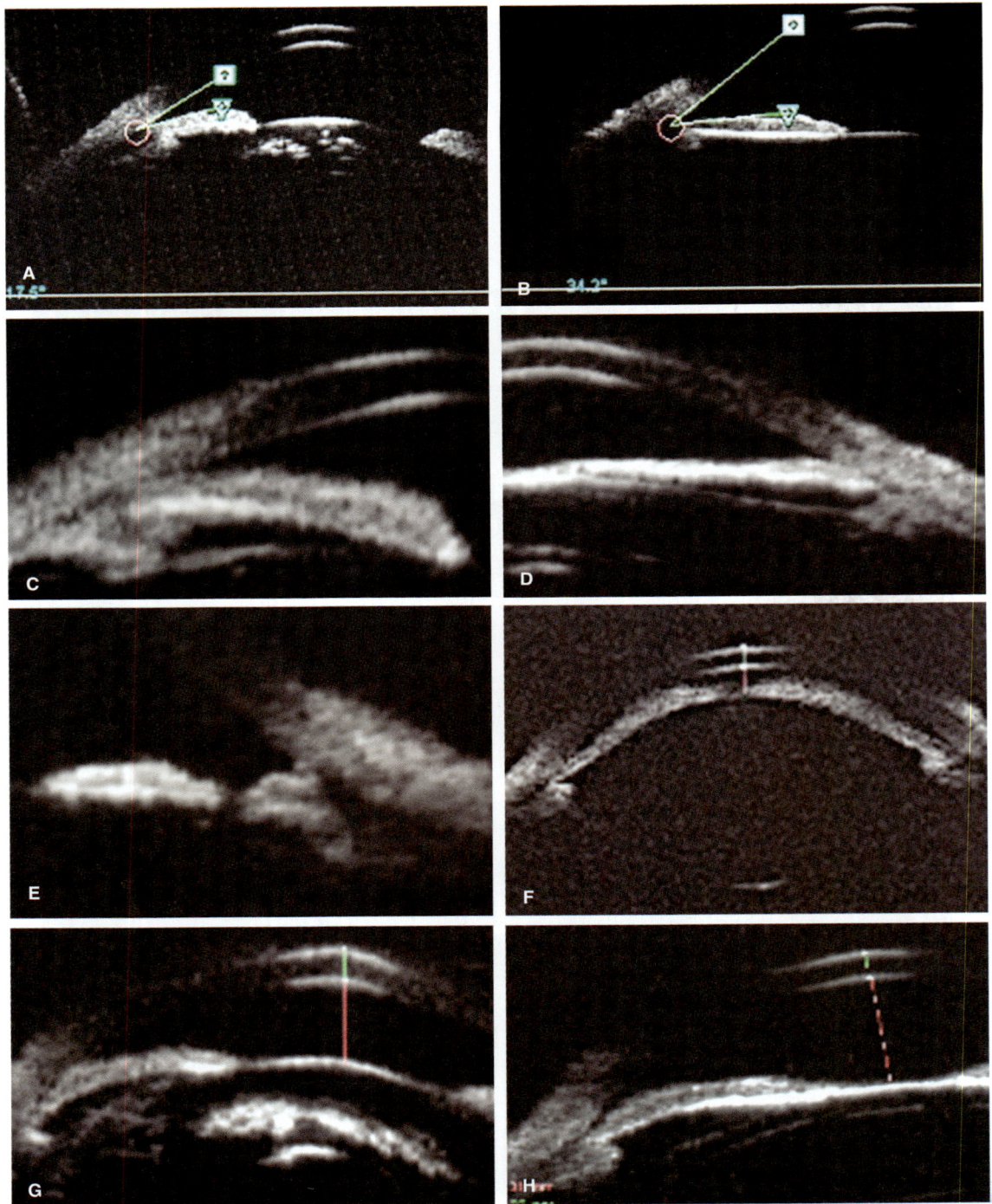

Fig. 33.8A to H: *Common UBM finding in patients with glaucoma: (A) Angle closure glaucoma; (B) Open angle glaucoma; (C) Slit like angle; (D) PAS; (E) LASER iridotomy; (F) Malignant glaucoma lens iris diaphragm pushed forward, no posterior chamber; (G) Phacomorphic glaucoma large cataractous lens, iris tightly apposed, posterior chamber absent; (H) Plateau iris ciliary process rotated anteriorly, double hump at angle due to ciliary body and iris.*

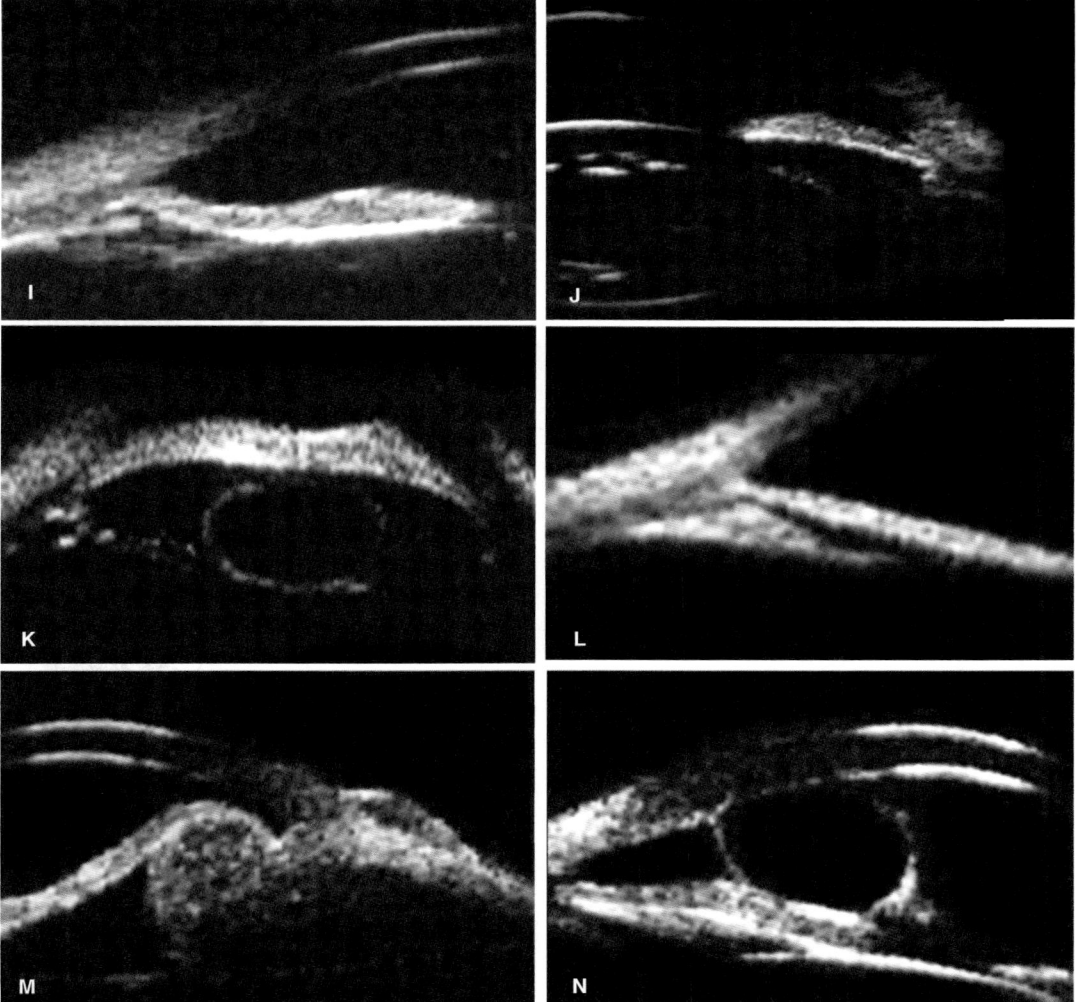

Fig. 33.8I to N: *Common UBM finding in patients with glaucoma: (I) Pigmentary glaucoma posterior bowing of mid peripheral iris rubbing zonula; (J) Pseudo exfoliation on lens and ciliary body; (K) Spherophakia, pupil block; (L) Buphthalmos long selender iris, finger like ciliary processes, deep anterior chamber; (M) Ciliary body mass pushing iris, invading angle and sclera; (N) Iris cyst blocking the angle.*

III. UBM in Uveitis

Signs of uveal inflammation like endothelial deposits, synechiae, exudate or membrane in AC, fibrosis and secondary lens changes are picked up on UBM (Fig. 33.10A to E).

Unexplained persistent mild ciliary congestion after cataract extraction usually turns out to be due to pars planitis as diagnosed by UBM (Fig. 33.10D).

IV. UBM before penetrating keratoplasty

Prognosis of the corneal graft can be predicted by assessing anatomical status of anterior segment preoperatively. In eyes with synechial angle closure graft is likely to fail. UBM aids in surgical planning for penetrating keratoplasty and anterior segment reconstruction[5] (Fig. 33.11A to F).

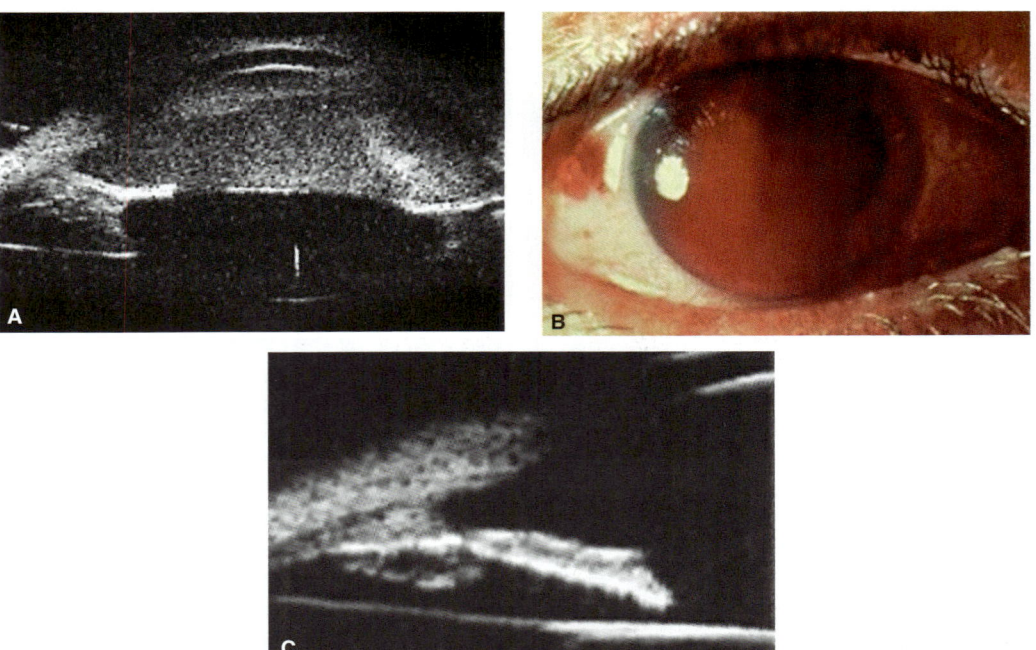

Fig. 33.9: *Common UBM finding in patients with post-traumatic glaucoma: (A) Blood in AC and PC; (B) Hyphaema; (C) Angle recession, CB receds from scleral spur, iris facts back.*

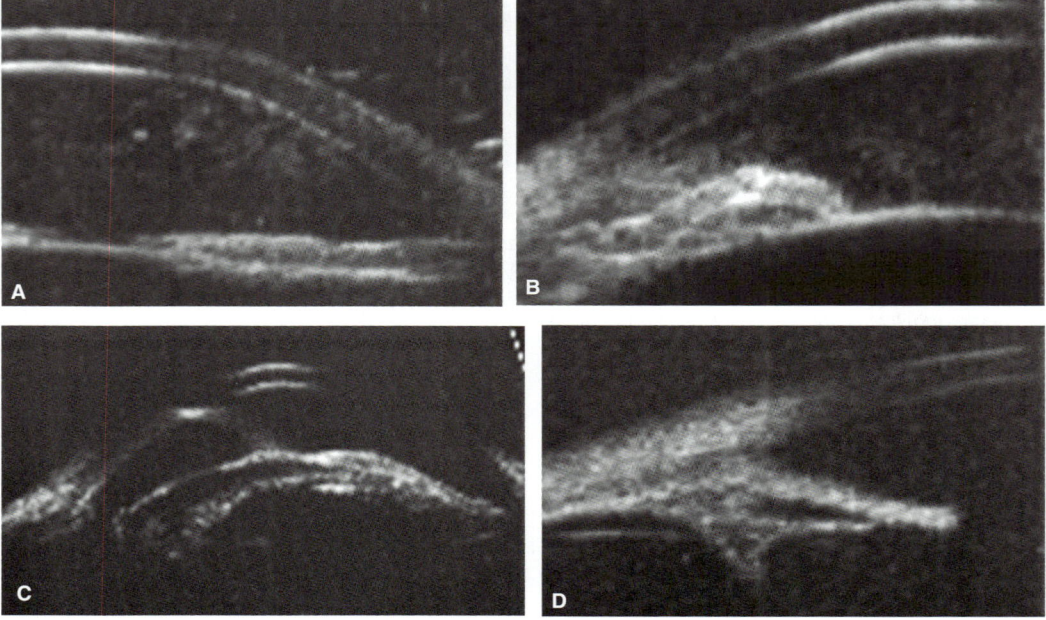

Fig. 33.10A to D: *Signs of uveal inflammation seen on UBM: (A) Total posterior synechiae iris adherent to lens, exudates in AC; (B) Ring synechiae, iris bombé, pupil margin adherent to lens, exudates in the angle; (C) Posterior synechiae iris bombé cataract; (D) Pars planitis, organized exudates near ciliary body.*

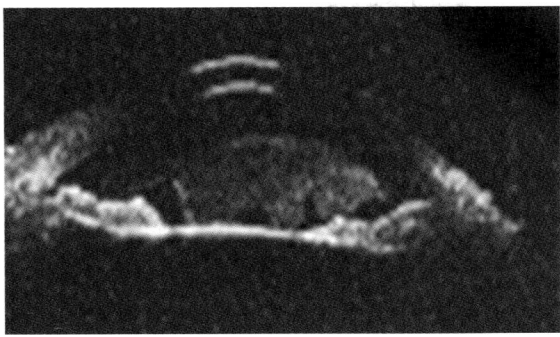

Fig. 33.10E: *Signs of uveal inflammation seen on UBM: Plastic uveitis, thick exudates in anterior chamber, irisoedema.*

V. UBM for evaluation of ocular trauma

UBM adds to the information derived from slit-lamp examination (SLE) or provides the anterior segment details when SLE is not possible. Integrity of posterior capsule can be made out and damage to the ciliary body and zonules is evident only by UBM. It provides useful information in evaluation of known and occult anterior segment foreign bodies[6,7] (Fig. 33.12A to L).

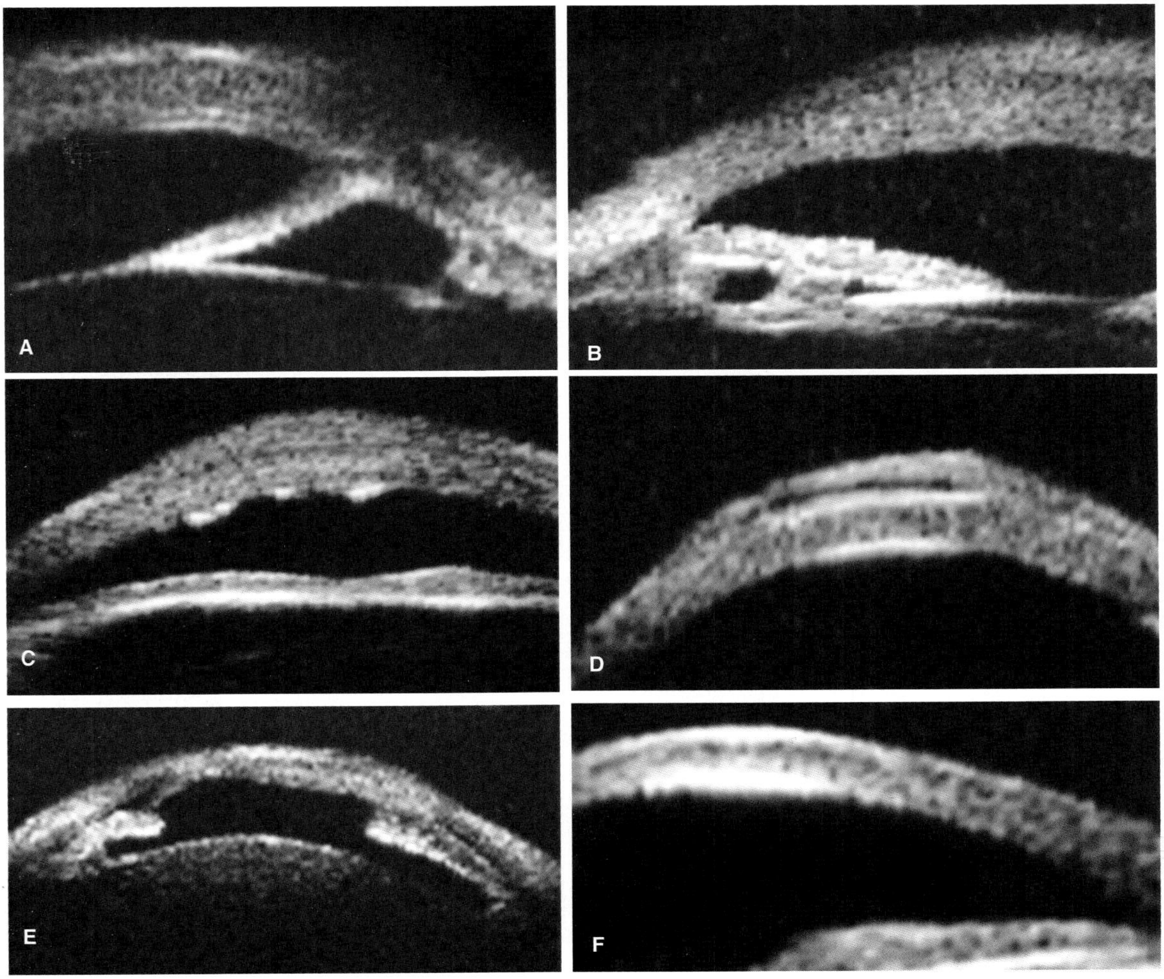

Fig. 33.11: *Common UBM finding seen in patients with cornea leucoma undergoing penetrating keratoplasty: (A) Angle closed, PAS; (B) Angle open IOL haptic but angled in iris IOL; (C) Fuch's dystrophy endothelial deposits; (D) Epithelial bulla with stromal hoze; (E) Cataract, anterior synechiae; (F) Corneal dystrophy, uniform thickness of cornea with echogonecity.*

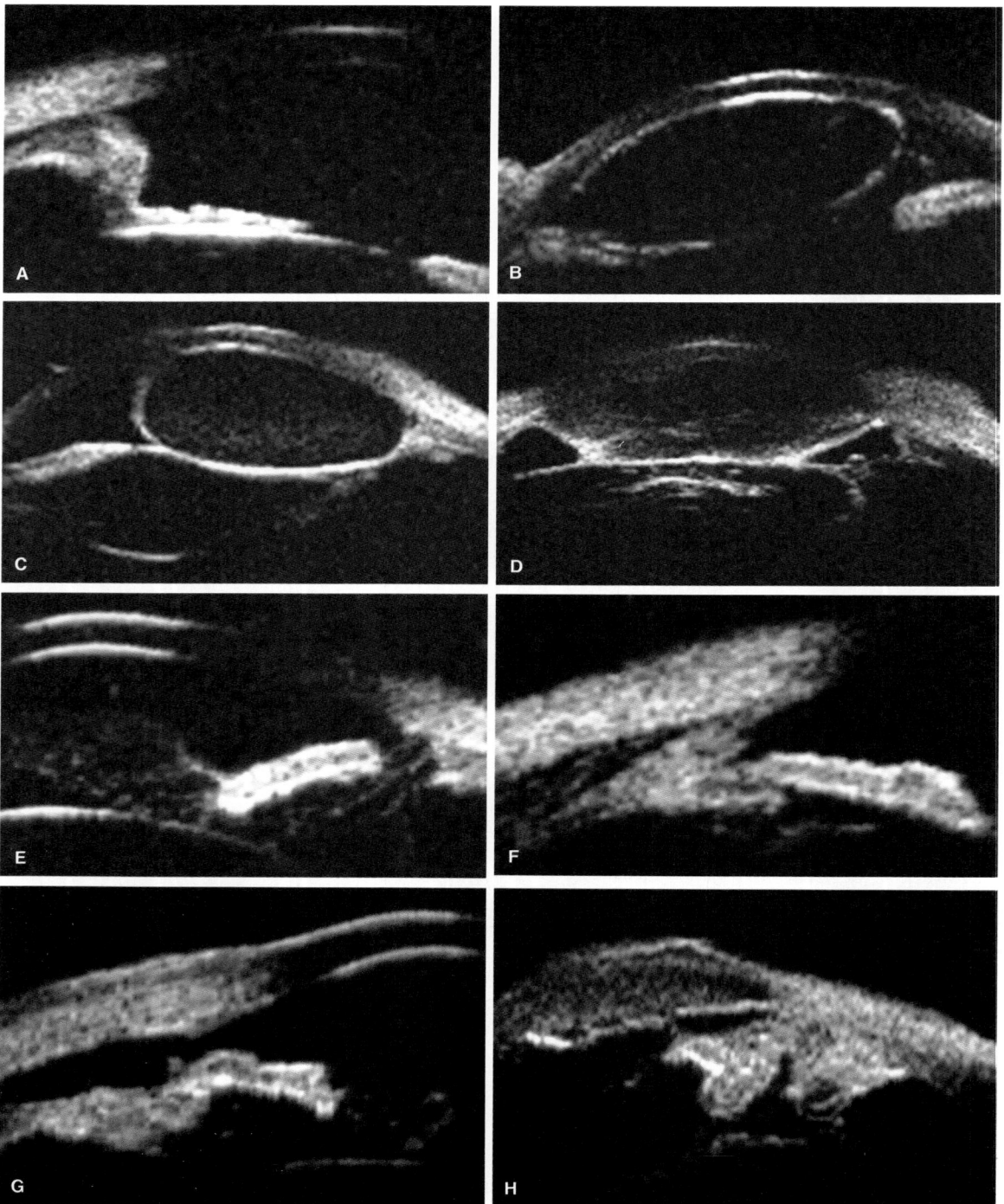

Fig. 33.12A to H: *UBM finding seen in patients with ocular trauma: (A) Posterior dislocation of lens; (B) Anterior dislocation of crystalline lens; (C) Iris cyst, following thorn injury; (D) Hyphaema, cataract, iris bombé; (E) Iridodialysis root of iris disinserted; (F) Cyclodialysis cleft; (G) Iridocyclodialysis detached iris and ciliary body; (H) Fire cracker injury very thick iris, ciliary body and cornea.*

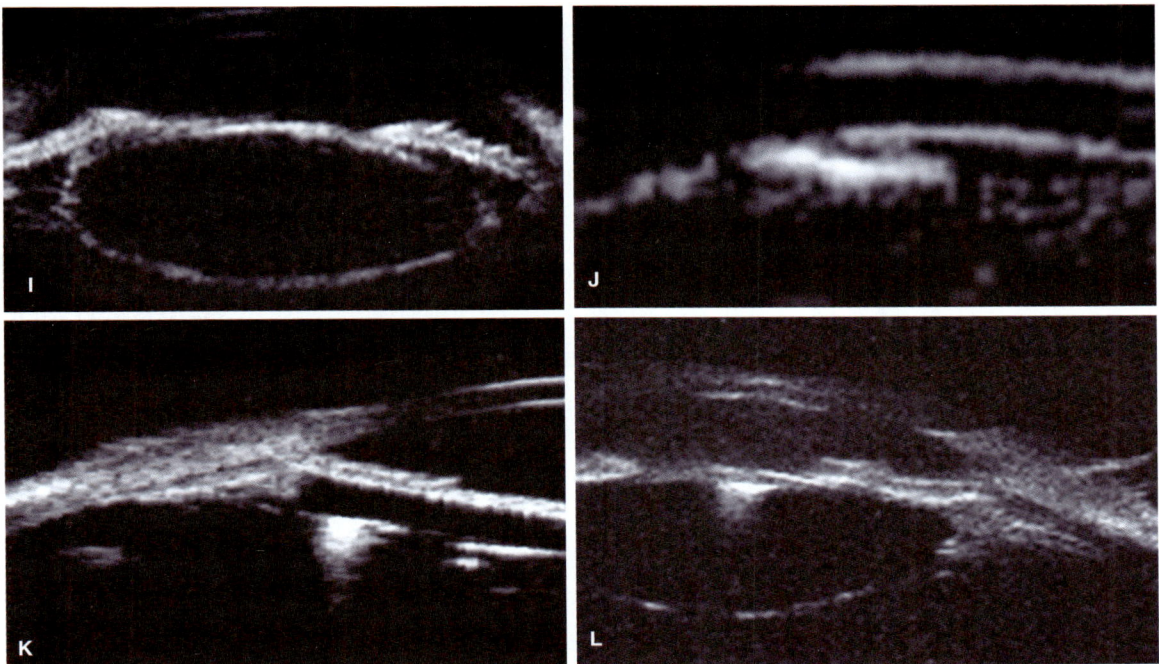

Fig. 33.12 I to L: *UBM finding seen in patients with ocular trauma: (I) Posterior capsule intact in traumatic cataract; (J) Wooden FB on endothelium; (K) Iron FB near zonules; (L) FB in the lens.*

VI. UBM for intraocular mass lesions

Very small (<4 mm) malignant melanoma of ciliary body are demonstrated only by UBM. Extension of the limbal growth is documented. Choroidal haemengioma leading to glaucoma can be seen in Sturge Weber syndrome. Small secondary deposits in anterior chamber from systemic or ocular malignancies are seen on UBM. UBM penetrates all tumours completely so is preferable for clinical anterior tumour assessment[8] as against AS OCT which does not show posterior aspects of pigmented mass lesions (Fig. 33.13A to J).

VII. UBM in paediatric patients

In children of any age UBM can be carried out under topical anaesthesia provided the palpebral aperture accommodates the eye cup. Congenital anterior segment anomalies, buphthalmos, dermoid and other mass lesions and effect of trauma can be studied with this technique (Fig. 33.14A to H).

VIII. Measurements with UBM

Central corneal thickness in open angle glaucoma, angle width and anterior chamber depth before and after iridotomy along with other parameters can be accurately measured with this technique. Size of the cystic and solid mass with their progression on successive visits can be measured (Fig. 33.15A to C).

IX. UBM after intraocular surgeries

Glaucoma surgery. Patency of sclerostomy and configuration of bleb after anti glaucoma surgery can be studied (Fig. 33.16A to C). Position of shunt in AC is visualized.

Keratoplasty. Grafts of various keratoplasties can be imaged (Fig. 33.17A and B).

Silicon oil blocking angle is well-documented even through opaque cornea (Fig. 33.18).

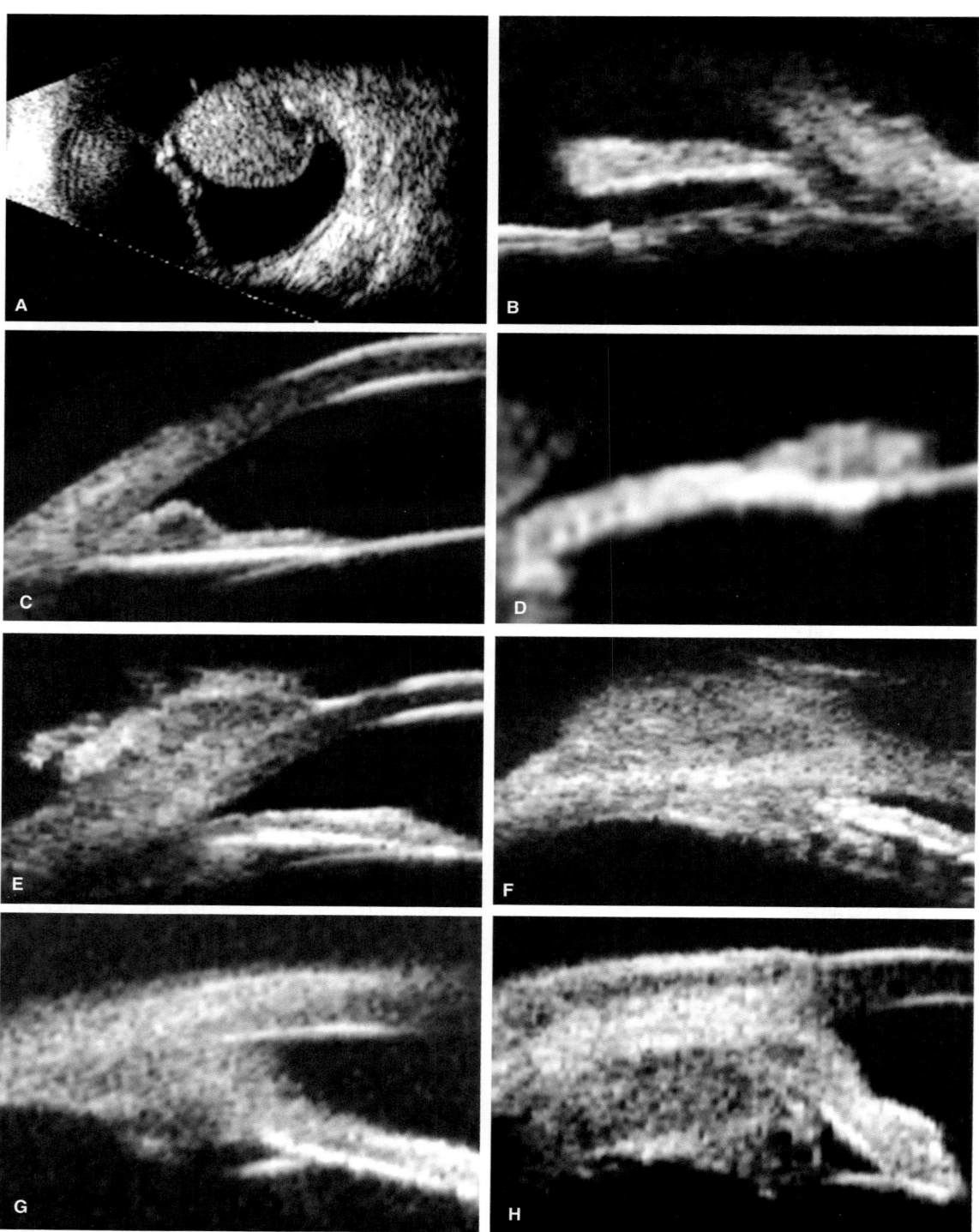

Fig. 33.13A to H: *UBM finding in patients with intraocular mass lesions: (A) Malignant melanoma seen at posterior pole on B scan; (B) Ciliary body deposit in same patient as A; (C) Deposit at iris root; (D) Deposit at pupil; (E) Superficial limbal mass; (F) Penitrating limbal mass; (G) CB haemangioma; (H) Deposits of leukaemia on iris and ciliary body.*

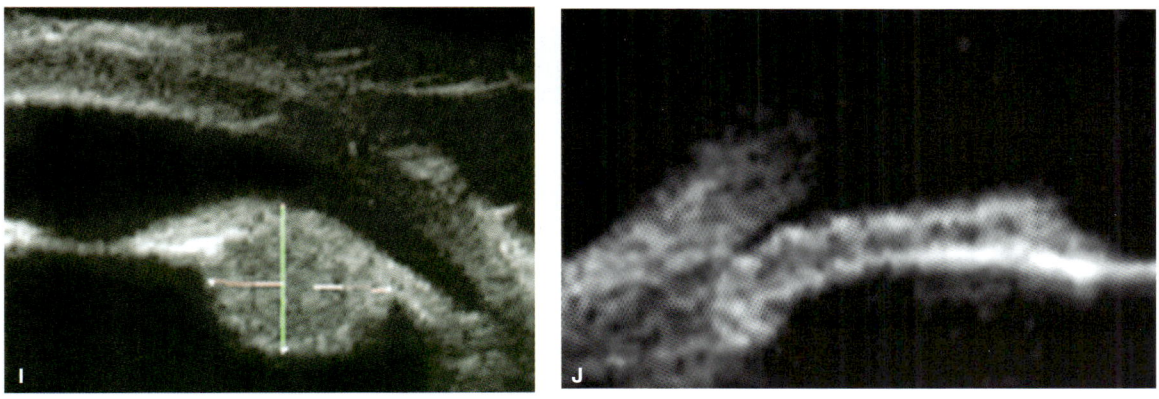

Fig. 33.13 I and J: *UBM finding in patients with intraocular mass lesions: (I) Posterior epithelial Iris mass; (J) Carcinoma cervix, deposits in the eye.*

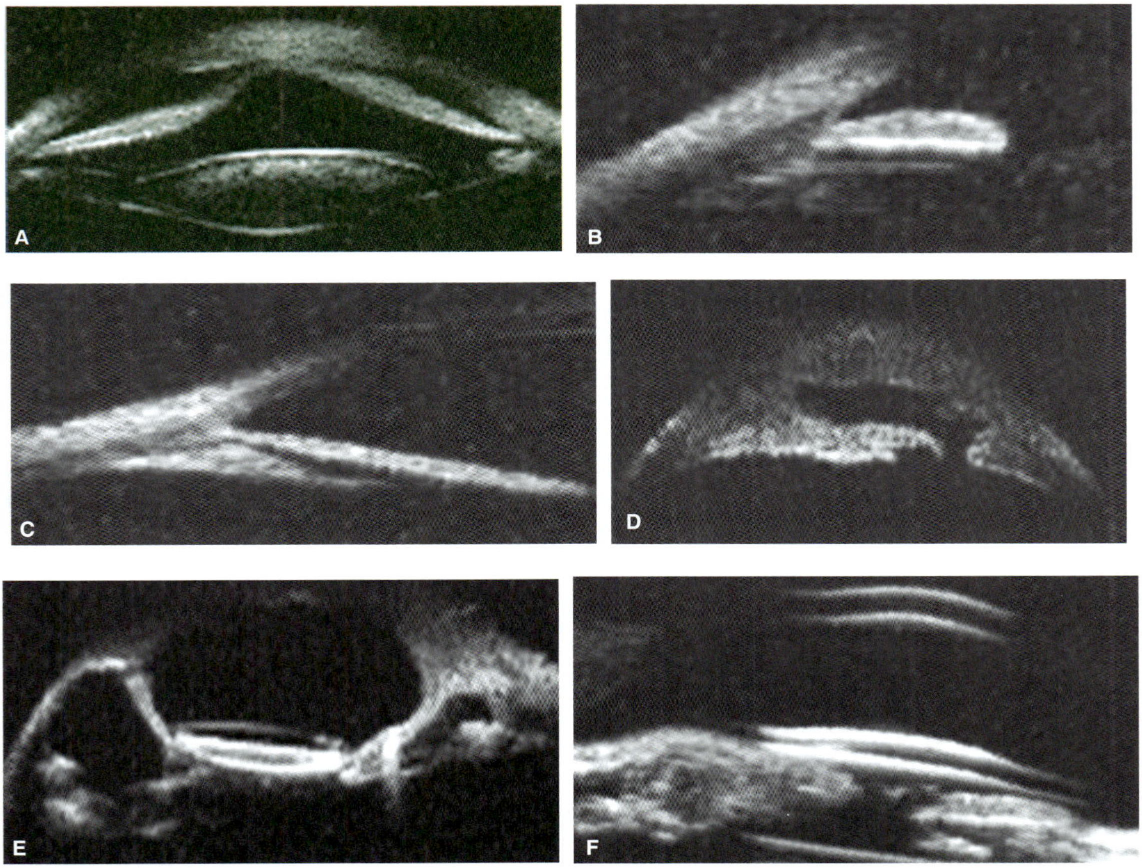

Fig. 33.14A to F: *UBM finding in paediatric ophthalmology patients: (A) Cataract and leucoma; (B) Membrane in angle; (C) Long ciliary process; (D) Anterior staphyloma dysgenesis; (E) Secondary glaucoma in pseudophakic eye; (F) AC IOL, after cataract .*

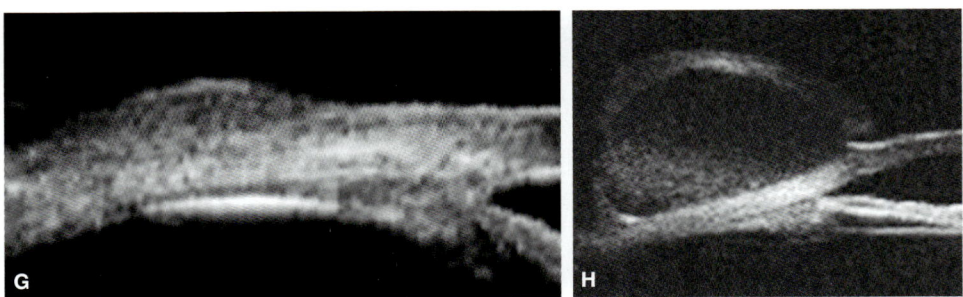

Fig. 33.14G and H: *UBM finding in paediatric ophthalmology patients: (G) Benign conjunctival melanoma hypoechoic surface lesion; (H) Conjunctival cyst with echogenic debris.*

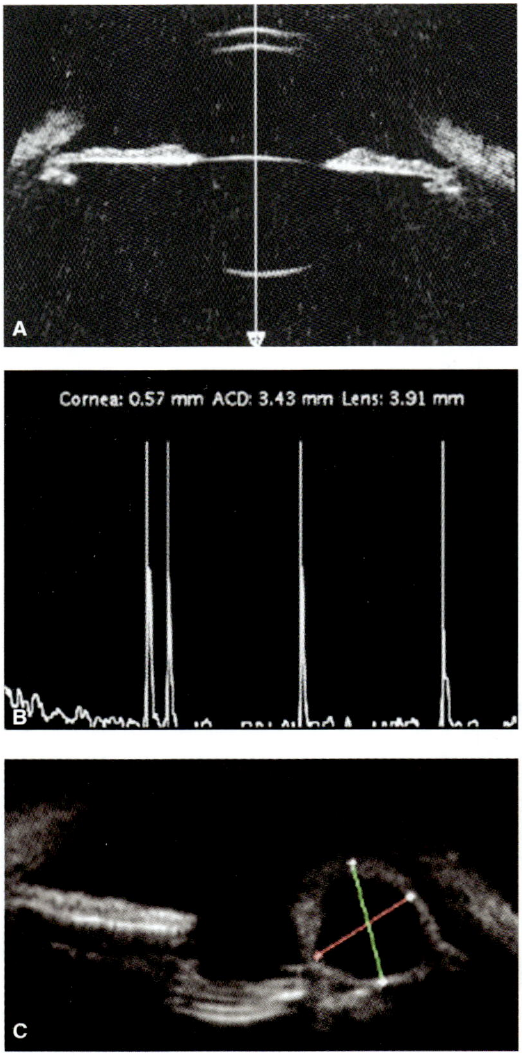

Fig. 33.15: *Measurements with UBM machine: (A) Anterior segment; (B) Biometry reading; (C) Iris cyst dimension.*

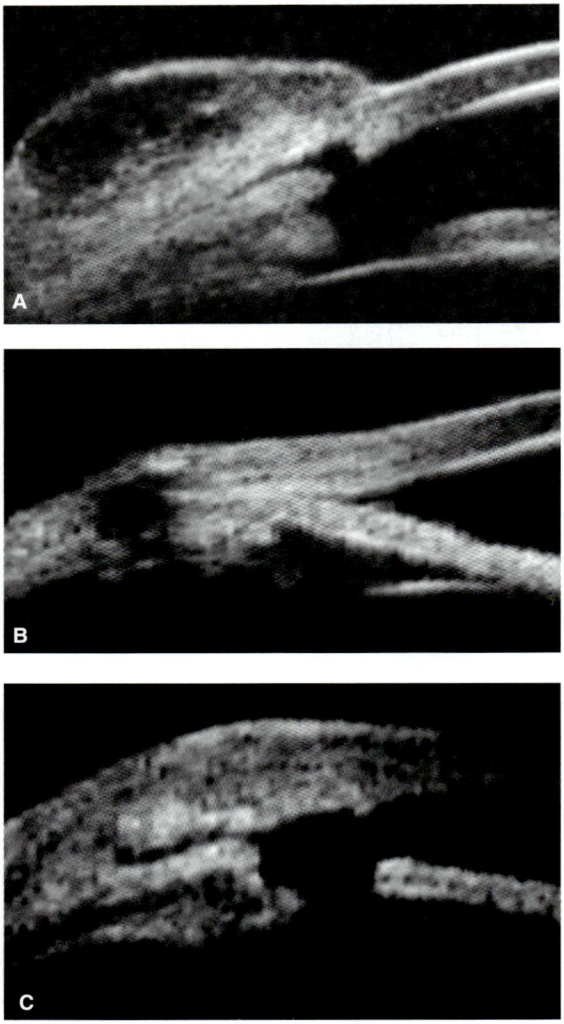

Fig. 33.16: *UBM finding in patients after glaucoma surgeries: (A) Diffuse bleb AGS; (B) Sclerostomy too posterior; (C) Insufficient sclerostomy.*

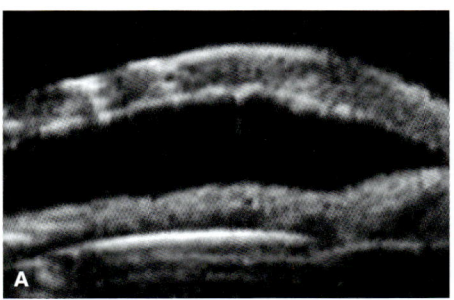 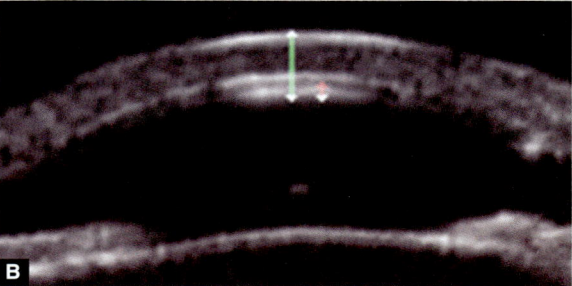

Fig. 33.17: *(A) Penetrating keratoplasty; (B) Deep endothelial keratoplasty.*

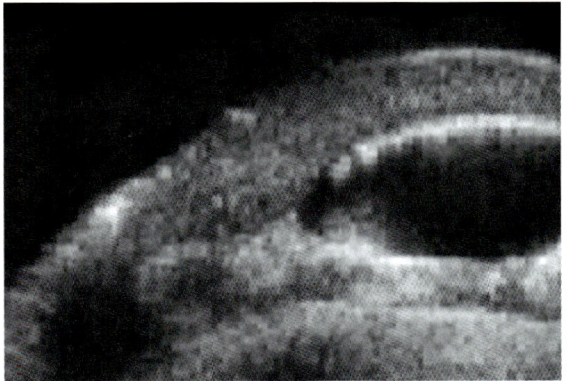

Fig. 33.18: *Silicon oil keratopathy.*

REFERENCES

1. Charles J Pavlin, Foster F Stuart. Ultrasound biomicroscopy. Radiological clinics of North America: 1998 Nov;36(6):1047–57.

2. Clinical use of UBM. Charles J Pavlin, Kasia Harasiewicz, Michael D Sherar, Stuart Foster. Ophthalmology 1991;98:287–95.

3. Kentaro Amino, Ryoji Yamakawa. Long term results of out of the bag IOL implantation. J Cataract Refract Surg 2000;26:266–70.

4. Jane R Mackimon, Hatem R Atta. Role of ultrasound biomicroscopy in managing Pseudohakic pupillary block glaucoma. Srinivasan Satish (Ed), J Cataract Refract Surg 2000;26:1836–8.

5. Milner MS, Liebmaan JM, Tello C, Speaker MG, Ritch R. High-resolution ultrasound biomicroscopy of the anterior segment in patients with dense corneal scars.

6. Daniel Laroche, Hiroshi Ishikawa, David Greenfield, Jeffery M Liebmaan, Robert ritch. Ultrasound biomicroscopic localization and evaluation of intraocular foreign bodies. Acta Ophthalmol. Scand. 1998;76:491–5.

7. Barash D, Goldenberg-Cohen N, Tzadok D, Lifshitz T, Yassur Y, Weinberger D. Ultrasound biomicroscopic detection of anterior ocular segment foreign body after trauma. Am J Ophthalmol. 1998 Aug;126(2):197–202.

8. Pavlin CJ, Vasquez LM, Lee R, Simpson ER, Ahmed II. Anterior segment optical coherence tomography and ultrasound biomicroscopy in the imaging of anterior segment tumours. Am J Ophthalmol, 2009 Feb;147(2):214–9.

Computed Tomography Scanning in Ophthalmology

Chapter Outline

GENERAL CONSIDERATIONS
- Definition
- Principle of CT scan
- CT scan machine
- Basic steps of CT scan imaging
- Advantages and disadvantages of CT scan
- Indications and contraindications of CT scan

SYSTEMATIC APPROACH TO CT SCAN AND NORMAL ORBITAL ANATOMY
- Systematic approach for reporting/interpretation of CT scan
- Normal orbital anatomy on CT scan

CT SCAN FINDINGS IN OCULAR AND ORBITAL LESIONS
Measurement of Proptosis on CT Scan
- Requirements for reliable assessment
- Methods of measuring proptosis

CT Scan Findings in Intraocular Lesions
- Congenital intraocular lesions
- Traumatic intraocular lesions
- Intraocular tumours
- Miscellaneous ocular conditions

CT Scan Findings in Intraorbital Lesions
- Congenital intraorbital lesions
- Traumatic intraorbital lesions
- Inflammatory/infective intraorbital lesions
- Vascular intraorbital lesions
- Orbital tumours
- Ocular adnexal lymphoma
- Lacrimal gland lesions

SPECIAL CT INVESTIGATIONS
- CT angiography
- CT venography
- SPECT and its role in ophthalmology

GENERAL CONSIDERATIONS

Computed tomography (CT) scanning is an indispensable imaging diagnostic tool in the evaluation of most orbital and ocular pathologies. It helps in the assessment of precise location, extent and configuration of the lesion and its effect on adjacent structures and thus helps to plan the proper surgical management of the patient.

DEFINITION

Computed tomography is an imaging technique where contrast differences are based on tissue density when X-ray beams are transmitted through the tissues. It involves the indirect measurement of attenuation of X-rays at numerous positions surrounding the patient. For each section, X-ray tube rotates around the patient to obtain preselected slice thickness. Most CT slices are oriented vertically to patient's body axis (axial or transverse sections). CT scan images are then reconstructed from a large number of measurements of X-ray transmission through the patient (called projection data). The resulting images are tomographic 'maps' of the X-ray linear attenuation coefficient.

PRINCIPLE OF CT SCAN

When X-ray beam is transmitted through tissues, the beam is attenuated as a function of both the atomic number of the element (or the effective atomic number of a complex structure) and the concentration of the substances forming the structure depending on the type of tissue they pass through. Images are acquired by rapid rotation of the X-ray tube 360° around the patient, the radiation is then measured by a ring of sensitive radiation detectors located on the gantry around the patient. Increasing the energy of the X-ray leads to a decrease in attenuation. These absorption values are converted into gray scale units and the reconstructed image is shown on a screen or reviewed on picture archiving and communication system (PACS). High density areas are arbitrarily depicted as white whereas low density areas appear black.

CT SCAN MACHINE

CT scan machine consists of a gantry, operating console and data acquisition system (Fig. 34.1). Gantry assembly is the largest and consists of patient support, positioning couch, mechanical support and scanner housing. It also contains the heart of the CAT scanner, the X-ray tube, as well as detectors that generate and detect X-rays. The operating console is the master control center of the CAT scanner. It is used to input all of the factors related to taking a scan. Typically, this console is made-up of a computer, a keyboard, and multiple monitors. Often there are two different control consoles, one used by the CAT scanner operator, and the other used by the physician. The operator's console controls such variables as the thickness of the imaged tissue slice, mechanical movement of the patient couch, and other radiographic technique factors.

STEPS OF CT SCAN

- The patient is placed on the CT scan table in a supine position and the tube rotates around the table in the gantry.
- CT scan image is produced by firing X-rays at a moving object which is then detected by an array of rotating detectors.
- The detected X-rays are then converted into a computerised signal which is used to produce a series of cross-sectional images.
- The raw data can be reconstructed into different imaging planes, i.e. axial, sagittal and coronal planes.
- The image produced is dependent on the differential densities of which the object is made up of. The computer could then reconstruct the image from the data points resulting from the attenuation of the X-ray beams.

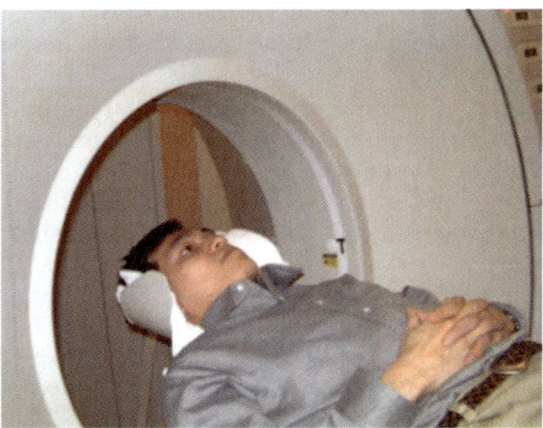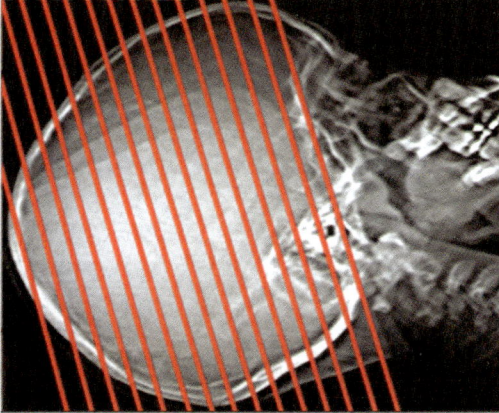

Fig. 34.1: *CT scanner.*

- These data points are represented as pixels of a numeric value, based on the attenuation noted.
- This attenuation seen on the two-dimensional (2D) pixel is based on the three-dimensional (3D) voxel.

CONTRAST ENHANCED CT SCAN

- The administration of intravenous contrast media is an important adjunct to CT scanning.
- The iodinated CT contrast material does not cross an intact blood–brain barrier and therefore there will be contrast material within the blood vessels, and if the blood–brain barrier is disrupted or absent, there will be visible contrast enhancement in the area of interest on CT scan.
- In some cases, the contrast is unnecessary or the risk outweighs the benefit for the administration of iodinated contrast material. For example, in the diagnosis of many orbital disorders (e.g. thyroid orbitopathy or orbital fracture).
- The major complications following the use of iodinated contrast media are renal toxicity and allergic reactions, both of which can be life-threatening.
- Non-contrast scans are usually taken in the orbital region as the abnormalities of BBB are rarely of clinical value. However, if intracranial extension of an orbital lesion is suspected, contrast study may be indicated.
- Contrast study is crucial in the evaluation of lesions in chiasmal and parachiasmal regions.
- The contrast material may be:
  - ◆ Iodinated contrast (Iodine—atomic no. 53 and atomic weight 127)
  - ◆ Ionic, combined with sodium and meglumine salts
  - ◆ Non-ionic.
- In general, the use of contrast improves the sensitivity and specificity of CT scan interpretation.

HELICAL/SPIRAL CT SCAN

- With helical CT, X-ray tube rotates continuously in one direction while the table on which the patient is lying is mechanically moved through the X-ray beam.
- X-ray beam from the CT scan traces a helical path. The helical path results in a three-dimensional data set, which can then be reconstructed into sequential images for a stack. Helical CT allows a scan to be performed in a single breath-hold.
- Advantages of helical CT include dramatically shortened examination times, improved visibility of vascular structures, better enhancement of parenchymal organs, the capability for retrospective imaging and three-dimensional (3D) vascular studies, and potential reduction in use of contrast material.

ADVANTAGES AND DISADVANTAGES OF CT SCAN

Advantages of CT scan

- Better imaging and depiction of bony pathology and calcification
- Comparatively cheaper
- Initial imaging modality of choice in cases of orbital trauma when intraocular foreign body is suspected
- Ideal for unstable patients as test duration is very short
- Lesser patient cooperation required.

Disadvantages of CT scan

- Exposure to ionising radiation.
- Iodine based dye contrast reactions.
- Lesser sensitive than MRI in imaging intracanalicular and intracranial optic nerve, cavernous sinus and diseases of white matter such as disseminated sclerosis.
- Also, the bony orbital wall can sometimes interfere with the interpretation of soft tissue orbital content.

INDICATIONS AND CONTRAINDICATIONS OF CT SCAN

Indications

- Unexplained proptosis, ophthalmoplegia or ptosis
- Palpable orbital mass
- Preseptal cellulitis with orbital signs

- Orbital signs associated with paranasal sinus disease
- Unexplained afferent dysfunction
- Ocular surface or lid tumour with suspected orbital spread
- Intraocular tumour with proptosis
- Orbital trauma.

Conditions in which CT scan is preferred over MRI

- Evaluation of proptosis if orbital space occupying lesion is suspected if calcification or bony erosion is suspected
- In retinoblastoma, calcification is better detected
- Bony fragment better delineated in traumatic optic neuropathy
- In penetrating trauma, if intraocular or intraorbital foreign body is suspected.

Contraindications

Contraindications for the use of iodinated contrast media:

- Allergy to iodine
- Toxic goitre of the thyroid
- Planned radioiodine treatment of thyroid cancer.

Contraindications against the use of ion-based contrast media in patients:

- Children below 2 years of age
- Pregnant women
- Patients over 60 years of age
- Patients with complications after the previous administration of a contrast medium
- Patients with acute and chronic circulatory and respiratory failure
- Patients with hepatic and renal failure (also dialyzed patients)
- Patients with asthma and pulmonary oedemas
- Patients with allergies
- Patients with insulin-dependent diabetes
- Patients with hypertension
- Patients with convulsions of cerebral aetiology.

SYSTEMATIC APPROACH AND NORMAL ORBITAL ANATOMY

SYSTEMATIC APPROACH TO INTERPRET CT SCAN

The density of the body tissue determines the degree to which the X-rays are attenuated. In turn, this affects the brightness and contrast of the imaged tissues. Those tissues with **high attenuation coefficients** (strong absorption) show up white, and those which absorb with low attenuation coefficients (weak absorption) show up black. This is quantified by the Hounsfield scale of radiodensity. All densities greater than bone, such as a metallic foreign body, also appear white. Because of this, tissues of different but similar densities may not be distinguishable on standard CT scan. Hounsefield number of various structures is as below:

- Air   :   – 1000 HU
- Fat   :   –100 HU
- Water   :   0 HU
- Soft tissue   :   +30 to +40 HU
- Haemorrhage   :   +70 to +80 HU
- Calcium   :   >100 HU
- Bone   :   >300 HU

CT SCAN VERSUS MRI SCAN

- First of all, it is important to judge is it a CT scan or MRI scan? One might confuse the CT and T1 MRI sequence. Both images display a structure that is white in the periphery and has CSF that is dark. On MRI this white structure represents the subcutaneous fat and on CT the bright structure is the skull.
- CT images are acquired only in the axial plane. The axial plane image data then can be used to reconstruct images in sagittal and coronal planes. MRI can be acquired in all the three axial, sagittal and coronal planes.
- In MRI scans the fat can be either white or dark in appearance, depending on the sequence either T1 or T2. In a CT scan image, fat and fluid never appears white, thus if either fat or fluid appears white, it is definitely a MRI scan.

- On CT scan bone is always white as calcium blocks the X-ray photons. The calcium does not emit a signal in MRI scans and thus both bone and bone marrow appears dark. If one can see that bony structures are of black or dark gray in colour, then one can be sure that it is a MRI scan.

PATIENT AND IMAGE DETAILS

- Name of the patient should match with the name written on the report.
- Time and date written on the reports should be checked to ensure that those reports are the latest and also for proper follow-up of patients in future. It is always worthwhile to confirm that you are looking at the correct CT of the specific patient, done at the specific time (in case of serial CT scans) before you begin to interpret.
- Check the laterality (right or left) of the patient you are visualising.

WHETHER THE CT SCAN IS CONTRAST ENHANCED?

- Note whether the plates provided are plain CT scans or contrast enhanced. Though the image brightness and the Hounsfield value enables us to identify the contrast images, it will be printed next to each image whether the scan is plain or contrast enhanced.

CT WINDOWING

- On CT scan, low density tissues are assigned darker (blacker) colours and high density structures are assigned brighter (whiter) colours. Because the human eye can perceive only a limited number of gray shades, the full range of density values is typically not displayed for a given image. Instead, the tissues of interest are highlighted by devoting the visible gray shades to a narrow portion of the full density range, a process called 'windowing'.
- The same image data can be displayed in different window settings to allow evaluation of injury to different tissues. Brain and orbit CT Scan are generally viewed on 'brain' or 'bone' windows to allow the most emergent pathology to be assessed. Window setting is done to represent the density of tissue of interest. The mean density level of window should be set as close as possible to the density level of tissue to be examined.
- *Brain windows* (Fig. 34.2A) allows evaluation of the brain parenchyma, haemorrhage, CSF spaces and soft tissues at the expense of bony

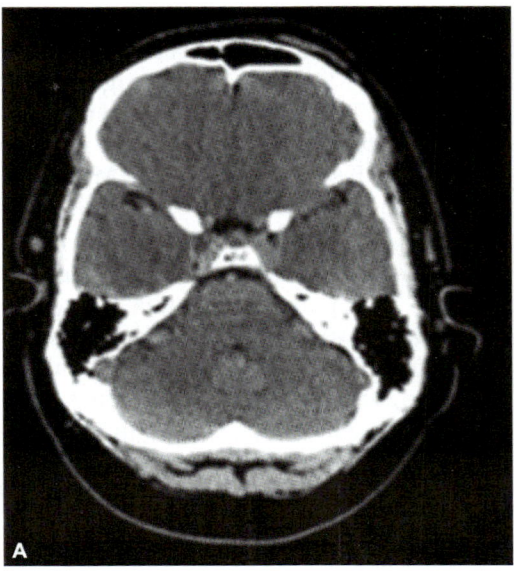 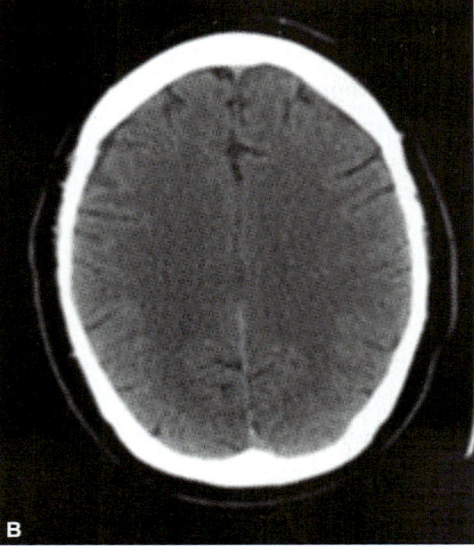

Fig. 34.2: *CT scan windows: (A) Brain window; (B) 2-bone window.*

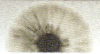

details. Only gross fractures can be visualised. 'Brain windows' are used to view a range of densities close to the average density of the soft tissues of the brain.

- *Bone windows* (Fig. 34.2B) are used to emphasise a narrow range of densities close to the density of bone. Bone windows allows detailed examination of fractures but obscure all soft tissue details. The bone window images provide no useful detail of brain structure.

NORMAL ORBITAL ANATOMY ON CT SCAN

APPEARANCE OF NORMAL ORBITAL AND PERIORBITAL STRUCTURES ON CT SCAN

Appearance of normal orbital and periorbital structures on CT scan is summarized in Table 34.1.

Figure 34.3A to D depicts the normal orbital anatomy seen on bone window.

Table 34.1 *Appearance of normal orbital and periorbital structures*

Tissue	Brain window	Bone window
Air	Black	Black
Calcification	White	Dark
Blood	Intermediate to dark	Very dark
Fat	Very dark	Very dark
Muscle	Intermediate	Dark
Optic nerve	Intermediate	Dark
Proteinaceous fluid	Intermediate	Dark
Sclera	Intermediate	Dark
Vitreous	Intermediate to dark	Dark
Water	Dark	Dark
White matter	Intermediate	Dark
Cortical grey matter	Intermediate	Dark

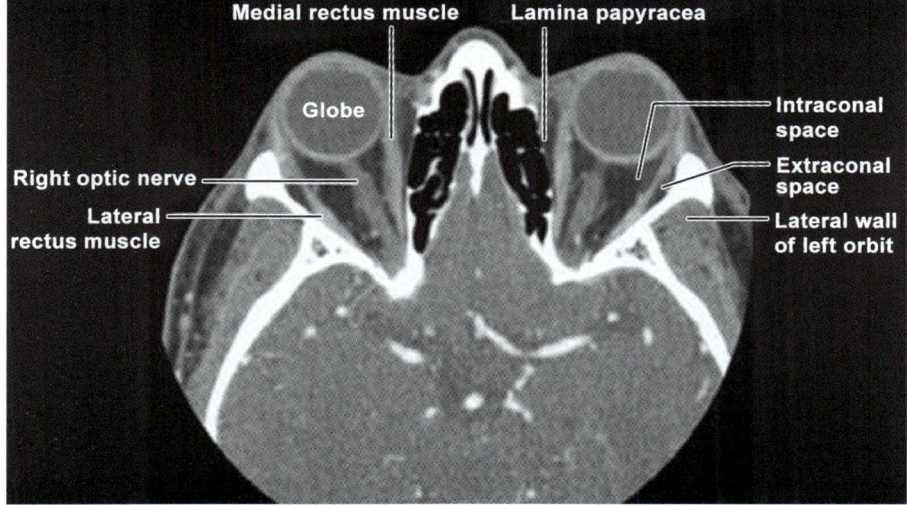

Fig. 34.3A: *Axial orbital CT images with contrast at level of the optic nerve.*

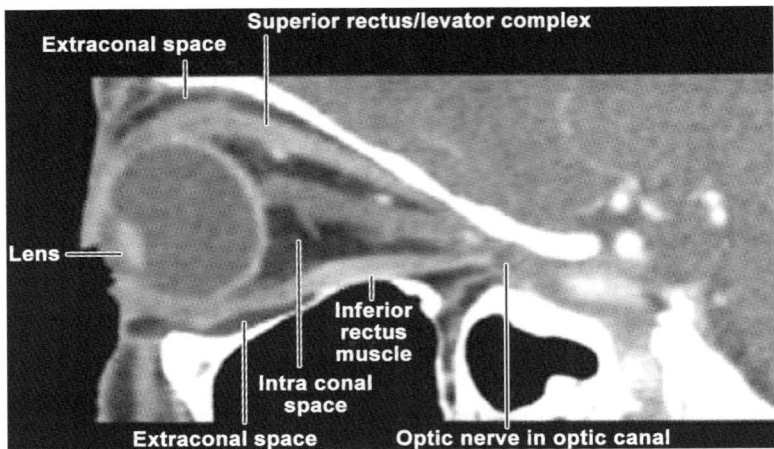

Fig. 34.3B: *Parasagittal orbital CT along the course of the optic nerve.*

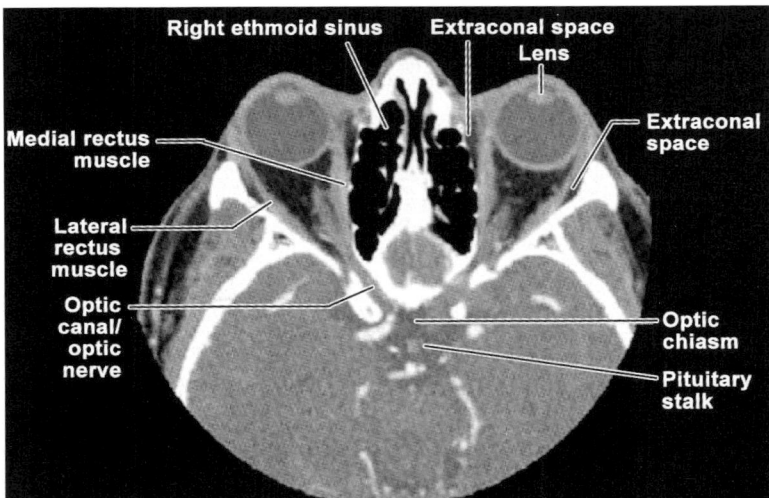

Fig. 34.3C: *Axial orbital CT images with contrast showing the optical canal.*

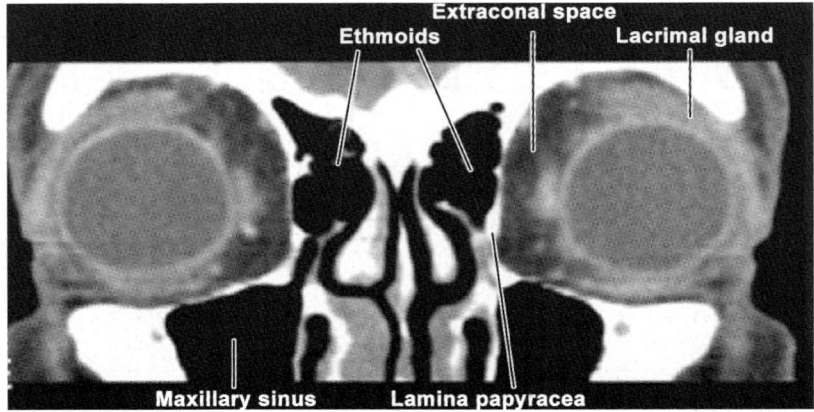

Fig. 34.3D: *Coronal orbital contrast enhanced CT scan at the equator level of the globe.*

CT SCAN BASED NORMATIVE VALUES FOR OCULAR AND ORBITAL MEASUREMENTS

- **Normal position of globe on CT scan.** Posterior margin of globe is 9.9 ± 1.7 mm behind the interzygomatic line
- **Width of ophthalmic vein** = 3–4 mm
- **Optic nerve (axial plane):**
  - Retrobulbar segment = 5.5 ± 0.8 mm
  - Narrowest point (at approximately mid-orbit) = 4.2 ± 0.6 mm.

CT FINDINGS IN OCULAR AND ORBITAL LESIONS

MEASUREMENT OF PROPTOSIS ON CT SCAN

Requirements for reliable assessment

Requirements for reliable assessment of proptosis on CT scan include:
- Plane of the scan must be parallel to the plane passing through the optic nerve head and lens.
- Eyelids must be open, with the patient looking straight ahead.

Methods of measuring proptosis

On CT scan, proptosis can be measured by following methods:

1. *By measuring distance from the anterior corneal surface to interzygomatic line (IZL).* A line between the bony lateral orbital margins drawn on the slice containing the optic nerve head and lens, and the distance of the cornea in front of this line is measured (Fig. 34.4).

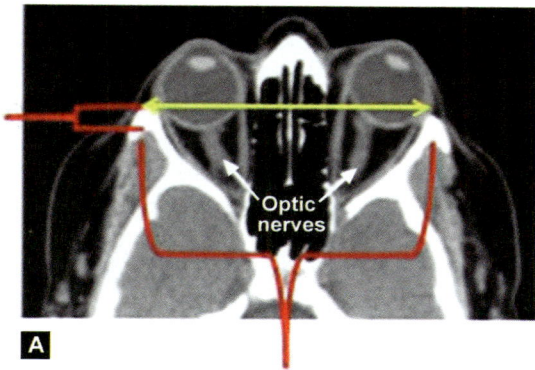

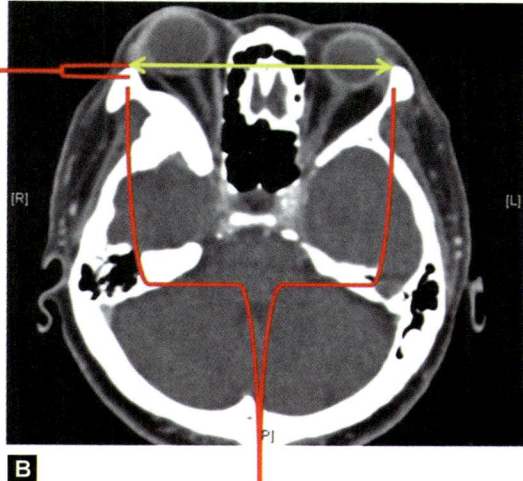

Fig. 34.5: *Measuring proptosis from distance between posterior scleral margin and interzygomatic line: (A) Normal person; (B) Patient with proptosis.*

2. *Distance from posterior scleral margin (PSM) to interzygomatic line (IZL)* can also be used to measure proptosis. Figure 34.5A depicts distance between PSM and IZL in a normal patient; which is decreased in a patient with proptosis (Fig. 34.5B).

CT SCAN FINDINGS IN INTRAOCULAR LESIONS

CONGENITAL INTRAOCULAR LESIONS

Persistent hyperplastic primary vitreous

Common CT scan findings in a patient with PHPV include (Fig. 34.6):
- Microphthalmia
- Increased vitreous attenuation

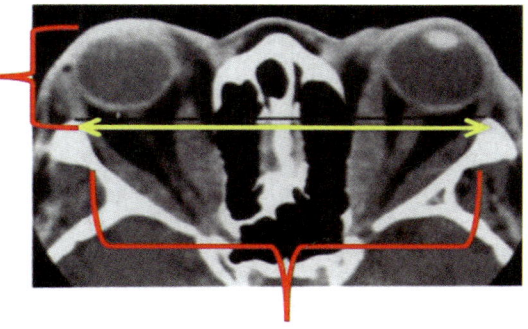

Fig. 34.4: *Measuring of proptosis on CT scan by distance from the anterior corneal surface to interzygomatic line.*

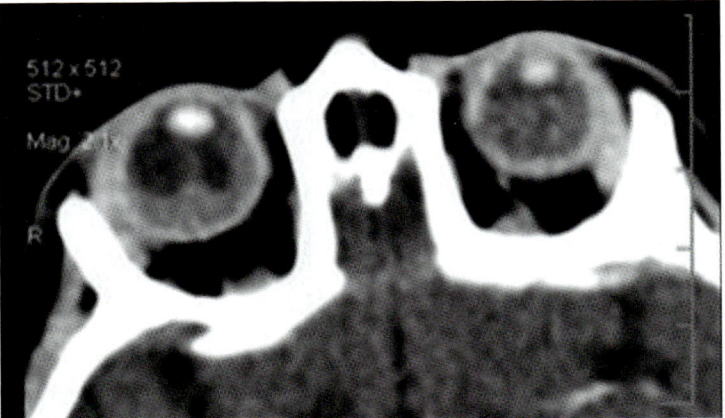

Fig. 34.6: *Axial CT scan image showing bilateral persistent hyperplastic primary vitreous.*

- Contrast enhancement of abnormal intra-vitreal tissue
- Fluid-fluid levels from breakdown of recurrent hemorrhage
- Lens may be small and irregular
- Often shallow anterior chamber (type I anterior PHPV)
- Optic nerve (ON) may be small
- No calcifications (as in retinoblastoma).

Colobomas

Common CT scan findings seen in a patient with ocular coloboma are summarised below (Fig. 34.7):

- Funnel-shaped excavation of posterior fundus at the optic disc. Flattening of posterior oculus.

- The globe is usually enlarged. However, colobomas that involve uvea tend to show microphthalmia with cyst formation. Focal posterior bulging shows no uveoscleral thinning or abnormal contrast enhancement.
- Cone-shaped or notch-shaped deformity.

Optic disc drusen

Common CT scan findings seen in a patient with optic disc drusen are summarised below (Fig. 34.8):

- Childhood drusen are small and non mineralized
- May see slight swelling and increased attenuation on CT

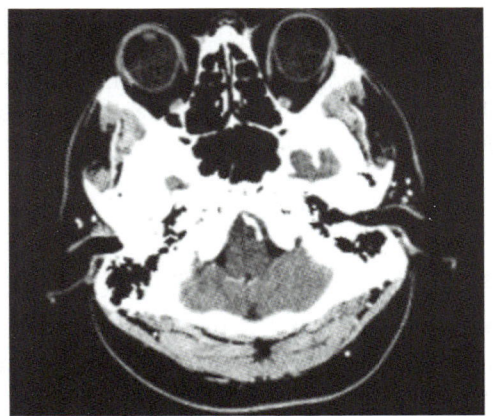

Fig. 34.7: *Axial CT scan image showing bilateral ocular coloboma.*

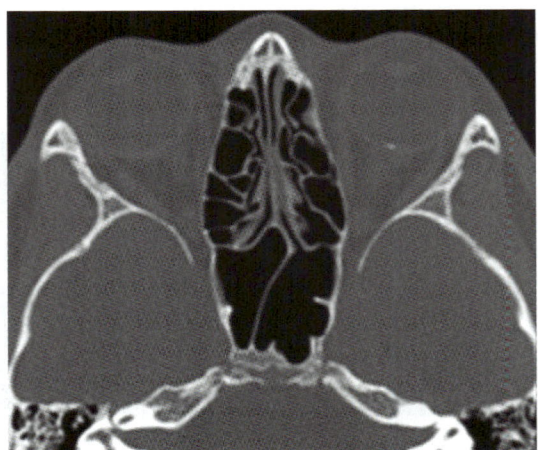

Fig. 34.8: *Axial CT scan image showing optic disc drusen, left eyeball.*

- Adult drusen demonstrate well-defined calcifications, a few millimeters in size
- ODDs are co-located with the optic disc
- Occasionally drusen may be away from the optic disc.

TRAUMATIC INTRAOCULAR LESIONS

Intraocular foreign body

Computed tomography (CT) is currently considered the 'gold standard' for the detection, localization and characterization of both metallic and nonmetallic IOFBs. Axial sections separated by 3 to 5 mm have been utilized as an initial screening study for IOFBs (Fig. 34.9).

Globe rupture

Common CT scan findings in a patient with globe rupture include (Fig. 34.10):
- Globe collapse may give a flat tire appearance
- May see intraocular air or FB

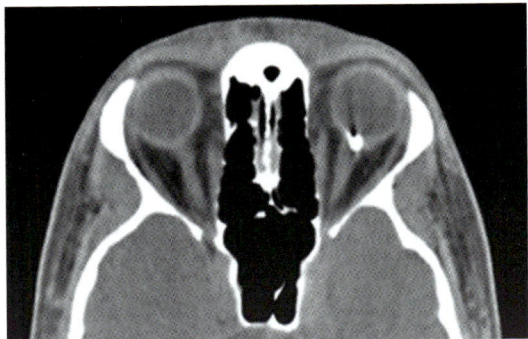

Fig. 34.9: *Axial CT scan image showing intraocular foreign body, left eyeball.*

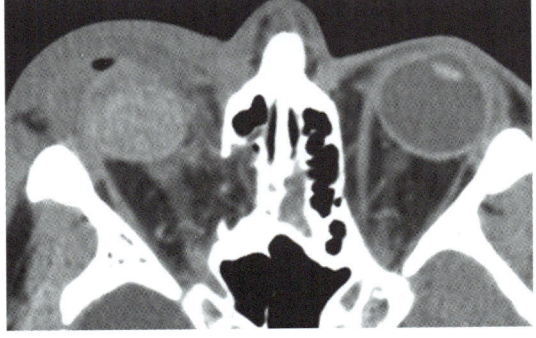

Fig. 34.10: *Axial CT scan image showing globe rupture, right eyeball.*

- Thickened posterior sclera
- Hazy outline of the globe
- Enlarged anterior chamber suggests posterior scleral rupture
- A discrepancy of at least 2 mm between anterior chamber depths raises the question of scleral rupture
- Traumatic posterior scleral rupture with vitreous decompression may allow lens retropulsion, thus deepening the anterior chamber
- Anterior chamber depth normally ranges from 2.5 to 3.5 mm, but varies according to age, sex, and measurement method
- Vitreous haemorrhage suggests retinal or choroidal tear, optic nerve avulsion, or foreign body
- Retinal tears, edema, detachment, and haemorrhage may be seen.

INTRAOCULAR TUMOURS

Retinoblastoma

Common CT scan findings in a patient with retinoblastoma include (Fig. 34.11):
- Calcified solid intraocular mass
- Posterior location, 90% have soft tissue mass with punctuate or finely speckled calcifications

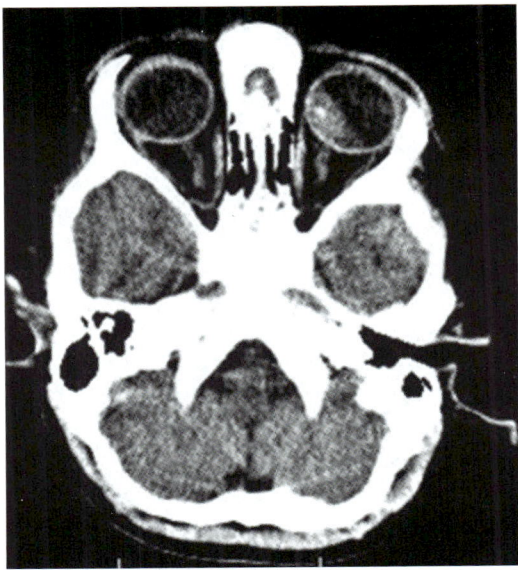

Fig. 34.11: *Axial CT scan image showing retinoblastoma, left eyeball.*

- Moderate or avid contrast enhancement
- Any intraocular calcifications in an infant or young child suggest RB until proved otherwise
- Retinal detachment common.

MISCELLANEOUS OCULAR CONDITIONS

Retinal Detachment

Common CT scan findings seen in a patient with retinal detachment are summarised below (Fig. 34.12):

- CT attenuation of the RD depends on what fluid is below the detachment
- The fluid beneath the RD often depends on the cause of the RD
- Recent haemorrhage demonstrates high attenuation
- Retinal tears may permit low-attenuation vitreous humour to burrow beneath the retina.

Phthisis Bulbi

CT scan findings in phthisis bulbi include (Fig. 34.13):

- The globe is small and shrunken with diffuse linear or mottled calcium deposits

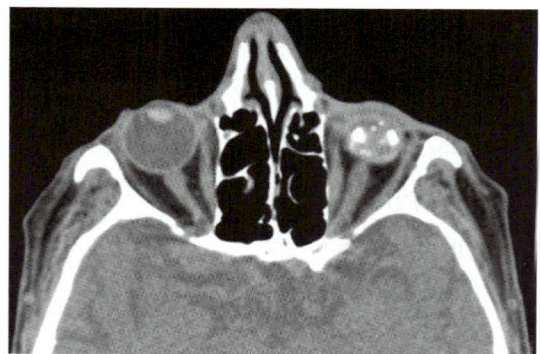

Fig. 34.13: *Axial CT scan image showing phthisis bulbi, left eyeball.*

- Scattered foci of calcium deposits and ossification in the sclera, cornea, lens, retina, and optic nerve
- Fibrotic scarring may cause an irregular globe contour with diffusely increased attenuation
- The globe is usually half to a third normal size as a result of reduced aqueous production
- Devitalized tissue may demonstrate ossification.

Posterior Ocular Staphyloma

Common CT scan findings in a patient with posterior ocular staphyloma include (Fig. 34 .14):

- Bulging of posterior aspect of the globe away from optic disc, usually on the temporal aspect

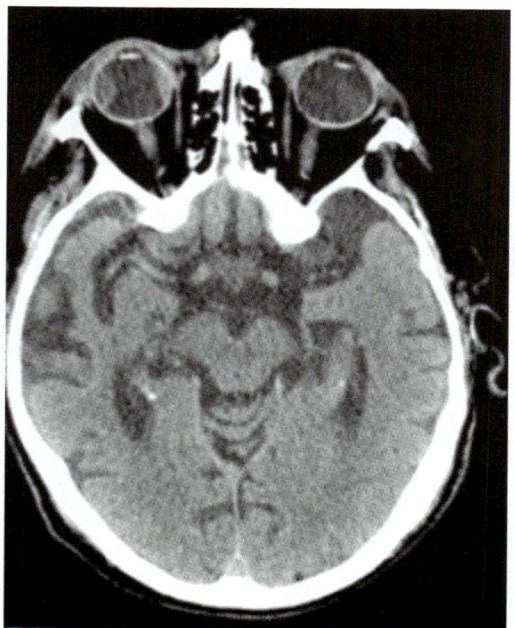

Fig. 34.12: *Axial CT scan image showing retinal detachment, right eyeball.*

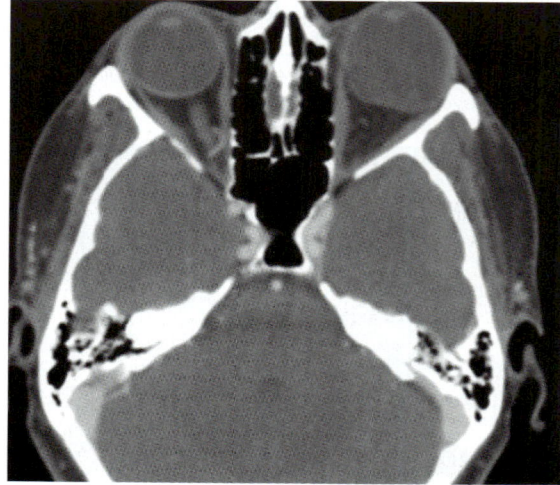

Fig. 34.14: *Axial CT scan image showing posterior ocular staphyloma, left eyeball.*

- Scleral thinning is associated with focal bulge
- May see associated retinal or choroidal detachment, with or without haemorrhage.

CT SCAN FINDINGS IN INTRAORBITAL LESIONS

CONGENITAL INTRAORBITAL LESIONS

Congenital intraorbital teratomas

Common CT scan findings seen in a patient with congenital orbital teratoma are summarised below (Fig. 34.15):

- Irregular, heterogeneous masses with solid and multiloculated cystic components
- Cystic areas may contain fat-fluid levels
- Calcifications common and may represent bone and teeth
- Bony orbit is typically enlarged
- Lesion may extend intracranially or into sinuses
- Moderate contrast enhancement of solid components.

TRAUMATIC INTRAORBITAL LESIONS

Intraorbital foreign body

CT is sensitive and is usually the first imaging test performed (Fig. 34.16).

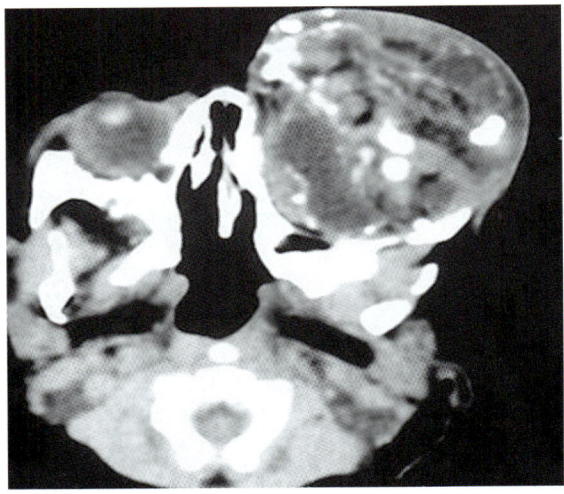

Fig. 34.15: *Axial CT scan image showing congenital orbital teratoma, left eyeball.*

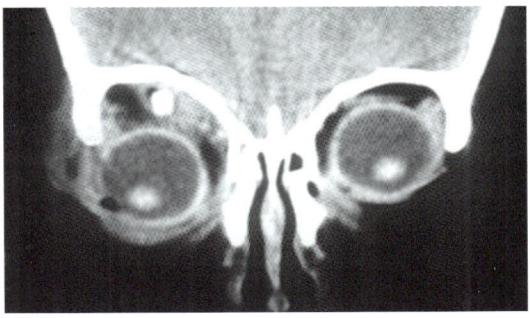

Fig. 34.16: *Axial CT scan revealing a pencil fragment in right superior orbit.*

Blowout orbital floor fractures

Common CT scan findings seen in a patient with blowout orbital fracture are summarised below (Fig. 34.17):

- Fracture involving the bony cortex with or without displacement
- Soft tissue mass extending into the roof of the adjacent maxillary sinus
- Herniated orbital contents usually contain orbital fat
- May have complete or partial opacification of the adjacent maxillary sinus as a result of haemorrhage and edema
- Herniation or entrapment of the extraocular muscles may cause limited ocular motion
- New fractures may cause associated fluid and/or air-fluid levels in the maxillary sinus
- May see intraorbital air and/or air-fluid levels.

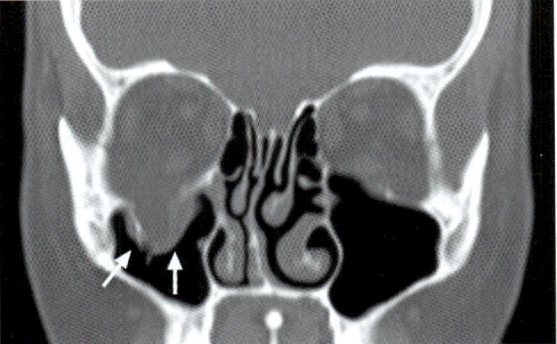

Fig. 34.17: *Coronal non-contrast CT scan orbit showing fracture floor of orbit with prolapsed of orbital contents in maxillary sinus.*

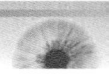

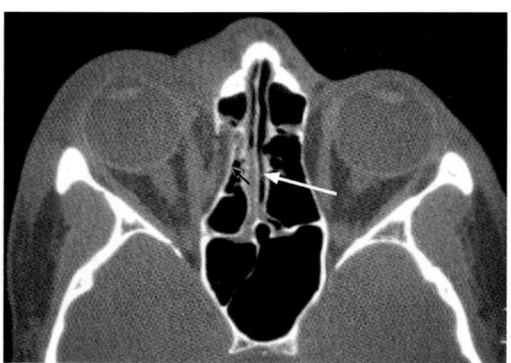

Fig. 34.18: *Axial non-contrast CT scan right orbit showing fracture medial wall of right orbit.*

Fracture of medial wall of orbit

Common CT scan findings seen in a patient with fracture medial wall of orbit are summarised below (Fig. 34.18):

- Medial bowing or displacement of the medial orbital wall
- Fracture may be visible through the bony cortex with or without displacement
- Air collections may be visible within the orbit and/or air-fluid levels.

INFLAMMATORY AND INFECTIVE INTRAORBITAL LESIONS

Graves ophthalmopathy

Common CT scan findings in a patient with Grave's ophthalmopathy include (Fig. 34.19):

- EOM enlargement and enhancement which is usually bilateral and symmetric
- Involved EOMs in decreasing frequency: Inferior, medial, superior, and lateral rectus muscles

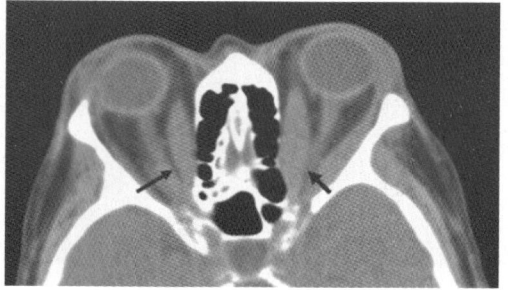

Fig. 34.19: *Axial CT scan showing thickened extraocular muscles in a case of Grave's ophthalmopathy.*

- Isolated muscle involvement most commonly involves superior rectus and levator palpebrae complex
- Classically, maximal swelling in muscle belly spares tendinous global attachment
- Smooth margins of involved muscles
- Increased retrobulbar fat volume
- Uveoscleral thickening
- Orbital apex crowding may cause dilated superior orbital veins
- Cerebrospinal fluid (CSF) trapping in sub-arachnoid space may increase diameter of ON sheath.

Idiopathic orbital Inflammatory disease

Common CT scan findings in a patient with idiopathic orbital inflammatory disease include (Fig. 34.20):

- Abnormal enhancement of retrobulbar fat
- May see lacrimal, EOM, or other intraorbital mass
- May be focal or infiltrative
- Lesions are poorly circumscribed
- Dynamic CT shows late phase increased attenuation increasing
- May show bone remodelling or erosion
- May see nonspecific structural thickening of sclera, episclera, Tenon's capsule, and uvea
- Can cause diffuse infiltration of orbital fat, globe, and ON sheath complex.

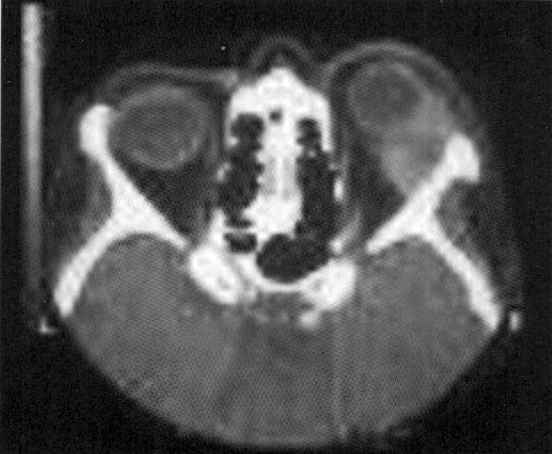

Fig. 34.20: *Axial CT scan image showing idiopathic orbital inflammatory disease, left eyeball.*

Orbital cysticercosis

CT scan in a patient with orbital cysticercosis shows a hypodense mass with a central hyperdensity suggestive of scolex (Fig. 34.21):

- Involved extraocular muscle may be thickened and have surrounding soft tissues inflammation.

Orbital echinococcosis

CT scan in a patient with orbital echinococcosis reveals a clear cystic structure with calcification on cyst wall (Fig. 34.22).

Orbital myositis

CT scan in a patient with orbital myositis shows enlargement of involved extraocular muscles with irregular muscle borders and diffuse inflammatory shadow which extends to tendon and orbital fat (Fig. 34.23).

Orbital abscess

Common CT scan findings in a patient with orbital abscess include (Fig. 34.24):

- Obliteration of fat planes
- Eccentric globe displacement suggests subperiosteal abscess
- Intraorbital gas or air-fluid level is strongly suggestive of OA

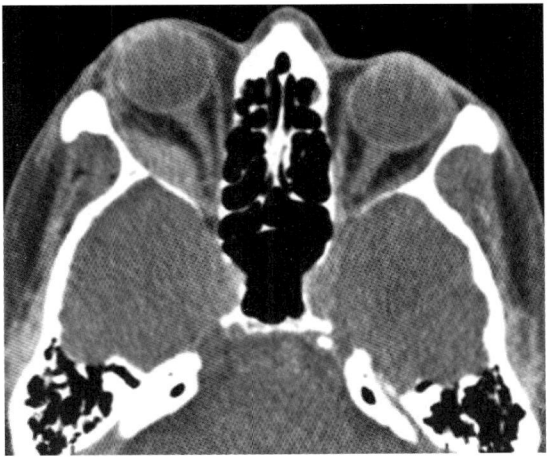

Fig. 34.23: *Axial CT scan image showing right orbital myositis.*

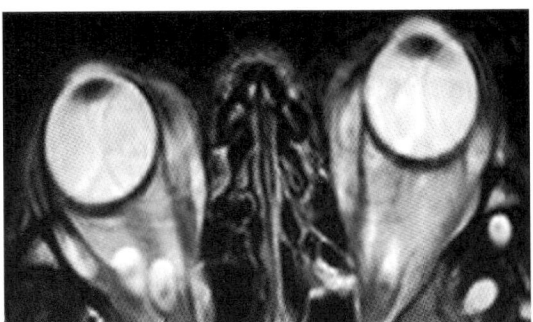

Fig. 34.21: *Axial CT scan image showing bilateral disseminated orbital cysticercosis.*

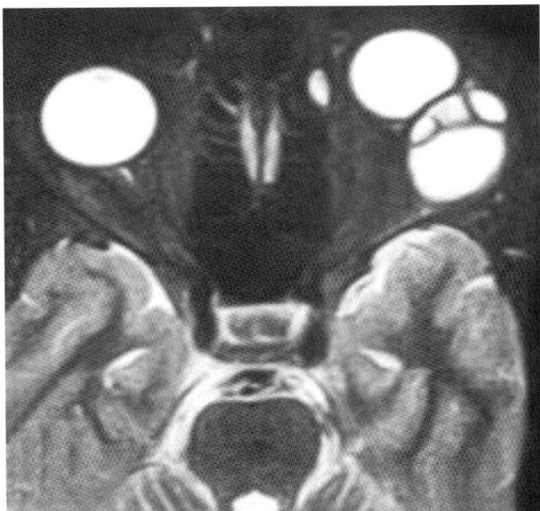

Fig. 34.22: *Axial CT scan image showing orbital echinococcosis, left eyeball.*

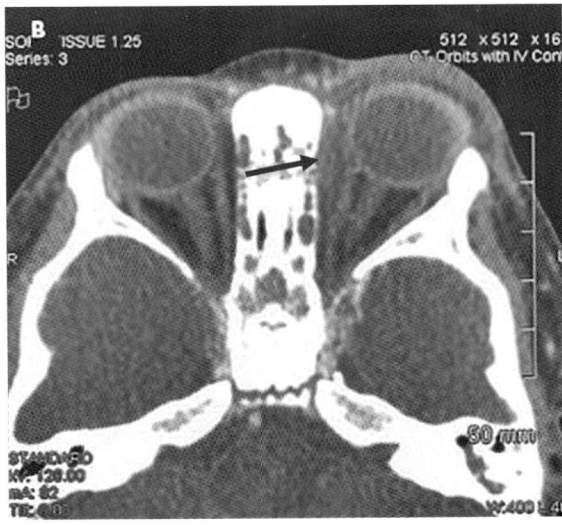

Fig. 34.24: *Axial CT scan orbit showing left orbital abscess.*

- Homogeneous or heterogeneous mass with enhancing margins
- Inflammation of sinuses and adjacent structures is usually well-demonstrated
- Associated CT findings include: sinusitis, cavernous sinus thrombosis, and subdural empyema
- Cellulitis displays a diffuse, homogeneously enhancing mass lesion
- 'Ring' enhancement or air bubbles herald the progression from cellulitis to suppuration and abscess development.

Pott's puffy tumour

Common CT scan findings seen in a patient with Pott's puffy tumour are summarised below (Fig. 34.25):

- Regional osteopenia with decreased bone density
- Periosteal reaction can cause Codman's triangle
- Focal bony lysis
- Loss of bony trabeculation
- Sequestra are better seen on computed tomography (CT)
- Typically see opacified frontal sinus with overlying scalp swelling
- Bone algorithms often better demonstrate sinus wall defect
- Often see obliteration of fat planes
- Cellulitis can display a diffuse homogeneously enhancing mass lesion
- Contrast can show focal abscess

- Eccentric globe displacement suggests subperiosteal OA
- Intraorbital gas or air-fluid level strongly suggests OA
- Inflammation of sinuses and adjacent structures is usually well-demonstrated
- 'Ring' enhancement or air bubbles herald the progression from cellulitis to suppuration and abscess development
- CT findings include sinusitis, cavernous sinus thrombosis, and subdural empyema.

VASCULAR INTRAORBITAL LESIONS

Orbital venous varix

Common CT scan findings in a patient with orbital venous varix include (Fig. 34.26):

- High-density mass with occasional phleboliths a characteristic feature
- Contrast-enhanced CT (CECT): Performed supine and prone or with the Valsalva maneuver
- Enhancing mass significantly larger when straining
- Enhances the same as other venous structures (e.g. cavernous sinus).

Cavernous sinus thrombosis

Common CT scan findings seen in a patient with cavernous sinus thrombosis are summarised below (Fig. 34.27):

- May see multiple irregular low attenuation filling defects within enhancing CS and occasionally SOV, as exhibited in case presented

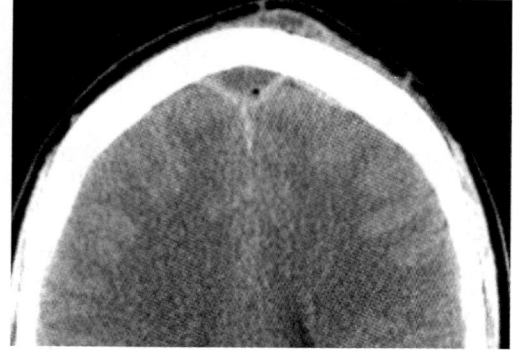

Fig. 34.25: *Coronal CT scan image showing Pott's puffy tumour.*

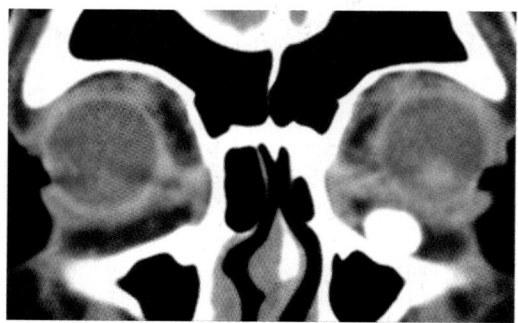

Fig. 34.26: *Coronal CT scan shows the presence of an irregular mass in the inferior with a hyperdense well-circumscribed lesion along the orbital floor.*

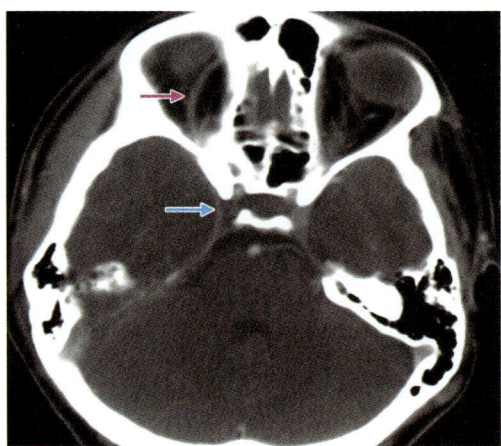

Fig. 34.27: *Axial CT scan image showing right cavernous sinus thrombosis.*

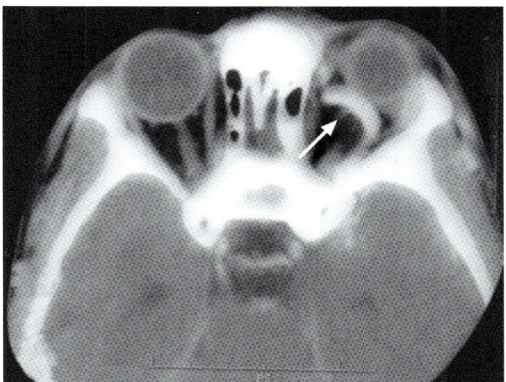

Fig. 34.28: *Axial CT scan of a patient showing prominent cavernous sinuses (L>R), dilated left superior ophthalmic vein, evidence of soft tissues swelling present in left retroorbital tissue.*

- May see SOV enlargement with hetero-geneous enhancement, proptosis, and periorbital swelling
- Rarely, cavernous internal carotid artery (ICA) narrowing or occlusion causing cerebral infarction
- Important to image and report status of cavernous ICA
- Inflammation of sinuses and adjacent structures usually well-demonstrated
- Associated CT finding include sinusitis, orbital abscess, and subdural empyema.

Carotid-cavernous fistula (CCF)

Common CT scan findings in a patient with carotid cavernous fistula include (Fig. 34.28):
- Enlarged superior ophthalmic vein
- Enlarged cavernous sinus
- Extraocular muscles (EOMs) may be enlarged
- Orbital edema
- Dilated superficial veins are an ominous sign of cortical venous drainage
- May show subarachnoid hemorrhage (SAH) or intracranial hemorrhage (ICH) from ruptured cortical vein.

ORBITAL TUMOURS

Orbital dermoid cyst

- CT scan in patient with orbital dermoid cyst shows a cystic lesion with enhancement of the

wall but no significant enhancement of lumen (Fig. 34.29).
- Also useful to assess any bony defect.

Optic nerve glioma (ONG)

Common CT scan findings in a patient with optic nerve glioma include (Fig. 34.30).
- Fusiform 'sausage-shaped' enlargement of the ON
- May detect subtle erosion of the optic canal
- Calcifications are rare.

Optic nerve meningioma

Common CT scan findings seen in a patient with optic nerve meningioma are summarised below (Fig. 34.31):
- High-density mass surrounding the ON

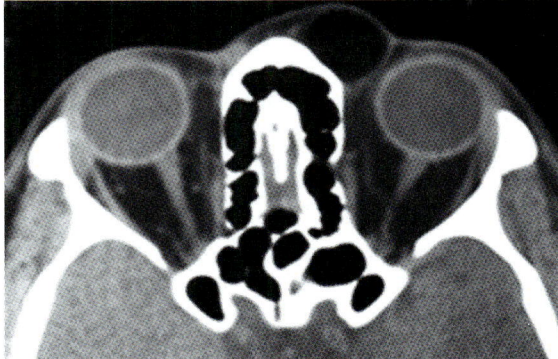

Fig. 34.29: *Axial CT scan orbit showing a cystic lesion in left superomedial orbit.*

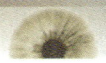

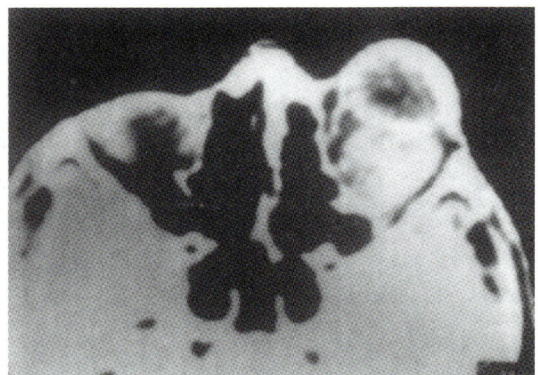

Fig. 34.30: *Axial CT scan image showing left optic nerve glioma.*

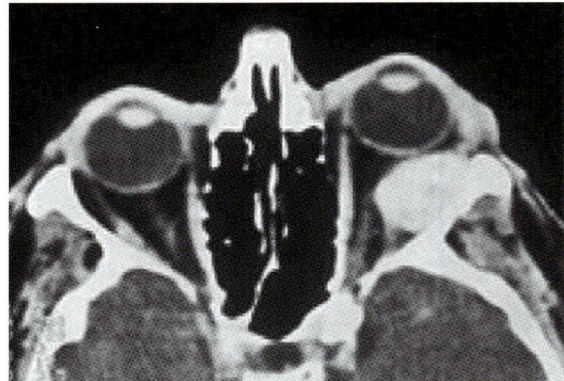

Fig. 34.32: *Axial CT scan image showing left orbital schwannoma.*

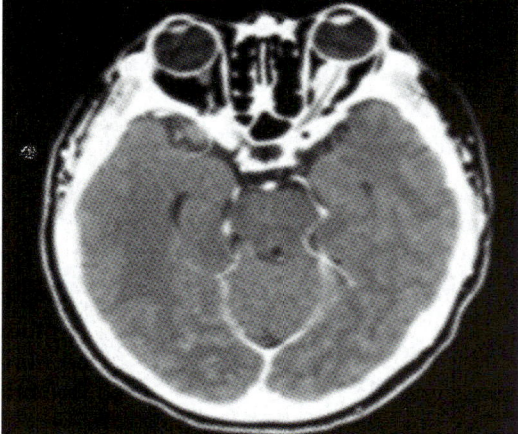

Fig. 34.31: *Axial CT scan image showing left optic nerve sheath meningioma.*

- Calcification in 20 to 50% of cases
- Postcontrast enhancement demonstrates the 'tram track' or 'sandwich' sign with the ON sandwiched between tumour masses
- Calcified ONMs may show the above appearance even without contrast
- Bony changes may include erosion and hyperostosis of the sphenoid and/or optic canal enlargement.

Orbital Schwannomas

Common CT scan findings in a patient with orbital schwannoma include (Fig. 34.32):

- Well-circumscribed, encapsulated mass
- Most OSs show mild enhancement on contrasted CT

- Enlargement of the superior orbital fissure or invasion of the cavernous sinus may be apparent.

Esthesioneuroblastoma

Common CT scan findings seen in a patient with esthesioneuroblastoma are summarised below (Fig. 34.33):

- Nonenhancing computed tomography (NECT) shows a soft tissue mass causing nasal cavity enlargement and remodeling.
- 'Figure-8' or dumbbell-shaped mass with a 'waist' at the cribriform plate.

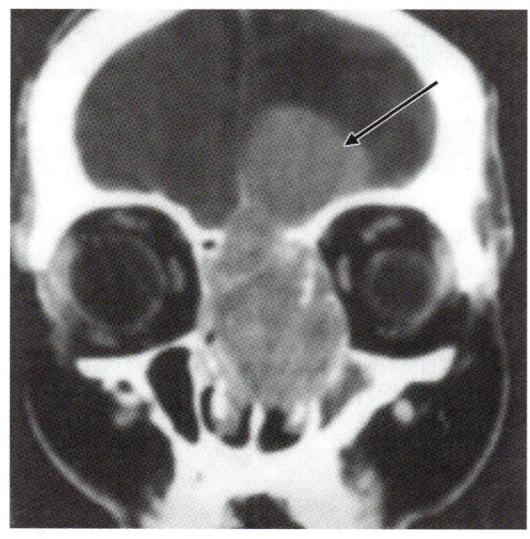

Fig. 34.33: *Axial CT scan image showing left orbital esthesioneuroblastoma.*

- Unilateral mass with its epicenter near the superior nasal wall.
- Depending on tumour phase, bone destruction may be seen and calcium deposition may sometimes be present showing a speckled pattern. Sometimes hyperostosis may be seen, suggesting slow growth.
- Bony changes particularly involve the cribriform plate.
- Contrast-enhanced CT (CECT) shows a homogeneous, enhancing soft tissue mass.
- Computed tomography angiography (CTA) shows a conspicuous vascular blush.

Rhabdomyosarcoma

Common CT scan findings in a patient with rhabdomyosarcoma include (Fig. 34.34):

- Typically homogeneous soft tissue mass isodense to normal muscle (but may rarely resemble a cystic lesion with areas of hemorrhage).
- Commonly appears as a well-circumscribed mass with irregular margins.
- The mass may extend into the eyelid, or invade through the bone into the ethmoid sinuses or the anterior cranial fossa.
- The tumour is not calcified.
- Hyperostosis of the adjacent orbital bones is virtually never present.
- CT and fluorodeoxyglucose (FDG) positron emission tomography (PET)/CT play major roles in evaluating metastatic disease.

Orbital lymphangioma

Common CT scan findings seen in a patient with orbital lymphangioma are summarised below (Fig. 34.35):

- Appear as a poorly defined masses with heterogeneous tumour density
- They have irregular margins, and show little or no contrast enhancement.

Orbital cavernous hemangioma

Common CT scan findings in a patient with orbital cavernous hemangioma include (Fig. 34.36):

- Precontrast hyperdensity related to microcalcifications
- Postcontrast hyperdensity calcifications appears as a well-demarcated contrast enhancing intraconal mass.

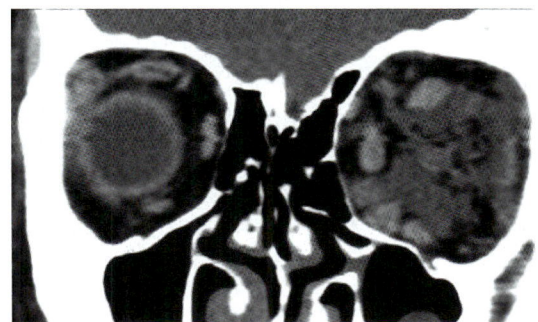

Fig. 34.35: *Axial CT scan image showing left orbital lymphangioma.*

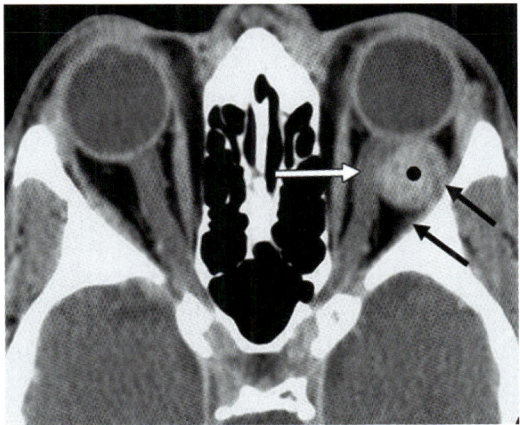

Fig. 34.36: *Axial CT scan image showing left orbital cavernous hemangioma.*

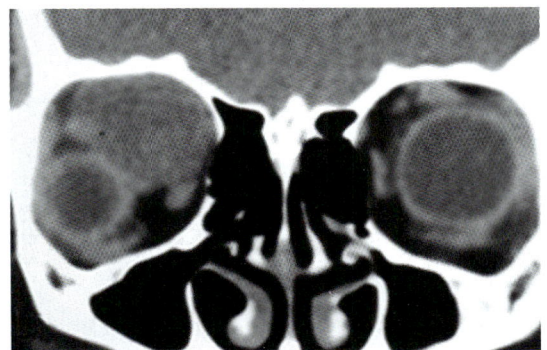

Fig. 34.34: *Coronal CT scan showing a large right superomedial orbital lesion displacing the globe downward and outward.*

Orbital capillary hemangioma

CT scan in a patient with orbital capillary hemangioma include a well-demarcated, homogeneous, contrast enhancing, extraconal mass occupying the periorbital soft tissue and anterior orbit (Fig. 34.37).

OCULAR ADNEXAL LYMPHOMA

Common CT scan findings in a patient with ocular adnexal lymphoma include (Fig. 34.38):

* Homogeneous. Isodense or slightly hyper-dense to extraocular muscles (EOMs)

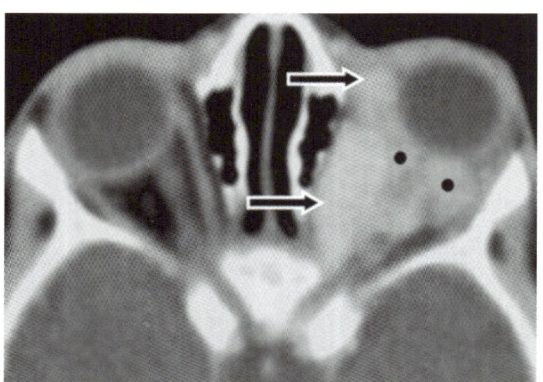

Fig. 34.37: *Axial CT scan image showing left orbital capillary hemangioma.*

* Lesions usually sculpt themselves to adjacent structures without bony erosion
* Heterogeneous lesions with bony destruction suggest high-grade histology
* Mild to moderate postcontrast enhancement similar to EOM or lacrimal gland (LG)
* Calcifications are rarely seen
* Usually has an extraconal epicenter but may extend intraconally
* May involve the lacrimal sac and EOMs
* Irregular infiltration of retrobulbar fat may cause a streaky or 'dirty fat' appearance
* Bilateral lesions suggest the presence of systemic disease.

LACRIMAL GLAND LESIONS

Dacryops

CT scan in a patient with dacryops reveals a cystic structure in the region of lacrimal gland without bony disruption (Fig. 34.39).

Lacrimal gland dermoids

Common CT scan findings in a patient with lacrimal gland dermoid include (Fig. 34.40):

* Unilateral well-defined cyst-like masses containing fluid or fat
* May contain calcifications
* Filled with hypodense material

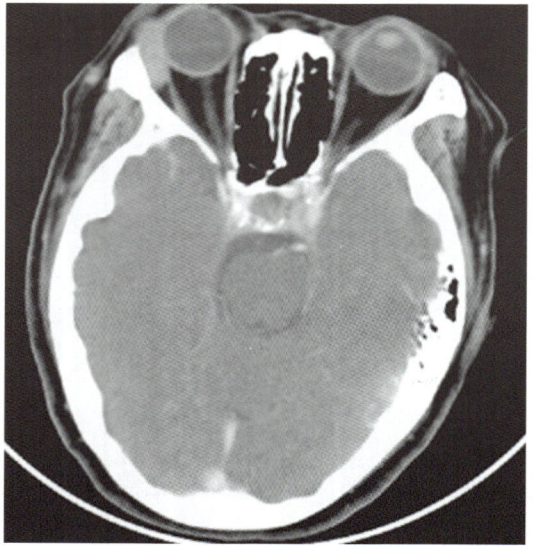

Fig. 34.38: *Axial CT scan image showing right ocular adnexal lymphoma.*

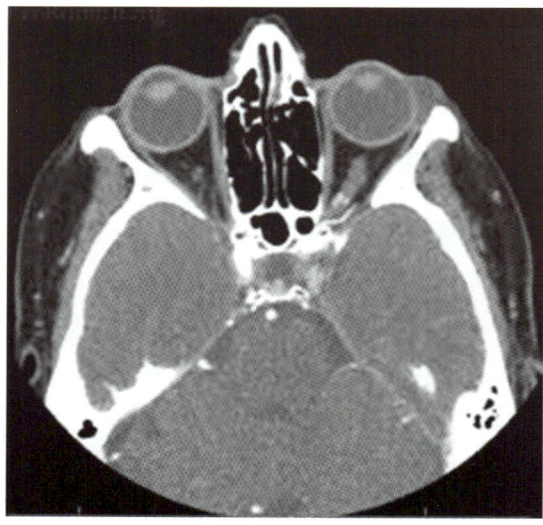

Fig. 34.39: *Axial CT scan orbit showing a cystic structure in region of lacrimal gland.*

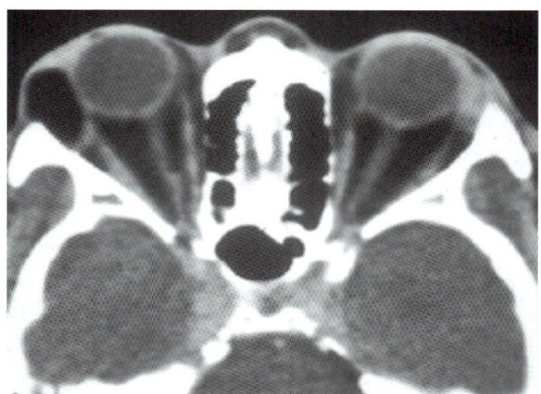

Fig. 34.40: *Axial CT scan image showing right lacrimal gland dermoid.*

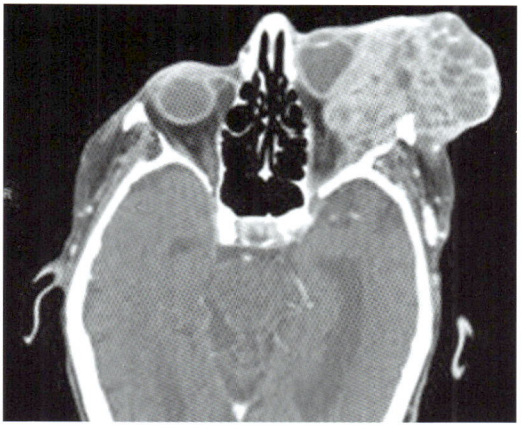

Fig. 34.42: *Axial CT scan image showing adenoid cystic carcinoma, left lacrimal gland.*

- Central cavity may contain keratin and other cystic debris
- Cause scalloping or sclerosis of adjacent bone
- May show 'dirty fat' appearance when infected.

Pleomorphic Adenomas

Common CT scan findings seen in a patient with pleomorphic adenoma are summarised below (Fig. 34.41):
- Nodular well-delineated lesions with moderate contrast enhancement
- They have smooth and well-defined margins, and local bony fossa formation is common.

Adenoid cystic carcinoma of lacrimal gland

Common CT scan findings seen in a patient with adenoid cystic carcinoma of lacrimal gland are summarised below (Fig. 34.42):

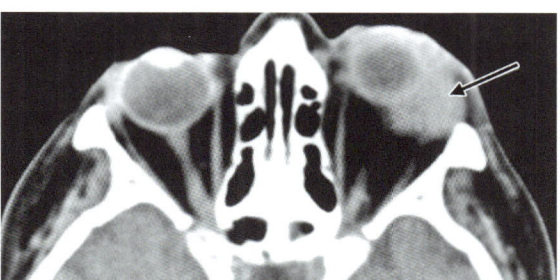

Fig. 34.43: *Axial CT scan image showing squamous cell carcinoma, left lacrimal gland.*

- Computed tomography (CT) shows an un-encapsulated, irregular, infiltrating, enhancing lacrimal gland mass
- Calcification is common.

Squamous cell carcinoma (SCC) of lacrimal gland

- Computed tomography (CT) in a patient with squamous cell carcinoma of lacrimal sac shows a lacrimal gland mass that may erode the lacrimal fossa and adjacent structures (Fig. 34.43).
- Bone destruction suggests a malignant etiology.

SPECIAL CT INVESTIGATIONS

CT ANGIOGRAPHY

Computed tomographic angiography (CTA) requires an injection of iodinated contrast,

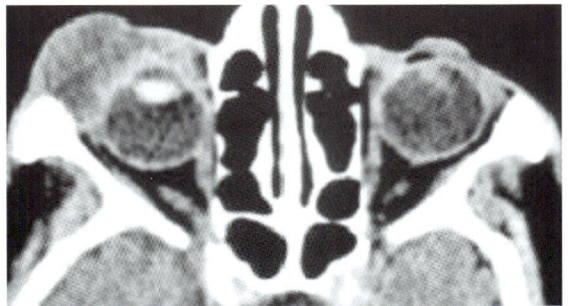

Fig. 34.41: *Axial CT scan image showing pleomorphic adenoma, right lacrimal gland.*

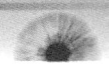

intravenously followed by high-speed spiral CT scan with computer-generated 3-dimensional images of medium-sized and large-sized arteries. It is sensitive to detect aneurysm of >3 mm and stenosis of >70 percent.

Advantages of CT angiography (CTA) over standard MR angiography

- Increased spatial resolution
- Takes less time to aquire images
- Less motion artifacts
- Images of the true lumen (rather than flow within a vessel)
- Detection of aneurysms as small as 1.7 mm
- Superior imaging of the aneurysm neck, better delineation of surgical anatomy
- Characterization of mural thrombi
- Detection of vasospasm
- Arterial stenosis, and carotid-cavernous fistulas
- Ability to be performed in patients with claustrophobia, pacemakers, and older aneurysm clips.

Drawbacks of CT angiography

- Difficult detection and delineation of cavernous sinus and posterior inferior cerebellar artery aneurysms, feeding vessels for dural carotid cavernous fistula.
- Risks involving radiation exposure and contrast agents.

CT VENOGRAPHY

- Computed tomography venography (CTV) is an excellent imaging modality for visualizing the cerebral venous system and is comparable to MRV.
- It is used for detecting cerebral venous thrombosis, which is both rapid and widely available. CTV can provide very detailed imaging of the venous system, which is superior to TOF MRV, and is at least as accurate for detecting thrombosis.
- Disadvantages to CTV include the use of iodinated contrast material, ionizing radiation exposure, and difficulty in reconstructing maximum intensity projection (MIP) images because of problems subtracting bone adjacent to the venous sinuses.

SINGLE-PHOTON EMISSION COMPUTED TOMOGRAPHY (SPECT)

SPECT is performed with systemically administered isotopes such as iodine-123 iodoamphetamine or technetium-99, incorporated into biologically active compounds, and CT plots their distribution. They are used to image biological processes that measure regional cerebral blood flow and glucose consumption and thus, indirectly, tissue metabolism. These techniques trace the transport and phosphorylation of glucose, and the glucose-linked positron emits two photons, which strike detectors placed around the head is an excellent agent to use for cerebral metabolism imaging. Tomographic images are obtained in a manner similar to those for MRI or CT scanning. Cerebral blood flow, oxygen utilization, and glucose utilization may be measured. SPECT can detect regional cerebral blood flow (rCBF) increase in the visual cortex with visual stimulation. The clinical utility of brain SPECT has also been documented in patients with cortical visual loss, even in those patients who had normal or non diagnostic MRI. Although the spatial resolution of SPECT is lower than that of PET, it is less expensive, more widely available and offers a more practical approach in routine clinical studies. Current applications of functional imaging include detection of hypermetabolic states associated with tumour, differentiation of tumour from areas of radiation-induced necrosis, localization of seizure foci, detection of ischaemic regions, evaluation of biochemical changes associated with cognitive and psychiatric abnormalities and their response to pharmaceutical intervention, and drug localization in the brain.

BIBLIOGRAPHY

1. Apfaltrer P, Hanna EL, Schoepf UJ, et al. Radiation dose and image quality at high-pitch CT angiography of the aorta: intra individual and inter individual comparisons with conventional CT angiography. AJR Am J Roentgenol 2012;199:1402–9.
2. Brenner DJ, Hall EJ. Computed tomography—an increasing source of radiation exposure. N Engl J Med 2007;357:2277–84.

3. Dong F, Davros W, Pozzuto J, et al. Optimization of kilovoltage and tube current-exposure time product based on abdominal circumference: an oval phantom study for pediatric abdominal CT. AJR Am J Roentgenol 2012;199:670–6.

4. Garrity JA, Forbes GS. Computed tomography of the orbit. In: Tasmman W, Jaeger EA, editors. Duane's Clinical Ophthalmology. Philadelphia: Lippincott-Raven 1997;2:1–16.

5. Gnannt R, Winklehner A, Eberli D, et al. Automated tube potential selection for standard chest and abdominal CT in follow-up patients with testicular cancer: comparison with fixed tube potential. Eur Radiol 2012;22:1937–45.

6. Halliburton SS, Abbara S, Chen MY, et al. SCCT guidelines on radiation dose and dose-optimization strategies in cardiovascular CT. J Cardiovasc Comput Tomogr 2011;5:198–224.

7. Hamberg LM, Rhea JT, Hunter GJ, et al. Multi-detector row CT: radiation dose characteristics. Radiology 2003;226:762–72.

8. Hilal SK, Trokel SL. Computerized tomography of the orbit using thin sections. Semin Roentgenol 1977;12:137–47.

9. Korn A, Fenchel M, Bender B, et al. High-pitch dual-source CT angiography of supraaortic arteries: assessment of image quality and radiation dose. Neuroradiology 2013;55:423–30.

10. Leipsic J, Labounty TM, Heilbron B, et al. Estimated radiation dose reduction using adaptive statistical iterative reconstruction in coronary CT angiography: the ERASIR study. AJR Am J Roentgenol 2010;195:655–60.

11. Mahesh M. CT physics: the basics of multi-detec-tor physics. Philadelphia: Lippincott Williams & Wilkins; 2009.

12. Martinsen AC, Saether HK, Hol PK, et al. Iterative reconstruction reduces abdominal CT dose. Eur J Radiol 2012;81:1483–7.

13. Nungent R, Rootman J, Robertson W. Applied investigative anatomy. In: Virginia Barishek (Ed). Diseases of the Orbit-A Multidisciplinary Approach. Part 1. Philadelphia: Lippincott Company; 1988, pp 35.

14. Patel H, Coughlin B, LaFrance T, et al. (Eds). Comparison of full chest CTA with limited CTA and triple rule-out CTA for PE detection and effective dose implications. Chicago, Illinois: Radiological Society of North America; 2007.

15. Raman SP, Johnson PT, Deshmukh S, et al. CT dose reduction applications: available tools on the latest generation of CT scanners. J Am Coll Radiol 2013;10:37–41.

16. Weir J, Abrahams PH, Spratt JD, et al. Mosby; 4 edition (2 Mar. 2010). Imaging Atlas of Human Anatomy.

17. Weisberg LA. Computed tomographic findings in carotid cavernous fistula. Comput Tomogr 1981;5:31–6.

Magnetic Resonance Imaging in Ophthalmology

Chapter Outline

GENERAL CONSIDERATIONS
- Definition
- Principle of MRI
- MRI machine
- Advantages and disadvantages of MRI
- Indications and contraindications of MRI
- Basic steps of MR imaging

SYSTEMATIC APPROACH FOR REPORTING/INTER-PRETATION OF MRI SCAN
- Scheme of interpretation
- Normal orbital anatomy on MRI

MRI FINDINGS IN OCULAR LESIONS

Congenital Ocular Lesions
- Persistent hyperplastic primary vitreous
- Congenital anophthalmos

Inflammatory/Infective Ocular Lesions
- Optic neuritis
- Endophthalmitis
- Scleritis
- Cytomegalovirus retinitis
- Uveal effusion syndrome

Intraocular Tumours
- Retinoblastoma
- Malignant melanoma

Miscellaneous Conditions
- Retinal detachment
- Phthisis bulbi

MRI FINDINGS IN ORBITAL LESIONS

Congenital Orbital Lesions
- Congenital orbital teratoma

Traumatic Orbital Lesions
- Intraorbital foreign body

Inflammatory/Infective Orbital Lesions
- Thyroid orbitopathy
- Idiopathic orbital inflammatory disease
- Orbital cysticercosis
- Orbital echinococcosis
- Orbital abscess
- Tolosa-Hunt syndrome

Vascular Orbital Lesions
- Orbital varix
- Cavernous sinus thrombosis
- Carotid cavernous fistula

Orbital Tumours
- Optic nerve glioma
- Optic nerve meningioma
- Orbital schwannoma
- Orbital lymphangioma
- Orbital cavernous hemangioma
- Orbital capillary hemangioma

Lacrimal Gland Lesions
- Lacrimal gland sarcoidosis
- Lacrimal gland lymphoma (LGL)
- Malignant epithelial lacrimal gland tumour

SPECIAL MRI INVESTIGATIONS
- Functional MRI
- MRI spectroscopy
- MR angiography
- MR venography

GENERAL CONSIDERATIONS

DEFINITION

MRI is a diagnostic technique that uses nuclear magnetic resonance and radiowaves to produce an extremely accurate and detailed cross-sectional images of the soft tissues of the body. It has become an indispensable imaging diagnostic tool in orbital and ocular anatomy and pathology as it produces images without use of ionizing radiation, has excellent contrast resolution and can obtain images in any plane without changing the position of the patient.

PRINCIPLE OF MRI

MRI is based on the electromagnetic activity of protons of nuclei of the body cells. Since hydrogen is abundant in the human body (as a component of water molecule), MRI can be used to image any part of human body. Every spinning proton has a small magnetic field around it. Different tissues of the body have differing magnetic properties and hence show different signals in different pulse sequences. Depending upon the time when this signal is recorded, different kinds of images, T1 and T2, can be acquired.

T1- and T2-weighted images: When radiofrequency (RF) pulse is switched off, longitudinal magnetisation (LM) starts increasing and transverse magnetisation (TM) starts reducing. The time taken by LM to recover to its original value after RF pulse is switched off is called longitudinal relaxation time or T1. The time taken by TM to reduce to its original value is transverse relaxation time or T2. The magnitude of LM indirectly determines the strength of MR signal. The tissues with short T1 regain their maximum LM in short-time after RF pulse is switched off. When the next RF pulse is sent, TM will be stronger and resultant signal will also be stronger. Therefore, material with short T1 have bright signal on T1-weighted images.

- Short TR and short TE gives T1-weighted images
- Long TR and long TE gives T2-weighted images

- T1W image has higher spatial resolution and better depicts anatomy of the orbit. T2W image, in contrast has higher contrast resolution and depicts the pathology better .

FLAIR (fluid attenuation inversion recovery): As the name suggests, the cerebrospinal fluid (CSF) signal is strongly attenuated, accentuating periventricular and extra-axial disease near the brain surface, thereby allowing visualization of the underlying pathology (e.g. white matter demyelination, posterior reversible encephalopathy) that might otherwise be obscured by the bright signal of normal CSF. FLAIR sequences help reveal demyelination or MS plaques in the central nervous system, tumours and ischaemic lesions that often are not visible on routine MR imaging.

Fat suppression is commonly used in magnetic resonance (MR) imaging to suppress the signal from adipose tissue or detect adipose tissues. It can be applied to both T1- and T2-weighted sequences by suppression of hyperintense signals from orbital fat and subcutaneous fat. Due to short relaxation times, fat has a high signal on magnetic resonance images (MRI). This high signal, easily recognised on MRI, may be useful to characterise a lesion. STIR (short tau inversion recovery) sequence can also be used to suppress the fat signal, but it has lesser resolution. Fat suppression is especially useful to image the orbit with post-contrast T1W images; this removes the inherently high signal of retrobulbar fat with which enhancing lesions may blend on T1W image.

Diffusion-weighted imaging (DWI) is a form of MR imaging based upon measuring the random Brownian motion of water molecules within a tissue. Highly cellular tissues or those with cellular swelling exhibit lower diffusion coefficients. Apparent diffusion coefficient is a measure of the diffusion. ADC is independent of magnetic field strength. The area with reduced ADC (restricted diffusion) will manifest as a bright area on the diffusion-weighted images (DWI) while the same area will turn dark on the ADC map, thus diffusion is particularly useful in tumour characterisation, abscess and cerebral ischaemia.

Use of contrast agent

- Intravenous gadolinium-diethylene-triamine-penta-acetic acid (Gd-DTPA) chelate is the routine contrast agent used with MRI. This agent shortens the T1 relaxation time and hence makes them appear bright. There is substantial improvement in lesion identification and characterization with Gd.
- It is most commonly used in the evaluation of optic nerve and other orbital pathologies. MR angiograms can also be performed using contrast and is useful in vascular lesions, e.g. in carotico cavernous fistula.
- Other contrast agents which can be used are iron oxide, Mn-DPDP, dysprosium chelates.
- Patient with history of allergy, asthma and previous reaction to drugs, iodinated contrast are more prone for the adverse reactions.
- Gadolinium-based contrast media administration in patients with renal failure can cause nephrogenic systemic fibrosis.
- Gadolinium is known to cross the placenta, so contrast medium should not be routinely injected in pregnant patient.
- Gadolinium is excreted in human milk. Breast milk should be expressed after injection and thrown away. Baby should not be breastfed for 36–48 hours.

MRI MACHINE

MRI scanner is a large tube (bore) that holds powerful magnets, gradient coil, radiofrequency coil (RF coil) and a computer. The biggest and most important component of an MRI system is the magnet. The magnets used are: superconducting, resistive and permanent magnet. But the most commonly used magnet is superconducting magnet. During the imaging process, the field must be distorted with gradients. A gradient is just a change in field strength from one point to another in the patient's body. The gradients are produced by a set of gradient coils, which are contained within the magnet assembly. The RF coils are located within the magnet assembly and relatively close to the patient's body. These coils function as the antennae for both transmitting signals to and receiving signals from the tissue. The scanning operation is controlled from a central computer. They perform functions of data collection and manipulation, image viewing, storage, retrieval and documentation.

Types of MRI machine

- Closed MRI
- Open MRI

Closed MRI machine is that which takes detailed images in a narrow cylindrical container normally spanning a bore diameter of 60 cm (Fig. 35.1A).

Open MRI (Fig. 35.1B) was created to offer an alternative to patients who either have symptoms of anxiety or suffer from claustrophobia or obesity due to the enclosed nature. While

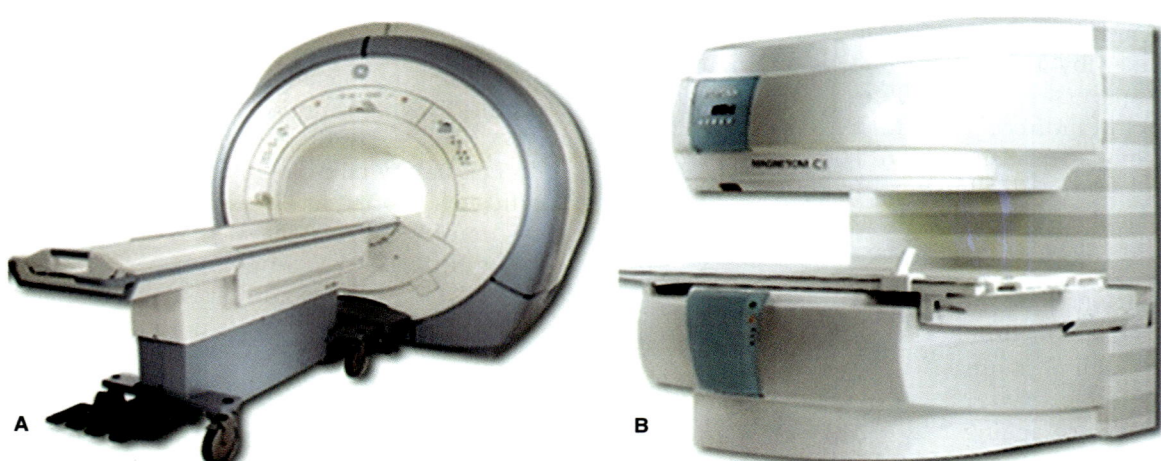

Fig. 35.1: *MRI scanners: (A) Closed type; (B) Open type.*

the open MRI excels at providing comfort, it does not provide the same level of detail as a closed MRI.

UNIT OF MRI

All MRI machines are calibrated in Tesla units. The strength of a magnetic field is measured in Tesla or Gauss units. The stronger the magnetic field, the stronger the amount of radiosignals which can be elicited from the body atoms and thus higher the quality of MRI images. Routinely MRI scanning is done with a 1.5 Tesla system . Now, with the availability of 3-T systems, orbital and ocular pathology imaging has improved drastically. This results from an increased signal to noise ratio (SNR) by this high strength system which can be used to increase the spatial resolution or reduce the scan time. This high strength system thus may play an increasingly important role in ophthalmic imaging in future.

ADVANTAGES AND DISADVNATAGES

Advantages of MRI

- Excellent soft tissue resolution of orbital contents
- No exposure to ionising radiations
- Better able to distinguish white from gray matter
- Better resolution of optic nerve and orbital apex.

Disadvantages of MRI

- Contrast dye reactions
- Expensive
- Systemic nephrogenic fibrosis can occur in patients with renal compromise.

INDICATIONS AND CONTRAINDICATIONS OF MRI IN OPHTHALMOLOGY

Indications

- Unexplained proptosis, ptosis or ophthalmoplegia
- Palpable orbital mass
- Orbital trauma after excluding ferromagnetic foreign body
- For screening and assessment of known or suspected optic neuritis
- For screening and evaluation of ocular tumor
- Unexplained afferent dysfunction—Orbital, intracanalicular, and prechiasmal optic pathways
- Papilledema
- For screening and evaluation of suspected orbital pseudotumor
- Tumor response after radiotherapy or chemotherapy
- Anophthalmic socket when orbital tumor recurrence is suspected.

Conditions in which MRI is preferred over CT scan

- Retinoblastoma to look for extent of optic nerve involvement/intracranial spread, for better evaluation of soft tissue involvement and to diagnose trilateral retinoblastoma/pinealoblastoma
- Dermoid cyst for delineating the intracranial spread
- As optic nerve and cavernous sinus are better studied on MRI, so in cases of multiple cranial nerve palsies, when cavernous sinus lesion or basal meningitis is suspected, T2-weighted MRI is preferred to depict intracranial course of nerves
- When optic neuritis is suspected, MRI is the preferred imaging modality for proper assessment of optic nerves and to look for associated white matter abnormality
- In cases of optic atrophy,intracranial and intracanalicular portions of optic nerve are better assessed on MRI.
- For evaluation of proptosis,
  - If thyroid orbitopathy or orbital cellulitis is suspected, MRI is preferred to look for involvement of orbital apex or cavernous sinus
  - If orbital varix is suspected, MRI in prone position can show distensibility of varix.

Contraindications

- Ferromagnetic foreign body/implants
- Cochlear implants
- Pacemakers
- Metallic cardiac implant

- Non MRI compatible intracranial aneurysm clips
- Claustrophobia

BASIC STEPS OF MR IMAGING

- Placing the patient in the centre of the bore of a large super-conducting magnet is done to perform MRI. This magnet has a unidirectional field and the protons of the body become aligned with it.
- Application of radiofrequency (RF) gradients is done by a coil which causes disturbance of the alignment of protons. This results in reduction in the longitudinal magnetization and increase in transverse magnetization.
- On termination of radiofrequency gradient, the excited protons return to the resting state and tend to align (relax) back to the main magnetic field. During this process, energy is released in the form of a signal (echo), which is received by a receiver coil.
- **Generation of MR image:** RF energy that is detected, localized, and then processed by a computer algorithm to produce a cross sectional tomographic anatomical image. This process of applying RF pulse and receiving a signal is repeated many times to generate a MR image.

Repetition time (TR) is the time interval between start of one RF pulse and start of the next RF pulse. Echo time (TE) is the time interval between start of RF pulse and reception of the signal (echo).

SYSTEMATIC APPROACH FOR REPORTING/INTERPRETATION OF MRI SCAN

SCHEME OF INTERPRETATION

Following points must always be kept in mind while interpretation of a MRI scan:

1. Is it a CT scan or MRI scan?

- First of all, it is important to judge is it a CT scan or MRI scan. One might confuse the CT and T1 MRI sequence. Both images display a structure that is white in the periphery and

has CSF that is dark. On MRI this white structure represents the subcutaneous fat and on CT the bright structure is the skull.

- CT images are acquired only in the axial plane. The axial plane image data then can be used to reconstruct images in sagittal and coronal planes. MRI can be acquired in all the three axial, sagittal and coronal planes.
- In MRI scans, the fat can be either white or dark in appearance, depending on the sequence either T1 or T2. In a CT scan image, fat and fluid never appears white, thus if either fat or fluid appears white, it is definitely a MRI scan.
- On CT scan bone is always white as calcium blocks the X-ray photons. The calcium does not emit a signal in MRI scans and thus both bone and bone marrow appears dark. If one can see that bony structures are black or dark gray in colour, then one can be sure that it is a MRI scan.

2. Patient and image details

- Name of the patient should match with the name written on the report.
- Time and date written on the reports should be checked to ensure that those reports are the latest and also for proper follow-up of patients in future.
- Check the laterality (right or left) of the patient you are visualising.

3. Check planes of all the images which are available

MRI images are commonly viewed in three planes:

Axial MRI scan: An axial MRI scan consists of a series of images which look at the brain and orbit from below starting at the chin and moving up to top of head (Fig. 35.2A).

Sagittal MRI scan: Sagittal MRI scan consists of a series of images which look at the brain and orbit from side to side, starting at one ear to other ear (Fig. 35.2B).

Coronal MRI scan: Coronal MRI scan consists of a series of images which look at the brain and orbit from behind, starting at the back of the head and moving up to the face (Fig. 35.2C).

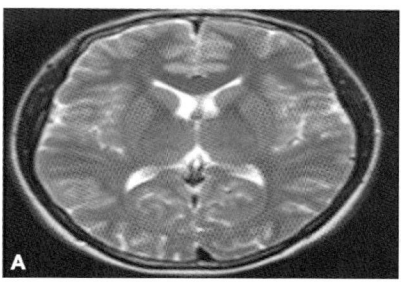 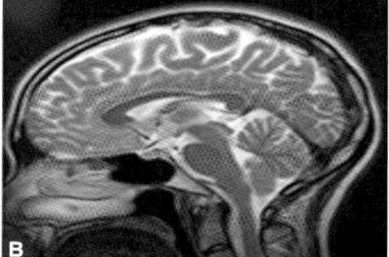 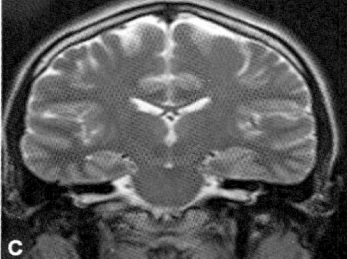

Fig. 35.2: *Three planes of MRI scan: (A) Axial; (B) Sagittal; (C) Coronal.*

4. Check if the image is with or without contrast

Gadolinium is the most common contrast agent used for MRI.

Abnormal tissue may enhance more after contrast administration and retain contrast for long than surrounding normal tissue.

Routine MRI is presented as black and white images and not in colour (Fig. 35.3A). The grey colour is represented in varying shades depending on their signal intensity. White colour is suggestive of contrast administration (Fig. 35.3B).

White signal in the blood vessel appears due to contrast. Contrast enhanced images are useful for vascular structures and in cases of breakdown of blood–brain barrier and blood retinal barrier.

5. Is it a T1- or T2-weighted image?

- **In T1-weighted images,** only **FAT appears bright** (Fig. 35.4, right orbit)
- **In T2-images,** both **FAT** and **WATER appear bright** (Fig. 35.4, left orbit)
- Generally T1- and T2-weighted images can be distinguished by looking at the CSF and vitreous humour. CSF and vitreous humour appear dark on T1 and bright on T2 as CSF and vitreous are fluid and contain no fat.

6. Abnormal MRI signal

- Look for abnormalities of MRI signal
- Determine the nature of the change in the signal that whether it is due to abnormal fat or fluid

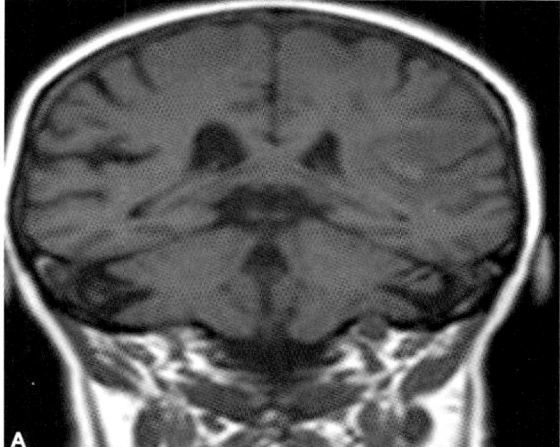

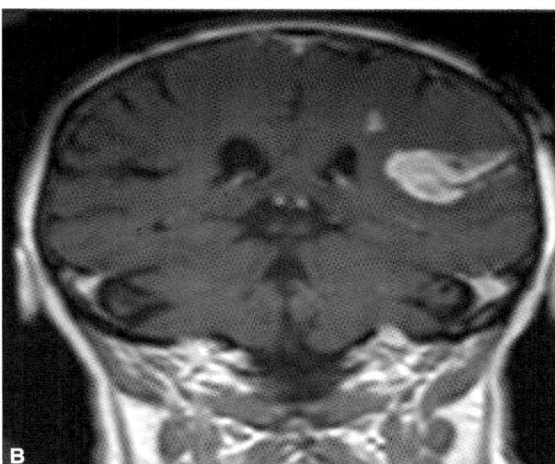

Fig. 35.3: *MRI scan (A) without and (B) with contrast.*

- Check whether the abnormal signal is hyper or hypointense
- Note the anatomical location, size and shape of the abnormality for diagnosis and further follow-up.

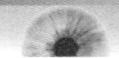

Lesions hyperintense on T1 and hypointense on T2

- Retinoblastoma
- Malignant choroidal melanoma
- Posterior orbital dermoid
- Wegener's granulomatosis.

Lesions hypointense on T1 and hyperintense on T2

- Optic nerve glioma
- Optic nerve sheath meningioma
- Orbital cavernous hemangioma
- Orbital schwannoma
- Malignant epithelial lacrimal gland tumours.

Lesions hypointense on T1 and T2

- Orbital lymphoma
- Nonmetallic intraorbital foreign body.

Lesions hyperintense on T1 and T2

- Cavernous sinus hemangioma.

NORMAL ORBITAL ANATOMY ON MRI

Normal orbital anatomy as seen in axial scan and coronal scan is depicted in Figs 35.4 and 35.5, respectively. Appearance of various ocular and orbital structures in T1- and T2-weighted image is depicted in Table 35.1

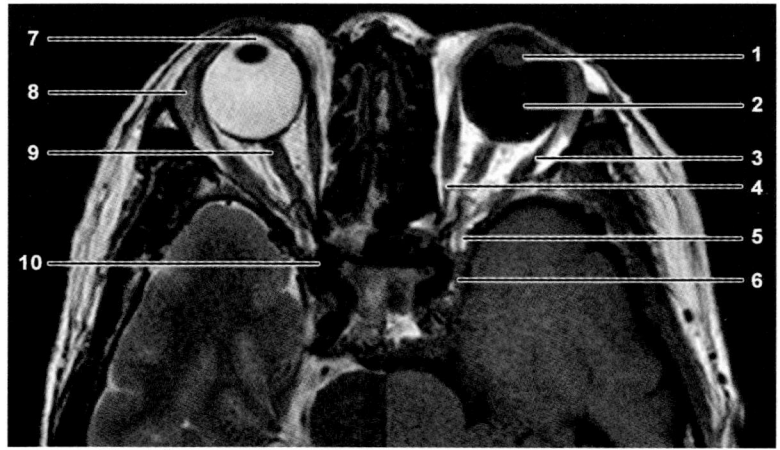

Fig. 35.4: Axial MRI scan comparing T1 (right) and T2 (left) images (1-lens, 2-vitreous, 3-lateral rectus, 4-medial rectus, 5-superior orbital fissure, 6-cavernous sinus, 7-anterior chamber, 8-lacrimal gland, 9-optic nerve, 10-internal carotid artery).

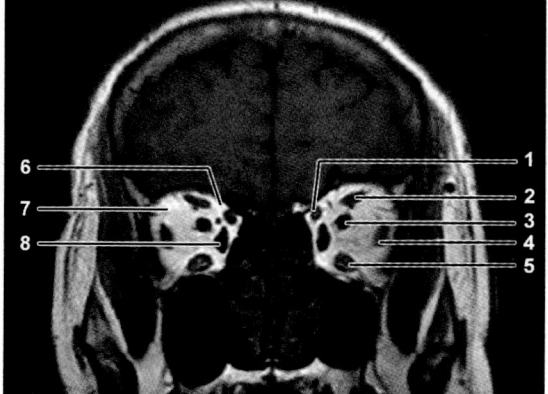

Fig. 35.5: Normal orbital anatomy as seen in coronal scan (1-superior oblique, 2-superior rectus, 3-optic nerve, 4-lateral rectus, 5-inferior rectus, 6-ophthalmic artery, 7- superior ophthalmic vein, 8-medial rectus).

Table 35.1 *Appearance of orbital tissues in T1- and T2-weighted image*

Tissue	*T1-weighted image*	*T2-weighted image*
Aqueous, vitreous and CSF	Dark	Bright
Lens	Bright	Dark
Scelera, choroid and retina	Bright	Dark
Extraocular muscles	Bright	Bright
Optic nerve	Bright	Bright
Optic nerve sheath	Dark	Bright
Inflammation (demyelination)	Dark	Bright

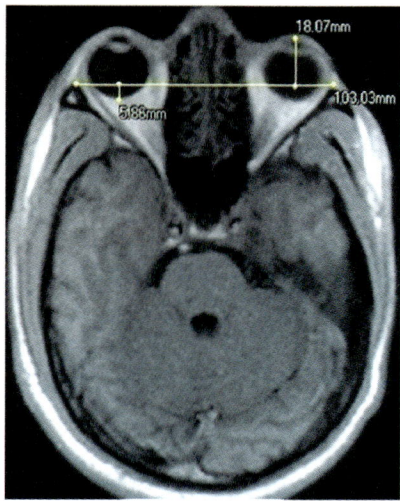

Fig. 35.6: *Axial T1-weighted MRI showing normal position of the globe.*

MRI based normative values for ocular and orbital measurements

Position of globe

• Distance from the anterior corneal surface to interzygomatic line 18.07 mm
• Distance from posterior sclera margin to interzygomatic line = 5.86 mm (Fig. 35.6)
• The mean optic nerve sheath diameter values with MRI on T2-weighted image when measured 3 mm behind the globe are 5.5 mm (Fig. 35.7).

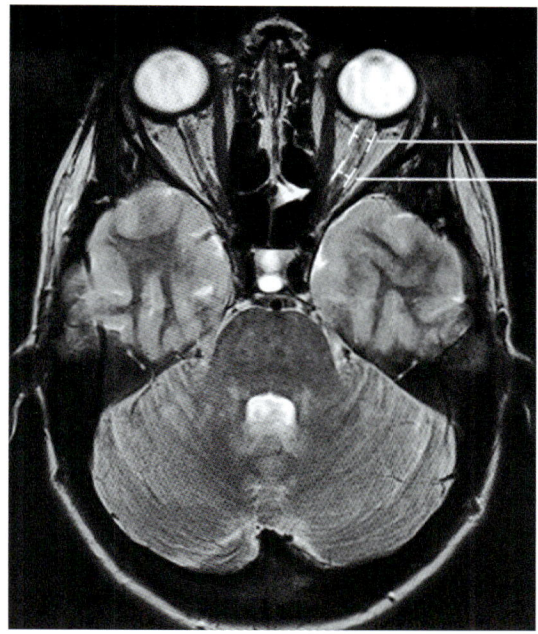

Fig. 35.7: *Axial T2-weighted MRI showing normal diameter of optic nerve sheath.*

MRI FINDINGS IN COMMON OCULAR LESIONS

MRI findings in common ocular lesions are described here briefly.

CONGENITAL OCULAR LESIONS

Persistent hyperplastic primary vitreous

• T1 axial MRI image shows conspicuous micropthalmia (Fig. 35.8)
• Hypointense to isointense thin triangular band extending from optic disc to lens suggest persistence of Cloquet's canal
• Characteristic hyperintense T2 signal differentiates this from retinoblastoma, which has hypointense T2 signal.

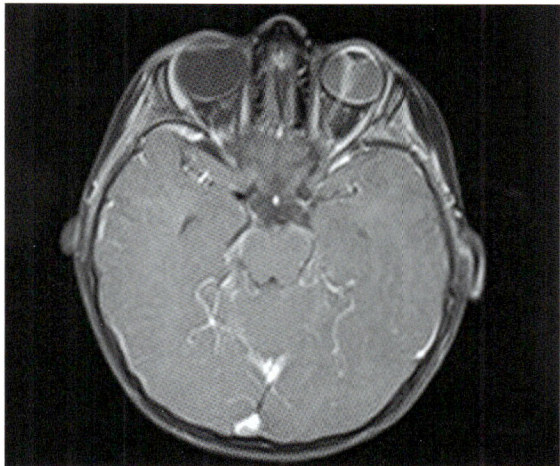

Fig. 35.8: *T1 axial scan of a patient with persistent hyperplastic primary vitreous left eyeball.*

Congenital anophthalmos

• Delineation of intraorbital contents, including rudimentary optic nerve (ON) and tracts (Fig. 35.9)
• Partial agenesis of the corpus callosum and microgyria of the calcarine cortex.

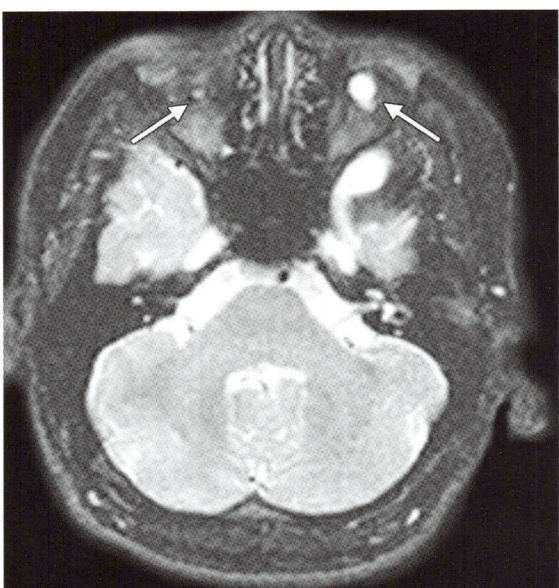

Fig. 35.9: *T1 axial scan of a patient with bilateral congenital anophthalmos.*

INFLAMMATORY/INFECTIVE OCULAR LESIONS

Optic neuritis

- Fat saturated T2-weighted and short TI inversion recovery (STIR) MRI brain and orbits shows swelling and increased signal intensity of optic nerve (Fig. 35.10)

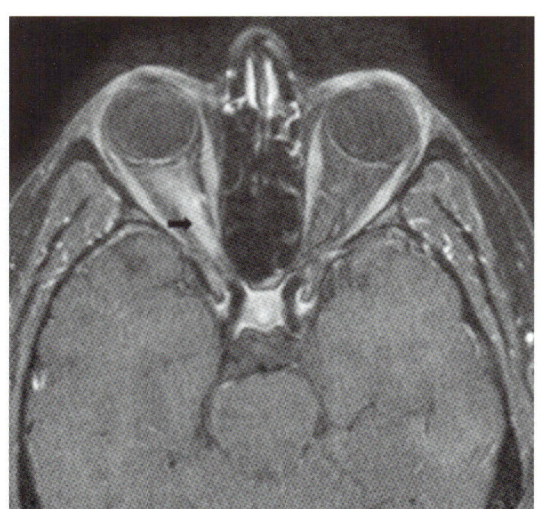

Fig. 35.10: *T1 axial scan orbit in a patient with right optic neuritis.*

- Fluid attenuation inversion recovery (FLAIR) sequences reveal demyelination of MS plaques often not visible on routine MRI imaging. CSF signal is strongly attenuated, accentuating periventricular and extra-axial disease near brain surface, allowing visualization of underlying pathology.

Endophthalmitis

- Aqueous and vitreous humour, being nearly completely water, demonstrate hyperintense T2 and hypointense T1 signal on MRI (Fig. 35.11).
- The uveal tract is difficult to separate from the adjacent bright signal in the vitreous on T2-WI.
- On T1-WI the uvea may be appreciated as a very thin, slightly hyperintense layer.
- The sclera, being fibrous, is hypointense on T1- and T2-WI.

Scleritis

Contrast enhanced T1-weighted image with fat suppression shows contrast enhancement of the outer aspect of the sclera extending to the optic nerve sheath (Fig. 35.12).

Cytomegalovirus retinitis

- Magnetic resonance imaging (MRI) demonstrates heterogeneous irregular uveal thickening and enhancement, retinal detachment, and retinal calcifications.
- The thickened, edematous retina is best appreciated on T1 with gadolinium enhancement (Fig. 35.13).

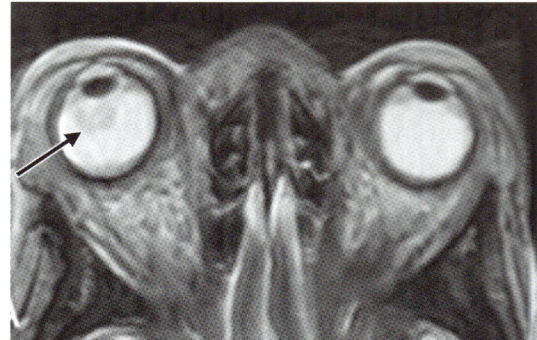

Fig. 35.11: *T1 axial scan orbit in a patient with bilateral endophthalmitis.*

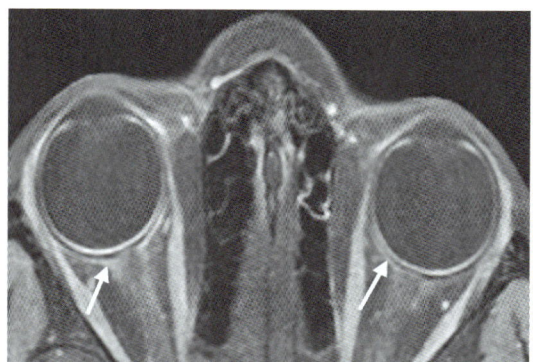

Fig. 35.12: *T1 contrast enhanced axial scan orbit in a patient with bilateral scleritis.*

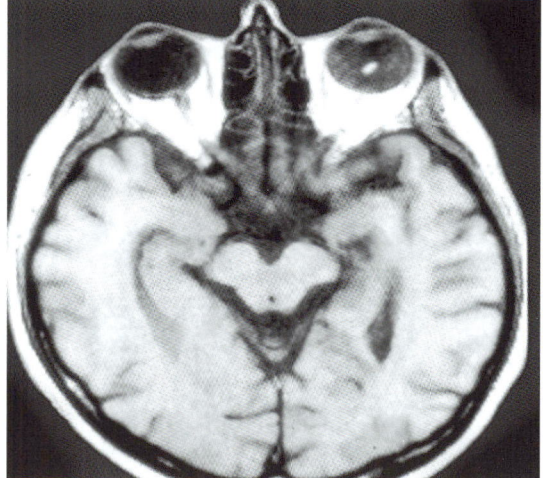

Fig. 35.13: *T1 contrast enhanced axial scan orbit in a patient with bilateral CMV retinitis.*

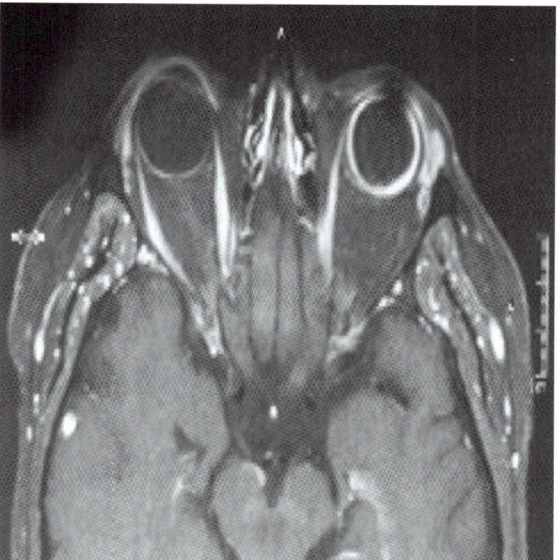

Fig. 35.14: *T1 contrast enhanced axial scan orbit in a patient with uveal effusion left eye.*

- T2 may show retinal detachment with fluid behind the retina.

Uveal effusion syndrome

- Axial contrast enhanced T1-weighted MRI show a diffuse enhancing lesion of the choroid. (Fig. 35.14)
- Uveal effusion mostly involves the peripheral choroid and ciliary body.

INTRAOCULAR TUMOURS

Retinoblastoma

- T1 image appears moderately hyperintense.
- T2 hypointense (Fig. 35.15).

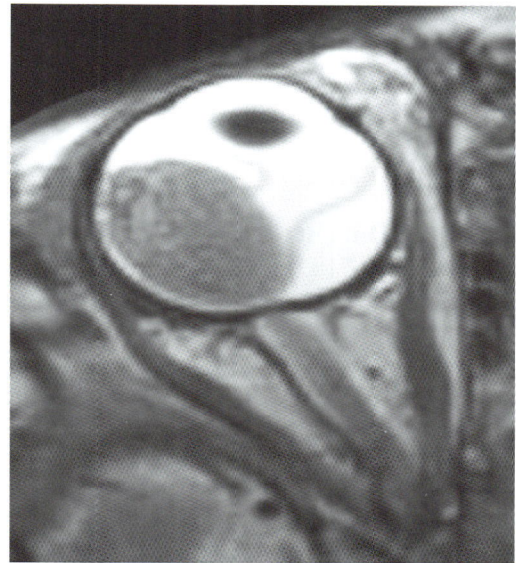

Fig. 35.15: *T2 axial scan orbit in a patient with retinoblastoma.*

- Conspicuous 'filling defect' relative to intra-ocular fluid.
- MR can demonstrates retro-orbital extension, involvement of optic nerve and intracranial involvement for detecting pinealoblastoma, and to aid differentiation from simulating conditions.

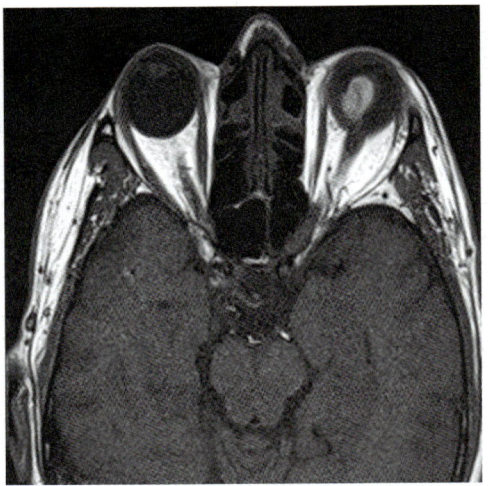

Fig. 35.16: *Contrast enhanced axial T1-weighted scan orbit in a patient with malignant melanoma left eyeball.*

Malignant melanoma

- T1 image appears hyperintense
- T2 hypointense (Fig. 35.16)
- **Contrast enhanced axial T1-weighted image** typically enhances in a peripheral rim pattern or a diffusely heterogeneous pattern.

MISCELLANEOUS CONDITIONS

Retinal detachment

- MRI signal of RD depends on characteristic of fluid below the detachment.
- Recent haemorrhage demonstrates high T1 signal (Fig. 35.17)
- RD containing an effusion typically has increased T1 signal related to increased protein levels.
- Effusions can generally be distinguished from tumours by T1 gadolinium enhancement, in which tumours appear bright, whereas effusions are not enhanced.

Phthisis bulbi

- T1-weighted image appears isointense to normal eye with heterogeneous areas of increased signal, depending on degree of calcification and haemorrhage.
- T2 shows heterogeneous vitreous containing dark 'filling defects' caused by coarse calcifications (Fig. 35.18).

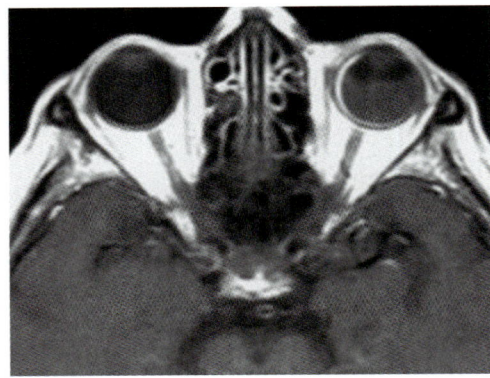

Fig. 35.17: *Contrast enhanced axial T1-weighted scan orbit in a patient with left retinal detachment*

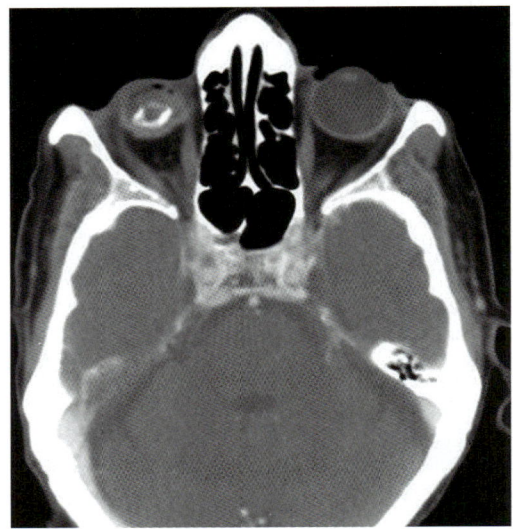

Fig. 35.18: *T1 axial scan orbit in a patient with phthisis bulbi right eyeball*

- Fluid-attenuated inversion recovery (FLAIR) sequences shows increased signal, which contrasts sharply with the dark contralateral globe.

MRI FINDINGS IN ORBITAL LESIONS

CONGENITAL ORBITAL LESIONS

Congenital orbital teratoma

- Magnetic resonance imaging (MRI) with gadolinium enhancement and fat suppression is preferred to define the extent of disease and follow-up.

- Gadolinium enhanced axial T1-weighted MRI image shows an orbital mass with a heterogeneous signal from cystic and solid elements (Fig. 35.19).

TRAUMATIC ORBITAL LESIONS

Intraorbital foreign body

- Ferromagnetic foreign body is the contraindication of magnetic resonance imaging (MRI) examination because its translocation under MRI may cause secondary damage to eye.
- MRI examination is of value when there is a high suspicion of nonmetallic IOFBs, especially wooden foreign body with a negative CT image (Fig. 35.20).
- Nonmetallic IOFBs show low signal on both T1- and T2-weighted sequences.

INFLAMMATORY/INFECTIVE ORBITAL LESIONS

Thyroid orbitopathy

- T1-weighted image shows hypointense signal due to vascularisation and hypointense signal in the middle of the muscle due to fat and inflammatory cell infiltration (Fig. 35.21)
- T2-weighted image shows hyperintense signal of the muscle
- Bilateral, spindle shaped thickening of extraocular recti muscles, with relative sparing of their tendinous insertion into the globe.

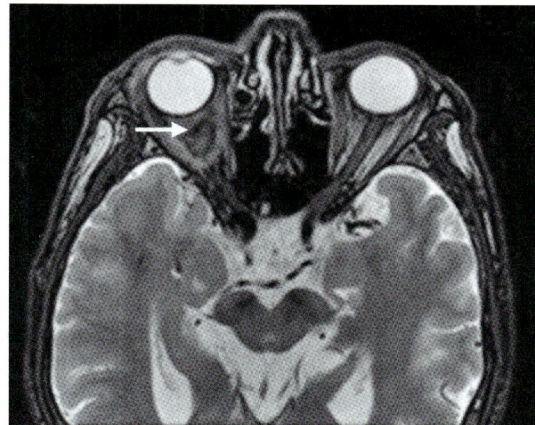

Fig. 35.20: *Axial T2-weighted MRI scan orbit in a patient with right intraorbital nonmagnetic foreign body.*

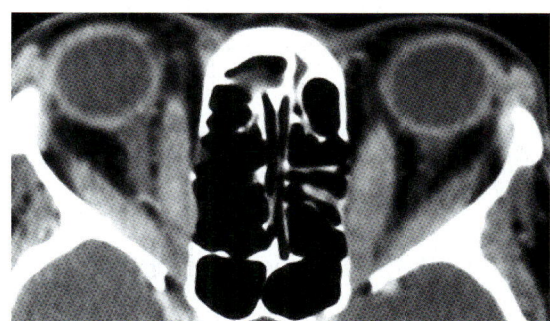

Fig. 35.21: *Axial T1-weighted MRI scan orbit in a patient with thyroid orbitopathy.*

Idiopathic orbital inflammatory disease

- MRI shows hypointense lesion with respect to extraocular muscle on T1 and hyperintense lesion with respect to extraocular muscle on T2 (Fig. 35.22).
- There occurs moderate enhancement with gadolinium.

Orbital cysticercosis

MRI reveals a cystic lesion within the extraocular muscle (Fig. 35.23).

Orbital echinococcosis

- MRI reveals a clear cystic structure with calcification on cyst wall (Fig. 35.24).
- Cyst appears as a low-intensity signal on T1-weighted image and as a high-intensity signal on T2-weighted image.

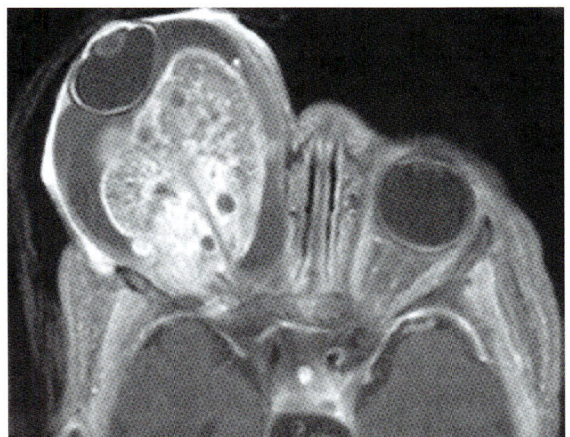

Fig. 35.19: *Axial T1-weighted MRI scan orbit in a patient with right orbital teratoma.*

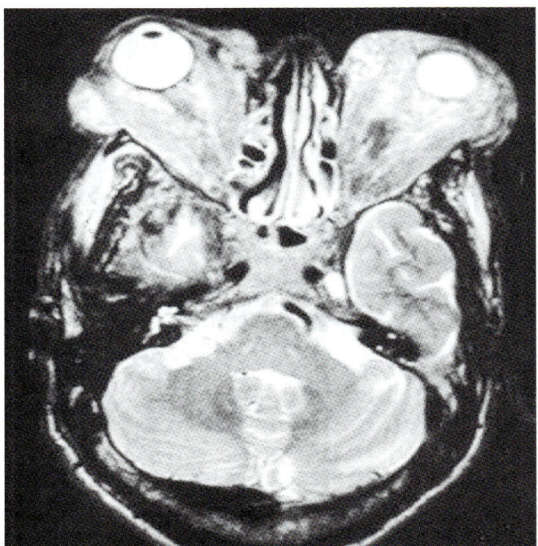

Fig. 35.22: *Axial T2-weighted MRI scan orbit in a patient with Idiopathic orbital inflammatory disease.*

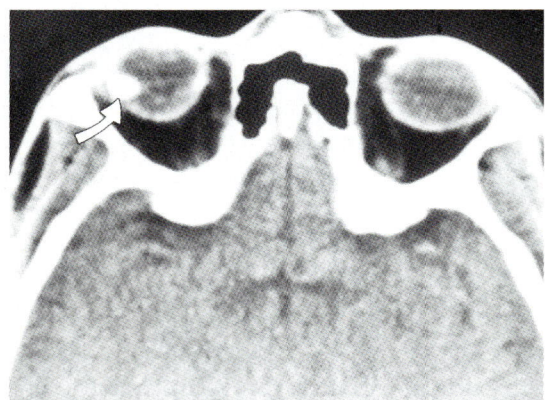

Fig. 35.23: *Axial T1-weighted MRI scan orbit in a patient with orbital cysticercosis, right eyeball.*

- Contrast enhanced T1-weighted MRI scan showed capsular contrast enhancement.

Orbital abscess

- Magnetic resonance imaging (MRI) is the preferred imaging procedure to define extension of disease into orbital apex, optic canal, and intracranially.
- Gadolinium enhanced and fat suppression MRI is the 'gold standard'.
- T1 image shows 'ring enhancement' around the periphery of the abscess.

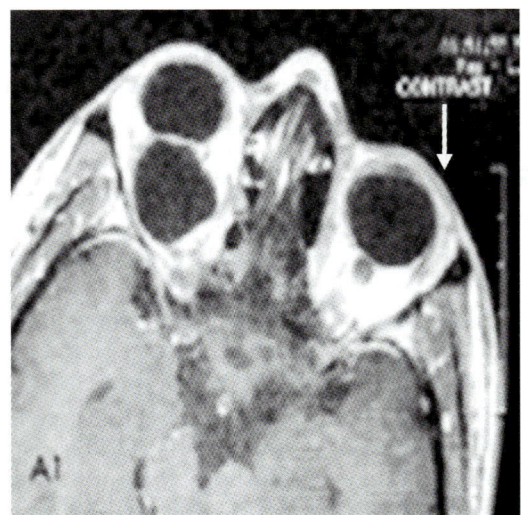

Fig. 35.24: *Axial T1-weighted MRI scan orbit in a patient with orbital echinococcosis, right eyeball.*

- Diffusion-weighted imaging (DWI) demonstrates restricted diffusion. Orbital abscess restricts diffusion appearing bright on DWI with dark appearance on corresponding apparent diffusion coefficient (ADC) image (Fig. 35.25).

Tolosa-Hunt syndrome

- In Tolosa-Hunt syndrome (THS), enhancement and fullness of anterior cavernous sinus

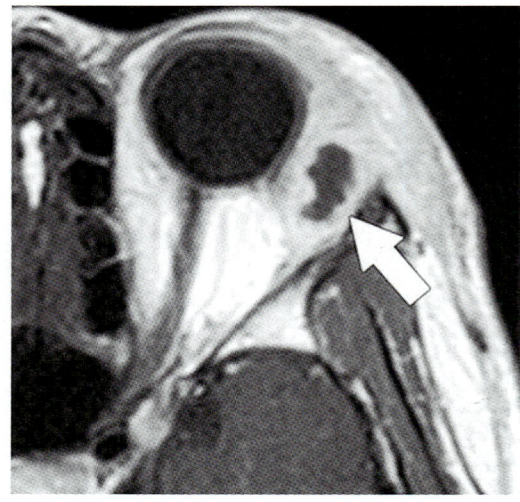

Fig. 35.25: *Axial T1-weighted MRI scan showing extraconal abscess corresponding with area of diffusion restriction.*

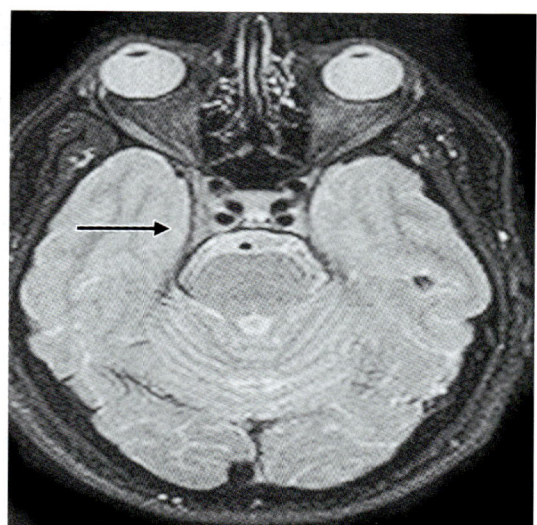

Fig. 35.26: *Axial T2-weighted MRI scan an enlarged right cavernous sinus.*

and superior orbital fissure (SOF) on gadolinium enhanced T1 image.

- T2 image shows enlarged cavernous sinus (Fig. 35.26).
- Magnetic resonance angiography (MRA) may show narrowing of cavernous internal carotid artery (ICA).

VASCULAR ORBITAL LESIONS

Orbital venous varix

- MRI is the imaging procedure of choice. In the absence of thrombus, T1 and T2 images are hypointense to extraocular muscles. If thrombus is present, T1 and T2 image is heterogeneous with areas of increased signal (Fig. 35.27).

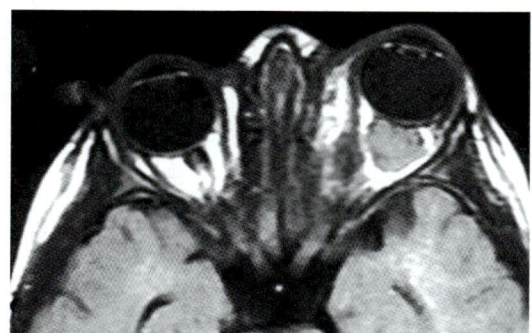

Fig. 35.27: *Axial T1-weighted fat suppressed MRI orbit shows the presence of an irregular left orbital mass.*

- The patient can be imaged supine and then prone to detect significant differences in size of mass as well as degree of exopthalmos.
- MRI should also be performed with Valsalva or straining.
- Magnetic resonance venogram (MRV) can be used to show extent of abnormal veins.

Cavernous sinus thrombosis

- Magnetic resonance imaging (MRI) may appreciate change in size, contour or signal of cavernous sinus (Fig. 35.28)
- Axial T1 MRI shows exopthalmos and enlarged cavernous sinus with thrombus isointense to muscle
- Magnetic resonance angiography shows an absence of flow void in thrombosed sinuses.

Carotid cavernous fistula

- Gadolinium enhanced coronal and axial T1-weighted image shows increased orbital edema with enhancement in extraocular muscles and other orbital soft tissues along with abnormal choroidal enhancement (Fig. 35.29).
- Dilatation of one or both cavernous sinuses and superior ophthalmic veins is characteristic.

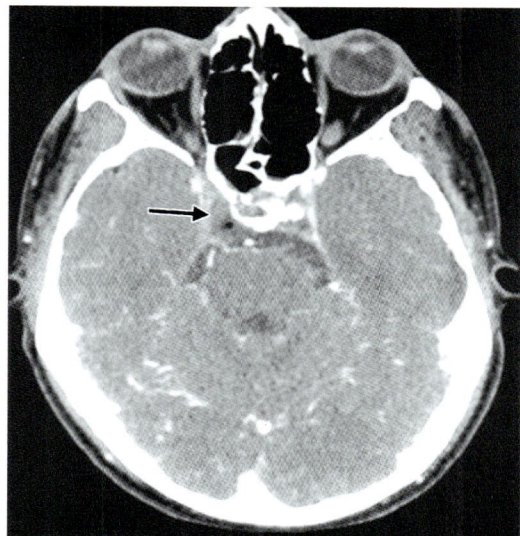

Fig. 35.28: *Axial T1-weighted MRI scan showing cavernous sinus thrombosis, right orbit.*

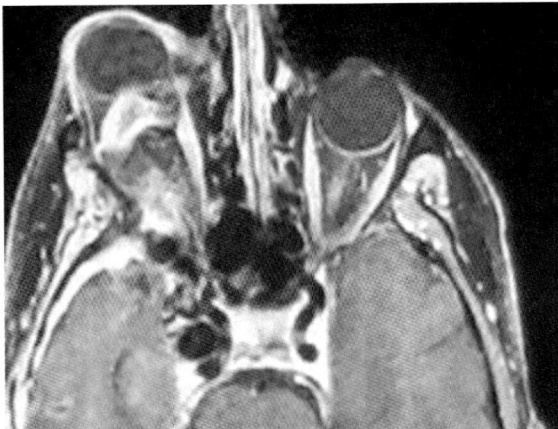

Fig. 35.29: *Axial T1-weighted MRI scan showing carotid cavernous fistula, right orbit.*

- MRA reveals enlargement of affected cavernous sinus, abnormal intracranial vessels dilatation of superior ophthalmic vein and enlarged extraocular muscles.

ORBITAL TUMOURS

Optic nerve glioma

- T1 axial MRI image shows fusiform enlargement of the optic nerve from globe through the orbital apex which shows homogeneous enhancement with contrast. The retrobulbar ON kinks and flattens posterior to the globe (Fig. 35.30).
- On T2-weighted image, optic nerve glioma is hyperintense to cerebral cortex and may appear heterogenous due to cystic degeneration.
- MRI is also useful in showing intracranial extension.

Optic nerve meningioma

- Contrast enhanced MRI with fat suppression is ideal for diagnosis.
- MRI demonstrate diffuse tubular thickening of optic nerve sheath encasing the optic nerve producing characteristic tram track appearance on axial scans and doughnut sign on coronal scans (Fig. 35.31).
- Areas of calcification are often seen in tumours.
- MRI is also useful for delineating extent of tumour and evaluating its intracranial extension.

Orbital schwannoma

- Axial T1 gadolinium enhanced MRI shows a large isointense mass with areas of 'ring' enhancement extending from the posterior globe to the orbital apex causing exophthalmos and hyperintense signal on T2 (Fig. 35.32).
- On dynamic MRI, there is a 'progressive' enhancement of an orbital schwannoma, which begins peripherally and progresses to centre.

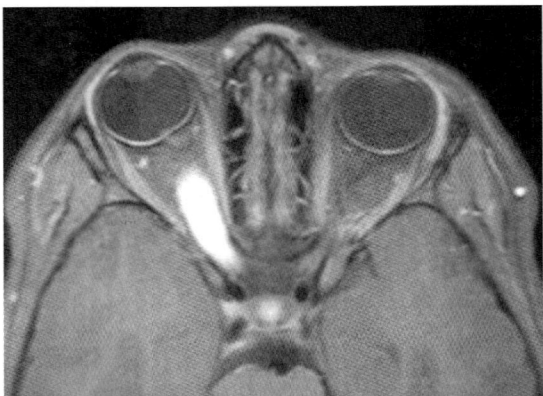

Fig. 35.30: *Contrast enhanced axial T1-weighted MRI scan showing optic nerve glioma, right orbit.*

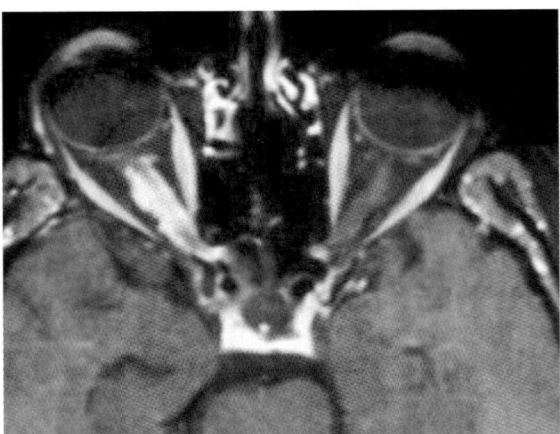

Fig. 35.31: *Contrast enhanced axial T1-weighted MRI scan showing optic nerve meningioma, right orbit.*

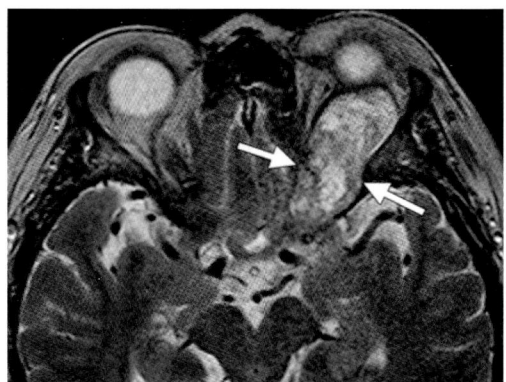

Fig. 35.32: *Axial T2-weighted MRI scan showing orbital schwannoma, left orbit.*

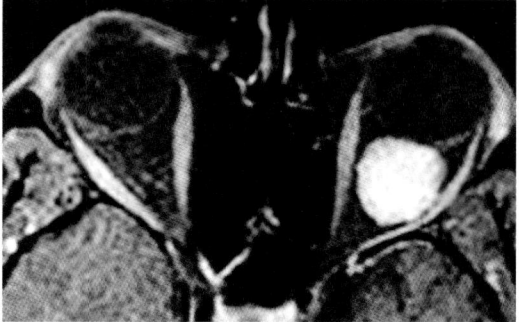

Fig. 35.34: *Axial T1-weighted fat suppressed contrast enhanced MRI orbit shows the presence of a well circumscribed left orbital intraconal mass.*

Orbital lymphangioma

- Axial T1-weighted fat suppressed post-contrast MRI orbit shows the a diffuse multicystic orbital lesion with both intraconal and extraconal components ,which enhances well with contrast (Fig. 35.33).
- Fluid level may be evident due to presence of blood and plasma.

Orbital cavernous haemangioma

- MRI is characteristic and pathognomonic. Axial T1-weighted MRI reveals a well-circumscribed intraconal homogeneous mass with a signal isointense to muscle and grey matter which shows a 'mulberry' pattern on gadolinium enhancement (Fig. 35.34).
- Axial T2-weighted MRI demonstrates signal hyperintense to brain and fat and a characteristic sharp, low-signal pseudocapsule. They

have a dark hemosiderin rim with 'blooming' artifact on MRI (susceptibility artifact due to presence of paramagnetic substance hemosiderin, blooming refers to the fact that lesions appear larger than they actually are).

Orbital capillary haemangioma

Contrast enhanced T2-weighted MRI shows a well-circumscribed diffuse mass which enhances well with contrast (Fig. 35.35).

LACRIMAL GLAND LESIONS

Lacrimal gland sarcoidosis

- T1 image shows hypointense signal in region of lacrimal gland (Fig. 35.36)
- T2 image shows hyperintense signal in region of lacrimal gland
- **Contrast enhanced axial T1-weighted image** typically enhances in heterogeneous pattern in region of lacrimal gland.

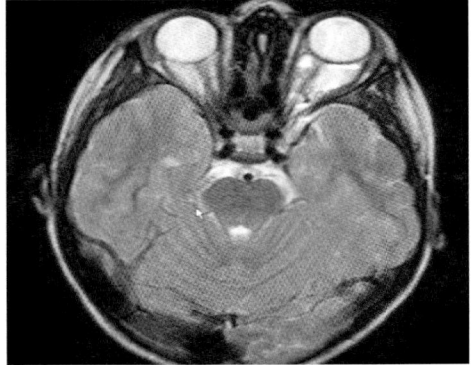

Fig. 35.33: *Axial T2-weighted MRI scan showing orbital lymphangioma, left orbit.*

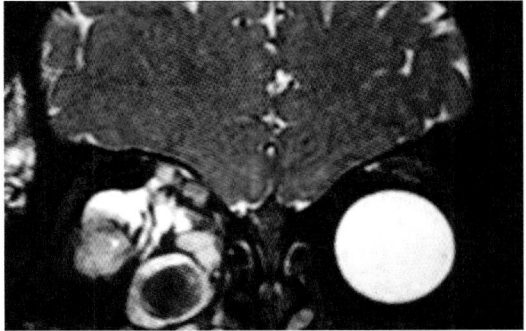

Fig. 35.35: *Coronal T2-weighted contrast enhanced MRI orbit revealing presence of a diffuse mass in deep right orbit.*

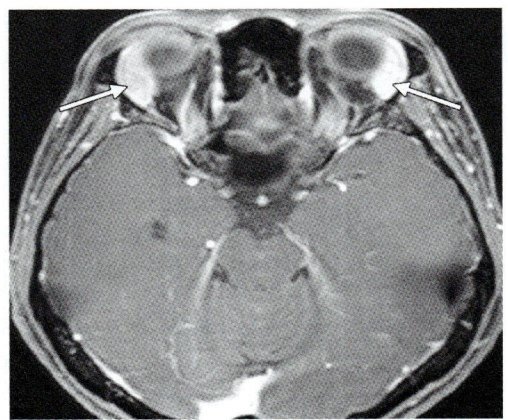

Fig. 35.36: *Contrast enhanced axial T1-weighted scan orbit in a patient with bilateral lacrimal gland sarcoidosis.*

Lacrimal gland lymphoma (LGL)

- T1 isointense to hypointense to extraocular muscle (EOM).
- T2 isointense to hyperintense to EOM (Fig. 35.37).
- Contrast enhanced T1 scan exhibits homogeneous enhancement.
- Lacrimal gland lymphoma (LGL) reveals restricted diffusion with diffusion weighted imaging (DWI) and decreased apparent diffusion coefficient (ADC) signal intensity.

Malignant epithelial lacrimal gland tumours

- T1 image shows hypointense signal in area of lacrimal gland.
- T2 image shows hyperintense signal in area of lacrimal gland (Fig. 35.38).

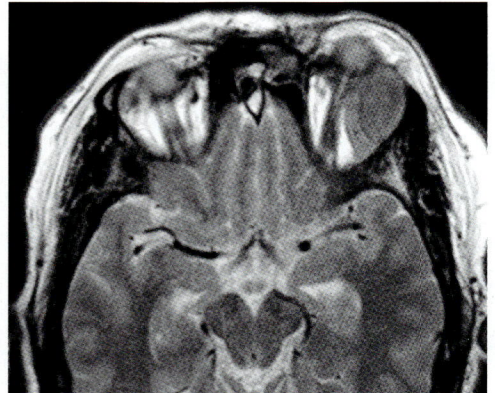

Fig. 35.37: *Axial T1-weighted scan orbit in a patient with left lacrimal gland lymphoma.*

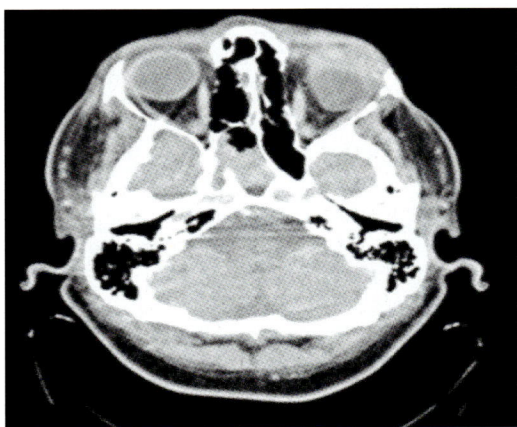

Fig. 35.38: *Contrast enhanced axial T1-weighted scan orbit in a patient with left adenoid cystic carcinoma of lacrimal gland tumour.*

SPECIAL MRI INVESTIGATIONS

FUNCTIONAL MRI

*f*MRI: Functional MRI: A noninvasive MR technique to map or localize brain areas which are responsible for a particular task. *f*MRI is based on the concept of blood oxygen level dependant (BOLD) imaging. Deoxyhemoglobin is paramagnetic while the oxyhemoglobin is diamagnetic relative to the surrounding tissues. Presence of deoxyhemoglobin causes microscopic field variation in and around the microvasculature resulting into signal drop on T2-weighted images. When any brain area is activated by the particular task blood flow to that area increases. This increase in the blood flow is much more than the metabolic demand with resultant increased amount of oxyhemoglobin and relatively less deoxyhemoglobin in that area. This leads to increased signal in the area from less deoxyhemoglobin. *f*MRI includes tasks to stimulate brain areas. Functional magnetic resonance imaging (*f*MRI) is used for mapping cerebral cortical activation in response to performing specific cognitive, sensory or motor tasks. *f*MRI is used for functional cortical mapping, psychophysical tests, brain tumour mapping and understanding the basis of higher visual functioning. Localized increases in neuronal activity from task-related brain activation produce increased cerebral blood flow and decreased deoxyhemoglobin, and this can be imaged with *f*MRI. Presurgical mapping of brain function, including localization of visual functions, has provided new insights into brain physiology. Functional MRI has many potential advantages because it does not require the injection of contrast agents and has relatively high spatial and temporal resolution. There are a few clinical indications for which the general ophthalmologist would require *f*MRI. Functional imaging studies show information about the physiology and metabolic function of brain. These functional studies might be particularly useful when structural imaging appears normal despite clinical findings that suggest underlying brain dysfunction. Localized increases in neuronal activity from task-related brain activation produce increased cerebral blood flow and decreased deoxyhemoglobin and this can be imaged with *f*MRI. Current applications of functional imaging include detection of hypermetabolic states associated with tumour, differentiation of tumour from areas of radiation-induced necrosis, localization of seizure foci, detection of ischaemic regions, evaluation of biochemical changes associated with cognitive and psychiatric abnormalities and their response to pharmaceutical intervention, and drug localization in the brain. In neuro ophthalmology, *f*MRI is a reliable technique allowing accurate visualization of the cortical areas involved in ocular motility, and of cortical retinotopy within the visual cortex. Besides being less expensive than positron emission tomography, *f*MRI has the additional advantages of faster imaging speed, higher spatial resolution, practical repeatability, and being less invasive. These advantages can be helpful not only in research but also in planning neurosurgical procedures to avoid eloquent areas of cerebral function such as those involved with language or vision.

MR SPECTROSCOPY

Magnetic resonance spectroscopy (MRS) is a noninvasive application of magnetic resonance imaging to assess various metabolites or biochemicals from the body tissues. This information is then used in diagnosis and monitoring of diseases and assessing response to the treatment. MRI scans are generally reconstructed from the signal from all protons in the tissue that is dominated by water and fat protons. The protons from other metabolites do not contribute to imaging because of their negligible concentration. In contrast to routine MRI, MRS detects these small metabolites. The commonly measured metabolites in MRS include N-acetyl aspartate (NAA), creatine and phosphocreatine (Cr), choline containing phospholipids (Cho), lactate, glutamate, glutamine, gamma amino butyric acid, myoinositol (MI) and fatty acids. MRS is used for diagnostic biochemistry *in vivo*. Pathologies documented by MRS include brain tumour, stroke, focal cerebral lesions, multiple sclerosis and intracranial haemorrhage. An acutely ischaemic brain produces lactate by anaerobic metabolism during the first 2–3 days after injury, which can be detected by MRS. The spectrum of MRS applications in neuro ophthalmology include ischaemic, neoplastic, demyelinating, radiation necrosis, inflammatory and mitochondrial disorders.

- In diffuse axonal injury, there is decrease in NAA/Cr ratio and absolute concentration of NAA.
- In MS plaques, there is decrease in NAA/Cr and increased Cho/Cr and MI/Cr. Active plaque shows elevated lipid, lactate, Cho/Cr ratio and MI. Progression can be monitored by NAA/Cr ratio.
- Abscess can be differentiated from neoplasm. The changes in MR spectra in abscess include visualization of amino acid peaks at 0.9 ppm. These amino acids include valine, leucine and isoleucine. The abscess may shows peaks representing acetate, pyruvate, lactate and succinate, which are end products arising from some microorganisms. In neoplasm, there is increase in Cho, lactate and lipids and reduction in NAA and creatinine.

MAGNETIC RESONANCE ANGIOGRAPHY

MR angiography is an excellent noninvasive technique for detecting asymptomatic aneurysms >5 mm in size. The technique of MRA relies on the flow-sensitive nature of the MR signal. On conventional MR, fast-moving blood appears dark on all sequences as a 'flow void'.

There are two basic types of MRA: (i) time-of-flight (TOF) MRA; and (ii) phase-contrast MRA. Both TOF and PC MRA can acquire data using either a 2-D or a 3-D scan. The addition of contrast enhances the MRA acquisition and optimizes visualization of possible dural venous sinus disease and is also useful for evaluating carotid stenosis.

Magnetic resonance angiography does not simply display vascular anatomy, as in contrast angiography. Instead, it extrapolates physiological data obtained from flow characteristics of protons to demonstrate anatomy. Thus, in MR angiography, the diameter of the blood vessels sometimes may appear smaller than that shown on conventional angiograms and tends to overestimate vascular stenosis.

Clinical applications of MRA

Evaluation of the
- Extracranial circulation (carotid artery stenosis, plaques, and dissections in the evaluation of transient visual loss)
- Intracranial circulation (aneurysms, AVMs, occlusive disease and carotid artery fistulas).

Limitations of MR angiography

- It cannot detect aneurysms <5 mm in diameter
- It can yield false-positive results in tightly wound vessel loops
- It has a tendency to exaggerate vessel stenosis.

Advantages of MRA over CTA

- Lack of ionizing radiation exposure
- Less nephrotoxic contrast material (i.e. gadolinium *vs* iodinated contrast)
- Increased signal-to-noise ratio
- Easier post processing techniques.

MR VENOGRAPHY

The major ophthalmic indication for performing a venogram is to exclude dural venous sinus thrombosis in patients presenting with papilloedema from increased intracranial pressure. Symptoms of cerebral venous sinus thrombosis may mimic those of idiopathic intracranial hypertension. A number of venographic techniques have been developed to better define sinus anatomy. These include phase contrast MRV (PC MRV), non-contrast time of flight (TOF) MRV, contrast enhanced MRV and CTV. An important pitfall on MRV is that flow gaps in a hypoplastic non-dominant transverse sinus can be misinterpreted as areas of venous thrombosis. In such cases, it is important to evaluate the ipsilateral jugular vein, as it will be smaller on the side of the hypoplastic sinus, and to correlate findings with the brain MRI. MRV may be helpful in excluding thrombosis within the dural venous sinuses, a condition that may cause papilloedema.

BIBLIOGRAPHY

1. Ahmed II, Feldman F, Kucharczyk W, Trope GE. Neuroradiologic screening in normal-pressure glaucoma: study results and literature review. J Glaucoma 2002;11(4):279–86.
2. Albers GW, Lansberg MG, Norbash AM, Tong DC, O'Brien MW, Woolfenden AR, Marks MP, Moseley ME. Yield of diffusion-weighted MRI for detection of potentially relevant findings in stroke patients. Neurology 2000;54(8):1562–7.
3. Atlas S, Galetta S. The orbit and visual system. In: Atlas S, (Ed). Magnetic resonance imaging of the Brain and Spine. Raven Press; New York: 1991.
4. Berkowitz BA, McDonald C, Ito Y, Tofts PS, Latif Z, Gross J. Measuring the human retinal oxygenation response to a hyperoxic challenge using MRI: eliminating blinking artifacts and demonstrating proof of concept. Magn Reson Med 2001;46(2):412–6.
5. Berkowitz BA, Roberts R, Goebel DJ, Luan H. Noninvasive and simultaneous imaging of layerspecific retinal functional adaptation by manganese-enhanced MRI. Invest Ophthalmol Vis Sci 2006;47(6):2668–74.
6. Bert RJ, Caruthers SD, Jara H, Krejza J, Melhem ER, Kolodny NH, Patz S, Freddo TF. Demonstration of an anterior diffusional pathway for solutes in the normal human eye with high spatial resolution contrast-enhanced dynamic MR imaging. Invest Ophthalmol Vis Sci 2006; 47(12):5153–62.
7. Bert RJ, Patz S, Ossiani M, Caruthers SD, Jara H, Krejza J, Freddo T. High-resolution MR imaging of the human eye 2005. Acad Radiol 2006;13(3):368–78.
8. Bilaniuk LT, Schenck JF, Zimmerman RA, Hart HR Jr, Foster TH, Edelstein WA, Goldberg HI, et al. Ocular and orbital lesions: surface coil MR imaging. Radiology1985;156(3):669–74.

9. Cheng H, Nair G, Walker TA, Kim MK, Pardue MT, Thule PM, Olson DE, Duong TQ. Structural and functional MRI reveals multiple retinal layers. Proc Natl Acad Sci USA 2006;103(46): 17525–30.

10. De Graaf P, Knol DL, Moll AC, Imhof SM, Schouten-van Meeteren AY, Castelijns JA. Eye size in retinoblastoma: MR imaging measurements in normal and affected eyes. Radiology 2007;244(1):273–80.

11. De Marco J, Bilaniuk LT. Magnetic resonance imaging: Technical aspects. In: Newton T, Bilaniuk LT (Eds). Radiology of the eye and orbit. Vol. 4. Clavadel Press; San Anselmo, CA: 1990.

12. De Potter P, Shields JA, Shields CA (Eds). MRI of the Eye and Orbit. JB Lippincott Company; Philadelphia, PA: 1995. p. 304.

13. Duong TQ, Ngan SC, Ugurbil K, Kim SG. Functional magnetic resonance imaging of the retina. Invest Ophthalmol Vis Sci 2002;43(4): 1176–81.

14. Georgouli T, James T, Tanner S, Shelley D, Nelson M, Chang B, Backhouse O, McGonagle D. High-resolution microscopy coil MR-Eye. Eye. 2007.

15. Greenfield DS, Siatkowski RM, Glaser JS, Schatz NJ, Parrish RK 2nd. The cupped disc. Who needs neuroimaging? Ophthalmology 1998;105(10):1866–74.

16. Harms S. The orbit. In: Edelman R, Hesselink J, (Eds). Clinical magnetic resonance imaging. WB Saunders; Philadelphia: 1990.

17. Ito Y, Berkowitz BA. MR studies of retinal oxygenation. Vision Res 2001;41(10–11): 1307–11.

18. Kashiwagi K, Okubo T, Tsukahara S. Association of magnetic resonance imaging of anterior optic pathway with glaucomatous visual field damage and optic disc cupping. J Glaucoma 2004;13(3): 189–95.

19. Kim SH, Galban CJ, Lutz RJ, Dedrick RL, Csaky KG, Lizak MJ, Wang NS, Tansey G, Robinson MR. Assessment of subconjunctival and intra-scleral drug delivery to the posterior segment using dynamic contrast-enhanced magnetic resonance imaging. Invest Ophthalmol Vis Sci 2007;48(2):808–14.

20. Mafee MF. Ocular manifestations of cat-scratch disease: role of MR imaging. AJNR Am J Neuroradiol 2005;26(6):1303–4.

21. Metrikin DC, Wilson CA, Berkowitz BA, Lam MK, Wood GK, Peshock RM. Measurement of blood-retinal barrier breakdown in endotoxin-induced endophthalmitis. Invest Ophthalmol Vis Sci 1995;36(7):1361–70.

22. O'Brien JM. Retinoblastoma: clinical presentation and the role of neuroimaging. AJNR Am J Neuroradiol 2001;22(3):426–8.

23. Pop-Fanea L, Vallespin SN, Hutchison JM, Forrester JV, Seton HC, Foster MA, Liversidge J. Evaluation of MRI for in vivo monitoring of retinal damage and detachment in experimental ocular inflammation. Magn Reson Med 2005; 53(1):61–8.

24. Reddy AK, Morriss MC, Ostrow GI, Stass-Isern M, Olitsky SE, Lowe LH. Utility of MR imaging in cat-scratch neuroretinitis. Pediatr Radio 2007;37(8):840–3.

25. Scheie H, Albert DM, (Eds). TB of Ophthalmology. WB Saunders Company; Philadelphia: 1977. p. 616.

26. Schenck JF, Leue W. Instrumentation: Magnets, coils, and hardware. In: Atlas S (Ed). Magnetic imaging of the brain and spine. Raven Press; New York: 1991.

27. Schmalfuss IM, Dean CW, Sistrom C, Bhatti MT. Optic neuropathy secondary to cat scratch disease: distinguishing MR imaging features from other types of optic neuropathies. AJNR Am J Neuroradiol 2005;26(6):1310–6.

28. Shen Q, Cheng H, Pardue MT, Chang TF, Nair G, Vo VT, Shonat RD, Duong TQ. Magnetic resonance imaging of tissue and vascular layers in the cat retina. J Magn Reson Imaging 2006; 23(4):465–72.

29. Sobel D, Mills C, Char D, Norman D, Brant-Zawadski M, Kaufman L, Crooks L. NMR of the normal and pathologic eye and orbit. Am J of Neuroradiology 1984;5: 345–350.

30. Tarver-Carr ME, Miller NR. Tilted optic discs visualized by magnetic resonance imaging. J Neuroophthalmol 2006;26(4):282–3.

31. Trick GL, Berkowitz BA. Retinal oxygenation response and retinopathy. Prog Retin Eye Res 2005;24(2):259–74.

32. Villablanca P, Curran J, Arnold A, Lufkin R. Orbit and optic nerve. Top Magn Reson Imaging 1996;8(2):87–110.

33. Wirtschafter J, Berman E, McDonald C. Magnetic resonance imaging and computed tomography. Vol. 6. American Academy of Ophthalmology; San Francisco: 1992.

34. Wollstein G, Paunescu LA, Ko TH, Fujimoto JG, Kowalevicz A, Hartl I, Beaton S, Ishikawa H, Mattox C, Singh O, Duker J, Drexler W, Schuman JS. Ultrahigh-resolution optical coherence tomography in glaucoma. Ophthalmo-logy 2005;112(2):229–37.

Section

X

Determination of Refractive Errors

36. Clinical Refraction: Determination of the Errors of Refraction

Clinical Refraction: Determination of the Errors of Refraction

Chapter Outline

INTRODUCTION

OBJECTIVE REFRACTION

Retinoscopy
- Principle
- Optics
- Prerequisites for retinoscopy
- Procedure
- Problems in retinoscopy

Autorefractometry
- Optical principles
- Modern refractometers

Photorefraction

Electrophysiologic Methods of Objective Refraction

SUBJECTIVE REFRACTION

Monocular Subjective Refraction
- Selection and verification of baseline starting point lenses
    - Refinement of spherical lenses
- Refinement and finalization of cylindrical lens
    - Finalization of spherical lens

Binocular Balancing

Correction for Near Vision

DETERMINATION OF THE MUSCLE BALANCE
- Modifications in the prescription

SUMMARY OF CLINICAL REFRACTION

INTRODUCTION

The procedure of determining and correcting refractive errors is termed *clinical refraction*. It is an art that can only be mastered by practice. The clinical refraction comprises two complementary methods:

- Objective refraction, and
- Subjective refraction.

However, in clinical practice, the refraction is incomplete without the estimation and correction of associated muscle imbalance. Therefore, in this chapter, the determination of muscle balance has also been dealt along with the determination of refractive errors.

OBJECTIVE REFRACTION

In objective refraction, the examiner determines the type and degree of refractive error without active participation of the patient. Objective refraction is not only useful but often essential, e.g. when examining young children and patients with poor communication due to mental or language difficulties. The findings of objective refraction should always, wherever possible, be checked subjectively, and the most comfortable lenses should be prescribed to the patient. The final refraction of the patient is much easier and is completed quickly, if it is based on an objective estimate instead of it being only the subjective technique.

Objective methods of refraction include the following:

A. Retinoscopy,
B. Autorefractometry,
C. Photorefraction, and
D. Electrophysiological method of objective refraction.

PRINCIPLE

Retinoscopy, introduced by Bowman in 1859, is also known as *skiascopy or shadow test or pupilloscopy or korescopy*. It is an objective method of finding out the error of refraction by utilizing the technique of neutralization. It is based on the fact that when light is reflected from a mirror into the eye, the direction in which the light will travel across the pupil will depend upon the refractive state of the eye.

OPTICS

In retinoscopy, an area of the fundus is illuminated by the light reflected into the patient's eye with the help of a retinoscope. This illuminated area serves as an object and the rays which emanate from this area illuminate the pupillary area (in practice, known as reflex or shadow in the pupillary area) and form its image at the far point of the eye. When the immediate source of light is moved across the eye, the behaviour of the luminous reflex in the pupil will depend upon the refractive status of the eye.

Thus, for the purpose of understanding, the detailed optics of retinoscopy can be considered in three stages:

1. Illumination of the subject's retina (*illumination stage*)
2. The reflex imagery of this illuminated area formed by the subject's dioptric apparatus (*reflex stage*)
3. The projection of the image by the observer (*projection stage*).

ILLUMINATION STAGE

The optics of illumination stage of retinoscopy is basically understanding of the concept of immediate source of light and the movement of the illuminated area of the fundus with the

movement of the reflecting mirror, as summarized below:

- *Immediate source of light* (S_1) refers to the image of original light source (S_0) formed by the reflecting mirror.
- *When a plane mirror is used to reflect the light,* the immediate source of light (S_1) moves against the movement of the mirror, i.e. when the mirror is moved upwards, the immediate source of light moves downwards (S'_1) and vice versa (Fig. 36.1).
- *When a concave mirror is used to reflect the light,* the immediate source of light (S_1) moves with the movements of the mirror; i.e. when the mirror is moved upwards, the immediate source of light also moves upwards (S'_1) and vice versa (Fig. 36.2).

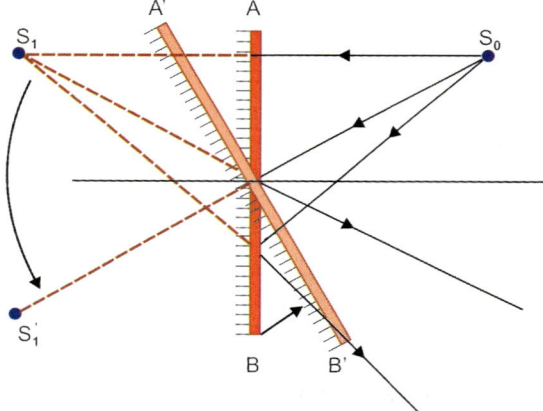

Fig. 36.1: *Movement of immediate source of light (S₁) in opposite direction to the movement of plane mirror.*

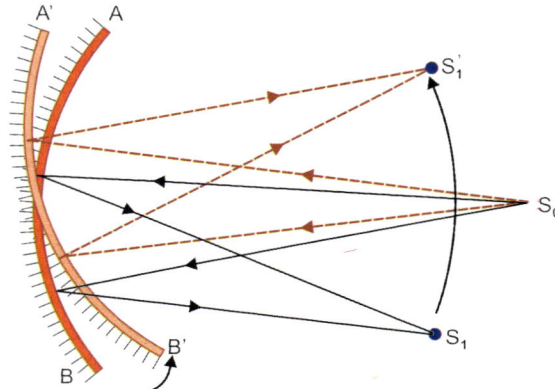

Fig. 36.2: *Movement of immediate source of light (S₁) to S'₁ in the same direction as that of concave mirror.*

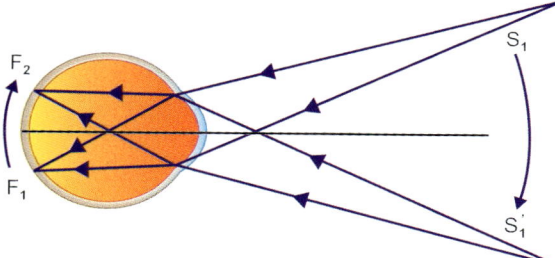

Fig. 36.3: *Movement of image of illuminated area of fundus with the movement of immediate source of light.*

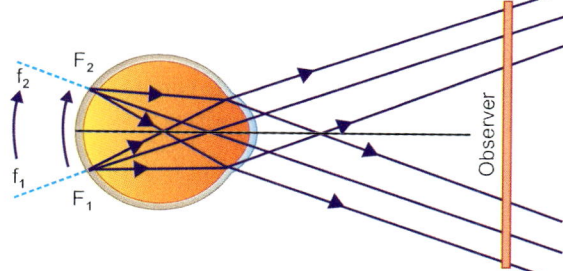

Fig. 36.4: *Movement of image of illuminated spot of fundus in emmetropia.*

- When the immediate source of light (S₁) moves downwards (S'₁) (with the upwards movement of plane mirror retinoscope), the illuminated spot of fundus (F₁) moves upwards (F₂) and vice versa (Fig. 36.3).

THE REFLEX STAGE AND PROJECTION STAGE

As mentioned earlier, the illuminated patch of fundus can now be considered as an object in its own right and will form an image at the far point of the subject's eye. The light rays reflected back from the illuminated area of fundus also form a reflex shadow in the pupillary area of the subject (*reflex stage*), which is observed by the examiner by aligning his or her eye with these light rays (*projection stage*).

The optics of reflex stage and projection stage of the retinoscopy (when performed using a plane mirror from a distance of 1 m from the subject), depending upon the refractive status of the eye, is as below.

Optics of movement of reflex in emmetropia

In emmetropia, the light rays emerging out of the eye from the illuminated spot on the fundus (F₁) are parallel to each other, and so the examiner projects the image of F₁ to f₁ and that of spot F₂ to f₂ (Fig. 36.4). Thus, when the spot F₁ moves to F₂ (upwards), the image f₁ also moves upwards to f₂, i.e. along the movement of the plane mirror.

Optics of movement of reflex in hypermetropia

In hypermetropia, the light rays emerging out of the eye from the illuminated spot on the fundus (F₁) are divergent and so the examiner projects the image of F₁ to f₁ and that of spot F₂ to f₂ (Fig. 36.5). Thus, when the spot F₁ moves to

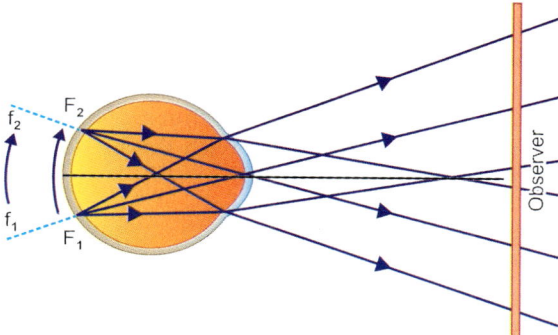

Fig. 36.5: *Movement of image of illuminated spot of fundus in hypermetropia.*

F₂ (upwards), the image f₁ also moves upwards to f₂, i.e. along the movement of the plane mirror.

Optics of movement of reflex in myopia of less than 1 D

In myopia of less than 1 D, the light rays emerging out of the eye from the illuminated spots on the fundus (F₁ and F₂) are convergent and meet at f₁ and f₂ behind the observer, sitting at 1 m from the patient (Fig. 36.6). Since these

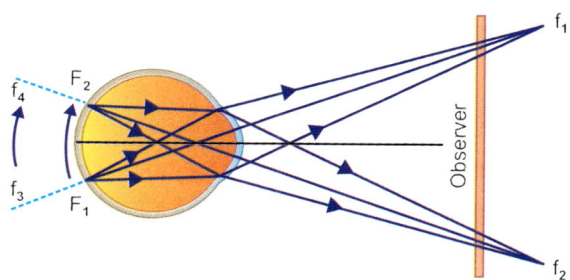

Fig. 36.6: *Movement of image of illuminated spot of fundus in myopia of less than 1 D.*

rays are intercepted by the examiner before they meet, so the examiner projects them along f_3 and f_4. Thus, when the spot F_1 moves to F_2 (upwards), the image f_3 also moves upwards to f_4, i.e. along the movement of the plane mirror.

Optics of movement of reflex in myopia of 1 D

In myopia of 1 D, the light rays emerging out of the patient's eye from the illuminated spots on the fundus (F_1 and F_2) are convergent and meet at a point 1 m in front of the patient, i.e. at the level of pupillary plane of the observer (Fig. 36.7). Thus, when the illuminated spot F_1 moves to F_2 (upwards), its image moves from f_1 to f_2. Since in both the positions, the image is formed at the pupillary plane, so the examiner does not appreciate any movement of the shadow. In other words, there occurs no movement of the shadow with the movement of the retinoscopic mirror.

Optics of movement of reflex in myopia of more than 1 D

In myopia of more than 1 D, the light rays emerging out of the patient's eye from the illuminated spots F_1 and F_2 are convergent and meet at f_1 and f_2 in the space between the patient and the observer. Thus, when the spot F_1 moves to F_2 (upwards), the image f_1 moves to f_2 (downwards), i.e. opposite to the movement of the plane mirror (Fig. 36.8).

PREREQUISITES FOR RETINOSCOPY

1. *A dark room*, preferably 6 m long, or that can be converted into 6 m by use of a plane mirror.
2. *A trial set*. A standard trial box usually consists of the following:

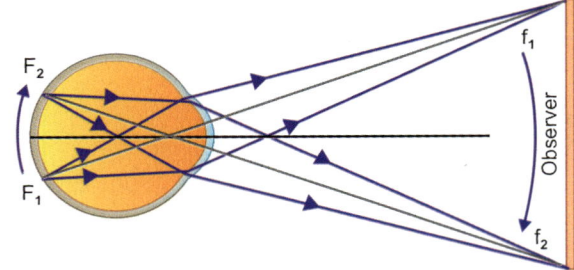

Fig. 36.8: *Movement of image of illuminated spot of fundus in myopia of more than 1 D.*

- Spherical lenses (plus and minus) of powers 0.12 D, 0.25–4.00 D in increments of 0.25 D, 4.5–6.0 D in increments of 0.5 D, 7–14 D in increments of 1 D, and 16–20 D in increments of 2 D.

    These test lenses should ideally conform as far as possible in form and thickness to the spectacle lenses to be worn subsequently. Practically, this is impossible. The reduced aperture lenses (thin lenses of small size, approximately 25 mm in diameter) probably give the best approximation. These should preferably be in planoconvex or planoconcave form.
- Cylindrical lenses (plus and minus) of powers 0.25–2.00 D in increments of 0.25 D, and 2.5– 6.0 D in increments of 0.5 D.
- Prisms up to 10 D with additional two of 15 and 20 D.
- Accessories such as plano lenses, opaque discs, pinhole, stenopaeic discs, Maddox rods and red and green glasses.
3. *A trial frame* (Fig. 36.9), which preferably should have following features:
- Light in weight with a comfortable fitting nose rest.
- Adjustable, both horizontally and vertically.

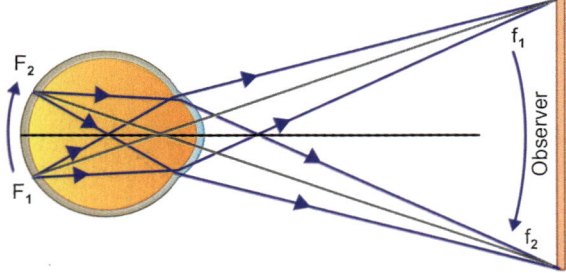

Fig. 36.7: *Movement of image of illuminated spot of fundus in myopia of 1 D.*

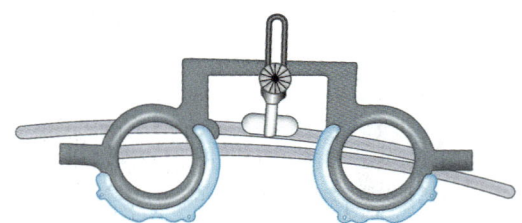

Fig. 36.9: *A trial frame.*

- Fitted with at least three compartments, one each, for lodging spherical lens, cylindrical lens and the occluder or any of the accessories.
- The compartment for the cylindrical lens should be capable of smooth and accurate rotation.
- The dial indicating the axis should be properly positioned to avoid error in the prescription of axis of cylindrical lens.
- The side pieces of the frame should be joint so that it could be tilted while testing for near vision, to align the optic axes of lenses with the line of vision.

4. *Phoropter* or *refractor* (Fig. 36.10), when available, saves lot of time with ease of manipulation. In it, the entire trial set of lenses and accessories are mounted on a circular wheel so that each lens can be brought before the aperture of the viewing system by merely turning a dial.

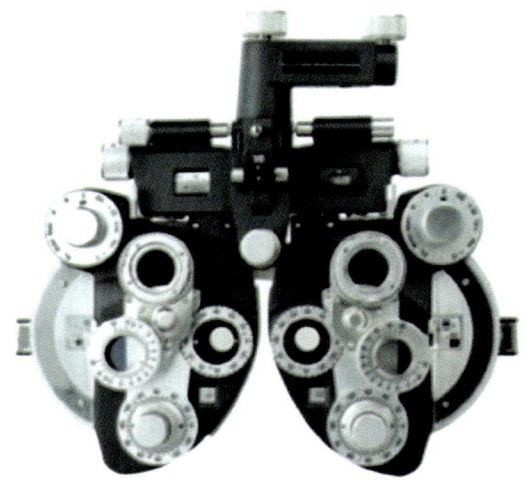

Fig. 36.10: *Phoropter or refractor.*

5. *Distance-vision chart.* A Snellen's self-illuminated vision box (Fig. 36.11A) is used commonly. The projector charts (Fig. 36.11B)

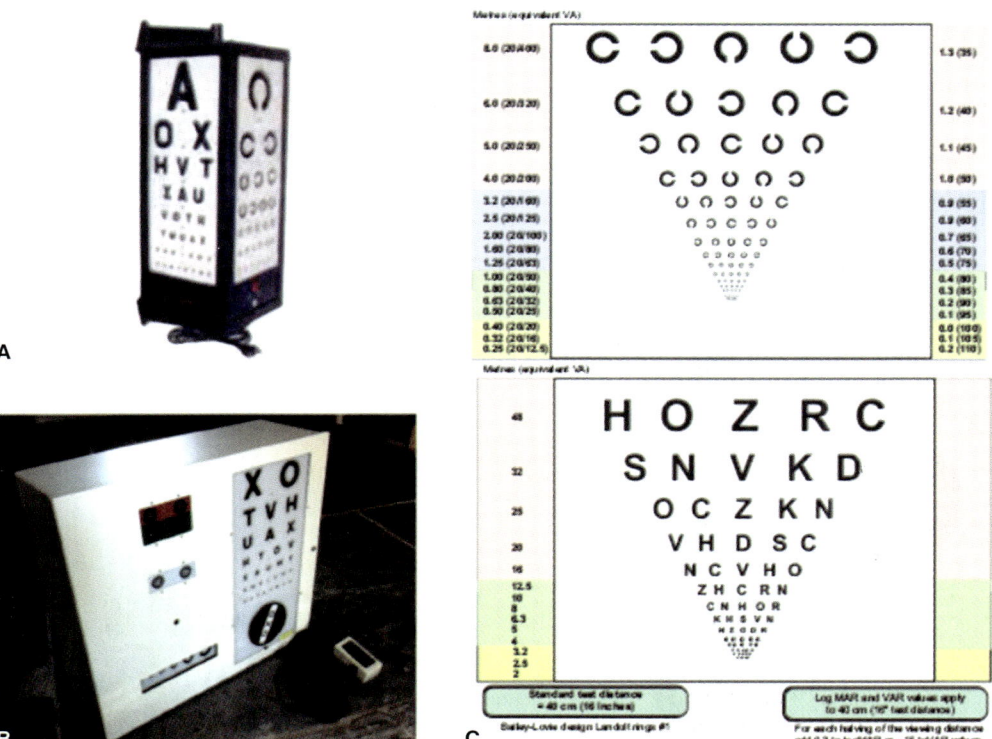

Fig. 36.11: *Distance vision charts: (A) Snellen's self-illuminated vision box; (B) Projector chart; (C) LogMAR vision chart (ETDRS chart).*

and LogMAR chart (ETDRS chart; Fig. 36.11C) have also become popular nowadays.

6. *Near-vision charts*, commonly used for testing near vision, are Jaeger's chart, reduced Snellen's test types and Times Roman type face.

7. *Retinoscope* is a simple device to perform the retinoscopy.

Types of retinoscope

1. *Reflecting (mirror) retinoscopes:* Reflecting (mirror) retinoscopes are cheap and at one time were the most commonly employed. However, presently these are sparingly used. A source of light is required when using mirror retinoscope, which is kept above and behind the head of the patient. The source of light used should be small, bright and enclosed; a pointolite is ideal. A mirror retinoscope may consist of a single plane mirror (Fig. 36.12A) or a combination of plane and concave mirrors (*Priestley-Smith* mirror; Fig. 36.12B).

Plane mirror gives comparatively more accurate results than the concave mirror. The central aperture in the mirror should be 3–4 mm in diameter so that a sufficient amount of light can enter the observer's eye. However, the advantages of a hole of this size are counterbalanced by the appearance of a circular dark patch in the centre of reflection corresponding to the hole, which reduces the illumination in pupillary area and confuses the retinoscopy. This difficulty is overcome by using a very slightly concave mirror wherein the focal length is greater than the distance between the examiner and the patient, that is at least 150 cm. For all practical purposes of retinoscopy, it acts as a plane mirror.

2. *Self-illuminated retinoscopes:* Self-illuminated retinoscopes are costly but handy. These have become more popular nowadays. Two types of self-illuminated retinoscope available are: (i) a spot retinoscope and (ii) a streak retinoscope (Fig. 36.13). The streak retinoscope is more popular, and most commonly used, since it is more sensitive than spot retinoscope in detecting astigmatism.

- *Spot self-illuminous retinoscope* consists of a bulb with a tiny wired filament about 1–2 mm in size. This is imaged by a convex lens of about 20 mm focal length to give a beam of light which is reflected by a mirror (at 45°) that is either totally silvered around a small circular unsilvered aperture (Fig. 36.14A) or half silvered (Fig. 36.14B).

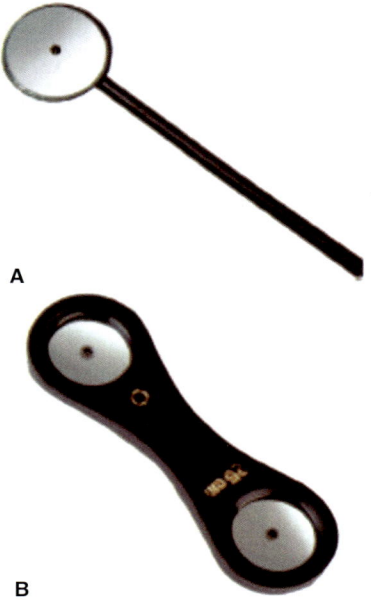

Fig. 36.12: *Mirror retinoscopes: (A) Plane mirror; (B) Priestley-Smith mirror.*

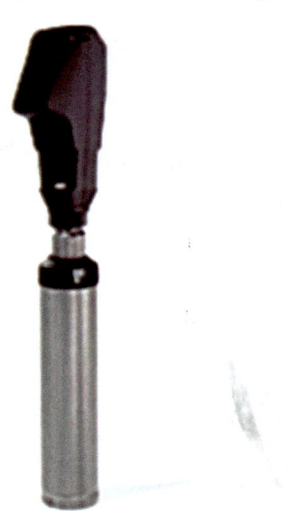

Fig. 36.13: *Self-illuminous streak retinoscope.*

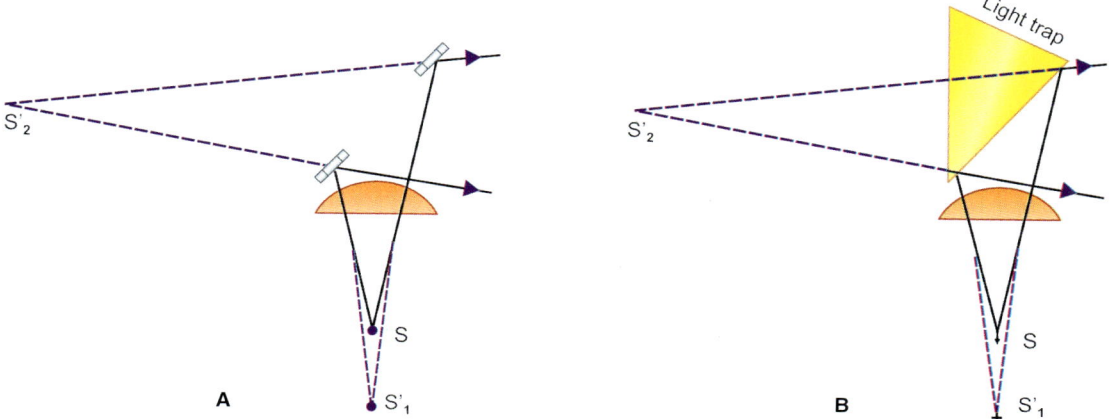

Fig. 36.14: *Ray diagram showing working principle of two types of self-illuminous retinoscopes: (A) an instrument with perforated mirror; (B) the instrument with a semisilvered reflector. The immediate source of light is the bulb image S'₂.*

- In *streak retinoscope,* the illumination is provided by a special bulb that has a straight filament, thus forming a 'streak' in its projection.

The filament may be moved in relation to convex lens in the system. If the light beam emerging from the lens is slightly divergent, it appears to come from a point behind the retinoscope—as if the light had been reflected off a plane mirror (*plane-mirror effect*) (Fig. 36.15A).

Alternatively, the distance between the convex lens and the bulb may be increased (by moving the sleeve on the handle), thus allowing converging light to be emitted. In this case, the image of the filament would be between the examiner and the patient—as if the light had been reflected off a concave mirror (*concave-mirror effect*) (Fig. 36.15B).

The axis of the streak of the retinoscope can be rotated by rotating the sleeve to align it with the axis of astigmatic error.

In practice, *plane-mirror effect* is used for retinoscopy. In patients with hazy media and high degree of ametropia, *concave-mirror effect* is more useful.

PROCEDURE

The patient is made to sit at a distance of 1 m (for ease of calculation) from the examiner (Fig. 36.16). However, a working distance of 2/3 m is more convenient and so is preferred in practice.

For non-cycloplegic refraction of patients who are not presbyopic (especially if they are myopic), *it is necessary to fog (blur) the fellow eye.* This involves placing a +1.50 or +2.00 spherical lens on top of the presumed refraction (estimated

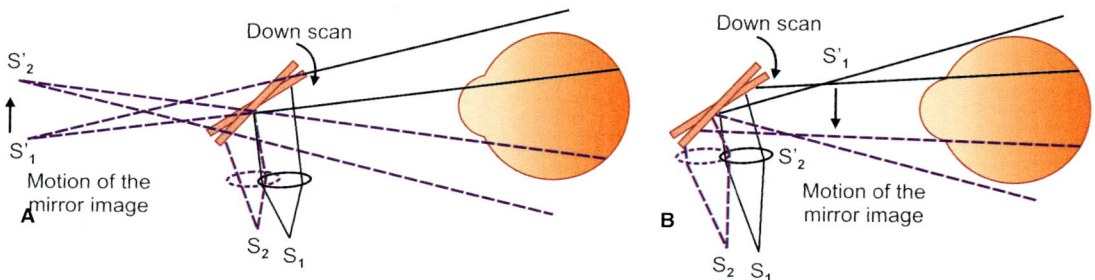

Fig. 36.15: *Illumination system of retinoscope, depicting:(A) position of the light source with plane mirror effect; (B) position of the light source with concave mirror effect.*

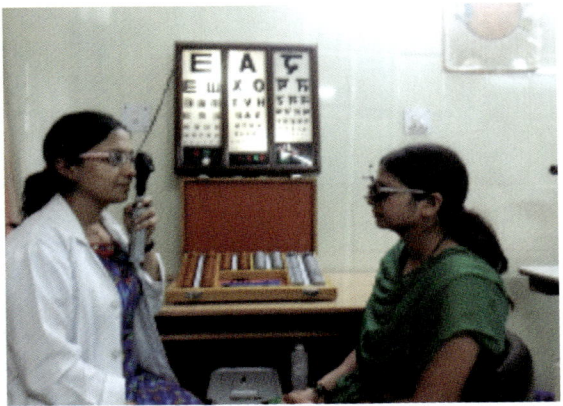

Fig. 36.16: *Procedure of retinoscopy.*

from their acuity, which you have just checked), so that the acuity is poorer than that of the eye being examined with the retinoscope. The reason why the fellow eye should be fogged is to reduce accommodation, which would give a false result when examining the fellow eye with the retinoscope.

This fogging induces less accommodation than simple occlusion with a black occluder, thus, ordinarily occlusion, should be avoided, as it stimulates more accommodation. However, *occlusion is required in the following situations*:

- When the eye being tested is densely amblyopic
- If the patient markeclly objects to fogging due to diplopia or asthenopia
- If you are unable to estirrnate acuity and provide an adequate fog lens.

With cycloplegic refraction (typically in children), there is no need to fog, since the accommodative component is removed by the cycloplegia.

To begin retinoscopy, with the help of a retinoscope, light is thrown onto the patient's eye, who is instructed to look at a far point (to relax the accommodation). However, when a cycloplegic has been used, the patient can look directly into the light and have the refraction assessed along the actual visual axis. Through a hole in the retinoscope's mirror, the examiner observes a red reflex in the pupillary area of the patient, which is seen as below:

- *With spot retinoscope*, whole of the pupil glows as red reflex.
- *With streak retinoscope*, red reflex is seen on a band of light (Fig. 36.17).

Then the retinoscope is moved in horizontal and vertical meridians, keeping a watch on the red reflex (which also moves when the retinoscope is moved). The characteristics of the moving retinal reflex are noted.

OBSERVATIONS AND INFERENCES

I. Direction of movement of red reflex

Depending upon the movement of the red reflex (when a plane mirror retinoscope is used at a distance of 1 m), the results are interpreted as follows:

1. *No movement* of red reflex indicates myopia of 1 D (Fig. 36.17A).

2. *With movement* of red reflex *along* the movement of the retinoscope indicates either

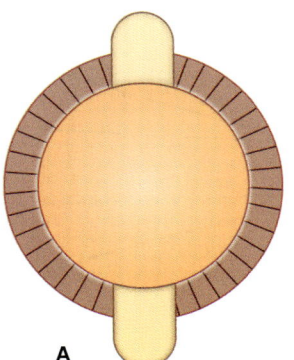
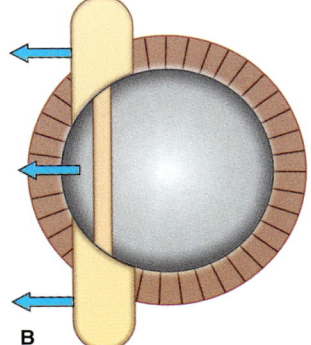
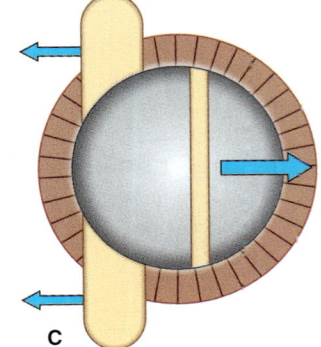

A   B   C

Fig. 36.17: *Red reflex during streak retinoscopy: (A) neutralization point; (B) with movement; (C) against movement.*

emmetropia or hypermetropia or myopia of less than 1 D (Fig. 36.17B).

3. *Against movement* of red reflex to the movement of the retinoscope implies myopia of more than 1 D (Fig. 36.17C).

The above assertions can be easily remembered from Fig. 36.18.

II. Brightness and speed of movement of red reflex

- *Bright and fast* shadow (red reflex) is seen in the pupillary area which moves rapidly with the movement of the mirror, in patients with low degrees of refractive errors.
- *Dull reflex* which moves slowly with the movement of mirror, is seen in patients with high degrees of ametropia.

III. Width of red reflex

Width of reflex, when using streak retinoscope, is narrow in high degrees of ametropia and wide in low degrees of ametropia. At the neutralization point, the entire pupil is filled with light.

IV. Orientation of red reflex

In the presence of astigmatism, when the axis does not correspond with the movement of the mirror, the shadow appears to swirl around. Following types of orientation of red reflex may be noted.

1. *Horizontal and vertical orientation* of the red reflex is observed when either there is no astigmatism or when the astigmatism is with the rule/against the rule. In these situations, ensure the slit is first vertical and then horizontal (by rotating the slit with the help of cuff of retinoscope), to nuetralise these meridians.

2. *Oblique orientation.* With oblique astigmatism, the principal meridians are still perpendicular but do not lie vertically and horizontally. Therefore, when a horizontal scope sweep is made with the slit orientated vertically, the orientation of the pupil reflex will be oblique and not lie vertically (it will lie between 45° and 90° or 90° and 135°). Similarly, if the scope slit was orientated horizontally and a sweep made vertically, the orientation of the pupil reflex will again be oblique and not be horizontal (it will lie between 0° and 45° or 135° and 180°). For oblique astigmatism, the scope slit should be rotated by turning the cuff slightly so the slit is parallel to the pupil reflex to aid subsequent neutralization. The perpendicular meridian can then be neutralized by rotating the slit 90° (e.g. if one meridian is at 120, the other be at 30°).

3. *Scissor reflex* or *some other problems* may be observed in the red reflex. These are described later (*see* page 716).

NEUTRALIZATION OF RED REFLEX

REFLECTING PLANE MIRROR (SPOT) RETINOSCOPY

Neutralization

To estimate the degree of refractive error, the movement of red reflex is neutralized by

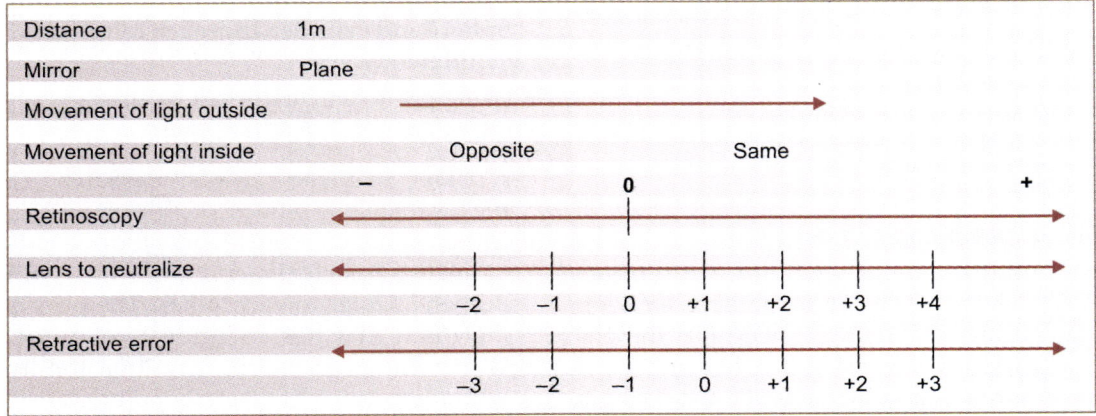

Fig. 36.18: *Diagrammatic depiction of the relation of movement of pupillary red reflex with the error of refraction.*

addition of increasingly convex (+) spherical lenses (when the red reflex was moving with the movement of plane mirror) or concave (−) spherical lenses (when the red reflex was moving against the movement of plane mirror). When a simple spherical error alone is present, the movements of red reflex will be neutralized in both vertical and the horizontal meridians.

However, in the presence of an astigmatic refractive error, the situation is not quite so simple. The examiner has to determine not only the different neutralization points of the two meridians but also the orientation of these. The relationship of the direction of external movement to that of the reflex has an important bearing on determination of axis of cylindrical error.

Finding the cylinder axis

The initial examination with retinoscope is always exploratory. In the presence of astigmatism, with its principal axis horizontal and vertical, one axis is neutralized with the appropriate spherical lens and the second axis (vertical or horizontal) still shows the movement of reflex in the direction of axis of astigmatism. In the presence of oblique astigmatism, close to neutralization point, the reflex may alter its plane of movement. Under such a situation, the examiner must again explore different planes of external movement of the light until they correspond to that of the retinoscopy reflexes.

Finding the cylinder power

Once the two principal meridians have been identified, each should be neutralized separately to find the cylindrical power by any of the following methods:
- With a sphere and a cylinder, or
- With spheres only, or
- With two cylinders.

1. With a sphere and cylinder

First neutralize one axis with an appropriate spherical lens (in order to be able to keep working using 'with reflexes', neutralize the lens plus axis first). Then with this spherical lens in place, neutralize the other axis 90° away with a cylindrical lens at the appropriate orientation.

The spherical–cylindrical gross retinoscopy may be read directly from the trial lens apparatus.

The main advantage of using spherocylinder combination over the two spheres is in verifying the position of axis. For this purpose, the appropriate sphere and a slight undercorrecting cylinder should be put in the trial frame. (For example, if the neutralizing spherocylindrical combination is 12 DS and 13 DC, then put 12.0 DS and 12.5 DC in the trial frame.) In this case, on moving the retinoscopic mirror at right angles to the axis of cylinder, the reflex should move exactly at right angles to the axis of cylinder (representing the 10.5 D of uncorrected hypermetropia). If the axis of the cylinder is not proper, this reflex will not move at right angles to the cylinder, but markedly obliquely (about six times). Let us suppose, in the above example, where the correction required is 12 DS and 13 DC at 85° and the examiner wrongly estimates that the direction of axis is 90°. In this case, when the cylinder is undercorrected by 10.5 D and placed at 90°, on moving the mirror horizontally, the reflex will obliquely move along 150° axis, i.e. 30° oblique. Thus the error in axis (5°) is multiplied six times. Since the obliquity of the shadow multiplies any error in the direction of the axis to such an enormous extent, a very small deviation from the true axis is easily detected. The angle that the oblique reflex now makes with the axis of cylinder should be assessed and the cylinder rotated through an angle one-sixth of this. The procedure should be repeated until the final and correct axis is obtained.

Sphere and cylinder approach can be used in two different ways:
- Using positive cylinder notation, or
- Using negative cylinder notation.

i. Using positive cylinder notation. This means that your retinoscopy result will be in a plus cylinder format. Identify the orientation of the two principal meridians, which will be perpendzicular to each other. The principal meridian that has an against reflex or, if both reflexes are with, it will be the least with reflex (which is fastest and brightest, as it nearest neutralization) is neutralized first with spheres. This will result in the other principal meridian giving a with reflex, which is then neutralized with positive cylinder (the axis on the lens in the same orientation as the scope slit). The resultant prescription will be the lenses in the trial frame.

ii. Using negative cylinder notation. This means that your retinoscopy result will be in a minus cylinder format. Identify the orientation of the two principal meridians, which will be perpendicular to each other. *First, neutralize the most with reflex with plus spheres then neutralize the perpendicular against reflex with minus cylinders.* The lenses in the trial frame will give the retinoscopy result in minus cylinder format, which must then be corrected for working distance.

2. With spheres only

It is possible to obtain an objective refractive result without using any cylindrical lenses first of all, identify the two principal meridians, then neutralize one of the meridians with a sphere and record the result and orientation of reflex. Following this, neutralize the perpendicular meridian with an appropriate sphere and record the result and orientation of the reflex. The magnitude of the cylinder is the difference between the two spheres. It is better to use a power cross to record the results and generate the resultant prescription. For example, if the 180° axis is neutralized with +2.0 sphere, and the 90° axis with +3.0 sphere, the power cross for gross retinoscopy will be: $^{(+2)}+_{(+3)}$

3. With two cylinders

Although it is possible to use two cylinders at right angles to each other for the gross retinoscopy, there seems to be no advantage of this variant over the spherocylinder combination. Which is the most preferred technique.

End point of retinoscopy

The end point of retinoscopy using a simple plane mirror retinoscope is neutralization of red reflex, i.e. no movement of the reflex in any meridian with the movement of the mirror. The end point of retinoscopy can be and should be verified by following manoeuvres:

- Overcorrection by 0.25 D should cause reversal of the movement.
- On altering the working distance, i.e. by slight forward movement of the head, the examiner should observe a 'with' movement and an 'against' movement by slight backward movement.

STREAK RETINOSCOPY

With streak retinoscope, the retinoscopy is performed in the usual way and a band of light appears in the pupillary area which moves 'with' or 'against' the movement of band of light outside the pupil (Fig. 36.17). The movement of the band of light is then neutralized by adding appropriate spherical lenses as described in reflecting mirror retinoscopy.

When a simple spherical error alone is present, at neutralization, the band-shaped reflex disappears and the pupil appears completely illuminated (Fig. 36.17A) or completely dark. However, in the presence of astigmatism, a band-shaped reflex will appear in the meridian still not neutralized.

Finding the cylinder axis

In a patient with regular astigmatism, two reflexes—one from each of the principal meridians—need to be neutralized. Before measuring the power in each of the principal meridians, one must determine the axes of the meridians.

Characteristics of the streak reflex that can aid in determining the axis are as follows:

1. *Break in the alignment between the reflex in the pupil and the band out side it* is observed (Fig. 36.19) when the streak is not parallel to one of the meridians. The band of light in pupillary area lies in a position intermediate between the band outside the pupil and that from axis of the cylinder. The axis, even in the case of low astigmatic errors, can thus be determined by rotating the streak until the break disappears. The correcting cylinder should be placed at this axis.

2. *Width of the streak varies as it is rotated around the correct axis.* It appears narrowest when the streak aligns with the true axis (Fig. 36.20).

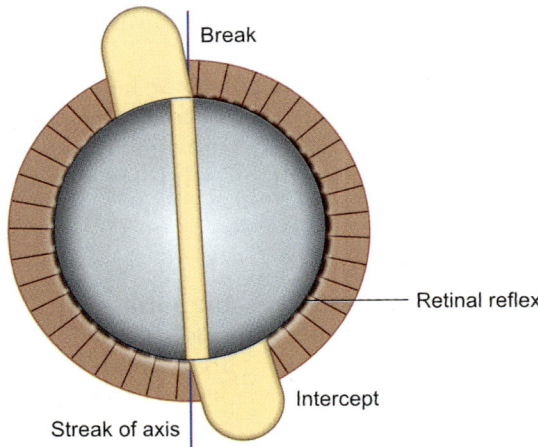

Fig. 36.19: *Break in the alignment between the reflex in the pupil and the band outside it when the streak is off the correct axis.*

3. *Intensity of the reflex band in pupil is brighter when the streak aligns with true axis.* This is a subtle finding, useful only in small cylinders.

4. *Skew (oblique motion of the streak reflex)* may be used to refine the axis in small cylinders. The streak and reflex will move in the same direction

only when streak is aligned with one of the principal meridians. Therefore, if the streak is not aligned with the true axis, skewing will be observed on movement of the streak (Fig. 36.21).

Confirmation of the axis. Finally, the axis of cylinder may be confirmed with a technique known as *straddling*. This is performed with approximately the correct cylinder in place. The retinoscope streak is turned 45° off axis in both directions. If the axis is correct, the width of the reflex should be equal in each of the two positions. If the axis is not correct, the widths will be unequal in the two positions (Fig. 36.22). In such a situation, the narrower reflex serves as the guide towards which the cylinder's axis should be turned (Fig. 36.22A).

Final localization of the axis on the protractor. Once the axis of cylinder is finally confirmed (Fig. 36.23A), to pinpoint it on the protractor, the sleeve of the retinoscope is adjusted to enhance the intercept until the reflex is seen as a fine line (Fig. 36.23B).

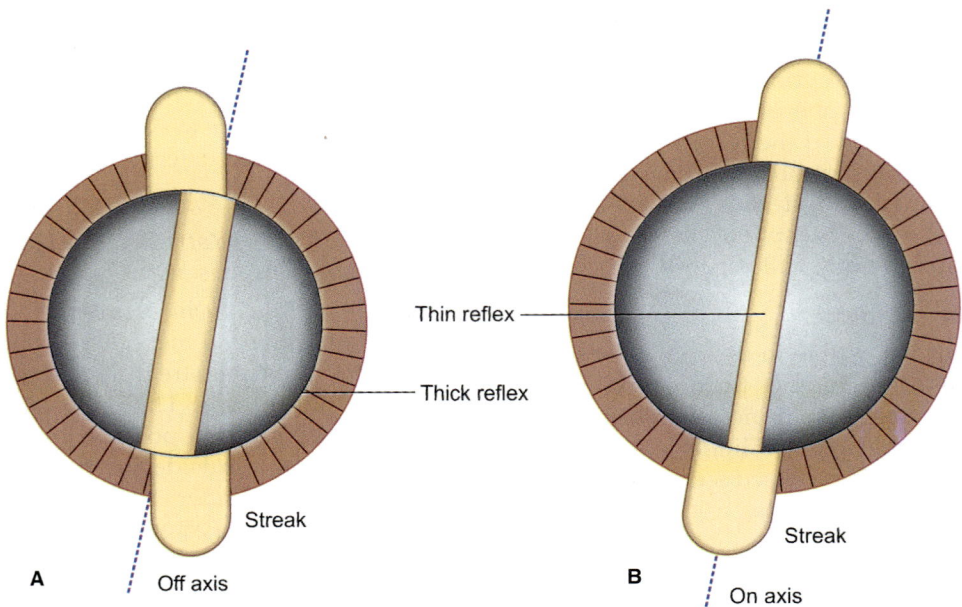

Fig. 36.20: *Width of the reflex in the pupil is narrowest when the streak is exactly aligned with the axis: (A) off axis, (B) on axis.*

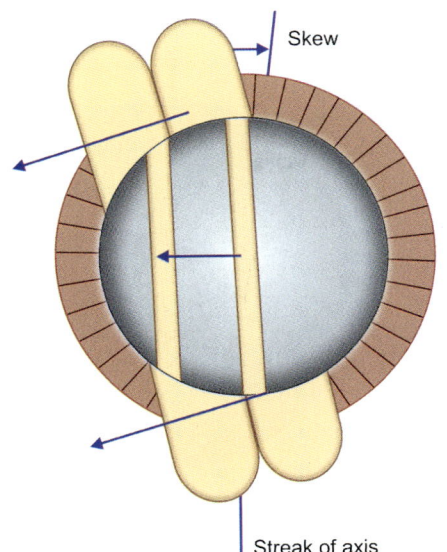

Fig. 36.21: *Skewing of the pupillary reflex and the band outside it when the streak is off axis.*

Finding the cylinder power

Once the two principal meridia have been identified, the cylindrical power can be determined in a manner similar to that described in reflecting mirror retinoscopy.

End point of neutralization

When streak retinoscopy is performed, the width of the reflex widens progressively as the neutralization is approached, and at the end point, streak disappears and the pupil appears completely illuminated (Fig. 36.17A) or completely dark.

The end point can be verified by the same methods as described in spot retinoscopy.

USE OF CYCLOPLEGICS IN RETINOSCOPY

Cycloplegics are the drugs that cause paralysis of accommodation and dilate the pupil. These are used for retinoscopy, when the examiner suspects that accommodation is abnormally active and will hinder the exact retinoscopy. Such a situation is encountered in young children and hypermetropes. When retinoscopy is performed after instilling cycloplegic drugs, it is termed as *wet retinoscopy* in converse to *dry retinoscopy* (without cycloplegics).

Commonly employed cycloplegics

*1. **Atropine** is indicated in children below the age of 5 years. It is used as 1% ointment thrice daily for 3 consecutive days before performing retinoscopy. Its effect lasts for 10–20 days.

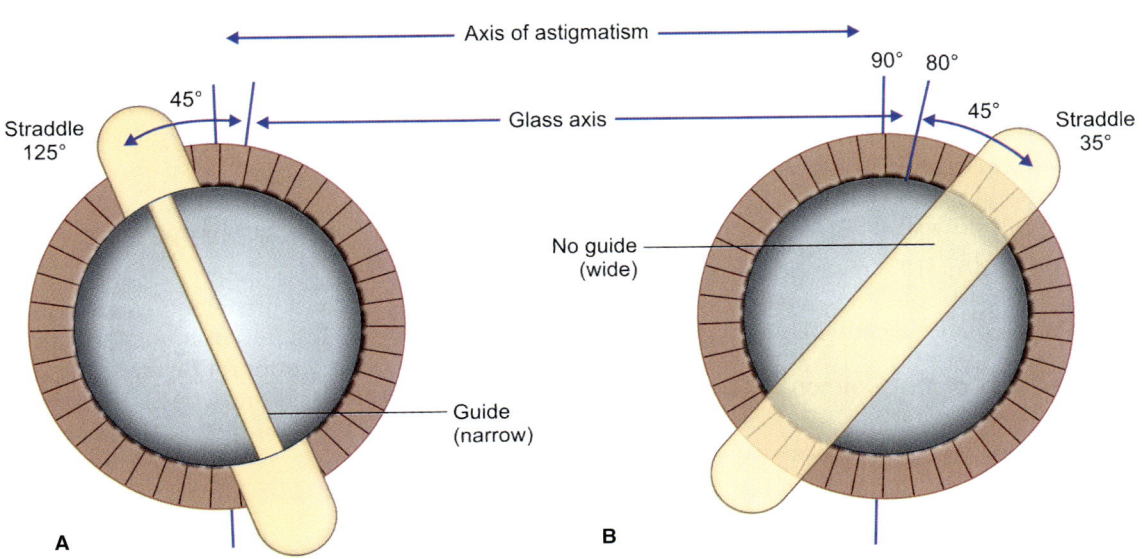

Fig. 36.22: *Technique of straddling showing narrow reflex (A) when the meridian is 45° off axis towards 125° from 80° and wide reflex; (B) when the meridian is 45° off axis towards 35° from 80°. The narrow reflex (A) is the guide towards which cylinder's axis should be turned.*

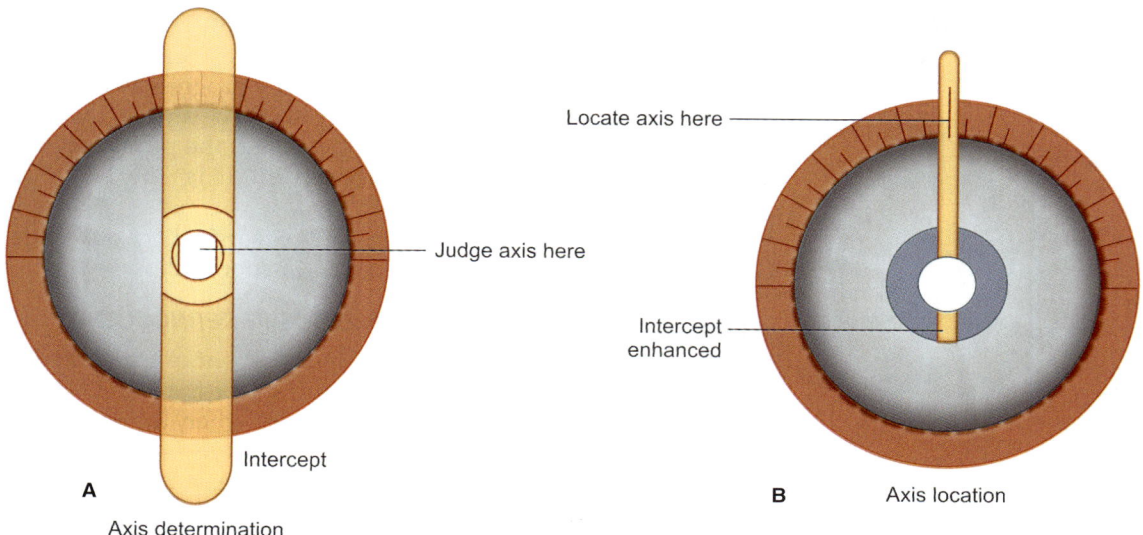

Locate axis here

Judge axis here

Intercept enhanced

A

Intercept

Axis determination

B   Axis location

Fig. 36.23: *Final localization of the axis on protractor. First the astigmatic axis is determined (A); and then the sleeve of the retinoscope is adjusted to enhance the intercept until the reflex is seen as a fine line pinpointing the axis (B).*

2. *Homatropine* is used as 2% drops. One drop is often instilled every 10 minutes for six times and the retinoscopy is performed after 1–2 hours. Its effect lasts for 48–72 hours. It is used for most of the hypermetropic individuals between 5 and 25 years of age.

3. *Cyclopentolate* is a short-acting cycloplegic. Its effect lasts for 6–18 hours. It is used as 1% eyedrops in patients between 8 and 20 years of age. One drop of cyclopentolate is instilled after every 10–15 minutes for three times (Havener's recommended dose) and the retinoscopy is preformed 1–1½ hour or 60–90 minutes later, after estimating the residual accommodation which should not exceed 1D.

4. *Only mydriatic* (10% phenylephrine) may be needed in elderly patients when the pupil is narrow or media is slightly hazy.

Salient features of the common cycloplegic and mydriatic drugs:

Salient features of the common cycloplegic and mydriatic drugs are summarized in Table 36.1.

Note. The mydriatics should be used with care in adults with shallow anterior chamber, owing to the danger of an attack of narrow angle glaucoma. In older people, mydriasis should be counteracted by the use of miotic drug (2% pilocarpine).

STATIC VERSUS DYNAMIC RETINOSCOPY

- *Static retinoscopy* refers to the procedure performed without active use of accommodation (as described above).
- *Dynamic retinoscopy* implies when the procedure is performed for near vision with active use of accommodation by the patient. However, usefulness of performing dynamic retinoscopy has not yet been established in refraction.

ROUGH ESTIMATE OF REFRACTIVE ERROR AFTER RETINOSCOPY

Objectively, a rough estimate of error of refraction is made by taking into account the retinoscopic findings, deductions for distance (e.g. 1 D for 1 m and 1.5 D when retinoscopy is performed at 2/3 m distance) and deduction for the cycloplegic when used (e.g. 1 D for atropine, 0.5 D for homatropine and 0.75 D for cyclopentolate).

Thus briefly,

Amount of refractive error = Retinoscopic findings – deduction for distance – tonus allowance for cycloplegic drug used.

Table 36.1 *Salient features of common cycloplegic and mydriatic drugs*

S. no.	Name of the drug	Age of the patient when indicated	Dosage of instillation	Peak effect	Time of performing retinoscopy	Duration of action	Period of post-cycloplegic test	Tonus allowance
1.	Atropine sulphate (1% ointment)	<5 years	TDS × 3 days	2–3 days	4th day	10–20 days	After 3 weeks of retinoscopy	1 D
2.	Homatropine-hydrobromide (2% drops)	5–8 years	One drop every 10 minutes for six times	60–90 min	After 90 min of instillation of first drop	48–72 hours	After 3 days of retinoscopy	0.5 D
3.	Cyclopentolate hydrochloride (1% drops)	8–20 years	One drop every 15 minutes for three times	80–90 min	After 90 min of instillation of first drop	6–18 hours	After 3 days of retinoscopy	0.75 D
4.	Tropicamide (0.5%, 1% drops)	Not used as cycloplegic for retinoscopy; used only as mydriatic	One drop every 15 minutes for three to four times	20–40 min		4–6 hours		—
5.	Phenylephrine (5%, 10% drops)	Used only as mydriatic alone or in combination with tropicamide	One drop every 15 minutes for three to four times	30–40 min		4–6 hours		—

Power cross

It is customary to do retinoscopy both vertically and horizontally and note the values separately (Fig. 36.24). In the power cross (Fig. 36.24A), X denotes retinoscopy value along the vertical meridian and Y denotes the value along the horizontal axis.

- *When retinoscopy values along horizontal and vertical meridiand are equal,* then there is no astigmatism and a spherical lens is required to correct the refractive error. *For example,* when retinoscopic finding is +7 DS, with the procedure preformed at 1 m distance, using atropine as cycloplegic, then appropriate refractive error will be 7–1 D (for distance) 2–1 D (tonus allowance for atropine) = + 5 DS (Fig. 36.24B).
- *When retinoscopy values along horizontal and vertical meridians* are unequal, then it denotes

presence of astigmatism, which is corrected by a cylindrical lens alone or in combination with a spherical lens (Figs 36.24C and D).

PROBLEMS IN RETINOSCOPY

Certain difficulties encountered during the procedure of retinoscopy are summarized below.

1. *Red reflex may not be visible or may be poor.* This may happen with small pupil, hazy media and high degree of refractive error. In most cases, this difficulty is overcome by causing mydriasis and/or use of converging light with concave mirror retinoscope.

2. *Changing retinoscopy findings* are observed due to abnormally active accommodation and this is corrected by following measures:

- *Fogging retinoscopy.* In this technique, plus lenses much higher than the expected

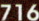

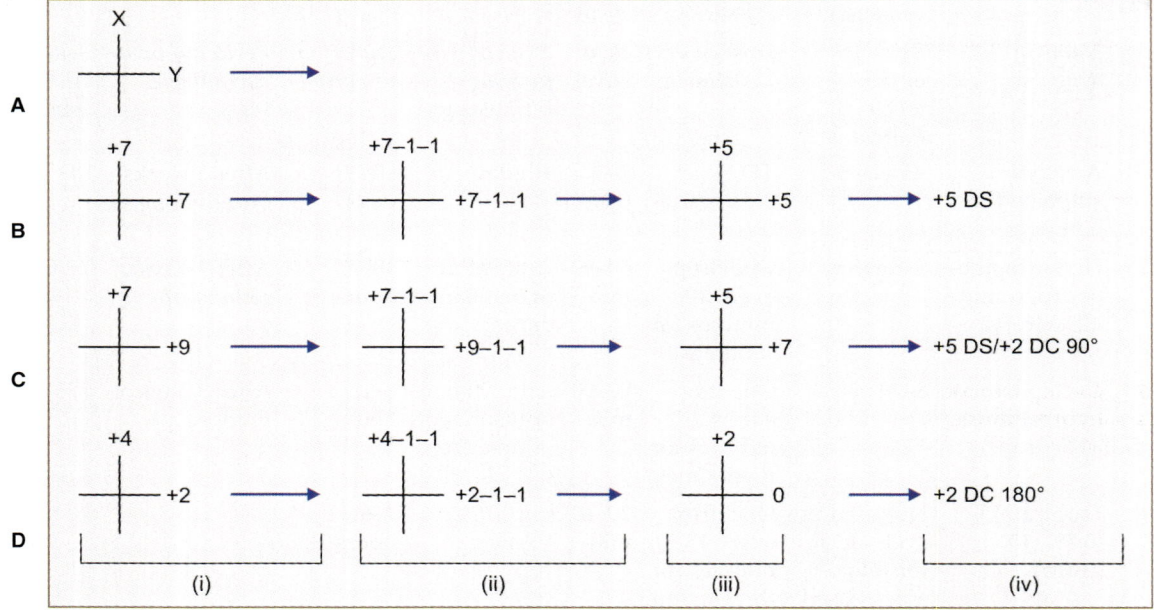

Fig. 36.24: *(A) Customary way of writing retinoscopic findings. (B, C, and D) Calculation for rough estimate of refractive error: (i) Retinoscopic findings, when performed at 1 m distance under atropine cycloplegia; (ii) deduction of 21 D for distance and 21 D for the atropine from the retinoscopic findings. (iii) Rough estimate of refractive error along horizontal and vertical meridians; and (iv) prescription required.*

retinoscopic findings are placed in front of both the eyes. The patient is instructed to look at a far distance target, without making efforts to see clearly. Retinoscopy is performed and the plus lenses are decreased successively till neutralization is achieved. Care is taken to insert the replacing lens before the replaced lens is removed.

- *Cycloplegic* may be required in young patients to control accommodation.

3. Scissoring shadows may sometimes be seen in patients with astigmatism (Fig. 36.25). In such a situation, two band reflexes appear which move towards and away from each other like the blades of scissors. It happens due to mixed aberration so that one-half of the reflex differs in its refractivity considerably in character from the other. The optics of this phenomenon is depicted in Fig. 36.26. Mostly this difficulty is diminished with the undilated pupil.

4. Spherical aberrations lead to variation of refraction in the centre and periphery of pupil. Such differences are accentuated with dilated

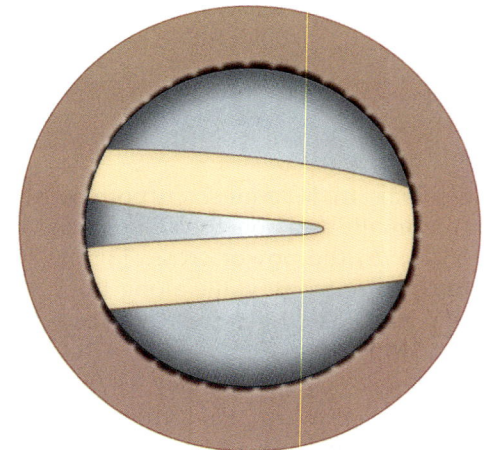

Fig. 36.25: *Scissor shadows.*

pupils. The spherical aberrations tend to cause an increase of brightness at the centre or the periphery of the pupillary reflex depending on whether the aberrations are positive or negative (Figs 36.27 and 36.28). The spherical aberrations may be seen in normal eyes, but are more marked in conditions like lenticular sclerosis.

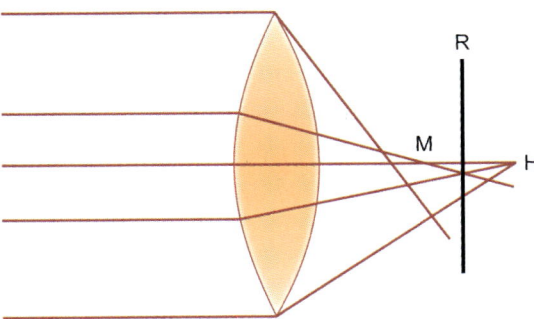

Fig. 36.26: *The optics of scissor shadows wherein at the plane of observation (R), one part of the aperture is relatively myopic (M) and the other relatively hypermetropic (H).*

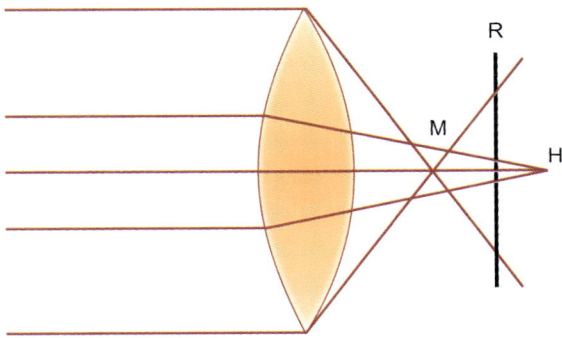

Fig. 36.29: *Optics of positive aberration. Central part shows myopic refraction (M), and peripheral part shows hypermetropic refraction (H); (R=Retina).*

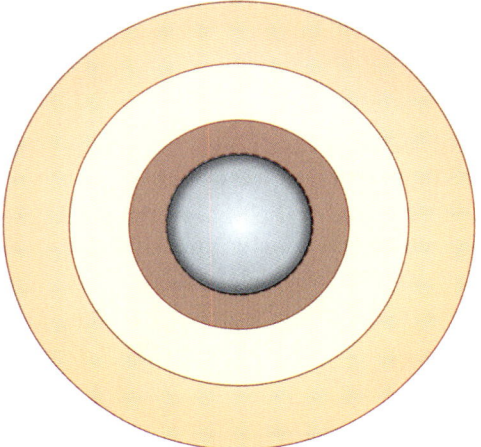

Fig. 36.27: *Positive aberration.*

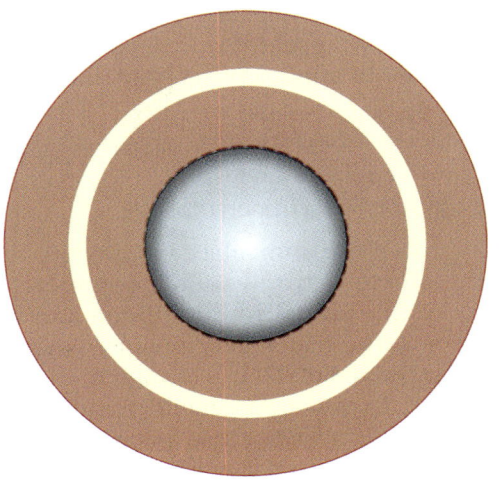

Fig. 36.28: *Negative aberration.*

The optics of spherical aberration is shown in Fig. 36.29.

5. ***Conflicting shadows*** moving in various directions in different parts of the pupillary area are seen in patients with irregular astigmatism.

6. ***Triangular shadow*** may be observed in patients with conical cornea.

B. AUTOREFRACTOMETRY

Refraction being the most commonly performed optical procedure has been widely developed. Though the conventional technique of retinoscopic refraction is an excellent method of objective refraction, it is a time-consuming procedure and not every practitioner manages to accomplish it accurately.

The refractometry (optometry) is an alternative method of finding out the error of refraction by use of an optical equipment called refractometer or optometer.

OPTICAL PRINCIPLES

The present day autorefractors (AR) are based on the principles used in earlier attempts for automation of the refraction. Most of the autorefractometers are essentially based on following two principles.

1. The Scheiner principle

Scheiner, in 1619, observed that refractive error of the eye can be determined by using double pinhole apertures before the pupils. Following are his observations:

- *The parallel rays of light entering the eye* from a distant object, which are normally focused on a point on the retina in an emmetropic patient (Fig. 36.30A), are limited to two small bundles when double pinhole apertures are placed in front of the pupil (Fig. 36.30B).
- *In a myopic eye*, the two ray bundles cross each other before reaching the retina and two small spots of light are seen (Fig. 36.30C).
- *In a hypermetropic eye*, the ray bundles are intercepted by the retina before they meet and thus again two small spots of light are seen (Fig. 36.30D).
- These two points of light can be coalesced to a single point by moving the double pinhole to the far point of eye.

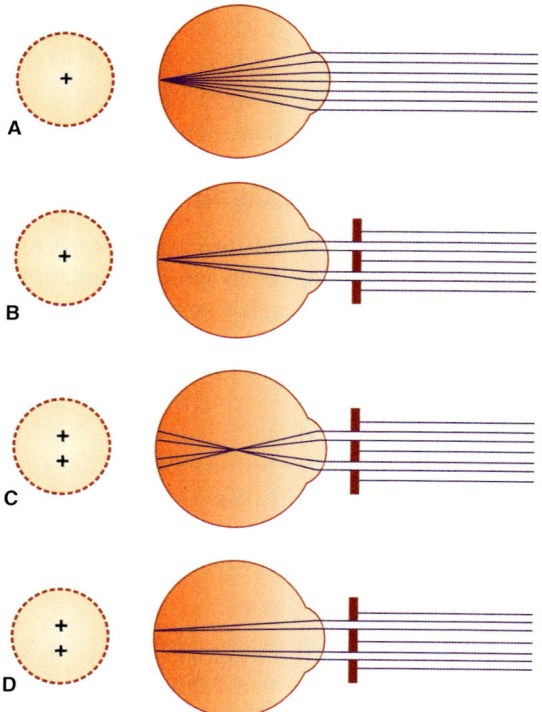

Fig. 36.30: *Scheiner's principle. Parallel rays of light entering an emmetropic eye are focused on the retina (A). Double apertures placed in front of the eye isolate two bundles of the light passing through the pupil, which are focused as a single spot on the retina in an emmetropic eye (B) and as two small spots of light in the myopic (C) as well as hypermetropic eye (D).*

- Thus, from the far point of the eye, the refractive error of the eye can be determined.

2. The optometer principle

Porterfield, in 1759, coined the term optometer to describe an instrument for measuring the limits of distinct vision. The optical principle on which this instrument was based is now known as *the optometer principle*. This principle permits continuous variation of power in the refracting instruments (Fig. 36.31).

- As shown in Fig. 36.31A, the autorefracto-meters based on this principle use a single converging lens placed at its focal length from the eye (or the spectacle plane) instead of interchangeable trial lenses.
- Light from the target on the far side of the lens enters the eye with vergence of different amounts, i.e. [zero (Fig. 36.31B), minus (Fig. 36.31C) or plus (Fig. 36.31D)] depending on the position of the target.
- The vergence of the light in the focal plane of the optometer lens is linearly related to the displacement of the target.
- A scale with equal spacing can thus be made which would show the number of dioptres of correction (Fig. 36.31E).

MODERN REFRACTOMETERS

With the rapid development in electronics and microcomputers, a number of innovative methods and instruments for automated clinical refraction have appeared since 1960. Efforts have been made to eliminate the limitations of old refractors.

The modern refractors can be grouped as below:
- Objective refractometers
- Subjective refractometers

Both objective and subjective modern auto-refractometers are available commercially (Fig. 36.32). A detailed description and comparison of the major instruments, which are currently on the market, is beyond the scope of this book. However, a general comparison of objective and subjective instruments and a brief description of some of the instruments presently in use are given.

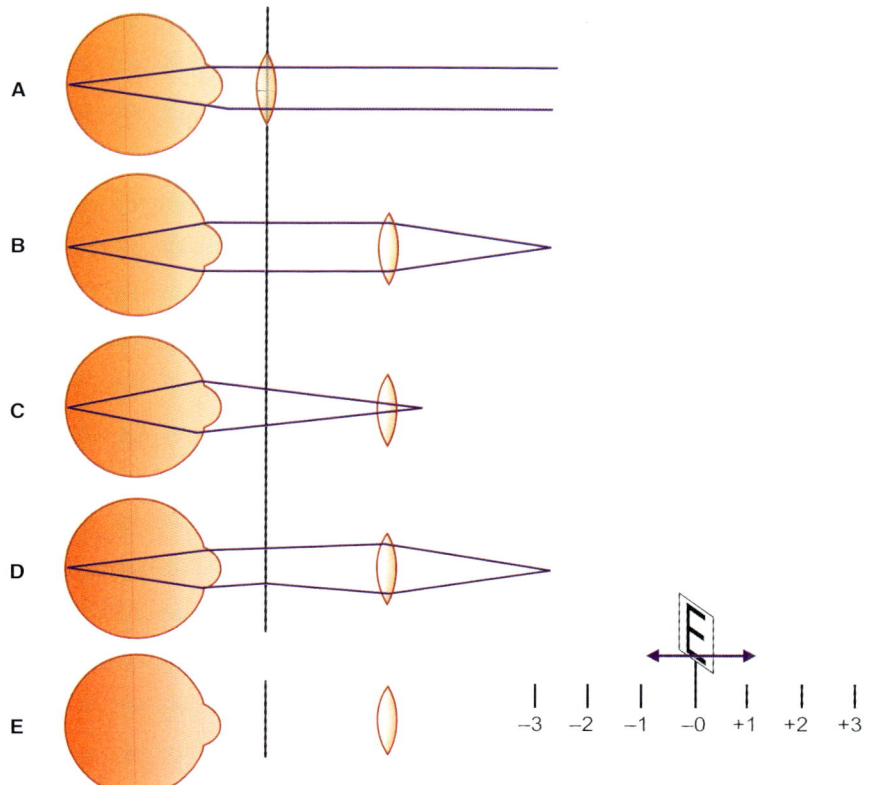

Fig. 36.31: *The optometer principle. Refractometer based on this principle uses a single converging lens (A), light from a target on the far side of the lens may enter with zero (B), minus (C) or plus (D) vergence. The scale used in optometers would show the amount of ametropia in dioptres (E).*

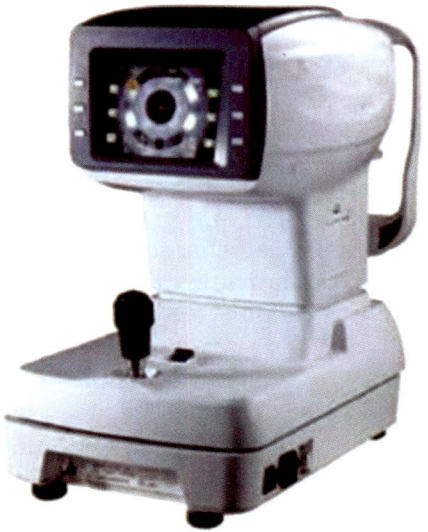

Fig. 36.32: *Computerized autorefractometer.*

GENERAL COMPARISON OF SUBJECTIVE AND OBJECTIVE INSTRUMENTS

1. *Source of light.* The objective refractometers use low levels of invisible infrared light to perform the refraction, while the subjective refractors use visible light. Thus subjective refractors are calibrated using visible light in a manner similar to calibration of lensometer. There occurs a substantial difference of about 0.75–1.50 D between the infrared refraction obtained by the objective refractometers and the visible light refraction that is desired. This difference can be explained by both the chromatic aberration of the eye and the fact that the infrared light is refracted not from the photoreceptor but from a different layer of retina. Therefore, a bias must be built into each instrument to account for this difference.

2. *Time required for refraction.* The objective refractometer usually takes 2–4 minutes, while subjective refractometer takes 4–8 minutes to refract from both eyes.

3. *Information provided.* The subjective refractometers supply more information, and the corrected visual acuity is obtained as part of the refracting procedure. The objective refractometers do not provide this information except for the Humphrey Automatic Refractor which provides visual acuity capability.

4. *Patient cooperation factors.* The objective refractometer requires less patient cooperation, since while refracting with these instruments the patients have simply to stay reasonably still and look straight ahead at a target. On the other hand, while refracting with subjective refractometers, in addition, the patients should be able to turn a knob to focus various targets or answer simple questions about the appearance of the targets.

In general, it has been observed that children above 5 years of age can be refracted with objective refractometers, while for subjective refractometer use the child should be about 8 years of age to obtain the desirable cooperation. Regardless of the instrument being used, children should be subjected to cycloplegic refraction.

5. *Ocular factors.* Ocular diseases may limit the performance of the refractometers as below:
- Objective refractors give better results than the subjective refractors in the presence of macular diseases with clear ocular media.
- Performance of objective and subjective refractometers is equal in the presence of hazy ocular media which cause decreased Snellen's visual acuity up to 6/18.
- In the presence of hazy ocular media causing a drop in visual acuity of more than 6/18, the objective refractors usually do not function properly, but rough refraction often still may be obtained with the subjective refractors.

6. *Over-refraction capability.* The over-refraction in patients using spectacles, contact lenses or intraocular lenses is comparatively difficult with objective refractors due to reflection. On the other hand, no such problem is encountered while over refracting with subjective refractors.

7. *Expected results.* The objective refractors provide only preliminary refractive findings. The practitioner has to refine these results. However, some of the subjective refractors, such as Vision Analyser and the SRN, provide refined subjective results. The 'Vision Analyser', in addition, provides binocular refraction capability for those practitioners who use binocular techniques.

C. PHOTOREFRACTION

Over the years, there has been increasing interest in methods of objectively refracting eyes with photographic and videographic techniques. There are now several photographic and videographic refractors commercially available that are used at distances of 0.5 to 2 metres from the patient. Often called *photorefractors*, these devices characteristically capture images of the fundus reflexes from the two eyes of a patient, simultaneously, and these images are produced either by a flash of visible white light or infrared radiation (IR) from a source centred in or adjacent to the camera's lens. The fundus reflexes can be captured on film, digitally, or by video, and they are then subjected to analysis.

At the present time, most photorefractive techniques are used in research laboratories, and only a few have found their way into clinical practice. Those that are found commercially are generally recommended for the screening of infants and children at schools or other sites away from the eye care practitioner's office, although traditional retinoscopy remains more accurate and informative when a professional takes the time to do screenings with a retinoscope.

Two different overall principles of photo-refraction can be distinguished:
1. Photorefractors based on a pointspread method, and
2. Photorefractors based on a retinoscopic-like method.

POINTSPREAD METHOD OF PHOTOREFRACTION

Two pointspread methods are available for photorefraction. The advantage of these methods is the very short time required for taking a measurement, i.e. the time required by a single flash exposure.

Howland and Howland method of pointspread photorefraction

The first method introduced by Howland and Howland (1974) uses a photographic method to deduce the refractive or accommodative state of the patient's eyes. Because the photographs can be taken immediately, the patient appears to be looking at the camera. This method can be used with young infants whose span of attention is too short for retinoscopy. In such cases, an automated objective optometer is equally unsuitable because the eye has to be positioned accurately in relation to the instrument. Atkinson and Braddick recommended photorefraction as a screening test for significant refractory errors in young infants.

The photorefractor consists essentially of a small source of light mounted in front of a suitable camera. The source is formed by an electronic flash, illuminating one end of a fibreoptic light guide, the other end being mounted centrally in front of the camera lens. It illuminates the patient's face and is imaged on the fundus of both eyes. The retinal image may be regarded as a secondary source giving rise to a fundus image in the plane conjugate with the retina.

If the eye is in focus for the source, the light leaving the eye returns to the source and is thus occluded from the camera lens. As a result, the pupil appears dark in the photograph. When the eye is out of focus, a blur circle or ellipse is formed on the fundus, producing in turn an illuminated zone around the source. The size of this zone varies with the ocular focusing error relative to the source.

Grolman's method of pointspread photorefraction

The second method, introduced by Grolman, is more accurate than the first. As shown in Fig. 36.33, this method uses an array of point

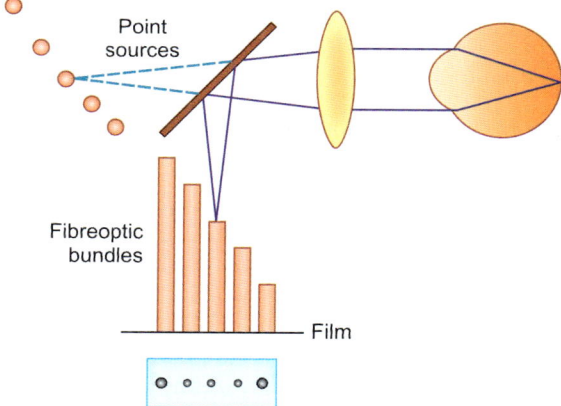

Fig. 36.33: *Grolman photographic system for objective refraction.*

sources of light spaced at varying dioptric distances from the patient's eye and flashed simultaneously. One end of a separate fibreoptic bundle is conjugate to each point source and receives the image point source as reflected from the patient's fundus. The image received by all fibreoptic bundles are recorded in a common plane on a strip of photographic film. The refractive error is judged by identifying the two sharpest ellipses and their orientation on the film.

RETINOSCOPIC-LIKE METHODS OF PHOTOREFRACTION

Synonyms of photoretinoscopy are eccentric photorefraction, photoskiascopy, and paraxial photorefraction. In photoretinoscopy, a light source close to the aperture of the camera is directed into the subject's eyes. The camera, which is focused on the subject's entrance pupils, records the pupils illuminated by their respective fundus reflexes. The light returned from the fundus returns into the camera aperture in a manner similar to that described in Static Streak Retinoscopy.

- *Stationary equivalent of retinoscopic "against motion"* occurs when the eye is focused myopically relative to the camera. In this case, the pupil appears illuminated on the same side as that of the light source.
- *Stationary equivalent of "with motion"* occurs, if the eye is hyperoptically focused relative to

the camera. The pupil will appear to be illuminated on the opposite side relative to the light source.

Techniques of retinoscopic photorefraction

Following techniques are there:

1. *Visible-light photoretinoscopy.* In visible-light photoretinoscopy, an exposure of the subject's pupils is achieved with a visible light source that is slightly eccentric (usually inferior) to the camera aperture. This results in an illumination of the pupils with red backscattered light from the fundi, which are the glowing "red eyes". When the radius of the pointspread image exceeds the eccentricity of the light source, a bright orange/yellow crescent appears in the periphery of the pupil as the red reflex becomes non-uniform in illumination.

2. *Infrared videoretinoscopy.* An IR source, consisiting of a row or several rows of IR-light emitting diodes (IR-LEDs), can be located below a knife-edge aperture similar to that of a visible light photoretinoscope. The IR-LEDs are mounted in front of a video camera, and the apparatus is called an infrared videoretinoscope. When the various rows of IR-LEDs are illuminated sequentially, a retinoscopic-like IR fundus reflex can be detected at the video screen as the fundus reflexes appear to move across the pupils of the subject's eyes. The optical principles of the infrared videoretinoscope are virtually the same as that of an ordinary retinoscope. As the eccentricity of the IR source is increased (i.e. as the IR-LED rows illuminate sequentially away from the knife-edge of the aperture), the size of the crescent detected in the subject's eye decreases. The crescent appears to move in a direction opposite to that of the IR source (in relative hyperopia) or in the same direction as the IR source (in relative myopia).

3. *Computer-assisted infrared videoretinoscopy.* The videoretinoscopy images could be captured in a computer frame store and processed by a computer. Although there are only three well-described instruments for this purpose, it appears likely that the next decades will see a proliferation of this technology as a result of steady improvement within the video and computer fields.

D. ELECTROPHYSIOLOGIC METHODS OF OBJECTIVE REFRACTION

This uses the visually evoked response for estimating automated clinical refraction. An advantage of this method is that it tests the entire visual system, from the cornea to the visual cortex. Spherical correction to the nearest 0.25 D is relatively easy to obtain. However, it does not measure the astigmatism very effectively.

SUBJECTIVE REFRACTION

Subjective refraction is meant for finding out the most suitable lenses to be prescribed. It can be carried out after objective refraction or even without that. However, preferably, it should always be carried out after getting a rough estimate of the refractive error by the objective refraction as described above. This practice is not only time saving but more accurate method of testing as well. However, in some instances, where it is impossible to obtain a satisfactory retinoscopy, usually on account of hazy media, the examiner may have to limit himself or herself to subjective testing only. When a cycloplegic has been used, the subjective refraction (post-mydriatic test) should be carried out preferably after 3–4 days (when homatropine or cyclo-pentolate is used) and 14 days (when atropine is used).

The technique of subjective refraction requires patient's cooperation in arriving at the proper estimation of the refractive error. Therefore, it may not be possible in very young children and in patients with lack of comprehension. Therefore, in such cases, the examiner has to prescribe on the basis of objective refraction (e.g. retinoscopy) alone.

Instrumentation for subjective refraction are as below:

- *Phoropter* or the so-called manual refractor (Fig. 36.10) should be the preferred unit.
- *Trial frame and loose lenses from the trial box* (Fig. 36.16), are, however, still the most frequently used in practice.

Steps of subjective refraction include:

A. Monocular subjective refraction,

B. Binocular balancing, and

C. Correction for near vision

A. MONOCULAR SUBJECTIVE REFRACTION

AIMS

Aims of monocular subjective refraction are to find out for each eye separately the:

- Cylindrical lens with exact power and axis, and
- The best vision sphere.

PROCEDURE

Many methods of monocular subjective refraction have been described. The widely accepted protocol, described here, includes following steps:

- I. Selection of baseline starting point lenses
- II. Refining the sphere
- III. Refinement and finalization of cylindrical lens axis and power
- IV. Further refirement and finalization of spherical lens.

I. SELECTION OF BASELINE STARTING POINT LENSES

The patient is seated at a distance of 6 m from the Snellen's vision chart. A trial frame is properly centred and adjusted on the face of the patient and the visual acuity is tested for both the eyes, separately.

Although a totally subjective refraction is possible, it is always better to first estimate the refraction objectively.

Baseline starting point lenses for objective refraction can be obtained from:

1. Retinoscopy, or
2. Autorefractometry, or
3. Evaluation of the patient's old glasses, or
4. From the level of visual accuity: While performing totally subjective refraction, a clue for the baseline starting point can be made from the relationship between the unaided vision and approximate amount of ametropia (Table 36.2).

- *The visual acuity* does not, however, suggest whether the patient is myopic or hyper-

Table 36.2 *Expected vision in various ametropic states*

Vision	Refractive error (D)	
	Spherical*	Astigmatic**
6/6 (20/20)	Small	Small
6/9 (20/30)	0.50	1.00
6/12 (20/40)	0.75	1.50
6/18 (20/60)	1.00	2.00
6/24 (20/80)	1.50	3.00
6/36 (20/120)	2.00	4.00
6/60 (20/200)	2.00–3.00	High

*Myopia or absolute hypermetropia.
**The predicted vision in astigmatism is on the assumption that the circles of least confusion lie on or close to the retina.

metropic. For example, if the patients unaided vision is 6/36, the estimated refractive error can be either around –2 DS or +2 DS.

- *To know whether patient is myopic or hypermetropic,* compare the unaided distance acuity and unaided near acuity. A myopic patient (–2 DS) will have poor distant vision but good near vision while a hypermetropic patient (+2 DS) will have poor vision for distance as well as near. This concept, however, is more useful in presbyopic patients, since otherwise the effect of accommodation confounds the estimation.

II. REFINING SPHERE

In subjective refraction, spherical lenses should be verified first. This technique employs use of trial of different spherical and cylindrical lenses as based on the baseline starting point mentioned above. As with retinoscopy, during subjective refraction, it remains important to fog the fellow eye or, if appropriate, occlude the fellow eye. This not only reduces accommodation in non-cycloplcgic refraction but also ensures that the patient's answers to your subjective refraction questions are based entirely on the eye being examined. In addition, as with retinoscopy, when changing a lens, always put the next lens into the trial frame before taking a lens out, to minimize the accommodation. The *'best vision sphere'*, i.e. the strongest convex lens and the weakest concave lens providing best vision should be chosen in patients with hypermetropia and myopia, respectively.

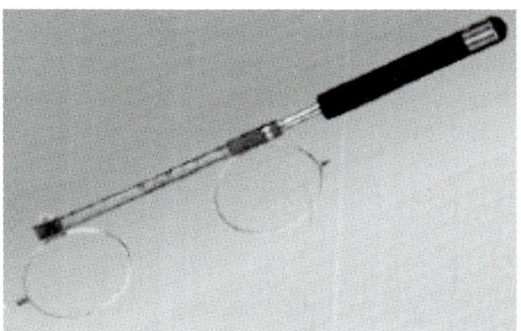

Fig. 36.34: *Weak spherical lenses mounted in a row used for easy manipulation.*

The procedure of finding best vision sphere can be made easy by having a mounted row of weak spheres of power 10.25, 10.5, 20.25 and 20.5 (Fig. 36.34) which can quickly be moved over the front of the trial lenses. There is always a need to advise the myopic patients to choose the lens that makes the letters more clear and note the one which makes the letters smaller and darker.

Note that when the 0.25 sphere is offered, only hold this up for a couple of seconds. If the patient does not make a decision quickly, remove the 0.25 sphere and reoffer them the lens the question. Do not simply hold the lens up waiting for a decision, since the quality of the decision will decrease with time and, in the case of this minus lens, the patient will accommodate. At this stage, do not panic, if the acuity is poor and cannot be improved. It may be that the patient has a large cylinder (a high degree of astigma-

tism). Therefore, move onto refining the cylinder when an end point is reached, rather than persevering only with spheres in the pursuit of perfect acuity.

III. REFINEMENT AND FINALIZATION OF CYLINDRICAL LENS AXIS AND POWER

An accurate determination of the spherical component is predicated on having fully corrected the astigmatic error to ensure that a point focus is obtained with the final correcting cylindrical lens. Therefore, in the presence of astigmatic error, it is mandatory to refine and finalize the cylindrical component before the spherical component.

The cylindrical lens can be finalized by using any one or more of the following techniques:
• Astigmatic clock dial and fogging technique
• Jackson's cross-cylinder technique
• Astigmatic fan and block technique.

1. Astigmatic clock dial and fogging technique

Steps of astigmatic clock dial and fogging technique are:
i. Obtain best visual acuity using sphere only in one eye, with other being occluded.
ii. Fog the eye (make artificially myopic) to about 20/50 by putting enough plus sphere before the eye to focus all meridians anterior to the retina, i.e. to bring forward compound, simple or mixed hyperopic meridians and thus create a state of compound myopic astigmatism (Fig. 36.35).

+ Spherical lens

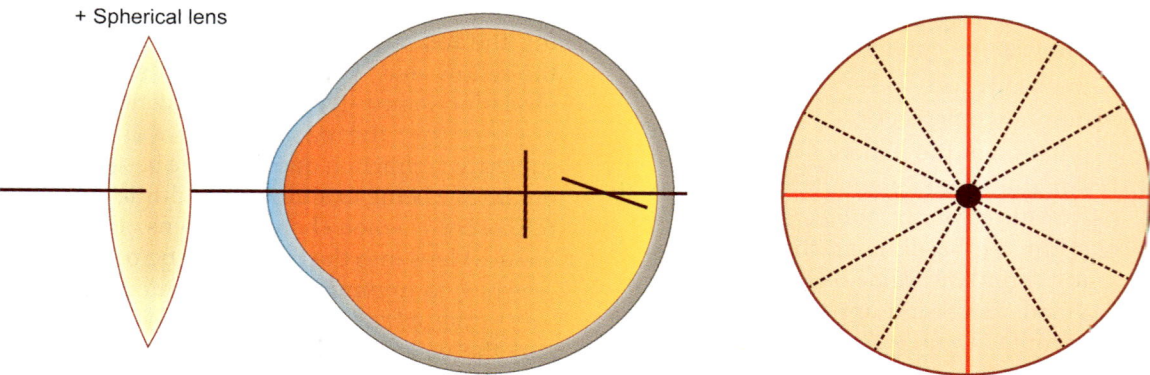

Fig. 36.35: *Fogging by plus spherical lens to create compound myopic astigmatism.*

With the eye fogged, accommodation can only blur the lines more, and the patient, therefore, tends to relax accommodation, thus stabilizing the refractive error of the eye.

iii. The patient is asked to look at the astigmatic dial and identify the 'darkest and sharpest' line. Let us suppose it is 3–9 o'clock line, i.e. 180° axis line (Fig. 36.36).

iv. Add minus cylinder of progressively increasing power with axis perpendicular to the blackest and sharpest line (i.e. at 90° as per above example) till all lines appear equal. A rotatable cross dial (Fig. 36.37) is often used for this step, aligned with principal meridian, for easy comparison of the two meridians. The 'rule of 30s' may be used to calculate the axis of the minus cylinder; i.e. multiply the lower number of the astigmatic dial clock with 30 to find the axis. If in the above example blackest line was that in 3–9 o'clock position, then the axis of minus cylinder was $3 \times 30 = 90°$. Similarly, if the darkest line seen is in 6–12 o'clock position, the axis of minus cylinder will be $6 \times 30 = 180°$. If the axis of darkest line falls between hours on the clock, multiply by lowest member plus half, i.e. between 1 and 2 o'clock = $1.5 \times 30° = 45°$.

As shown in Fig. 36.38, by adding minus cylinders the vertical focal line has been moved back to the position of the horizontal focal line. Thus, as the interval of Sturm is collapsed, the focal lines disappear into a point focus.

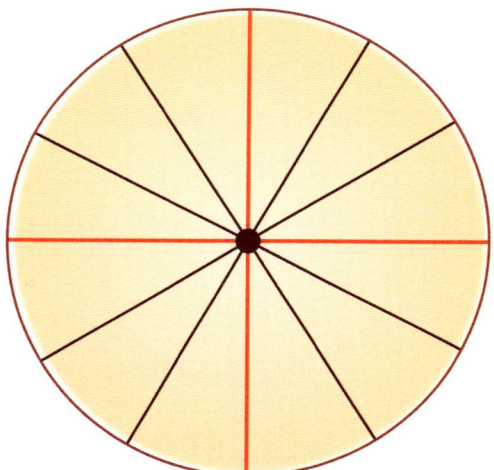

Fig. 36.36: *Clock dial as seen by 'fogged' patient with astigmatic error, 3–9 axis appears darker.*

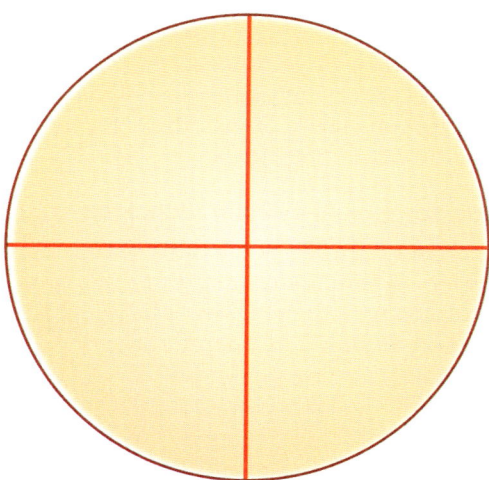

Fig. 36.37: *Two-line rotating dial is set at 3–9 position. Axis of correcting minus cylinder is 90° (3 × 30).*

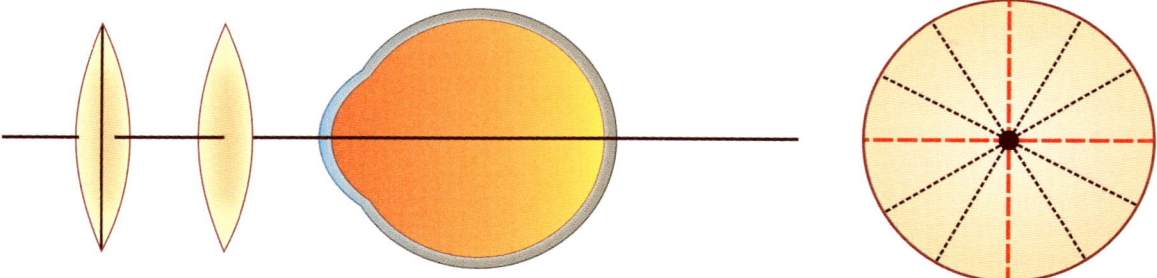

Fig. 36.38: *The vertical focal line has been moved back to the position of the horizontal focal line and collapsed to a point by adding a minus cylinder with axis at 90°.*

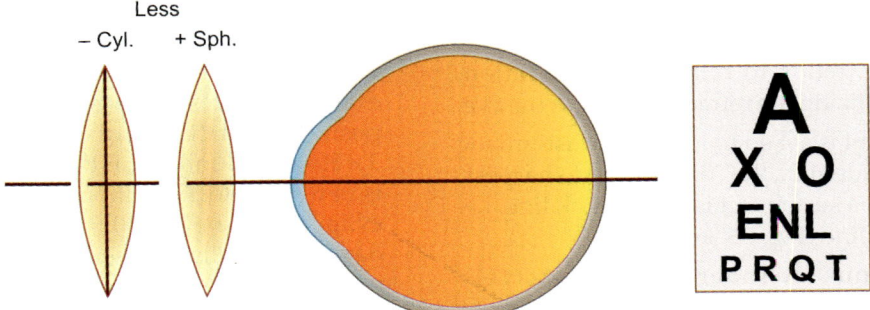

Less
– Cyl. + Sph.

A
X O
ENL
PRQT

Fig. 36.39: *Focus is on the retina after defogging*

v. Now all the lines of the astigmatic dial appear equally black (since astigmatism has been neutralized), but still are not in perfect focus (blurred), for eye is still fogged. At this juncture, switch to a distance-vision chart and reduce plus spheres (and add minus spheres, if required) until the patient achieves maximum clarity of vision; i.e. focus is now on the retina (Fig. 36.39).

2. Jackson's cross-cylinder technique

The cross-cylinder is a combination of two cylinders of equal strength, but with opposite sign placed with their axis at right angles to each other and mounted in a handle (Fig. 36.40). The commonly used cross-cylinders are of ± 0.25 and ± 0.5 D. The Jackson cross-cylinder, in Edward Jackson's words, is probably 'far more useful and, far more used' than any other lens in clinical refraction. Every ophthalmologist should be familiar with the principles involved in its use. Although the cross-cylinder is usually used to refine the cylinder axis and power of a refraction already obtained, it may also be used for the entire astigmatic refraction.

Steps of cross-cylinder refraction are as below:

- *Adjust sphere to the most plus or least minus* that gives best visual acuity. This is done by fogging the eye (adding plus sphere before the eye), while viewing a visual acuity chart, and then decreasing the fog until best visual acuity is obtained. The goal, if astigmatism is present, is to place the circle of least diffusion of the conoid of Sturm on the retina, thus creating mixed astigmatism.

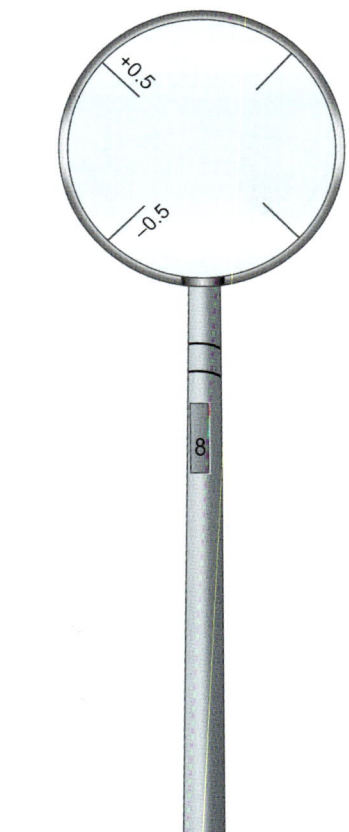

Fig. 36.40: *Jackson's cross-cylinder*

- *Baseline cylindrical lens*, discovered on retinoscopy and/or autorefractrometry, is then placed in the trial frame at the axis discovered. Refinement of the axis and then of the power of the cylindrical lens is done with Jacleson cross-cylinder.

- *Refinement of the axis* is always done first. This is because the correct axis can be found in the presence of an incorrect power, but the full cylinder power will not be found in the presence of an incorrect axis. To refine the axis, cross-cylinder (±0.5 D) is placed before the eye with its handle parallel (along the same line) to the axis of cylindrical axis in the trial frame, i.e. with its axis at 45° to the axis of cylinder in trial frame (first with +0.5 D cylinder in Fig. 36.41 and then −0.5 D cylinder or vice versa in Fig. 36.41) and the patient is asked to tell about any change in the visual acuity. If the patient notices no difference between the two positions, the axis of the correcting cylinder in the trial frame is correct. However,

if the visual improvement is attained in one of the positions, a 'plus' correcting cylinder should be rotated in the direction of the plus cylindrical components of the cross-cylinder (and vice versa). The test is then repeated several times until the neutral point is reached.

- *Refinement of cylinder power.* To check the power of the cylinder, the cross-cylinder of ± 0.25 D is placed, with its axis parallel to the axis of the cylinder in the trial frame, first with the same sign in Fig. 36.42 and then with opposite sign in Fig. 36.42. In the first position, the cylindrical correction is enhanced by 0.25 D and in the second it is diminished by the same amount. When the visual acuity does not improve in either of the positions,

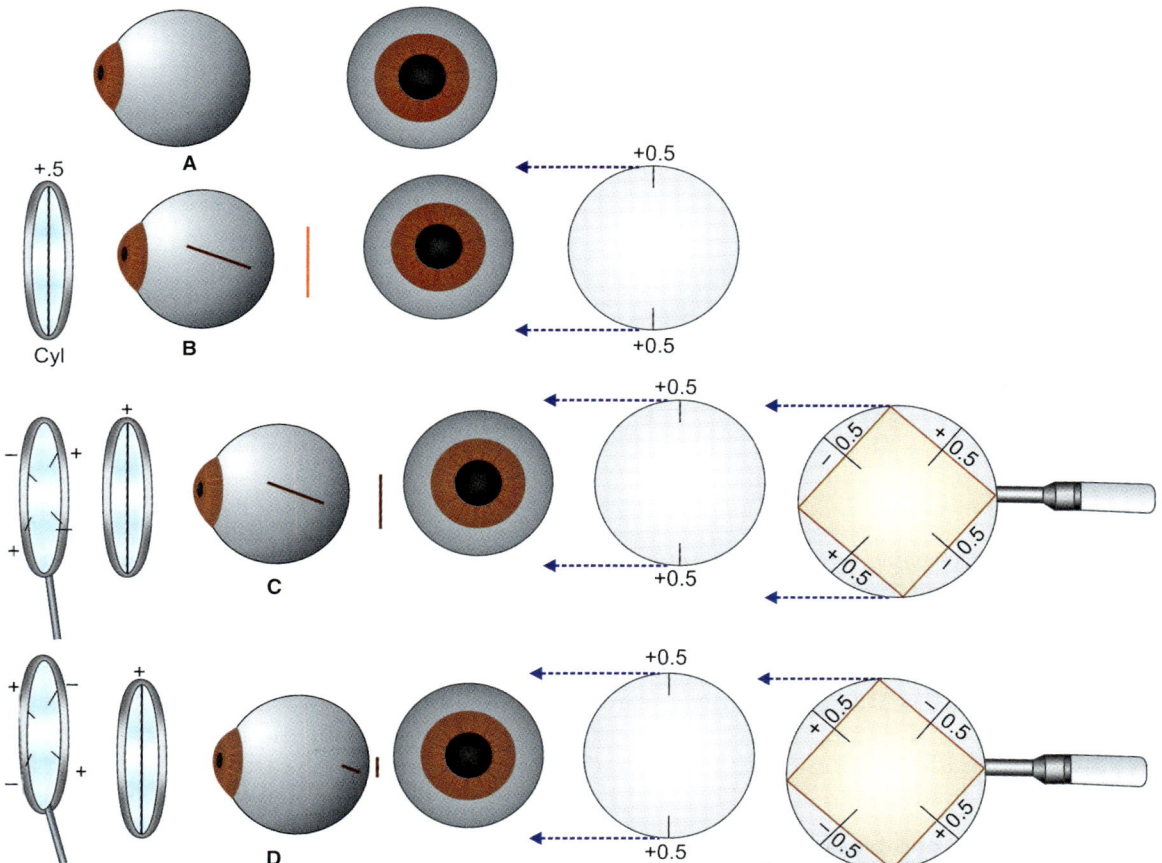

Fig. 36.41: *Use of Jackson's cross-cylinder (JCC) to refine the axis of astigmatism: (A) side and front view of patient's eye; (B) correcting cylindrical lens (say +0.5 DC at 90°) is placed in front of the patient's eye; (C) JCC is placed with −0.5 DC at 45° to the axis of correcting cylindrical lens; and (D) JCC is placed with +0.5 DC at 45° to the axis of correcting cylindrical lens.*

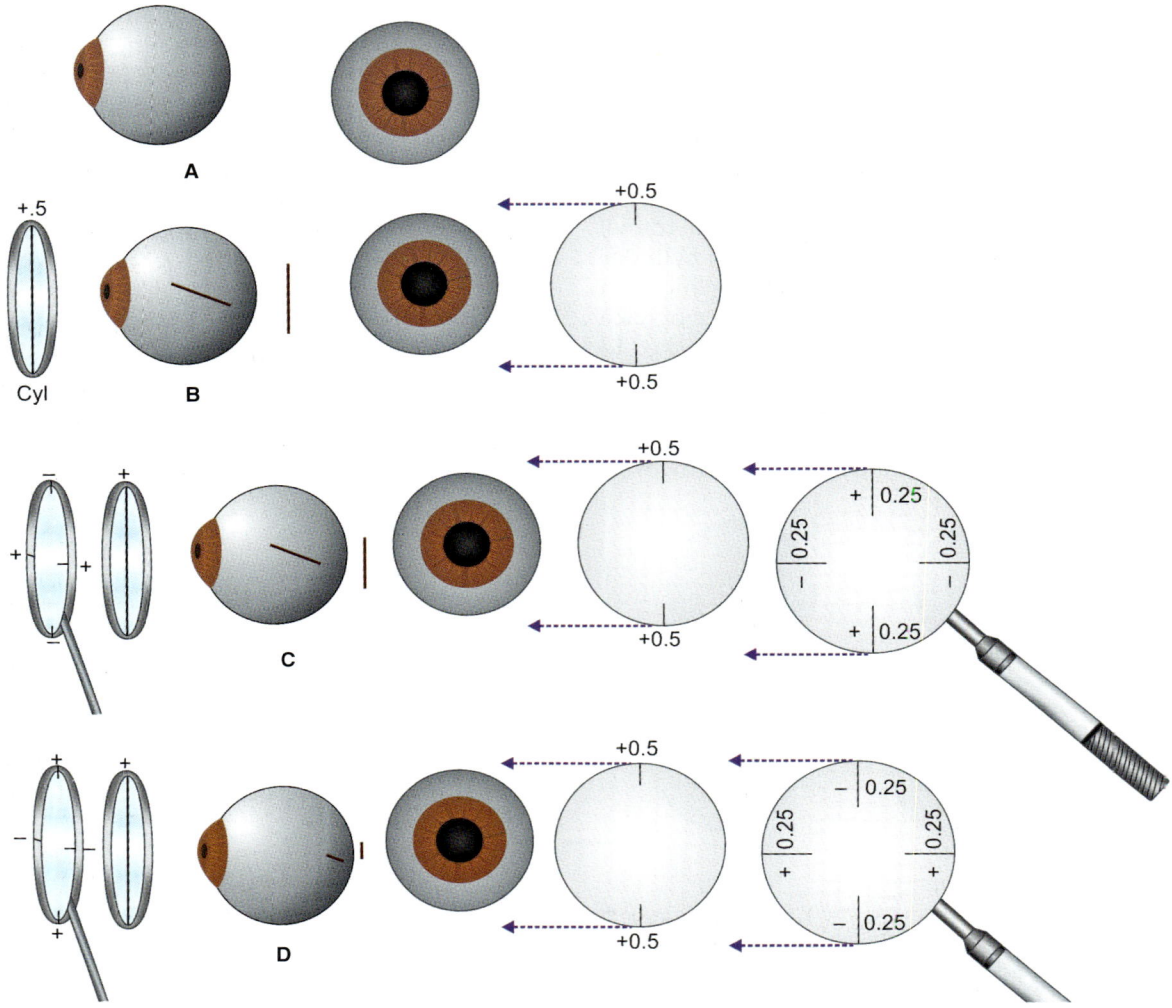

Fig. 36.42: *Use of Jacks's cross-cylinder (JCC) to refine power of the astigmatic cylinder: (A) side and front view of patient's eye; (B) correcting cylindrical lens (say +0.5 DC) at 90° is placed infront of patient's eye; (C) JCC of 0.25 DC is placed with axis parallel to the axis of correcting lens; (D) JCC of –0.25 DC is placed with axis parallel to the correcting cylindrical axis.*

the power of cylinder in trial frame is correct. However, if the visual acuity improves in any of the positions, a corresponding correction should be made and reverified till final correction is attained.

3. Astigmatic fan and block technique

It is not always easy for the patients to respond satisfactorily with cross-cylinder testing. Therefore, it is useful to employ the older technique of fan and block method, or the so-called Maddox V test.

The fan and block consists of a series of radiating lines spaced at 10° interval and arranged after the manner of the rays of a rising sun around a central panel carrying a V and two sets of mutually perpendicular lines (the blocks) (Fig. 36.43). The V and the block simultaneously can be rotated through 180°.

Steps of the fan and block technique are as follows:

1. *Obtain the best visual acuity using sphere only (best vision sphere).* It is assumed that the best

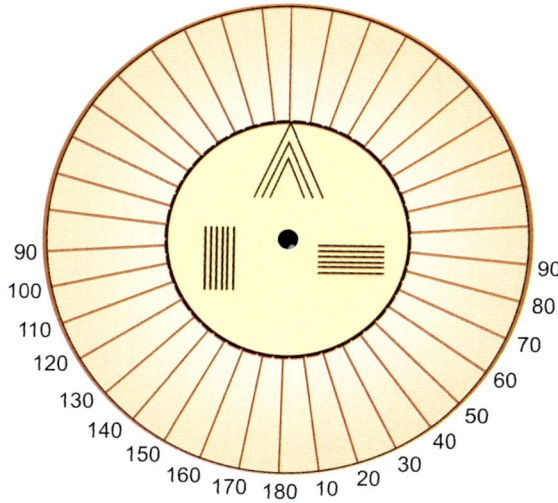

Fig. 36.43: *Fan and block dial (Maddox V test).*

vision sphere puts the circle of least diffusion on the retina.

2. *Add a positive sphere* equal to half of the estimated amount of astigmatism in order to bring the eye into a state of simple myopic astigmatism.

3. *Refer the patient to the fan chart and ask which line or group of lines appear clearest and darkest.* This gives the approximate direction of the astigmatic error. However, a simple check test should be made by temporarily adding an extra −0.50 DS in order to confirm that the eye is in a state of simple myopic astigmatism. The blackest lines should blur, but if not, more positive sphere should be added until they do. (In some cases, the clearest lines will change through 90°, indicating that the eye had been in a state of simple hypermetropic astigmatism, with the anterior focal line near the retina. In this case, continue adding positive sphere until this new set of lines just begins to blur.)

4. *Direct the attention to the Maddox arrow* and rotate it away from its blacker limb until both limbs appear equally blurred. This gives the axis of the astigmatism, but care must be taken to ensure that the patient's head is upright.

5. *Directing attention now to the blocks, add negative cylinder* at the appropriate axis until the second becomes as clear as the first. If this is not quite

possible, it is better to just undercorrect than overcorrect the astigmatic error, that is, leaving the first group of lines, the clearer or blacker of the two.

6. *Make a second check test by again adding −0.50 DS*, or, if the patient is a critical observer, −0.25 DS. Both blocks should blur equally, but if the blackest lines change over, the astigmatism has been overcorrected. If the originally darker block again becomes blacker, the original sphere from step 3 was wrong and must be rechecked. Return to the letter chart and determine the sphere giving best acuity, the cylindrical element remaining as just determined. As usual a positive lens should be tried first, but a weak minus lens will most frequently be required.

If in step 3 no lines appear blacker than the other, there may be no astigmatism present, but other possibilities are that the eye is excessively fogged, has the circles of least diffusion on the retina or is in a state of compound hypermetropic astigmatism. The −0.50 DS check test will show up either of these last two conditions, by making some lines darker. On the other hand, if the eye is already fogged, extra positive power will blur the lines even more, whereas the addition of minus power will make some lines blacker in the presence of astigmatism, or all equally black, if there is no astigmatism.

IV. FURTHER REFINEMENT AND FINALIZATION OF THE SPHERICAL LENS

After the cylinder power and axis have been refined, the final step in monocular refraction is refining of the sphere which can be done by fogging technique using Snellen's visual acuity chart and can be verified by duochrome test and pinhole test.

1. Finalizing sphere with fogging technique using Snellen's visual acuity chart

A simple criterion for initially establishing the end point for the spherical correction is to fog the eye after the cylindrical correction has been finalized and then unfog by reducing every time −0.25 DS till the best Snellen's visual acuity is attained. Some doubt, however, may exist at the very end point because the steps from one line of acuity to the next are rather large, particularly in the smaller letters. Thus, one lens may result in 6/6 acuity, and unfogging another 0.25 D may still only record 6/6 because the vision is unable to reach the 6/5 line. It may not be possible to determine by the Snellen's chart which lens truly represents *best acuity*, and the examiner may face the quandary of either slightly fogging the eye with one choice or undercorrecting with the other. At this juncture, attempts to verify the best endpoint or ultimate correction point of the spherical component can be made by duochrome test.

2. Duochrome test

It is based on the principle of chromatic aberration. It has been found that in emmetropes yellow light (570 nm) is focused on the retina, while red (620 nm) and green light (535 nm) are focused 0.24 D behind and 0.20 D in front of the retina, respectively (Fig. 36.44). In duochrome test, the patient is asked to read the letters graded from 6/18 to 6/5 with red and green background (Fig. 36.45). As in an emmetropic eye, the green rays are focused slightly anterior and red rays slightly posterior to the retina. Therefore, to an emmetropic patient, letters of both colours look equally sharp. When the patient tells that he or she sees red letters more clear than the green, it indicates that one is slightly myopic. His or her spherical lenses should be adjusted such that one sees letters of both colours with equal clarity.

Note that, although the duochrome test is easily and rapidly performed, it has the inherent weakness that it does not relax accommodation. This test should always be introduced, therefore,

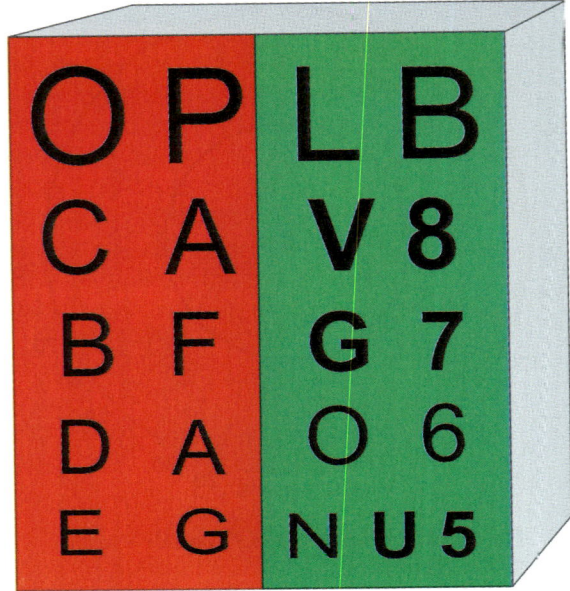

Fig. 36.45: *Duochrome test box consisting of Snellen's 6/18 to 6/5 visual acuity letters with red and green background.*

with the patient slightly fogged. The letters on the red side should appear clearer and minus sphere should be added until the letters with red and green background are equally clear.

The duochrome test is not much useful with visual acuities worse than 6/9 (20/30), for the 0.5D difference between the two sides becomes difficult to distinguish.

3. Pinhole testing

A pinhole test at this juncture helps in confirming whether the optical correction in the trial frame is correct or not. An improvement in visual acuity while looking through a pinhole (Fig. 36.46) indicates that optical correction in the trial frame is incorrect.

SPECTACLE PRESCRIPTION: NOTATION AND TRANSPOSITION

NOTATION

After subjective refraction the writing of spectacle prescription is known as notation:

Types of notation. The spectacle/contact lens prescription can be written in any of the two

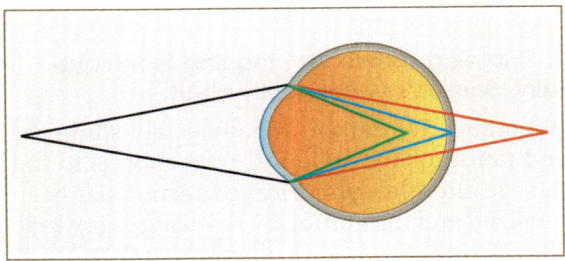

Fig. 36.44: *Optical principle of duochrome test (for explanation see text).*

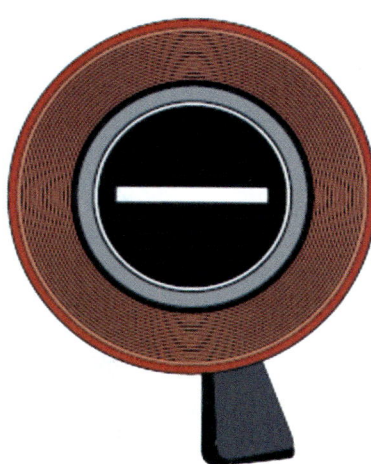

Fig. 36.46: *Pinhole.*

equivalent notations in which any single refractive error can be corrected. These notations are:

- *Plus cylinder notation*, e.g. –2 DS/+ 1 DC 180°
- *Minus cylinder notation* of the above prescription will be: –1 DS/– 1 DC 90°

Note

- Both plus and minus cylinder notations are acceptable, so either may be used and is correct.
- However, always ensure that for any single patient both eyes are prescribed in the same cylinder notation, i.e. both eyes in either plus or minus cylinder notation.

TRANSPOSITION OF NOTATION

To obtain equivalent notation, one form has to be transposed to the other form, i.e. plus cylinder notation can be changed to minus cylinder notation or vice versa.

Steps of transposition. Transposition involves three steps:

- *Add the cylinder to sphere* to give new sphere
- *Change the sign of cylinder* to give new cylinder power
- *New axis of cylinder* is perpendicular to the old axis.

Examples of transposition are given below:

Example 1: Transposition of plus cylinder notation will be as below:

Plus cylinder notation: –2 DS/+1 DC 180°
- New sphere = –2+1 = –1 DS
- *New cylinder = –1 DC*
- *Axis of cylinder = 90°*

Minus cylinder notation, so, will be: –1 DS/–1 DC 90°.

Example 2: Plus cylinder notation: + 1 DS + 1 DC 180°
- *New sphere:* +1+1 = +2 DS
- *New cylinder:* –1 DC
- *Axis of new cylinder = –1 DC 90°*

Minus cylinder notation, so, will be: +2 DS/– 1 DC 90°.

Example 3: Minus cylinder notation : +2 DS/–1 DC 180°
- *New sphere*: (–2) + (–1) = –3 DS
- *New cylinder = +1 DC*
- *Axis of new cylinder = +1 DC 90°*
- *Plus cylinder notation,* so, will be: –3 DS/+ 1 DC 90°.

Example 4: Minus cylinder notation: +2 DS/ –1 DC 180°
- *New sphere* : (+2) + (–1) = +1 DS
- *New cylinder* : + 1 DC
- *Axis of new eye* : +1 DC 90°
- *Plus cylinder notation,* so, will be: +1 DS/+1 DC 90°.

Example 5: Minus cylinder notation: +2DS/–4DC 180°
- *New sphere:* (+2) + (–4) = –2 DS
- *New cylinder:* + 4 DC
- *Axis of new cylinder:* +4 DC 90°
- *Plus cylinder notation,* so, will be: –2 DS/+4 DC 90°.

B. BINOCULAR BALANCING

The final step in the subjective refraction is 'binocular balancing'—a process sometimes known as 'equalizing the accommodative effort' or 'equalization of vision'. This allows both eyes to have the retinal image simultaneously in focus. An imbalanced correction often leads to asthenopia because of unstable accommodation. Several methods have been described for binocular balancing. Most of the methods require that correctable visual acuity be essentially equal in the two eyes. A few commonly used methods are described here.

1. FOGGING AND ALTERNATE OCCLUSION METHOD

With the best accepted lenses in trial frame, both eyes are fogged with +1.0 DS, reducing the vision. Then a rapid alternate cover test is performed and the patient is asked to tell about the eye showing comparatively clearer image. If the eyes are in balance, the patient will report equal blur in both eyes. If the eyes are not in balance, +0.25 D sphere should be added to the better seeing eye until balance is achieved and both eyes are equally blurred. Now slowly defog both eyes simultaneously until patient can read the 6/6 line.

2. DUOCHROME TEST WITH FOGGING

With the best correcting lenses in trial frame, each eye observes the vision chart in turn while its fellow eye is fogged with a +1.0 DS. The sphere before the observing eye is then adjusted to give equally red preference or green preference as felt appropriate by the refractionist.

3. PRISM DISSOCIATION METHOD

With the best correcting lenses in trial frame, both eyes are fogged with +1.0 DS and a vertical prism of 3 or 4 D is placed with base down in front of right eye and base up in front of left eye. Then a single line, usually 6/12, is projected on the chart. The patient will be able to see the same line with both eyes simultaneously. If the patient reports difference in the clarity between the upper and lower lines, seen as two separate images, then, +0.25 sphere is placed before the eye with better vision. This is done until the two lines are equally distinct for the two eyes. Having established a balance between the two eyes, the prism is removed and the fog is then reduced binocularly until maximum vision is reached with the highest plus or lowest minus spheres.

It is considered the most sensitive method of binocular balance and so is practised more commonly.

4. TURVILLE INFINITY BALANCE TECHNIQUE

A set of letters is seen with a septum in the middle which masks some letters from each eye. If all the letters are seen clearly and equally, this implies a binocular balance.

5. POLAROID FILTERS

With a set of letters visible to one eye and the other set through the other eye also help in binocular balancing.

C. CORRECTION FOR NEAR VISION

Correction for near vision is indicated usually after the age of 40 years. When the distance vision has been satisfactorily corrected, the visual acuity at working distance of the patient should be estimated using any of the near-vision charts (Jaeger's chart, Snellen's reading test types or number points types standardized by the faculty of ophthalmologists N5 to N48). In case near vision is defective, further testing should proceed as follows:

1. The determination of near point of accommodation and amplitude of accommodation

The near point should always be determined with the distance correction in place. Determination of amplitude of accommodation is essential for presbyopic corrections. For details of assessment of accommodation *see* page 396.

Average accommodative amplitudes for different ages are summarized in Table 36.3. In general, it must be remembered that:

- From the age of 8 years onwards the accommodation decreases by 1 D for every 4 years till the age of 40 years.
- From 40–48 years of age, accommodation decreases by 1.5 D for every 4 years.
- From age 48 years onwards, the accommodation decreases by 0.5 D for every 4 years.

2. The determination of near point of convergence

While correcting near vision, the assessment of convergence is essential and needs consideration. For details *see* page 395.

3. Dynamic retinoscopy

The dynamic retinoscopy (*see* page 714) provides an objective basis for the optical condition when

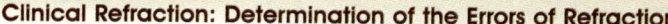

Table 36.3 *Average accommodation amplitude for different ages*	
Age (years)	**Average accommodative amplitude (D)**
8	14 ±2
12	13 ±2
16	12 ±2
20	11 ±2
24	10 ±2
28	9 ±2
32	8 ±2
36	7 ±2
40	6 ±2
44	4.5 ±1.5
48	3.0 ±1.5
52	2.5 ±1.5
56	2.0 ±1.0
60	1.5 ±1.0
64	1.0 ±0.5
68	0.5 ±0.5

the eye is focused for near vision. In other words, it is an attempt to give an objective accuracy to measurement of accommodation. However, in practice, this matter has been left entirely to subjective testing.

4. Determination of near add

A suitable convex lens addition should be made over the distant correction. The presbyopic spectacles should never be prescribed mechanically by ordering an approximate addition, varying with the age of the patient. Each patient should be tested individually (and each eye separately), for the individual, variation is large. The near adds ordered should give the most serviceable and comfortable (not necessarily the clearest) vision for the particular work for which the lenses are intended.

Rule of thumb, that has gained wide acceptance, is that the near add at a given distance should allow half of the patient's accommodative amplitude to remain in reserve.

DETERMINATION OF THE MUSCLE BALANCE

Before the final prescription is given, it is always desirable to test for the oculomotor balance, both for distant vision and near vision, with and without the correction in front of the eyes.

For details of the work-up of a patient for oculomotor balance, the readers are referred to the manuscript on 'Squint and Orthoptics'. However, it must be emphasized that before dispensing, one must ascertain for the presence of:

- Any manifest deviation
- Heterophoria, type and degree
- Convergence insufficiency
- Fusional reserves

The oculomotor imbalance, when discovered, should be given a due attention, since it can be a potent cause of the symptoms of eye strain.

MODIFICATIONS IN THE PRESCRIPTION

Modifications in the prescription which may sometimes be required to take care of the associated oculomotor imbalance are as follows:

1. *A full cycloplegic correction,* without making any tonus allowance for the cycloplegic used, should be given in children having refractive error with associated manifest deviation.

2. *An undercorrection of hypermetropic* error is recommended to reduce the degree of consecutive exotropia. However, this should not be at the cost of asthenopic symptoms.

3. *A slight overcorrection of myopia* may sometimes help in controlling the intermittent exotropia.

4. *An overcorrection by +1 to +3 D* of the amblyopic eye has been advocated by some workers as penalization treatment.

5. *Bifocal glasses* are quite useful in controlling deviation of patients having non-refractive accommodative esotropia.

6. *In exophoria,* both eyes may be undercorrected by an equal amount of spherical plus power. This forces the patient to accommodate constantly and accordingly induces accommodative convergence. However, it should be kept in mind that constant accommodation itself may lead to eye strain.

7. *In esophoria,* the patient should receive as much spherical plus correction as is compatible with his or her best visual acuity. Bifocal glasses decrease or eliminate the need for accommodation during near vision and thus may be

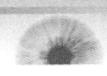

useful in patients having esophoria of convergence excess type. Bifocals should be used as a temporary aid to orthoptic treatment aiming to reduce the focal segment as soon as possible.

8. In hyperphoria, if feasible, the lenses of the patient's optical correction may be decentred to achieve a prismatic effect, thus relieving the stress on patient's vertical vergence control.

9. In cyclophoria, best possible efforts should be made to discover and correct the associated astigmatic refractive error.

10. Prisms may need to be incorporated in glasses sometimes in the presence of phorias as below:

• *Role of prisms as a permanent correction in horizontal phorias is debatable.* They should be considered only after other measures have failed to relieve the symptoms. For exophoria base-in prisms and for esophoria base-out prisms are incorporated into the glasses.

• *Prisms are quite useful as a permanent correction in the treatment of comitant vertical phorias.* A vertical prismatic correction of 10 D is the maximum amount that can be tolerated. There is no fixed rule as to the amount of prism correction to be given in a particular patient. However, in practice, prisms are prescribed with apex towards the phoria to correct only half or at the most two-thirds of total heterophoria.

SUMMARY OF CLINICAL REFRACTION

The technique of determination of errors of refraction described in this chapter may give the impression that, perhaps, clinical refraction is a cumbersome and lengthy procedure. On the contrary, it is not so. In fact, the technique takes longer to describe than to perform. However, it does emphasize that the refractionist must be fully aware of the theory as well as art of performing refraction.

Steps of clinical refraction

Steps of clinical refraction can be summarized as follows:

1. *History* of visual symptoms complained of by the patient should be elicited quickly and meticulously.

2. *Visual acuity* should be tested, uniocularly and binocularly, both with and without any correction, for distance as well as near.

3. *External examination*, preferably with a slit-lamp, should be carried out, especially to rule out diseases of cornea and lens.

4. *Ophthalmoscopic examination* should be carried out to rule out opacities in the media and diseases of fundus responsible for low vision.

5. *Cover tests* to detect latent and manifest deviations may best be done at this stage, before the trial frames are put on. A manifest deviation may account for marked loss of vision in that eye.

6. *Retinoscopy*, and its verification with the spherocylindrical combination, provides the best objective refraction. Alternatively, *autorefractometry* observations may be used as objective refraction.

7. *Subjective refinement of sphere* should be carried out first.

8. *Subjective refinement and finalization of cylindrical lens* axis first and then power should be carried out using either astigmatic dial clock fogging technique or cross-cylinder, or astigmatic fan and block method. Most practical and thus common approach is use of Jackson's cross cylinder.

9. *Further subjective refinement and finalization of sphere* should then be done using fogging technique, duochrome test, and pinhole test.

10. *Equalization of vision (binocular balancing)* should always be carried out to avoid asthenopic symptoms due to unstable accommodation. Prism dissociation method of binocular balancing is perhaps the most sensitive one.

11. *Near vision correction* should be carried out in patients with presbyopia. It should always be verified by evaluating the range.

12. *Muscle balance* should be tested with full correction both for distance and near vision. Adjustment in trial frame correction, if required, may be made accordingly.

BIBLIOGRAPHY

1. Allen RJ, Fletcher R, Still DC (Eds). Eye Examination and Refraction. Blackwell Scientific Publications, Oxford: 93.

2. Benett Jeffrey R, et al. Comparison of refractive assessment by wavefront aberrometry, auto-refraction, and subjective refraction. Journal of Optometry 2015; pp. 109–15.

3. Benjamin William J. Borish's Clinical Refraction. St Louis: Elsevier Health Sciences, 2007. ISBN 13:978-0-7506-7524-6.

4. Bennett AG. An historical review of optometric principles and techniques. Ophthalmic and Physiological Optics 1986;6:3–21.

5. Choong YF, Chen AH, Goh PP. A comparison of autorefraction and subjective refraction with and without cycloplegia in primary school children. Am J Ophthalmol. 2006 Jul;142(1): 68–74.

6. Freeman H. Working method–subjective refraction. British Journal of Physiological Optics 1955;12:20–30.

7. Jennings JAM, Charman WN. A comparison of errors in some methods of subjective refraction. Ophthalmic Optics 1973;13:8.

8. Jorge J, Queiros A, Almeida JB, Parafita MA. "Retinoscopy/autorefraction: which is the best starting point for a noncycloplegic refraction?" Optom Vis Sci. 2005 Jan;82(1):64–8.

9. Khurana AK. Determination of the errors of refraction. Theory and Practice of Optic and Refraction. Elsevier India, 2013.

10. Michaels DD. Visual Optics and Refraction: A Clinical Approach (2nd ed). Missouri: CV Mosby Company. 1980; p379–83.

Index

Aberrations 213
   Ray aberrations 214
   wave aberrations 214
   Zernick's terms 214
   Zernike's polynomials 214
Aberrometry and wavefront technology 213
Abnormal head posture 439
   examination for 398
Absolute exophthalmometry 497
AC/A ratio, assessment of 397
Accommodation, assessment of 396
Acquired myogenic ptosis 475
Active force generation test 452
Air-puff tonometer 240
Allen Thorpe gonioprism 249
Amblyopia, evaluation for 415
   neutral density filter test 416
AmbP iNet Program 430
Ancillary tests in uveitis 352
Anomaloscopes 49
Anterior segment optical coherence tomo-
      graphy 154, 302
Aponeurotic ptosis 474
Applanation tonometry 237
Assessment of ocular movements 391
   ductions 391
   vergences 393
   versions 392
Automated keratometer 186
Automated perimetry 310
Autorefractometry 717
   optical principles of 717
     Scheiner principle 717
   optometer principle 718

Bagolini's striated glass test 414
Barrett universal II formula 539
Bausch and Lomb keratometer 181
Bell's phenomenon 470
Berke's method 469
Bielschowsky three-step test 443
Bielschowsky's after image test 410

Bielschowsky's head tilt test 404
Bielschowsky's phenomenon Test 404
Binocular balancing 731
Binocular indirect ophthalmoscopy 72
Biometric gonioscopy 257
Biometry 531
Blink reflex test 33
Bruckner pupillary red reflex test 382
Brückner's red reflex test 36, 382

C scan ultrasound 637
Campimetry 307
Catford drum test 37
Cheiroscope 426
Clinical approach to uveitis 329
Clinical methods in ophthalmology 1
Clinical refraction 701
   binocular balancing 731
   monocular 723
   objective 701
   subjective 722
Colour doppler imaging 628
Colour vision, tests for 48
   anomaloscopes 49
   Ishihara test 48
   lantern tests 50
Comparative exophthalmometry 497
Computed tomography scanning in ophthalmo-
      logy 656
   in intraocular lesions 663
   in intraorbital lesions 667
   measurement of proptosis 663
   normal orbital anatomy 661
Computed tomography 108, 121
Computer vergence system (CVS) 429
Computer-based orthoptic programs and instru-
      ments 428
   neurovision therapy programs 431
     neurovision rehabilitator 432
     revital vision 431
   optodrum 428
   vision therapy programs 429

Confocal microscopy 152, 167
Confocal scanning laser ophthalmoscopy 90, 284
Confoscan 169
Congenital ptosis 471
Contrast enhanced ultrasonography 636
Contrast sensitivity 45, 118
Convergence spasm 126
Corneal aesthesiometry 157
Corneal biopsy 160
Corneal hysteresis 177
Corneal sensations 14, 140
Corneal topography 152
Corneal vascularization 14
Corneal wavefront map 216
Correction for near vision 732
CT angiography 675
CT venography 676
Cup–disc ratio 266

4**D** base-out prism test 412
Dacryocystography 485
Diatom transpalpebral tonometer 242
Digital subtraction-dacryocystography 485
Diplopia charting 398
Diplopia test 407
Diplopia test or red glass test 414
Diploscope 424
Direct gonioscopy 248
Direct ophthalmoscopy 66
Disc damage likelihood score 266
Distant direct ophthalmoscopy 66
Double prism test 390
Ductions, assessment of 391
Dynamic IOL optimization 547

Electronystagmography 460
Electrooculogram 594
Electrooculography 460
Electrophysiological tests in ophthalmology 590
    electrooculogram 594
    electroretinogram 591
    visual evoked potential 595
Electroretinogram 591
Enophthalmos 511
    nontraumatic 512
    traumatic 512
Epiphora 482
Euthyscope 423

Evaluation for ocular deviation 380
    Bruckner pupillary red reflex test 382
    double prism test 390
    haploscopic tests 391
    Hirschberg corneal reflex test 382
    Maddox rod test 386
    Maddox wing test 388
    prism and alternate cover test 382
    prism reflex test 385
    simultaneous prism cover test 386
Evaluation of a case of strabismus 378
    history and preliminary examination 378
    motor evaluation 380
    sensory evaluation 405
Exaggerated traction test 452
Exophthalmometers 497
    Hertel's 497
    Luedde's 497
    Mutch 498
Exophthalmometry 497
    absolute 497
    comparative 497
    FASTPAC 312
    postural 497
    relative 497

Field of binocular fixation 404
Fixation behavior, test for 406
Flicker-defined form perimetry 325
Fluorescein dye disappearance test 483
Fluorescein staining 15
Forced duction test 129
Frequency doubling perimetry 324
Friedenwald nomogram 245
    full threshold testing 312
Functional MRI 694
Fundus autofluorescence 569
Fundus camera 83
Fundus fluorescein angiography 553

Gaze palsies 124
GDx VCC nerve fiber layer analyser 99
Genetic testing in glaucoma 231
Glaucoma hemifield test 317
Goldmann applanation tonometer 238
Goldmann single-mirror gonioprism 249
Goldmann three-mirror gonioprism 248
Goldmann two-mirror gonioprism 249

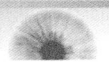
Gonioprisms 248
  Allen Thorpe 249
  Goldmann single-mirror 249
  Goldmann three-mirror 248
  Goldmann two-mirror 249
  Posner 250
  Sussman lens 250
  Tokel 250
  Zeiss four-mirror 250
Gonioscopy 26, 230, 246
  direct 248
  indirect 248
  manipulative 252
Grading of angle of anterior chamber
  modified gonioscopic grading 256
  RP centre gonioscopic grading 256
  Scheie's grading 255
  Shaffer's grading 255

Hand-held slit-lamp 63
Haploscopic tests 391, 399
  Hess screen test 400
  Lancaster red-green test 399
  Lees screen test 402
Hartmann-Shack aberrometry 217
Heidelberg retina tomography 90
Heidelberg retinal tomograph 3 169
Helmholtz keratometer 180
Hertel's exophthalmometer 497
Hess screen test 400
High pass resolution perimetry 325
Hill–RBF formula 539
Hirschberg corneal reflex test 382
Hoffer H-5 Formula 539
Hoffer's Q formula 538
Holladay I formula 538
Holladay II formula 538
Hruby lens biomicroscopy 78
HTS iNet/computer vergence system (CVS) 432
Hyperacuity 31
Hyperlacrimation 481

Icare or rebound tonometer 242
IDEM lenses 530
Illif's test 469
Incomitant squint 435
Indentation tonometry 234
  Schiötz tonometer 235
Indirect fundus biomicroscopy 80

Indirect gonioscopy 248
Indocyanine green angiography 564
Intermittent proptosis 491
Internuclear ophthalmoplegia 124
Intraoperative, real-time wavefront guided aberro-
  metry 221
Investigations in uvzeitis 339
  ancillary tests 352
  haematological 340
  nuclear medicine study 352
  pathological diagnostic tests 365
  radiological tests 350
  skin tests 349
IOL master 533
IOL power, formulae for 535
  Barrett universal II formula 539
  Hill–RBF formula 539
  Hoffer H-5 formula 539
  Hoffer's Q formula 538
  Holladay I formula 538
  Holladay II formula 538
  Olsen formula 539
  SRK II formula 537
  SRK/T formula 538
Ishihara test 48
Itrace system 219

Jaeger's chart 43
Javal–Schiötz keratometer 183
Jerk nystagmus 456
Jones dye tests 484

Keratometry 151, 179
  automated keratometer 186
  Bausch and Lomb keratometer 181
  Helmholtz keratometer 180
  Javal–Schiötz keratometer 183
Kinetic perimetry 308

Lancaster red-green test 399
Landolt C test 39
Lantern tests 50
Lees screen test 402
LenStar 534
Levator function, assessment of 469
  Berke's method 469
  Illif's test 469
  Putterman's method 469

Livingston binocular gauge 422
LogMAR visual acuity charts 43
Loupe and lens examination 25
Luedde's exophthalmometer 497

MacKay-Marg tonometer 241
   pneumotonometer 241
   tono-pen 241
Maddox rod test 130, 386
Maddox wing test 388
Magnetic resonance angiography 695
Magnetic resonance imaging 109, 121
   in ocular lesions 685
   in ophthalmology 678
   in orbital lesions 688
Maklakov tonometer 237
Manipulative gonioscopy 252
Manometry 233
Marble game test 38
Marcus Gunn jaw-winking syndrome 473
Menace reflex test 36
Minimum discriminable 31
Minimum visible 31
Monocular indirect ophthalmoscopy 71
Monocular subjective refraction 723
Motion detection perimetry 324
MR spectroscopy 695
MR venography 696
Muscle sequelae 438
Mutch exophthalmometer 498

Naffziger's method 495
Nasal endoscopy 484
Near point of convergence, measurement of 395
Neostigmine/Tensilon test 471
Nerve fibre layer defects 268
Neurogenic ptosis 474
Neuroimaging 121
   computed tomography 121
   magnetic resonance imaging 121
Neutral density filter test 416
Nystagmus 456
   Jerk 456
   Pendular 456

Objective refraction 701
   autorefractometry 717
   photorefraction 720
   retinoscopy 702

Oblique illumination 25
   loupe and lens examination 25
   slit-lamp examination 26
Octopus printout 320
Ocular examination 7
   fluorescein staining 15
   gonioscopy 26
   loupe and lens examination 25
   oblique illumination 25
   perimetry 27
   swinging flash light test 17
   testing of visual acuity 7
   tonometry 26
Ocular movements, assessment of 391
Ocular rigidity 243
Ocular ultrasound-guided anaesthesia 635
Ocular wavefront 216
Olsen formula 539
Ophthalmoscopy 66
   binocular indirect 72
   direct 66
   distant direct 66
   monocular indirect 71
Optic disc changes in glaucoma 264
Optic nerve head evaluation 230
Optical biometers 533
Optical coherence tomography 577
   spectral domain 579
   time domain 577
Optical coherence tomography in glaucoma 273
   spectral domain OCT 279
   time domain (stratus) OCT 273
     RNFL thickness protocol 274
     screening protocols 273
Optical pachymetry 173
   specular microscopy pachymetry 174
Optimization of IOL power 546
Optodrum 428
Optokinetic nystagmus 35
Orbital imaging 107
   computed tomography 108
   magnetic resonance imaging 109
   plain radiography 107
   ultrasonography 109
Orbscan III 203
Orthoptic instruments 418
   cheiroscope 426
   conventional orthoptic instruments 418

diploscope 424
euthyscope 423
livingston binocular gauge 422
reading bars 426
remy separator 426
synoptophore 419
Tibb's binocular trainer 427
visuscope 423

Pachymeters, ultrasound-based 172
Pachymetry 150, 172
    optical 173
    ultrasound-based pachymeters 172
    with corneal topographers 175
Paediatric biometry 543
Pascal dynamic contour tonometer 242
Passive forced duction test 449
Pathological diagnostic tests in uveitis 365
Pendular nystagmus 456
Pentacam 206
Perceptual visual tracking program (PVT) 429
Perimetry 27, 306
    kinetic 308
    static 310
Perkin's applanation tonometer 240
Photoacoustic imaging 638
Photorefraction 720
Placido-disc-based corneal topography systems 192
Pneumotonometer 241
Posner gonioprism 250
Postural exophthalmometry 497
Preferential looking test 37
Preoperative evaluation for cataract surgery 521
Prism and alternate cover test 382
Prism bar and red filter test 409
Proptosis 489
    acute 491
    bilateral 490
    intermittent 491
    pulsatile 491
    unilateral 490
Proptosis, investigations for 499
    carotid angiography 507
    contrast orbitography 507
    CT scan 501
    histopathologic studies 507
    laboratory investigations 499
    magnetic resonance imaging 506
    orbital imaging techniques 499

plain X-rays examination 500
    ultrasonography 503
Pseudoproptosis 494
Psychophysical tests in glaucoma 323
Ptosis 467
    acquired myogenic 475
    aponeurotic 474
    congenital 471
    Marcus Gunn jaw-winking syndrome 473
    neurogenic 474
Pulsar perimetry 325
Pulsatile proptosis 491

Radiography, plain 107
Ray aberrations 214
Ray-tracing aberrometry 219
    iTrace system 219
Reading bars 426
Reichert's ocular response analyser 242
Relative exophthalmometry 497
Remote and robotic ultrasound 638
Remy separator 426
Retcam 86
Retinal correspondence, test for 406
    Bielschowsky's after image test 410
    Cupper's binocular visuscope test 411
    diplopia test 407
    prism bar and red filter test 409
    striated glass test (Bagolini test) 406
    synoptophore test 409
    Worth's four-dot test 409
Retinal correspondence, tests for 406
Retinal thickness analyser 95
Retinoscopy 702
Revital vision 431

Scanning laser ophthalmoscopy 89
Scanning laser polarimetry 98, 291
Scheimpflug imaging based corneal topography
        systems 205
    pentacam 206
Schiötz tonometer 235
Sensory adaptations 441
Sensory evaluation 405
Sheridan's ball test 39
Short wavelength automated perimetry 324
Simultaneous prism cover test 386
Skew deviation 125
Slit-lamp examination 53

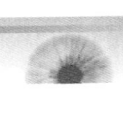

Slit-scanning corneal tomography system 203
  orbscan III 203
Spectral domain OCT 579
Specular microscopy pachymetry 174
Specular microscopy 152, 162
Spring-back balance test 452
SRK II formula 537
SRK/T formula 538
Static perimetry 310
Striated glass test (Bagolini test) 406
Subjective refraction 722
  binocular balancing 731
  monocular subjective refraction 723
  correction for near vision 732
Sussman lens 250
Swinging flash light test 17, 116
Synoptophore 419
Synoptophore test 409, 414

Teller acuity cards 37
  testing programmes 312
  testing strategies 311
Three- and four-dimensional ultrasound 636
Tibb's binocular trainer 427
Time domain (TD) OCT 577
Tokel gonioprism 250
Tonometers 235
  air-puff 240
  diatom transpalpebral 242
  Goldmann applanation 238
  ICARE or rebound 242
  MacKay-Marg 241
  Maklakov 237
  Pascal dynamic contour 242
  Perkin's applanation 240
  pneumotonometer 241
  Reichert's ocular response analyser 242
  tono-pen 241
Tonometry 26, 230, 233
  applanation 237
  indentation 234
Tono-pen 241
Transient visual loss 112
TrYe (train your eyes) 432
Tscherning aberroscope 218

Ultrasonography in ophthalmology 608
  colour doppler imaging 628

  in intraocular lesions 613
  in orbital lesions 623
Ultrasonography 109
Ultrasound based special tnvestigations 634
  C scan ultrasound 637
  contrast enhanced ultrasonography 636
  fusion imaging 637
  ocular ultrasound-guided anaesthesia 635
  photoacoustic imaging 638
  remote and robotic ultrasound 638
  three- and four-dimensional ultrasound 636
  ultrasound biomicroscopy 634
  ultrasound elastography 637
  ultrasound guided fine needle aspiration
    biopsy 635
Ultrasound biomicroscopy 296, 634, 640
  after intraocular surgeries 651
  appearance of normal eye 642
  for intraocular mass lesions 651
  in glaucoma 645
  in uveitis 647
  machine 640
Ultrasound elastography 637
Ultrasound guided fine needle aspiration biopsy 635

Vergences, measurement of 393
Versions, assessment of 392
Vestibulo-ocular reflex 34
Videokeratography 156
Videonystagmography 461
Vision therapy programs 429
Vision, milestones in development of 32
Visual acuity, measurement of 32
  blink reflex test 33
  Brückner's red reflex test 36
  Catford drum test 37
  Landolt C test 39
  marble game test 38
  Menace reflex test 36
  optokinetic nystagmus test 34
  preferential looking test 37
  Sheridan's ball test 39
  Teller acuity cards 37
  Vestibulo-ocular reflex test 34
Visual acuity, testing of 7
Visual acuity 30
Visual angle 30
Visual evoked potential 595

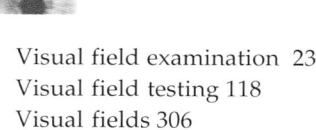

Visual field examination 231
Visual field testing 118
Visual fields 306
    central 307
    peripheral 307
Visuscope 423

Wave aberrations 214
Wavefront aberrometry 217
    Hartmann-Shack aberrometry 217
    intraoperative, real-time wavefront guided
        aberrometry 221
    ray-tracing aberrometry 219

Tscherning aberroscope 218
Worth's four-dot test 409, 411

X-rays in ophthalmology 601
    base view 602
    Caldwell view 602
    lateral view 602
    Rhese view 602
    Townes projection 602
    Water's view 602

Zeiss four-mirror gonioprism 250
Zernick's terms 214
Zernike's polynomials 214